Cancer Consult

Cancer Consult

Expertise in Clinical Practice, Second Edition

Volume 2: Neoplastic Hematology & Cellular Therapy

Edited by

Syed A. Abutalib, Maurie Markman, James O. Armitage, and Kenneth C. Anderson

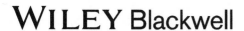

Contents

Editors Volume 2

Syed A. Abutalib, MD2
Medical Director
Hematologic Malignancies and
Transplantation and Cellular Therapy
Aurora St. Luke's Medical Center
Advocate Aurora Health Care
Milwaukee, Wisconsin

Maurie Markman, MD
Professor, Department of Medical
Oncology and Therapeutics Research
City of Hope

President, Medicine & Science, City of
Hope Atlanta, Chicago, Phoenix

Kenneth C. Anderson, MD
Program Director, Jerome Lipper Multiple
Myeloma Center and LeBow Institute for
Myeloma Therapeutics
Kraft Family Professor of Medicine
Harvard Medical School
Dana Farber Cancer Institute, Boston, MA

James O. Armitage, MD
Joe Shapiro Professor of Medicine,
University of Nebraska Medical Center
Omaha, NE

Editors Volume 1

Syed A. Abutalib, MD2
Medical Director, Malignant Hematology,
Transplantation and Cellular Therapy
Aurora St. Luke's Medical Center
Advocate Aurora Health
Milwaukee, Wisconsin

Maurie Markman, MD
Professor, Department of Medical
Oncology and Therapeutics Research
City of Hope

President, Medicine & Science
City of Hope Atlanta
Chicago, Phoenix

Al B. Benson III, MD FACP FASCO
Professor of Medicine
Associate Director for Cooperative Groups
Robert H. Lurie Comprehensive Cancer
Center of Northwestern University

Hope S. Rugo, MD, FASCO
Professor of Medicine
Director, Breast Oncology and Clinical
Trials Education
University of California San Francisco
Helen Diller Family Comprehensive
Cancer Center

Preface

It is commonplace in the oncology arena for patients to request a "second opinion."

But it is equally usual for oncologists to discuss with a colleague a complex or unusual case, or a patient with serious comorbidities, to insure that a particular individual is given the greatest opportunity to experience the benefits of therapy while minimizing the risks of possible treatment- related harm. Such discussions occur both within a particular specialty (e.g., surgery, radiation, or medical oncology) and between various specialties.

And as cancer management becomes more multimodal in nature, with an increasing focus on both maximizing the opportunity for extended survival and at the same time optimizing quality of life, the requirement for essential communication between individual specialists with their own unique knowledge and experience of critically relevant components of care becomes ever more important.

It is with these thoughts in mind that the editors conceived of an oncology text that would focus on the "expert perspectives" of oncology professionals. The intent was to have each individual book chapter be viewed as a "miniconsultation" provided by a specialist regarding a specific, highly clinically relevant issue in cancer management.

Considering the specific purpose and focus of the material presented, the book is written without detailed references (although a few selected readings are included at the end of each chapter). However, many of the authors have prepared a more extensive reference list, and the editors will be happy to email any reader the more detailed reference lists for individual book chapters, if so requested.

The chapters that follow have been written by clinicians selected for their recognized clinical expertise and experience. It is hoped that those reading this book will find the material of value in their own interactions with their patients.

Syed A. Abutalib, Maurie Markman Markman, James O. Armitage, and
Kenneth C. Anderson

Author Bios

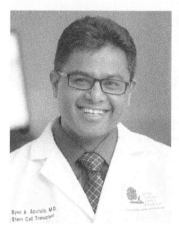

Syed A. Abutalib, MD2, is Medical Director of Malignant Hematology, Transplantation and Cellular Therapy at Aurora St. Luke's Medical Center, Milwaukee, Wisconsin. He also serves as active member of Executive Committee on Education for American Society of Transplantation and Cellular therapy (ASTCT®) and is one of the Associate Editors for The ASCO Post®. Dr. Abutalib is the Founding Editor of Advances in Cell and Gene Therapy, a Wiley Journal. In addition, he is Associate Professor of Medicine at Rosalind Franklin University of Medicine and Science. Dr. Abutalib has co-edited 10 Hematology/Oncology and Cellular/Gene therapy books over a short span of 6 years and has published in a number of cancer magazines, journals, and textbooks. He continues to collaborate with most cancer experts worldwide in the area of Hematology/Oncology and stem cell transplantation to explore and develop innovative ideas and breakthroughs in Medical Education with a prime focus to improve patient care.

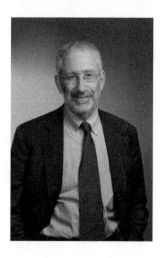

Maurie Markman, MD, is Professor of Oncology and Therapeutics Research, City of Hope and President of Medicine & Science, City of Hope Atlanta, Chicago, Phoenix. A nationally renowned oncologist, Dr. Markman has more than 20 years of experience in cancer treatment and gynecologic research at some of the country's most recognized facilities. Dr. Markman has served as the Vice President for Clinical Research and Chairman of the Department of Gynecologic Medical Oncology at M.D. Anderson Cancer Center in Houston, Texas. Prior to that, Dr. Markman spent 11 years as Chairman of the Department of Hematology/Oncology and Director of the Taussig Cancer Center at the Cleveland Clinic Foundation. He also spent five years as Vice Chairman of the Department of Medicine at Memorial Sloan-Kettering Cancer Center in New York.

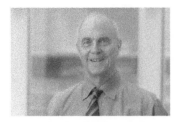

James O. Armitage, MD, is a graduate of the University of Nebraska Medical Center, completed his internship and residency in internal medicine at Nebraska, a fellowship in hematology oncology at the University of Iowa and spent 2 years in private practice. He returned to the University of Iowa and developed and directed the Bone Marrow Transplant program. At the University of Nebraska Medical Center, he developed the Bone Marrow Transplant program and the Nebraska Lymphoma Study Group. At Nebraska he has served as Vice-Chair of Internal Medicine, Chief of the Section of Oncology and Hematology, Chair of the Department of Internal Medicine, and Dean of the College of Medicine. He currently is the Joe Shapiro Professor of Medicine at the University of Nebraska Medical Center. Dr. Armitage is board certified in internal medicine, medical oncology, and hematology, and a Fellow of both the American and the Royal College of Physicians, a Fellow of ASCO, and a Fellow of the American Association for the Advancement of Science, and a Fellow of ASTCT (American Society for Transplantation and Cellular Therapy). He has served on many national/international oncology committees including the United States National Cancer Advisory Board and the French National Cancer Advisory Board. He is past president of both the American Society of Clinical Oncology and the American Society of Blood and Marrow Transplantation. He has received numerous honors including the Claude Jacquillat Award for achievement in Clinical Oncology from Paris, the San Salvatore Foundation Research Award from Lugano, Switzerland, the Richard and Hinda Rosenthal Foundation Award from the American Association of Cancer Research, the Heath Memorial Award from the University of Texas MD Anderson Cancer Center, the Robert A. Kyle Award for Outstanding Clinical Scientist from the Mayo Clinic, the Special Recognition Award from ASCO, and election to the Association of American Physicians. Dr. Armitage has published more than 600 papers, written 115 chapters, and is editor/co-editor of 33 books. He currently edits the ASCO Post.

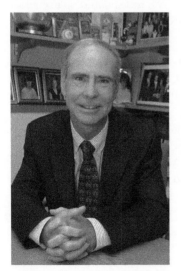

Kenneth Anderson, MD, is the Kraft Family Professor of Medicine at Harvard Medical School, as well as Director of the LeBow Institute for Myeloma Therapeutics and Jerome Lipper Multiple Myeloma Center at Dana-Farber Cancer Institute. Over the last four decades, he has developed laboratory and animal models of myeloma in its microenvironment which have allowed for both identification of novel targets and validation of novel targeted therapies. He has then rapidly translated these studies to clinical trials culminating in FDA approval of novel targeted therapies, which have markedly improved patient outcome. He received the American Society of Hematology William Dameshek Prize, the American Association for Cancer Research Joseph H. Burchenal Award, the American Society of Clinical Oncology David A. Karnofsky Award, and the Harvard Medical School Warren Alpert Prize. He is a member of the National Academy of Medicine, and past President of the International Myeloma Society and the American Society of Hematology.

Acknowledgement

Syed A. Abutalib, I am immensely grateful to God for providing me with the inspiration, and strength throughout this endeavor. I would like to extend my heartfelt acknowledgment to the timeless wisdom of Ali Ibne Abutalib (PBUH), who once said, "Knowledge is a companion that will never betray you, an ornament that will enhance your worth, a friend that will be with you in solitude, and a guide that will lead you to righteousness." Inspired by these profound words, I express my gratitude to the co-editors, and esteem contributors. Their expertise, and dedication have significantly enhanced the breadth and depth of the content in this book series. Also, I would like to remember my grandparents, Hamid and Laila Jafry for their unwavering support. Their love and belief in me have been a constant source of motivation. Lastly, I would like to extend my appreciation to the courageous cancer patients and their families.

Maurie Markman, To my grandsons, James, William and Conrad.

James O. Armitage, Thanks to my wife, Shirley.

Kenneth C. Anderson, The rapid pace of bench to bedside progress has transformed the treatment paradigm, and Cancer Consult will assure that both caregivers and patients have access to these advances, ultimately overcoming disparity in cancer care and improving outcomes for patients and their families. I extend my heartfelt thanks to the many contributing colleagues, I am inspired by the commitment of Dr. Abutalib and my co-editors and honored to have been part of this great team. Without the loving support of our families, none of this would be possible.

Part 1

Acute Lymphoblastic Leukemia in Adults

1

Prognostic Markers and Models in Acute Lymphoblastic Leukemia

Dieter Hoelzer

University of Frankfurt, Germany

Introduction

Acute lymphoblastic leukemia (ALL) is a heterogeneous disease characterized by subgroups with different biological and clinical features and cure rates. They have prognostic impact for the achievement of remission or the remission duration. There are two phases to evaluate prognostic factors: (1) Patient's characteristics at diagnosis, and (2) patient's response to treatment (Table 1.1). Pretherapeutic prognostic features are age, initial white blood cell (WBC) count, immunophenotype, and abnormal cytogenetics or molecular genetics. Response parameters are achievement of complete remission, particularly molecular remission, and time to achieve a complete remission and molecular remission. The aim of evaluating prognostic factors in ALL is to stratify patients into good and poor risk groups and to adapt different treatment strategies accordingly. One important decision in adult ALL is, thereby, whether a patient should have an allogeneic hematopoietic cell transplantation (allo-HCT) in first complete remission or not.

1) **What is the prognostic value of patient's age at diagnosis in adult ALL, and what are the therapeutic implications?**

Expert Perspective: Advancing age is undoubtedly associated with poorer outcome in all studies. In adolescents and young adults (AYAs, i.e. adults up to age 40), pediatric-inspired intensive protocols are applied. Thereafter, the protocol intensity is decreased. Currently, treatment protocols for elderly (> 60 years) are with less intensive chemotherapy backbone combined with immunotherapies and/or with tyrosine kinase inhibitors (TKIs) in Ph+ ALL (discussed in chapters on treatment in B- and T-ALL). Patients older than age 60 years have a substantially poorer outcome due to comorbidities and an increasing incidence of adverse risk factors. All patients are subject to CNS screening by flow cytometry and prophylaxis.

Cancer Consult: Expertise in Clinical Practice, Volume 2: Neoplastic Hematology & Cellular Therapy, Second Edition. Edited by Syed A. Abutalib, Maurie Markman, James O. Armitage, and Kenneth C. Anderson. © 2024 John Wiley & Sons Ltd. Published 2024 by John Wiley & Sons Ltd.

Table 1.1 Prognostic factors for risk stratification of adult acute lymphoblastic leukemia (ALL)[1].

Prognostic factors	B-lineage			T-lineage	
Pretherapeutic parameters	**Good**	**Intermediate**	**Adverse**	**Good**	**Adverse**
• Age	**< 35 years**	35–50 years	**> 55–60 years** **> 70 years elderly/frail**		
• White blood cell count	**< 30,000/μL**		**> 30,000/μL**		
• Organ involvement[3]					
• Immunophenotype				Thymic (CD1a+, TAL/LMO)	Early T (CD1a−, sCD3−) Mature T (CD1a−, sCD3+)
• Molecular/subgroups cytogenetics	**Ph+/BCR–ABL1 t(9;22) (q34;q11.2)** IgH-MYC+, t(8,14)(q24;q32) TEL–AML1 (?) HOX11[2] NOTCH1[2] (?)	*IKZF1*-Deletion 7p focal deletions/ mutations MLL rearranged	**Ph-like** **ALL1–AF4 / t(4;11)** t(1;19)/E2A–PBX (?) Complex aberrations (?)		HOXA aberrations CALM-AF10 Complex aberrations (?)
Treatment response					
Prednisone response	Good		Poor		
Time to complete remission	**Early (<2–3 weeks)**		**Late (> 3–4 weeks)**		
MRD[4] after induction	**Negative < 10^{-4}**		**Positive > 10^{-4}**		

[1]Generally accepted factors are printed in **bold**.
[2]Overexpression of genes.
[3]Organ involvement, particularly central nervous system involvement, and mediastinal tumors have lost their adverse impact with recent treatment strategies.
[4]MRD, measurable residual disease.

2) Does WBC at diagnosis still have a prognostic impact in B-ALL and T-ALL?

Expert Perspective: Elevated WBC at diagnosis ($> 30,000$–$50,000$/mL) is a poor prognostic feature, especially deleterious in precursor B-cell ALL. Subtype Ph-like ALL (provisional category 2016 WHO classification) has higher WBC count at presentation, higher measurable residual disease at the end of induction therapy and inferior overall survival (Chapter 2). In T-ALL a high WBC $> 100,000$ was considered a poor prognostic factor but with an ongoing more-intensive protocol these adverse factors seem to be abrogated (Chapter 3).

3) What is the relevance of cytogenetic and molecular markers for treatment decisions?

Expert Perspective: Ph+ ALL with the t(9;22) translocation and the BCR–ABL fusion transcript is the most prevalent cytogenetic abnormality in adults with B-ALL, increasing from $< 3\%$ in children up to 40–50% in adults over the age of 50–60 years. Ph+ ALL was so far the poorest ALL subtype, with a survival rate at 5 years of $< 10\%$ with chemotherapy and $< 30\%$ with allo-HCT. Targeted therapy with tyrosine kinase inhibitors (TKIs) in combination with chemotherapy has changed the prognosis landscape dramatically; now the complete remission rates approach levels $> 90\%$ and survival > 50–70% in most series. Allo-HCT is still a curative approach with a survival rate of 50–70% for ALL.

4) Which of the following statements about Ph-like ALL is correct?

    a) It is more common in adults than in children.
    b) It is associated with superior outcomes without allogeneic transplant.
    c) There is no role of *JAK-2* inhibitor therapy in B-ALL.
    d) All of the above.

Expert Perspective: Ph-like ALL is characterized by a gene-expression profile like that of *BCR::ABL1*-positive ALL but lacks the *BCR::ABL1* fusion protein, or t(9;22), by cytogenetic, FISH, or molecular analysis and alterations of lymphoid transcription factor genes. It is associated with poor prognosis and is seen in 10–20% of pediatric cases and 20–30% of adult cases of B-ALL. It is included as a provisional entity in the 2016 WHO Classification. A variety of different genetic abnormalities are identified in this entity, but they all converge on pathways that are potentially responsive targeted therapy added to conventional chemotherapy, one of them being *JAK-2* inhibitor therapy (more on this topic in Chapter 2).

Tyrosine Kinase Rearrangements

A feature of Ph-like ALL is the presence of fusion genes involving a tyrosine kinase: the *ABL*-class and *JAK2* arrangements. In adolescents and adults, *ABL*-class rearrangements occur in about 10% and *JAK2* rearrangements are detected in 7–8%. Patients with *ABL*-class rearrangements should receive additional TKI therapy. Patients with *JAK2* rearrangements may be candidates for additional *JAK2*-inhibitor therapy.

Diagnosis of Ph-like ALL

Diagnosis of a Ph-like ALL is difficult. There are low density classifiers (LDA) to identify predictor genes assays of either 8 or 9 gene signatures. Since the diagnosis of Ph-like ALL is not trivial and is not available at first diagnosis, commonly specific drugs are added later. There are, however, studies to identify Ph-like ALL genetics stratification at diagnosis as in the COG trial (Chapter 2).

Ph-like ALL has poor prognosis, and patients often present with adverse features such as high WBC. These patients should be considered for frontline allo-HCT. Whether the addition of immunotherapy as in Ph+ ALL improves the poor outcome of Ph-like ALL remains an open question (Chapter 5).

Correct Answer: A

5) In current clinical practice, what are the targetable surface antigens in B-ALL?

Expert Perspective: A variety of targeted monoclonal antibody therapies directed against surface antigens, particularly CD20 (rituximab and other anti-CD 20 antibodies), CD19 (blinatumomab and chimeric antigen receptors T cells), and CD22 (inotuzumab ozogamicin). These targeted antibodies have been and are further being explored (Chapter 2).

6) What is the prognostic value of CD20, CD22, and CD19 surface expression in B-ALL?

Expert Perspective: The question arises of whether antigen expression itself within an immunologically defined subtype is a prognostic marker.

- **Surface CD20 expression**, observed in about 40% of adult pre-B-ALL and common B-ALL, had an adverse prognostic impact, but the therapy with rituximab has apparently overcome the potential adverse influence.
- **Surface CD22** is expressed on leukemic blasts in 90–100% of B-ALL and is an excellent target for the inotuzumab ozogamicin. It seems, however, that the antigen expression of CD22 per cell as a prognostic impact has a better outcome for highly expressed CD22 as long as therapy against CD22 is utilized. In the INO-VATE study, the rate of complete remission was higher with inotuzumab ozogamicin than with standard therapy, and a higher percentage of patients in the inotuzumab ozogamicin group had results below the threshold for MRD. Both progression-free and overall survival were longer with inotuzumab ozogamicin. However, veno-occlusive liver disease was a major adverse event associated with inotuzumab ozogamicin. This agent is a humanized CD22-directed monoclonal antibody-drug conjugate, which is composed of the IgG4 kappa antibody inotuzumab (which is specific for human CD22), a calicheamicin component (a cytotoxic agent that causes double-stranded DNA breaks), and an acid-cleavable linker that covalently binds the calicheamicin to inotuzumab. After the antibody-drug conjugate binds to CD22, the CD22-conjugate complex is internalized and releases calicheamicin. Calicheamicin binds to the minor groove of DNA to induce double strand cleavage and subsequent cell cycle arrest and apoptosis.
- **Surface CD19** is also expressed on nearly 100% B cells. Blinatumomab is a bispecific T-cell engager (BiTE) that binds to CD19 expressed on B cells and CD3 expressed on T cells. It

activates endogenous T cells by connecting CD3 in the T-cell receptor complex with CD19 on B cells (malignant and benign), thus forming a cytolytic synapse between a cytotoxic T cell and the cancer target B cell. Blinatumomab mediates the production of cytolytic proteins, release of inflammatory cytokines, and proliferation of T cells, which result in lysis of CD19-positive cells. In the TOWER study, treatment with blinatumomab resulted in significantly longer OS than chemotherapy among adult patients with relapsed or refractory B-cell precursor ALL. CD19 is also target of *ex vivo* gene therapy, namely chimeric antigen receptor T cells. Although the CD19-antigen expression per cell is of prognostic relevance, the greater impact is the loss of CD19 antigen after this therapy, which is associated with failure of targeted therapies and poor outcome (see Chapter 2 for further discussion).

Response Parameters in B-ALL

7) Is achievement of first complete remission a prognostic marker for overall outcome, and how important is time to achieve complete remission?

Expert Perspective: Some response parameters after induction therapy are highly predictive for outcomes. For example, time to achieve a complete remission within 3–4 weeks or a molecular complete remission after 14–16 weeks are important. The rate of complete remission is prognostically less relevant since > 95% of children and > 90% of adults achieve a complete remission. Despite favorable complete remission rates in adults, 40–50% eventually relapse. One of the reasons is the limited sensitivity to measure the leukemic cell reduction by cytomorphology. Complete remission is, however, still an important goal and first step toward ensuring success. Therefore, achievement of complete remission is still commonly accepted as endpoint for studies. (See Chapters 2, 4, and 5.)

Risk Stratification in B-ALL

8) What is the purpose of stratification into risk groups?

Expert Perspective: Similar to childhood ALL, several large ALL study groups have defined risk groups in adults. Pretherapeutic prognostic factors and response parameters are used to define risk groups; standard-risk (SR) patients are generally defined as those without any adverse risk factors, whereas high-risk (HR) patients have one or more risk factors (Table 1.1). The aim of these still important prognostic strategies is to identify an SR group with a good outcome (e.g. with an expected > 50% survival probability at five years in adults) and the HR patient group with a less favorable outcome. High-risk patients are generally candidates for an immediate allo-HCT in first complete remission, whereas standard-risk patients in most studies continue with consolidation cycles ± reinduction and maintenance therapy (see Chapter 6). In several study groups, there was also the definition of a very-high-risk (VHR) group in adults, preferentially patients with Ph+ ALL or Ph-like ALL. The prognosis of this Ph+ALL has completely changed with better outcomes using various combinations of chemotherapy, TKIs, immunotherapy ± allo-HCT in first complete remission (Figure 1.1).

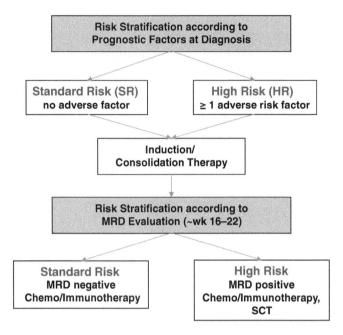

- Minimal residual disease after Ind/Cons is the most important prognostic factor and relevant for treatment decision

- Targeted Therapy Applied in B-lineage ALL
  - Surface Antigens CD19, CD20, CD22 → Immunotherapy
  - Ph+/Ph-like → Tyrosine Kinase Inhibitors (TKI) ± Immunotherapy

Figure 1.1 Practical approach for treatment stratification in adult B-cell acute lymphoblastic leukemia (ALL).
SCT—allogeneic stem cell transplantation
MRD—measurable residual disease

9) Will the prognostic impact of pretherapeutic risk factors and stratification into risk groups be replaced by measurable residual disease?

Expert Perspective: Clearly not; standard-risk patients have high complete remission rates of 90%, supported by a high rate of MRD clearance, and are spared for allo-HCT. High-risk patients still have lower rates of complete remission by 50–60%, also with a lower MRD rate. They are candidates for allo-HCT in first complete remission, but with the targeted therapy to reduce MRD load further before transplant (see Chapter 2).

The achievement of a complete remission is also relevant since not all patients, for several reasons, have access to MRD evaluation (~15% don't have). Furthermore, many hospitals and treatment centers around the world do not have experienced lab to follow MRD (also for cost reasons), and therefore, the conventional response parameters such as complete remission and CRi (incomplete hematological remission) are still of high prognostic relevance.

Whether the increasing use of immunotherapy will change the prognosis of specific B-ALL subtypes and thereby the indications for allo-HCT also remains currently an open question (see Chapters 2 and 3).

T-lineage ALL

Based on immunophenotyping, T-ALL comprises the subtypes of early T-ALL, thymic (cortical) T-ALL, and mature T-ALL. In the GMALL studies these subtypes were the most relevant prognostic factors.

- **Thymic T-ALL** is CD1a-positive and constitutes about half of the adult T-ALL patients; it has the best prognosis, with complete remission rates ≥95% and overall survival at five years of 60–80% (Table 1.1).
- The other subtypes, early T-ALL and mature T-ALL, have lower rates of complete remission and poorer survivals; both subtypes profit from an allo-HCT in first complete remission (although opinion among experts varies!). However, within the early T-ALL a new subtype has been identified as Early progenitor T-ALL (ETP-ALL), which has the least favorable outcomes (discussed in depth in Chapter 3).

10) Is ETP-ALL clinically and prognostically relevant?

Expert Perspective: ETP-ALL is a newly described provisional entity. The immunophenotype is CDy1a-, CD8-, or CD5 weak or negative. It is characterized by stem cell markers such as CD34, HLA-DR, CD117, and/or myeloid antigens (CD 13, CD33, CD65s). The mutational status of ETP vs non-ETP early T-ALL is characterized by *FLT3 (ITD)* with 25% vs 0% and *NOTCH* mutations with a lower rate of 7% vs 53%, respectively. Importantly, ETP-ALL has poor prognostic marker, although in some studies there is no difference in overall survival between ETP and non-ETP early T-ALL. Some groups observed inferior outcomes for early T-ALL with co-expression of CD13, CD33, and/or CD34; a high expression of the transcription factors *ERG* and/or *BAALC*; and overexpression of *HOX11-L2* and *SIL-TAL1*-positive ALL (Chapter 3).

11) What is the prognostic relevance of molecular markers in relation to the immunophenotypic T-ALL subtypes?

Expert Perspective: The overexpression of *HOX11*, *HOX11L2*, *SIL-TAL1*, and *CALM–AF10* is associated with described subtypes since it represents the maturation states of thymocytes.

- **Low expression of *ERG* and *BAALC*** was associated with favorable outcome as well as overexpression of *HOX11*, which is associated with thymic T-ALL.
- ***NOTCH1*-activating mutations**, which are identified in up to 50% of T-ALL cases, so far have an unclear prognostic relevance. Attempt to be targeted by γ-secretase inhibitors have largely failed due to toxicity. Five percent of T-ALL shows the *NUP214–ABL1* aberration, which may identify a target population for imatinib therapy. Altogether there have been many attempts to stratify T-ALL by genetic markers, mostly based on retrospective analysis, but the impact on prospective risk stratification and different treatment strategies is limited (see Chapter 3).

Recommended Readings

Chiaretti, S., Messina, M., and Foà, R. (2019). BCR/ABL1–like acute lymphoblastic leukemia: how to diagnose and treat? *Cancer* 125: 194–204.

Chiaretti, S., Elias, J., and Dieter, H. (2018). ""Society of Hematologic Oncology (SOHO) State of the Art Updates and Next Questions"-Treatment of ALL". *Clin Lymphoma Myeloma Leuk* 18 (5): 301–310.

Cordo' V., van der Zwet J.C.G., Cante-Barrett K., Pieters R., and Meijerink JPP. (2012). T-cell Acute Lymphoblastic Leukemia; A Roadmap to Targeted Therapies. *Blood Cancer Discov* 2 (1): 19–31. (Accessed 13 January 2012)

Coustan-Smith, E., Mullighan, C.G., Onciu, M. et al. (2009). Early T-cell precursor leukaemia: a subtype of very high-risk acute lymphoblastic leukaemia. *Lancet Oncol* 10: 147–156.

Den Boer, M.L. et al. (2009). A subtype of childhood acute lymphoblastic leukaemia with poor treatment outcome: a genome-wide classification study. *Lancet Oncol* 10 (2): 125–134.

Gokbuget, N. (2021). MRD in adult Ph/BCR-ABL-negative ALL: how best to eradicate? *Hematol Am Soc Hemat Educ Prog* (1): 718–725.

Harvey R.C. and Tasian S.K. (2020). Clinical diagnostics and treatment strategies for Philadelphia chromosome-like acute lymphoblastic leukaemia. *Blood Adv* 4 (1): 218–228. (Accessed 14 January 2020)

Hoelzer, D., Bassan, R., Dombret, H., Fielding, A., Ribera, J.M., and Buske, C. ESMO Guidelines Committee (2016 September). Acute lymphoblastic leukaemia in adult patients: ESMO Clinical Practice Guidelines for diagnosis, treatment and follow-up. *Ann Oncol* 27 (suppl 5): v69–v82.

Hoelzer, D. (2017). Clinical Applications and pitfalls of MRD in ALL. *Clin Lymphoma Myeloma Leuk* 17: S9–S11.

Hoelzer, D., Thiel, E., Loffler, H. et al. (1988). Prognostic factors in a multicenter study for treatment of acute lymphoblastic leukemia in adults. *Blood* 71 (1): 123–131.

Kimble E.L. and Cassaday R.D. (2021). Antibody and cellular immunotheripes for acute lymphoblastic leukemia in adults. *Leukemia & Lymphoma* 62 (14): 3333–33347.

Malard F. and Mohty M. (2020). Acute lymphoblastic leukaemia. *The Lancet* 395 (10230): 1146–1162.

Mullighan, C.G., Su, X., Zhang, J. et al., Children's Oncology Group (2009 January 29). Deletion of IKZF1 and prognosis in acute lymphoblastic leukemia. *N Engl J Med* 360 (5): 470–480.

Neumann, M., Heesch, S., Gökbuget, N. et al. (2012). Clinical and molecular characterization of early T-cell precursor leukemia: a high-risk subgroup in adult T-ALL with a high frequency of FLT3 mutations. *Blood Cancer J* 2 (1): e55.

Roberts, K.G., Li, Y., Payne-Turner, D. et al. (2014). Targetable kinase-activating lesions in Ph-like acute lymphoblastic leukemia. *N Engl J Med* 371 (11): 1005–1015.

2

Acute Lymphoblastic Leukemia—Treatment and Outcomes in B-ALL

Vijaya Raj Bhatt[1], Prajwal Dhakal[2], and Syed A. Abutalib[3]

[1] University of Nebraska Medical Center, Omaha, NE, USA
[2] University of Iowa Health Care, Iowa City, IA, USA
[3] Aurora St. Luke's Medical Center, Milwaukee, WI

Introduction

B-cell acute lymphoblastic leukemia (B-ALL) represents around 70–75% of cases of ALL, with T-ALL and T-LBL constituting the remaining cases (discussed in Chapter 3). Incidence rates in the USA are 17.3 cases per million; the highest incidence is seen in early childhood, with a second smaller increase in adults over the age of 60 (bimodal distribution). Large studies have typically not included patients over the age of sixty-five, and this may be one of the reasons that survival in older patients has not improved. This leads to a particular unmet need, since the median age of adults with ALL is above 60 years. Population-based registry studies report complete remission rates of 20–51% in adults over 60, with five-year survival rates of only 5–12%.

In younger adults, the overall survival of B-ALL patients has improved over the last few decades. The treatment approach has incorporated time-specific measurable residual disease (MRD) assessment to continuously evolving, genomic parameters which has led to better disease stratification and prognostication. The detection of MRD in ALL has implications for consolidation strategies and transplantation. It has long been established that failure to achieve MRD negativity portents ALL relapse, although the exact timing of when to assess MRD, and the cut-off values for MRD positivity, varies among studies. Also, patients with negative MRD also relapse. Additionally, adults with Philadelphia negative B-ALL (Ph-ALL) are now approached as either NIH-defined "adolescents and young adults (AYA)" or non-AYA, highlighting the sobering fact that not all AYA patients are candidates for intensive pediatric-inspired protocol. With this background, it important to acknowledge that conventional therapy results in remission rates greater than 60% in adults, but relapse remains a major barrier in curing these patients, and allogeneic hematopoietic cell transplant (allo-HCT), preferably myeloablative, remains an important curative modality along with recent addition of CAR T cell therapy. Blinatumomab offers significant promise in achieving deeper first remissions with the goal of preventing relapses in newly diagnosed B-ALL.

Cancer Consult: Expertise in Clinical Practice, Volume 2: Neoplastic Hematology & Cellular Therapy,
Second Edition. Edited by Syed A. Abutalib, Maurie Markman, James O. Armitage, and Kenneth C. Anderson.
© 2024 John Wiley & Sons Ltd. Published 2024 by John Wiley & Sons Ltd.

About 20% of adults have primary refractory disease. Currently, the five-year overall survival rates for all adults are between 20 and 60% with wide variability due in part to higher-risk disease features and intolerability to currently available regimens in older adults. Our chapter will focus on overall management approach, its challenges, controversies, and future prospects of treating adults with this heterogenous disease. In-depth discussion of risk stratification, MRD, and cellular therapies including allogeneic hematopoietic cell transplantation (allo-HCT) in ALL is available in the preceding and following chapters (Chapters 1,4, and 5, respectively).

1) **What is the standard of care for front-line management of Philadelphia chromosome–negative (Ph-) B-cell acute lymphoblastic leukemia (B-ALL)?**

Expert Perspective: The front-line strategy for the management of "fit" adult with B-ALL requires induction, multiple cycles of consolidation, maintenance phase, and successive prophylaxis intrathecal injections of chemotherapy. Most protocols include approximately three years of therapy in the absence of allo-HCT indication (allo-HCT is discussed in Chapter 5). There are several accepted regimens, and most involve the same key elements of vincristine, anthracycline (e.g. doxorubicin or daunorubicin), dexamethasone, with or without L-asparaginase (e.g. PEG-asparaginase), CNS prophylaxis using systemic chemotherapy such as cytarabine, methotrexate, and intrathecal chemotherapy and intravenous or subcutaneous rituximab (provided CD20+ and age ≤ 60 [GRAALL-2005/R]).

Best treatment selection depends on multiple factors including age, comorbidity index, MRD status, allogeneic transplant donor availability, and institutional and patient preferences.

- **Adolescents and young adults** (AYA) benefit most from a pediatric-inspired regimens for example, CALGB 10403 (ages 16–39 years old) which incorporates more extensive use of glucocorticoids, vincristine, and pegylated asparaginase with intensive and prolonged CNS prophylaxis. AYA patients treated with a pediatric-type regimen, who achieve protocol-defined MRD negative status (at least 10^{-4}) have excellent outcomes without allo-HCT provided Ph-like ALL is excluded at diagnostic evaluation. In the CALGB 10403, three-year overall survival was 73%, compared with earlier CALGB studies, where overall survival for this age group was 55% at three years. The treatment-related mortality was 3%. Richard-Carpentier and colleagues (2019) have reported (n = 27) promising early results of a phase II study employing sequential use of hyper-CVAD and blinatumomab in patients with ages 18–57 years. The regimen consists of four cycles of Hyper-CVAD followed by four cycles of blinatumomab. Earlier incorporation of blinatumomab after two cycles of chemotherapy is allowed for patients at high risk for early relapse, particularly those with Ph-like ALL (discussed later), complex karyotype, t(4;11), low-hypodiploidy/near triploidy, or persistent MRD (Table 2.1). Four cycles of blinatumomab were also incorporated within 12 cycles of POMP (prednisone, vincristine, methotrexate, and 6-mercaptopurine) maintenance therapy. The one-year relapse-free survival and overall survival were 76% and 89%, respectively. A randomized phase III trial recently reported results of chemotherapy with or without blinatumomab in the front-line setting for patients between the ages of 30 to 70 years (ECOG-ACRIN

Table 2.1 Genomic risk categories in B-ALL.

Risk categories	Genetic abnormalities
Standard risk	Hyperdiploidy (51–65 chromosomes, often with trisomy of chromosomes 4, 10, and 17) t(12;21) (p13;q22): *ETV6-RUNX1*
High risk	Hypodiploidy (< 44 chromosomes) *KMT2A* rearranged t(v;14q32)/IgH Philadelphia chromosome positive Ph-like B-ALL with variety of molecular abnormalities (see text) Complex karyotype Intrachromosomal amplification of chromosome 21 t(17;19): *TCF3-HLF* fusion *IKZF1* alterations (without *DUX4r*)

E1910). This study demonstrated significant improvement in overall survival with upfront addition of blinatumomab to consolidation chemotherapy in patients with Ph-ALL, who have achieved MRD negative status following chemotherapy. Potential benefits of adding inotuzumab ozogamicin to the pediatric-inspired CALGB 10403 chemotherapy protocol are under investigation in a phase III multicenter trial (NCT03150693), aiming to recruit 310 patients, aged between 18 and 39, with newly diagnosed patients with B-ALL.

- **Adults between ages 40–50 years**, depending on overall fitness and comorbidity index, may or may not tolerate a pediatric-type regimen. In addition to data described above for AYA, the Dana–Farber (2015) and GRAALL-2005 (2018) studies allowed older patients but observed more treatment-associated toxicity, as well as poorer outcomes in those with age above 55 years. The Nordic ALL2008 study (2018) recruited patients ages between 1 and 45 years. The adult cohort suffered more treatment-associated toxicity in terms of thrombosis, pancreatitis, and osteonecrosis. For these reasons, most older adults receive "adult-type ALL regimens," i.e. hyper-CVAD regimen +/– anti-CD20 antibody, which employs the combination of hyperfractionated cyclophosphamide, vincristine, doxorubicin, and dexamethasone alternating with high-dose methotrexate and cytarabine along with CNS prophylaxis. Cycles are repeated approximately monthly for eight cycles, at which point patients move to the maintenance therapy. In patients eligible for allo-HCT, chemotherapy is usually terminated early in favor of allograft.

- **Older adults above the age of 60–65 years** have a significant risk of toxicities and poor survival with traditional chemotherapy regimens. These patients suffer with the worst outcomes (five-year overall survival < 15%) mainly due to unfavorable clinical and biologic characteristics. Emerging data indicate benefits of incorporating novel drugs with mini-hyper-CVAD. A phase II study from MDACC updated their results of sequential combination of inotuzumab ozogamicin with mini-hyper-CVAD (cyclophosphamide and dexamethasone at 50% dose reduction, no anthracycline, methotrexate at 75% dose reduction, cytarabine at 0.5 g/m^2 × 4 doses) followed by blinatumomab in patients with ages 60 to 87 years (n = 74). The complete remission rate was 98%, and the MRD negativity rate was 95%. The three-year complete remission duration and overall survival rate were 76% and 54%, respectively. With a median follow-up of 56 months (range: 1–111 months), the five-year continuous remission and overall survival rates were 76% and 47%, respectively. Outcomes were superior for those 60–69 years of age versus those who were ≥ 70 years (five-year overall survival rates: 58% and 31%, respectively; $P = 0.04$) and for those without poor-risk cytogenetics versus with poor-risk cytogenetics (5-year OS rates: 56% and 25%, respectively; $P = 0.01$; Table 2.1). A propensity match score showed significant improvement compared to the historical three-year overall survival rate of 32% with hyper-CVAD in this older population ($P = 0.007$). Although no early death occurred in induction, the rate of death in remission was 33% and was significantly higher in those with ages ≥ 70 years compared to those with ages 60–69 years (50% versus 22%, respectively; $P = 0.02$). In order to mitigate the significant toxicity in this older population, the protocol was amended to decrease the number of mini-hyper-CVAD plus inotuzumab ozogamicin cycles from four to two and to replace POMP maintenance with blinatumomab monotherapy for patients ≥ 70 years of age. Most recently, SWOG 1318 (2022) evaluated chemotherapy-free induction and consolidation with blinatumomab (total of four to five cycles) followed by POMP maintenance in patients (n = 29) with ages 66–84 years. The three-year disease-free survival and overall survival estimates were 37% (95% CI 17–57) and 37% (95% CI 20–55), respectively. The results of UKALL60+/HOVON 117 (NCT01616238) prospective, non-randomized multi-pathway observational study (including a choice of pathway intensity) are awaited. Results of ECOG-ACRIN E1910 are discussed in previous section. Figure 2.1 outlines a general approach in treating patients with B-ALL.

2) Is immunogenicity an issue with L-asparaginase treatment?

Expert Perspective: Yes. L-asparaginase is an important component of the ALL regimens for children and AYA leading to superior complete remission and disease-free-survival rates. L-asparaginase, is an enzyme used to deprive lymphoblasts of the nonessential amino acid, asparagine. Due to its benefit, now it is also included in several adult ALL regimens (e.g. modified hyper-CVAD), but the cumulative dose is generally lower than that of the pediatric programs. A pegylated form of the drug (PEG-asparaginase; half-life of six days) has advantage over L-asparafinase of continuous exposure over a period of one to two weeks (dependent on the dose), reducing the number of infusions or intramuscular injections (intramuscular administration is less likely to cause anaphylactic reactions). Patients who develop an anaphylactic reaction to one preparation may be considered for treatment with another preparation. PEG-asparaginase is the preferred preparation for most circumstances because it appears to be less immunogenic. If asparaginase serum levels are nondetectable with one preparation, an alternative preparation may be more effective. More recently, calaspargase pegol was approved by the FDA for treatment of ALL in pediatric and young adult patients with ages 1 month to 21 years based on achievement and maintenance of nadir

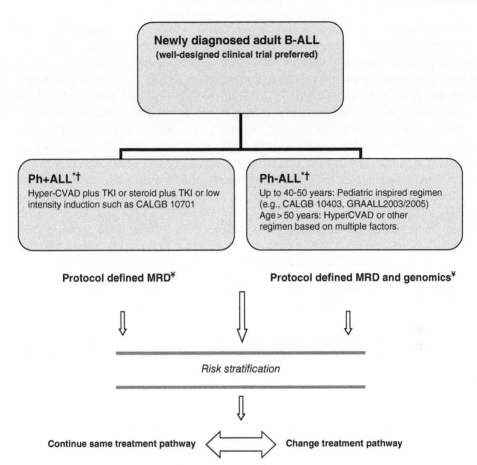

Figure 2.1 Simplified algorithm of proposed treatment approaches for adults with B-ALL.
*In general, rituximab is added if B-ALL expresses CD20 antigen
† Some cases of Ph-like ALL depending on type of mutation (ABL versus non-ABL)
¥ See Chapter 4

serum asparaginase activity > 0.1 units/mL at a dose of 2,500 units/m^2 intravenously every three weeks.

3) What are some of the important toxicities of asparaginase?

Expert Perspective: Potential important toxicities that pose a problem include transaminitis, pancreatitis, thrombosis, allergic reactions, hyperglycemia, and hypofibrinogenemia. A detailed review of asparaginase toxicity and its management has been published by a group of experts and is also available at the National Comprehensive Cancer Network Guidelines.

4) What is the role of anti-CD20 immunotherapy in the treatment of B-ALL?

Expert Perspective: Approximately 30–50% of patients' leukemic blasts express the CD20 antigen. The prognostic role of CD20 expression in B-ALL is controversial, but it is an actionable target. Several studies including the GRAALL-2005/R randomized control trial have demonstrated that the addition of rituximab (16–18 infusions) to multiagent chemotherapy improves survival in younger adults (age range 18–60 years). The study showed improvement in the two-year overall survival rates from 64 to 71% ($P = 0.095$; with censoring for allo-HCT, $P = 0.018$). Although rituximab was incorporated when CD20 expression was 20% or greater, anti-CD20 therapy may be beneficial even if expression is lower.

Thomas and colleagues from MDACC reported 10% cutoff had significant prognostic value. Interestingly, unlike other studies in adult ALL, where CD20 expression has been associated with inferior survival, CALGB 10403 found equivalent outcomes regardless of CD20 expression. Given the results from the MDACC and GRAALL-2005/R studies, it is common to incorporate rituximab in all patients with CD20+ B-ALL. Also, in patients with low or very low CD20 expression levels at baseline, the use of higher-affinity anti-CD20 antibodies, such as obinutuzumab or ofatumumab, might offer an attractive alternative. The UKALL14 (NCT01085617; 2022) study has given rituximab (× 4 doses) regardless of CD20 expression level in older adults with B-ALL.

5) What are the options for front-line management of Philadelphia chromosome–positive (Ph+) ALL?

Expert Perspective: The Ph+ ALL is the most common chromosomal abnormality in adult ALL, with increasing incidence with age, reaching up to 50% in patients above the age of 60 years. The treatment strategy for Ph+ ALL is evolving. The goal of therapy in Ph+ ALL is to achieve complete molecular response early (~three months) into treatment. The choice of TKI depends on the treatment protocol; authors prefer to use either dasatinib or ponatinib. The optimal duration of TKI therapy is not well established. Clinical trials have used rituximab in addition to TKI for CD20+ Ph+ ALL Use of blinatumomab with ponatinib or dasatinib is excellent chemotherapy free approach especially in older adults is another excellent option.

Conventional chemotherapy plus TKI

- Imatinib combined with conventional chemotherapy has been proven to be superior to chemotherapy alone in several trials. For example, addition of imatinib to hyper-CVAD in the MDACC study (2015), improved complete remission rates to about 93% with long-term overall survival rate of 43%, which compared very favorably to the historical long-term overall survival of < 20% in the pre-TKI era. In the UKALLXII/ECOG2993 study adding imatinib to standard therapy improved complete remission rate and long-term overall survival. A major concern is resistance to imatinib with acquisition of point mutations within the *BCR::ABL1* kinase domain, including development of gatekeeper mutation, *T315I*. Other *BCR::ABL1*-independent mechanisms of resistance include decreased drug influx and activation of other downstream or parallel cell-signaling pathways that promote cell proliferation and survival, such as the Src family of kinases (see Chapter 16). Dasatinib is a second-generation TKI that is about 325-fold more potent than imatinib, with additional ability to block the SFKs (dual *BCR::ABL1* and SRC kinase inhibitor). Dasatinib was combined with hyper-CVAD in two phase II trials (MDACC and US Intergroup), showing greater improvement over imatinib, with a complete response rate of 96%, complete molecular response rate of 56%, and three-year disease-free survival and overall survival rates of 60–62% and 64–69%, respectively. A Korean leukemia group studied nilotinib plus chemotherapy backbone (n = 90). Similarly, they reported favorable two-year OS rate of 72%. *T315I* (threonine to isoleucine at position 315) mutations of the *ABL1* kinase domain have been described in up to 75% of relapsed patients after treatment with first- or second-generation TKIs. This led to studies using ponatinib with an amended dose de-escalation of 30 mg daily after achievement of complete remission and to 15 mg daily after achievement of complete molecular remission. The meta-analysis by Sasaki and colleagues (2016), favored hyper-CVAD plus ponatinib (n = 47) over hyper-CVAD plus dasatinib (n = 63). With propensity score matching, the three-year event-free survival rates for patients treated with hyper-CVAD plus ponatinib and hyper-CVAD plus dasatinib were 69% and 46%, respectively ($P = 0.04$), and the three-year overall survival rates were 83% and 56%, respectively ($P = 0.03$).

De-escalation of chemotherapy

- Phase II CALGB 10701 (2016) demonstrated high rates of complete remission and a lower induction mortality using low-intensity chemotherapy plus dasatinib (n = 66). Median age was 60 years (age range 22–87 years). They combined dasatinib with prednisone in induction and then added minimal chemotherapy in consolidation; complete remission rates of 86% were observed, allowing a third of patients to undergo allo-HCT, among whom no relapses occurred at a median follow-up of 23 months. Dasatinib maintenance was feasible after allo-HCT, autologous transplant, and chemotherapy alone with no missed doses in 59%, 83%, and 63% of cycles, respectively. Similarly, the combination of dasatinib with prednisone was evaluated in younger patients in the GIMEMA LAL1509 trial (2021). Median age was 42 years (age range 19–59 years, n = 60). Patients who did not achieve complete molecular remission by day 85 (82% of the study population) subsequently received chemotherapy, with or without transplant, whereas those who achieved complete molecular remission continued with dasatinib alone. Among non-complete molecular responders (n = 47), 22 underwent an allo-HCT. With a median follow-up of 57.4 months (range: 4.2–75.6), overall survival and disease-free survival were 56.3% and 47.2%, respectively. A better disease-free survival was observed in patients who obtained a molecular response at day 85 compared to cases who did not. The presence of additional copy number aberrations—*IKZF1* plus *CDKN2A/B* and/or *PAX5* deletions—was the most important unfavorable prognostic factor on overall and disease-free survival ($P = 0.005$ and $P = 0.0008$). In addition, the authors concluded that p210+ patients may require an intensified approach, given the lower rates of complete molecular remission and higher relapse rates in this group of patients with Ph+ALL.

Chemotherapy-free approach using steroids and TKI

- With just steroids and TKI, deep responses are rarely attained, remissions are short, and relapses are common resulting in poor long-term survival, signaling that additional agent(s) are required to achieve and maintain responses. Such strategy of steroids and TKI, was initially studied in the GIMEMA LAL0201-B trial is reasonable in Ph+ALL patients ineligible for cytotoxic chemotherapy. While it is clear that rates of complete molecular remission are higher with successive generations of TKIs (e.g. 46% with ponatinib, 18% with dasatinib, and 4% with imatinib), the toxicity profile of ponatinib may be prohibitive especially in patients with cardiovascular disease. The phase II, GIMEMA LAL1811 study (2017) analyzed efficacy and safety of steroids plus ponatinib in elderly or unfit patients with Ph+ALL (n = 42). Median age was 68 years (age ranged from 27 to 85 years). Nine out of 42 patients were < 60 years and were considered unfit. Complete molecular remission and one-year overall survival rates were 46% and 88%, respectively. At week 24, 15 of 42 patients still received 45 mg of ponatinib daily, and only 4 of 42 patients permanently withdrew from the study. Moving forward, blinatumomab is being studied on the backbone of a glucocorticoid, dasatinib (or ponatinib), and prophylactic intrathecal chemotherapy. Early results of SWOG 1318 are encouraging using blinatumomab, in combination with dasatinib and steroids. Patients 65 years of age or older with Ph+ or Ph-like ALL (with dasatinib sensitive fusions/ mutations) were eligible and could be newly diagnosed or relapsed/ refractory. With a median of 2.7 years of follow up, 3-year overall survival and disease-free survival were 87% (95% CI 64%-96%) and 77% (95% CI 54%-90%), respectively. (NCT02143414). The MRD-based studies in Ph+ALL suggest that reducing induction intensity results in reduced initial mortality, without compromising overall cure rates.

Allo-HCT in Ph+ALL, an area of uncertainty: Allo-HCT is generally considered a standard of care for young adult patients with Ph+ALL; however, a certain group of patients such as those younger than 21 years or those achieving complete molecular response may have long-term remission without allo-HCT. Patients who do not undergo allo-HCT receive a combination of chemotherapy and TKI as maintenance, whereas post-transplant remission is generally maintained with TKI only. Maintenance therapy is often continued for at least two years, but the precise duration is based on the treatment protocol. The optimal duration of post-transplant TKI maintenance therapy is unknown. The role of allo-HCT and post-transplant maintenance TKI therapy is discussed in Chapter 5.

In summary, the outcomes of patients with Ph+ALL continue to improve with a multifaceted approach with second- or third-generation TKIs, immunotherapy, and intrathecal chemotherapy with and without less intense multiagent chemotherapy. Interestingly, emerging data indicate that chemotherapy may be omitted or significantly decreased with incorporation of novel and highly effective agents such as blinatumomab. In addition, the role of allo-HCT might be of less value due to superior long-term outcomes in highly selected patients who achieve rapid complete molecular response. MRD negativity at protocol-defined time points seems to be a good surrogate marker for superior long-term outcomes. Nonetheless, relapse remains a problem in a subset of patient with MRD-negative disease; therefore, besides MRD detection there might be other biologic determinants (e.g. *IFZF1^{plus}*) that portend inferior outcomes requiring allo-HCT or novel approaches. The GRAALL 2022, EWALL-Ph-03, and GIMIMA ALL 2820, among others are few important trials testing the role of low-intensity chemotherapy, chemotherapy-free, and allogeneic transplant-free management approaches. Figure 2.1 outlines a general approach in treating patients with B-ALL.

6) **What is the diagnostic approach and testing limitations to properly diagnose Philadelphia chromosome–like acute lymphoblastic leukemia (Ph-like ALL)?**

Expert Perspective: Philadelphia chromosome–like ALL (Ph-like ALL) accounts for 15–30% of B-ALL depending on which subsets of B-ALL patients are reviewed. Due to unknown reasons there seems to be higher frequency among Hispanics.

- **Diagnostic approaches:** Whenever possible (preferably always!), patients with Ph-negative B-ALL should be evaluated for known alterations that define Ph-like ALL with FISH or validated special testing. Increased expression of TLSPR (thymic stromal lymphopoietin receptor) by flow cytometric immunophenotyping should prompt reflex *CRLF2* gene rearrangement testing. TSLPR$^+$ specimens with negative *CRLF2* (cytokine receptor-like factor 2) rearrangement FISH should trigger for *P2RY8-CRLF2* fusion analysis via RT-PCR or fusion panel testing. The most common kinase fusions are divided into 4 major categories based upon the presumed 3′ functional fusion partner: (i) ABL (Abelson kinase) class (*ABL1, ABL2, CSF1R* [colony-stimulating factor 1 receptor], *PDGFRA* [platelet-derived growth factor A], and *PDGFRB* [platelet-derived growth factor B]) rearrangements, (ii) *CRLF2* (cytokine receptor–like factor 2 rearrangements), (iii) *EPOR* (erythropoietin receptor) rearrangements, and (iv) *JAK2* (distinct from the canonical *JAK2 V617F* mutation) rearrangements. The categorization is based on the similarity of functions of these partners and their potential sensitivity to kinase inhibitors (e.g. *SRC/ABL/PDGFR* inhibitors for ABL class fusions and *JAK* inhibitors for *CRLF2, EPOR*, and *JAK2* rearrangements). Other rare Ph-like ALL–associated alterations (2.4%) have been reported, such as SH2B3 deletions potentially targetable by the JAK inhibitor ruxolitinib and *NTRK* fusions potentially targetable by the TRK inhibitors crizotinib and larotrectinib. *IKZF1* gene deletion is a common co–genetic abnormality that was seen in almost 60% of these patients. This topic is elegantly reviewed in a recent paper by Harvey and colleagues (see Recommended Readings).
- **Limitations:** Real-time diagnosis of patients can be quite challenging, and the best therapy for these patients is unclear due to remarkable genetic heterogeneity (> 70 discrete alterations reported) and the often cytogenetically cryptic nature of Ph-like ALL-associated alterations. Alteration in *CRLF2* is the most frequent abnormality (64%) in Ph-like ALL followed by *ABL* class (18.7%), *JAK2* (9.0%), and *EPOR* (5.7%) rearrangements. Of further interest, few cases with *CRLF2* gene rearrangement, particularly in children, lack the Ph-like ALL gene signature.

7) **What are the therapeutic challenges of Ph-like ALL?**

Expert Perspective: A growing body of evidence suggests that the presence of Ph-like ALL is a high-risk subtype associated with high rates of MRD positivity and treatment failures (Table 2.1). Identifying these patients early in diagnosis is becoming increasingly important. In the CALGB 10403, 31% of evaluable patients had Ph-like fusion, and these patients had significantly worse outcomes, with estimated three-year event-free survival of only 42% (95% CI 29–61%), in contrast to 69% (95% CI 60–80%) for those without these fusions (HR, 2.06; log-rank $P = 0.008$). As discussed, a majority of patients with Ph-like ALL have aberrant *CRLF2* expression, resulting in activation of the *JAK-STAT* pathway, and particularly poor outcomes, with a threefold increased risk of death (HR, 2.97; $P = 0.001$). Similarly, the MDACC study (n = 56) has shown inferior outcomes using hyper-CVAD–based therapies (all age groups) or an augmented BFM regimen (age < 40 years). Patients with Ph-like ALL who do not achieve MRD-negative complete remission post-induction may benefit from blinatumomab for MRD eradication followed by allo-HCT. Clinical trials are assessing the efficacy of the addition of TKIs and JAK inhibitors to mul-tiagent chemotherapy in patients with Ph-like ALL harboring ABL class translocations or *CRLF2* rearrangements, respectively (NCT02420717).

8) What is the value of CNS prophylaxis in B-ALL?

Expert Perspective: Intrathecal therapy is an essential component of every protocol for ALL and should be started during induction therapy. The design of the CNS prophylactic regimens is often quite empiric. This aspect of ALL has not been studied in a randomized fashion; rather, each group has adopted a regimen, and this has been maintained in succes-sive studies. For example, the hyper-CVAD regimen employs eight intrathecal chemo-therapy doses for standard-risk ALL, and 12 for Ph+ALL, a risk-adapted approach that has resulted in a CNS recurrence rate < 5%. The most common agent used for intrathecal pro-phylaxis is methotrexate. Other agents, given concurrently or separately, are cytarabine, methylprednisolone, and liposomal cytarabine. CNS prophylaxis with cranial radiation is an uncommon strategy in adults due to prohibitive toxicity and is reserved for patients who present with CNS disease or if there is a recurrence in the CNS that is not controlled with less toxic methods.

9) What are options in patients with relapsed and refractory B-ALL?

Expert Perspective: The prognosis of adults with relapsed or refractory B-ALL is gener-ally poor, with median overall survival ranging between four and seven months. Patients who are resistant to initial induction therapy, or those who have a complete remission duration of less than 12 months, have a particularly unfavorable prognosis.

Traditionally, salvage therapies included intensive chemotherapy regimens such as fludarabine, high-dose cytarabine, and granulocyte colony-stimulating factor (FLAG) with or without anthracycline, and high-dose cytarabine- or clofarabine-based regimens. A combination regimen including methotrexate, vincristine, PEG-asparaginase and dexa-methasone, and intrathecal chemotherapy with rituximab for CD20-positive disease, has also been used in R/R Ph-ALL. Liposomal vincristine is approved by the FDA for the treatment of R/R Ph-ALL. Liposomal formulation of vincristine generally produces less neurotoxicity and increased efficacy compared with the conventional formulation. Although capping doses of conventional vincristine at 2 mg has become common practice, it could be administered without dose capping. Patients with R/R Ph+ ALL can be treated with successive generations of TKIs often in combination with chemotherapy and/or ino-tuzumab ozogamicin. Allo-HCT, if possible, should be performed in patients who achieve response; however, only few patients are able to undergo allo-HCT because of poor disease responses and overall health. The higher risk of post-transplant sinusoidal obstruction syn-drome (SOS) with inotuzumab ozogamicin should be considered during the decision-making process.

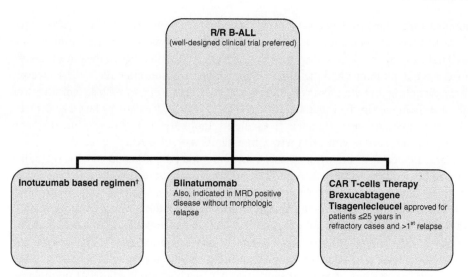

Figure 2.2 Simplified algorithm of treatment in relapsed or refractory or MRD-positive B-ALL. Consolidative transplant is generally recommended for suitable candidates who achieve remission. *†In cases with surface (not cytoplasmic!) CD22 positivity CRS: cytokine release syndrome; MRD: measurable residual disease; SOS: sinusoidal obstruction syndrome.*

In recent years, newer treatment options have been approved by the US FDA for the treatment of R/R Ph- and Ph+ ALL (Figure 2.2). These treatments include inotuzumab ozogamicin, blinatumomab (also approved for patients with minimal residual disease based on the results of BLAST study; Chapter 4), and chimeric antigen receptor (CAR) T-cell therapy (see Chapter 5). Currently two CARs against the CD19 antigen are approved for use in R/R ALL. Tisagenlecleucel (Tisa-cel) is indicated for the treatment of patients up to age 25 years with B-cell precursor ALL that is refractory or in second or later relapse. Brexucabtagene autoleucel for adult patients with relapsed or refractory B-ALL. Other developments include bispecific CARs, with receptors against both CD19 and CD22, designed to address the phenomenon of CD19-negative disease escape.

Anti-CD22 Antibody

Surface CD22 expression (not cytoplasmic) occurs in more than 90% of patients with ALL. The rapid internalization of CD22 upon receptor binding makes it an excellent target for monoclonal antibody–cytotoxic chemotherapy conjugates. Once internalized, the toxic component is released, causing cell destruction and death. Inotuzumab ozogamicin is a monoclonal antibody against CD22 that is linked to calicheamicin, a potent cytotoxin that induces double-stranded DNA breaks. In phase III of the randomized controlled INO-VATE study, inotuzumab ozogamicin was compared to standard chemotherapy in patients with relapsed or refractory ALL. The study reported excellent outcomes with inotuzumab ozogamicin compared to chemotherapy, including high complete remission rates (80% vs 29%), high MRD negative status (78% vs 28% among patients who achieved complete remission) and two-year overall survival (23% vs 10%; HR 0.75; one-sided $P = 0.01$). Forty-one percent underwent allo-HCT after treatment with inotuzumab compared to 11% with chemotherapy. There was no significant difference in the rate of relapse between the inotuzumab and the standard chemotherapy arms after allo-HCT. However, it is worth noting that the 100-day cumulative incidence rate of non-relapse mortality was significantly higher in the inotuzumab arm (21.8% vs 6.5%, $P = 0.01$). The SOS occurred in 19% in this cohort and was fatal in five patients. Inotuzumab ozogamicin has also been studied in combination with TKI therapy in patients with Ph+ ALL.

Patients treated with inotuzumab ozogamicin are at a risk of hepatotoxicity, including fatal and life-threatening SOS, also called hepatic veno-occlusive disease (VOD; about 11% incidence). The risk of SOS is greater in patients who undergo allo-HCT after inotuzumab ozogamicin treatment, have total bilirubin level ≥ upper limit of normal before allo-HCT, and receive allo-HCT conditioning regimens containing two alkylating agents. Other risk factors for SOS may include ongoing or prior liver disease, prior allo-HCT, increased age, later salvage lines, and a greater number of inotuzumab ozogamicin treatment cycles. Patients who receive inotuzumab ozogamicin also have a higher post-allo-HCT non-relapse mortality rate. An expert panel guideline recommends several measures to reduce the risk of SOS such as avoidance of allo-HCT conditioning regimens containing dual alkylating agents, thiotepa, or both; avoidance of hepatotoxic agents including an azole antifungal drug in combination with high-dose alkylator-conditioning regimen; and use of protective agents such as ursodiol. Additionally, it is recommended to limit treatment with inotuzumab to two cycles in patients eligible for allo-HCT. The efficacy of inotuzumab ozogamicin for MRD-positive B-ALL is also currently being evaluated in two clinical trials (NCT03610438 and NCT03441061).

Anti-CD19 Antibody

CD19 is another surface receptor with nearly universal expression on B-ALL cells. The receptor also internalizes sufficiently upon binding, making it an excellent target for immunoconjugate compounds. Harnessing one's immune system as a cancer-fighting modality has been studied extensively. Recruiting T-cells directly to leukemic blasts using monoclonal antibody technology may lead to synergistic effects and improved outcomes.

Blinatumomab is in a class known as the bispecific T-cell engaging (BiTE) molecules that contain components of two monoclonal antibodies. One arm of blinatumomab is designed to bind to CD3+ cytotoxic T-cells, while the other recognizes CD19. Upon binding to CD19, the T-cell becomes activated, thereby leading to the death of the malignant cell. Because of its short half-life, blinatumomab is given as a continuous infusion for four weeks, followed by a two-week treatment break.

- **Phase III TOWER study** in patients with relapsed or refractory B-ALL reported excellent results with blinatumomab, a bispecific T-cell engager (BiTE) anti-CD3/CD19 monoclonal antibody. Blinatumomab, compared to standard chemotherapy, produced complete remission rate of 34% versus 16% ($P < 0.001$), high MRD negative status (76% vs 48% among patients who achieved complete remission), and a median overall survival of 7.7 versus 4 months ($P = 0.001$), respectively. In all, 24% of patients in both blinatumomab and chemotherapy arms underwent subsequent allo-HCT. Adverse events of grade 3 or higher were reported in 87% of the patients in the blinatumomab group and in 92% of the patients in the chemotherapy group.

- **Single-arm multicenter phase II trial** of blinatumomab (n = 45) in Ph+ALL patients (50% with prior exposure to ponatinib and 27% with *T315I* mutation) was studied. The drug achieved complete remission and complete remission with partial hematologic recovery rates of 36% (95% CI 22–51%) during the first two cycles with 88% of responders achieving MRD negativity. Responses were observed regardless of *T315I* mutation status. Half of patients were able to undergo allo-HCT. Median relapse-free survival and overall survival were 6.7 and 7.1 months, respectively.

Important risks with blinatumomab include risks of cytokine release syndrome (CRS) and neurologic events, which require brief hospitalization for monitoring, and mild to moderate adverse events can generally be managed with treatment interruptions. The risks of CRS and neurotoxicity may be lower in patients with lower tumor burden; hence, cytoreduction with drugs such as dexamethasone or cyclophosphamide prior to initiation of blinatumomab may be helpful in patients with high tumor burden (see Chapter 59).

10) What are the future directions and perspectives in the treatment of front-line and relapsed B-ALL?

Expert Perspective: The incorporation of monoclonal antibodies is changing the treatment paradigm for adults with ALL. Studies have demonstrated the benefit of adding rituximab to an up-front chemotherapy regimen. The use of monoclonal antibodies against CD20 is potentially hampered by the varying degrees of expression of this antigen on lymphoblasts. An interesting concept that has been studied is the potential for corticosteroid-induced upregulation of CD20 expression, which would broaden the applicability in favor of using anti-CD20 agents.

Inotuzumab ozogamicin and blinatumomab can induce molecular remission in a high number of patients, which is critical to improving outcomes. Monoclonal antibodies also appear to be less toxic than conventional cytotoxic agents, making them particularly interesting for patients who are ineligible for intensive chemotherapy. Given excellent results in relapsed and refractory B-ALL, inotuzumab and blinatumomab are being incorporated in the up-front setting with or without reduced doses of intensive chemotherapy or TKI (in Ph+ALL). In fact, a strategy utilizing inotuzumab as a first-line therapy in combination with mini-hyper-CVAD with or without rituximab has already shown favorable results. The anthracycline infusion (doxorubicin) is omitted completely from this protocol, as it tends to cause significant problems for this age group and calicheamicin component in inotuzumab ozogamicin is an anthracycline. Calicheamicin binds to the minor groove of DNA to induce double strand cleavage and subsequent cell cycle arrest and apoptosis. Clinical trials are also underway using inotuzumab induction followed by consolidation with blinatumomab. Recently, excellent phase II data from MDACC (2022) was presented combining ponatinib with blinatumomab in front-line and relapse or refractory Ph+ALL. Use of blinatumomab and ponatinib in 40 patients with newly diagnosed Ph+ALL resulted in high complete remission and complete molecular response rates and estimated OS of 95% at 2 years. In addition, therapeutic developments in newly diagnosed Ph-negative ALL were also reported recently by ECOG-ACRIN E1910 investigators. After about 3.5 years of follow-up, 83% of the patients who went on to receive additional standard consolidation chemotherapy plus experimental blinatumomab were alive versus 65% of those who received chemotherapy only.

The progress in managing B-ALL is likely to accelerate further with parallel efforts in search of genetic abnormalities that drive the growth of B-ALL and serve as new targets. Examples would be the use of targeted therapies against specific molecular markers. Ph-like ALL, whose gene expression is like Ph+ALL despite lacking *BCR::ABL1* fusion gene, have *CRLF2* or various kinds of kinase-activating alterations involving *JAK2*, *ABL1*, *ABL2*, *CSF1R*, *PDGFRB*, *EPOR*, in addition to other mutations. The use of targeted agents with TKIs and JAK2 inhibitors can be beneficial in Ph-like ALL and are undergoing testing in clinical trials. Small molecules that inhibit DOT1L have been found to decrease the expression of *MLL* fusion target genes, inducing apoptosis selectively in leukemia cell lines derived from *MLL*-rearranged leukemia patients. Venetoclax, a selective small-molecule inhibitor of B-cell lymphoma-2 proteins in blast cells, has shown encouraging results in combination with mini-hyper-CVD chemotherapy in an early phase trial. Further testing in clinical trials and use of novel agents in various combinations will continue to improve outcomes of B-ALL in the future. Additional aspects of cellular therapy including transplant is discussed in the next chapter.

Recommended Readings

Advani, A.S., Moseley, A., O'Dwyer, K.M. et al. (2022 November 2). Dasatinib/Prednisone induction followed by Blinatumomab/Dasatinib in Ph+ acute Lymphoblastic Leukemia. *Blood Adv* 2022 Nov 2. doi: 10.1182/bloodadvances.2022008216. Epub ahead of print. PMID: 36322825.

Chiaretti, S., Ansuinelli, M., Vitale, A. et al. (2021 July 1). A multicenter total therapy strategy for *de novo* adult Philadelphia chromosome positive acute lymphoblastic leukemia patients: final results of the GIMEMA LAL1509 protocol. *Haematologica* 106 (7): 1828–1838. doi: 10.3324/haematol.2020.260935. PMID: 33538150; PMCID: PMC8252956.

Harvey, R.C. and Tasian, S.K. (2020 January 14). Clinical diagnostics and treatment strategies for Philadelphia chromosome-like acute lymphoblastic leukemia. *Blood Adv* 4 (1): 218–228. doi: 10.1182/bloodadvances.2019000163. PMID: 31935290; PMCID: PMC6960477.

Jabbour, E., Sasaki, K., Ravandi, F. et al. (2018 October 15). Chemoimmunotherapy with inotuzumab ozogamicin combined with mini-hyper-CVD, with or without blinatumomab, is highly effective in patients with Philadelphia chromosome-negative acute lymphoblastic leukemia in first salvage. *Cancer* 124 (20): 4044–4055. doi: 10.1002/cncr.31720. Epub 2018 Oct 11. PMID: 30307611; PMCID: PMC6515924.

Jain, N., Roberts, K.G., Jabbour, E. et al. (2017 February 2). Ph-like acute lymphoblastic leukemia: a high-risk subtype in adults. *Blood* 129 (5): 572–581. doi: 10.1182/blood-2016-07-726588. Epub 2016 Dec 5. PMID: 27919910; PMCID: PMC5290985.

Kantarjian, H., Stein, A., Gokbuget, N. et al. (2017). Blinatumomab versus chemotherapy for advanced acute lymphoblastic leukemia. *N Engl J Med* 376: 836–847.

Kantarjian, H.M., DeAngelo, D.J., Stelljes, M. et al. (2016). Inotuzumab ozogamicin versus standard therapy for acute lymphoblastic leukemia. *N Engl J Med* 375: 740–753.

Martinelli, G., Piciocchi, A., Papayannidis, C., Paolini, S., Robustelli, V., Soverini, S. et al. (2017). First report of the Gimema LAL1811 phase II prospective study of the combination of steroids with ponatinib as frontline therapy of elderly or unfit patients with Philadelphia chromosome-positive acute lymphoblastic leukemia. *Blood* 130 (Supplement 1): 99.

Maury, S., Chevret, S., Thomas, X. et al. (2016 September 15). Rituximab in B-lineage adult acute lymphoblastic leukemia. *N Engl J Med* 375 (11): 1044–1053.

Ravandi, F., Othus, M., O'Brien, S.M., Forman, S.J., Ha, C.S., Wong, J.Y.C., Tallman, M.S., Paietta, E., Racevskis, J., Uy, G.L., Horowitz, M., Takebe, N., Little, R., Borate, U., Kebriaei, P., Kingsbury, L., Kantarjian, H.M., Radich, J.P., Erba, H.P., and Appelbaum, F.R. (2016 December 27). US intergroup study of chemotherapy plus dasatinib and allogeneic stem cell transplant in Philadelphia chromosome positive ALL. *Blood Adv* 1 (3): 250–259. doi: 10.1182/bloodadvances.2016001495. PMID: 29046900; PMCID: PMC5642915.

Roberts, K.G., Li, Y., Payne-Turner, D. et al. (2014 September 11). Targetable kinase-activating lesions in Ph-like acute lymphoblastic leukemia. *N Engl J Med* 371 (11): 1005–1015. doi: 10.1056/NEJMoa1403088. PMID: 25207766; PMCID: PMC4191900.

Rowe, J.M., Buck, G., Burnett, A.K. et al. (2005 December 1). ECOG; MRC/NCRI Adult Leukemia Working Party. Induction therapy for adults with acute lymphoblastic leukemia: results of more than 1500 patients from the international ALL trial: MRC UKALL XII/ ECOG E2993. *Blood* 106 (12): 3760–3767. doi: 10.1182/blood-2005-04-1623. Epub 2005 Aug 16. PMID: 16105981.

Sasaki, K., Jabbour, E.J., Ravandi, F. et al. (2016 December 1). Hyper-CVAD plus ponatinib versus hyper-CVAD plus dasatinib as frontline therapy for patients with Philadelphia chromosome-positive acute lymphoblastic leukemia: a propensity score analysis. *Cancer* 122 (23): 3650–3656. doi: 10.1002/cncr.30231. Epub 2016 Aug 1. PMID: 27479888; PMCID: PMC5321539.

Stock, W., Luger, S.M., Advani, A.S. et al. (2019). A pediatric regimen for older adolescents and young adults with acute lymphoblastic leukemia: results of CALGB 10403. *Blood* 133 (14): 1548–1559.

Wieduwilt, M.J., Yin, J., Wetzler, M. et al. (2016). A phase II study of dasatinib and dexamethasone as primary therapy followed by hematopoietic cell transplantation for adults with Philadelphia chromosome-positive acute lymphoblastic leukemia: CALGB study 10701 (Alliance). *Blood* 128 (22): 2782.

3

T Cell Acute Lymphoblastic Leukemia and Acute Lymphoblastic Lymphoma

Syed A. Abutalib[1] and Daniel J. DeAngelo[2]

[1] *Aurora St. Luke's Medical Center, Milwaukee, WI*
[2] *Dana-Farber Cancer Institute, Harvard Medical School, Boston, MA, USA*

Introduction

T-cell acute lymphoblastic leukemia/lymphoma (T-ALL/BL) is an aggressive precursor lymphoid neoplasm, driven by malignant transformation and expansion of T-cell progenitors. T-ALL/LBL is composed of small to medium-sized blast cells with scant cytoplasm, moderately condensed to dispersed chromatin, and inconspicuous nucleoli, involving bone marrow and blood (Figure 3.1) often presenting with involvement of the thymus, nodal, or extranodal sites. The diagnosis of T-ALL versus T-LBL is arbitrarily distinguished by the presence of 25% blasts in the bone marrow or peripheral blood. Since most patients present with a mass lesion as well as lymphoblasts in the marrow, the distinction between leukemia and lymphoma is arbitrary.

Current treatment of T-ALL/BL consists of a high-intensity combination chemotherapy in suitable candidates. For young adult patients under 40 years of age, the AYA (adolescent and young adult) age group, risk-adapted pediatric, or pediatric-inspired regimens are often administered with a resulting high overall survival of 70 to 80%. However, not all adult patients are suitable candidates for AYA regimens, and conventional ALL adult regimens such as hyper-CVAD or other BFM (Berlin-Munich-Frankfurt) containing regimens with an overall survival of 50 to 60% are used. Despite the high complete remission rates, about 20% of pediatric and 40% of adult patients will relapse. Different from B-1 ALL, relapses in T-ALL/LBL tend to occur early and often during therapy resulting in a higher frequency of refractory disease. Furthermore, effective monoclonal antibodies as well as approved chimeric antigen receptor (CAR) T-cells are lacking in T-ALL/LBL. Nelarabine is the only FDA approved agent specifically for relapsed/refractory disease. Unfortunately, response rates for relapsed or refractory T-ALL/LBL remain low, and the overall prognosis is extremely dismal. The role of transplantation (detail discussion in Chapter 5), and measurable residual disease (MRD; also see discussion in Chapters 1 and 4) directed therapy is evolving. These among other important clinical issues, challenges, and controversies in the treatment of T-ALL/LBL will be discussed in this chapter.

Cancer Consult: Expertise in Clinical Practice, Volume 2: Neoplastic Hematology & Cellular Therapy,
Second Edition. Edited by Syed A. Abutalib, Maurie Markman, James O. Armitage, and Kenneth C. Anderson.
© 2024 John Wiley & Sons Ltd. Published 2024 by John Wiley & Sons Ltd.

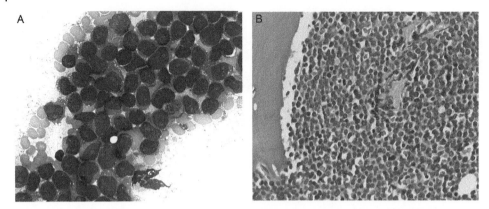

Figure 3.1 **A.** Bone marrow aspirate smear showing numerous blasts with prominent nucleoli and a high nucleus:cytoplasm ratio. **B.** Bone marrow biopsy specimen showing complete replacement of the medullary space by lymphoblasts. A bone trabecula is present at the left of the field. (Courtesy of L. Jeffrey Medeiros, MD, The University of Texas MD Anderson Cancer Center).

Case Study 1

A 20-year-old male patient presents with a two-week history of dyspnea on exertion and fatigue. A chest radiograph reveals a large mediastinal mass that is confirmed by computed tomography (CT) scan. The presenting leukocyte count is 20×10^9/L with 58% lymphoblasts. He also has a hemoglobin level of 12.3 g/dL and a platelet count of 110×10^9/L. A bone marrow aspirate reveals 26% lymphoblasts with an immunophenotype positive for CD34, TdT, cytoplasmic CD3, CD1a, CD5, and CD7. The blasts were negative for myeloperoxidase and other B-cell and myeloid markers. The cytogenetics revealed a normal 46XY karyotype. The findings are consistent with T-ALL.

The patient comes to you for a second opinion and asks about the diagnosis, therapy, and prognosis.

1) What is the epidemiology of T-ALL and T-LBL?
    A) T-ALL and T-LBL are more common in males than in females.
    B) T-ALL accounts for approximately 25% of cases of adult ALL.
    C) The incidence of T-LBL is higher in children than adults.
    D) There are genetic and gene expression differences between T-ALL and T-LBL.
    E) All of the above.

Expert Perspective: T-ALL accounts for about 15% of childhood ALL cases; it is more common in adolescents than in younger children and more common in males than in females. T-ALL accounts for approximately 25% of cases of adult ALL. T-LBL accounts for 85–90% of all LBLs; like its leukemic counterpart, it is most frequent in adolescent males. The incidence of T-LBL is higher in children and constitutes about 30% of the non-Hodgkin lymphoma (NHL). While T-ALL and T-LBL show many similarities in their genetics and gene expression, key differences exist, which may be related to the requirements for oncogenesis and survival in nodal and extranodal tissues. Basso and colleagues (2011) compared genome-wide gene expression and copy number alteration analysis in T-ALL and T-LBL and found differential expression of genes involved in chemotaxis and angiogenesis. A recent study by (Kroeze and colleagues 2020) demonstrated genetic and gene expression differences between T-ALL and T-LBL.

Correct Answer: E

2) **Which of the following statements about clinical presentation of T-ALL and T-LBL is correct?**
   A) T-ALL should not have extramedullary involvement.
   B) T-LBL always involves lymph nodes or one or more extranodal solid mass with lymphoblasts.
   C) T-LBL does not have circulating peripheral blasts.
   D) Mediastinal tumors do not cause pleural effusions.

Expert Perspective: If the patient presents with a mass lesion and lymphoblasts in the marrow, the distinction between leukemia and lymphoma is arbitrary. T-LBL, by definition, always involves lymph nodes or one or more extranodal solid mass but without < 25% abnormal lymphoblasts (unlike this case). T-ALL may also have extramedullary involvement. Of note, according to current WHO classification, patients with < 25% lymphoblasts in the absence of extramedullary disease will be classified as T-ALL. Circulating blasts in the peripheral blood are common in T-LBL. Mediastinal tumors may be associated with pleural effusions in 40% of T-LBL and in 10% of T-ALL. Few T-ALL/LBL patients present with pericardial effusions, which often necessitates an emergent pericardiocentesis.

Correct Answer: B

3) **Which of the following statements about karyotype abnormalities in T-ALL and T-LBL is correct?**
   A) Abnormal karyotype is detected in about 50% of cases.
   B) The prognostic implication of most chromosomal translocations is well defined.
   C) t(1;14) (p32;q11) translocation is detected in 20% of T-ALL cases.
   D) Detection of complex karyotype has no bearing on prognosis.

Expert Perspective: An abnormal karyotype is detected in 50 to 70% of cases of T-ALL/LBL. However, there are several different T-cell oncogenes (e.g. *HOX11*, *TAL1*, *LYL1*, *LMO1*, and *LMO2*) that may be aberrantly expressed in the absence of chromosomal abnormalities. The *TAL1* gene is altered as a consequence of the t(1;14) (p32;q11) chromosome translocation and is observed in 3% of patients with T-ALL (not 20%). As a consequence of the translocation, *TAL1* gene is transposed from its normal location on chromosome 1 into the T cell receptor (TCR) α/δ chain locus on chromosome 14. Brown and colleagues reported additional 25% of T-ALL patients bearing *TAL1* gene rearrangements that were not detected by karyotype analysis (discussed later). Surprisingly, the rearrangements observed in different patients were identical, i.e. all of them arose from a precise 90 kb deletion that disrupts the coding region of *TAL1* in a manner analogous to the t(1; 14)(p32;q11) translocation. The *TAL1* gene on chromosome 1 encodes a hematopoietic transcription factor. In general, the prognostic implication of genomic mutations and fusions are less well defined in T-ALL/LBL compared to B-ALL. In the UKALL XII/ECOG 2993 study, complex cytogenetics (≥ 5 abnormalities) was observed in about 8% of cases, and its presence negatively influenced the prognosis compared to its absence (five-year overall survival of 19 versus 51%, respectively, P = 0.006). Interestingly, the study found an association between CD2+ and complex karyotypes.

Correct Answer: A

4) **Which of the following statements about the front-line therapy in adults with T-ALL (our patient) is correct?**
   A) There is agreement that young adults with T-ALL should be treated on intensive pediatric-inspired protocols; however, clarity on how we define AYA (adolescents and young adults) is lacking.
   B) Definition of what constitutes a pediatric-inspired protocol is not clear in the modern era where adult protocols are also based on an MRD risk-based stratification.
   C) A subset of AYA patients might benefit from allogeneic hematopoietic cell transplantation in first complete remission.
   D) All of the above.

Expert Perspective: Increasing age is one of the most important adverse prognostic factors. The five-year disease-free survival is approximately 80% for children and 30–50% for adults with ALL. Given the dismal prognosis for recurrent T-ALL/BL, there have been rigorous efforts to improve overall survival by way of optimization of conventional agent(s) and integration of new agents (e.g. nelarabine or bortezomib) in selected AYA patients as a risk adapted approach. But still, some patients do remain either frankly refractory or MRD positive requiring allo-HCT.

   Overview of therapy: The goal of induction therapy in adult ALL is to achieve a reliable and accurate MRD-negative remission with low treatment-related toxicity/mortality and rapid hematologic recovery to enable prompt reinitiation of successive therapy. Although induction regimens vary, most use T-ALL–based pediatric-inspired regimens in suitable patients (e.g. ages 18 to 40 years, such as our patient), which include intensive use of the non-myelosuppressive agents (glucocorticoids, L-asparaginase, and vincristine), earlier and rigorous use of central nervous system (CNS) prophylaxis, delayed intensification and stringent maintenance therapy with 6-mercaptopurine and methotrexate, pulses of vincristine and steroids, and additional intrathecal CNS prophylaxis. While recognizing that differing disease biology between pediatric and adult ALL means we are unlike to match the exceptional overall survival seen within the pediatric cohort, this observation has led medical oncologists treating adult patients to question whether the benefits of the pediatric approach might extend beyond the traditional age cutoff of 25-years! NIH defines AYA as age range between 15 through 39 years. In addition to the obvious treatment differences between adult and pediatric trials, there has been much debate about the potential differences in adherence to therapy protocols among pediatric and adult medical hematologists and the patients whom they treat. Front-line myeloablative allo-HCT should be considered for high-risk T-ALL/LBL (this topic is further discussed in Chapter 5).

But what defines "high-risk disease" varies among study groups and is an area of uncertainty and controversy.

ALL-based pediatric-inspired regimens

- **Dana-Farber Cancer Institute** reported excellent results with pediatric-inspired regimen in adults up to age 50 years with three-year overall survival of 75%.
- **CALGB 10403:** This US Intergroup large phase II trial for younger adults up to age 39 years (n = 295) tested the successful approach used by the Children Oncology Group (COG) AALL0232 for treatment of high-risk adolescents with ALL. Use of the pediatric-inspired regimen was safe; overall treatment-related mortality was 3%, and there were only two post-remission deaths. The median event-free survival was 78.1 months (95% CI, 41.8–not reached), which was more than double the historical control of 30 months (95% CI, 22–38 months). Rates of estimated three-year overall survival were 73% (95% CI, 68–78) and event-free survival 59% (95% CI, 54–65); median overall survival was not reached after follow-up of 64 months. Obesity was a pretreatment risk factor associated with worse treatment outcomes.

There are additional intensive pediatric-inspired protocols (e.g. CALGB 8811/9111, GRAALL 2003, GRAALL 2005, augmented/intensified Berlin Frankfurt Munster [BFM]) in ALL; the preference of one regimen over the other is influenced by toxicity profile and institutional and patient's preference.

Patients who are unable to receive ALL pediatric-inspired protocol
(Let us assume that our patient in case study 1 is 55 years of age)
Many adults (especially age ≥ 40 years or younger with comorbidities) are not suitable for an intensive pediatric-inspired approach due, in part, to their inability to tolerate the intensive L-asparaginase, glucocorticoid, and vincristine dosing schedules along with intense CNS prophylaxis. In such patients, less-intense, and shorter-duration combination chemotherapy such as the hyper-CVAD, CALGB 8811 Larson regimen, GRAALL-2005, Linker 4-drug regimen, or UK XII/ECOG 2993 regimens are reasonable options.

Two most commonly utilized regimens are discussed below.

- **UK XII/ECOG 2993:** In all, 356 patients with T-lineage ALL were uniformly treated. Twenty (5.6%) of the 356 T-ALL patients failed to achieve complete remission (16 died during induction and 4 did not enter remission) and two patients had a transplantation without remission. Thus, 334 evaluable patients, i.e. 94%, achieved first complete remission. Subsequent therapy was sibling allograft (n = 88), autologous hematopoietic cell transplantation (n = 47), unrelated donor allograft (n = 14), other type of allograft (four mismatched and one allograft with reduced intensity conditioning), unknown type of transplantation (n = 2), and chemotherapy (n = 178). Ninety-nine patients were randomized between chemotherapy and autograft. Of the 45 patients randomized to chemotherapy, none were transplanted. The role of sibling donor allograft was assessed by a comparison with those without a sibling donor. A total of 253 patients were tissue typed of whom 110 had a related donor and 139 did not (and four are unknown). Of the 54 patients randomized to autograft, 33 had an autograft, 19 had chemotherapy, one had an unrelated donor allograft, and one patient received a transplantation from an unknown donor (assumed to be unrelated). For 99 patients randomized between autograft and chemotherapy, five-year survival was 51% in each arm. A total of 123 patients relapsed (37%). The OS at five years was 48% (95% CI, 42–53%). Of note, this study defined a high-risk group based on three factors in T-ALL/LBL: age > 35 years old, > 4 weeks to complete remission, and WBC count above 100×10^9/L. Biologic adverse factors are discussed in the next question. Older patients (> 35 years) and females had a poorer outcome (P = 0.004 and 0.05, respectively) and may require different strategies. In all, 27% of patients presented with a WBC at diagnosis more than 100×10^9/L; these patients had slightly inferior survival. Thirty-two patients had CNS involvement at diagnosis (9%); this did not affect five-year OS significantly (46% vs 48%, P = 0.8).

- **Hyper-CVAD** was developed by MD Anderson Cancer Center and uses hyperfractionated cyclophosphamide, dexamethasone, vincristine, and doxorubicin without asparaginase alternating with high-dose cytarabine and methotrexate. The complete response rate of hyper-CVAD is 91% with three- and five-year disease-free survival of rates of 50% and 38%, respectively. The MDACC group has developed augmented hyper-CVAD, which incorporates L-asparaginase, but this is not widely used.

There is a paucity of data concerning the best consolidation therapy in adults with T-ALL/LBL. Surely, a subgroup of AYA patients with T-cell ALL/BL are likely to benefit from allogeneic hematopoietic cell transplantation (allo-HCT) in first complete remission; however, widely accepted risk stratification models to identify such group of patients at diagnosis or early during treatment course are lacking. Maintenance therapy for two–three years is administered after induction and consolidation except in patients who undergo allogeneic transplantation; there is some role of delayed intensification in few non-transplant protocols. There is no role for maintenance therapy post allo-HCT in T-ALL/BL.

Correct Answer: D

5) **Which of the following statements about UKALL/ECOG2993 uniformly treated adult patients with T-ALL/LBL is correct?**
   A) Complex karyotypes had a significantly inferior survival.
   B) *TLX1* overexpression/translocations had an inferior outcome.
   C) Relapse was the problem for CD1a⁻ patients and death in remission for CD13⁺ patients.
   D) A and C.

Expert Perspective: This study (n = 356) also identified biologic factors associated with a poor outcome, namely, complex cytogenetics, CD13 positivity, and CD1a negativity. Achieving remission was not an issue in these poorer prognosis patients; relapse was the problem for CD1a⁻ patients and death in remission for CD13⁺ patients. These patients are candidates for trials of aggressive therapy, such as alternative donor (besides HLA-matched sibling donor) allografting in first complete remission or the use of nelarabine to consolidate remissions or if suitable candidates should be considered for ALL pediatric-type protocol. The study was unable to establish that *TLX1* overexpression/translocations (n = 21) and deletion of *CDKN2A* were not associated with superior outcomes.

This discrepancy could be the result of differential response to varied protocols. Patients with a mutation in the *NOTCH* pathway (*NOTCH-1* and/or *FBXW7*) had higher event-free survival versus those without 51% (±14%) versus 27% (±19%), but this was not statistically significant (*P* = 0.1).

Correct Answer: D

6) **Which of the following statements about prophylactic CNS-directed therapy in T-ALL/ LBL is correct?**
   A) Prophylactic cranial radiation therapy can be safely omitted given improvement in current T-ALL treatment.
   B) Asparaginase inclusion to escalating methotrexate in AALL0434 study showed to be effective in reducing CNS relapses.
   C) Lumbar puncture and intrathecal therapy at the time of diagnosis is performed in most adult patients with T-ALL/BL.
   D) A and B.

Expert Perspective: CNS involvement at diagnosis is more likely in T- than in B-ALL (9.6 vs 4.4%, P = 0.001), although less than 10% of adults with ALL will present with CNS involvement. In the UKALL XII/E2993 trial, patients presenting with CNS disease had inferior five-year OS of 42% compared with patients without CNS involvement of 29% due to an increased risk of both systemic and CNS relapses. Without CNS-directed therapy, CNS relapse will occur in 35 to 75% of patients at one year. A lumbar puncture at the time of ALL diagnosis is always performed in pediatric studies, but this is typically delayed in most adult ALL regimens.

Symptoms of CNS disease may include headache, meningismus, fever, or cranial nerve palsies. However, some patients are asymptomatic. If symptomatic CNS disease is present at diagnosis, such as focal cranial nerve palsies, concurrent radiation therapy and intrathecal chemotherapy are administered. An alternative combination strategy that uses intrathecal chemotherapy without radiation has also been investigated. This treatment regimen includes a so-called triple therapy that uses intrathecal methotrexate, cytarabine, and corticosteroids without radiation. High-dose methotrexate (HD-MTX) has also been used; however, its utility has been questioned. In the COG's AALL0434 a 2 × 2 randomization that compared the COG-augmented BFM regimen with either consolidation-methotrexate (included pegaspargase) or high-dose methotrexate (HD-MTX) during the eight-week interim maintenance phase. All patients with T-ALL, except for those with low-risk features, received prophylactic (12 Gy) or therapeutic (18 Gy) cranial irradiation during either the consolidation (second month of therapy) or delayed intensification (HD-MTX; seventh month of therapy) phase. The five-year disease-free survival and overall survival rates were 91.5% and 93.7% for consolidation methotrexate and 85.3% and 89.4% for HD-MTX, respectively. Of note, the timing of administration of prophylactic cranial radiation therapy was different between the groups and was delivered at week four in the escalating/consolidation methotrexate group vs week 26 in the HD-MTX group. Further, two additional doses of PEG-asparaginase were administered in the escalating methotrexate group, although all these differences in the randomized regimens could have also contributed to the superiority of the escalating methotrexate group.

Correct Answer: D

7) Which of the following statements about incorporation of nelarabine in front-line T-ALL and T-LBL therapy is correct?
A) All patients should receive nelarabine in front-line setting.
B) A selected subgroup of young adults have improved disease-free survival with its addition in front-line setting.
C) Patients who receive nelarabine in front-line setting must undergo up-front allogeneic transplantation.
D) B and C.

Expert Perspective: Nelarabine's encouraging results in relapsed T-ALL/LBL stimulated interest in its use in the front-line therapy of T-cell ALL and T-LBL.

Here we highlight two important studies,

- **COG (AALL0434) experience:** A pilot study from the COG added nelarabine to an intensified BFM protocol for children and young adults, initially reserving this therapy for slow early responders. Equivalent outcomes for the slow early responders who received nelarabine (73% with five-year event-free survival) and the rapid early responders who did not receive nelarabine (69% with five-year event-free survival, $P = 0.64$) were reported. Recently, (Dunsmore and colleagues 2020) on behalf of COG (AALL0434) published the results of a randomized phase III trial investigating the addition of nelarabine to the augmented BFM treatment with a 2 × 2 pseudo-factorial randomizations to receive escalating-dose methotrexate without leucovorin rescue plus PEG-asparaginase or HD-MTX with leucovorin rescue. Intermediate- and high-risk patients with T-ALL were randomly assigned after induction to receive or not six five-day courses of nelarabine in addition to an augmented BFM treatment regimen (upper age limit of 31 years). The addition of nelarabine improved the five-year disease-free survival of 91% (n = 147), but not the overall survival rate. The increased disease-free survival rate as well as the decreased CNS relapse rate without excessive toxicity support the inclusion of nelarabine into front-line therapy for pediatric or young adult patients with T-ALL, especially for patients with high-risk disease. Up-front allo-HCT did not seem to further improve the outcomes in the nelarabine treated patients.
- **MDACC experience in older adults:** A single-arm phase II study from MDACC of nelarabine addition to front-line or minimally pretreated (failure to one induction course or achieving complete remission after ≤ 2 cycles) hyper-CVAD regimen in 67 patients (age range 18 to 78 years; median 37 years) failed to improve complete remission duration or overall survival rates compared to historical controls treated with hyper-CVAD.

The combination of nelarabine with standard intensive induction chemotherapy (25 to 65 years) is in evaluation in a phase II randomized trial (UKALL14; NCT01085617).

Correct Answer: B

Case Study 2

A 20-year-old male patient presents with a two-week history of dyspnea on exertion and fatigue. A chest radiograph reveals a large (12.8 cm) mediastinal mass that is confirmed by computed tomography (CT) scan. The presenting leukocyte count is 20×10^9/L with 58% lymphoblasts. He also has a hemoglobin level of 12.3 g/dL and a platelet count of 110×10^9/L. A bone marrow aspirate reveals 0% lymphoblasts. The mediastinal mass biopsy shows immunophenotype positive for CD34, TdT, cytoplasmic CD3, CD1a, CD5, and CD7. The blasts were negative for myeloperoxidase and other B-cell and myeloid markers. The cytogenetics revealed a normal 46XY karyotype. The findings are consistent with T-LBL.

8) Should patients who present with T-LBL undergo a different treatment approach compared to the approach for T-ALL?

Expert Perspective: T-LBL represents approximately 2% and 30% of adult and pediatric NHLs, respectively. The peak incidence is in the second decade of life, with a smaller peak in adults > 40 years of age (bimodal distribution). As discussed, males are affected twice as often as females. The immunophenotype of T-LBL overlaps (is identical) with that of T-ALL. The clinical distinction between these two entities is arbitrarily defined. Bone marrow infiltration below 25% is considered T-LBL and above, T-ALL (operational versus biologic separation?). The lymphoblasts can be detected in the bone marrow in about 20% of patients with T-ALL/BL using conventional morphologic examination of bilateral bone marrow aspirates and biopsies. Using a flow cytometric method that allows the detection of one lymphoblast cell among 10,000 normal cells, marrow involvement is present in 72% of children with newly diagnosed T-LBL, a proportion that is much higher than that previously established by morphologic examination. The levels of involvement ranged from 0.01% to 31.6%. Moreover, high levels of marrow disease (defined as ≥ 1%) is associated with a poorer event-free survival. Of note, some patient may present without any evidence of marrow involvement, and such patients might be considered for autologous transplant (refer to MRD discussion and next chapter on transplant in T-ALL/LBL) especially in the absence of suitable allogeneic transplant donor.

Moreover, T-LBL is less likely to involve the CNS at diagnosis or at relapse compared to T-ALL, which led the AALL0434 study to exclude prophylactic cranial irradiation and HD-MTX prophylaxis in this group. Risk stratification in T-LBL is primarily based on marrow MRD (if involved) and based on PET response (e.g. at end-induction and end-consolidation on AALL1231 study). The role of marrow MRD in T-LBL is less clear even in patients treated on the AALL0434 study. It is important to realize that MRD assessment is not feasible in all the patients with either T-ALL or T-LBL (see Chapter 4). Response data in T-LBL are less robust, and COG experts recommend that patients with T-LBL who are not in remission by the end of consolidation be considered for allo-HCT once they achieve remission. The role of consolidative mediastinal irradiation is also diminishing with the advent of PET-guided assessment; however, this remains an area of controversy and investigation. Based on the German Multicenter Study Group for Adult ALL (GMALL) experience, mediastinal irradiation (as consolidation) with 24 Gy dose is suboptimal. Systemic relapses occurred in T-LBL patients with complete resolution of mediastinal tumors as well as in those with residual tumors after induction therapy. In pediatric T-LBL, low mediastinal recurrence rates are observed by intensive chemotherapy.

Besides these points, the treatment strategy for lymphoblastic lymphoma is similar to T-ALL. Data selective to adult T-LBL is scarce due to the rarity of the disease. Intensive multi-agent systemic chemotherapy regimens incorporating CNS-directed therapy have resulted in event-free survival rates of 75 to 90% in children and 40 to 80% in adults. Future studies are needed to determine whether there is an MRD cutoff at diagnosis or after initiating therapy (reliable time points of PET scan with different regimens!) with sufficient prognostic significance to justify changing therapy in T-LBL.

Case Study 3

A 28-year-old female patient presents with a one-month history of bruising and fatigue. A complete blood count (CBC) reveals a leukocyte count of 32×10^9/L with 62% lymphoblasts. She also has a hemoglobin level of 9.7 g/dL and a platelet count of 42×10^9/L. A bone marrow aspirate reveals 58% lymphoblasts with an immunophenotype shown in Figure 3.2. The findings are consistent with the diagnosis of ETP-ALL. CT scans that are performed on the chest, abdomen, and pelvis reveal a 6 cm mediastinal mass and scattered lymphadenopathy. The liver and spleen appear normal. The cytogenetics revealed a normal 46XX karyotype.

How the approach and treatment of this patient would differ compared to the patients in case studies 1 and 2 will be the focus of our discussion

9) **Which of the following statements about immunophenotyping of T-ALL and T-LBL is correct?**
   A) Immunophenotype subtypes of T-ALL reflect the different stages of differentiation of normal thymocytes.
   B) The 2016 revision of the WHO classification added a provisional entity called early T-cell precursor (ETP) ALL.
   C) Thymic subtype expresses CD1a, with or without surface CD3 expression, and expresses CD2 and CD4 or CD8.
   D) All of the above.

Expert Perspective: Immunophenotype subtypes of T-ALL reflect the different stages of differentiation of normal thymocytes based mainly on membrane expression of various antigens. According to the European Group for the Immunologic Classification of Leukemia (EGIL) classification, there are four subtypes of T (TdT+, cyCD3+, CD7) ALL: pro–T-ALL, pre–T-ALL, cortical/thymic T-ALL, and mature T-ALL. In most recent T-ALL/LBL trials, pro-T and pre-T phenotypes are combined together as early T-ALL making three distinct immunologic subtypes, differentiated by IHC parameters (Table 3.1) as follows:

• **ETP:** The 2016 revision of the WHO classification added a provisional entity called ETP ALL. It accounts for 15% of all T-cell ALL in children and about 35% in adult T-cell

Early T-cell Precursor Acute Lymphoblastic Leukemia
Flow cytometry

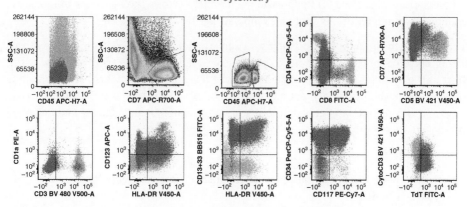

Figure 3.2 Flow cytometry immunophenotypic analysis of a case of early T-cell precursor acute lymphoblastic leukemia. The blasts are positive for CD4 (partial), CD7, CD13+33, CD34, CD117(partial), CD123, and TdT and are negative for CD1a, CD3 (cytoplasmic and surface), CD5, and CD8. (*Source:* Courtesy of Sanam Loghavi, MD, The University of Texas MD Anderson Cancer Center).

Table 3.1 Three distinct immunologic subtypes, differentiated by IHC parameters.

T-ALL/LBL subtypes	Immunophenotype
T-Lineage	TdT+, cytoplasmic CD3+, CD7+
A) Early	CD2–, surface CD3–, CD1a– plus myeloid marker(s) except MPO
B) Thymic	CD1a+, surface CD3±
C) Mature	Surface CD3+, CD1a–

ALL/LBL. ETP-ALL expresses CD7 but lacks or has low expression of CD5 and is negative for CD1a. In addition, ETP-ALL is often positive for one or more of the myeloid cell markers CD117, CD13, CD33, CD11b, and CD65 but not myeloperoxidase (MPO). ETP ALL is also characterized by lack of expression of CD4 and CD8 and presence of the "double negative 1" (DN1) thymocyte. ETP-ALL has been associated with a poorer prognosis in both children and adults, but with newer risk adapted approaches, the outcomes for patients with ETP-ALL is similar to those with classical T-ALL/LBL (Chapter 1).

- **Thymic:** Classical or thymic T-ALL/LBL usually expresses CD1a, with or without surface CD3 expression, and expresses CD2 and CD4 or CD8. This subtype is more common in children than adults and has the superior prognosis compared to other immunologic subtypes. In general, this subtype responds well to therapy and seems to do well, in most cases without transplantation in first complete remission.

- **Mature:** This is the rarest subtype and occurs often in older adults. Mature T-ALL/LBL is characterized by surface CD3 expression while CD1a is lost. The incidence of mediastinal tumors is higher in this subtype compared to ETP-ALL.

In adult T-ALL the immunophenotype distinction is an important prognostic factor with an inferior outcome for early and mature T-ALL and a superior outcome for thymic T-ALL; the effect of the immunophenotype in adult T-LBL remains unclear. Of note, immunophenotyping is not always possible in patients with T-LBL due to the scarcity of available tissue. The prognostic distinction between these subtypes is variable and is likely influenced by different treatment protocols.

Correct Answer: D

10) **What is known about the molecular spectrum of different immunologic subtypes of T-ALL and T-LBL?**
   A) Fusion gene transcripts without chromosomal rearrangements are observed in about 20% of T-ALL cases.
   B) Cytogenetic and global transcriptomic analyses have led to the classification of T-ALL into molecular subgroups.
   C) The molecular characterization has provided a strong rationale for targeted therapies in T-ALL.
   D) All of the above.

Expert Perspective: Significant number of T-ALLs cases have genomic aberrations especially in the oncogenic transcription factors by T cell specific enhancers, resulting in overexpression of numerous oncogenes, including *TAL1, TAL2, LYL1, OLIG2, LMO1, LMO2, TLX1 (HOX11), TLX3 (HOX11L2), NKX2-1, NKX2-2, NKX2-5, HOXA* genes, *MYC, MYB, and TAN1*. In addition, recurrent chimeric protein fusions include rearrangements of *KMT2A (AFDN [AF6], MLLT1, ELL), SET-NUP214, ABL1 (NUP214::ABL1, BCR::ABL1), MLLT10 (PICALM, DDX3X, NAP1L1, XPO1)*, and the ETS family (*SPI* and *ETV6*). Similar oncogene-associated translocations and/or chimeric protein fusions have been found in pediatric T-LBL patients compared to T-ALL patients, although their prevalence and significance is less clear. It is impossible to integrate these vast molecular abnormalities in risk models, but their discovery has allowed better understanding of pathogenetic taxonomy and therapeutic targets.

Meijerink and colleagues clustered T-ALL in four main subtypes with characteristic oncogenic aberrations, namely (i) early thymocyte progenitor (ETP)/immature-ALL (described previously), (ii) *TLX*, (iii) *TLX1/NKX2.1* (originally denoted as proliferative subgroup), and (iv) *TAL/LMO* (Figure 3.3).

Brief summary of the data and its implications

i) **Molecular spectrum of ETP-ALL:** This subtype (10% of T-ALL) is driven by aberrant *MEF2C (SPI1, RUNX1, ETV6::NCOA2,* and *NKX2.5)* or *HOXA* gene expression, presents frequent mutations in the IL7 signaling cascade, and shows self-renewal genes including *LMO2, LYL1,* and *HHEX,* and the antiapoptotic BCL2. *HOXA* locus activating events have been correlated to chemoresistance and inferior outcome in adult ETP-ALL. Interestingly, ETP-ALL blasts have higher mutational loads compared with blasts of other T-ALL subtypes. The distinct mutational profile from other T-ALLs, has fewer

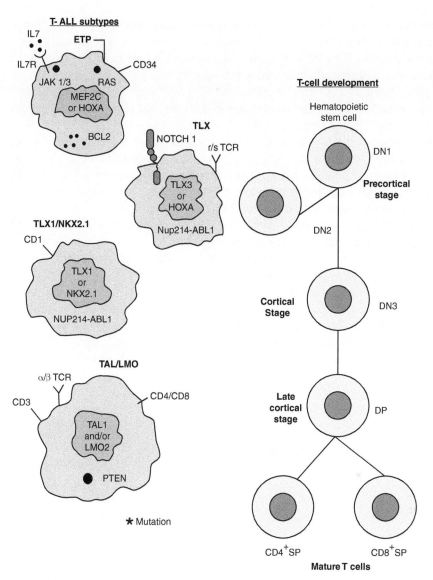

Figure 3.3 Relationship of four T-ALL subtypes with T-cell development (credit of artwork to T. and K. Schiera and adapted from Cordo' et al. 2020).

NOTCH pathway-activating mutations and *CDKN1I2* mutations with relatively high prevalence of mutations in *acute myeloid leukemia-associated genes* such as *KIT, GATA2,* and *CEBPA, IDH1, IDH2, DNMT3A, FLT3, JAK1, JAK3* and *NRAS*; whether these genetic characteristics are shared by ETP-LBL is not known. In addition, recurrent 5q deletions result in deletion of the *NR3C1* locus, conferring resistance to steroids, which has also been observed. According to the COG experience, in our opinion, suitable patients with ETP ALL should be treated the same as their non-ETP counterparts on a contemporary MRD response-adapted pediatric-inspired regimen whenever possible. Of clinical importance, the kinetics of MRD response appears to be quite different in ETP-ALL compared with other T-ALL (slow MRD clearance!); however, on intensive COG regimens the ultimate outcome with appropriate therapy appears to be the same. Does this favorable outcome also hold true with treatment in AYA and older adults?

ii) **TLX**, driven by either *TLX3* (translocation with *BCL11B*)- or *HOXA*- (like ETP-ALL) activating events. This subgroup includes immature cases that either lack a functional T-cell receptor (TCR) or present a γ/δ TCR, which is in line with early or γ/δ T-cell lineage development (double negative 2 [DN2] stage). *TLX3*-rearranged T-ALLs often have *NOTCH1*-activating mutations and aberrations (better prognosis) in epigenetic regulators such as PHF6 and CTCF. Interestingly, a recent study in children by Pui and colleagues suggests that patients with γ/δ T-ALL have higher MRD levels after induction chemotherapy compared with other T-ALL cases.

iii) **TLX1/NKX2.1** is driven by either *NKX2.1* or *TLX1* aberrations, CD1 expression, and differentiation arrest at the cortical (DN3-DP) stage of T-cell development. *TLX*-rearranged cases can present the oncogenic *NUP214::ABL1* fusion, a target for *ABL1/Src*-family kinase inhibitors. This subgroup has better prognosis.

iv) **TAL/LMO**, which is characterized by ectopic expression of TAL1 (either via translocation or *SIL–TAL1* deletion), *TAL2*, *LYL1*, *LMO1*, *LMO2*, or *LMO3*, includes the most mature T-ALL cases. As for late cortical T-cell progenitors, TAL/LMO blasts express mature T-cell surface markers such as CD4+, CD8+, CD3+, and α/β TCR. In addition, PIK3R1- or PIK3CG-activating lesions are frequent within this cluster. *PTEN* mutations are most common in this subgroup and have been associated with poor outcome in childhood T-ALL/LBL. Moreover, *TAL1*-rearranged cases often have mutations in the ubiquitin-specific protease USP7, which regulates MDM2 and TP53 stability (Chapter 1).

Most recently, Stemle and colleagues (2022) identified fusion gene transcripts in 20% (without chromosomal rearrangements) of T-ALL cases (n = 522). *PICALM::MLLT10* (4%, n = 23), *NUP214::ABL1* (3%, n = 19), and *SET::NUP214* (3%, n = 18) were the most frequent. The clinico-biological characteristics linked to fusion transcripts in a subset of 235 patients (138 adults in the GRAALL2003/05 trials and 97 children from the FRALLE2000 trial) were analyzed to identify their prognosis impact. Patients with *HOXA* trans-deregulated T-ALLs with *MLLT10*, *KMT2A*, and *SET* fusion transcripts (17%, 39 of 235) had a worse prognosis with a five-year event-free survival of 35.7% vs 63.7% (HR = 1.63, P = 0.04) and a trend for a higher cumulative incidence of relapse (five-year cumulative incidence of relapse = 45.7% vs 25.2%, HR = 1.6, P = 0.11).

The molecular characterization provided a strong rationale for targeted therapies in T-ALL, such as drugs directed against JAK, NOTCH1, BCL-2, or PI3-AKT signaling pathways facilitating pathway for precision medicine (Figure 3.4).

Correct Answer: D

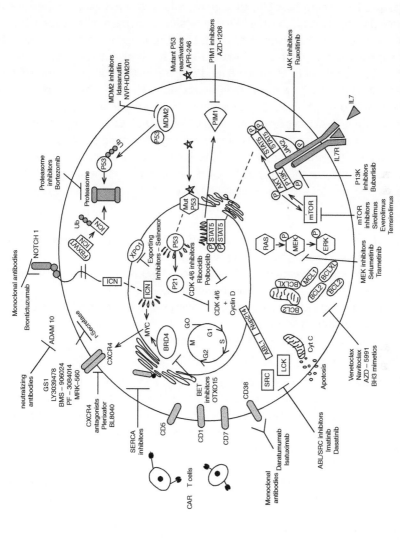

Figure 3.4 T-ALL/LBL and potential targets (*Source*: credit of artwork to T. and K. Schiera and adapted from Cordo' et al. 2020).

Case Study continued: Our patient is started on CALGB 10403 protocol

11) **Which of the following is a widely accepted factor as an indication for allogeneic transplant in patients treated on an intensive pediatric-inspired protocol?**
    A) MRD > 1×10^{-4} after two courses of therapy.
    B) Complex cytogenetics $\geqslant$ 5 abnormalities.
    C) Early T-cell precursor ALL.
    D) Presenting WBC > 100×10^9/L.

Expert Perspective: Where possible, all patients with T-cell ALL (and T-LBL) should be treated on a prospective clinical trial. Outside of a clinical trial, the indication of allogeneic transplant varies on the type of protocol being used among other variables. Given that this patient is being treated on CALGB 10403, the best answer is option A. Nonetheless, the precise relevance of option B (and sometimes C) for allo-HCT even if patient achieves MRD negativity (at defined time points) is unclear in adults with T-ALL/LBL. Most experts would not transplant the patient who achieves MRD negativity (at defined time points) with ETP-ALL or presenting WBC > 100×10^9/L. Equally important is to consider and compare the long-term outcomes of the regimen being used, its relapse risk in subgroups, patients' overall condition, and specific transplant outcomes. If survival with chemotherapy is better or the same as for transplantation, then the transplant should be deferred.

Correct Answer: A

12) **Which of the following statements about MRD detection on a pediatric or pediatric-inspired regimen in adults with T-ALL/BL is correct?**
    A) Several studies have confirmed early MRD response as a powerful predictor of long-term survival in adult patients with T-ALL/BL.
    B) There is discrepancy among experts on how best to interpret MRD detection when it comes to altering therapy.
    C) There are variable definitions of MRD detection.
    D) All of the above.

Expert Perspective: Numerous studies have confirmed "early" MRD response as a powerful predictor of long-term survival in adult patients with ALL. What defines "early" with the exception of few regimens defining it, otherwise remain unclear. Molecular-based and flow cytometry–based techniques allow reliable assessment of MRD, whose monitoring at precise time points is the standard of care for ALL patients treated with curative intent (see Chapter 4 on MRD in ALL).

Based on the poor outcome with high MRD (United States > 0.1%; United Kingdom >0.05%) at the end of consolidation, most experts would recommend allo-HCT. In addition, in the United Kingdom, experts recommend allo-HCT in patients with end-induction MRD $\geqslant$ 5% except those under 16 years with negative (< 10^{-4}) end-of-consolidation MRD.

Following are major studies with MRD assessment and its implications

- German: GMALL examined MRD at nine time points in adults receiving GMALL 09/99 ALL therapy and showed that, using their treatment protocols, molecular MRD quantification after two courses of therapy (10 to 16 weeks from diagnosis) was the most predictive of outcomes with patients failing to achieve molecular remission (MRD > 10^{-4}) post-induction having inferior survival compared with patients who were MRD-negative (MRD < 10^{-4}) (42% vs 80%, P < 0.001). Seventy-two of the 196 patients (37%) within this study had T-cell disease.
- French: GRAALL analyzed the prognostic significance of MRD at six weeks from the initiation of induction therapy on the pediatric-inspired GRAALL 2003 and 2005 trials in 163 patients with T-cell ALL (n = 423). They defined a high-risk group as those with an MRD level ⩾ 10^{-4} and unfavorable cytogenetics (no *NOTCH/ FBXW7* mutation and/ or *N/K-RAS* mutation and/or *PTEN* mutation). The patients in this high-risk group (59%) had markedly inferior overall survival compared with the good-risk group (62% vs 91% at five years, respectively).
- Hough et al. reported overall survival outcomes of 72% at five years for AYA patients aged 16 to 25 years treated on a risk-adapted pediatric protocol where the strongest predictor for survival was immunoglobulin heavy chain (B-ALL) gene or T-cell receptor-defined (T-ALL/LBL) MRD status after induction. Patients with low-risk MRD (< 0.01%) had a 93% event-free survival at five years compared with 64% event-free survival at five years for those with high-risk MRD (at least 0.01%). Over 75% of AYA patients with T-cell ALL had high-risk or indeterminate MRD post-induction in this study.

Although it is reasonable to recommend allo-HCT for patients with persistent MRD while in first complete remission, there are currently no data to show that intervention with novel agents or allogeneic transplantation can overcome the relapse risk.

Correct Answer: D

Case Study continued: Our patient is MRD+ and has a healthy HLA-matched sibling donor.

13) **Which of the following statements about UKALL XII/E2993 and allogeneic transplants for T-ALL and T-LBL are correct?**
   A) This trial assessed the role of an HLA-matched sibling donor allo-HCT by a comparison of outcomes in those with versus those without an HLA-matched sibling donor.
   B) The results of this study suggest that myeloablative allo-HCT is an effective therapy in adults and can be considered for patients with high-risk T-ALL/LBL.
   C) HLA-matched sibling donor is preferred over HLA-matched unrelated donor for patients with high-risk T-ALL/BL.
   D) All of the above.

Expert perspective: Determining whether T-ALL and T-LBL patients may also benefit from allogeneic transplant in first complete remission continues to be area of active debate and investigation.

- **UKALL XII/E2993** (2009): Myeloablative conditioning of etoposide and total body irradiation (13.2 Gy in eight fractions) was used. The results of this study suggest that myeloablative allo-HCT is an effective therapy in adults and can be considered for patients with high-risk T-cell disease. In the UKALL XII/E2993 study, sibling donor halved the chance of relapse (25% vs 51%, $P < 0.0001$), but modestly increased non-relapse mortality (22% vs 12%, $P = 0.06$) was observed. The overall survival at five years was 46% (38 to 55%) for the no donor group and 61% (51 to 70%) for the donor group (log rank $P = 0.07$, χ^2 test of difference at five years, $P = 0.02$); this difference was maintained at 10 years. HLA-matched sibling donor is preferred over HLA matched unrelated donor for patients with high-risk T-cell disease.

Correct Answer: D

14) **Which of the following statements about UKALL14 study and allogeneic transplants for T-ALL and T-LBL are correct?**
    A) Study reported that a sufficient number of patients were analyzed.
    B) Like UKALL XII/E2993, a myeloablative regimen was utilized.
    C) Patients with MRD > 10^{-4} at allo-HCT had a lower event-free survival.
    D) All of the above.

Expert Perspective: Compared to reduced intensity conditioning regimen, myeloablative conditioning regimen allows better disease control but at the cost of higher treatment-related mortality especially in older adults (defined as age > 40 years).

- The UKALL14 study (2022) used reduced intensity conditioning (intravenous fludarabine 30 mg/m^2 on days −6 to −2, melphalan 140 mg/m^2 on day −2, and alemtuzumab 30 mg on day −1 [sibling donor] and days −2 and −1 [8/8 unrelated donor]) in patients (aged ⩾ 41 years) with ALL, and although the number of T-cell patients was insufficient to be analyzed separately, the risk of relapse was increased. Donor lymphocyte infusions was given from six months for mixed chimerism or MRD. Patients with MRD > 10^{-4} at allo-HCT had a lower event-free survival (primary endpoint, HR 2.75, $P = 0.047$) compared with those that were MRD-negative ⩽ 10^{-4}). This patient subgroup may require additional pre-transplant therapy to achieve MRD negativity before transplant.

Further exploration of the optimal conditioning regimen to reduce relapse is the focus of research in the UKALL reduced intensity conditioning study (NCT03821610). Also refer to the subsequent chapter for further discussion.

Correct Answer: C

15) **Which of the following statements about relapsed and refractory T-ALL and T-LBL is correct?**
    A) About 80% of relapses occur within two years of diagnosis.
    B) The five-year survival rate is < 10%.
    C) Once the patient relapses, subsequent cure is unlikely.
    D) All of the above.

Expert Perspective: About 81% of relapses occur within two years of diagnosis. In the UKALL XII/E2993 study, the five-year survival rate was only 5% for these patients. Once the patient relapses, subsequent cure is unlikely whatever the initial therapy may have been. The survival rates are clearly much lower than for those treated on this study with transplant in first complete remission: 42% for autograft, 45% for HLA-matched unrelated donor allograft, and 52% for sibling allograft, which suggests, unsurprisingly, that allo-HCT is much more beneficial if used in first complete remission rather than being delayed according to this protocol. See Chapter 5 for further detailed discussion about transplant in T-ALL/BL.

Correct Answer: D

Case Study 4

A 28-year-old male patient presents with a history of T-ALL that was diagnosed seven months ago; he is currently receiving maintenance chemotherapy and returns for a regular appointment feeling well. On routine laboratory assessment, the leukocyte count is 2.1×10^9/L with 28% lymphoblasts. He also has a hemoglobin level of 8.9 g/dL and a platelet count of 57×10^9/L. A bone marrow aspirate reveals 42% lymphoblasts with an immunophenotype positive for CD34, TdT, cytoplasmic CD3, CD1a, weak CD5, and CD7. The blasts were negative for myeloperoxidase and other B-cell and myeloid markers. The cytogenetics revealed a normal 46XY karyotype. The findings are like the initial presentation and consistent with recurrent T-ALL. He did not receive nelarabine in the front-line therapy. The patient and his family wish to know what treatment options are available.

16) **What is the most appropriate initial therapy for this patient with relapsed/refractory T-ALL?**
   A) Nelarabine.
   B) Allogeneic transplantation.
   C) Clofarabine.
   D) Single-agent PEG-asparaginase.

Expert Perspective: Although the majority of adult ALL patients reach complete remission, many will eventually relapse and subsequently be much less responsive to salvage therapy. First relapse typically occurs within the first two years after induction, and remissions lasting longer than 18 months are associated with improved response to salvage regimens. The complete remission rates for salvage regimens range from 31 to 78%, and survival for these patients remains poor.

Nelarabine, a T-specific purine (deoxyguanosine) analog prodrug, is approved as single-agent therapy for both pediatric and adult patients. Upon demethoxylation and intracellular phosphorylation, it is converted to ara-G triphosphate preferentially accumulating in T-lymphoblasts inhibiting DNA replication and subsequently causing cell death.

Following are the data for nelarabine in relapsed/refractory T-ALL/BL

- CALGB 19801 (2007) administered nelarabine to treat relapsed and refractory patients and demonstrated a complete remission rate of 41% and overall survival rate of 28% at one year. These results were especially impressive given that many of the patients had failed two or more inductions or had not achieved complete remission with their last induction regimen. Similar data were seen in the COG study in pediatric patients with relapsed or refractory T-ALL. The use of nelarabine has allowed a greater number of patients to receive curative, allo-HCT.

- GMALL (2011): Patients received nelarabine 1.5 g/m^2 on days one, three, and five for either one or two 21-day cycles. At the start of the study, allo-HCT was recommended as soon as a complete remission was achieved; later, a second cycle of nelarabine was advised to reduce pre-allo-HCT MRD levels. After either one or two cycles, 36% of patients (45 of 126) achieved a complete remission, 10% (12 of 126) a partial response, and 55% (62 of 126) were refractory. Overall survival was 24% at one year. An impressive 80% of patients who achieved a complete remission proceeded to allo-HCT, with a three-year relapse-free survival of 37%. These results were in line with those from the smaller CALGB 19801 study. The exact number of cycles prior to allo-HCT is unknown.

Correct Answer: A

The clinical dilemma is what should one do in relapsed or refractory T-ALL/BL patients who are previously exposed to nelarabine (COG AALL0434) especially in the frontline setting. This brings us to our next question.

Targetable genetic lesions

17) **Which of the following agents or strategies are or have been focus of clinical trials in patients with relapsed and refractory T-ALL/LBL?**
    A) Venetoclax.
    B) Navitoclax.
    C) Bortezomib.
    D) Crenigacestat.
    E) Selumetinib.
    F) Daratumumab.
    G) OBI-3424.
    H) Ruxolitinib.
    I) Imatinib.
    J) CAR T cell therapy.
    K) All of the above.

Expert Perspective: Advances have been limited in the management of relapsed and refractory T-ALL/LBL. The insight in the genomic landscape has paved the way for novel targeted drugs, and *ex vivo* gene therapy (Figure 3.4) Some of the novel agents and CAR T cell therapy targets are discussed below:

- **Venetoclax and navitoclax** (BH3 Mimetics): BH3 (e.g. BCL2, BCLXL, and/or MCL1) profiling of T-ALL cell lines and patient blasts identified a dependency on BCL2 in ETP-ALL and BCLXL in the remaining subtypes of T-ALL. Consequently, immature/ETP-ALL cells are most responsive to venetoclax, whereas other T-ALL subtypes are more sensitive to navitoclax (ABT-263; BCL2/BCLW/BCLXL inhibitor) treatment, respectively. The MCL1 inhibitor S63845 also induces efficient cell death in various T-ALL cell lines as single treatment (39), therefore serving as an interesting alternative to venetoclax, especially given the limited dependency on BCL2 in most patients with T-ALL.

- **Bortezomib:** Early data using bortezomib in combination with intensive chemotherapy has demonstrated promising results leading to its further development in ALL.

- **Crenigacestat and BMS-906024** (NOTCH1 Inhibitors): Over 70% of T-ALL cases present *NOTCH1*-activating mutations (gain of function), and up to 25% of patients harbor mutations in the *FBXW7* gene, which mediates the proteasomal degradation of *NOTCH1*. Despite promising preclinical results, γ-secretase inhibitors failed during clinical trials due to insufficient efficacy (even in presence of *NOTCH1* mutations) and excessive gastrointestinal toxicity. Preclinical data showed that simultaneous corticosteroid administration can relieve gastrointestinal toxicity and enhance the GSI antitumor activity. In a phase I study, crenigacestat with dexamethasone (2021) demonstrated limited activity. Alternative strategies are also being developed to alleviate the GI toxicity from γ-secretase inhibitors and to target *NOTCH1*-activating mutations via different mechanisms.

- **Selumetinib** (MEK inhibitor): In the phase I/II of the SeluDex study (NCT03705507), selumetinib will be given in combination with dexamethasone to a planned 42 adult and pediatric participants with relapsed B- and T-ALL with evidence of RAS-pathway mutations.

- **Daratumumab:** CD38 is frequently expressed on both pediatric and adult B- and T-ALL blasts (78% and 91%, respectively). The efficacy of daratumumab in combination with chemotherapy in treating relapsed B- and T-ALL in patients aged up to 30 years is under investigation in the phase II multicenter Delphinius trial (NCT03384654).

- **OBI-3424:** This is a first-in-class targeted treatment for liquid and solid tumors that overexpress the Aldo-Keto Reductase 1 c3 (AKR1C3) enzyme. AKR1C3 is also expressed in T-ALL, with the exclusion of *TLX1/3*-rearranged cases. In September 2017, OBI-3424 received FDA orphan drug designation for AKR1C3-expressing tumors, including ALL.

- **Ruxolitinib:** This agent shows efficacy, in combination with dexamethasone in IL7-responsive T-ALL and ETP-ALL.

- **Imatinib/Dasatinib** (ABL1/Src-Family Kinase Inhibitors): The most common *ABL1* aberration in T-ALL is the *NUP214::ABL1* fusion due to an episomal amplification of the 9q34 region, which was one of the few discovered T-ALL lesions that can be directly targeted by a kinase inhibitor. Interestingly, in 2017, Frismantas and colleagues identified a subgroup of patients with T-ALL who are highly sensitive to dasatinib treatment in vitro despite the absence of ABL1 aberrations, suggesting a role for the SRC kinase as a putative novel target for therapy.

- **CAR T cell therapy:** A clinical trial using these modified anti-CD7 CAR T cells for treating CD7-positive T-ALL/LBL has been designed (NCT03690011).

Other targets include BET Inhibitors, PIM1 Inhibitors, proteosome inhibitors, PI3K–AKT–mTOR Inhibitors, cell-cycle Inhibitors, p53, *FLT3*-inhibitors and immunotherapy, among others.

Recommended Readings

Beldjord, K., Chevret, S., Asnafi, V. et al. (2014). Group for Research on Adult Acute Lymphoblastic Leukemia (GRAALL). Oncogenetics and minimal residual disease are independent outcome predictors in adult patients with acute lymphoblastic leukemia. *Blood* 123 (24): 3739–3749.

Chiesa, R., Georgiadis, C., Syed, F., et al. (2023 June 14). Base-Edited CAR T Group. Base-Edited CAR7 T Cells for Relapsed T-Cell Acute Lymphoblastic Leukemia. N Engl J Med. doi: 10.1056/NEJMoa2300709. Epub ahead of print. PMID: 37314354.

Cordo', V., van der Zwet, J.C.G., Canté-Barrett, K., Pieters, R., and Meijerink, J.P.P. (2020 November 24). T-cell acute lymphoblastic leukemia: a roadmap to targeted therapies. *Blood Cancer Discov* 2 (1): 19–31. doi: 10.1158/2643-3230.BCD-20-0093. PMID: 34661151; PMCID: PMC8447273.

DeAngelo, D.J., Yu, D., Johnson, J.L. et al. (2007). Nelarabine induces complete remissions in adults with relapsed or refractory T-lineage acute lymphoblastic leukemia or lymphoblastic lymphoma: Cancer and Leukemia Group B study 19801. *Blood* 109: 5136–5142.

Dunsmore, K.P., Winter, S.S., Devidas, M. et al. (2020 October 1). Children's Oncology Group AALL0434: a phase III randomized clinical trial testing nelarabine in newly diagnosed T-cell acute lymphoblastic leukemia. *J Clin Oncol* 38 (28): 3282–3293. doi: 10.1200/JCO.20.00256. Epub 2020 Aug 19. PMID: 32813610; PMCID: PMC7526719.

Fielding, A.K., Richards, S.M., Chopra, R., Lazarus, H.M., Litzow, M.R., Buck, G. et al. (2007). Outcome of 609 adults after relapse of acute lymphoblastic leukemia (ALL); an MRC UKALL12/ECOG 2993 study. *Blood* 109: 944–950. doi: 10.1182/blood-2006-05-018192.

Gokbuget, N., Basara, N., Baurmann, H. et al. (2011). High single drug activity of nelarabine in relapsed T-lymphoblastic leukemia/lymphoma offers curative option with subsequent stem cell transplantation. *Blood* 118 (13): 3503–1.

Hoelzer, D. and Gökbuget, N. (2009). T-cell lymphoblastic lymphoma and T-cell acute lymphoblastic leukemia: a separate entity? *Clin Lymphoma Myeloma* 9 (Suppl 3): S214–S221. doi: 10.3816/CLM.2009.s.015. PMID: 19778844.

Hough, R., Rowntree, C., Goulden, N. et al. (2016). Efficacy and toxicity of a paediatric protocol in teenagers and young adults with Philadelphia chromosome negative acute lymphoblastic leukaemia: results from UKALL 2003. *Br J Haematol* 172 (3): 439–451.

Khanam, T., Sandmann, S., Seggewiss, J. et al. (2020). Integrative genomic analysis of pediatric T- cell lymphoblastic lymphoma reveals candidates of clinical significance. *Blood*. 2021 Apr 29;137(17):2347-2359. doi: 10.1182/blood.2020005381. PMID: 33152759; PMCID: PMC8759350.

Kline, K.A.F., Kallen, M.E., Duong, V.H., and Law, J.Y. (2021 October). Acute lymphoblastic leukemia and acute lymphoblastic lymphoma: same disease spectrum but two distinct diagnoses. *Curr Hematol Malig Rep* 16 (5): 384–393. doi: 10.1007/s11899-021-00648-y. Epub 2021 Aug 21. PMID: 34417955.

Kroeze, E., Loeffen, J.L.C., Poort, V.M., and Meijerink, J.P.P. (2020). T-cell lymphoblastic lymphoma and leukemia: different diseases from a common premalignant progenitor? *Blood Adv* 4 (14): 3466–3473.

Marks, D.I., Clifton-Hadley, L., Copland, M. et al. (2022 April). In-vivo T-cell depleted reduced-intensity conditioned allogeneic haematopoietic stem-cell transplantation for patients with acute lymphoblastic leukaemia in first remission: results from the prospective, single-arm evaluation of the UKALL14 trial. *Lancet Haematol* 9 (4): e276–e288. doi: 10.1016/S2352-3026(22)00036-9. PMID: 35358442; PMCID: PMC8969058.

Marks, D.I., Paietta, E.M., Moorman, A.V. et al. (2009). T-cell acute lymphoblastic leukemia in adults: clinical features, immunophenotype, cytogenetics, and outcome from the large randomized prospective trial (UKALL XII/ECOG 2993). *Blood* 114: 5136–5145. doi: 10.1182/blood-2009-08-231217.

Morita, K., Jain, N., Kantarjian, H. et al. (2021 May 1). Outcome of T-cell acute lymphoblastic leukemia/lymphoma: focus on near-ETP phenotype and differential impact of nelarabine. *Am J Hematol* 96 (5): 589–598. doi: 10.1002/ajh.26144. Epub 2021 Mar 18. PMID: 33639000.

Steimlé, T., Dourthe, M.E., Alcantara, M. et al. (2022 January 26). Clinico-biological features of T-cell acute lymphoblastic leukemia with fusion proteins. *Blood Cancer J* 12 (1): 14. doi: 10.1038/s41408-022-00613-9. PMID: 35082269; PMCID: PMC8791998.

4

Minimal Residual Disease in Acute Lymphoblastic Leukemia

Caner Saygin, Sarah Monick, and Wendy Stock

Introduction

Detection of measurable residual disease (MRD) after therapy is prognostic in acute lympho-blastic leukemia (ALL) and should be considered when making therapeutic decisions. MRD in ALL can be measured based on leukemia-associated immunophenotypes (i.e. flow cytometry), expression of gene fusions (e.g. reverse transcriptase polymerase chain reaction, RT-PCR), and clonal rearrangement of immunoglobulin or T-cell receptor genes (with quantitative PCR or next-generation sequencing, NGS). In general, MRD positivity in a patient with morphologic complete remission is defined by the presence of 0.01% or more ALL cells, and the risk of relapse is proportional to the level of MRD. Recent technologic advances enabled detection of MRD at a higher resolution, reaching sensitivity as low as 10^{-6} with NGS-based MRD detection. In this chapter, we review the clinical significance of MRD, different MRD methods, and incorporation of MRD data in decision making for management of adult patients with ALL. The interactive case-based discussions are based on commonly encountered scenarios in oncology practice.

B-Cell Acute Lymphoblastic Leukemia

Case Study 1

A 40-year-old previously healthy male was recently diagnosed with precursor B-lineage acute lymphoblastic leukemia (pre-B-ALL) without CNS involvement. At time of diagnosis, he was found to have a peripheral WBC count of 50×10^9/L with 92% blasts, and cytoge-netics demonstrated *BCR::ABL1* translocation. He has completed induction therapy on CALGB 10701 (dasatinib, prednisone, and intrathecal chemotherapy) and is due for a post-induction bone marrow biopsy for response assessment.

1) **What is the optimal bone marrow aspiration technique for the assessment of measur-able residual disease (MRD)?**

   A) Aspiration of up to 3 cc via first pull.
   B) Aspiration of greater than 3 cc via first pull.
   C) Aspiration of up to 3 cc via second pull.
   D) Aspiration of greater than 3 cc via second pull.

Cancer Consult: Expertise in Clinical Practice, Volume 2: Neoplastic Hematology & Cellular Therapy, Second Edition. Edited by Syed A. Abutalib, Maurie Markman, James O. Armitage, and Kenneth C. Anderson. © 2024 John Wiley & Sons Ltd. Published 2024 by John Wiley & Sons Ltd.

Expert Perspective: Measurable residual disease (MRD) refers to the subclinical leukemic cells remaining in the bone marrow or peripheral blood after achievement of morphologic remission. The most common technical error associated with MRD quantification is the hemodilution from peripheral blood during sample collection. To reduce hemodilution, the optimal aspiration technique is via an initial pull of no more than 3 mL of bone marrow aspirate. Signs of hemodilution include aspicular sample and > 90% neutrophils in the sample. MRD testing in a hemodiluted sample is less sensitive.

MRD is highly sensitive to hemodilution given that it is reported as the proportion of leukemic cells to total cell number. Thus, the impact of hemodilution on MRD quantification is an underestimate of MRD, resulting in potential false negatives and inferior care.

Accurate quantification of MRD has important therapeutic implications. Pediatric and adult studies demonstrate MRD negativity is strongly associated with favorable outcomes independent of other risk factors. These studies show an increased risk of relapse in patients with MRD positivity $\geq 0.01\%$ ($\geq 10^{-4}$) after induction therapy or if detected in later post-remission treatment samples.

Correct Answer: A

Case Study 2

A 34-year-old female was recently diagnosed with pre-B-ALL without CNS involvement. At time of diagnosis, she was found to have a peripheral WBC count of 23×10^9/L with 80% blasts, and cytogenetics demonstrated *TCF3::PBX1* rearrangement. Fluorescence in-situ hybridization (FISH) for *BCR::ABL1* translocation was negative. She completed induction therapy on CALGB 10403 (an intensive pediatric regimen) and underwent bone marrow biopsy for response assessment. There was no morphologic evidence of leukemia, and further testing was performed for MRD assessment.

1) **Which of the following MRD assessment methods has the highest sensitivity and specificity in B- and T- cell ALL?**

   A) Multi-color flow cytometry.
   B) Reverse transcriptase polymerase chain reaction (RT-PCR) for *TCF3::PBX1* rearrangement detection.
   C) Immunoglobulin (IGH) or T-cell receptor (TCR) gene rearrangement real-time quantitative PCR (qPCR).
   D) IG/TCR rearrangement-based next-generation sequencing (NGS).
   E) All are acceptable methods to detect MRD.

Expert Perspective: ALL is uniquely suitable for MRD quantification by various techniques, including multiparameter flow cytometry (MFC), quantitative PCR-based assays for allele-specific *IG/TCR* rearrangements or specific fusion gene transcripts, and *IG/TCR* next-generation sequencing (NGS) (Table 4.1). The choice of technique depends on clinical trial design, disease biomarker, and resource availability. Regardless of the method used, a sensitivity of at least 10^{-4} must be reached for adequate MRD assessment. Thus, any of these methods are acceptable (RT-PCR is useful only if there is a trackable fusion transcript present) and validated when assayed in an accredited laboratory.

- **Types of MFC:** MFC utilizes fluorochrome-conjugate antibodies to identify specific aberrant leukemia-associated immunophenotypes (LAIPs). These LAIPs are identified in diagnostic samples and then used to look for residual disease in a case-specific manner. A second MFC approach is to identify leukemic cells by assessing how they deviate from normal hematopoietic cell counterparts using a defined set of antigens. This is called different-from-normal (DfN) approach, which does not rely on using the diagnostic sample and can identify new phenotypic aberrations acquired at the time of relapse. MFC is the most commonly used method in the United States. It is quick (hours), can be utilized in > 90% of cases, and has reliable sensitivity of 10^{-4} when four or more fluorochromes are utilized. It is important to note that standard clinical immunophenotyping using MFC does not achieve adequate sensitivity (0.1% [10−3]) for quantifying MRD. Limitations include the need for 500,000 to 1 million cells for analysis, quick sample analysis to avoid cell death, presence of false positives resulting from regeneration of normal lymphoid cells co-expressing ALL-type antigens (hematogones), and phenotypic switches resulting in erroneous interpretations.
- **Translocation RT-PCR:** RT-PCR (RNA)–based quantification of fusion transcripts can be utilized in 40–50% of patients carrying commonly recurring chromosomal translocations/gene fusions such as *BCR::ABL1, ETV6::RUNX1, KMT2A::AFF1, TCF3::PBX1*, translocations associated with *ABL1*, or *TAL1* deletions. RNA is the preferred substrate to detect these translocations as opposed to DNA since the exact breakpoint/fusion site occurs in different intronic regions spanning large segments of DNA, making it challenging to determine for each patient. The spliced mRNA product is translated into a fusion protein which is similar between patients, enabling the use of universal RT-PCR primers for mRNA quantitation. It is easy to perform, inexpensive, and has a sensitivity of detection of 10^{-4} to 10^{-5}. It does not require patient-specific assay development. Limitations are inability to perform in patients lacking chromosomal translocations resulting in chimeric transcripts and variable mRNA transcript expression in blasts.

Table 4.1 Comparison of methods for measurable residual disease (MRD) detection.

	Multicolor flow cytometry	Translocation RT-PCR	IG or TCR real-time PCR	Next-generation sequencing
Sensitivity	10^{-4}	10^{-4}–10^{-5}	10^{-4}–10^{-5}	10^{-6}–10^{-7}
Substrate	Cell suspension	RNA	DNA	DNA
Principle	LAIP/DfN approach	Leukemia-specific fusion transcript	Clone-specific VDJ rearrangement	Clone-specific VDJ rearrangement
Requires patient-specific optimization	Yes for LAIP, no for DfN approach	No	Yes	No
Applicability	> 90% (fresh sample required)	40–50%	> 90%	> 90%

DfN, different-from-normal; IG, immunoglobulin; LAIP, leukemia-associated immunophenotype; PCR, polymerase chain reaction; RT-PCR, reverse-transcriptase PCR; TCR, T-cell receptor

- **IG or TCR real-time PCR:** The antigen binding regions of the IG and TCR are made up of V (variable), D (diversity), and J (joining) segments. During lymphoid commitment and maturation, DNA encoding these genes undergoes a V(D)J rearrangement in order to increase the repertoire of antigen specificity. Lymphoblasts exhibit clonality and often originate from a single B or T cell clone; thus their V(D)J repertoire is also monoclonal, representing their fingerprint. Leveraging this unique biologic feature, PCR-based methods have been used to track *IG* or *TCR* rearrangements for MRD detection. First, the rearranged region is amplified by using primers for conserved V-family framework regions and J-family reverse primer. This amplified product is then sequenced to identify patient-specific rearrangements as well as unique junctional regions between V-D and D-J segments. To amplify the target regions in subsequent samples, patient-specific primers are designed. Therefore, the MRD assessment with qPCR in remission samples relies on comparison with the diagnostic sample. The qPCR-based quantitation of *IG* or *TCR* gene rearrangements can be utilized in > 90% of cases and has a reliable sensitivity of $10-4$ to $10-5$. Limitations include that these assays need to be optimized for each individual case, making them labor and cost intensive. Moreover, new subclones with different IG or TCR rearrangements may arise at the time of relapse, which would be missed with the qPCR method relying on diagnostic sequences. The assay is also not applicable for most patients with early T-precursor (ETP)-ALL, which arises from a progenitor/stem-like cell that lacks *TCR* rearrangement.
- **Next-generation sequencing:** NGS (DNA)–based quantification of *IG* or *TCR* gene rearrangements and of gene fusions have sought to overcome many of the limitations associated with qPCR and RT-PCR–based quantification, respectively. This method requires identification of patient-specific V(D)J rearrangement sequence at diagnosis for subsequent tracking of these clones throughout disease course. Its difference from the *IGH* or *TCR* qPCR method is that NGS amplifies DNA by multiplexed PCR using a combination of universal primers that amplify all areas of interest. It eliminates labor-intensive optimization steps required for each patient-specific assay design for qPCR and can detect subclones with new V(D)J sequences at relapse. It can be utilized in > 90% of cases, and its sensitivity depends on the amount of DNA used, ranging from $10-4$ to $10-7$. NGS can also be used to identify chromosomal translocations, using RNA as a substrate (RNA-seq). Studies have demonstrated that NGS is more sensitive than MFC and more specific than both qPCR and MFC in detecting relapsed disease after both induction and allogeneic hematopoietic cell transplantation (HCT). Cost is a major limitation.

Correct Answer: E

Case Study continued: She achieves remission and her marrow demonstrates complete response (CR), a normal female karyotype but detectable MRD at 0.2% via flow cytometry of an aberrant clone consistent with B-ALL as measured by flow cytometry. She then receives post-remission consolidation therapy per the 10403 regimen (approximately eight weeks of intensive treatment) and at week 14 post initiation of therapy, a repeat bone marrow aspiration and biopsy reveal low level persistent MRD at 0.05%.

2) **Which of the following is accurate regarding her prognosis?**

   A) Her prognosis remains favorable due to favorable cytogenetics and other clinical features at diagnosis.

B) Despite morphologic remission after induction and consolidation, persistence of MRD following consolidation therapy confers an increased risk of relapse.

C) You reassure the patient that her marrow indicates a slow early response and that the persistence of MRD at this point is of no concern.

Expert Perspective: MRD status after intensive chemotherapy has been identified as a significant prognosticator for relapse-free survival and overall survival in patients with ALL achieving CR. An MRD threshold of ≥ 0.01% confers an increased risk of relapse, regardless of risk stratification at time of diagnosis. Similarly, despite this patient's initial "standard risk" stratification based on WBC count and cytogenetics at time of diagnosis, her MRD positivity re-stratifies her at higher risk for disease relapse. Thus, quantification of MRD facilitates both risk re-stratification and determining the appropriateness of intensified therapies.

The landmark meta-analysis by Berry et al. demonstrated persistent and powerful strong associations between negative MRD status and positive clinical outcomes in both pediatric and adult populations regardless of MRD detection method, MRD threshold, MRD detection period, cell phenotype, Ph status, or treatment regimen. Pediatric and adult patients achieving MRD negativity had superior 10-year event-free survival compared to those with positive MRD (77% versus 32% for pediatrics; HR, 0.23; and 64% versus 21% for adults; HR, 0.28) and identical respective HRs for OS (0.28 and 0.28).

Multiple studies support the findings of Berry et al. For example, GMALL demonstrated the importance of MRD positivity in predicting disease relapse in adults with standard risk ALL (n = 196). Patient were re-stratified into MRD low-risk (MRD-negative on day 11 and 24), MRD high-risk (MRD-positive on day 11 and week 16), and MRD intermediate (remainder of patients not fitting in low- or high-risk groups) categories based on MRD status at middle of induction (day 11), end of induction (day 24), and end consolidation (week 16). Three-year risk of relapse was 0%, 47%, 94% in low-, intermediate-, and high-risk groups, respectively. Similarly, Vidriales et al showed the importance of MRD status for prognostication in adolescent and young adults with ALL (n = 102) after attaining CR post-induction. Patients with MRD > 0.1% on day 35 experienced relapse within two years, and those with MRD < 0.05% had significantly longer relapse-free survival than those with > 0.05% (42 versus 16 months; P = 0.001). The North Italy Leukemia Group (NILG) demonstrated that MRD positivity > 10^{-4} was a stronger predictor of relapse than cytogenetic or clinical features (HR, 5.33; P = 0.001). Patients were stratified to either standard chemotherapy or allogeneic HCT based on MRD status after consolidation. The three-year disease-free survival and overall survival were 72% and 75%, respectively, in MRD-negative group versus 14% and 13%, respectively, in the MRD-positive group.

Correct Answer: B

3) After hearing her prognosis, the patient is eager to discuss potential treatment options. What do you tell her?

A) You recommend continuing with current treatment.

B) You recommend re-induction with chemotherapy.

C) You recommend immediate allogeneic HCT.

D) You recommend starting blinatumomab.

Expert Perspective: In March 2018, blinatumomab was approved for additional indication by the US Food and Drug Administration (FDA) for the treatment of both adult and pediatric patients with ALL in first and second remission but with persistent MRD defined as disease ⩾ 0.1%. Blinatumomab is a bispecific T-cell engager (BiTE) monoclonal antibody constructed with dual specificity for CD19 and CD3. Crosslinking of autologous CD3-positive cytotoxic T-cells with CD-19 positive B-cells actives cytotoxic signaling cascades resulting in T-cell mediated perforin/granzyme lysis of both malignant and normal B-cells. Blinatumomab is also approved for the treatment of Ph-negative relapsed or refractory B-cell precursor ALL (see Chapter 2.)

The phase II BLAST trial (n = 116) studied blinatumomab in patients with MRD-positive (⩾ 10−3) B-ALL in CR. Seventy-eight percent of patients achieved MRD negativity (< 10−4), with MRD responders having longer event-free survival (23.6 vs 5.7 months; P = 0.002) and OS (38.9 vs 12.5 months; P = 0.002) compared to non-responders. Subgroup analysis of Ph- B-ALL (n = 110) again demonstrated MRD responders had longer relapse-free survival (23.6 vs 5.7; P = 0.002) and OS (38.9 vs 12.5 months; P = 0.002). Subsequently, most of the MRD-negative patients went on to receive an allogeneic hematopoietic cell transplant (see Chapter 5). The most common adverse reactions to blinatumomab in at least 20% of patients were pyrexia, infusion-related reactions, headache, infections (pathogen unspecified), tremor, and chills. (See Chapter 59 for identification and management of CRS and neurotoxicity associated with bispecific antibodies and CAR T cell therapy.)

Case Study 3

A 50-year-old male is diagnosed with pre-B-ALL based on peripheral blood flow cytometry showing TdT+ CD19+ CD20− CD22− blast population, representing 60% of blood cells. RT-PCR for *BCR::ABL1* at diagnosis was positive for p190 transcript. He starts induction therapy with course 1A of hyper-CVAD (cyclophosphamide, vincristine, adriamycin, dexamethasone) plus dasatinib.

4) When should he get his first MRD assessment?

    A) At the end of course 1A hyper-CVAD (day 28).
    B) At the end of course 1B hyper-CVAD.
    C) After approximately three months of therapy.
    D) Prior to proceeding with allogeneic HCT.

Expert Perspective: Consensus recommendations exist for the timing of bone marrow MRD assessments. For adults with ALL undergoing front-line treatment, MRD should be assessed after induction, in early consolidation (after approximately three months of therapy), and every three months for at least three years (five years for Ph+ ALL patients who do not undergo allogeneic HCT in first remission). Patients undergoing allogeneic HCT should have MRD assessed immediately before transplant and serially roughly every three months after transplant. For adults with relapsed ALL receiving salvage therapy, MRD should be assessed at time of morphologic remission and at the end of treatment.

Correct Answer: A

Case Study continued: His post-induction bone marrow biopsy shows morphologic CR with undetectable *BCR::ABL1* transcript. He proceeds with course 1B, and at three months of therapy, his bone marrow biopsy shows morphologic CR, but *BCR::ABL1* transcript level is detectable at 0.23%. He also gets MFC-based MRD testing in the marrow, which detects 0.1% leukemic cells based on LAIP approach.

5) What is your recommendation?

A) Proceed with course 2 of hyper-CVAD and repeat MRD assessment after next cycle.
B) Stop hyper-CVAD and switch to inotuzumab with dasatinib.
C) Send *ABL1* kinase domain mutation testing.
D) Immediately proceed with matched sibling allogeneic HCT.

Expert Perspective: Mutation testing for the *ABL1* kinase domain is recommended in patients with Ph+ ALL who have relapsed or are refractory to initial tyrosine kinase inhibitor (TKI)−containing therapy in order to guide treatment options based on *ABL1* status. It is important to identify potential kinase domain mutations for patients with resistance to TKI therapy. In patients who develop resistance to dasatinib, *T315I* mutations are common and can be targeted by switching to ponatinib (Table 4.2; also see Table 20.3 in Chapter 20). Although no single *ABL* mutant has been observed to confer resistance against ponatinib, compound mutations in the same *ABL* allele have been implicated in treatment failure. Additionally, studies have identified ponatinib to target several other kinase families implicated in hematologic malignancies including *FGFR, VEGFR, PDGFR, c-SRC, c-KIT*, and *FLT3*, suggesting an anti-leukemic effect independent of BCR-ABL inhibition.

Recent clinical trials have explored the use of ponatinib plus chemotherapy as a front-line regimen for Ph+ ALL. Jabbour et al. demonstrated the promising effect of combination hyper-CVAD with ponatinib as first line therapy for Ph+ ALL. An initial analysis of the ongoing phase II clinical trial revealed a 70% three-year event-free survival (95% CI 56−80), suggesting that chemotherapy plus ponatinib is both well tolerated and effective in achieving long-term remission in patients with newly diagnosed Ph+ ALL. However, phase III randomized controlled studies comparing outcomes of front-line chemotherapy plus ponatinib versus chemotherapy plus earlier generation TKIs are needed before it supplants current standard of care (see Chapter 2).

Case Study continued: Since this patient's ALL was CD22 negative, the CD22 antibody-drug conjugate inotuzumab is unlikely to be effective in achieving remission. This patient is a candidate for allogeneic HCT, ideally from HLA-matched sibling donor, but it should be done after achieving MRD-negative remission to improve long-term success.

Correct Answer: C

Table 4.2 Second generation TKIs and *ABL1* kinase resistance mutations.

Second-generation TKI	Mutations associated with resistance
Bosutinib	T315I, V299L, G250E, F317L
Dasatinib	T315I/A, F317L/V/I/C, V299L
Nilotinib	T315I, Y253H, E255K/V, F359V/C/I, G250E

Case Study continued: Patient undergoes matched sibling allogeneic HCT. His day 30 bone marrow biopsy shows 100% donor chimerism in all compartments, both *BCR::ABL1* RT-PCR and NGS-MRD are undetectable.

6) **What is the recommended interval and source of MRD assessment during the first three years?**

   A) Bone marrow biopsy every three months with *BCR::ABL1* MRD testing.
   B) Peripheral blood sampling every three months with *BCR::ABL1* MRD testing.
   C) Combined bone marrow and peripheral blood sampling every three months with *BCR::ABL1* MRD testing.
   D) Bone marrow biopsy every three months with NGS-MRD testing.

Expert Perspective: Patients with Ph+ ALL who undergo allogeneic HCT should have MRD testing performed every three months for the first few years. Both peripheral blood and bone marrow samples are acceptable for *BCR::ABL1* MRD testing. Several studies have shown concordance between the two, making blood sample an acceptable, less-invasive source for monitorization. Similarly, a strong correlation has been shown between peripheral blood and bone marrow NGS MRD results in ALL, favoring non-invasive monitoring of peripheral blood–based MRD in ALL patients undergoing curative intent cellular therapies.

Correct Answer: B

Case Study 4

An 18-year-old female with refractory *KMT2A*-rearranged (*KMT2A*-r, or previously, *MLL*-rearranged [*MLLr*]) B-ALL is treated with CD-19-specific chimeric antigen receptor (CAR)–modified T-cells. Her pre-CART marrow demonstrates abnormal B-lymphoblasts expressing CD19, CD38, CD58, CD22 (dim), HLA-DR, CD34 and CD45. FISH detects a *KMT2A* fusion, and cytogenetic analysis demonstrates 46XY, t(4;11)(q21.3;q23.3). Day +30 bone marrow biopsy post-CAR-T therapy demonstrates morphologic CR, MFC-based MRD is negative, but RT-PCR for MLLr is positive. The patient undergoes surveillance bone marrow biopsy three months after CAR-T infusion, and MFC reveals 3% blast population expressing MPO, CD56, CD64, CD13, CD33, CD38, HLA-DR, CD34, CD45, and CD71. She has persistent *KMT2Ar* by FISH. No abnormal B-lineage populations are identified.

7) **What is your interpretation?**

   A) Concern for sampling error.
   B) Concern for mixed-phenotype acute leukemia.
   C) Concern for therapy-related AML.
   D) Concern for phenotypic switch to myeloid leukemia.

Expert Perspective: MFC is unique in its ability to detect phenotypic switches compared to other methods of MRD testing. MFC utilizes immunophenotyping to identify populations of cells with atypical surface antigens, combinations of antigens, or quantities of antigens. Immunophenotyping identifies variable expression of clusters of differentiation (CDs) antigens to define both specific cell lineages and state of maturation. For example, the presence of immature T cells found outside the thymus is a marker of MRD in T-ALL (see Chapter 3), whereas in B-ALL markers must be utilized to distinguish blasts from precursor cells.

Lineage switching has been described as a method of evasion from CD-19 targeted immunotherapies including CAR T cell and BiTE (i.e. blinatumomab) therapies. Multiple adult and pediatric cases reports describe *KMT2A* B-ALL recurring as a myeloid relapse after receiving CD-19 targeted immunotherapies. Interestingly, the phenotypic switch in *MLLr* B-ALL is often clonal, suggesting the inherent plasticity of *KMT2A* B-ALL may predispose to phenotypic switch under selective pressure of targeted immune therapies.

Correct Answer: D

Case Study continued: At follow-up, she develops a nodular rash on her forehead, and biopsy reveals granulocytic sarcoma (i.e. chloroma). She has 5% circulating blasts with MPO+ CD33+ phenotype.

8) What is the best treatment approach in this case?

    A) Blinatumomab.
    B) Radiation to the affected area.
    C) Cytarabine-mitoxantrone.
    D) Pembrolizumab.

Expert Perspective: Patients who relapse with phenotype switch after CD19-directed therapy should receive agents effective in AML. This patient has systemic disease as determined with both peripheral blood and bone marrow analyses; therefore, a local radiation approach is not sufficient. Cytarabine-doublet chemotherapy is an effective approach for myeloid leukemias.

Correct Answer: C

T Cell Lymphoblastic Leukemia/Lymphoma

Case Study 5

A 30-year-old male presents with dyspnea and chest pain. CT scan reveals a 6.5 cm mediastinal mass along with retroperitoneal lymphadenopathy. Biopsy of the mediastinal mass is consistent with T-lymphoblastic lymphoma (T-LBL), and the NGS testing from the tissue identifies a V(D)J sequence to track this malignant clone. His bone marrow biopsy did not show morphologic evidence of T-ALL, but MFC of the marrow reveals CD7+ CD4+ CD8+ TdT+ CD34+(variable) lymphoblasts at 0.5%. He starts treatment with CALGB 10403 regimen.

9) After the induction therapy, what is the best approach for MRD assessment?

    A) PET/CT scan and NGS-MRD testing in bone marrow.
    B) PET/CT scan and MFC-MRD testing in blood.
    C) PET/CT scan alone.
    D) CT scan with MFC-MRD testing in bone marrow.

Expert Perspective: Patients with T-LBL should be monitored with PET/CT scan to improve the sensitivity of detecting systemic bulky disease. The patient in this question had small amount of disease in bone marrow, and subsequent response assessments should include bone marrow biopsy. As he had a detectable clone by NGS testing at diagnosis, NGS-MRD can be used to monitor systemic disease with high sensitivity (also see Chapter 3).

Correct Answer: A

Case Study continued: Post-induction PET scan was without evidence of disease, and bone marrow biopsy showed CR with negative NGS-MRD. He proceeded with consolidation chemotherapy, and subsequent peripheral blood NGS-MRD was positive with 25 cells in 1 million. PET/CT remains unremarkable with Deauville score of 1.

10) What is the best treatment approach?

    A) If bone marrow biopsy is without morphologic evidence of leukemia, proceed with the interim maintenance of CALGB 10403.

    B) Add nelarabine with close NGS-MRD monitoring and subsequent allogeneic HCT.

    C) Increase the number of intrathecal chemotherapies to prevent CNS relapse.

    D) Plan for salvage radiation therapy for mediastinum and retroperitoneal nodal areas.

Expert Perspective: As in patients with pre-B-ALL, positivity of NGS-MRD after initial chemotherapy predicts poor prognosis in T-ALL/LBL patients. Nelarabine is an active drug for T-ALL/LBL and can be an effective way to erase MRD in this case. In the options provided, allogeneic HCT should be strongly considered given limited number of effective FDA-approved therapies for relapsed T-ALL/LBL. Early phase studies showed promising results for daratumumab (in CD38-positive disease) and newer BH3 mimetics (venetoclax and navitoclax) in T-ALL/LBL, but their efficacy in eradicating MRD should be investigated further in larger studies.

Correct Answer: B

Recommended Readings

Akabane, H. and Logan, A. (2020). Clinical significance and management of MRD in adults with acute lymphoblastic leukemia. *Clin Adv Hematol Oncol* 18 (7): 413–422.

Bartram, J., Patel, B., and Fielding, A.K. (2020). Monitoring MRD in ALL: methodologies, technical aspects and optimal time points for measurement. *Semin Hematol* 57 (3): 142–148.

Berry, D.A., Zhou, S., Higley, H. et al. (2017). Association of minimal residual disease with clinical outcome in pediatric and adult acute lymphoblastic leukemia: a meta-analysis. *JAMA Oncol* 3 (7): e170580.

Brüggemann, M. and Kotrova, M. (2017). Minimal residual disease in adult ALL: technical aspects and implications for correct clinical interpretation. *Blood Adv* 1 (25): 2456–2466.

Gökbuget, N., Dombret, H., Bonifacio, M. et al. (2018). Blinatumomab for minimal residual disease in adults with B-cell precursor acute lymphoblastic leukemia [published correction appears in Blood 2019 Jun 13;133(24):2625]. *Blood* 131 (14): 1522–1531.

Hovorkova, L., Zaliova, M., Venn, N.C. et al. (2017). Monitoring of childhood ALL using BCR-ABL1 genomic breakpoints identifies a subgroup with CML-like biology. *Blood* 129 (20): 2771–2781.

Jabbour, E., Short, N.J., Ravandi, F. et al. (2018). Combination of hyper-CVAD with ponatinib as first-line therapy for patients with Philadelphia chromosome-positive acute lymphoblastic leukaemia: long-term follow-up of a single-centre, phase 2 study. *Lancet Haematol* 5 (12): e618–627.

Kantarjian, H., Stein, A., Gökbuget, N. et al. (2017). Blinatumomab versus chemotherapy for advanced acute lymphoblastic leukemia. *N Engl J Med* 376 (9): 836–847.

Kim, I.S. (2020). Minimal residual disease in acute lymphoblastic leukemia: technical aspects and implications for clinical interpretation. *Blood Res* 55 (S1): S19–S26.

Liang, E.C., Dekker, S.E., Sabile. J.M.G., Torelli. S., Zhang, A., Miller, K., Shiraz, P., Hayes-Lattin, B., Leonard, J.T., and Muffly. L. (2023 Jul 25). Next-generation sequencing-based MRD in adults with ALL undergoing hematopoietic cell transplantation. *Blood Adv* 7 (14): 3395–3402. doi: 10.1182/bloodadvances.2023009856. PMID: 37196642; PMCID: PMC10345845.

Liao, W., Kohler, M.E., Fry, T., and Ernst, P. (2021 Aug). Does lineage plasticity enable escape from CAR-T cell therapy? Lessons from MLL-r leukemia [published online ahead of print, 2021 Jul 21]. *Exp Hematol* 100:1–11. S0301-472X(21)00248-4.

Soverini, S., Martelli, M., Bavaro, L. et al. (2021). BCR-ABL1 compound mutants: prevalence, spectrum and correlation with tyrosine kinase inhibitor resistance in a consecutive series of Philadelphia chromosome-positive leukemia patients analyzed by NGS. *Leukemia* 35 (7): 2102–2107.

5

Hematopoietic Transplantation and Cellular Therapy in Acute Lymphoblastic Leukemia

Yael Morgenstern[1], Netanel A. Horowitz[1,2], and Jacob M. Rowe[3]

[1] Department of Hematology and Bone Marrow Transplantation, Rambam Health Care Campus, Haifa, Israel
[2] The Ruth and Bruce Rappaport Faculty of Medicine, Technion, Israel Institute of Technology, Haifa, Israel
[3] Department of Hematology, Rambam Health Care Campus, Department of Hematology, Shaare Zedek Medical Center, Israel

Introduction

Treatment of acute lymphoblastic leukemia (ALL) in adults presents a formidable challenge. While overall results have improved over the past three decades, the current long-term survival is in the range of 50–60% in patients with precursor B-cell ALL, 50–60% with T-cell ALL, and 80% with mature B-cell ALL. The historic lack of clear-cut biological prognostic factors has led to over- or under-treatment of some patients. Response to initial therapy is an important prognosticator of outcome based on disease biology, as well as pharmacogenetics, which include the patient's response to drugs given. The more wide-spread availability of allogeneic transplantation and reduced-intensity regimens for older patients have opened up this curative modality to a greater number of patients. Hopefully, those options, as well as novel targeted agents and cellular therapy, i.e. chimeric antigen receptor (CAR) T cell therapy, will cure a greater proportion of adults with ALL. Our chapter will discuss in some detail and summarize the available data for the most important factors affecting therapeutic decision-making.

Case Study 1

A 29-year-old male presents with complaints of fever and increasing fatigue. The complete blood count shows a white blood cell count of 45,000/µL, most of which are lymphoblasts; hemoglobin of 7 g/dL; and platelets of 7000/µL. Further workup reveals retroperitoneal adenopathy, an elevated lactate dehydrogenase of 516 U/L, and a markedly hypercellular bone marrow. He is diagnosed with CD20-positive, precursor B-cell acute lymphoblastic leukemia (ALL). Cytogenetics and molecular diagnostic tests disclosed Philadelphia chromosome with *BCR::ABL1* fusion gene. The cerebrospinal fluid (CSF) evaluation is unremarkable. He achieves complete morphologic, cytogenetic, and molecular remission after the first round of chemoimmunotherapy. While you plan for a second session of therapy for this patient, he and his family request you to comment on the following questions.

1) What is the optimal treatment before proceeding with allogeneic transplantation?

Expert Perspective: The case presented in the vignette concerns a young patient recently diagnosed with Philadelphia chromosome (Ph)–positive ALL. The Ph chromosome is the most frequent genetic abnormality in adult ALL; its prevalence in the 18–35 age group is reported to vary between 12% and 30%, and it is associated with a highly unfavorable prognosis. That is why, for the past five decades, the standard recommended consolidation therapy after achieving complete remission (CR) has been a matched related or matched unrelated stem cell transplantation, depending on finding an appropriate histocompatible donor. The introduction of tyrosine kinase inhibitors (TKIs) into the therapy of Ph-positive ALL has very significantly improved patient survival. For instance, in the large international ALL study UKALL12/E2993, the combination of imatinib-based induction followed by allogeneic stem cell transplantation (allo-SCT) resulted in a four-year overall survival (OS) rate of 50% (Fielding et al. 2014). In a study conducted by the GMALL group, the OS rate at three years was 72%. Nevertheless, even after incorporation of imatinib as front-line treatment, a high relapse rate was observed with a four-year RFS of only 40%, highlighting the need for deepening response using new treatments. Currently, new-generation TKIs are being tested in clinical trials. As prospective studies comparing different TKIs have not been conducted in adult patients, the choice of the optimal TKI remains controversial. A number of non-randomized trials evaluated treatment with the second-generation TKI dasatinib as front-line treatment in combination with chemotherapy and resulted in clinical outcomes comparable to those achieved with imatinib. In contrast to previous results, in a recent randomized controlled trial comparing treatment with imatinib versus dasatinib in the pediatric Ph-positive ALL patient population, dasatinib treatment demonstrated superiority over imatinib with four-year event-free survival (EFS), OS, and risk of relapse of 49%, 84%, and 20%, respectively. Acquisition of a *T315I* mutation in *BCR* was found to be the central mechanism conferring resistance to older-generation TKIs, suggesting a potential advantage for the use of a third-generation TKI such as ponatinib. Indeed, in a recent phase II study, a combination of ponatinib with hyper-CVAD as front-line treatment attained encouraging results including 100% CMR and five-year OS and EFS of 76% and 70%, respectively. Notably, in this study, a long-term survival was observed also in patients who did not proceed to allo-SCT, underscoring the prognostic significance of MRD eradication, which may serve as a future tool to guide the decision regarding necessity of allo-SCT. Nonetheless, cardiovascular toxicity associated with ponatinib warrants special caution when employing it in first line, particularly in the older patient population.

Further to the discussion regarding the optimal TKI to use, during recent years a chemotherapy-free approach consisting of TKI, steroids, and immunotherapy was suggested as an alternative treatment strategy for front-line therapy of Ph+ ALL patients. In the D-ALBA, GIMEMA LAL2116 study (Foà et al. 2020) a combination based on steroids and dasatinib for induction followed by consolidation with the bispecific monoclonal antibody blinatumomab resulted in 41% complete molecular response and 95% OS at a median follow-up of 18 months with few relapses and a low mortality rate. Interestingly, treatment with blinatumomab appeared to successfully overcome the appearance of

T315I mutations and subsequent relapse. Another trial addressing the necessity of chemo-therapy in the treatment of Ph-positive ALL is the recently activated ECOG-ACRIN EA9181 (NCT04530565) study, which is an ongoing prospective randomized phase III study, eval-uating efficacy of a chemotherapy-free induction treatment consisting of TKI, steroids, and blinatumomab versus TKI, steroids, and hyper-CVAD, whose results are anticipated eagerly. The recommendation for this patient would be to enter a clinical trial evaluating the use of chemotherapy-free induction. In the absence of the availability of such a trial, an institutional-preferred standard B-ALL induction regimen should be used, followed by CNS prophylaxis, together with a TKI such as imatinib, dasatinib, or nilotinib.

2) When is the optimal time to proceed with allogeneic transplantation?

Expert Perspective: Previous studies reported a poor outcome with short relapse-free survival (RFS) and OS when transplantation was not performed in CR1. There are several well-established protocols for the treatment of ALL, all of them with very high rates of post-induction CR. However, in all of these well-known studies, allo-SCT is never per-formed before completion of all phases of induction and two–three cycles of CNS pro-phylaxis, even if CR is achieved early in the treatment course, although this has never been prospectively studied. Nevertheless, prognostically the most important factor for performing a successful allo-SCT is achieving minimal/measurable residual disease (MRD) negativity prior to SCT. In Ph-positive ALL, MRD is assessed by *BCR::ABL* transcript quan-tification. Persistence of MRD is associated with a higher relapse risk and lower OS. In a recent phase II study, MRD-positive Ph-positive ALL patients were treated with TKI and the bispecific antibody blinatumomab resulting in conversion to MRD negativity in 75% of patients with two-year RFS and OS of 62% and 76%, respectively, compared to 40% two-year RFS and OS in patients who remained MRD-positive. The patient presented above should preferably only proceed to an allo-SCT after achieving MRD eradication. If MRD remains positive, we would recommend giving treatment with blinatumomab for MRD eradication before transplantation.

3) How many sessions of prophylactic intrathecal chemotherapy are considered optimal prior to and following allogeneic transplantation?

Expert Perspective: Reports from a variety of studies indicate that 5–10% of adult ALL patients have central nervous system (CNS) involvement at presentation (Cortes et al. 1995, Lazarus et al. 2006). Factors associated with CNS disease at presentation include a higher white blood cell (WBC) count at diagnosis, T-cell immunophenotype, and presence of a mediastinal mass. In the largest clinical trial performed so far in adult ALL, the presence of Ph positivity was not found to be a risk factor for CNS involvement (Lazarus et al. 2006). Moreover, the rate of CNS involvement in Ph-positive ALL was not signif-icantly higher than in Ph-negative ALL. The administration of CNS penetrating agents such as cytarabine and high-dose methotrexate (MTX) as prophylactic therapy to prevent CNS involvement is an inherent part of all established protocols for ALL. In this regard, dasatinib has a theoretic advantage over imatinib treatment since it has the ability to cross the blood-brain barrier and thus augment the existing armamentarium for prophy-laxis against CNS relapse. However, despite common usage, the superiority of dasatinib over other TKIs has not been demonstrated in Ph-positive ALL. Most protocols use repeat intrathecal (I.T.) administration of MTX, or triple therapy (i.e. MTX, cytarabine, and dexamethasone) as part of this prophylactic strategy (Fielding et al. 2014). However, there are no comparative studies regarding the optimal number of prophylactic I.T. courses before proceeding to allo-SCT. In the absence of such data, for a patient with no evidence of CNS involvement at presentation, based on the UKALL12/E2993 study, we would recommend administering up to eight courses of IT as CNS prophylaxis with triple therapy. Clearly, any protocol-specific variation is reasonable.

4) Should he continue treatment till the time of myeloablative preparative regimen?

Expert Perspective: TKI inhibitors are an integral part of induction regimens for newly diagnosed Ph-positive ALL. Previous studies demonstrated that treating patients with TKIs as a single drug regimen (combined only with steroids) resulted in a high rate of CR; however, the duration of response was short with a high rate of relapse. In a recent study of elderly patients, TKI treatment was combined with a low dose of standard ALL induction chemotherapy, resulting in a 90% CR rate, but a high rate of relapse was observed, with median OS of 27 months. Therefore, for young patients, TKIs should be combined with intensive chemotherapy-based induction regimens. The optimal intensity of chemotherapy that is required to achieve the best clinical results with minimal therapy-related morbidity and mortality is unknown. Ongoing studies are evaluating incorporation of novel agents in front-line therapy as a strategy to de-escalate or omit chemotherapy and reduce toxicity. Nevertheless, until more data accumulate, current ALL treatment protocols integrate TKIs with intensive regimens (Fielding et al. 2014). For example, in the hyper-CVAD protocol, dasatinib is given for the first 14 days of each course. The main issue with continuous administration of TKIs is prolonged myelotoxicity. The question of how long before allo-SCT TKIs are to be administered has never been studied in clinical trials; however, we administer TKIs once the blood count recovers after completion of induction phases and continue thereafter until the initiation of conditioning therapy for transplant.

5) When should he resume tyrosine kinase inhibitor (TKI) treatment following allogeneic transplantation?

Expert Perspective: This is a very important yet unanswered question. Existing data regarding this complex issue date to the early imatinib clinical trials. Some studies reported that resuming imatinib treatment after allo-SCT is associated with high rates of drug discontinuation or dose reduction due to severe toxicity, particularly myelosuppression. In the PET-HEMA trial, only 62% of patients were able to resume imatinib treatment at a median of 3.9 months after myeloablative allo-SCT (Ribera et al. 2010). In the GMALL study, patients were randomized to up-front imatinib, resuming three months after allo-SCT, or starting imatinib upon any *BCR::ABL* transcript reappearance. The up-front approach resulted in poor tolerance, and no difference in clinical outcome has yet been observed between the two approaches (Pfeifer et al. 2013). In contrast, retrospective studies from the EBMT and the MD Anderson Cancer Center demonstrated improved clinical outcomes, including OS, disease-free survival (DFS), and RFS, in patients who can tolerate imatinib pre- and post-allo-SCT (Bachanova et al. 2014, Saini et al. 2020). Data regarding the efficacy of treatment with newer-generation TKIs as maintenance therapy post-allo-SCT are limited.

Nevertheless, since mutations in *BCR* remain the main cause of relapse, newer-generation TKIs that overcome these mutations might be advantageous in cases of MRD persistence. In this relatively young, very high-risk patient, we would recommend resuming dasatinib administration early after allo-SCT and not later than three months post-transplant, depending on the rate of engraftment. The optimal duration for TKI maintenance post-allo-SCT remains unclear, and regular quantitative *BCR::ABL* monitoring policy is mandatory. In a recent retrospective study (Saini et al. 2020), the benefit of treatment with TKI maintenance after allo-SCT was observed only in patients who received this therapy for at least two years. At this time, we would continue the TKI therapy for at least two years with strict MRD monitoring, awaiting studies that indicate that TKIs could be safely discontinued at some point.

Case Study 2

The patient presented in the previous clinical vignette undergoes successful myeloablative fully HLA-matched sibling donor (MSD) transplantation. Approximately, two years later, he remains in morphologic and cytogenetic CR; however, *BCR::ABL* fusion gene levels have become detectable in the bone marrow aspirate. He is now 31 years of age, with a Karnofsky performance score of 90% and has a calculated hematopoietic cell transplantation comorbidity index (HCT-CI) of 0. He was treated with imatinib as maintenance therapy following allogeneic transplantation. He does not have chronic graft-versus-host disease (GvHD) but does have a brief history of steroid-sensitive grade II acute skin GvHD.

6) Should this patient undergo a second allogeneic transplantation, assuming that he achieves second molecular remission with single-agent therapy?

Since this patient was treated with a first-generation TKI before molecular relapse, ponatinib should be started immediately in order to achieve a second CR (CR2). A *BCR::ABL* mutational screen is required to predict the optimal TKI for the prevention of disease relapse. This patient did not have GvHD, which strongly suggests a lack of alloreactivity of the transplant against the leukemia cells. That is why an extensive search should be initiated for another donor, including a matched sibling or a matched unrelated donor. Transplant from a haploidentical donor is also a very reasonable option. In addition to new-generation TKIs, another consideration is the use of one of the new agents including blinatumomab or inotuzumab ozogamicin (InO) before transplantation. Currently, no prospective randomized study has been conducted to compare head-to-head between these two agents. Results of blinatumomab treatment reported in the ALCANTARA study demonstrated a 36% ORR and a median OS of 7.1 months compared to a 78% ORR and a median OS of 7.7 months observed after treatment with InO (Kantarjian et al. 2016). Of note, difference in patient populations between these studies precludes comparisons of treatment efficacy. Data regarding patients who achieved MRD negativity with one of the new agents and did not proceed to allo-SCT are scarce. Thus, until long-term follow-up data on patients in whom a second allo-SCT was deferred are available, the current recommendation is to proceed to a second allo-SCT.

Case Study 3

A 54-year-old previously healthy male is diagnosed with pre-B-ALL. PCR for *BCR::ABL* is negative. He is started on steroid therapy to be given for seven days, with subsequent induction according to the ECOG protocol. FISH analysis identifies a translocation involving *PDGRFB*. The patient is diagnosed with Ph-like ALL.

7) What is the optimal treatment for this patient with Ph-like ALL?

Expert Perspective: Ph-like ALL constitutes around 25% of adult ALL cases, is a high-risk ALL subgroup, and is associated with high relapse rate and short OS. It was originally defined by a gene expression signature similar to Ph-positive ALL, except without the *BCR::ABL* fusion transcript. Nevertheless, currently there is no universal consensus regarding the diagnosis of Ph-like ALL. At the molecular level, Ph-like ALL patients express diverse genetic variants activating kinase or cytokine receptors pathways. Around 50% of Ph-like ALL patients harbor translocations involving *CRLF2* and approximately 10–15% of patients express *ABL*-class fusions, involving *ABL1, ABL2, CSF1R,* and *PDGRFB.* Pre-clinical studies support a synergistic effect of chemotherapy combined with JAK inhibitor or dasatinib in Ph-like ALL patients harboring genetic variants activating *JAK-STAT* or *ABL* pathways, respectively. Notably, Ph-like ALL is associated with low rates of MRD clearance and a poor prognosis irrespective of the induction protocol (pediatric-inspired vs adult) or MRD eradication, highlighting the need for new treatment strategies. The presence of genetic alterations inducing tyrosine kinase activation raised great interest in adding TKIs for these patients as a targeted therapy approach. Indeed, case series studies demonstrated that incorporation of dasatinib in Ph-like ALL patients harboring *ABL*-class genetic alterations resulted in sustained CR and a low relapse rate. Currently, there is limited evidence regarding treatment with *JAK* inhibitors (ruxolitinib) in the front-line treatment of Ph-like ALL patients with genetic alteration activating the *JAK-STAT* pathway. Several ongoing clinical trials are studying the optimal combination therapy for Ph-like ALL patients, including treatment with TKIs or ruxolitinib in the front-line setting for Ph-like patients and incorporation of novel agents including blinatumomab or inotuzumab ozogamicin during induction. The clinical case describes a patient diagnosed with Ph-like ALL with an *ABL*-class translocation. Although the addition of TKIs to front-line standard chemotherapy treatment is still being evaluated in clinical studies and considered experimental, given their established safety and outstanding results in Ph+ ALL, it seems reasonable to combine them with standard chemotherapy. In this patient we would recommend treatment with dasatinib combined with chemotherapy and follow MRD kinetics along treatment as assessed by FISH or RT-PCR. Given the high relapse rate observed even in patients achieving MRD negativity, we would consider proceeding to allo-SCT in this patient and continue maintenance therapy post SCT with TKI.

8) Which of the following patient(s) should be considered for up-front allogeneic transplantation assuming availability of MSD for all of the patients?

   A) 16-year-old female with precursor B-cell ALL, positive *BCR::ABL* fusion gene, and in molecular remission.
   B) 56-year-old female with precursor B-cell ALL, positive *BCR::ABL* fusion gene, and in molecular remission.

C) 35-year-old male with precursor B-cell ALL and normal cytogenetics, who presented with a WBC count of 15,000/µL. Bone marrow evaluation at the end of induction showed CR with MRD (10^{-4}) positivity.

D) 35-year-old male with precursor B-cell ALL, *MLL::AF4* gene fusion, and in molecular remission following four weeks of therapy.

E) 44-year-old male with precursor B-cell ALL and normal cytogenetics, who presented with a WBC count of 15,000/µL. Bone marrow evaluation at the end of induction showed CR with MRD < 10^{-4}.

Expert Perspective: Before discussing each case separately, a short discussion regarding standard and high-risk ALL is appropriate. The generally accepted prognostic factors defining high risk are age, WBC count, immunophenotyping, and high-risk cytogenetics or molecular determinants. The OS ranges from 34 to 57% for patients less than 30 years old compared with only 15 to 17% for patients older than 50 years old. A WBC count greater than 30,000/µL or 50,000/µL for B-lineage ALL and, to a lesser extent > 100,000/µL for T-ALL, are associated with poor prognosis (see Chapters 1 and 2). T-lineage ALL also appears to have better outcomes than B-lineage ALL. The presence of the Ph chromosome or t(4; 11)(q21; q23) has been associated with inferior survival in multiple large series Moorman et al. 2007). Additionally, the presence of the t(8;14)(q24.1;q32), complex karyotype defined as ≥ 5 chromosomal abnormalities, or low hypodiploidy (< 44 chromosomes) / near triploidy were noted to have poor survival in the UKALL XII/ECOG 2993 trial (Moorman et al. 2007). However, even in the standard risk group the relapse rate approaches 40–55%. During recent years, persistent MRD > 10^{-4}, as assessed by flow cytometry or molecular analysis emerged as an independent prognostic factor for OS, irrespective of preexisting conventional risk factors. Employing MRD as a tool for making clinical therapeutic decisions regarding therapy intensification is currently incorporated in all clinical trials. Further to persistence of MRD, the kinetics of MRD eradication during different time points after induction and during consolidation was identified as a critical prognostic factor; however, there is still no consensus regarding the exact MRD level and time points in which it should be evaluated. The presence of MRD positivity as a prognostic tool may indeed supersede other established prognostics markers. As discussed previously, patients diagnosed with Ph-positive ALL are considered at high risk and recommended to proceed to allo-SCT in CR1. Nevertheless, the COG AALL0031 and AALL0622 studies, conducted in adolescents and young adults (AYA) with Ph-positive ALL, evaluated treatment with TKI combined with a pediatric-inspired chemotherapy regimen with or without allo-SCT. Interestingly, although considered a high-risk group, in this relatively small study, no benefit for allo-SCT in terms of OS and EFS was observed in patients who responded with rapid MRD kinetics and achieved MRD eradication compared to patients who did not proceed to SCT.

Our perspective on choices discussed in the question:

A) The 16-year-old female with Ph-positive B-cell ALL in molecular remission should be treated up front with TKI and chemotherapy. If she achieves molecular remission with MRD negativity, it may be reasonable to defer allo-SCT at this point and continue therapy with TKI maintenance and periodic monitoring of BCR-ABL MRD levels.

B) The second case of a 56-year-old female with the same clinical scenario is more challenging. In the UKALL XII/ECOG 2993 trial, performing a myeloablative allo-SCT in the high-risk group (most of these patients were older than 35 years) did not translate into improved OS due to high rates of non-relapse mortality, most of them due to GvHD or infections (Goldstone et al. 2008). However, the rate of relapse was significantly lower in the high-risk group who were transplanted in first CR. The availability of reduced intensity conditioning (RIC) protocols has made allo-SCT an attractive therapeutic option for elderly patients with Ph-positive ALL. In the relatively small single-center study conducted in high-risk ALL patients (median age 56 years), the subgroup of Ph-positive ALL patients receiving a non-myeloablative conditioning at first CR had a three-year OS of 62% with a relapse rate of 32% (Goldstone et al. 2008). Recent clinical studies using new combinations as front-line therapy such as steroids, dasatinib, and blinatumomab (Foà et al. 2020) or ponatinib, steroids, and hyper-CVAD suggest promising results with low relapse rates and long OS, possibly obviating the need for allo-SCT. Results from randomized prospective trials are urgently needed. However, in the meantime, considering that beyond first CR, allo-SCT is curative in only a minority of patients, we recommend that this patient should be treated with an up-front RIC allo-SCT and continuing with TKI maintenance therapy post transplantation.

C) The third patient is considered an AYA patient with pre-therapy standard risk. Several studies reported that treatment with a pediatric-inspired protocol in this patient group resulted in remarkable improvement of clinical outcomes compared to historical controls, with three-year OS and EFS of 73% and 59%, respectively (Tosi et al. 2021). Notably, in terms of relapse-free survival, a benefit for allo-SCT was observed in this group only for patients with persistent MRD. Prospective ongoing trials are evaluating treatment with the bispecific antibody blinatumomab in MRD-positive patients as a potential approach to eradicate MRD and avert the need for allo-SCT. The patient described in this case is MRD-positive with high risk for relapse; thus, we would recommend on up-front allo-SCT.

D) The fourth patient belongs to the AYA group and has the cytogenetic translocation t(4:11), which is associated with an adverse prognosis. However, after four weeks of induction therapy he is in complete molecular response. Does MRD negativity after four weeks of induction therapy supersede the adverse prognosis of t(4:11)? This question is very hard to answer as patients with rare adverse prognostic factors are usually diluted within the whole ALL population. In the recent ALL-HR-11 study, high-risk Ph-negative ALL patients who achieved MRD eradication after induction and consolidation were given treatment with delayed consolidation and maintenance without allo-SCT, resulting in cumulative incidence of relapse and OS rates of 45% and 59%, respectively (Ribera et al. 2021). Nevertheless, despite achieving MRD negativity, patients with 11q23 rearrangement exhibited poor OS results without allo-SCT. Currently there are no data regarding MRD-based intervention in t(4:11) ALL patients. Therefore, we conclude that outside the setting of clinical trial, this patient should be offered the option of an up-front allo-SCT, particularly if he has a matched sibling donor.

E) The fifth patient presents with baseline disease parameters and a clinical course similar to patient #3. However, because of his older age, a pediatric-inspired protocol associated with high toxicity is not suitable in his case. Hence, this patient is at high risk, and we would recommend treatment with induction and intensification, subsequently continuing to allo-SCT. Nevertheless, the high non-relapse mortality (NRM) associated with allo-SCT in this patient population raises the need for new treatment strategies. Indeed, the recently completed phase III ECOG-ACRIN E1910 study demonstrated a significant improvement in overall survival upon upfront addition of the bi-specific antibody blinatumomab to consolidation chemotherapy therapy in patients who were MRD negative after intensification therapy. Ultimately, this may obviate the need for an allo-SCT, thus reducing the toxicity and NRM in adult Ph-negative ALL patients.

Case Study 4

You are seeing a 38-year-old female with Philadelphia chromosome–positive precursor B-cell ALL with your transplant fellow. The patient is in complete remission. You plan and discuss the role of myeloablative allogeneic transplantation with the patient.

9) Your fellow requests you to help him understand the best myeloablative and immuno-suppressive regimen in this disease and why you would not consider reduced intensity conditioning (RIC) regimen for this patient.

Expert Perspective: Standard myeloablative conditioning regimens are based on total body irradiation (TBI) combined with cyclophosphamide or etoposide. According to the EBMT registry, the use of reduced toxicity myeloablative regimens, for example intravenous busulfan, to avoid TBI-related short- and long-term toxicity, is gaining popularity.

Direct comparisons between different myeloablative conditioning regimens in the setting of ALL have never been studied in clinical trials; therefore, a firm recommendation regarding specific myeloablative regimens cannot be made. This decision should be based on institutional preference, mainly extensive experience with a specific protocol. The traditional immunosuppressive therapy is based on the historic methotrexate and cyclosporine regimen.

Data regarding RIC for ALL patients is sparse relative to myeloid or other low grade lymphoid malignancies. In a study from the CIBMTR (Marks et al. 2010), Ph-negative ALL patients were analyzed (Marks et al. 2010). Ninety-three RIC patients were compared with 1428 myeloablative allo-SCT counterparts. Interestingly, regimen intensity has no impact on transplant-related mortality or relapse risk on a multivariate analysis. In a similar analysis from the EBMT (Mohty et al. 2010), RIC patients experienced a significantly decreased risk for non-relapse mortality and an increased risk for relapse (Mohty et al. 2010). The risk for relapse is significantly higher in RIC conditioning than in a full myeloablative regimen. RIC was evaluated in the prospective UKALL14 study in which all patients > 41 years old were treated with a RIC regimen (Okasha 2021). Data from this study reported fairly good results with a two-year OS and EFS of 63% and 56%, respectively, in MRD-negative patients. In contrast, a high rate of relapse with two-year EFS of 28% was observed in patients who remained MRD positive post-induction. However, for the young patient with ALL, evidence concerning RIC SCT is scanty and premature. Thus, although lacking unequivocal data, for this young patient, existing data suggest that a myeloablative regimen followed by a matched sibling SCT is the therapy of choice.

Case Study 5

A 48-year-old female is being prepared to undergo allogeneic transplantation for Ph-negative ALL in CR1. The patient is MRD-negative. No matched sibling donor (MSD) or matched unrelated donor (MUD) is found. However, the patient's son is found as a potential haploidentical donor. You discuss the transplantation options with the patient using a haploidentical donor (son).

10) What is the evidence for haploidentical transplantation in adult ALL?

Expert Perspective: Allo-SCT is the treatment of choice enabling disease cure in adult ALL patients in CR1. Less than one-third of patients who need transplant will have a matched sibling donor (MSD). For other patients a search for an alternative donor should be performed. Matched unrelated donor (MUD) and haploidentical donors are reasonable options. In recent years, data regarding the efficacy and safety of MUD transplant is accumulating and showing promising results. A multicenter large retrospective study reported no significant difference in five-year DFS in 221 high-risk ALL patients transplanted from a matched related vs matched unrelated donor. Data from the CIBMTR had shown no difference in leukemia-free survival (LFS) or transplant-related mortality between sibling and MUD allo-SCT in 672 ALL patients. However, such data need to be cautiously interpreted as there is an inherent selection bias in deciding who should undergo MUD transplant. For ALL patients with no matched related or unrelated donor, over recent years, haploidentical transplant using post-transplant cyclophosphamide as GVHD prophylaxis has emerged as a suitable alternative. In fact, in several large centers this has now become the preferred transplant modality. As reported by the EBMT registry, in terms of LFS, OS, and graft-versus-host–free survival (GRFS), haplo-transplanted patients showed similar outcomes as observed in MSD (Nagler et al. 2021) and MUD (Shem-Tov et al. 2020) transplantations. Notably, comparison of haplo-SCT to MSD transplantations showed a reduction in relapse incidence (26% vs 31.6%) and increased NRM (22.9% vs 13%), attributed mainly to the high rate of infections. However, no difference in relapse or NRM was detected in comparison to outcomes of MUD transplantations. These studies demonstrate haplo-SCT is feasible and efficacious and is increasingly used in the absence of a well-matched related or unrelated donor. For the patient described in the question, if no matched related or unrelated donor was found, we would recommend proceeding to haplo-SCT.

11) In your opinion, how crucial is (i) determination of intrathymic (pro-T, pre-T, cortical-T, or medullary-T) differentiation status, and (ii) identification of specific cytogenetic/ molecular abnormalities in appropriately selecting patients for front-line allogeneic transplantation for precursor T-cell leukemia/lymphoma?

Expert Perspective: The immunophenotyping definition of intra-thymic differentiation status of leukemic cells is based on the commonly used European Group for the Immunological Characterization of Leukemias (EGIL) classification system (Okasha 2021). Several studies have shown an association between T cell developmental subgroups and prognosis. In both pediatric and adult ALL clinical trials, lower remission rates, early relapses, and shortened OS were associated with immunophenotypically immature T-ALL (Vitale et al. 2006). For instance, In the GIMEMA LAL 0496 study, 91% of the cortical mature group achieved CR relative to only 56% in the early pro/pre T group (Vitale et al. 2006). CD1a is a biomarker expressed in the cortical thymocyte stage and not in the earlier pro-T/pre-T stages. In the UKALL XII/ECOG 2993 study, patients with positive CD1a expression at diagnosis had a better five-year OS (64%) compared with CD1a-negative patients (39%) (Vitale et al. 2006). Early T-cell precursor (ETP) ALL, defined by $CD1a^{neg}$, $CD8^{neg}$, and $CD5^{neg/dim}$ and positivity for one or more myeloid/stem cell markers, was recently identified as a high-risk ALL subgroup (see Chapter 1). Notably, ETP ALL was associated with significantly worse prognosis than other T-ALL subtypes with-high MRD persistence and median event-free survival and OS of 14 and 20 months, respectively, after treatment with hyper-CVAD or augmented BFM protocol. Analysis of ETP ALL patients from the GRAALL-2003 and -2005 studies, in which a high percentage of ETP ALL patients exhibited resistance to induction therapy and proceeded to allo-HCT in CR1, showed a trend toward better OS after up-front allo-HCT in this group of patients (Asnafi et al. 2017). The survival benefit of up-front allo-HCT in ETP ALL patients was further demonstrated in a recent retrospective study from the MD Anderson with five-year EFS rates of 36% versus 18%, underscoring the role of allo-SCT in first remission in this high-risk group. Interestingly, in this study, no advantage for allo-HCT was observed in non-ETP patients, raising the question of whether allo-HCT can be omitted in T-ALL patients achieving MRD negativity (see Chapters 3 and 4).

While many clinical trials evaluated the impact of immunophenotypically characterized T-ALL subtypes, cytogenetic aberrations, and molecular profile, on disease clinical outcomes, none of these studies used these variables as clinical tools for making therapeutic decisions regarding the best consolidative or maintenance therapy. Therefore, outside of well-conducted clinical trials, all young T-ALL patients with a matched histocompatible sibling should be offered myeloablative conditioning followed by SCT regardless of their intrathymic differentiation status or specific cytogenetic aberrations.

Case Study 6

You are scheduled to see two patients with T-ALL/lymphoblastic lymphoma (LBL). Both are 38-year-old males in first CR following four weeks into front-line therapy.

- A) The first patient (patient 1) presented with symptomatic mediastinal mass and has T cell-LBL (without marrow involvement).
- B) The second patient (patient 2) has T cell-ALL and has negative bone marrow biopsy 3.5 weeks into induction therapy.

Both patients had a negative CSF evaluation and presented with a WBC of 45,000/μL with predominant lymphocytes.

12) Which of the following are acceptable treatment option(s) for patient 1 (T-LBL) and patient 2 (T-ALL)?

- A) Maintenance POMP therapy.
- B) High-dose chemotherapy followed by autologous rescue.
- C) Allogeneic transplantation.

Expert Perspective: T-LBL is a neoplasm of immature T cells arising from precursor thymic T cells at varying stages of differentiation. In the past, LBL and ALL were considered the same disease with different clinical presentations. The word lymphoma is used where there is a bulky mass in the mediastinum or elsewhere and up to 25% blasts in the bone marrow. New data suggested different molecular profiles of T-ALL and T-LBL. From a clinical point of view, therapeutic aspects seem to differ among these two acute leukemia subtypes. For example mediastinal irradiation is recommended in addition to chemotherapy for T-LBL while mediastinal masses in T-ALL will respond to a chemotherapy-only regimen. In the GRAALL-LYSA LL03 study of T-LBL, high LDH and mutation status of *NOTCH1/FBXW7/RAS/PTEN* were the only risk factors for OS (Asnafi et al. 2009). In the MD Anderson series only CNS involvement at diagnosis was associated with poor outcome. Recently, and as discussed previously, the role of MRD monitoring as a validated tool for making therapeutic decisions has emerged in ALL, despite the difficulty of immunophenotypically defining MRD in T-ALL when compared with B-ALL. Whether this approach is relevant in patients with LBL remains to be defined. LBL patients should be treated with an ALL-type regimen in order to achieve a high rate of CR and disease-free survival. Since the rate of mediastinal relapse is high among T-LBL patients, most authors recommend consolidating patients with mediastinal irradiation given after a dose-intensive ALL treatment. The management of post therapy residual mediastinal mass is controversial and beyond the scope of this discussion. The role of autologous hematopoietic cell transplantation (auto-HCT) as a consolidation strategy for LBL has been studied in few small series, all of which suggested a disease-free survival benefit (Milpied et al. 1989, Santini et al. 1991). A single, relatively small (119 patients) study conducted by the EBMT and the United Kingdom Lymphoma Group prospectively randomized LBL patients (68% with T-LBL) to auto-HCT or conventional chemotherapy (Sweetenham et al. 2001). Performing auto-HCT in first CR resulted in a trend for improved relapse-free survival (24% vs 55% $P = 0.065$) but did not translate into improved OS compared with conventional-dose therapy (45% vs 56%). The role of allo- vs. auto-HCT in this setting has been evaluated in a large retrospective series (Sweetenham et al. 2001). In this study, allo-HCT was associated with fewer relapses than auto-HCT (at five-year, 34% vs 56%; $P = 0.004$) but higher treatment-related mortality (at six months, 18% vs 3%; $P = 0.002$), which masked any potential survival advantage. So far, no OS benefit has been demonstrated for auto- or allo-HCT over conventional chemotherapy regimen. Current ongoing clinical trials are evaluating risk factors and clear indications for performing transplant at first CR. Therefore, for the patient with T-LBL in first CR, maintenance therapy, based on methotrexate/mercaptopurine, is the recommended mode of treatment. In T-ALL (excluding T-LBL), auto-HCT has no advantage over conventional chemotherapy as has been shown by the large international UKALL XII/ECOG 2993 trial (Marks et al. 2009).

Traditional risk factors for high-risk T-ALL are: WBC > 100,000/μL at presentation, adverse cytogenetics, and ETP-ALL. Absence of mutations in NOTCH1 or FBXW1 were identified as additional poor prognostic factors. These risk factors are taken into consideration when considering allo-HCT for T-ALL patients. Myeloablative allo-HCT has been incorporated in several small studies, all of which use various risk factors to assign patients to allo-HCT. In the largest study reporting on T-ALL patients, a donor vs no donor randomization was implemented, and all T-ALL patients with a histocompatible sibling donor were assigned for allo-HCT regardless of the presence of traditional high-risk factors (Marks et al. 2009).

The OS at five years was 46% for the no donor group and 61% for the donor group, a difference maintained at 10 years. Therefore, for the young patient with T-ALL, allo-HCT is recommended if a suitable family donor is available.

13) **You are discussing the management of two patients with Ph-negative presenting with relapsed disease after achieving prior remission.**

   A) A 28-year-old patient diagnosed with disease relapse one year after completing treatment, which consisted of induction, consolidation, and two-year maintenance. At diagnosis of relapse, the patient presents with 70% blasts positive for CD19 and CD22 in bone marrow and CNS involvement as shown by CSF analysis.

   B) A 23-year-old patient, diagnosed five years ago with high-risk Ph-negative ALL. He was given treatment with induction and consolidation after which MRD was still positive. He then was given two cycles of blinatumomab with conversion to MRD-negative and proceeded to allo-HCT. Currently, the patient has no signs of active GVHD and presents now with a 0.5% MRD after previous MRD measurements were negative. Bone marrow examinations show 0.3% blasts CD19-positive and CD22-negative.

Expert Perspective: Relapsed ALL, particularly following allo-HCT, is one of the most difficult clinical scenarios to manage. Allo-HCT is the only curative strategy for relapsed ALL, irrespective of whether the patient had undergone a previous transplant. Historically, the rate of CR was about 50%, and even for a patient who achieved CR the median remission duration is extremely short and estimated to be three–four months. That is why a second allo-HCT is the treatment of choice. Nevertheless, recent progress in development of targeted therapies including the bispecific monoclonal antibody blinatumomab, antibody-drug conjugate inotuzumab ozogamicin (InO), and CAR-T cell therapies (tisagenlecleucel and brexucabtagene autoleucel; see also chapter 2) has revolutionized treatment options in the setting of relapsed disease. Nevertheless, in order to choose the optimal treatment, it is imperative to consider patient comorbidities, disease burden, CNS involvement, previous treatments, immunophenotype, and eligibility for stem cell transplant. Assessment of CD19 and CD22 positivity is critical in order to employ a targeted therapy approach using one of the novel agents including blinatumomab directed to CD19, InO (an anti-CD22 monoclonal antibody conjugated to the drug calicheamicin), or CD19-directed CAR T cells. In the setting of relapsed disease, regarding outcomes of OS, overall response rate, relapse-free survival, achieving MRD negativity, and percentage of patients who proceeded to allo-HCT, novel agents demonstrated superiority over standard of care chemotherapy. In the phase III TOWER trial, treatment with blinatumomab resulted in a median OS and overall response rate of 7.7 months and 44%, respectively, compared to four months and 25% in the group that received SoC (Kantarjian et al. 2017). Notably, in the blinatumomab group, reduced relapse-free survival and OS were observed in patients with high disease burden at relapse compared to patients with low disease burden. Additionally, the presence of CNS involvement was associated with a high rate of neurotoxicity in patients who received blinatumomab. Results regarding InO treatment in the setting of relapsed disease were reported in the phase III INO-VATE study with a median OS and CR rate of 7.7 months and 81%, respectively, compared to 6.7 months and 29% in the standard of care arm (Kantarjian et al. 2016). The two-year survival rate was 23% versus 10% in the InO and standard of care groups, respectively. However, although a significant reduction of mortality was observed, one of the major non-hematological adverse effects observed in the InO group was a high rate (11%) of veno-occlusive disease (VOD) translating to high nonrelapse mortality.

Patient no. 1 is an AYA who presented with an early relapse with high disease burden (> 50% blasts in marrow) and CNS involvement. This patient should receive InO, with the hope of attaining MRD negativity as a bridge to subsequent allo-HCT. Choice of the conditioning regimen for allo-SCT should consider the increased risk for VOD in this patient, possibly avoiding dual alkylator therapy.

The second clinical case presents a patient with late relapse after allo-HCT. Despite prior treatment with blinatumomab, disease cells at relapse remained CD19-positive, raising the option for treatment with CD19 CAR T cells. Infusion of tisagenlecleucel CAR T cells demonstrated remarkable results with overall response rate of 81% of whom all patients with response attained MRD negativity (Maude et al. 2018). Two-year relapse-free survival was 62% with a median OS of 12.9 months. Notably, event-free survival and OS were inversely correlated to disease burden with low burden disease (< 5% blasts) patients achieving a median event-free survival of 11 months and median OS of 20 months (Maude et al. 2018). Improvement in event-free survival was observed in patients who were bridged to allo-HCT after CAR T cell therapy. Another anti-CD19 CAR T cell product, brexucabtagene autoleucel is FDA approved for adult patients with relapsed or refractory B-cell precursor ALL. Its efficacy was evaluated in ZUMA-3 (NCT02614066), a single-arm multicenter trial. Patients received a single infusion of brexucabtagene autoleucel following completion of lymphodepleting chemotherapy. The efficacy outcome measures used to support approval were CR achieved within 3 months from infusion and duration of CR. Of the 54 patients evaluable for efficacy, 28 (52%; 95% CI: 38, 66) achieved CR within 3 months. With a median follow-up for responders of 7.1 months, the median duration of CR was not reached; the duration of CR was estimated to exceed 12 months for more than half the patients. A recent update after 26.8-months median follow-up, the overall CR rate (CR + CR with incomplete hematological recovery) among treated patients (N = 55) in phase 2 was 71% (56% CR rate); medians for duration of remission and overall survival (OS) were 14.6 and 25.4 months, respectively. Most patients responded to brexucabtagene autoleucel regardless of age or baseline bone marrow blast percentage, but less so in patients with > 75% blasts. No new safety signals were observed. In patients with high burden disease, CAR T cell therapy is not always applicable as such patients require urgent treatment and cannot withstand waiting for CART cell production. Additionally, these patients with high disease burden experienced high rate of adverse events including cytokine release syndrome (CRS) and neurotoxicity. The patient described in case no. 2 presents with a low burden disease (MRD 0.5%) thus allowing suspending treatment until CAR T cell manufacture (~one month). Patient no. 2 should receive CAR T cells followed by allo-HCT, preferably from a different donor.

Current evidence supports using the novel agents' armamentarium in R/R ALL as a bridge to bone marrow transplant. Information regarding eliminating the need for allo-HCT in patients who achieved MRD negativity is limited. Thus, until more data from long-term follow-up are available, these novel agents should be used with the aim of reaching MRD negativity and subsequently proceeding to allo-HCT.

Recommended Readings

Asnafi, V., Bond, J., Graux, C., Lhermitte, L., Lara, D., Cluzeau, T. et al. (2017). Early response–based therapy stratification improves survival in adult early thymic precursor acute lymphoblastic leukemia: a group for research on adult acute lymphoblastic leukemia study. *J Clin Oncol* 35: 2683–2691.

Asnafi, V., Buzyn, A., Le Noir, S., Baleydier, F., Simon, A., Beldjord, K. et al. (2009). NOTCH1/FBXW7 mutation identifies a large subgroup with favorable outcome in adult T-cell acute lymphoblastic leukemia (T-ALL): a Group for Research on Adult Acute Lymphoblastic Leukemia (GRAALL) study. *Blood* 113: 3918–3924.

Cortes, J., O'Brien, S.M., Pierce, S., Keating, M.J., Freireich, E.J., and Kantarjian, H.M. (1995). The value of high-dose systemic chemotherapy and intrathecal therapy for central nervous system prophylaxis in different risk groups of adult acute lymphoblastic leukemia. *Blood* 86: 2091–2097.

Fielding, A.K., Rowe, J.M., Buck, G., Foroni, L., Gerrard, G., Litzow, M.R. et al. (2014). UKALLXII/ECOG2993: addition of imatinib to a standard treatment regimen enhances long-term outcomes in Philadelphia positive acute lymphoblastic leukemia. *Blood* 123: 843–850.

Goldstone, A.H., Richards, S.M., Lazarus, H.M., Tallman, M.S., Buck, G., Fielding, A.K. et al. (2008). In adults with standard-risk acute lymphoblastic leukemia, the greatest benefit is achieved from a matched sibling allogeneic transplantation in first complete remission, and an autologous transplantation is less effective than conventional consolidation/maintenance chemotherapy in all patients:final results of the International ALL Trial (MRC UKALLXII/ECOG E2993). *Blood* 111.1827-1833

Kantarjian, H., Stein, A., Gökbuget, N., Fielding, A.K., Schuh, A.C., Ribera, J.-M. et al. (2017). Blinatumomab versus chemotherapy for advanced acute lymphoblastic leukemia. *N Engl J Med* 376: 836–847.

Kantarjian, H.M., DeAngelo, D.J., Stelljes, M., Martinelli, G., Liedtke, M., Stock, W. et al. (2016). Inotuzumab ozogamicin versus standard therapy for acute lymphoblastic leukemia. *N Engl J Med* 375: 740–753.

Litzow, M.R., Sun, Z., Paietta, E., Mattison, R.J., Lazarus, H.M., Rowe, J.M. et al. (2022). Consolidation Therapy with Blinatumomab Improves Overall Survival in Newly Diagnosed Adult Patients with B-Lineage Acute Lymphoblastic Leukemia in Measurable Residual Disease Negative Remission: Results from the ECOG-ACRIN E1910 Randomized Phase III National Cooperative Clinical Trials Network Trial. *Blood* 140 (Supplement 2): LBA-1.

Marks, D.I., Paietta, E.M., Moorman, A.V., Richards, S.M., Buck, G., DeWald, G. et al. (2009). T-cell acute lymphoblastic leukemia in adults: clinical features, immunophenotype, cytogenetics, and outcome from the large randomized prospective trial (UKALL XII/ECOG 2993). *Blood* 114: 5136–5145.

Maude, S.L., Laetsch, T.W., Buechner, J., Rives, S., Boyer, M., Bittencourt, H. et al. (2018). Tisagenlecleucel in children and young adults with B-cell lymphoblastic leukemia. *N Engl J Med* 378: 439–448.

Milpied, N., Ifrah, N., Kuentz, M., Maraninchi, D., Colombat, P., Blaise, D. et al. (1989). Bone marrow transplantation for adult poor prognosis lymphoblastic lymphoma in first complete remission. *Br J Haematol* 73: 82–87.

Moorman, A.V., Harrison, C.J., Buck, G.A.N., Richards, S.M., Secker-Walker, L.M., Martineau, M. et al. (2007). Karyotype is an independent prognostic factor in adult acute lymphoblastic leukemia (ALL): analysis of cytogenetic data from patients treated on the Medical Research Council (MRC) UKALLXII/Eastern Cooperative Oncology Group (ECOG) 2993 trial. *Blood* 109: 3189–3197.

Nagler, A., Labopin, M., Houhou, M., Aljurf, M., Mousavi, A., Hamladji, R.M. et al. (2021). Outcome of haploidentical versus matched sibling donors in hematopoietic stem cell transplantation for adult patients with acute lymphoblastic leukemia: a study from the Acute Leukemia Working Party of the European Society for Blood and Marrow Transplantation. *J Hematol Oncol* 14: 53.

Pfeifer, H., Wassmann, B., Bethge, W., Dengler, J., Bornhäuser, M., Stadler, M. et al. (2013). Randomized comparison of prophylactic and minimal residual disease-triggered imatinib after allogeneic stem cell transplantation for BCR-ABL1-positive acute lymphoblastic leukemia. *Leukemia* 27: 1254–1262.

Ribera, J.M.J., Morgades, M., Ciudad, J., Montesinos, P., Esteve, J., Genescà, E. et al. (2021). Chemotherapy or allogeneic transplantation in high-risk Philadelphia chromosome–negative adult lymphoblastic leukemia. *Blood* 137.

Saini, N., Marin, D., Ledesma, C., Delgado, R., Rondon, G., Popat, U.R. et al. (2020). Impact of TKIs post-allogeneic hematopoietic cell transplantation in Philadelphia chromosome-positive ALL. *Blood* 136: 1786–1789.

Santini, G., Coser, P., Chisesi, T., Porcellini, A., Sertoli, R., Contu, A. et al. (1991). Autologous bone marrow transplantation for advanced stage adult lymphoblastic lymphoma in first complete remission. *Bone Marrow Transplant* 4: 181–185.

Shah, B.D., Ghobadi, A., Oluwole, O.O., Logan, A.C., Boissel, N., Cassaday, R.D., Leguay, T., Bishop, M.R., Topp, M.S., Tzachanis, D., O'Dwyer, K.M., Arellano, M.L., Lin, Y., Baer, M.R., Schiller, G.J., Park, J.H., Subklewe, M., Abedi, M., Mi nnema, M.C., Wierda, W.G., DeAngelo, D.J., Stiff, P., Jeyakumar, D., Feng, C., Dong, J., Shen, T., Milletti, F., Rossi, J.M., Vezan, R., Masouleh, B.K., and Houot, R. (2021 August 7). KTE X19 for relapsed or refractory adult B cell acute lymphoblastic leuk aemia: phase 2 results of the single arm, open label, multicentre ZUMA 3 study. *Lancet* 398 (10299): 491–502. doi: 10.1016/S0140 6736(21)01222 8. Epub 2021 Jun 4. PMID: 34097852.

Shah, B.D., Ghobadi, A., Oluwole, O.O., Logan, A.C., Boissel, N., Cassaday, R .D., Leguay, T., Bishop, M.R., Topp, M.S., Tzachanis, D., O'Dwyer, K.M., Arellano, M.L., Lin, Y., Baer, M.R., Schiller, G.J., Park, J.H., Subklewe, M., Abedi, M., Minnema, M.C., Wierda, W.G., DeAngelo, D.J., Stiff, P., Jeyakumar, D., Dong, J., Adhikary, S. S., Zhou, L., Schuberth, P.C., Faghmous, I., Masouleh, B.K., and Houot, R. (2022 December 10). Two year follow up of KTE X19 in patients with relapsed or refractory adult B cell acute lymphoblastic leukemia in ZUMA 3 and its contextualization with SCHOLAR 3, an external historical control study. *J Hematol Oncol* 15 (1): 170. doi: 10.1186/s13045 022 01379 0. PMID: 36494725; PMCID: PMC9734710.

Shem-Tov, N., Peczynski, C., Labopin, M., Itälä-Remes, M., Blaise, D., Labussière-Wallet, H. et al. (2020). Haploidentical vs. unrelated allogeneic stem cell transplantation for acute lymphoblastic leukemia in first complete remission: on behalf of the ALWP of the EBMT. *Leukemia* 34: 283–292.

Tosi, M., Spinelli, O., Leoncin, M., Cavagna, R., Pavoni, C., Lussana, F. et al. (2021). MRD-based therapeutic decisions in genetically defined subsets of adolescents and young adult philadelphia-negative all. *Cancers (Basel)* 13: 2108.

Vitale, A., Guarini, A., Ariola, C., Mancini, M., Mecucci, C., Cuneo, A. et al. (2006). Adult T-cell acute lymphoblastic leukemia: biologic profile at presentation and correlation with response to induction treatment in patients enrolled in the GIMEMA LAL 0496 protocol. *Blood* 107: 473–479.

Part 2

Acute Myeloid Leukemia in Adults

6

Prognosis in Acute Myeloid Leukemia: Beyond Cytogenetics

Caner Saygin[1] and Lucy A. Godley[2]

[1] University of Chicago, Chicago, IL
[2] Northwestern University Feinberg School of Medicine, Chicago, IL

Case Study 1

A 32-year-old woman presents to her primary doctor with fever and sore throat of 10 days' duration. On physical exam, she has gingival hyperplasia and petecchiae. A complete blood cell count (CBC) shows a total white blood cell (WBC) count of 80,000/μL with 40% blasts. The patient is referred to the hematology/oncology department with a suspected diagnosis of acute myeloid leukemia (AML).

1) When should I order cytogenetic and fluorescent in situ hybridization (FISH) analysis ?

A) I should always order only FISH.

B) I should always order only cytogenetic analysis.

C) I should always order both tests.

D) I should order only molecular tests.

Expert Perspective: Chromosomal abnormalities (e.g. deletions, duplications, gain and loss of chromosome material, translocations, and inversions) are common drivers of pathogenesis. Conventional chromosome analysis is a critical part of laboratory workup for acute myeloid leukemia (AML), as it can provide: (i) diagnostic information; (ii) information useful for classification, staging, and prognostication; (iii) information to guide an appropriate choice of therapy; and (iv) evidence of remission or relapse. Karyotyping (performed on metaphase chromosomes) can detect both balanced (translocations and inversions) and unbalanced (deletions and duplications) rearrangements at any chromosomal location, and it is irreplaceable at diagnosis, when no information is available about the abnormalities that might be present in the sample. It is also widely available and affordable.

FISH (performed on interphase chromosomes) is a highly sensitive, targeted test for known chromosome rearrangements. The method does not, however, provide the genome-wide screen obtainable by classical cytogenetic analysis. At diagnosis, FISH can be a useful adjunct to karyotyping in specific situations, if a particular chromosomal abnormality is strongly suspected based on the morphology or clinical picture. For example, it is faster to confirm the presence of the t(15;17)-*PML::RARA* (promyelocytic leukemia and retinoic acid receptor alpha) in suspected acute promyelocytic leukemia (APL) by FISH than by karyotyping. FISH may also be faster than molecular diagnostics, depending on the laboratory. In addition, the inv(16) should always be confirmed by FISH, since it causes a subtle change in the chromosome 16 banding pattern and is therefore often difficult to recognize reliably by karyotyping, especially in samples with poor morphology. When a variant translocation is seen by karyotyping, FISH should be used to verify the presence of the expected gene rearrangement. However, the most important application of FISH is not at diagnosis but rather to evaluate follow-up samples for residual disease, assuming that a FISH assay is available for the cytogenetic abnormality that was detected at diagnosis. FISH is useful particularly for cases in which it is not possible to monitor residual disease by another, more sensitive method (e.g. flow cytometry or polymerase chain reaction [PCR]). Furthermore, in cases that will be monitored for residual disease by FISH, it is advisable to perform the analysis on the diagnostic sample to verify the signal pattern for future comparison (see Chapter 10).

With the advent of whole genome sequencing (WGS), it is possible to discern chromosomal rearrangements by sequencing of entire tumor cell genomes. In some cases, WGS can detect chromosomal abnormalities that are below the level of detection of karyotyping. Currently, most centers are not implementing clinical chromosome analysis via WGS due to cost—both up-front investment in equipment to perform such analysis and sample processing costs. However, incorporation of this approach may be imminent as sequencing costs decrease and bioinformatic pipelines become fully automated.

Correct Answer: C

2) What additional studies should be done for prognostication of AML?

   A) CT chest/abdomen/pelvis to investigate extramedullary disease.
   B) V(D)J gene rearrangement study to identify malignant clone for future MRD detection.
   C) Lumbar puncture at diagnosis to investigate central nervous system (CNS) disease.
   D) Next-generation sequencing (NGS) panel for genes that are frequently mutated in AML.

Expert Perspective: In addition to cytogenetic abnormalities, several molecular abnormalities have been shown to have prognostic importance in patients with AML. The current National Comprehensive Cancer Network (NCCN) and European LeukemiaNet guidelines for diagnosis, prognostic assessment, and therapeutic decision recommend panel testing for frequently mutated genes in AML, including *BCOR, EZH2, SF3B1, SRSF2, STAG2, U2AF1, ZRSR2, FLT3, NPM1, CEBPA, KIT, ASXL1, RUNX1, TP53, IDH1*, and *IDH2*. These mutations have been incorporated into the most recent European LeukemiaNet (ELN) 2022 prognostic risk stratification. Mutations of *NPM1* and biallelic *CEBPA* are associated with favorable prognosis, whereas *RUNX1, ASXL1*, and *TP53* mutations are associated with adverse prognosis. In this case, lumbar puncture is indicated due to hyperleukocytosis (WBC > 40,000/μL) at diagnosis according to NCCN guidelines, but the presence of CNS disease is not a prognostic variable in ELN risk stratification. V(D)J gene arrangements are seen in lymphoid malignancies and thus are not indicated for myeloid neoplasms.

Correct Answer: D

3) **Do you need to perform multiple tests that assess the same molecular rearrangement? For example, for a patient with APL, do you need to order FISH, cytogenetic analysis, and reverse transcription PCR (RT-PCR) for *PML::RARA*?**

A) You need to order routine chromosome analysis only.
B) You should order FISH first and keep RT-PCR in reserve.
C) Both A and B.
D) It is important to use an appropriate combination of tests for each patient.

Expert Perspective: No single genetic testing procedure fulfills all the needs of clinical care for patients with AML. It is important to use a combination of testing methods that are best suited for each clinical situation. At diagnosis of AML, conventional chromosome analysis is essential for initial identification of chromosome abnormalities. If abnormalities identified by karyotyping cannot be tracked by FISH or RT-PCR due to a lack of suitable probes or primers, conventional cytogenetic analysis becomes the sole method for detecting the presence of genetically abnormal clones in follow-up samples. However, many common chromosome abnormalities associated with AML [e.g. t(9;22), t(15;17), inv(16), and t(8;21)] can be detected by all three clinically used methods: chromosome analysis, FISH, and RT-PCR. In these cases, the genetic test of choice should be selected according to the clinical situation, turnaround time, and cost. Conventional cytogenetic analysis should be repeated whenever there is a concern for disease progression or relapse, since it can detect additional abnormalities that were not present at diagnosis and are consistent with clonal evolution and disease progression. However, FISH and RT-PCR are superior to karyotyping for monitoring patients who are believed to be in remission, since these methods are more sensitive and quantitative. RT-PCR is the most sensitive of the three assays, and when available, it might be the method of choice. It has proven useful to test for very low levels of the *BCR::ABL1* and other fusion transcripts in patients after treatment or post bone marrow transplantation. Due to its quantitative nature, RT-PCR is the standard method to monitor responses to tyrosine kinase inhibitor therapy in chronic myeloid leukemia. For abnormalities for which RT-PCR assay is not available, FISH can be a viable alternative for confirming that a patient remains in remission. For patients in molecular remission from APL, appearance of the *PML::RARA* transcript by RT-PCR or the t(15;17) by FISH or chromosomal karyotyping indicates impending relapse and is an indicated for initiating re-induction chemotherapy.

Correct Answer: D

4) **Which statement about chromosomal and molecular tests is correct?**

A) Karyotyping can give false-negative results, but molecular methods are always accurate.
B) FISH can give false-negative results, but karyotyping and molecular methods are always accurate.
C) Molecular methods can give false-negative results, but karyotyping and FISH are always accurate.
D) Each method can sometimes give false-negative results.

Expert Perspective: A possible reason for obtaining false-negative results by chromosome analysis is a failure of tumor cells to grow in tissue culture. When malignant cells do not proliferate *in vitro*, a normal karyotype is typically obtained from nonmalignant, actively dividing cells in the bone marrow sample, and without further studies, it is impossible to decipher whether leukemic cells failed to be analyzed or were indeed cytogenetically normal. Although rarely a problem in acute leukemias, this is a major limitation for cytogenetic testing of indolent diseases such as plasma cell malignancies and chronic lymphocytic leukemia.

The presence of submicroscopic (cryptic) abnormalities, which are not detectable by karyotyping due to its limited resolution, is another potential cause for obtaining false-negative results by conventional cytogenetics.

FISH testing will occasionally give false-negative results in cases of atypical chromosomal rearrangements. Fusion genes can sometimes be generated by small interstitial insertions of chromosomal material, which may be undetectable by clinically used FISH probes. Additionally, although FISH has much higher resolution than karyotyping, some microdeletions (which remove only a part of the region targeted by a FISH probe) will be too small for detection by FISH.

PCR assays developed for detection of fusion genes may give false-negative results due to breakpoint heterogeneity. PCR assays are typically optimized to detect fusion transcripts generated through the most frequent breakpoints, and therefore, cases with less common breakpoints within one or both partner genes will be missed by most clinically available PCR tests. Polymorphisms within PCR primer binding sites can lead to allelic dropout and therefore, serve as a source of false-negative results for any PCR-based molecular test. For this reason, it is important for clinical laboratories to design PCR probes in genomic regions that lack genomic polymorphisms. Finally, mutations present in a very small fraction of cells are usually undetected by traditional Sanger sequencing, due to its limited sensitivity.

Correct Answer: D

5) **Which result do you believe if there are discordant results from FISH versus karyotype analysis?**

   A) A discrepancy is not a reason to disregard either result.
   B) You should only believe karyotyping, since it is a "gold standard."
   C) You should only believe FISH, since it is more targeted.
   D) If the results are discordant, neither method should be believed.

Expert Perspective: Karyotype analysis and FISH have different indications, strengths, and weaknesses, and they do not always provide the same answers. Discrepancies that occasionally occur between a karyotype and a FISH result do not imply that either assay failed or is not reliable. A normal karyotype in a case with a clearly abnormal FISH result may be observed for multiple reasons, including (i) low or no yield of metaphase chromosomes from tumor cells, (ii) tumor cells with a very poor chromosome morphology, or (iii) deletions, duplications, translocations, and other structural abnormalities involving small chromosomal regions so that the resolution of conventional analysis is insufficient for their identification.

Possible explanations for a negative FISH result when an abnormality is observed by karyotyping may include: (i) an abnormality that looks by G-banding like a particular translocation or other specific structural rearrangement identifiable by FISH [e.g. t(15;17), t(9;22), inv(3), etc.] but actually involves different chromosomal regions and different breakpoints; and (ii) a chromosome or a chromosomal region appears to be missing by conventional analysis, but is actually present within marker chromosomes and other unidentifiable chromosomal segments in the karyotype.

When thinking about FISH, it is very important to remember its targeted nature. A negative FISH result does not mean an absence of chromosomal abnormalities in leukemic cells. It only indicates that specific abnormalities tested for by the selected FISH probes are not present.

Correct Answer: A

Case Study 2

A 52-year-old man is admitted to the Leukemia Service with AML. Cytogenetic analysis reveals a normal male karyotype, and a myeloid malignancy-specific NGS panel detects mutations in *NPM1 exon 12* (variant allelic frequency [VAF] of 48%), and *FLT3-ITD*.

6) What is the risk group of this leukemia based on ELN22 stratification?

A) Favorable.
B) Intermediate.
C) Adverse.
D) Not classifiable.

Expert Perspective: The recently proposed ELN22 classification stratifies AML into three risk groups based on cytogenetic abnormalities and the presence of certain myeloid mutations (Table 6.1). In this stratification, *NPM1* mutations are associated with favorable prognosis and can be seen in 20–30% of AML patients. Somatic mutations in *FLT3*, or *FMS-like tyrosine kinase 3*, lead to constitutively active signaling in myeloblasts that drives accelerated growth and survival of leukemia cells. Two main classes of mutations include internal tandem duplication (ITD) mutations and *tyrosine kinase domain (TKD)* point mutations. *ITD* and *TKD* mutations can be seen in 25–30% of AML patients, and often co-occur with *NPM1* mutation. These patients often present with a high WBC count at presentation. Concomitant presence of *NPM1* and *FLT3-ITD* mutations would be classified in "intermediate-risk" category of ELN 2022. Combination of a *FLT3*-targeting tyrosine kinase inhibitor (e.g. midostaurin) with induction chemotherapy improves survival in patients with *FLT3* mutations. Given the high relapse risk associated with a high allelic ratio, allogeneic hematopoietic cell transplantation (allo-HCT) at the time of first complete remission (CR1) is recommended for eligible patients (see Chapter 11).

Correct Answer: B

Table 6.1 2022 ELN risk stratification by genetics in AML.

Risk category	Genetic abnormality
Favorable	t(8;21)(q22;q22.1)/*RUNX1::RUNX1T1*
	inv(16)(p13.1q22) or t(16;16)(p13.1;q22)/*CBFB::MYH11*
	Mutated *NPM1* without *FLT3-ITD*
	bZIP in-frame mutated CEBPA
Intermediate	Mutated *NPM1* with *FLT3-ITD*
	Wild-type *NPM1* with *FLT3-ITD*
	t(9;11)(p21.3;q23.3)/*MLLT3::KMT2A*
	Cytogenetic and/or molecular abnormalities not classified as favorable or adverse
Adverse	t(6;9)(p23;q34.1)/*DEK::NUP214*
	t(v;11q23.3)/*KMT2A*-rearranged
	t(9;22)(q34.1;q11.2)/*BCR::ABL1*
	t(8;16)(p11;p13)/KAT6A::CREBBP
	inv(3)(q21.3q26.2) or t(3;3)(q21.3;q26.2)/GATA2, MECOM(EVI1)
	t(3q26.2;v)/MECOM(EVI1)-rearranged
	−5 or del(5q); −7; −17/abn(17p)
	Complex karyotype, monosomal karyotype
	Mutated *ASXL1, BCOR, EZH2, RUNX1, SF3B1, SRSF2, STAG2, U2AF1,* or *ZRSR2*
	Mutated *TP53*

Case Study 3

A 62-year-old woman presents with AML and is found to have a normal karyotype and bi-allelic *CEBPA* mutations at VAF of 45% and 48%. She has an excellent performance status and is recommended to proceed with standard induction chemotherapy.

7) What is the clinical significance of biallelic *CEBPA* mutations?

  A) There is no clinical significance to biallelic *CEBPA* mutations.
  B) They confer a poor prognosis.
  C) They are often found in acute promyelocytic leukemia.
  D) They may be seen in a familial predisposition syndrome in which patients inherit one mutated *CEBPA* allele.

Expert Perspective: About 10% of patients who have biallelic *CEBPA* mutations have inherited one of the mutated alleles as a germline mutation. It is important to identify such individuals because allo-HCT should be considered in these individuals and there may be other family members who carry the familial germline mutation and would benefit from genetic counseling, mutation testing, and potentially increased surveillance (see Chapter 14). In the case of familial biallelic *CEBPA* mutations, often the germline mutation is found within the 5′-end of the gene, and development of AML is accompanied by acquisition of a second somatic mutation, usually within the 3′-end of the gene. Notably though, germline 3′ *CEBPA* mutations have also been identified. Familial AML with mutated *CEBPA* is inherited in an autosomal dominant fashion, and it appears to confer nearly complete penetrance for the development of AML. Biallelic *CEBPA* mutations confer a relatively favorable prognosis and chemosensitive disease.

Correct Answer D

8) **She achieves CR after induction chemotherapy with anthracycline and cytarabine. She also undergoes skin biopsy, which identifies a germline *CEBPA* mutation. What is the significance of this finding?**

   A) Patients with inherited *CEBPA* mutations may develop independent *de novo* AMLs in their lifetime.
   B) The clinical presentation and the course of disease do not differ between patients with germline vs somatic biallelic *CEBPA* mutations.
   C) Patient should also be counseled about an increased risk of solid tumors, including breast and ovarian cancer.
   D) Germline *CEBPA* mutations are often *de novo*, and therefore it is unlikely for her parents to carry the same deleterious variant.

Expert Perspective: All patients with biallelic *CEBPA* mutated AML should be offered skin biopsy for germline testing, since about 10% of them will have a germline mutation, typically the 5′-end mutation. Skin fibroblasts can be cultured and DNA extracted to determine if either *CEBPA* allele is germline. Germline testing from blood or saliva (which is heavily contaminated with blood cells) is not reliable for leukemia patients given the nature of disease. Patients with an inherited germline *CEBPA* mutation often acquire an additional somatic mutation in the normal allele, and present with AML containing biallelic mutations. These patients can achieve remission with standard chemotherapy but are at risk for developing independent AMLs later in their life, as evidenced by unique somatic 3′-end *CEBPA* mutations. Therefore, consideration for allo-HCT in first CR should be discussed with such individuals, and the risks and benefits weighed on an individual basis. If both *CEBPA* mutations are determined to be somatic, then outcomes for patients with biallelic *CEBPA* mutations remain excellent when treated with chemotherapy only.

Correct Answer: A

Case Study 4

A 75-year-old woman complains to her primary doctor that she feels tired. A CBC shows a hemoglobin of 7 g/dL, and a bone marrow biopsy shows 5q– syndrome.

9) **If 5q– syndrome is a "good prognosis" MDS, then why is deletion or loss of chromosome 5 considered as a "bad" prognostic marker for AML?**

   A) Deletions in MDS and AML affect different critical regions of 5q.
   B) Different genes and pathways play a role in pathogenesis.
   C) Different outcomes are related to the presence or absence of associated genetic abnormalities.
   D) All of the above.

Expert Perspective: A deletion of the long arm of chromosome 5 is one of the most frequent cytogenetic abnormalities in MDS and AML, occurring in 10–15% of cases. The 5q– syndrome is a distinct type of MDS defined by a medullary blast count of less than 5% and the deletion of 5q [del(5q)] as the sole karyotypic abnormality. It is characterized by macrocytosis, anemia, a normal or high platelet count, hypolobulated megakaryocytes in the bone marrow, a female preponderance, and a good prognosis, with approximately 10% of patients transforming to AML (see Chapters 12 and 13). In contrast, cases of non-5q– syndrome myeloid disorders with losses of genetic material involving chromosome 5 have consistently been associated with poor prognosis.

The commonly deleted regions (CDRs) in 5q disorders have been extensively studied, with two distinct CDRs mapped to 5q33.1 (more telomeric) in 5q– syndrome, and 5q31.1 (more centromeric) in non-5q– syndrome MDS and AML.

Major advances have been made in understanding the molecular pathogenesis of the 5q– syndrome by the demonstration that haploinsufficiency for the ribosomal gene RPS14 results in ribosomal deficiency, further causing p53 activation and defective erythropoiesis.

Completely different molecular pathways seem to play a role in the pathogenesis of non-5q– syndrome MDS and AML. The 1–1.5-Mb CDR at 5q31 identified in these disorders includes two main candidate genes for the role in pathogenesis: *EGR1* and *CTNNA1*.

Critical differences between 5q– syndrome and non-5q– syndrome MDS and AML also lie with mutations and genomic aberrations on chromosomal regions outside 5q. Importantly, the del(5q) in non-5q– syndrome MDS and AML, particularly secondary AML, invariably occurs together with other karyotypic abnormalities and frequently as part of a complex karyotype. Additionally, mutations with loss of function of p53 are significantly associated with the del(5q) in therapy-related MDS and therapy-related AML after previous treatment with alkylating agents.

Correct Answer: D

Case Study 5

A 75-year-old man is diagnosed with AML. Cytogenetic analysis reveals trisomy 8, and a myeloid malignancy NGS panel identifies mutations in *DNMT3A R882H* (VAF 40%), *SRSF2 P95H* (VAF 46%), and *IDH2 R140Q* (VAF 45%). He is recommended to receive azacitidine plus venetoclax for first-line management of his disease.

10) Which of the following statements about prognosis is correct?

   A) *DNMT3A* mutations are associated with favorable risk disease.
   B) Patients with *IDH2* mutations have inferior outcomes when treated with the combination of azacitidine and venetoclax.
   C) Mutations in *IDH* genes do not have an independent effect in predicting overall survival in AML.
   D) All of the above.

Expert Perspective: *DNMT3A* and *SRSF2* mutations are common ancestral mutations in AML and can also be seen as part of clonal hematopoiesis (CH). Mutations in *SRSF2* and *IDH2* genes often co-occur. Several reports indicate that *DNMT3A* and *SRSF2* mutations may be associated with high-risk disease. Mutations in *IDH1* or *IDH2* disrupt the normal function of the isocitrate dehydrogenase enzyme and confer a neomorphic enzymatic activity that leads to the conversion of isocitrate to 2-hydroxyglutarate, which acts as an oncometabolite. Mutations in the *IDH* genes do not have a strong impact on overall survival in AML patients, but patients with these mutations tend to have higher rates of response to the combination of azacitidine and venetoclax, as shown in the VIALE-A study

Correct Answer: C

Case Study continued: The patient achieves first CR with azacitidine and venetoclax, but the disease relapses after eight cycles of therapy. Given the continued presence of the *IDH2* mutation, he starts enasidenib monotherapy.

11) **Which of the following mutations acquired at relapse may be associated with a poor response to enasidenib?**

   A) *PTPN11*
   B) *TET2*
   C) *WT1*
   D) Monosomy 7

Expert Perspective: Enasidenib has been approved by FDA for management of relapsed AML with *IDH2* mutations (see Chapters 7 and 8). It has been reported that the presence of RAS pathway mutations, including *NRAS*, *KRAS*, and *PTPN11* are associated with lower response to enasidenib. Therefore, repeating the genetic studies at the time of relapse can provide important prognostic and predictive information for clinical decision-making.

Correct Answer: A

Recommended Readings

Amatangelo, M.D., Quek, L., Shih, A. et al. (2017). Enasidenib induces acute myeloid leukemia cell differentiation to promote clinical response. *Blood* 130 (6): 732–741.

Döhner, H., Estey, E.H., Grimwade, D. et al. (2017). Diagnosis and management of AML in adults: 2017 ELN recommendations from an international expert panel. *Blood* 129: 424–447.

Döhner H, Wei AH, Appelbaum FR, et al. Diagnosis and Management of AML in Adults: 2022 ELN Recommendations from an International Expert Panel. Blood. 2022 Jul;7. doi: 10.1182/blood.2022016867. Epub ahead of print. PMID: 35797463.

Duncavage, E.J., Schroeder, M.C., O'Laughlin, M. et al. (2021). Genome sequencing as an alternative to cytogenetic analysis in myeloid cancers. *N Eng J Med* 384: 924–935.

Godley, L.A. (2021). Germline mutations in MDS/AML predisposition disorders. *Curr Opin Hematol* 28 (2): 86–93.

Jourdan, E., Boissel, N., Chevret, S. et al. (2013). Prospective evaluation of gene mutations and minimal residual disease in patients with core binding factor acute myeloid leukemia. *Blood* 121 (12): 2213–2223.

Khoury JD, Solary E, Abla O, et al. The 5th edition of the World Health Organization Classification of Haematolymphoid Tumours: Myeloid and Histiocytic/Dendritic Neoplasms. Leukemia. 2022 Jul;36(7):1703-1719. doi: 10.1038/s41375-022-01613-1. Epub 2022 Jun 22. PMID: 35732831; PMCID: PMC9252913.

Marcucci, G., Haferlach, T., and Dohner, H. (2011). Molecular genetics of adult acute myeloid leukemia: Prognostic and therapeutic implications. *J Clin Oncol* 29: 475–486.

O'Donnell, M.R., Abboud, C.N., Altman, J. et al. (2012). Acute myeloid leukemia. *J Natl Compr Canc Netw* 10: 984–1021.

Papaemmanuil, E., Gerstung, M., Bullinger, L. et al. (2016). Genomic classification and prognosis in acute myeloid leukemia. *N Eng J Med* 374: 2209–2221.

Stubbins, R.J., Asom, A.S., Wang, P. et al. (2023 May 4). Germline loss of function BRCA1 and BRCA2 mutations and risk of de novo hematopoietic malignancies. *Haematologica*. doi: 10.3324/haematol.2022.281580. Epub ahead of print. PMID: 37139596.

Patel, J.P., Gonen, M., and Figueroa, M.E. (2012). Prognostic relevance of integrated genetic profiling in acute myeloid leukemia. *N Engl J Med* 366: 1079–1089.

Tawana, K., Wang, J., Renneville, A. et al. (2015). Disease evolution and outcomes in familial AML with germline CEBPA mutations. *Blood* 126 (10): 1214–1223.

7

Young Adults with Acute Myeloid Leukemia

Sangeetha Venugopal[1] and Farhad Ravandi[2]

[1] *University of Miami Health System*
[2] *The University of Texas – MD Anderson Cancer Center Texas*

Introduction

Acute myeloid leukemia (AML) is a disease of older age with a median age of 68 years at diagnosis. Advances in next-generation sequencing and better understanding of the molecular pathogenesis of AML has revealed the existence of age-related differences in AML biology. Until recently, almost all patients with AML received relatively similar treatment regardless of their ability to receive intensive therapy. On October 16, 2020, venetoclax in combination with hypomethylating agents was approved for newly diagnosed AML in adults older than 75 years or not eligible to receive intensive chemotherapy. Since then, the AML treatment paradigm has become distinctly bisected into those who are able to receive intensive chemotherapy and those who are not eligible. In general leukemia parlance, "young adults" typically refer to those aged 15–39 years; however, the focus of our discussion will be adults younger than 60 years who are eligible to receive intensive chemotherapy.

A Central European study of 5,564 patients with *de novo* AML spanning infancy through adulthood has demonstrated that the incidence of favorable cytomolecular aberrations decreases with increasing age. Adults younger than 60 years are more likely to harbor core binding factor (CBF) cytogenetic abnormalities [inv (16), t(8;21)], mutations in the nucleophosmin (*NPM1*), and *NPM1*/fms-related tyrosine kinase 3–internal tandem duplication (*FLT3-ITD*) genes and less likely to harbor adverse cytogenetics and/or mutations in *TP53*.

1) What constitutes standard induction therapy in AML?

Expert Perspective: The standard induction therapy for AML is typically referred to as the "7 + 3" regimen incorporating a combination of seven days of cytarabine (ara-C: 100mg/m^2/d) with an anthracycline (daunorubicin 60 mg/m^2 or idarubicin 12 mg/m^2 on days 1–3). Upon achieving complete remission (CR), the response is consolidated with three to four cycles of high-dose ara-C. Based on this approach, Mayer et al. reported a CR rate of 64%, and four-year disease-free survival and overall survival (OS) rates of 39% and 46%, respectively. Multiple randomized trials have attempted to improve response rates and survival using newer agents, variations in doses, and addition of third agents. Important areas of investigation have included (i) dose of anthracycline, (ii) choice of anthracycline,

(iii) dose of ara-C, and (iv) additional nucleoside analogs to implement three drug combinations. More recent trials are focusing on the addition of molecularly targeted agents.

2) What is the optimal dose of anthracycline? Is the choice of anthracycline for induction in AML important?

Expert Perspective:

- **Optimal dose of anthracycline**: Dose intensification of daunorubicin has been suggested as means to achieve higher CR rates and prolonged OS. The ECOG study evaluated daunorubicin 45 mg/m^2/d × 3 days versus 90 mg/m^2/d × 3 days, each in combination with ara-C 100 mg/m^2/d × 7 days in patients aged ≤ 60 years, with newly diagnosed AML. Higher dose daunorubicin (90 mg/m^2/d) demonstrated significantly better CR rates (57% vs 71%; $P < 0.001$) and median OS (15.7 vs 23.7 months; $P = 0.003$) than the lower dose with no differences in the side effect profile. The European group investigated the same question but in patients aged ≥ 60 years. Higher-dose daunorubicin demonstrated higher CR rates (65% vs 54%; $P = 0.002$), but there was no difference in OS ($P = 0.16$) compared to lower dose. However, a post hoc analysis showed an OS benefit in patients aged 60–65 years. Furthermore, the UK NCRI AML17 trial evaluated 60 and 90 mg/m^2 doses of daunorubicin, each in combination with ara-C 100 mg/m^2/d × 7 days. A planned interim analysis showed a significant increase in day 60 mortality in the 90 mg/m^2 arm, leading to premature trial termination.
- **Choice of anthracycline:** Following the question of dose intensity of anthracycline during induction therapy of AML comes the question of choice between daunorubicin and idarubicin. The Acute Leukemia French Association (ALFA) 9801 study compared daunorubicin (80 mg/m^2 × 3 days) to idarubicin [12 mg/m^2 for 3 (IDA3) or 4 days (IDA4)] each with cytarabine at 200 mg/m^2/d for seven days as induction therapy. Remission rates were high in IDA3 arm, but there was no difference in survival outcomes between daunorubicin and standard and dose-intensified idarubicin. Grade 3 or 4 mucositis was most common in the four days of idarubicin arm. There was an advantage in event-free survival and OS in the IDA4 arm, although not statistically significant.

Based on these data, either daunorubicin 60 mg/m^2/d or idarubicin 12 mg/m^2 for three days is used to treat younger patients with newly diagnosed AML.

3) Is the dose of cytarabine (ara-C) during induction of AML important? Is there an optimal dose?

Expert Perspective: Ara-C is the most active agent in the treatment of AML and the backbone for many of the standard and investigational combination regimens.

- **Dose of cytarabine:** Standard doses of ara-C range from 100 to 200 mg/m^2 and high-dose ara-C (HiDAC) typically refers to doses > 1000 mg/m^2. The utility of HiDAC in induction regimens of AML is less clear. SWOG study randomized AML patients < 65 years to standard-dose ara-C of 200 mg/m^2/d × 7 to high-dose ara-C (HiDAC) of 2000 mg/m^2 every 12 hours × 12 doses, each in combination with daunorubicin (45 mg/m^2/d × 3 days). Although there was no difference in CR rates and four-year OS across all age groups, four-year relapse-free survival was better following HiDAC induction in patients < 50 years, and those aged between 50 and 64 years but was associated with significantly increased neurologic toxicity. An Australian study randomized patients aged ≤ 60 years to either HiDAC (3000 mg/m² Q12 × 8 doses) or standard-dose ara-C (defined here as 100 mg/m²/d × 7 days) in combination with daunorubicin 50 mg/m²/d × 3 and etoposide 75 mg/m²/d × 7 days. Similarly, there was no significant difference in the CR rate or OS but five-year relapse-free survival in the HiDAC arm was better (49% vs 24% standard dose of ara-C). The HiDAC arm was associated with comparatively increased rates of myelosuppression and ocular toxicity but similar rates of neurotoxicity. A meta-analysis of three randomized trials of standard-dose ara-C versus HiDAC for induction therapy of AML showed that relapse-free survival and OS were better with HiDAC in patients aged < 60 years, but the higher burden of toxicities may attenuate some of the OS benefit.

- **Optimal dose of cytarabine:** Studies performed by Plunkett et al. (1987) have established that higher doses up to 3 g/m² may be beyond the dose necessary to saturate ara-C uptake and maximal cellular ara-C-triphosphate (ara-CTP) levels (the active product of ara-C that is incorporated into DNA and is responsible for its cytotoxic effects). Therefore, escalation of the dose of ara-C can be beneficial but only up to the point before these maximal levels are surpassed. One can consider an optimal ara-C dose able to achieve maximal cellular ara-CTP levels and not result in unwanted toxicity. Clinically, ara-C doses between 1,000 and 2,000 mg/m²/d has demonstrated tolerability in regimens such as FLAG-Ida incorporating fludarabine, cytarabine (2 g/m²), granulocyte colony-stimulating factor, and idarubicin. In the EORTC-GIMEMA AML-12 randomized trial of standard dose ara-C versus HiDAC for induction in AML patients aged 15–60 years, patients randomized to the HiDAC treatment arm had a significant survival benefit, which was more pronounced in those aged ≤ 45 years with a six-year OS rate of 52%. In the authors' practice, we routinely use ara-C doses of 1,000 to 1,500 mg/m²/d for induction to achieve improved relapse-free survival and OS.

4) Is there a role for adding a second nucleoside analog, i.e. triple nucleoside regimen, in AML induction?

Expert Perspective: The cytotoxicity of ara-C is directly related to the intracellular concentration of its metabolite ara-CTP. Several purine nucleoside analogs (fludarabine, cladribine, and clofarabine) have been shown to be synergistic in combination with ara-C by increasing intracellular ara-CTP, thereby potentiating leukemia cell kill. In the MRC AML 15 trial, FLAG-Ida regimen (Fludarabine 30 mg/m² days 2–6, cytarabine 2 g/m² starting four hours after fludarabine on days 2–6, G-CSF days 1–7, and idarubicin 8 mg/m² IV on days 4–6) demonstrated higher CR rates and reduced relapse risk in patients with newly diagnosed AML with no significant difference in early mortality but with delayed count recovery.

Based on several positive single-arm studies combining cladribine with standard chemotherapy, the Polish Acute Leukemia Group (PALG) randomized 400 patients with newly diagnosed AML to receive daunorubicin and ara-C combination, with or without cladribine. In the three-drug arm, the CR rates (64% vs 47%; $P = 0.0009$) and leukemia-free survival (44% vs 28%; $P = 0.05$) was significantly higher with three drugs than the two-drug arm. In a follow-up study of 652 untreated AML patients, the PALG compared outcomes of either fludarabine (DAF) or cladribine (DAC) added to daunorubicin and ara-C (DA). Compared to DAF, DAC was associated with a significantly higher CR rate (67.5% vs 56%; $P = 0.01$) and better three-year OS (45% vs 33%; $P = 0.02$), suggesting an advantage for the three-drug combinations over the standard doublet of ara-C + anthracycline.

We at the MD Anderson Cancer center have shown that CLIA regimen (cladribine 5 mg/m^2 IV on days 1–5, followed by ara-C 1,500 mg/m^2 IV on days 1–5, and idarubicin 10 mg/m^2 IV on days 1–3) is safe and tolerable in patients aged $\leq$ 60 years with newly diagnosed AML. CLIA regimen demonstrated an overall response rate of 81% and a six-month OS estimate of 89% with 0% and 4%, four- and eight-week mortality, respectively. In the absence of eligibility for clinical trial, we routinely employ CLIA-based regimen for younger patients with newly diagnosed AML.

5) How to optimize remission induction strategy in CBF (core binding factor) AML?

Expert Perspective: CBF AML is considered relatively favorable risk owing to their high CR rates > 90%, survival rates of 50–70%, and lower relapse risk. Several randomized trials have affirmed the chemosensitivity of CBF AML to cytarabine-based chemotherapy, either with "7 + 3" or fludarabine, cytarabine, and G-CSF (FLAG)–based regimens. Addition of gemtuzumab ozogamicin (GO: anti-CD33 monoclonal antibody conjugated to the potent cytotoxin calicheamicin) to conventional chemotherapy improved upon the survival benefit accorded by the chemotherapy. Although the initial clinical development of GO was troubled due to early deaths, the benefit of GO was resolutely proved by the meta-analysis of five randomized trials, which showed that the addition of GO in lower fractionated doses to remission induction therapy provided an absolute survival benefit of 20.7% (odds ratio 0.47, 0.31–0.73; $P = 0.0006$) in CBF AML. Similarly, adding GO to FLAG regimen has demonstrated three-year OS and relapse-free survival rates of 78% and 85%, respectively, in an ongoing study of FLAG-GO (3 mg/m^2 of GO single dose during induction). Therefore, in the authors' clinical practice, we incorporate GO in the FLAG-based remission induction to maximize the survival benefit in CBF AML.

6) What is the prognostic role of measurable residual disease (MRD) in CBF (core binding factor) AML?

Expert Perspective: Highly sensitive real-time quantitative PCR (RT-qPCR) techniques enable the detection of *RUNX1::RUNX1T1* and *CBFB::MYH11* transcripts in CBF AML thereby permitting to track the kinetics of response as well as identify early relapse. The United Kingdom MRC AML 15 trial prospectively assessed the CBF transcripts in 278 patients at the end of induction and consolidation. At the end of induction, > 3 log reduction in *RUNX1::RUNX1T1* transcripts in bone marrow in t(8;21) patients, and < 10 copy numbers of *CBFB::MYH11* transcripts in peripheral blood in inv(16) patients predicted for superior relapse-free survival. Furthermore, ascending transcripts or copy numbers of fusion genes on serial monitoring portended hematologic relapse. Data from MD Anderson confirmed that a $\geq$ 3 log reduction of transcripts in the bone marrow at end of induction in addition to > 4 log reduction after two to three courses of consolidation were associated with less likelihood of relapse. RT-qPCR–based MRD monitoring for CBF AML is not routinely available due to the lack of standardization techniques and technological expertise for qPCR and the lack of consensus on optimal sample (bone marrow vs peripheral blood) for MRD monitoring (see Chapter 10). Although serial MRD monitoring identifies the patients at risk of relapse, currently there is no data for MRD-guided treatment decision-making in CBF AML.

7) Is there a role for hematopoietic cell transplantation in CBF AML in first remission?

Expert Perspective: Given the excellent long-term prognosis associated with CBF leukemias, hematopoietic cell transplantation (HCT) is typically not considered for patients in first remission; however, relapse is the major cause of treatment failure in CBF AML. Risk factors for relapse include age, type of CBF subunit involved, additional molecular or cytogenetic abnormalities, and dynamics of MRD. Allogeneic transplantation is reserved for those with relapsing CBF AML achieving second CR. Perhaps with MRD monitoring, patients at risk for early relapse could be identified, and preemptive allogeneic transplantation may be a viable strategy in such patients.

8) How to treat *FLT3* mutated AML?

Expert Perspective: $FLT3^{mut}$ are either a point mutation in the *tyrosine kinase domain (TKD)* or an internal *tandem duplication mutation* (ITD) in the juxtamembrane domain leading to constitutive activation of the receptor tyrosine kinase. The prognosis of FLT3-TKD is variable, whereas a high ratio of mutant (*FLT3-ITD*) to wild-type *FLT3* alleles (allele ratio) presages poor prognosis due to high relapse rates and inferior OS. Midostaurin, gilteritinib, quizartinib and sorafenib are orally administered small-molecule tyrosine kinase inhibitors targeted against $FLT3^{mut}$AML. While midostaurin and sorafenib are first-generation multitargeted kinase inhibitors that account for its off-target side effect profile, gilteritinib and quizartinib are potent and specific second-generation FLT3 inhibitors (FLT3i) with better tolerability. Additionally, FLT3i are classified into type I (midostaurin, gilteritinib), which targets both *ITD* and *TKD* mutations, and type II (sorafenib, quizartinib), which is active against *ITD* but not *TKD* mutations.

Midostaurin is approved to treat patients with newly diagnosed $FLT3^{mut}$ AML in combination with standard cytarabine and daunorubicin induction and cytarabine consolidation. In the placebo-controlled randomized phase III CALGB RATIFY trial, newly diagnosed $FLT3^{mut}$ AML patients were randomized to receive either midostaurin 50 mg twice daily or placebo on days 8–21 in combination with "7 + 3" for up to two cycles of induction and in combination with high-dose cytarabine for up to four cycles of consolidation, followed by continuous midostaurin or placebo for up to 12 28-day cycles as maintenance. At a median follow-up of 59 months, there was no significant difference in CR rates (58.9% midostaurin vs 53.5% placebo), but midostaurin was associated with significantly longer OS (HR 0.78, $P = 0.009$) and event-free survival (HR 0.78, $P = 0.002$) regardless of allelic ratio or mutation subtype. The difference in OS was significant in the initial six months of treatment after which the curves plateaued. Notably, the median duration of midostaurin exposure was three months, and 28% of these patients received allo-HCT in first CR limiting midostaurin exposure up to three cycles of therapy, which also contributed to the OS difference, thereby validating the role of HCT in post remission therapy for $FLT3^{mut}$ AML.

Most common midostaurin associated adverse events include nausea, vomiting, skin rash, and anemia attributed to its multitarget kinase inhibitory effect.

Gilteritinib is approved as a monotherapy to treat relapsed or refractory $FLT3^{mut}$ AML (*ITD* or *TKD*). The phase III ADMIRAL study randomized patients to receive either gilteritinib 120 mg daily or standard chemotherapy, with a primary endpoint of OS. At a median follow-up of 17.8 months, patients treated with gilteritinib demonstrated higher CR with full or partial hematologic recovery rates (CR + CRh: 34.0% gilteritinib vs 15.3% chemotherapy group) and longer OS (HR, 0.64; one-sided $P = 0.0004$; median OS, 9.3 vs 5.6 months) compared to chemotherapy regardless of the intensity of therapy.

Quizartinib is approved with standard cytarabine and anthracycline induction and cytarabine consolidation, and as maintenance monotherapy following consolidation chemotherapy, for the treatment of adult patients with newly diagnosed *FLT3*-ITD-positive AML (QuANTUM-First).

Our approach to patients with $FLT3^{mut}$ AML involves risk stratification based on *FLT3* mutation subtype, enrolling in an investigational trial incorporating an *FLT3* inhibitor, and early evaluation for allo-HCT, when eligible. (See Chapter 8 for best therapy $FLT3^{mut}$ AML patients unsuitable for intensive therapy.)

9) Is there a role for *FLT3* inhibitors as maintenance therapy post allogeneic transplantation?

Expert Perspective: Yes. Currently no FLT3i is approved as maintenance therapy. However, sorafenib was shown to be synergistic with post-HCT alloimmune effects, which led to the evaluation of sorafenib as post-HCT maintenance therapy in patients with $FLT3$-ITD^{mut} AML who have undergone HCT (SORMAIN, placebo-controlled phase II trial). At a median follow-up of 42 months, sorafenib demonstrated significantly improved two-year relapse-free survival (85% vs 53.3%, $P = 0.002$) and OS (90.5% vs 66.2%, $P = 0.007$) compared to placebo. Although the toxicity-related drug discontinuation rate was low (22%), higher rates of graft-versus-host disease and skin toxicity were observed with sorafenib treated patients (see Chapter 11). Perl et al. (2022) reported the landmark analysis (day + 60 post HCT) of ADMIRAL trial favoring resumption of gilteritinib in patients with *FLT3*-ITD. BMT CTN 1506 (NCT02997202) evaluated post-HCT gilteritinib maintenance in *FLT3*-ITD AML in larger number of patients. While the study failed to reach its primary end point for relapse-free survival (RFS), patients treated with gilteritinib achieved a numerical but not statistically significant improvement in RFS (HR, 0.679; 95% CI, 0.459–1.005; 2-sided P = .0518).

10) How can risk-adapted strategies be used to select post-remission therapy for younger adults with AML?

Expert Perspective: Risk-adapted strategies consider a patient's anticipated risk of relapse (favorable risk) in the absence of HCT and their anticipated risk of non-relapse mortality (adverse risk) with HCT. Although there is wide variation in consolidation regimens across different cooperative groups, current guidelines suggest the use of a risk-adapted strategy emphasizing the use of consolidation chemotherapy for patients with favorable-risk disease and allo-HCT for patients with adverse-risk disease across the spectrum. Of note, these risk groups were based on data sets on newly diagnosed young, fit patients treated only with intensive chemotherapy (generally "7 + 3" or similar chemotherapy, followed by high-dose cytarabine consolidation). Given the ongoing progress in AML therapy, many prognostic factors derived from the era of conventional chemotherapy may become extraneous. Post-remission therapy guidelines do not account for age, targeted therapy, or intensity of therapy. For example, the addition of FLT3 inhibitors to front-line regimens may overcome the historically poor prognosis associated with $FLT3^{mut}$-ITD AML. Risk-adapted post remission treatment strategy is an area of ongoing investigation. Other than those with favorable-risk AML, we evaluate all the other patients for their eligibility to undergo HCT.

11) What is the standard post-remission consolidation chemotherapy for younger patients with AML in first CR?

Expert Perspective: The most commonly used post-remission regimen is HiDAC, which consists of 3,000 mg/m^2 every 12 hours of cytarabine given on days 1, 3, and 5 for three to four total cycles. There is, however, significant evidence that regimens utilizing lower cytarabine doses of 2,000 mg/m^2 every 12 hours on days 1–5, or even 1,000 mg/m^2 every 12 hours on days 1–6 may produce similar outcomes. Standard dose post-remission regimens use cytarabine at doses between 100 mg/m^2 and 400 mg/m^2 for five days combined with two doses of anthracycline. Such regimens may be a reasonable option for patients with intermediate- or poor-risk disease who are ineligible for transplant and are deemed unable to tolerate HiDAC therapy. Last, the addition of gemtuzumab ozogamicin to conventional regimens results in improved survival in patients with favorable-risk AML.

There also remains significant debate regarding the optimal number of cycles of post-remission therapy. The majority of trials to date have utilized a total of three cycles of therapy (either as a single induction followed by two consolidation cycles or as a double induction followed by a single consolidation cycle). However, controversy still remains. Data from Cancer and Leukemia Group B (CALGB) studies suggest that three to four cycles of HiDAC consolidation (after a single induction) are superior to one HiDAC consolidation for favorable cytogenetic risk. The CALGB also retrospectively compared four total cycles to five total cycles (single induction plus three or four courses of HDAC) for patients with normal-karyotype AML and demonstrated a significant relapse-free survival benefit of the fourth HiDAC cycle in this group. An alternative approach was taken by the Australasian Leukemia and Lymphoma Group (ALLG), which utilized a highly dose-intense, HiDAC-based induction (idarubicin, cytarabine, and etoposide) followed by randomization to either a second identical cycle or two cycles of standard-dose cytarabine consolidation therapy. There was no difference in the outcomes between the consolidation treatment arms suggesting that further use of HiDAC during consolidation may not confer additional benefit. The Finnish Leukemia Group compared four total cycles of therapy (double induction plus two HiDAC consolidations) to eight total cycles (double induction plus six consolidations) and demonstrated no benefit to the additional consolidation cycles. However, this study included only a small number of patients with favorable-risk cytogenetics (6%). In summary, up to four cycles of therapy may be ideal for younger patients; however, fewer cycles may yield comparable outcomes if a sufficiently dose-intense HiDAC regimen is used for induction.

12) Is there a role for maintenance therapy in younger patients with AML in first CR who are not candidates for allo-HCT?

Expert Perspective: On September 1, 2020, oral azacitidine (CC-486 not bioequivalent to injectable azacitidine) was approved as remission maintenance therapy in patients with AML who achieved first CR or CR with incomplete blood count recovery (CRi) following intensive induction chemotherapy and are not able to complete intensive curative therapy. The phase III, randomized, double-blind, placebo-controlled QUAZAR AML-001 study evaluated oral azacitidine (300 mg daily for 14 days per 28-day cycle) in 472 patients aged ≥ 55 years in CR or CRi following conventional chemotherapy who are not candidates for curative intent therapy. Oral azacitidine demonstrated significantly increased OS (24.7 months vs 14.8 months-placebo, $P = 0.0009$) and relapse-free survival (10.2 months vs 4.8 months; $P = 0.0001$), regardless of cytogenetic risk, receipt of consolidation therapy, and presence or absence of MRD at study entry. Adverse events were mostly gastrointestinal, and oral azacitidine was fairly well tolerated.

Oral azacitidine will not replace consolidation chemotherapy, but it's an option in adults who are unable to receive post-remission chemotherapy.

13) What is the role of measurable residual disease monitoring in AML?

Expert Perspective: Measurable residual disease (MRD) indicates the persistence of leukemic cells below the level of routine methods of morphological detection in patients who have achieved morphologic remission. MRD is monitored using more sensitive ($1:10^4$–$1:10^6$ leukemic cells) techniques such as multiparameter flow cytometry (MFC) or RT-qPCR for mutated transcripts. MRD is a powerful predictor for survival outcomes as shown by a systematic review and meta-analysis on 11,151 patients with AML. This systematic review of 81 publications showed that the estimated five-year disease-free survival and OS were 64% and 68% in patients who achieved MRD negativity, and 25% and 34% for those who did not, respectively. Additionally, those who achieved MRD negativity had 64% lesser chance of death, suggesting that MRD status may be a valid surrogate endpoint for both disease-free survival and OS in AML. However, the lack of quantitation and standardization of MRD assays remain an obstacle for its use in general clinical practice. While RT-qPCR for MRD monitoring in CBF AML (as previously discussed) and *NPM1* mutations in peripheral blood are commercially available, MRD monitoring by MFC is largely restricted to academic settings. Bulk next-generation sequencing (NGS) has also been used for MRD monitoring looking for mutation clearance but has lower sensitivity. Currently, MRD status does not guide treatment decision-making outside of clinical trials. However, routine MRD monitoring and development of MRD eradication strategies would allow us to intervene before a frank relapse occurs. For example, in a patient with favorable-risk CBF AML, serial rise in transcript levels would allow us to plan for preemptive therapy, be it chemotherapy or allo-HCT.

In the authors' clinical practice, we routinely use MRD monitoring by MFC, and/or RT-qPCR when applicable, at various time points including the end of induction and consolidation and as a part of pretransplant evaluation (See chapter 10).

Recommended Readings

Boddu, P., Gurguis, C., Sanford, D., Cortes, J., Akosile, M., Ravandi, F. et al. (2018 December). Response kinetics and factors predicting survival in core-binding factor leukemia. *Leukemia* 32 (12): 2698–2701. PMID: 29884905.

Burchert, A. et al. (2021). Sorafenib maintenance after allogeneic hematopoietic stem cell transplantation for acute myeloid leukemia With FLT3 Internal tandem duplication mutation (SORMAIN). *J Clin Oncol* 39: 1412–1413.

DiNardo, C.D., Lachowiez, C.A., Takahashi, K., Loghavi, S., Xiao, L., Kadia, T. et al. (2021 September 1). Venetoclax combined with FLAG-IDA induction and consolidation in newly diagnosed and relapsed or refractory acute myeloid leukemia. *J Clin Oncol* 39 (25): 2768–2778. PMID: 34043428; PMCID: PMC8407653.

Hills, R.K., Castaigne, S., Appelbaum, F.R., Delaunay, J., Petersdorf, S., Othus, M. et al. (2014 August). Addition of gemtuzumab ozogamicin to induction chemotherapy in adult patients with acute myeloid leukaemia: a meta-analysis of individual patient data from randomised controlled trials. *Lancet Oncol* 15 (9): 986–996. PMID: 25008258; PMCID: PMC4137593.

Ivey, A., Hills, R.K., Simpson, M.A., Jovanovic, J.V., Gilkes, A., Grech, A. et al. (2016 February 4). UK National Cancer Research Institute AML Working Group. Assessment of minimal residual disease in standard-risk AML. *N Engl J Med* 374 (5): 422–433. PMID: 26789727.

Jongen-Lavrencic, M., Grob, T., Hanekamp, D., Kavelaars, F.G., Al Hinai, A., Zeilemaker, A. et al. (2018 March 29). Molecular minimal residual disease in acute myeloid leukemia. *N Engl J Med* 378 (13): 1189–1199. PMID: 29601269.

Kadia, T.M., Reville, P.K., Borthakur, G., Yilmaz, M., Kornblau, S., Alvarado, Y. et al. (2021 August). Venetoclax plus intensive chemotherapy with cladribine, idarubicin, and cytarabine in patients with newly diagnosed acute myeloid leukaemia or high-risk myelodysplastic syndrome: a cohort from a single-centre, single-arm, phase 2 trial. *Lancet Haematol* 8 (8): e552–e561. PMID: 34329576.

Maziarz, R. T. et al. (2020) Midostaurin after allogeneic stem cell transplant in patients with FLT3-internal tandem duplication-positive acute myeloid leukemia. *Bone Marrow Transplant* 129, 424–10.

Perl, A.E., Martinelli, G., Cortes, J.E., Neubauer, A., Berman, E., Paolini, S. et al. (2019 October 31). Gilteritinib or chemotherapy for relapsed or refractory FLT3-mutated AML. *N Engl J Med* 381 (18): 1728–1740. PMID: 31665578.

Short, N.J., Zhou, S., Fu, C., Berry, D.A., Walter, R.B., Freeman, S.D. et al. (2020 December 1). Association of measurable residual disease with survival outcomes in patients with acute myeloid leukemia: a systematic review and meta-analysis. *JAMA Oncol* 6 (12): 1890–1899. PMID: 33030517; PMCID: PMC7545346.

Walter, R.B., Appelbaum, F.R., and Estey, E.H. (2021 February). Optimal dosing of cytarabine in induction and post-remission therapy of acute myeloid leukemia. *Leukemia* 35 (2): 295–298. PMID: 33328603.

Wei, A.H., Döhner, H., Pocock, C., Montesinos, P., Afanasyev, B., Dombret, H., Ravandi, F. et al. (2020 December 24). QUAZAR AML-001 trial investigators. Oral azacitidine maintenance therapy for acute myeloid leukemia in first remission. *N Engl J Med* 383 (26): 2526–2537. doi: 10.1056/NEJMoa2004444. PMID: 33369355.

Xuan, L. et al. (2020) Sorafenib maintenance in patients with FLT3-ITD acute myeloid leukaemia undergoing allogeneic haematopoietic stem-cell transplantation: an open-label, multicentre, randomised phase 3 trial. *Lancet Oncol.* 21, 1201–1212.

8

Older Adults with Acute Myeloid Leukemia

Mary-Elizabeth Percival[1] and Elihu Estey[2,†]

[1] University of Washington, Seattle, WA, USA
[2] Fred Hutchinson Cancer Center, Seattle, WA, USA

Introduction

Incidence of AML increases with age, with a median age at diagnosis in the late 60s. However, it remains an uncommon malignancy in the general population, representing only 1% of all cancer diagnoses based on approximately 20,000 new cases annually in the United States. The disease has a slight male predominance. Between 10% and 20% of newly diagnosed patients have an antecedent exposure contributing to development of AML, most commonly prior chemotherapy or radiation. Others have an antecedent hematologic disorder such as myelodysplastic syndrome or myeloproliferative neoplasm. The role of inherited susceptibility is less in older patients, but a gene mutation in *DDX41* seems to cause myeloid malignancies more commonly in patients over 50, making a detailed family history important at any age (see Chapter 14).

Case Study 1

A 62-year-old woman presents for an annual visit with her primary care physician. She has a history of type 2 diabetes mellitus and hypothyroidism. She has no current complaints. She notes that she is an avid tennis player who regularly competes in senior tournaments. A complete blood count (CBC) indicates mild thrombocytopenia with a platelet count of 122,000 cells/μL; the remainder of the laboratory studies are within normal limits. At a regular checkup two years later, when she is 64 years old, she continues to feel well. However, her CBC with differential demonstrates a white blood cell count of 1,100 cells/μL, absolute neutrophil count 600 cells/μL, hemoglobin 9.9 g/dL, hematocrit 31%, and platelet count 86,000 cells/μL.

The patient is referred to hematology for bone marrow aspirate and biopsy, which reveals 29% abnormal myeloid blasts. Karyotype shows monosomy 7 in 13 cells. Molecular

† Deceased

Cancer Consult: Expertise in Clinical Practice, Volume 2: Neoplastic Hematology & Cellular Therapy,
Second Edition. Edited by Syed A. Abutalib, Maurie Markman, James O. Armitage, and Kenneth C. Anderson.
© 2024 John Wiley & Sons Ltd. Published 2024 by John Wiley & Sons Ltd.

analysis using a myeloid gene panel demonstrates mutations in *DNMT3A, TET2, ASXL1,* and *IDH2*.

1) How should the patient's disease be risk stratified?

Expert Perspective: At the time of diagnosis of AML, all patients should undergo immunophenotyping by flow cytometry, karyotyping using conventional metaphase cytogenetic analysis, and molecular testing using a myeloid gene panel. Additionally, fluorescence *in situ* hybridization can sometimes aid in rapid identification of particular chromosomal findings that may change management. Results from karyotype and molecular testing can be combined to stratify the disease as favorable, intermediate, or adverse risk using the European LeukemiaNet (ELN) guidelines (see Chapter 6). This patient's AML would fall into the adverse risk category based on the presence of monosomy 7; she has an additional adverse risk marker with the presence of a mutation in *ASXL1*.

2) Does the patient have secondary AML?

Expert Perspective: Secondary AML occurs when a patient with an antecedent hematologic disorder subsequently develops AML. The patient in the vignette likely had an antecedent hematologic disorder given her mild thrombocytopenia two years before diagnosis of AML, though she never had a bone marrow evaluation to establish such. At a minimum, she may have had clonal hematopoiesis of indeterminate prognosis (CHIP) or idiopathic cytopenia of undetermined significance (ICUS); she could also have had frank myelodysplastic syndrome (MDS), since disease presentation and severity vary widely (see Chapter 12). Danish registry data indicate that the presence of secondary AML is associated with poorer overall survival, with the worst outcomes in patients with non-MDS secondary AML. Areas of uncertainty are the extent to which secondary AML worsens prognosis after accounting for ELN risk and whether marrow documentation of MPN or MDS, rather than just abnormal blood counts, is prerequisite for a diagnosis of secondary AML.

3) What methods exist to risk-stratify the functional status of older patients?

Expert Perspective: The median age at diagnosis for AML is 68 years old based on data from the Surveillance, Epidemiology, and End Results (SEER) registry of the National Cancer Institute. "Older" AML patients are often defined as being 60 years or older at the time of diagnosis, which encompasses the large majority of newly diagnosed patients. Disease characteristics skew towards an adverse-risk pattern for older patients, but it is also important to determine the functional status of the patient. The Eastern Cooperative Oncology Group (ECOG) performance status can be combined with other baseline factors, including age, platelet count, albumin, presence of secondary AML, white blood cell count, peripheral blood blast percentage, and creatinine, to generate a prediction of likelihood of death within 28 days from initiation of intensive chemotherapy (https://trmcalculator.fredhutch.org). A comprehensive geriatric assessment, including evaluation of cognition, depression, distress, physical function, and comorbidity, is a more sensitive way to predict survival for older patients in particular. Uptake of geriatric assessment has been limited in clinical practice due to the perceived cumbersome nature of administering the physical and mental function tests. Though the ECOG performance status for the patient in the vignette is not specified, it is likely to be 0 or 1 given the description of her asymptomatic presentation and exercise habit of playing regular tennis. All methods of risk stratification in AML typically result in prognostic ability approximately intermediate between certainty and a coin flip.

4) What options exist for less intensive treatment?

Expert Perspective: The de facto standard of care for older patients in recent years has become the hypomethylating agent azacitidine plus the BCL2 inhibitor, venetoclax. Venetoclax received an accelerated approval in 2018 from the United States Food and Drug Administration (FDA) for the treatment of AML in combination with hypomethylating agent therapy or low-dose cytarabine following favorable results from a phase II trial. More recently, the phase III VIALE-A trial randomized untreated patients considered unfit for standard intensive induction chemotherapy to receive either azacitidine alone or azacitidine-venetoclax. Though fitness for intensive chemotherapy is often decided arbitrarily, the study considered patients eligible for enrollment if they were 75 years of age or older or if they had at least one of the following conditions: history of congestive heart failure requiring treatment, ejection fraction of 50% or less, chronic stable angina, diffusing capacity of the lung for carbon monoxide of 65% or less, forced expiratory volume in 1 second of 65% of less, or ECOG performance status of 2 or 3.

Azacitidine-venetoclax: The complete remission (CR) rate was 37% in the azacitidine-venetoclax arm vs 18% in the azacitidine alone arm ($P < 0.001$); the composite CR rate, which also included CR with incomplete hematologic recovery (CRi), was 66% vs 28% ($P < 0.001$). The primary endpoint was overall survival (OS), with median of 14.7 months in the combination group and 9.6 months in the control group ($P < 0.001$). The principal factor associated with longer survival was age < 75 (hazard ratio 0.54; 95% CI 0.39–0.73).

Glasdegib + low-dose cytarabine: Another less intensive regimen with efficacy in older adults is the combination of low-dose cytarabine (LDAC) with the hedgehog pathway inhibitor glasdegib. Glasdegib was approved by the FDA in 2018 following favorable results from the phase II, randomized, open-label, multicenter trial for patients with AML or high-risk MDS considered unsuitable for intensive chemotherapy. The definition of ineligibility for intensive chemotherapy varied somewhat from that of the VIALE-A trial and required at least one of: age of 75 years or older, creatinine > 1.3 mg/dL, ejection fraction < 45%, or ECOG performance status of 2. The median overall survival in the glasdegib-LDAC arm was 8.8 months compared to 4.9 months in the LDAC arm ($P = 0.0004$). Use of glasdegib has been limited, likely related to the choice of LDAC as the agent to be combined with glasdegib. Specifically, the overall response rate, combining CR plus CRi plus morphologic leukemia-free state, was only 5% with LDAC alone vs 27% for the combination.

Isocitrate dehydrogenase (IDH) inhibitors: FDA has also approved isocitrate dehydrogenase (IDH) inhibitors. Mutations in *IDH1* and *IDH2* occur in approximately 10–20% of AML cases and are more common in older patients. The accumulation of the oncometabolite 2-hydroxyglutarate leads to a block in differentiation; the IDH inhibitors ivosidenib and olutasidenib (targeting IDH1) and enasidenib (targeting IDH2) overcome the differentiation block by restoring functionality of the mutated IDH proteins. Both drugs are approved for patients with relapsed and refractory AML, but only ivosidenib is approved in newly diagnosed AML patients who are ineligible for intensive chemotherapy. Ivosidenib has recently been approved in combination with the hypomethylating agent azacitidine based on randomized data. Notably, the randomized phase II IDHENTIFY trial was stopped early due to lack of efficacy in the enasidenib arm. Since the patient in the vignette has an *IDH2* mutation, not an *IDH1* mutation, up-front *IDH* inhibitor treatment would not be supported by evidence.

5) How long should the less intensive combination be continued?

Expert Perspective: Less intensive treatment regimens, including both azacitidine-venetoclax and LDAC-glasdegib, should be continued as long as the patient is both tolerating the drugs and receiving clinical benefit. How should the latter be defined? One possibility is extending survival. Since there is strong association between the latter and response, largely due to response achievement per se, one approach is to continue until it is likely response will not be forthcoming or has been lost. Remission, if achieved, occurs quickly with azacitidine-venetoclax; the median time to CR or CRi with this regimen in the VIALE-A trial was 1.3 months (range 0.6 to 9.9 months). Time to response was not reported in the LDAC-glasdegib study. An important research question is whether the survival benefits of all responses are equivalent. With intensive therapy it appears that responses less than CR are associated with less survival benefit. This is less clear with less intense therapy. Nonetheless if prolonging survival is the principal goal, it seems reasonable to change therapy if response has not occurred after 3–4 courses. Naturally there are patients who are less concerned with quantity of life than with its quality. Here it might be contended that treatment should be continued as long as patients are tolerating treatment without excess inconvenience.

6) What are the expected side effects of less intensive treatment?

Expert Perspective: Though hypomethylating agents and LDAC are considered less intensive than inpatient induction chemotherapy, toxicity sustained during treatment can be considerable. Since these regimens target hematopoietic cells, it can be difficult to adjudicate the etiology of adverse events that occur during treatment. Though regimens that will be administered indefinitely must be tolerable, the toxicity from untreated or undertreated AML is very high. Indeed, the great majority of people who die as a direct effect of treatment can be shown to have residual AML in the last marrow obtained before death, suggesting their life expectancy would be limited even without occurrence of treatment-related mortality.

In the azacitidine-venetoclax group of the VIALE-A trial, the rate of grade 3 or higher adverse events was 99%. Most were hematologic adverse events, with grade 3 or higher adverse events including thrombocytopenia, neutropenia, febrile neutropenia, anemia, and leukopenia occurring in 82% of patients. Though many subjects had nonhematologic adverse events of all grades, such as nausea (44%), constipation (43%), diarrhea (41%), and vomiting (30%), the rates of grade 3 or higher nonhematologic adverse events were generally less than 10%. In the LDAC-glasdegib study, the glasdegib arm similarly had a high rate of grade 3–4 hematologic adverse events, including anemia (41.7%), febrile neutropenia (35.7%), and thrombocytopenia (31%). Similar to what was observed with the combination of azacitidine and venetoclax, the nonhematologic adverse events were common but lower grade than the hematologic adverse events. Appropriate antimicrobial prophylaxis should be initiated for patients with a sustained duration of neutropenia to decrease the risk of infectious complications. For patients receiving venetoclax in combination with an antifungal such as posaconazole or voriconazole, the venetoclax prescribing information details recommended dose reductions (that is, from venetoclax 400 mg daily to a dose of 70 mg daily if in combination with posaconazole, or to 100 mg daily if in combination with voriconazole).

7) Is there evidence supporting use of more intensive treatment in older patients?

Expert Perspective: Thus far, the discussion has focused on less intensive regimens used to treat newly diagnosed AML. However, the patient in the vignette is likely a candidate for intensive induction chemotherapy given her age, good performance status, and lack of co-morbidities. The ELN 2017 criteria suggest that patients should have older age plus another factor to receive non-intense therapy. These criteria include patient-related factors, such as an ECOG performance status of 3-4 or significant co-morbidities not related to AML, or disease-related factors, such as adverse-risk genetics. Ideally, such patients who are not eligible or appropriate for intensive therapy would be enrolled on a clinical trial since standard options are unlikely to be successful. Additionally, one might note that less intensive trials often exclude patients with a poor performance status; for example, the glasdegib-LDAC trial did not include patients with an ECOG performance status > 2, and the VIALE-A trial had a majority of patients with an ECOG performance status of 0 or 1 (55%). In general, there are no generally accepted or validated criteria to consider a patient ineligible for intensive chemotherapy.

The patient in the vignette may therefore be eligible for intensive treatment. The induction backbone of so-called 7 + 3, consisting of seven days of continuous cytarabine infusion combined with three days of anthracycline, was first described in 1973. Initial studies focused on administering induction therapy with 7 + 3 only to patients who were 60 or younger because of generally poorer outcomes in older patients (see Chapter 7). Clinical trials from the National Cancer Research Institute in the United Kingdom using the combination of fludarabine, cytarabine, filgrastim, and idarubicin (FLAG-ida) have generally limited participation to younger patients as well. However, retrospective population-based analyses from Sweden indicate that the survival of patients who receive intensive therapy is generally better than those who do not. Other intensive regimens, including a high-dose cytarabine regimen similar to FLAG-ida known as CLAG-M (cladribine, cytarabine, filgrastim, and mitoxantrone), have been successfully utilized in older previously untreated patients. Together, these findings suggest that fit older patients should be offered intense induction regimens, with a recent study by Sorror et al. suggesting patients achieved no survival or "quality of life" benefits from less intensive induction, which however did not include venetoclax. Trials randomizing patients age 40 or above to venetoclax + azacitidine or 7 + 3 may shed further light on this issue.

Another option for the patient in the vignette would be the liposomal formulation of cytarabine and daunorubicin (CPX-351). The formulation includes the drugs in a fixed 5:1 molar ratio and was approved by the FDA in 2017 based on a randomized phase III clinical trial that compared overall survival using CPX-351 vs standard 7 + 3. The study enrolled patients who were age 60–75 years with newly diagnosed adverse-risk AML, defined as having therapy-related AML, AML with antecedent MDS or chronic myelomonocytic leukemia, or *de novo* AML with MDS-related cytogenetic abnormalities using the 2008 World Health Organization criteria. The primary endpoint was overall survival, which was statistically significantly improved in the CPX-351 arm at 9.56 months vs 5.95 months in the 7 + 3 arm. The overall CR rate was significantly higher in the CPX-351 arm as well, at 47.7% vs 33.3%. CPX-351 appears to be a more effective treatment in this patient population, but some hoped that it would also be a more tolerable treatment given the slow release of drugs from the liposomes over time. However, notably, the rate of grade 3 or higher adverse events was similar and high in both groups; for example, the rate of febrile neutropenia was 68.0% in the CPX-351 arm and 70.9% in the 7 + 3 arm. Though CPX-351 appears effective, combination studies with CPX-351 and other drugs are ongoing. The patient in the vignette would be a candidate for CPX-351 given her AML with MDS-related cytogenetic abnormalities.

8) Should maintenance therapy be considered after intensive treatment?

Expert Perspective: The goal of initial induction therapy is to achieve CR. Most patients who achieve CR with intensive induction treatment will go on to receive further cycles of consolidation or post-remission treatment, often with high-dose cytarabine. The cytarabine dose is sometimes empirically reduced in older patients given an increased risk of neurotoxicity, which typically manifests as cerebellar ataxia in affected individuals, but the risk of neurotoxicity needs to be balanced with the risk of inadequately treated AML. Significant cytopenia is expected after cytarabine-based consolidation, but it can be mitigated by use of filgrastim. The optimal number of post-remission cycles is unknown but is likely lower in older patients than in younger patients (who are usually recommended to receive 3–4 cycles). It is very plausible that there is no single optimal number, with decisions for further courses based on how well the prior course was tolerated (see Chapter 7).

Maintenance therapy is less intense than consolidation therapy. The former's use in AML has been questioned until recent randomized trials examining azacitidine in its traditional subcutaneous formulation and its new oral form. A reduced dose of subcutaneous azacitidine (50 mg/m^2 on days 1–5 of a 28-day cycle administered until relapse or for a maximum of 12 cycles) was utilized by the Dutch-Belgian Hemato-Oncology Cooperative Group (HOVON) for older patients in remission after intensive induction. Eligible patients were 60 years of age or older, with an ECOG performance status of 2 or less and fewer than 5% bone marrow blasts after two cycles of induction chemotherapy. Patients could be in a CR or CRi, but they needed to have an absolute neutrophil count greater than 0.5 × 10^9/L and a platelet count greater than 50 × 10^9/L. Patients (n = 126) were then randomized to an observation group or to the azacitidine maintenance group. The primary endpoint was improvement in disease-free survival, which at 12 months was 64% with azacitidine and 42% with placebo. Azacitidine reduced the risk of relapse or death: hazard ratio of 0.62 (95% CI 0.41–0.95). Multivariable Cox regression analysis indicated that a platelet count > 100 × 10^9/L predicted a significantly better disease-free survival, but none of the other factors tested were significant, including presence of poor-risk cytogenetic abnormalities, age, time to response, or performance status. The disease-free survival improvement did not lead to an OS improvement.

More recently, oral azacitidine tablets (CC-486) were studied in a similar population of patients in CR or CRi after at least once cycle of intensive chemotherapy. Additional eligibility criteria included age 55 years or older, AML with intermediate- or poor-risk cytogenetic characteristics, ineligibility for allogeneic transplant, ECOG performance status of 3 or lower, absolute neutrophil count greater than 0.5×10^9/L, and platelet count greater than 20×10^9/L. 472 patients were randomized in a 1:1 fashion between CC-486 300 mg once daily for 14 days (out of a 28-day cycle) or placebo. The primary endpoint was overall survival, which was significantly longer in the CC-486 group at 24.7 months vs 14.8 months. Relapse-free survival was also improved in the CC-486 group. Gastrointestinal toxicity was high in the CC-486 group, including nausea (65%), vomiting (60%), and diarrhea (50%). The rate of neutropenia was also high, with grade 3 or 4 neutropenia in 41% of patients in the CC-486 arm compared to only 24% in the placebo arm. Formally assessed quality of life was not significantly different between the two arms. As opposed to the subcutaneous azacitidine administered in the HOVON trial for a maximum of 12 cycles, CC-486 was continued indefinitely.

If the patient in the vignette receives intensive induction chemotherapy and achieves CR or CRi after 1–2 cycles, she would be eligible for maintenance chemotherapy with azacitidine. Given the improvement in OS with the oral azacitidine tablets (CC-486), this regimen would be favored. The oral formulation of azacitidine is not identical to (and therefore not interchangeable with) subcutaneous or intravenous formulations, with different pharmacokinetic and pharmacodynamic characteristics. Because of these differences, the usage for oral azacitidine is limited only to maintenance therapy in older adults who have achieved CR or CRi after 1–2 cycles of intensive induction chemotherapy. Further studies are ongoing, which may expand the indications for use of oral azacitidine.

9) What is the role of allogeneic transplant in older patients?

Expert Perspective: Use of azacitidine has been said to be limited to patients who are not eligible for allogeneic hematopoietic cell transplant (allo-HCT). However, it is important to consider that allo-HCT is often considered the option most likely to produce cure in adverse-risk AML. Further, no upper age limit exists for allo-HCT, though typically the risk-benefit ratio becomes less favorable for those of age over 75 years. Data from the Center for International Blood and Marrow Transplantation Research indicate that the use of allo-HCT is rising in patients 70 years and older in the United States, with corresponding improvements in OS and progression-free survival. Data from the Fred Hutchinson Cancer Center suggest that despite its increasing use, HCT-related mortality and morbidity are decreasing. Multivariable analysis indicated that certain characteristics were associated with decreased OS, namely higher allo-HCT comorbidity index, umbilical cord blood graft, and myeloablative conditioning. The advent of nonmyeloablative conditioning regimens (so-called mini transplants, often consisting of low-dose total body irradiation with fludarabine 90 mg/m^2) has expanded the availability of the allo-HCT procedure to an increasing number of older patients.

The patient in the vignette has an age that is borderline for a myeloablative conditioning regimen (64 years). Given her adverse-risk disease by the ELN criteria, she should be considered for an allo-HCT, likely with a nonmyeloablative or reduced-intensity conditioning regimen once she achieves CR/CRi after chemotherapy. A multicenter analysis of patients receiving nonmyeloablative conditioning revealed a five-year OS of 35% and progression-free survival of 32%. Unsurprisingly, a low relapse risk was associated with an improvement in OS, since a major complication is relapse (41% of patients at five years) vs a nonrelapse mortality rate of 27% at five years (see Chapter 11).

10) What is the significance of measurable residual disease?

Expert Perspective: Measurable residual disease, or MRD, refers to disease that is detectable below the 5% morphologic blast threshold in the marrow that typically denotes persistent disease or relapse. The ELN 2017 guidelines for the first time established criteria for CR without MRD, noting that patients who met this stringent category needed to have a CR along with having a pretreatment marker of disease that was now negative. Assays considered sensitive enough to quantify MRD include multiparameter flow cytometry and molecular assays (typically using polymerase chain reaction). Multiple retrospective analyses indicate that outcomes after chemotherapy and allo-HCT are worse for patients with MRD compared to those without. Additionally, it has become clear that not all detectable disease carries the same significance; in particular, continued ability to detect the DTA mutations (i.e. *DNMT3A*, *TET2*, and *ASXL1*) is not prognostic for survival outcomes, as demonstrated by the HOVON group. This is likely related to the fact that these mutations occur as part of CHIP; chemotherapy may have successfully eradicated the myeloid blasts, but early stem cells in the marrow may still harbor CHIP mutations.

Many unanswered questions remain about MRD, particularly with regards to treatment options. Most clinical trials ignore patients with MRD, preferring to focus on traditional morphologic blast thresholds, and optimal therapy for patients with MRD is unknown (see Chapter 10).

11) What treatment options exist for older patients who relapse after initial treatment?

Expert Perspective: Older AML patients are less likely to respond to treatment and more likely to relapse. For patients who fail azacitidine-venetoclax, the outcomes are very poor. A retrospective analysis identified 33 patients who relapsed after initial response and eight with primary refractory disease; the median OS after failure of hypomethylating agent combined with venetoclax was only 2.4 months. Because of the small cohort size and heterogeneity of the population, no conclusions could be drawn about optimal therapy after failure of the venetoclax-based regimen. These data may be important for counseling regarding initial treatment choices, especially given that some patients choose less intensive regimens up front because they believe they can pivot to a more intensive regimen later. For those patients who receive intensive treatment initially, optimal salvage is also unknown and likely varies based on risk stratification, duration of first CR, and receipt of prior allo-HCT, among other variables. More clinical trials are needed to improve outcomes for older patients, especially those with adverse-risk disease like the one described in the vignette.

12) When should older patients be referred for clinical trials?

Expert Perspective: The fundamental decision when seeing an older patient with AML is whether the patient should receive standard therapy, such as venetoclax + azacitidine/decitabine, or be considered for a clinical trial. As implied by the word, the outcomes of any trial are largely unknown when the decision must be made. Most trials have been unsuccessful, reflecting the lack of knowledge of differences between the AML cell and its normal counterpart. Hence the reason to enroll on a clinical trial must be dissatisfaction with the results of standard treatment. For example, the median survival with venetoclax plus azacitidine in the VIALE-A trial was 16 months. Obviously, some patients do better and some worse than the median, but, as stated above, our ability to identify these is more limited than we probably care to admit. Knowing this median survival, one 75-year-old may choose venetoclax + azacitidine, wondering whether the results of a trial might not be worse and might not allow him to see his granddaughter graduate medical school next year. Another 75-year-old informed of US Social Security Administration data indicating the average 75-year-old can expect to live 9–10 years in contrast to the 1.5-year median with azacitidine and venetoclax might opt for a trial. It is incumbent on physicians to provide this type of information if consent to enroll on a trial is to be truly informed.

Recommended Readings

Cortes, J.E., Heidel, F.H., Hellmann, A. et al. (2019). Randomized comparison of low dose cytarabine with or without glasdegib in patients with newly diagnosed acute myeloid leukemia or high-risk myelodysplastic syndrome. *Leukemia* 33: 379–389.

DiNardo, C.D., Jonas, B.A., Pullarkat, V. et al. (2020). Azacitidine and venetoclax in previously untreated acute myeloid leukemia. *N Engl J Med* 383: 617–629.

Dohner H., Wei A.H., Appelbaum F.R. et al. (2022). Diagnosis and management of AML in adults: 2022 recommendations from an international expert panel on behalf of the ELN. *Blood* 140:1345–1377.

Granfeldt Ostgard, L.S., Medeiros, B.C., Sengelov, H. et al. (2015). Epidemiology and clinical significance of secondary and therapy-related acute myeloid leukemia: a national population-based cohort study. *J Clin Oncol* 33: 3641–3649.

Huls, G., Chitu, D.A., Havelange, V. et al. (2019). Azacitidine maintenance after intensive chemotherapy improves DFS in older AML patients. *Blood* 133: 1457–1464.

Jongen-Lavrencic, M., Grob, T., Hanekamp, D. et al. (2018). Molecular minimal residual disease in acute myeloid leukemia. *N Engl J Med* 378: 1189–1199.

Juliusson, G., Antunovic, P., Derolf, A. et al. (2009). Age and acute myeloid leukemia: real world data on decision to treat and outcomes from the Swedish acute leukemia registry. *Blood* 113: 4179–4187.

Klepin, H.D., Geiger, A.M., Tooze, J.A. et al. (2013). Geriatric assessment predicts survival for older adults receiving induction chemotherapy for acute myelogenous leukemia. *Blood* 121: 4287–4294.

Lancet, J.E., Uy, G.L., Cortes, J.E. et al. (2018). CPX-351 (cytarabine and daunorubicin) liposome for injection versus conventional cytarabine plus daunorubicin in older patients with newly diagnosed secondary acute myeloid leukemia. *J Clin Oncol* 36: 2684–2692.

Maiti, A., Rausch, C.R., Cortes, J.E. et al. (2021). Outcomes of relapsed or refractory acute myeloid leukemia after frontline hypomethylating agent and venetoclax regimens. *Haematologica* 106: 894–898.

Muffly, L., Pasquini, M.C., Martens, M. et al. (2017). Increasing use of allogeneic hematopoietic cell transplantation in patients aged 70 years and older in the United States. *Blood* 130: 1156–1164.

Sierra, J., Montesinos, P., Thomas, X. et al. (2023 August 15). Midostaurin plus daunorubicin or idarubicin for young and elderly adults with FLT3-mutated AML: a Phase 3b trial. *Blood Adv.* bloodadvances.2023009847. doi: 10.1182/bloodadvances.2023009847. Epub ahead of print. PMID: 37581981.

Schiffer, C.A. (2019). An important gap in informed consent documents for oncology clinical trials: lack of quantitative details about expected treatment outcomes. *JAMA Oncol* 5: 1399–1400.

Sorror, M.L., Storer, B.E., Fathi, A.T. et al. (2021). Multisite 11-year experience of less-intensive vs intensive therapies in acute myeloid leukemia. *Blood* 138: 387–400.

Walter, R.B., Kantarjian, H.M., Huang, X. et al. (2010). Effect of complete remission and responses less than complete remission on survival in acute myeloid leukemia: a combined Eastern cooperative oncology group, Southwest oncology group, and M. D. Anderson cancer center study. *J Clin Oncol* 28: 1766–1771.

Wei, A.H., Dohner, H., Pocock, C. et al. (2020). Oral azacitidine maintenance therapy for acute myeloid leukemia in first remission. *N Engl J Med* 383: 2526–2537.

9

Acute Promyelocytic Leukemia

Eytan M. Stein[1] and Martin S. Tallman[2]

[1] *Memorial Sloan Kettering Cancer Center, New York, NY*
[2] *Northwestern University Feinberg School of Medicine, Chicago, IL*

Introduction

Acute Promyelocytic Leukemia (APL) is rare. APL occurs in approximately 2,000 patients per year in the United States and represents 10% of all AML cases. Compared with most patients with AML, patients with APL tend to be younger, in their third or fourth decade of life. While rare, APL is now the most curable subtype of AML, as differentiation therapy with all-trans-retinoic acid (ATRA) and arsenic trioxide (ATO) leads to cure in nearly 100% of treated cases. Early recognition of APL and prompt treatment avoids the complications of the characteristic coagulopathy that can lead to morbidity and mortality before treatment is initiated. Remaining important issues in the management of APL is whether oral ATO can substitute for intravenous ATO, whether ATRA and ATO—without chemotherapy or gemtuzumab ozogamicin—is equally effective in high-risk disease as it is in low-risk disease, and whether the amount of ATO given can be shortened to two days/week from five days/week.

Case Study 1

A 32-year-old Hispanic woman presents to the emergency room with severe menorrhagia, bruising, and shortness of breath for six days. The complete blood count shows a white blood cell (WBC) count of 8,000/μL, hemoglobin of 6.5 g/dL, and platelets of 6000/μL. Further laboratory evaluation shows hypofibrinogenemia, with elevated prothrombin and partial thromboplastin times. You suspect acute promyelocytic leukemia (APL). All-trans retinoic acid (ATRA) is started, and bone marrow examination is done. Several days into therapy, a noticeable improvement in the patient's condition is noted. The bone marrow findings are suggestive of APL, but the cytogenetics are reported as normal.

1) **What should be the best management strategy at this time**: To continue APL-focused therapy until molecular tests are available, discontinue ATRA and initiate acute myeloid leukemia (AML) induction therapy with 7 + 3, or repeat bone marrow aspirate?

Cancer Consult: Expertise in Clinical Practice, Volume 2: Neoplastic Hematology & Cellular Therapy,
Second Edition. Edited by Syed A. Abutalib, Maurie Markman, James O. Armitage, and Kenneth C. Anderson.
© 2024 John Wiley & Sons Ltd. Published 2024 by John Wiley & Sons Ltd.

Expert Perspective: The correct answer is to continue APL-focused therapy until molecular tests are available. APL is a unique subtype of AML characterized by a block at the promyelocyte stage of hematopoiesis. The original description and recognition of APL as a unique subtype of AML are credited to *Leif Hillestad*, a Scandinavian physician who reported three patients with rapidly progressive leukemia and a profound coagulopathy. This coagulopathy, like disseminated intravascular coagulation (DIC), produces a prolonged prothrombin time and partial thromboplastin time and hypofibrinogenemia. However, the coagulopathy extends beyond DIC to include fibrinolysis and proteolysis. The patient described in this vignette has clearly developed a bleeding diathesis, with severe menorrhagia and shortness of breath that are attributable to anemia or perhaps pulmonary hemorrhage.

The *sine qua non* of APL is a recurrent reciprocal translocation between chromosomes 15 and 17. This translocation, first described by Janet Rowley and colleagues, fuses the promyelocytic leukemia gene (PML) with the retinoic acid receptor alpha gene (RARα) and leads to the promyelocytic leukemia phenotype. In routine practice, this translocation is easily visualized with standard chromosomal analysis. However, cases have been described in the literature of cryptic translocations that fuse PML and RARα but are nevertheless not detectable on standard chromosomal analysis.

Because of the high clinical suspicion of APL, the first test done was a bone marrow aspiration and biopsy. Although we are not told the results of the bone marrow examination, APL patients typically have an abundance of promyelocytes with multiple granules that often coalesce and take the appearance of a bundle of sticks (so-called *faggot cells*). Based on the clinical history and bone marrow examination, the physician chose to initiate ATRA at the first suspicion of APL. Although the cure rates for APL are remarkable, early death (often defined as death within 30 days of diagnosis) remains the major cause of treatment failure. In clinical trials, the induction death rate ranges between 5% and 9%. In population-based studies, the early death rate ranges between 17% and 30%, and it is considerably higher in older patients. Indeed, the early death rate has not changed significantly since the introduction of ATRA. Emerging data suggest that early death may be related to delays in receiving ATRA once patients present to the hospital. In a retrospective analysis of 194 patients, most patients (69%) had ATRA administered two days or more after presentation. Although the early death rate was not increased, the percentage of patients who died from hemorrhage was markedly increased when ATRA was delayed for more than two days. In addition, the results of this retrospective analysis confirmed that high-risk patients with APL who received their first dose of ATRA three or four days after they were suspected of having APL had an early death rate of 80%, compared with a rate of only 18% in high-risk patients who received ATRA on days 0, 1, or 2.

Our Patient: Because the patient is improving on ATRA-based therapy and the clinical picture is consistent with APL, the treating physician should wait for the results of sensitive molecular genetics tests for the *PML::RARα* fusion product.

Case Study 2

A 45-year-old male presents with severe fatigue, shortness of breath, and epistaxis. Examination demonstrates diffuse petecchiae. The complete blood count shows a WBC count of 14,000/μL with 50% promyelocytes, hemoglobin of 5.3 g/dL, and platelets of 4,000/μL.

Further laboratory evaluation shows a fibrinogen level of 38, with prothrombin and partial thromboplastin times of 48 and 67, respectively. You plan to start APL induction therapy.

2) What is the preferred treatment for patients with low-risk APL?

Expert Perspective: Patients with APL are risk stratified based on their white blood count (WBC) at the time of diagnosis; those with a WBC of 10,000 or higher are classified as having high-risk disease, while those with a white blood count lower than 10,000 are classified as having low-risk disease. The treatment paradigm for patients with low-risk APL is now the combination of ATRA and ATO, based on the results of a phase III APL 0406 conducted by the GIMEMA and AMLSG study groups that randomized patients to receive repeated cycles of ATRA and ATO for induction and consolidation or ATRA with chemotherapy. ATRA and ATO was non-inferior to ATRA with chemotherapy and in fact showed possible superiority. Event-free survival was 97% in the ATRA and ATO arm, and overall survival in the ATRA and ATO group was 99%. These survival statistics persisted out past five years of follow-up. Patients who develop leukocytosis while taking ATRA and ATO as part of the differentiation effect of these two agents used hydroxyurea for cytoreduction. Prednisone was used for prophylaxis from differentiation syndrome in every patient from the start of ATRA and ATO through the completion of induction. Treatment with ATO can be complicated by QT-interval prolongation and, rarely, by sudden death. Therefore, before initiating treatment with ATO and periodically thereafter, any electrolyte imbalances should be corrected, especially hypomagnesemia and hypocalcemia; other drugs that can prolong the QT interval should be discontinued.

3) What is the role of ATRA and ATO combination therapy for high-risk APL?

Expert Perspective: The AML17 trial conducted by the Medical Research Council in the United Kingdom randomized patients, both with high-risk and low-risk APL, to receive ATRA with chemotherapy or ATRA and ATO. Patients randomized to ATRA and ATO could receive one dose of the anti-CD33 antibody-drug conjugate gemutuzmab ozogamicin for cytoreduction for those with high-risk disease. Maintenance was not given to patients with high-risk disease, whether on the standard arm or the investigational arm of ATRA with ATO. The outcomes with ATRA plus ATO for patients with high-risk APL was excellent, with four-year overall survival of 87%. The APML4 protocol utilized ATRA, ATO, and idarubicin for induction, consolidation with ATRA and ATO for two cycles of consolidation, and two years of maintenance therapy with ATRA, oral methotrexate, and 6-mercaptopurine. The five-year disease-free survival was 95%, and overall survival was 94%.

4) Should a bone marrow biopsy be performed following induction therapy?

Expert Perspective: Following induction chemotherapy, the leukemia promyelocytes differentiate into mature neutrophils. This differentiation process can take weeks, and therefore performing a bone marrow biopsy after induction often leads to confusion rather than clarity, with immature forms seen in the marrow. In addition, primary resistance to induction therapy in APL has only very rarely been reported. For both reasons, we do not perform a bone marrow biopsy until 4–6 weeks after induction chemotherapy has been completed. Patients who are in a hematologic remission after induction may not become molecularly negative for the *PML::RARα* fusion product until one or two cycles of consolidation are completed.

Case Study continued: On day 16 of therapy for APL, the patient develops fever, cough, pulmonary infiltrates, and right-sided pleural effusion. The oxygen saturation decreases to 88%. He is transferred to the intensive care unit with a presumptive diagnosis of pneumonia.

5) How is a diagnosis of APL differentiation syndrome established?

6) Would prophylactic steroids have prevented this complication?

7) What is the treatment of APL differentiation syndrome?

Expert Perspective: After administering ATRA, the astute physician must be vigilant for APL differentiation syndrome. The differentiation syndrome, first described with the use of ATRA but also seen with the use of arsenic triooxide (ATO), is manifested clinically as noncardiogenic pulmonary edema that can cause respiratory failure requiring intubation and mechanical ventilation. Its etiology is poorly understood. It is thought to be caused by a capillary leak syndrome induced by the rapid differentiation of leukemic promyelocytes. The treatment, dexamethasone at 10 mg twice daily, should be prescribed immediately to patients who are thought to be developing the differentiation syndrome. Temporary discontinuation of ATRA or ATO may be required for patients in very poor clinical condition. In our practice, we administer dexamethasone prophylactically for 10 to 14 days to patients with high-risk APL.

8) Is maintenance needed?

9) Should maintenance therapy be tailored according to the risk groups?

10) Should a bone marrow biopsy be performed after maintenance therapy?

Expert Perspective: The need for prolonged maintenance therapy after induction and consolidation for APL in the modern front-line treatment (i.e. ATRA + ATO) of high-risk APL is controversial. This controversy stems from conflicting results from randomized clinical trials. In addition, all the maintenance trials enrolled patients in CR, but some trials, before the widespread adoption of sensitive polymerase chain reaction (PCR) tests, used hematologic CR to define remission, whereas others used the more sensitive molecular CR. Finally, the induction and consolidation regimens in trials that evaluated maintenance therapy were varied, making it difficult to draw any conclusions between trials about the overall benefit of maintenance.

In 2007, the JALSG study reported the results of a clinical trial that randomized patients with APL who were PCR negative for the *PML::RARα* fusion transcript after induction and consolidation to intensified maintenance with combination chemotherapy or observation. The induction regimen in this trial used a risk-adapted approach: patients with a low WBC count (less than 3×10^9) received ATRA monotherapy, while those with a higher WBC count received idarubicin and cytarabine in combination with ATRA during induction. Consolidation consisted of three cycles of multidrug chemotherapy (without ATRA). Patients randomized to the intensified maintenance arm received six cycles of multidrug chemotherapy without ATRA. At a median follow-up of 49 months, 28% of patients in the intensified maintenance group had relapsed and 15% had died as compared to only 20% of patients relapsing in the observation group and only 3% dying. The results of JALSG study suggested that intensified maintenance after induction with ATRA and consolidation with combination chemotherapy may be harmful.

As discussed earlier, one question addressed by the North American Intergroup was the role of maintenance ATRA after achieving CR. In the long-term outcome data published in 2002, there was a distinct disease-free survival advantage for patients assigned to ATRA maintenance; disease-free survival in the ATRA maintenance group (regardless of induction regimen) was 61% and was only 36% in the observation arm. Those patients who received both ATRA in induction and ATRA maintenance had a disease-free survival of 74% compared to a disease-free survival of only 16% for those who received chemotherapy and observation.

In the European APL trial, patients who were in hematologic CR after consolidation were randomized to one of four maintenance arms: observation, ATRA (45 mg/m^2/day for 15 days once every three months), chemotherapy (methotrexate 15 mg/m^2/week and 6-MP 90 mg/m^2/day), or ATRA with chemotherapy for a total of two years, with chemotherapy dose modifications based on blood counts. In the final analysis, the 10-year event-free survival and OS in the concurrent chemotherapy–ATRA and chemotherapy-alone maintenance groups were significantly better than the results in the ATRA and observation arms. The cumulative incidence of relapse was lowest in the ATRA–chemotherapy group (13.4%), followed by the chemotherapy group (23.4%), ATRA group (33.0%), and observation group (43.2%).

The AIDA 0493 trial used a similar maintenance scheme as the European APL trial, but it only enrolled patients who were in a molecular CR at the end of consolidation. Interestingly, this trial saw no benefit to the use of ATRA maintenance for those patients in molecular CR at the end of consolidation, contradicting the results of the previous European and first North American Intergroup trials. Despite the negative results, subsequent, modern trials have adopted the widespread use of maintenance with ATRA, 6-mercaptopurine, and methotrexate after consolidation. In addition, the utility of maintenance therapy in the era when ATRA is given during consolidation has never been prospectively evaluated.

Case Study continued: Approximately a year following completion of maintenance therapy, the patient is diagnosed with molecular relapse.

11) Does molecular relapse portend hematologic relapse?

12) What is the best treatment for relapsed APL?

13) Should screening lumbar puncture be done at relapse?

Expert Perspective: Patients with molecular relapse of APL will likely develop overt hematologic relapse. Because of this, intervention when the *PML::RARα* transcript level is rising is the accepted approach for patients with evidence of relapse. In general, ATO is used for the treatment of relapsed disease, followed by high-dose chemotherapy with autologous stem cell rescue provided CSF is negative for leukemia. De Botton and colleagues retrospectively analyzed the outcomes of 122 patients in two successive multicenter APL trials conducted by the European Acute Promyelocytic Leukemia Group with first relapse APL who received an autologous or allogeneic stem cell transplant after achieving a second hematologic CR with chemotherapy. Of those receiving an autologous transplant, the seven-year overall survival was 59.8% with 6% transplant-related mortality. In the patients who received an allogeneic transplant, seven-year overall survival was 51.8% with a substantial transplant-related mortality of 39%. Based on these and other data, we generally recommend an autologous transplant for patients with first relapse of APL after achievement of second molecular remission.

14) What is the role of screening for CNS disease in relapsed APL?

Expert Perspective: Several patients with relapsed APL will have central nervous system (CNS) involvement at the time of relapse. Because of this, we perform a screening lumbar puncture and strongly consider empirical administration of intrathecal chemotherapy for CNS prophylaxis for six courses of intrathecal therapy. However, the role of prophylactic CNS treatment in relapsed APL remains controversial, and the benefit on overall survival is unclear.

Recommended Readings

Burnett, A.K., Russell, N.H., Hills, R.K., Bowen, D., Kell, J., Knapper, S., Morgan, Y.G., Lok, J., Grech, A., Jones, G., Khwaja, A., Friis, L., McMullin, M.F., Hunter, A., Clark, R.E., and Grimwade, D. (2015 October). UK National Cancer Research Institute Acute Myeloid Leukaemia Working Group. Arsenic trioxide and all-trans retinoic acid treatment for acute promyelocytic leukaemia in all risk groups (AML17): results of a randomised, controlled, phase 3 trial. *Lancet Oncol* 16 (13): 1295–1305. doi: 10.1016/S1470-2045(15)00193-X. Epub 2015 Sep 14.PMID: 26384238.

Cicconi, L., Platzbecker, U., Avvisati, G., Paoloni, F., Thiede, C., Vignetti, M., Fazi, P., Ferrara, F., Divona, M., Albano, F., Efficace, F., Sborgia, M., Di Bona, E., Breccia, M., Borlenghi, E., Cairoli, R., Rambaldi, A., Melillo, L., La Nasa, G., Fiedler, W., Brossart, P., Hertenstein, B., Salih, H.R., Annibali, O., Wattad, M., Lubbert, M., Brandts, C.H., Hanel, M., Rollig, C., Schmitz, N., Link, H., Frairia, C., Fozza, C., Maria D'Arco, A., Di Renzo, N., Cortelezzi, A., Fabbiano, F., Dohner, K., Ganser, A., Dohner, H., Amadori, S., Mandelli, F., Voso, M.T., Ehninger, G., Schlenk, R.F., and Lo-Coco, F. (2020 March). Long-term results of all-trans retinoic acid and arsenic trioxide in non-high-risk acute promyelocytic leukemia: update of the APL0406 Italian-German randomized trial. *Leukemia* 34 (3): 914–918. doi: 10.1038/s41375-019-0589-3.

de Botton, S., Fawaz, A., Chevret, S. et al. (2005). Autologous and allogeneic stem-cell transplantation as salvage treatment of acute promyelocytic leukemia initially treated with all-trans-retinoic acid: a retrospective analysis of the European acute promyelocytic leukemia group. *J Clin Oncol* 23 (1): 120–126.

Iland, H.J., Collins, M., Bradstock, K., Supple, S.G., Catalano, A., Hertzberg, M., Browett, P., Grigg, A., Firkin, F., Campbell, L.J., Hugman, A., Reynolds, J., Di Iulio, J., Tiley, C., Taylor, K., Filshie, R., Seldon, M., Taper, J., Szer, J., Moore, J., Bashford, J., and Seymour, J.F. (2015 September). Australasian Leukaemia and Lymphoma Group. Use of arsenic trioxide in remission induction and consolidation therapy for acute promyelocytic leukaemia in the Australasian Leukaemia and Lymphoma Group (ALLG) APML4 study: a non-randomised phase 2 trial. *Lancet Haematol* 2 (9): e357–e366. doi: 10.1016/S2352-3026(15)00115-5. Epub 2015 Aug 20. PMID: 26685769.

Lo-Coco, F., Avvisati, G., Vignetti, M. et al. (2010). Front-line treatment of acute promyelocytic leukemia with AIDA induction followed by risk-adapted consolidation for adults younger than 61 years: Powell BL, Moser B, Stock W, et al. Arsenic trioxide improves event-free and overall survival for adults with acute promyelocytic leukemia: North American Leukemia Intergroup Study C9710. *Blood* 116 (19): 3751–3757.

Lo-Coco, F., Avvisati, G., Vignetti, M., Thiede, C., Orlando, S.M., Iacobelli, S., Ferrara, F., Fazi, P., Cicconi, L., Di Bona, E., Specchia, G., Sica, S., Divona, M., Levis, A., Fiedler, W., Cerqui, E., Breccia, M., Fioritoni, G., Salih, H.R., Cazzola, M., Melillo, L., Carella, A.M., Brandts, C.H., Morra, E., von Lilienfeld-Toal, M., Hertenstein, B., Wattad, M., Lübbert, M., Hänel, M., Schmitz, N., Link, H., Kropp, M.G., Rambaldi, A., La Nasa, G., Luppi, M., Ciceri, F., Finizio, O., Venditti, A., Fabbiano, F., Döhner, K., Sauer, M., Ganser, A., Amadori, S., Mandelli, F., Döhner, H., Ehninger, G., Schlenk, R.F., and Platzbecker, U. (2013 July 11). Gruppo Italiano Malattie Ematologiche dell'Adulto; German-Austrian Acute Myeloid Leukemia Study Group; Study Alliance Leukemia. Retinoic acid and arsenic trioxide for acute promyelocytic leukemia. *N Engl J Med* 369 (2): 111–121. doi: 10.1056/NEJMoa1300874. PMID: 23841729.

Sanz, M.A., Montesinos, P., Vellenga, E. et al. (2008). Risk-adapted treatment of acute promyelocytic leukemia with all-trans retinoic acid and anthracycline monochemotherapy: long-term outcome of the LPA 99 multicenter study by the PETHEMA Group. *Blood* 112 (8): 3130–3134.

Tallman, M.S., Andersen, J.W., Schiffer, C.A. et al. (1997). All-trans-retinoic acid in acute promyelocytic leukemia. *New Engl J Med* 337 (15): 1021–1028.

10

Measurable Residual Disease in Acute Myeloid Leukemia

Marie Bill and Hans Beier Ommen

Department of Hematology, Aarhus University Hospital, Denmark

Introduction

Evaluation of treatment response in acute myeloid leukemia (AML) has traditionally been based on cytomorphology, and complete remission (CR) is continuously defined as less than 5% myeloblasts in the bone marrow after induction chemotherapy. However, relapse occurs in more than 50% of AML patients who obtain morphologically defined CR. From this it follows that a minor fraction of leukemic cells can persist in the marrow during treatment and propagate the neoplasm at a later time point. Modern sensitive laboratory techniques can reveal such residual leukemic cells by detecting leukemia-associated genetic abnormalities or aberrant immunophenotypes, termed measurable residual disease (MRD). The presence of MRD after induction chemotherapy is strongly associated with an increased risk of relapse and shorter survival in AML (refer to Chapters 7, 8, and 11).

Case Study 1

A 64-year-old sales manager experienced lack of appetite and energy, weight loss (8–10 kg), low-grade fever, and sweating spells. The general practitioner found elevated liver enzymes and moderate but progressive pancytopenia. A computed tomography scan of the abdomen showed no liver-related findings. Bone marrow examination showed 72% immature blasts with an immunophenotype suggestive of acute myelomonocytic leukemia (CD45lowCD34-CD117-CD64+CD14-CD13+CD33+HLA-DR+CD56highCD4+). Cytogenetics including fluorescence in situ hybridization (FISH) showed a normal karyotype and no AML-related cytogenetic abnormalities. Fast *NPM1/FLT3-ITD* testing detected a mutation in the *NPM1* gene but no *FLT3-ITD* abnormality. Elevated liver enzymes were considered leukemic infiltration, and the patient received protocolized anti-leukemic therapy with CPX-351 (liposomal cytarabine and daunorubicin). His condition improved upon antibiotic and anti-leukemic therapy, and he was followed during the neutropenic period in a semi-ambulatory setting. Targeted next-generation sequencing (NGS) of marrow cells confirmed the presence of the *NPM1* mutation and additionally revealed a *DNMT3A* mutation.

1) Which techniques are available for MRD detection in AML?

Expert Perspective: Any technique with sensitivity higher than classic immunohistochemistry will yield information regarding the depth of the achieved remission. In general, MRD detection is based on the principle that leukemic cells display genetic and/or immunophenotypical features different from healthy hematopoiesis. Due to the genetic heterogeneity of AML no single MRD detection technique or MRD target is useful in all patients. Thus, selection of the optimal technique and target is highly individual—and each MRD detection platform has advantages and limitations. Multicolor flow cytometry exploits the fact that most AML cells display aberrant immunophenotypic profiles, i.e. surface expression of leukocyte differentiation antigens present in either abnormal combinations or densities. These leukemia-associated immunophenotypes (LAIPs) are present in > 90 % of AML cases, and thus, they are widely applicable. In Case Study 1, the leukemic blasts displayed an abnormally high expression of CD56, and when combined with a backbone of myelomonocytic markers this compose a highly specific LAIP (CD45lowCD64+CD14-CD13+CD56high), which can be used for MRD detection during treatment. Multicolor flow cytometry is fast (results can be ready in 4–6 hours), and if optimally performed, sensitivity can reach 10^{-4}. However, the technique requires skilled and experienced interpretation, and another potential drawback is the fact that LAIPs are not necessarily stable over time. In Case Study 1, the leukemic cells also harbored an NPM1 mutation. This particular mutation is ideal for detection with real-time quantitative polymerase chain reaction (qPCR). The qPCR technique targets RNA or DNA sequences, which are derived from fusion genes, mutated genes, or genes overexpressed in AML cells and can reach sensitivity around 10^{-6}. Thus, the NPM1 mutation (detected with qPCR) was selected as MRD marker in this patient. Recently, digital droplet PCR (ddPCR) and NGS-based techniques are gaining ground as MRD detection tools. While ddPCR is superior to qPCR by yielding more stable and reproducible results, NGS has the advantage of being able to detect more than one mutation simultaneously. As such, by analyzing variant allele frequencies (VAF) of different somatic mutations within a particular patient sample, it is possible to study the interrelationship between subclones (Figure 10.1). Of note, not all mutations are suitable as MRD markers. For instance, mutations in *DNMT3A*, *ASXL1*, and *TET2* ("DAT") are commonly found in healthy individuals and most often represent preleukemic clonal hematopoiesis and not relapse-initiating cells.

2) How are MRD measurements useful in response evaluation?

Expert Perspective: While the intention of induction chemotherapy in AML is to obtain CR, consolidation therapy aims to minimize the risk of relapse. The most effective anti-relapse treatment is allogeneic hematopoietic cell transplantation (allo-HCT). However, allo-HCT comes with the cost of a not insignificant risk of transplant-related mortality and morbidity. Expert opinion differs regarding how high the relapse risk should be in order to perform allo-HCT after obtaining CR, but figures between 30% and 50% are typically mentioned (Chapter 11). Thus, precise relapse risk determination using both diagnostic genetic information and MRD surveillance during treatment is very often integrated in clinical decision-making and guide whether or not to recommend allo-HCT. Of note, a direct study

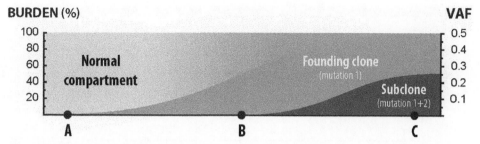

Figure 10.1 Schematic presentation of the rationale for employing VAF as indication of clonal evolution. At time point A, no mutations are evident, and the BM consists of 100% normal cells (light gray). At time point B, a heterozygous mutation has emerged, now representing the founding clone (medium gray). As 50% of the cells are mutated, this founding mutation will have a VAF of 25%. At time point C two mutations are present; the founding clone (medium gray) harboring mutation 1 has replaced the normal compartment and now has a VAF of 50%. Meanwhile, mutation 2 has emerged and is present in 50% of cells resulting in a VAF of 25%. As mutation 2 emerged from a cell harboring mutation 1, the subclone (dark gray) contains both mutations 1 and 2.

of whether to transplant or not has not been feasible as few physicians or patients have been willing to accept the transplant decision to be dependent on randomization.

In *NPM1*-mutated AML, a considerable amount of data exists regarding the relapse risk, which has proven to be much dependent on age and co-mutations. For patients below the age of 60 years who have co-mutation of *NPM1* and *DNMT3A* it has been shown that *NPM1*-based MRD negativity in blood after two courses of induction chemotherapy results in a relapse risk of 52% compared to 29% in NPM1-positive patients without co-mutated *DNMT3A*. In another study, looking at younger NPM1-mutated patients (< 60 years), and including both *FLT3 wild-type* and *FLT3-mutated* patients, MRD negativity in marrow after two courses of induction chemotherapy yielded a relapse risk of 6%. A third study of the same age group examined patients with co-mutation of *NPM1* and *FLT-ITD*, who have an inherently higher relapse risk due to the *FLT3* aberration. In this patient cohort, a reduction in MRD in blood by a factor of 10,000 after the first course of chemotherapy resulted in a better outcome without transplantation. As such, in *NPM1*-mutated AML patients below the age of 60, evidence supports to avoid allo-HCT in patients who become MRD negative after the second series of induction chemotherapy.

Similar evidence exists for patients with *RUNX1::RUNX1T1* t(8;21) and *CBFB::MYH11* inv(16) abnormalities. However, for older patients > 60 years, evidence of MRD negativity as a predictor of relapse risk remains sparse. Nevertheless, for patients such as in Case Study 1, who have an excellent MRD marker such as *NPM1*, and present with excellent MRD results, e.g. marrow negativity after one course of chemotherapy (Figure 10.2), considerations to waive the transplant would be appropriate, especially if chemotherapy has reduced the patients' fitness for transplantation.

3) Which markers can be used for MRD measurements, and are all markers equally useful?

Expert Perspective: Several factors should be considered when selecting the optimal MRD marker. First of all, the intra- and interpatient genetic heterogeneity of AML entails

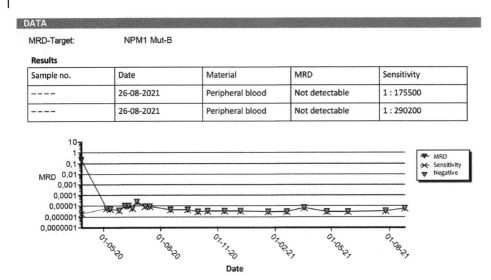

DATA

MRD-Target: NPM1 Mut-B

Results

Sample no.	Date	Material	MRD	Sensitivity
- - - -	26-08-2021	Peripheral blood	Not detectable	1 : 175500
- - - -	26-08-2021	Peripheral blood	Not detectable	1 : 290200

Figure 10.2 Longitudinal MRD assessment in Case Study 1.

that MRD measuring is equally diverse. While genetic aberrations such as fusion genes or point mutations in canonical AML-related genes (such as *NPM1*) are highly relevant MRD markers for PCR-based techniques, these are only present in up to 50% of AML patients (and less than 35% in the elderly). Also, while optimizing sensitivity of the MRD assay is thought to enable physicians to maximize discrimination between patients who are prone to relapse and patients who are not, it must be remembered that some MRD-negative patients actually do relapse. Thus, choosing the most relevant marker that represents biologically relevant and leukemia-propagating cells continues to be challenging in many patients. In line with this, the stability of a given MRD marker during the course of disease was of great concern during the earlier days of MRD technique development. Loss of MRD markers remains a concern when detecting impending relapse during long-term follow-up, but it seems to be of less concern during initial therapy, where MRD detection is used for decisions regarding consolidation therapy. Importantly, the degree to which MRD represents leukemic cells with actual relapse-generating potential has to be considered. For example, the pre-leukemic *DNMT3A* mutation is known to persist in remission, as was indeed the case in Case Study 1.

Case Study 1, continued after the first course of chemotherapy, the patient was in morphological CR and had achieved negativity for NPM1 in both blood and marrow. However, during regeneration he developed a sudden abducens nerve palsy. Magnetic resonance imaging of the brain was without any findings, and the cerebrospinal fluid was acellular. However, the cerebrospinal fluid (CSF) was found to be *NPM1* positive by qPCR. The patient was treated with intrathecal chemotherapy, and the abducens nerve palsy improved within days. The patient was taken off protocol and treated with high-dose cytarabine and etoposide, two drugs that cross the blood-brain barrier. The patient was severely ill during the neutropenic period and only restituted very slowly. For this reason, neither further chemotherapy nor allo-HCT was performed. The patient remained MRD negative in peripheral blood, CSF, and marrow during the next months and regained his pre-leukemia performance status. At this time point he did not want further treatment, and close surveillance with *NPM1* was performed to allow preemptive treatment and transplantation in second molecular remission, if necessary.

4) Which pitfalls should be considered in routine MRD detection?

Expert Perspective: As evident from Case Study 1, MRD cannot be detected in tissues that are not sampled! Both myeloid sarcomas and leukemias in the central nervous system are rare, but not unseen, and standard MRD determinations in blood and marrow only detect leukemic cells in these tissues. On the other hand, patients with myeloid sarcomas are often MRD positive in blood and marrow (personal observation). As such, the MRD tool can be valuable in detection of minute amounts of leukemia in other tissues (most often CSF, ascites, or pleural exudates). Note that in these cases, contamination with peripheral blood may produce false-positive results.

Case Study 2

A 62-year-old woman with no prior medical history was referred to the university hospital with abnormal blood counts and swelling of the gums. A complete blood count revealed leukocytosis of 47×10^9/L, anemia with hemoglobin of 5.7 mmol/L, and thrombocytopenia 39×10^9/L. Lactate dehydrogenase was elevated three times above the upper limit. A peripheral blood smear showed dominance of large, immature blastic cells without granules. Morphologic examination of BM confirmed a diagnosis of AML with 95% infiltration of myeloblasts. Immunophenotypically, the myeloblasts were CD45lowCD34+CD117+CD33+HLA-DR+CLEC12A+. Standard cytogenetic karyotyping showed a normal karyotype (46,XX), while fluorescence in situ hybridization (FISH) could detect an inversion of chromosome 16 resulting in a fusion gene between the core binding factor B (CBFB) and the *myosin heavy chain 11 gene (MYH11)*. Targeted NGS detected a mutation in the *ASXL1* gene with a VAF of 45%. The inv16A aberration was chosen as MRD marker, and MRD surveillance was performed by qPCR. The patient was treated with standard induction and consolidation chemotherapy together with an anti-CD33 antibody-drug conjugate directed against CD33 (gemtuzumab-ozogamicin). She obtained morphologic CR after the first course of chemotherapy and MRD negativity after a total of three chemotherapy courses. She was followed with monthly MRD measurements and after one year she experienced a molecular relapse with detectable and rising MRD levels in peripheral blood and marrow. Salvage chemotherapy was initiated, and the patient went on to an allo-HCT. She remains well and in continuous molecular remission (Figure 10.3).

5) Can overt relapse be prevented using MRD surveillance?

Expert Perspective: The patient in Case Study 2 experienced a molecular relapse (defined as rising MRD levels of one log in 2 measurements at least two weeks apart) more than one year after initial AML treatment. She never experienced an overt clinical relapse (deterioration of marrow function and more than 5% blasts morphologically in marrow). This illustrates that surveillance of MRD during follow-up of AML patients allows for early detection of impending relapse. First of all, this will allow the clinician time to consider an appropriate (and maybe even personalized) treatment strategy, including the

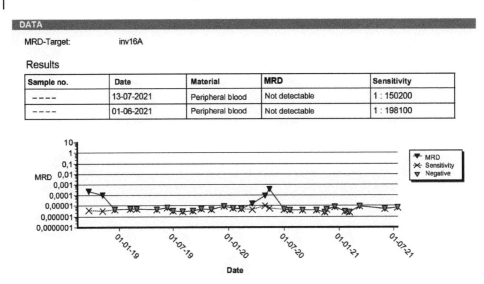

Figure 10.3 Longitudinal MRD assessment in Case Study 2.

time-consuming workup of finding a suitable donor for allo-HCT. Furthermore, detecting a molecular relapse enables initiation of preemptive treatment with, e.g. further chemotherapy, a hypomethylating agent, or targeted therapy directed against a known genetic abnormality. Such preemptive treatment can serve as bridging to a subsequent allo-HCT or slow down the momentum of the leukemia as a palliative strategy in cases where treatment options are otherwise exhausted. Several minor, unrandomized studies have addressed the impact of preemptive therapy in AML. One study investigated the use of 5-azacytidine as a preemptive treatment for molecular relapse in both transplanted and un-transplanted AML patients. Twenty patients were treated, and morphologic relapse was avoided in seven patients. However, further prospective, randomized studies are underway, and results are highly awaited.

6) Does detection of MRD always result in a subsequent relapse?

Expert Perspective: This is an important clinical question at the center of the ongoing evaluation of the value of MRD in AML. Even for highly disease-specific markers such as fusion transcript or mutated gene–based qPCR [e.g. t(8;21) and *NPM1*] several groups have reported scant positive MRD samplings not followed by a subsequent relapse. These MRD reversals not followed by a clinical relapse are most often seen immediately after cessation of chemotherapy but can be seen at later time points or even in the post-allogeneic setting. Generally, these MRD samples are positive at very low and stable levels. This is most probably a reflection of temporary changes in disease levels at the time when both normal and malignant hematopoiesis are in the rebound phase. In addition, it is becoming increasingly evident that factors of the marrow microenvironment such as the spatial localization of the neoplastic cells and the interplay with non-malignant cells, e.g. mesenchymal cells, are of great importance to leukemogenesis and might influence whether minute amounts of leukemic cells will lead to outgrowth of relapse or not. A strict follow-up program with repeated MRD measurements 2–3 weeks apart can be employed to delineate a significant increase.

7) Are there any ethical considerations when employing MRD monitoring?

Expert Perspective: Evidence remains sparse on whether initiating salvage therapy at the time of molecular relapse compared to the time of overt relapse actually improves outcome for these AML patients. This raises important ethical considerations as detecting MRD can cause a significant amount of anxiety in patients, who otherwise feel healthy and have normal blood counts. Thus, there is a high need for further studies in this area—not least in order to avoid unnecessary treatment (including possible unwanted side effects) in patients who could have had several months with high quality of life before starting treatment if treatment had not been initiated until blood counts started deteriorating. Utmost care is necessary when conveying the information regarding the positive MRD measurement and its consequences. Importantly, MRD surveillance in the follow-up setting is only indicated in AML patients for whom a realistic treatment option exists in the case of relapse.

Case Study 3

A 55-year-old man, who had received a combined kidney-pancreas transplant 2.5 years earlier due to diabetic nephropathy, developed moderate pancytopenia despite reduction in immunosuppressive drugs. Bone marrow examination showed AML, 35% blasts with a myeloid immunophenotype. The karyotype was normal (46, XY). Targeted NGS revealed a *DNMT3A* and a *RUNX1* mutation together with a *FLT3-ITD* aberration. The patient was treated with daunorubicin and cytarabine with midostaurin during the neutropenic periods. The *RUNX1* mutation was selected as MRD marker, and a personalized ddPCR assay was designed for MRD detection. After four courses of chemotherapy and midostaurin the patient was in CR, and the *RUNX1* mutation was undetectable by ddPCR with a sensitivity of 0.01%. An ASCT was waived in first remission based on concerns for the kidney-pancreas graft, and the patient was followed by *RUNX1*-targeted ddPCR. After two months ddPCR in PB became positive. Based on the molecular relapse, preemptive treatment with high-dose chemotherapy was initiated (FLAG-Ida). After this treatment, only a minor decrease in MRD was observed (Figure 10.3).

8) Is MRD negativity a prerequisite for allogeneic hematopoietic cell transplantation?

Expert Perspective: Several studies have shown that MRD-positive patients can be cured by allo-HCT. However, the same studies unequivocally show that the post-transplant prognosis is much better for patients who are MRD negative before transplantation (Chapter 11). This leads to the question of whether it is better to transplant early, i.e. after two courses of chemotherapy (thus avoiding treatment-related mortality from course three and four), even if the patient is MRD positive, or administer extra courses of chemotherapy in an attempt to achieve MRD negativity. No randomized studies have evaluated this question. The majority of studies examining pre-transplant MRD have been retrospective studies, and these are not well suited to provide answers to this dilemma. However, in practical hematology, the dichotomy of transplanting earlier or later is often less tangible. As soon as the decision to move forward to an allo-HCT has been taken, physicians and patients will often want to proceed to transplant as quickly as possible. However, requisites of finding an available donor and timing the transplant often result in postponement of the transplant to after the second, third, or in some cases fourth course of chemotherapy. Indeed, even if early transplant was shown to be better, it would often not be feasible.

The patient proceeded with an ASCT despite pre-transplant MRD positivity and achieved ddPCR negativity in both PB and BM at the three months' post-transplant status. However, four months post transplant, he became MRD positive for the *RUNX1* mutation by ddPCR, and treatment with azacitidine and venetoclax was initiated. If unsuccessful, special permission for the use of gilteritinib will be considered (Figure 10.4).

9) What is the role of MRD in the post-transplant setting?

Expert Perspective: Preemptive therapy based on molecular relapse has been studied in the post-transplant setting as well as in patients not transplanted. While the goal of such treatment in younger, non-transplanted patients is renewed leukemia control and bridging to an allo-HCT, the goal in transplanted patients is to hamper the leukemia enough to allow for the full development of the graft-versus-leukemia effect. In the post-transplant setting, available treatment modalities for molecular relapse include enhancement of graft-versus-leukemia effect by tapering of immunosuppressant or donor lymphocyte infusions (only if the patient is free of graft-versus-host disease). Thus, treatment strategies in the post-transplant setting often include less intensive cytoreduction such as hypomethylating agents and targeted treatments.

DATA

Results		MRD target = RUNX1: p.S303*	
Sample no.	Date	Material	MRD (%)
– – – –	05-08-2021	Peripheral blood	0.48
– – – –	05-08-2021	Bone marrow	0.72
– – – –	08-07-2021	Peripheral blood	0.20
– – – –	09-06-2021	Peripheral blood	0.10
– – – –	11-05-2021	Peripheral blood	0.01

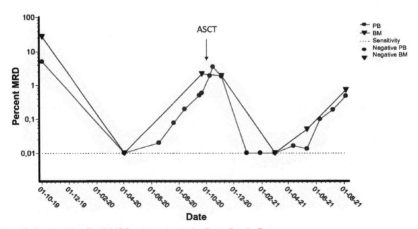

Figure 10.4 Longitudinal MRD assessment in Case Study 3.

Case Study 4

A 63-year-old male with a past medical history of alcohol abuse was transferred to the university hospital in June 2014 with newly diagnosed AML. Bone marrow morphology showed approximately 50% myeloblasts. Cytogenetic examination showed a normal karyotype (46,XY), and molecular testing revealed no AML-related fusion transcripts. However, overexpression of the *Wilms' tumor 1 (WT1)* gene could be demonstrated by qPCR analysis. The patient received four courses of standard chemotherapy and achieved a morphological CR and MRD negativity based on the WT1 assay. In 2014, panel sequencing for recurrently mutated genes was not available as part of the routine workup of AML. Three years later, the patient experienced a relapse of AML with 65% myeloblasts in the marrow; by flow cytometry these were CD45lowCD34+CD117+CD13+CD123+HLA-DR+. The karyotype was persistently normal. The patient was not found eligible for further intensive treatment regimens and received four cycles of 5-azacitidine with no anti-leukemic effect. He was observed for approximately one year without treatment and had stable cytopenias with anemia at the level of 6 mmol/L, neutropenia around 1×10^9/L, and a thrombocyte count about 30×10^9/L. Around this time point, an NGS panel of 30 recurrently mutated myeloid genes became available, and cryopreserved marrow samples from both 2014 and 2017 were analyzed. In both samples, mutations were detected in *IDH2, ASXL1,* and *SRSF2* together with three different *RUNX1* mutations. The patient was offered protocolled treatment with an oral *IDH2*-inhibitor (enasidenib), and after a few months of treatment his blood counts normalized. The patient has a good quality of life and is continuously receiving the *IDH2*-inhibitor. However, two years after initiation of enasidenib, dark clouds are on the horizon. The thrombocyte count is slowly decreasing, and by flow cytometry, MRD levels are slowly increasing. Furthermore, an immunophenotypic shift has occurred, as the myeloblasts have become aberrantly CD7 positive.

10) How many MRD markers are meaningful for surveillance?

Expert Perspective: Acute myeloid leukemia is generally regarded as a stem- and progenitor-cell disorder with a high degree of heterogeneity. This heterogeneity has long been known to clinicians, pathologists, and cytogeneticists. However, during the past decades, it has become increasingly evident that numerous different clones coexist with normal marrow cells at different time points during the disease course. In contrast to, e.g. CML, where a specific reciprocal translocation between chromosome 9 and 22 resulting in the *BCR::ABL1* fusion gene is present, no common malignant clone has been identified across AML patients. On the contrary, the genetic and immunophenotypical characteristics of the disease-propagating AML clones vary between patients, and on average each patient harbor 13 different mutations. Obviously, this remains a huge challenge in the setting of MRD surveillance. As previously mentioned, is it not recommended to follow mutations known to be of pre-leukemic nature, as these most often represent clonal hematopoiesis and persist during CR. It must be realized that local financial factors and the amount of available technical expertise and hardware can limit the possibilities for detecting more than one MRD marker during treatment and follow-up. However, recognizing the diverse nature of AML and the fact that separate subclones might respond very differently to therapy, for patients with many different leukemogenic abnormalities, monitoring several (or all) of these simultaneously would allow for detailed tracking of subclones. Such multi-target strategy is gaining feasibility as NGS emerges as the standard technical platform for MRD detection and is furthermore justified by the ongoing development of new targeted therapeutic options for patients with a sub-clonal relapse.

11) **Can MRD be of value in the elderly AML population treated with palliative strategies?**

Expert Perspective: It is generally accepted that MRD surveillance is a useful tool to evaluate the depth of response to intensive chemotherapy. However, the usefulness of MRD measurements in older patients treated with palliative strategies such as hypomethylating agents or—as in Case Study 4—with, e.g. an *IDH2*-inhibitor, remains controversial. For many patients, treatment with a hypomethylating agent does not necessarily even translate into morphological CR but might still keep the disease stable and controllable and thereby improve survival. Naturally, in these cases, MRD measurements are pointless. However, as new treatments are emerging (e.g. the add-on of a Bcl-2 inhibitor to hypomethylating agents), MRD is gaining attention in the elderly AML population, as obtaining MRD negativity actually has become a realistic treatment goal. To date, only a few prospective clinical studies have evaluated MRD in elderly AML patients, but more are under way. As the biology of *de novo* AML in the younger population is much different from AML in the elderly population who often have antecedent myelodysplastic syndrome, there will undoubtedly be other pitfalls to consider. The genetic complexity is much higher in elderly AML patients, and pre-leukemic, non-proliferating clones can be highly aberrant, e.g. by flow cytometry, making interpretation of MRD results quite challenging (see Chapter 8).

Recommended Readings

Balsat, M., Renneville, A., Thomas, X. et al. (2017). Postinduction minimal residual disease predicts outcome and benefit from allogeneic stem cell transplantation in acute myeloid leukemia with NPM1 mutation: a study by the acute leukemia french association group. *J Clin Oncol* 35 (2): 185–193.

Boyiadzis, M., Zhang, M.J., Chen, K., et al. (2023 May). Impact of pre transplant induction and consolidation cycles on AML allogeneic transplant outcomes: a CIBMTR analysis in 3113 AML patients. *Leukemia* 37 (5): 1006–1017. doi: 10.1038/s41375 022 01738 3. Epub 2022 Oct 30. Erratum in: (2023 March 22). *Leukemia* PMID: 36310182; PMCID: PMC10148918.

Buccisano, F., Dillon, R., Freeman, S.D., and Venditti, A. (2018). Role of minimal (measurable) residual disease assessment in older patients with acute myeloid leukemia. *Cancers (Basel)* 10 (7): 215.

Craddock, C. and Raghavan, M. (2019). Which patients with acute myeloid leukemia in CR1 can be spared an allogeneic transplant? *Curr Opin Hematol* 26 (2): 58–64.

Dillon, R., Hills, R., Freeman, S. et al. (2020). Molecular MRD status and outcome after transplantation in NPM1-mutated AML. *Blood* 135 (9): 680–688.

Döhner, H., Wei, A.H., Appelbaum, F.R., et al (2022). Diagnosis and Management of AML in Adults: 2022 ELN Recommendations from an International Expert Panel. *Blood* 7:blood.2022016867. Epub ahead of print.

Freeman, S.D., Hills, R.K., Virgo, P. et al. (2018). Measurable residual disease at induction redefines partial response in acute myeloid leukemia and stratifies outcomes in patients at standard risk without NPM1 mutations. *J Clin Oncol* 36 (15): 1486–1497.

Hokland, P., Ommen, H.B., Nyvold, C.G., and Roug, A.S. (2012). Sensitivity of minimal residual disease in acute myeloid leukaemia in first remission–methodologies in relation to their clinical situation. *Br J Haematol* 158 (5): 569–580.

Krönke, J., Schlenk, R.F., Jensen, K.-O. et al. (2011). Monitoring of minimal residual disease in NPM1-mutated acute myeloid leukemia: a study from the German-Austrian acute myeloid leukemia study group. *J Clin Oncol* 29 (19): 2709–2716.

Khoury, J.D., Solary, E., Abla, O. et al. (2022). The 5th edition of the World Health Organization Classification of Haematolymphoid Tumours: Myeloid and Histiocytic/Dendritic Neoplasms. *Leukemia* 36 (7):1703–1719.

Ommen, H.B. (2016). Monitoring minimal residual disease in acute myeloid leukaemia: a review of the current evolving strategies. *Ther Adv Hematol* 7 (1): 3–16.

Platzbecker, U., Wermke, M., Radke, J. et al. (2012). Azacitidine for treatment of imminent relapse in MDS or AML patients after allogeneic HSCT: results of the RELAZA trial. *Leukemia* 26 (3): 381–389.

Roug, A.S. and Ommen, H.B. (2019). Clinical use of measurable residual disease in acute myeloid leukemia. *Curr Treat Options Oncol* 20 (4): 28.

Schuurhuis, G.J., Heuser, M., Freeman, S. et al. (2018). Minimal/measurable residual disease in AML: a consensus document from the European LeukemiaNet MRD working party. *Blood* 131 (12): 1275–1291.

Shimony, S., Stahl, M., and Stone, R.M. (2023 March). Acute myeloid leukemia: 2023 update on diagnosis, risk stratification, and management. *Am J Hematol* 98 (3): 502–526. doi: 10.1002/ajh.26822. Epub 2023 Jan 13. PMID: 36594187.

Walter, R.B., Ofran, Y., Wierzbowska, A. et al. (2021). Measurable residual disease as a biomarker in acute myeloid leukemia: theoretical and practical considerations. *Leukemia* 35 (6): 1529–1538.

Wong, Z.C., Dillon, L.W., and Hourigan, C.S. (2023 June). Measurable residual disease in patients undergoing allogeneic transplant for acute myeloid leukemia. *Best Pract Res Clin Haematol* 36 (2): 101468. doi: 10.1016/j.beha.2023.101468. Epub 2023 Apr 18. PMID: 37353292; PMCID: PMC10291441.

11

Hematopoietic Cell Transplantation and Cellular Therapy in Acute Myeloid Leukemia

Piyanuch Kongtim and Stefan O. Ciurea

University of California, Irvine, CA

Introduction

Acute myeloid leukemia (AML) is a heterogeneous disease characterized by a variety of underlying genetic aberrations, which are associated with distinct prognostic features. Even though several targeted drugs along with intensive chemotherapy have been shown to induce high response rates, a significant proportion of patients eventually relapse (see Chapters 6, 7, and 8). Allogeneic hematopoietic cell transplant (allo-HCT) is a standard post-induction remission therapy for patients with intermediate- or high-risk AML both in first CR and with advanced disease. This treatment modality offers the benefit of more intense conditioning chemotherapy in appropriate candidates as well as graft-versus-leukemia (GVL) effect from donor T- and NK-cells, which better help eradicate leukemic clones than conventional chemotherapy. Several advances in transplant procedures and supportive care, as well as the use of alternative donors, have dramatically increased transplant numbers performed worldwide with significant improvement in survival outcomes (see Chapters 60 and 61). According to data from the Center for International Blood and Marrow Transplant Research (CIBMTR) more than 3,000 transplants have been performed for patients with AML in the United States in 2019. The benefits of allo-HCT, however, comes with the risk of transplant-related mortality (TRM). It is therefore critical to identify AML patients with high risk for disease relapse whose benefit outweighs the risks, as well as to customize the transplant procedure for each patient based on comorbidities and disease.

In this chapter, we present a representative number of AML case studies with different scenarios and guidance on transplant procedure selection based on the current available evidence.

Cancer Consult: Expertise in Clinical Practice, Volume 2: Neoplastic Hematology & Cellular Therapy,
Second Edition. Edited by Syed A. Abutalib, Maurie Markman, James O. Armitage, and Kenneth C. Anderson.
© 2024 John Wiley & Sons Ltd. Published 2024 by John Wiley & Sons Ltd.

Case Study 1

A 24-year-old female presented with low-grade fever and shortness of breath. Her initial WBC was 62 × 10^9/L, hemoglobin 5.9 g/dL, and platelets of 35 × 10^9/L. Bone marrow examination revealed AML with 83% myeloblasts. Genomic analysis revealed a normal diploid karyotype with *FLT3* internal tandem duplication mutations (*FLT3–ITD*) and *NPM1* mutation. She achieved a complete morphologic remission following induction therapy with the 7 + 3 regimen plus midostaurin.

She has a sibling who is a half (5/10) HLA match. An unrelated donor search yielded multiple 8/10 HLA match unrelated donors and 4/6 HLA matched umbilical cord blood (UCB) units. She recently completed her first consolidation with intermediate-dose cytarabine combined with midostaurin and remains in complete morphologic and molecular remission. Her Karnofsky performance status was 90% without significant comorbidities.

1) **What would be the best approach at this time?**
    A) Maintenance with midostaurin.
    B) Complete three cycles of intermediate-dose cytarabine plus midostaurin.
    C) Double UCB transplantation.
    D) 8/10 matched unrelated donor transplantation.
    E) Haploidentical transplantation.

Expert Perspective: Cytogenetics at diagnosis remains the most important prognostic factor in AML, and the benefit of aggressive consolidation strategies such as allo-HCT in first remission (CR1) in patients with high-risk cytogenetics is well established (see Chapter 6). Using newer technologies such as PCR or next-generation sequencing (NGS), a number of molecular mutations have been found to be significantly associated with the development and prognosis of AML and have been used to further refine AML prognosis. *NPM1* and *FLT3-ITD* represent two of the most common molecular alterations found in AML with normal cytogenetics (CN-AML). It has been shown that *NPM1* mutation conveys a favorable prognosis only in the absence of a *FLT3-ITD*, whereas the presence of *FLT3-ITD* mutations is widely accepted as a poor prognostic factor in CN-AML owing to its chemoresistance, high risk of relapse, and short relapse-free survival.

Several *FLT3* inhibitors have been studied; however, quizartinib and midostaurin has been approved for the treatment of newly diagnosed *FLT3*-mutated AML patients. The approval of midostaurin was based on the phase III RATIFY/CALGB 10603 trial, which demonstrated improved survival with the addition of midostaurin to intensive chemotherapy followed by single-agent maintenance therapy in patients aged younger than 60 years with newly diagnosed *FLT3*-mutated AML. In this study post-remission consolidation with allo-HCT was allowed, and more than half of the patients received allo-HCT at some point during the disease course. Efficacy of quizartinib with chemotherapy was evaluated in QuANTUM-First (NCT02668653), a randomized, double-blind, placebo-controlled trial of 539 patients with newly diagnosed FLT3-ITD positive AML. Patients were randomized (1:1) to receive quizartinib (n=268) or placebo (n=271) with induction and consolidation therapy and as maintenance monotherapy according to the initial assignment. There was no re-randomization at the initiation of post-consolidation therapy. Patients who proceeded to allo-HCT initiated maintenance therapy after allo-HCT recovery. The primary analysis was conducted after a minimum follow-up of 24 months after the last patient was randomized. The trial demonstrated a statistically significant improvement in OS for the quizartinib arm [hazard ratio (HR) 0.78; 95% CI: 0.62, 0.98; 2-sided p=0.0324]. The CR rate in the quizartinib arm was 55% (95% CI: 48.7, 60.9) with a median duration of 38.6 months (95% CI: 21.9, NE), and the CR rate in those receiving placebo was 55% (95% CI: 49.2, 61.4) with a median duration of 12.4 months (95% CI: 8.8, 22.7). There is no evidence to support that midostaurin or quizartinib consolidation or maintenance should replace allo-HCT in transplant candidates.

Although there is no prospective trial demonstrating that allo-HCT improves overall survival (OS) in *FLT3–ITD*-mutated patients, multiple retrospective series have shown that survival was significantly improved when allo-HCT was performed in first CR compared to nontransplant alternatives such as high-dose cytarabine and targeted therapy. In a study from Johns Hopkins, DeZern and colleagues (2011) showed a significantly better relapse-free survival of *FLT3-ITD*-mutated AML patients treated with allo-HCT as compared to non-transplant group (54 months vs 8.6 months). This series included patients who underwent allo-HCT from various donor types, including with haploidentical donors. Oran et al. (2016) compared post-remission treatment with consolidation chemotherapy and allo-HCT in 227 *FLT3*-mutated AML patients who achieved first CR after induction chemotherapy. Result from this study showed that allo-HCT reduced risk of relapse and improved both RFS and OS regardless of *NPM1* mutation status and *FLT3* allelic ratio. The OS and relapse-free survival at three years were 18% and 24%, respectively, for patients receiving chemotherapy and 46% and 54%, respectively, for those undergoing allo-HCT.

Moreover, Gaballa et al. (2017) analyzed outcomes of 200 *FLT3*-mutated AML patients (either *ITD* or *TKD* mutations) treated with allo-HCT with various donor types including haploidentical donor transplants. This study showed a dramatic increase in relapse rate and progressively worse progression-free survival (PFS) for patients transplanted beyond first CR, suggesting that patients benefit the most by receiving allo-HCT in first remission, and that lack of an HLA-matched donor type should not be a limitation transplantation, as they found that haploidentical transplants had similar survival compared with HLA-matched donor transplants.

Over the past decade, there have been remarkable developments in the field of haploidentical allo-HCT with significant improvements in TRM and transplant outcomes. These results have demonstrated that barriers associated with transplantation using major HLA-mismatched donors can be overcome, extending donor availability to virtually all patients in need, with outcomes comparable with HLA-matched transplantations. Using data of AML patients from the CIBMTR, showed that among patients receiving myeloablative conditioning (MAC) regimens, three-year probabilities of OS were 45% and 50% after haploidentical and matched unrelated donor transplants (*P* = 0.38). Corresponding rates after reduced intensity conditioning (RIC) transplants were 46% and 44% (*P* = 0.71), respectively.

Moreover, result from parallel phase II prospective studies from MD Anderson Cancer Center showed one-year OS and PFS rates of 70% and 60%, respectively, in patients receiving a haploidentical transplant and 60% and 47%, respectively, in those receiving allo-HCT from a 9/10 matched unrelated donor. Although this was a nonrandomized study and could not serve as a direct comparison between the two groups, haploidentical allo-HCT should be a preferred option over a mismatched unrelated donor, not only because of more promising outcomes but also its prompt availability, especially for patients with high risk of disease relapse who need to proceed urgently to allo-HCT, as in our patient.

Outcomes of haploidentical and double UCB transplants using a RIC regimen in adult patients with high-risk hematologic malignancies were also compared in a BMT CTN 1101 randomized controlled trial. Results from this study showed a significantly lower TRM (11% vs 18%) and significantly better OS (57% vs 46%) in patients who received a haploidentical transplant (Fuchs et al. 2021).

Taken together, available evidence suggests that allo-HCT ameliorates the negative prognostic impact of *FLT3-ITD* mutations by lowering relapse rate and is the preferred consolidation treatment for younger AML patients with *FLT3-ITD* mutations after achieving first complete remission. The use of haploidentical donors has expanded donor availability to virtually all patients in need and should be considered a preferred alternative option for patients without an HLA-matched donor or those who urgently need a transplant to prevent disease relapse.

Correct Answer: E

Case Study 2

A 45-year-old male presented with dyspnea on exertion and fatigue for two weeks before admission. His WBC was 30×10^9/L with 65% blasts, hemoglobin 7 g/dL, and platelets 12×10^9/L. The bone marrow study revealed 75% myeloblasts that were immunophenotypically CD34+, CD117+, CD13+, and CD33+. The karyotyping study showed a normal diploid karyotype while molecular profiling revealed *IDH1* and *NRAS* mutations. Patient achieved morphologic remission after induction with 7 + 3 regimen and completed the first consolidation with intermediate-dose cytarabine and remains in complete morphologic remission. Repeat NGS study shows persistence of both *IDH1* and *NRAS* mutations after induction as well as after first consolidation. He has hematopoietic cell transplant comorbidity index (HCT-CI) of 2 due to BMI > 35 and diabetes. His Karnofsky performance status is 90%. He has an HLA-matched brother who is ready to proceed with the stem cell donation.

2) What would be the most appropriate further management in this patient?
   A) Complete three cycles of consolidation with intermediate-dose cytarabine.
   B) Ivosidenib 500 mg orally daily.
   C) Allogeneic transplantation using myeloablative conditioning (MAC) regimen.
   D) Allogeneic transplantation using reduced intensity conditioning (RIC) regimen.
   E) Autologous stem cell transplant.

Expert Perspective: Measurable/minimal residual disease (MRD) after treatment measured by either multiparametric flow cytometry (MFC-MRD), quantitative PCR (RQ-PCR), or NGS has been shown to predict relapse and survival of patients with AML (see Chapter 10). However, method and timing of MRD test have not been well established and standardized. The decision on optimal MRD monitoring method depends on the presence of leukemia-specific genetic abnormality or immunophenotypic feature of leukemic clone. It has been shown that persistent MRD (MRD+) after induction therapy is strongly associated with an increased risk of relapse and poor survival regardless of cytogenetic risk group or type of induction treatment. Using multiparametric flow cytometry (MFC) to detect MRD in 547 patients with AML in CR1, showed that OS and relapse-free survival were significantly better in patients without MRD after completed induction treatment compared with MRD-positive patients. Multivariable analysis with adjustment for covariables demonstrated that the incidence of relapse was significantly reduced after allo-HCT compared with chemotherapy or autologous hematopoietic stem cell transplantation (hazard ratio [HR] 0.36; $P < 0.001$).

In the GIMEMA AML1310 study, patients with National Comprehensive Cancer Network (NCCN) 2009 intermediate-risk AML were treated with allo-HCT if they have positive MFC-MRD after one cycle of consolidation while those with negative MFC-MRD received autologous stem cell transplantation. Using this risk-adapted approach, no difference in survival was observed between MRD+ and MRD groups, suggesting that allo-HCT can overcome poor prognosis of MRD positivity. Based on the currently available evidence, MRD monitoring has been recommended as a standard practice to tailor post-induction treatment. According to the current NCCN guidelines (NCCN V3.2022) and the most recent European LeukemiaNet (ELN) recommendations (Döhner et al. 2022), allo-HCT should be considered in favorable or intermediate genetic risk AML patients with positive MRD after remission induction.

Regarding type of conditioning regimen for allo-HCT, ultra-deep DNA sequencing were used to measure MRD from blood samples from patients treated in the BMT CTN 0901 study (a phase III randomized clinical trial that compared outcomes by conditioning intensity in adult patients with myeloid malignancy undergoing an allo-HCT while in morphologic CR). Result from this study revealed a higher relapse rate and inferior OS and RFS in patients with persistent MRD before transplant who received allo-HCT using RIC compared with MAC regimens (Hourigan et al. 2020).

Our patient has persistent MRD positivity after completed induction and after consolidation, which indicates chemoresistance nature of the leukemic clone. This patient would benefit from myeloablative conditioning and the GVL effect of allo-HCT.

Correct Answer: C

Case Study 3

A 32-year-old man with relapsed AML following an HLA-matched-related allo-HCT was referred to your clinic for further treatment recommendations. Three years ago, he was diagnosed with AML-M4 with diploid cytogenetics, *FLT3-ITD* mutation negative, and *NPM1* mutation positive. He achieved a CR1 after standard induction therapy with the 7 + 3 regimen and proceeded with four cycles of high-dose cytarabine consolidation. After relapsing nine months later, the patient underwent re-induction therapy, again achieved a CR, and received an allo-HCT using stem cells from his HLA-matched brother. The post-transplant course was uncomplicated, and his immunosuppressive therapy has been discontinued without evidence of GvHD. Unfortunately, he relapsed on day +380 with findings of 90% blasts in the bone marrow. Unsorted chimerism study at the time to relapse showed 70% donor cells. He achieved a complete morphologic remission following salvage with a clofarabine-based regimen. On his most recent evaluation, a mutation in exon 12 of the *NPM1* gene was still detectable by PCR. He has 0 score on HCT-CI scale with a Karnofsky performance status of 90%.

3) What is the best treatment strategy at this time?
   A) Supportive care and close clinical observation.
   B) Donor lymphocyte infusion (DLI) from his prior sibling donor.
   C) A second matched related donor transplant using a different conditioning regimen.

D) A cord blood transplant.

E) Azacitidine maintenance indefinitely.

Expert Perspective: Outcomes of AML patients with relapsed disease post allo-HCT are dismal and remains a major therapeutic challenge since the current available treatment options are limited. Patients who developed significant toxic effects from the first allo-HCT are generally offered supportive care or low-intensity treatment. A small proportion of patients will achieve another remission with salvage therapy and are considered for a second allo-HCT or DLI.

In a retrospective CIBMTR study of 1,788 AML patients who relapsed after the first allo-HCT, the three-year OS correlated with time from first allo-HCT to relapse (4% for relapse during the 1-to-6-month period, 12% during the six-month to two-year period, 26% during the 2-to-3-year period, and 38% for ⩾ 3 years). Median survival was seven months (range, 1 to 177 months) among patients receiving DLI and 12 months (1–150 months) among those receiving second allo-HCT. In multivariable analysis, lower mortality was significantly associated with longer time from allo-HCT to relapse and a first allo-HCT using RIC, while age > 40 years, active GvHD, adverse cytogenetics, mismatched unrelated donor, and use of UCB for first allo-HCT were significantly associated with poor survival (Bejanyan et al. 2015). Another retrospective analysis from the European Society for Blood and Marrow Transplantation (EBMT) comparing outcomes of AML relapsing after first allo-HCT among those who did or did not receive DLI as part of post-relapse treatment showed a significantly improved OS with DLI (21% vs 9% at two years, P < 0.001). Two-year survival was 56% if DLI was performed in remission or with favorable karyotype and 15% if DLI was given in aplasia or with active disease (Schmid et al. 2007).

Currently, there is no randomized clinical trial comparing outcomes of a second allo-HCT *vs.* DLI in this setting. Several factors can influence the treatment decision such as remission status after relapse, donor availability, patient performance status, and presence of significant comorbidities or GvHD, as well as physician preference.

The EBMT group retrospectively compared outcomes of second allo-HCT vs DLI in AML patients with relapsed disease after first allo-HCT. In this study, there was no apparent difference in OS whether a second allo-HCT or DLI was prescribed (two-year OS 26% with allo-HCT vs 25% with DLI, P = 0.86). Moreover, result from subgroup analysis of patients who received a second allo-HCT did not show a significant difference in OS and NRM between patients transplanted using the same or different donor (Kharfan-Dabaja et al. 2018).

Our patient has more than six-month remission duration after the first transplant. He would benefit from cellular therapy either second allo-HCT or DLI. Even though there is no available evidence to support a second allo-HCT over DLI, in younger and physically fit patients, using a readily available donor and different conditioning regimen is preferred.

Correct Answer: C

Case Study 4

An active and otherwise healthy 68-year-old man was recently diagnosed with AML and referred to you after completion of induction chemotherapy. The patient originally presented after atypical cells were incidentally found on a preoperative workup before an elective surgical procedure two months ago. A bone marrow biopsy demonstrated the presence of leukemic blasts occupying 22% of total nucleated cells; karyotype revealed deletion of chromosome 8 in 8/20 metaphases. *ASXL1* mutations was detected by NGS. Patient received induction therapy with cytarabine 200 mg/m^2 and daunorubicin 45 mg/m^2. He achieved a complete morphologic remission. However, MFC-MRD remains positive at four weeks after induction therapy. He is an only child and has three healthy adult sons. A potential full HLA-matched unrelated donor was identified within the donor registry. The patient and his family are inquiring about the best curative approach currently. He denies comorbidity, and Karnofsky performance status is 90%.

4) What is your recommendation for this patient?
   A) Standard-dose cytarabine (200 mg/m^2) +/– daunorubicin.
   B) Azacitidine + venetoclax.
   C) Haploidentical transplant from his youngest son.
   D) Unrelated donor allogeneic transplantation.
   E) Close observation.

Expert Perspective: AML more frequently affect elderly patients with a median age at diagnosis of 70 years. Elderly patients with AML usually have a worse prognosis than those in the younger population primarily due to multiple comorbidities and intrinsic biologic factors underlying disease resistance. Despite achieving a CR with conventional chemo-therapy, response is typically short, and majority of patients relapse within six months without allo-HCT. The development of RIC and advances in supportive care have dramat-ically decreased TRM, improved survival, and expanded allo-HCT access to the elderly population during the past decades.

Using data of AML/MDS patients 40 years of age or older who received RIC allo-HCT from the CIBMTR, McClune et al. (2010) found that there were no significant differences in outcomes among allo-HCT recipients aged 40 to 50 years versus those older than 65 years.

Moreover, a retrospective analysis of AML/MDS patients older than 60 years demon-strated a PFS benefit in patients treated with post-induction allo-HCT compared with no allo-HCT. A meta-analysis of 13 studies of allo-HCT in elderly (> 60 years) AML patients showed relapse-free survival at six months, one, two, and three years of 62%, 47%, 44%, and 35%, respectively. The corresponding numbers for OS were 73%, 58%, 45%, and 38%, respectively (Rashidi et al. 2016). Taken together, these encouraging outcomes of allo-HCT in elderly AML patients indicate that age alone should not be an absolute contraindication to proceed with allo-HCT when pursuing a curative approach. A significant proportion of elderly patients who are physically fit may expect to be alive for a period of over three years after allo-HCT.

Regarding donor choice, encouraging outcomes have been reported using a haploidenti-cal allo-HCT in elderly patients (> 55 years or older) with AML and MDS with two-year PFS incidence for patients in CR1/2 of 63% (Ciurea et al. 2018). Moreover, haploidentical trans-plants with melphalan-based conditioning has been shown to overcome negative impact of MRD positivity before transplant. In a study by Srour et al. (2019), there was no survival differences in AML patients in CR with and without MRD who were treated with a haploi-dentical allo-HCT.

With the use of post-transplant cyclophosphamide for GvHD prophylaxis, several studies have shown that outcome of haploidentical allo-HCT are now comparable with

HLA-matched allo-HCT. Additionally, the rapid availability of a haploidentical donor is a major advantage over an HLA-matched unrelated donor especially for patients with high risk of disease relapse who need to proceed urgently to allo-HCT.

The case described in this vignette is not an uncommon scenario since adverse genetic risk is more frequently found in older patients. The best treatment approach for this patient, who is physically fit and looking to pursue a cure, is consolidation with an allo-HCT from a haploidentical donor with a RIC regimen as soon as possible given that the patient has high-risk disease and persistent MRD positivity.

Correct Answer: C

Case Study 5

A 39-year-old female was diagnosed with AML. Bone marrow cytogenetic study revealed > 3 clonal abnormalities including monosomy 7. She achieved CR after standard 7 + 3 induction chemotherapy and subsequently underwent a matched-sibling donor allo-HCT consolidation with MAC regimen. Tacrolimus and methotrexate were used for GvHD prophylaxis. The post-transplant course was uncomplicated. She achieved neutrophil and platelet engraftment at day +12 and +16 post-transplant, respectively. The disease reevaluation at day +30 revealed a complete morphologic remission with normal diploid karyotype and 100% donor chimerism. Post-transplant MRD was not detected by both MFC and NGS study. She is currently at 60 days post transplant and remains on tacrolimus without evidence of GvHD.

5) What would be the best further management for this patient?
   A) Early immunosuppression discontinuation.
   B) Low-dose 5-azacitidine maintenance.
   C) Low-dose decitabine maintenance until disease progression.
   D) Prophylactic DLI.
   E) Clinical trial of maintenance therapy post transplant.

Expert Perspective: Outcomes of patients with AML are strongly influenced by genetic factors. Among the unfavorable cytogenetic group, the presence of at least three unrelated clonal cytogenetic abnormalities, often designated as a complex karyotype, generally has been considered as associated with one of the worst outcomes both following conventional chemotherapy and allo-HCT (Döhner et al. 2022). Disease relapse is the most common cause of treatment failure for patients with complex karyotype AML after transplantation. A joint retrospective study of 1,342 patients with complex karyotype AML treated with allo-HCT by the Acute Leukemia Working Party (ALWP) of the EBMT and MD Anderson Cancer Center showed that approximately half of the patients experienced disease relapse within two years post transplant. The cumulative incidence of relapse at two years for patients in CR1, CR2, and with active disease at transplantation was 46%, 48%, and 63%, respectively ($P < 0.001$). The probabilities of leukemia free survival, OS, and GvHD and relapse-free survival at two years post transplantation were 31.3%, 36.8%, and 19.8%, respectively. Age, active disease at transplant, secondary AML, and presence of deletion/monosomy 5 or 7 were important predictors for high risk of relapse and poor survival (Ciurea et al. 2018).

Given the dismal prognosis of patients who have disease relapse after allo-HCT, various approaches aimed at preventing disease relapse in high-risk AML patients have been studied. Immune suppression discontinuation is a common practice after allo-HCT. This approach is based on the hypothesis that early discontinuation will allow a stronger GVL effect mediated by donor T and NK cells. However, this strategy could potentially put patients at risk of development of GvHD as well as mortality.

Using data of patients from two of phase III BMT-CTN studies (n = 827), Pidala and colleagues (2020) showed that earlier discontinuation of immune suppression was associated with approximately 40% of development of GvHD, without lower relapse rate and did not confer survival benefit.

It has been shown that hypomethylating agents (HMAs) such as 5-azacitidine and decitabine have efficacy against AML and MDS clone through epigenetic modification. Owing to their tolerable safety profile, HMAs are the most commonly adopted non-targeted strategy for relapse prevention post transplant with several early phase studies reporting their potential benefit. However, a recent phase III randomized study failed to demonstrate improvement in relapse and survival benefit of maintenance therapy with low-dose 5-azacitadine over no maintenance in high-risk AML and MDS patients who achieved a CR after transplant (Oran et al. 2020).

Another phase II, open-label, multicenter, randomized controlled trial conducted in China showed a significantly lower relapse rate, better leukemia-free survival, and OS in high-risk AML patients with MRD-negative CR after transplant who received minimal dose of decitabine (5 mg/m^2 for 5 days) in combination with G-CSF compared with no maintenance therapy. In this study, two-year cumulative incidence of relapse was 15% in decitabine +G-CSF group compared with 38% in control group (HR 0.32, $P < 0.01$) and the corresponding leukemia-free survival was 82% vs 61% (HR 0.38, $P < 0.01$). Approximately 97% of patients tolerated at least four cycles, and 96% of patients completed all four cycles. This regimen was very well tolerated with only 13% of the patients developing grade 3–4 neutropenia or thrombocytopenia requiring growth factor supports. Despite the promising outcomes, this combination has not been approved as a standard post-transplant maintenance.

To increase GVL effect after allo-HCT, the efficacy of DLI given either preemptively in patients who had MRD positivity after transplant or prophylaxis in high-risk patients with complete chimerism and negative MRD has been reported in several small studies. (Jedlickova et al. (2016) reported the results of a retrospective analysis assessing the safety and efficacy of prophylactic DLI following RIC allo-HCT in a cohort of 46 high-risk AML patients. Patients receiving DLI were in CR for at least 120 days from transplantation, being off immunosuppression for at least 30 days, being free of GvHD, without history of acute GvHD grade III–IV, and having no severe infection. Seven patients were given one, 15 patients two, and 24 patients three infusions. Compared with control group, relapse rate was significantly lower in the DLI group (22% vs 53%, $P = 0.004$), resulted in a superior OS (67% vs 31% at seven years, $P < 0.001$), and leukemia-free survival (68% vs 38% at six years, $P = 0.01$). Grade II–IV acute GvHD and extensive chronic GvHD was seen in 9% and 11%, respectively.

The ALWP of the EBMT recently reported outcomes of 318 adult patients with acute leukemia receiving preemptive (n = 192) or prophylactic DLI (n = 126) after HLA-matched donor allo-HCT.

For the prophylactic DLI cohort, the five-year non-relapse mortality, relapse, leukemia-free survival, and OS were 10%, 28%, 62%, and 68%, respectively. The respective results after preemptive DLI for MRD positivity were 9%, 44%, 47%, and 51% and for preemptive DLI for mixed chimerism were 15%, 28%, 57%, and 63%, respectively. The cumulative incidence of clinically relevant acute GvHD or chronic GvHD was 33.7% at five years.

Even though the results of several post-transplant strategies to prevent relapse in high-risk AML patients are promising, prospective randomized studies are needed to confirm the benefit and establish the standard initiation time post transplant of these approaches. Until then, patients with high-risk disease, such as our patient, should be treated on well-designed clinical trials.

Correct Answer: E

6) **What is the role of post-transplant sorafenib maintenance in patients with *FLT3* positive AML?**
   A) Sorafenib maintenance post allo-HCT improves progression-free-survival but not overall survival.
   B) Sorafenib maintenance post allo-HCT improves relapse-free-survival and overall survival.
   C) Sorafenib maintenance post allo-HCT improves relapse-free-survival but not overall survival.
   D) Sorafenib maintenance post allo-HCT in patients with *FLT3* positive AML has not been tested in a randomized trial.

Expert Perspective: *FLT3*-mutated AML patients have a high risk of relapse after allo-HCT. Two recent prospectively randomized controlled trials have shown a benefit from sorafenib maintenance after allo-HCT: (i) the placebo-controlled SORMAIN trial, and (ii) an open-label phase III trial from China. Both trials demonstrated that sorafenib maintenance post allo-HCT improves PFS and OS in *FLT3-ITD*-mutated AML. The primary endpoint in SORMAIN and the Chinese trial was RFS. After a median follow-up of 41.8 months in SORMAIN, median RFS was not reached with sorafenib versus 30.9 months with placebo (HR 0.39, 95% CI 0.18–0.85; P = 0.013). Sorafenib reduced the risk of relapse or death by 75% (HR 0.25, P = 0.002) in SORMAIN. In the Chinese phase III trial, the median follow-up duration is 21.3 months. The two-year leukemia-free survival was 78.9% versus 56.6% (HR 0.37, 95% CI 0.22–0.63; P < 0.0001). At 24 months, OS was higher with sorafenib versus placebo in SORMAIN (90.5% versus 66.2%; HR 0.24, 95% CI 0.08–0.74; P = 0.007) and also the phase III trial (82.1% versus 68.0%, HR 0.48, 95% CI 0.27–0.86; P = 0.012). Thus, for *FLT3-ITD*-mutated AML, there is strong evidence for a post allo-HCT maintenance therapy with sorafenib.

Correct Answer: B

Case Study 6

A 60-year-old woman was diagnosed with AML after initially presenting with fevers and gingival bleeding. Diagnostic workup revealed pancytopenia and a hypercellular marrow with significant dysplastic megakaryocytes and 58% myeloblasts. She had normal diploid cytogenetics. NGS was positive for *TP53* mutation. Her past medical history was positive for breast cancer, which has been in remission for five years after surgery and adjuvant chemotherapy, which consisted of cyclophosphamide, doxorubicin, and paclitaxel. Regarding AML, she achieved a CR with negative MRD by flow cytometry after two cycles of induction chemotherapy with CPX351 (a fixed combination of liposomal formulation of daunorubicin and cytarabine). She has KPS of 90% and HCT-CI of 3 due to history of breast cancer. She has a brother who is an HLA match. Multiple 5/6 cord blood units are available.

7) Which consolidation strategy would you recommend at this time?
    A) Consolidation with two cycles of high-dose cytarabine.
    B) Consolidation with two more cycles of CPX351.
    C) Decitabine maintenance.
    D) Urgent transplant using the HLA-matched donor.
    E) Umbilical cord blood transplantation due to lower relapse rate.

Expert Perspective: According to the 5th edition of the WHO classification, AML arising in patients exposed to cytotoxic (DNA-damaging) therapy for an unrelated condition is categorized as myeloid neoplasms post cytotoxic therapy (MN-pCT) (Khoury et al. 2022).

AML-pCT accounts for approximately 5–20% of all AML cases, commonly associated with adverse genetic alterations such as complex karyotypes or *TP53* mutations while normal karyotype among t-AML is found in approximately 20% of all AML-pCT cases.

Outcomes of patients with AML-pCT are generally poor compared to *de novo* AML because its adverse disease biology results in suboptimal responses to conventional chemotherapy despite having normal karyotype. According to data of 742 patients with newly diagnosed AML and normal karyotype from MD Anderson Cancer Center, outcomes were significantly inferior in patients with AML-pCT compared with *de novo* AML with a median RFS of 12 months and 15 months, respectively (HR 1.55; $P = 0.02$).

AML/MDS patients with *TP53* mutation have a particularly poor prognosis including with transplantation. However, urgent transplantation with a readily available donor for patients with good performance status and low HCT-CI has been shown to be associated with better survival (Ciurea et al. 2018).

CPX351 (liposomal formulation of cytarabine and daunorubicin in a 5:1 ratio), has been recently approved as induction treatment for patients with cytotoxic therapy-related or secondary AML, age 60–75 years (for all age groups in Europe). The approval was based on results of an open-label, randomized, phase III trial, which demonstrated superior response rates and survival benefit of CPX351 over the conventional 7 + 3 regimen (Lancet et al. 2018). In this study, consolidation with allo-HCT was allowed, and results from the post hoc analyses showed that median OS of patients who achieved a CR or CRi (complete remission with incomplete count recovery) and underwent allo-HCT was not reached in the CPX351 arm compared with 11.6 months from allo-HCT in the 7 + 3 arm (HR 0.43;

95% CI 0.21–0.89; Lin et al. 2021). Even though there was no direct comparison between allo-HCT and no allo-HCT group, these results indicate that older patients with AML-pCT who achieve a CR after CPX351 induction can achieve long-term survival after allo-HCT consolidation. Patients who are deemed as candidates for allo-HCT and who have an available donor should be transplanted in first remission.

A recent study of 1,531 patients with AML-pCT (n = 759) or t-AML (n = 772) who were treated with allo-HCT between 2000 and 2014 by the CIBMTR demonstrated disease-free survival and OS at five years of 23% and 25%, respectively, for AML-pCT. Probability of five-year disease-free survival of AML-pCT patients receiving allo-HCT in CR1 was 30% and 8%, respectively, for those transplanted in beyond first CR. Regarding donor type, in multivariable analysis, allo-HCT using mismatched unrelated donors or UCB were associated with significantly higher risk of non-relapse mortality (Metheny et al. 2021).

Correct Answer: D

Recommended Readings

Bejanyan, N., Weisdorf, D.J. et al. (2015). Survival of patients with acute myeloid leukemia relapsing after allogeneic hematopoietic cell transplantation: a center for international blood and marrow transplant research study. *Biol Blood Marrow Transplant* 21 (3): 454–459.

Bolaños-Meade, J., Hamadani, M., Wu, J. et al. (2023 June 22). BMT CTN 1703 investigators. Post-transplantation cyclophosphamide-based graft-versus-host disease prophylaxis. *N Engl J Med* 388 (25): 2338–2348. doi: 10.1056/NEJMoa2215943. PMID: 37342922.

Burchert, A. et al. (2021). Sorafenib maintenance after allogeneic hematopoietic stem cell transplantation for acute myeloid leukemia with FLT3-internal tandem duplication mutation (SORMAIN). *J Clin Oncol* 39: 1412–1413.

Ciurea, S.O. et al. (2018). Haploidentical transplantation for older patients with acute myeloid leukemia and myelodysplastic syndrome. *Biol Blood Marrow Transplant* 24 (6): 1232–1236.

Ciurea, S.O., Zhang, M.J., Bacigalupo, A.A. et al. (2015). Haploidentical transplant with posttransplant cyclophosphamide vs matched unrelated donor transplant for acute myeloid leukemia. *Blood* 126 (8): 1033–1040.

DeZern, A.E., Sung, A., Kim, S. et al. (2011). Role of allogeneic transplantation for FLT3/ITD acute myeloid leukemia: outcomes from 133 consecutive newly diagnosed patients from a single institution. *Biol Blood Marrow Transplant* 17 (9): 1404–1409.

Dholaria, B. et al. (2021). Hematopoietic cell transplantation in the treatment of newly diagnosed adult acute myeloid leukemia: an evidence-based review from the american society of transplantation and cellular therapy. *Transplant Cell Ther* 27 (1): 6–20.

Döhner, H., Wei, A.H., Appelbaum, F.R. et al. (2022). Diagnosis and management of AML in adults: 2022 recommendations from an international expert panel on behalf of the ELN. *Blood* 140 (12): 1345–77.

Fuchs, E.J., O'Donnell, P.V. et al. (2021). Double unrelated umbilical cord blood vs HLA-haploidentical bone marrow transplantation: the BMT CTN 1101 trial. *Blood* 137 (3): 420–428.

Gaballa, S,, Saliba, R. et al. (2017). Relapse risk and survival in patients with FLT3 mutated acute myeloid leukemia undergoing stem cell transplantation. *Am J Hematol* 92 (4): 331–337.

Hourigan, C.S., Dillon, L.W. et al. (2020). Impact of conditioning intensity of allogeneic transplantation for acute myeloid leukemia with genomic evidence of residual disease. *J Clin Oncol* 38 (12): 1273–1283.

Jedlickova, Z., Schmid, C. et al. (2016). Long-term results of adjuvant donor lymphocyte transfusion in AML after allogeneic stem cell transplantation. *Bone Marrow Transplant* 51 (5): 663–667.

Kharfan-Dabaja, M.A. et al. (2018). Association of second allogeneic hematopoietic cell transplant vs donor lymphocyte infusion with overall survival in patients with acute myeloid leukemia relapse. *JAMA Oncol* 4 (9): 1245–1253.

Kharfan-Dabaja, M.A., Labopin, M. et al. (2018). Association of second allogeneic hematopoietic cell transplant vs donor lymphocyte infusion with overall survival in patients with acute myeloid leukemia relapse. *JAMA Oncol* 4 (9): 1245–1253.

Khoury, J.D., Solary, E. et al. (2022). The 5th edition of the world health organization classification of haematolymphoid tumours: myeloid and histiocytic/dendritic neoplasms. *Leukemia* 36 (7): 1703–19.

Lancet, J.E., Uy, G.L. et al. (2018). CPX-351 (cytarabine and daunorubicin) liposome for injection versus conventional cytarabine plus daunorubicin in older patients with newly diagnosed secondary acute myeloid leukemia. *J Clin Oncol* 36 (26): 2684–2692.

Lin, T.L., Rizzieri, D.A. et al. (2021). Older adults with newly diagnosed high-risk/secondary AML who achieved remission with CPX-351: phase 3 post hoc analyses. *Blood Adv* 5 (6): 1719–1728.

McClune, B.L., Weisdorf, D.J. et al. (2010). Effect of age on outcome of reduced-intensity hematopoietic cell transplantation for older patients with acute myeloid leukemia in first complete remission or with myelodysplastic syndrome. *J Clin Oncol* 28 (11): 1878–1887.

Metheny, L. et al. (2021). Allogeneic transplantation to treat therapy-related myelodysplastic syndrome and acute myelogenous leukemia in adults. *Transplant Cell Ther* 27 (11): 923. e1–923.e12.

Metheny, L., Callander, N.S. et al. (2021). Allogeneic transplantation to treat therapy-related myelodysplastic syndrome and acute myelogenous leukemia in adults. *Transplant Cell Ther* 27 (11): 923.e921–923.e912.

Oran, B., Cortes, J. et al. (2016). Allogeneic transplantation in first remission improves outcomes irrespective of FLT3-ITD allelic ratio in FLT3-ITD-positive acute myelogenous leukemia. *Biol Blood Marrow Transplant* 22 (7): 1218–1226.

Oran, B., de Lima, M. et al. (2020). A phase 3 randomized study of 5-azacitidine maintenance vs observation after transplant in high-risk AML and MDS patients. *Blood Adv* 4 (21): 5580–5588.

Pidala, J., Martens, M., Anasetti, C., Carreras, J., Horowitz, M., Lee, S.J., Antin, J., Cutler, C., and Logan, B. (2020 January 1). Factors associated with successful discontinuation of immune suppression after allogeneic hematopoietic cell transplantation. *JAMA Oncol* 6 (1): e192974. doi: 10.1001/jamaoncol.2019.2974. Epub 2020 Jan 9. PMID: 31556923; PMCID: PMC6763979.

Rashidi, A., Ebadi, M. et al. (2016). Outcomes of allogeneic stem cell transplantation in elderly patients with acute myeloid leukemia: a systematic review and meta-analysis. *Biol Blood Marrow Transplant* 22 (4): 651–657.

Schmid, C., Labopin, M. et al. (2007). Donor lymphocyte infusion in the treatment of first hematological relapse after allogeneic stem-cell transplantation in adults with acute myeloid leukemia: a retrospective risk factors analysis and comparison with other strategies by the EBMT acute leukemia working party. *J Clin Oncol* 25 (31): 4938–4945.

Srour, S.A., Saliba, R.M. et al. (2019). Haploidentical transplantation for acute myeloid leukemia patients with minimal/measurable residual disease at transplantation. *Am J Hematol* 94 (12): 1382–1387.

Part 3

Myelodysplastic Syndromes and Familial Myeloid Neoplasms

12

Diagnosis of Myelodysplastic Syndromes

Jay Yang, Vijendra Singh, Ali Gabali, and Charles A. Schiffer

Wayne State University School of Medicine and Karmanos Cancer Institute, Detroit, MI

Introduction

Myelodysplastic syndromes (MDS) are a heterogeneous group of clonal stem cell diseases characterized by peripheral cytopenias, ineffective hematopoiesis, and dysplasia in one or more major myeloid cell lines. With a median age at diagnosis of 70 years, MDS largely affects older individuals with a slight male predominance. While the diagnosis is often straightforward, it can also be difficult when cardinal features of MDS are lacking. This can lead to delayed or incorrect diagnoses and considerable frustration for physician and the patient.

Molecular genetics have greatly improved our understanding of MDS. Advancements in next-generation sequencing (NGS) technologies have increased the practicality and enthusiasm for its routine use. NGS testing has been proposed as an important adjunct to aid in the diagnosis, classification, and assessment of prognosis in MDS patients. However, in our experience, there is some sophistication needed to use and appropriately interpret the test results.

The newest and fifth edition of the WHO classification has been published. MDS entities are now grouped based on whether they have defining genetic abnormalities and whether they are morphologically defined. Accordingly, this chapter will include these updated changes but also acknowledge the nomenclature of the prior version to avoid confusion for the reader.

Here we present eight cases that illustrate some of the complexities we have encountered in the clinic and our diagnostic approach.

Case Study 1

A 50-year-old male was found to have a bicytopenia with a hemoglobin of 10 g/dL and a platelet count of 75,000/μL; the mean corpuscular volume (MCV) was 105. All secondary causes of macrocytic anemia were excluded. The bone marrow biopsy was mildly hypercellular without lymphoid infiltrates. The aspirate smear showed "megaloblastoid" changes in < 10% of the erythroid precursors. Myeloid precursors and megakaryocytes showed no evidence of dysplasia. Conventional metaphase cytogenetics revealed a clone with deletion of the Y chromosome (-Y).

Cancer Consult: Expertise in Clinical Practice, Volume 2: Neoplastic Hematology & Cellular Therapy,
Second Edition. Edited by Syed A. Abutalib, Maurie Markman, James O. Armitage, and Kenneth C. Anderson.
© 2024 John Wiley & Sons Ltd. Published 2024 by John Wiley & Sons Ltd.

1) What is the diagnosis?

A) MDS with single-lineage dysplasia (now MDS with low blasts, MDS-LB, according to WHO 5th edition).

B) Idiopathic cytopenias of undetermined significance (ICUS).

C) Clonal cytopenias of undetermined significance (CCUS).

Expert Perspective: According to the World Health Organization (WHO) classification, the morphologic diagnosis of myelodysplastic syndrome requires evidence of dysplasia in at least 10% of cells in a cell line for the dysplasia to be considered significant. These recommendations come with a caveat that high-quality marrow sample preparations are not always available for accurate assessment of dysplasia and are hampered by poor preparations, poor staining, or hemodilute samples. Samples that have been exposed to anticoagulants for more than two hours are often unsatisfactory, and this can be an issue with marrow aspirates that are mailed overnight to centralized laboratories. Even using well-prepared samples, intra-observer variability in the assessment of dysplasia can be substantial.

Persistent cytopenias without significant marrow dysplasia can be diagnosed as a myelodysplastic syndrome in the presence of a specific cytogenetic abnormality considered typical of MDS. This excludes del(20q), trisomy 8, and -Y, which, although common in MDS, are not defining cytogenetic abnormalities because they have also been present in patients with aplastic anemia and other cytopenic syndromes that have not progressed to MDS with extended follow-up. In addition, loss of the Y chromosome is well-described in normal bone marrow cells with aging.

Persistent cytopenias without dysplasia and without a defining cytogenetic abnormality can be described as ICUS (this case). While not recognized as a distinct entity in the WHO classification, ICUS serves as a useful and descriptive placeholder for patients who do not meet the diagnostic criteria for MDS.

Correct Answer: B

2) What is the next best step?

A) Start therapy for MDS.

B) Transfuse the patient.

C) Close observation with serial counts.

D) All of the above.

Expert Perspective: It is premature to recommend treatment given the mild nature of the cytopenias and the lack of a confirmed diagnosis. Transfusions are not required at this time. Although the clinical course is not predictable and many patients can have stable counts for months and sometimes years, there is appreciable concern that his cytopenias can worsen and that his disease can progress to MDS. Therefore, he should carefully be followed with serial blood counts. A repeat marrow aspirate should be done if the cytopenias worsen.

Correct Answer: C

3) A next-generation sequencing (NGS) panel of 54 target myeloid genes most commonly mutated in MDS was performed. The testing identified *TET2* (VAF 33%) and *U2AF1* (VAF 29%) variants.

What is the diagnosis now?
A) MDS with single-lineage dysplasia.
B) ICUS.
C) Clonal cytopenias of undetermined significance (CCUS).
D) Clonal hematopoiesis of undetermined potential (CHIP).

Expert Perspective: Many recurrent somatic DNA mutations have been identified in patients with MDS. These entail genes involved in chromatin modification, RNA splicing, signal transduction, epigenetic regulation, transcription, and DNA repair. The commonly mutated genes in MDS include *SF3B1, TET2, ASXL1, SRSF2, DNMT3A, RUNX1, U2AF1,* and *TP53.* Depending on the number of genes tested in an assay, about 60–90% of patients with MDS will harbor at least one mutation, and the median number of mutations in an MDS patient is three. No single gene mutation is diagnostic of MDS; however, the presence of an identifiable mutation in a patient such as this with ICUS establishes clonality and greatly increases the chances of an eventual diagnosis of MDS, particularly if the variant allele frequency (VAF) is > 10% or if there are two or more mutations. This patient can formally be considered as CCUS with a presumptive diagnosis of MDS. This information (Figure 12.1) can be tremendously helpful when counseling patients and determining frequency of follow-up. CCUS has been formally recognized as a distinct entity in the WHO 5th edition.

Correct Answer: C

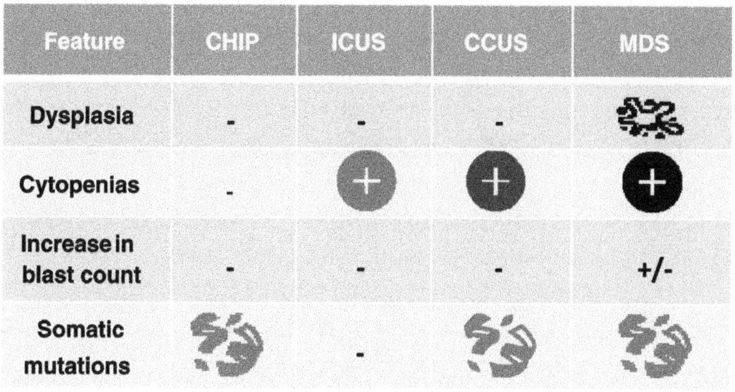

Feature	CHIP	ICUS	CCUS	MDS
Dysplasia	-	-	-	+
Cytopenias	-	+	+	+
Increase in blast count	-	-	-	+/-
Somatic mutations	+	-	+	+

Figure 12.1 Distinguishing CHIP, ICUS, CCUS, and MDS.

Case Study 2

A 67-year-old man is admitted with fever and found to have pancytopenia. He had been told that he was moderately anemic a few months ago. Now a complete blood count (CBC) showed a white blood cell (WBC) count of 2400/μL, an absolute neutrophil count of 800/μL, hemoglobin of 8.0 gm/dL, and platelets of 72,000/µL. A bone marrow aspirate was hyper-cellular with evidence of trilineage dysplasia and 18% blasts by morphologic assessment. The blasts appeared to be myeloid and had modest amounts of cytoplasmic granules. Flow cytometry was done and reported that 24% of the mononuclear cells were blasts positive for CD117 and CD34. Cytogenetics are reported as 46,XY. He is in good health otherwise and is eligible for treatment on a clinical trial evaluating a new intensive regimen for older patients with acute myeloid leukemia (AML).

4) You would tell him that:
- A) he is eligible for the AML protocol because he has ≥ 20% blasts.
- B) he is eligible for a protocol enrolling patients with high-risk MDS because he has < 20% blasts.
- C) a myeloid NGS panel will distinguish between MDS and AML.

Expert Perspective: This case highlights the common challenge that derives from the arguably arbitrary blast cutoff separating the diagnosis of myelodysplasia (MDS) with increased blasts from AML. It is quite common for older patients such as this to report poorly documented "anemia" of unknown duration before their initial definitive evalua-tion. Similarly, although the presence of dysplasia might be suggestive of AML evolving from prior MDS, it can also be present in apparently *de novo* AML. The normal karyotype is not informative in making this distinction, although the presence of a more typical "MDS karyotype," involving loss of part or all of chromosomes 5 and/or 7, would also not defi-nitely differentiate between MDS and AML.

In the not-so-distant past, the diagnosis of AML required the identification of ≥ 30% blasts, usually based on a count of 500 nucleated marrow cells. The definition was mod-ified by the WHO in 2002 to a cutoff of ≥ 20% blasts based on rather soft evidence after the review of a few trials that peripherally addressed this issue. Both definitions were based on morphologic assessments by experienced hematopathologists of blast percentage in good-quality bone marrow smears. Obviously, there is no difference in the biology and expected response to treatment of MDS and AML if a marrow has 19% ver-sus 21% blasts (or, in the past, 29% vs 31% blasts). Indeed, it is not easy to reproducibly do blast counts to this degree of accuracy. It is often difficult to distinguish undifferen-tiated myeloid blasts from dysplastic immature pronormoblasts, dysplastic myelocytes, or sometimes reactive lymphoid cells. Nonetheless, such categorization is important in defining populations of patients for protocol research studies to permit comparisons across studies.

It is now routine for laboratories to report marrow blast percentage based on flow cyto-metric analysis with the inference that this provides a more accurate quantification. Fre-quently, this information is provided even if the test had not been ordered by the clinician, and the results, because they are often discrepant from the morphologic assessment, can be confusing. Although the flow "differential" is the result of characterization of thousands of cells, there is no standardization of the definition of blast "gate" or the quantification of the population of other nucleated cells. In addition, although CD34 and/or CD117 expres-sion is used to identify myeloid blasts, there can be considerable heterogeneity in the expression of these antigens in an individual patient's leukemia. Thus, although flow char-acterization of the number of blasts is intuitively more objective, further standardization is still needed using this technique and should not be used as the primary method of quantifying blast percentages.

So does our patient have MDS or AML, and is he eligible for the research protocol? And, if he is entered into an AML protocol, does it make sense to consider his disease the same as that of a patient with a more proliferative AML with an elevated WBC count and a cellular marrow with 80% blasts? In fact, current (and past) AML studies grouped patients with "MDS" AML with the more proliferative disease, and it is very difficult to assess the relative number of patients in these two general categories in published studies, hence making comparisons of outcomes more complicated.

The 2022 WHO classification has changed the terminology from "MDS with excess blasts" to "MDS with increased blasts." The manuscript acknowledges the challenges of making a firm distinction between MDS-IB and low-blast count AML. And while the cutoff of 20% was not changed, the authors agreed that MDS-IB2 (10–19% blasts in the bone marrow) can be considered equivalent to low-blast count AML therapeutically.

Certain mutations may be much more likely to be found in AML (*FLT3* and *NPM1*) and other mutations more likely in MDS (examples listed in Case 1). And while there is considerable overlap, there are distinct genetic abnormalities that define AML even with a blast count of less than 20%. The most common example would be *NPM1* since studies have shown than MDS with *NPM1* mutation typically rapidly progresses to AML. While NGS testing may not often definitively delineate between MDS and AML, it is still warranted as certain variants may be important and may provide actionable targets.

Correct Answer: B

Case Study 3

A 42-year-old female was referred for evaluation of pancytopenia. Although she continued to work full time, she has noticed increased fatigue during the past six months as well as diffuse bruising and what she felt was "fragile" skin. She has had a weight decrease of 9 kg over the past two years. Physical examination was normal except for occasional ecchymoses on the arms. She appeared very thin with minimal subcutaneous tissue; she weighed 45 kg, and her BMI was 15.2.

CBC showed a WBC of 1600/µL, an absolute neutrophil count of 900/µL, hemoglobin of 13.6 gm/dL, MCV of 102, and platelets of 162,000/µL. The peripheral blood smear was morphologically unremarkable. Blood chemistries were unremarkable, with normal bilirubin and transaminases; the albumin was 4.1 g/dL. Vitamin B_{12} and red blood cell folate levels, serum copper and zinc levels, thyroid-stimulating hormone, ferritin, hepatitis serology, HIV antibody, and antinuclear antibody testing were normal.

A bone marrow aspirate and biopsy were done and showed a hypocellular (20%) marrow with decreased but maturing hematopoiesis. There was no increase in myeloblasts, and the karyotype was normal. There were multiple areas consistent with serous atrophy.

5) What is the most likely diagnosis?
   A) Malnutrition.
   B) Amyloidosis.
   C) Gaucher disease.

Expert Perspective: After the results became available, a more detailed nutrition history was obtained. She acknowledged that she ate inconsistently, eating very small portions "on the run," and rarely cooked meals for herself at home. She was referred to a nutritionist. Her CBC improved over the next two years with normalization of the MCV and neutrophil counts.

Serous atrophy of the bone marrow (gelatinous transformation) is a disorder characterized by weight loss and cytopenias. Bone marrow specimens exhibit fat cell atrophy, marrow hypoplasia, and the deposition of an extracellular amorphous substance that has been identified as mucopolysaccharides, which is rich in hyaluronic acid (Figure 12.2). This has been confused with marrow necrosis or amyloid. The pathogenesis of serous atrophy is unknown, but it has been associated with conditions resulting in cachexia, such as anorexia nervosa, acute febrile states, alcoholism, AIDS, carcinomas, and lymphomas. The bone marrow changes and cytopenias can be reversed by treating the underlying condition.

Gaucher disease is a lysosomal storage disease caused by an inborn error of metabolism that results in the accumulation of glucocerebroside. It should be considered in a patient presenting with unexplained anemia, thrombocytopenia, splenomegaly, particularly if there is a family history. Gaucher is more frequent in the Ashkenazi Jewish population. A bone marrow biopsy will identify Gaucher cells, macrophages filled with a lipid material that gives them a "wrinkled tissue paper" appearance.

Correct Answer: A

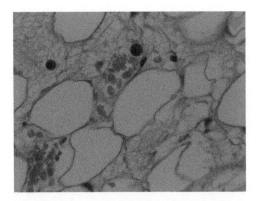

Figure 12.2   Serous atrophy. This bone marrow biopsy shows serous atrophy characterized by marrow hypoplasia, fat atrophy, and deposition of extracellular gelatinous material.

Case Study 4

A 36-year-old male with a history of gastric bypass surgery is referred to you because of transfusion-dependent anemia and neutropenia. Iron and B_{12} deficiency have been excluded. Bone marrow biopsy and aspiration reveal dysplasia and vacuolization in the myeloid precursors and an increase in ring sideroblasts. Conventional cytogenetic analysis reveals a normal karyotype. NGS testing did not detect any variants. He mentions numbness and cold sensitivity in his feet for the past several months, and examination is consistent with a distal sensory peripheral neuropathy.

6) Checking the levels of which of the following is least likely to assist with the diagnosis?
   A) Copper level.
   B) Zinc level.
   C) Lead level.
   D) Ceruloplasmin level.

Expert Perspective: Copper deficiency is probably an under-recognized cause of cytopenias. It may mimic MDS and can be easily misdiagnosed as such due to shared clinical and hematopathological findings. Patients have even been diagnosed with copper deficiency while undergoing evaluation for allogeneic hematopoietic stem cell transplantation for presumed MDS.

Anemia is almost universal at presentation, and coexisting leukopenia and neutropenia can also be seen. Significant thrombocytopenia is less common, and isolated thrombocytopenia has not been reported to our knowledge. The red cell indices can be microcytic, normocytic, or macrocytic. Histologic descriptions of bone marrows have included variable cellularity, an increase in ring sideroblasts, and dysplasia in the myeloid and erythroid series. Two of the most common features of copper deficiency are cytoplasmic vacuolization in granulocyte and erythroid precursors and the presence of stainable iron within macrophages and plasma cells, as in this case.

Many patients with copper deficiency have a myeloneuropathy that can be seen with or without the hematological changes but often precede them. Neurological findings may include an abnormal gait, sensory ataxia, dorsal column dysfunction, lower extremity spastic paraparesis, and a polyneuropathy. This may mimic subacute combined degeneration from vitamin B_{12} deficiency. The exact pathophysiology of these symptoms is unclear, but oxidative damage leading to demyelination and axonal degeneration has been hypothesized.

Absorption of copper occurs mainly in the stomach and proximal intestine. Therefore, the most common cause of copper deficiency is decreased gastrointestinal absorption in patients with a history of bariatric surgery or gastric resection. Copper deficiency can also be a result of excess ingestion of zinc, which inhibits the intestinal absorption of copper. Cases of copper deficiency have been described due to the use of zinc-containing denture creams or the overzealous use of zinc supplements. We have also witnessed a patient with a psychiatric condition who became copper deficient due to the surreptitious ingestion of pennies, which are ironically primarily composed of zinc.

The diagnosis of copper deficiency can be confirmed by the measurement of serum copper levels. In our laboratory, serum copper levels lower than 70 mcg/dL are considered diagnostic. Most patients also have decreased serum ceruloplasmin levels, but Wilson's disease, another cause of hypocupremia, must also be excluded. Twenty-four-hour urine copper excretion does not appear to correlate well with serum copper levels, and the use of this test is not encouraged. Zinc levels are often elevated, many times without an obvious explanation.

In summary, clinicians and hematopathologists should consider copper deficiency in the appropriate clinical scenario, including patients who have been given the diagnosis of low-risk MDS (without increased blasts). In this case, both the normal karyotype and the negative NGS panel would be consistent with a non-malignant cause of cytopenias.

Correct Answer: C

7) What is the treatment of choice?
    A) Oral copper.
    B) Intravenous copper.
    C) Ethylenediaminetetraacetic acid (EDTA).

Expert Perspective: Dosing of copper is empiric, but we typically treat with copper gluconate using 2 mg tablets, starting at three times daily with tapering over the next several weeks. Many patients will need a maintenance dose of 2 mg daily. Despite poor absorption, most patients are responsive to oral formulations of copper, so intravenous copper is reserved for cases in which copper repletion cannot be achieved by the oral route. Rarely, we have resorted to zinc chelation with EDTA in cases of zinc over-ingestion.

Hematological responses tend to be rapid with improvements seen within a few weeks and normalization of cytopenias within a few months of treatment. Marrow responses have also been reported. Neurological symptoms often do not reverse, but stabilization can be expected.

Correct Answer: A

Case Study 5

A 75-year-old female is found to have pancytopenia. Bone marrow biopsy shows a cellularity of 15%. Evaluation of morphology is limited due to the aparticulate nature of the aspirate, but dysplastic changes in the myeloid lineage are seen in less than 10% of cells. Cytogenetics and an MDS fluorescent in situ hybridization (FISH) panel are normal.

8) How should this be classified?
    A) Aplastic anemia.
    B) Hypoplastic MDS.
    C) Uncertain.

Expert Perspective: Although most patients with MDS have normo- to hypercellular bone marrows, MDS with hypocellular bone marrows is a well-recognized entity and one that has been recently incorporated into the WHO classification, fifth edition (MDS, hypoplastic). It may be exceedingly difficult and even impossible at times to confidently distinguish between aplastic anemia and MDS with marrow hypoplasia. Indeed, a biologic and clinicopathologic overlap may exist, as suggested by the effectiveness of immunosuppressive therapy (IST) in some patients with MDS.

The presence of dysplastic changes favors MDS, but the low cellularity in the aspirates may make morphologic analysis difficult. Structural and perhaps evolving cytogenetic abnormalities also favor MDS but are present in less than one-half of MDS cases. In addition, conventional karyotyping in hypocellular marrows may be limited by the low number of viable cells that can be induced into metaphase.

The quality of the bone marrow biopsy and aspirate is critical. Trephine bone marrow specimens may exhibit variable cellularity that may also confound the diagnosis, particularly when the sample is subcortical (Figure 12.3). Continued clinical correlation and repeat high-quality bone marrow evaluations may be necessary. In this patient, we were not able to give a firm diagnosis based on the initial bone marrow examination. However, persistent, and progressive cytopenias over the next four months prompted another bone marrow biopsy and aspirate, which was again hypocellular with only mild dysplasia. Nevertheless, the cytogenetic analysis revealed a new abnormality—a deletion of chromosome 5 in 15 of 20 cells—that ultimately favored the diagnosis of MDS.

We do not often use flow cytometry in the evaluation and diagnosis of MDS unless otherwise indicated (e.g. because of lymphadenopathy, abnormal or increased numbers of lymphocytes on the peripheral smear, or lymphoid aggregates seen in bone marrow). Flow cytometry should not replace a careful manual differential of high-quality bone marrow aspirates for the quantification of blasts (see the discussion from Case 2). Multiparameter flow cytometry has also been suggested as an adjunctive diagnostic and prognostic tool for MDS because myeloid and progenitor cells can exhibit abnormal differentiation patterns and aberrant antigen expression. Although progress has been made, the techniques, the antibody panels used, and their interpretation have not been rigorously standardized, and thus the use of flow cytometry cannot be routinely recommended for this purpose.

Flow cytometry may be helpful, however, if large granular lymphocytosis (LGL) disease is suspected. Patients with LGL leukemia frequently manifest cytopenias, particularly neutropenia, and it should be suspected if morphologically characteristic cells are seen in the peripheral blood or marrow, as well as in patients with a history of rheumatologic disorders and those with palpable splenomegaly.

Correct Answer: C

9) What other diagnostic testing should be considered?
   A) Flow cytometry for lymphoproliferative disorders.
   B) Multiparameter flow cytometry with fluorescent aerolysin (FLAER) assay for paroxysmal nocturnal hemoglobinuria (PNH).
   C) Flow cytometry for MDS.

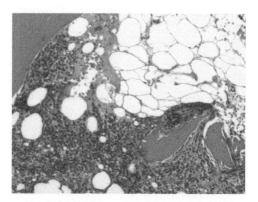

Figure 12.3 Variable cellularity. This bone marrow biopsy is subcortical and shows variable cellularity ranging from less than 5% cellularity (directly subcortical) to 40% cellularity.

Expert Perspective: Small populations of PNH clones can be found in approximately 20% of patients with aplastic anemia and MDS, particularly those with hypoplastic marrows and low-grade disease (without excess blasts). Flow cytometry is the preferred diagnostic test for PNH using antibodies against GPI-anchored proteins (i.e. CD55 and CD59), which are deficient in granulocytes and erythrocytes in patients with PNH. Sensitivity is increased further using multiparameter flow cytometry using a FLAER assay. Detection of a PNH clone in this context may help to confirm the diagnosis of a bone marrow failure syndrome.

PNH in the setting of a bone marrow failure syndrome is typically subclinical and is not associated with overt hemolytic disease. The clinical significance of the PNH clone remains unclear. Although not entirely consistent across studies, there is a suggestion of a greater benefit for immunosuppressive therapy with anti-thymocyte globulin and/or cyclosporine in patients with MDS and selected characteristics such as the presence of a PNH clone, marrow hypoplasia, HLA-DR15 histocompatibility type, younger age, normal cytogenetics, shorter duration of cytopenias, less than 5% blasts, and low-grade MDS. Even if the originally detected PNH clone size is small, it is recommended to periodically monitor the size since they can later expand and become symptomatic.

Correct Answer: C

Case Study 6

A 65-year-old male is found to be anemic with a hemoglobin of 7.6 g/dL. His WBC count is 3500/μL, and his platelet count is 512,000/μL. Bone marrow aspirate differential reveals erythroid dysplasia, 23% ring sideroblasts, normal cytogenetics, and adequate iron stores. He has been given the diagnosis of MDS with ringed sideroblasts (MDS-RS).

10) **Which of the following tests is least likely to be of benefit?**
    A) PCR for *JAK2V617F* mutation.
    B) Gene sequencing for *TET2* mutations.
    C) A FISH–MDS panel.
    D) PCR for *SF3B1* mutation.

Expert Perspective: This patient fulfills the criteria for "Myelodysplastic/myeloproliferative neoplasm with SF3B1 mutation and thrombocytosis," an entity that was previously considered provisional before the current 2022 WHO classification. It is currently classified as an MDS/MPN because it shares characteristics of both MDS and essential thrombocytosis (ET) as well as myelofibrosis to a lesser extent. Patients typically present with anemia and unusually high platelet counts (≥ 450,000/μL). Bone marrow aspirates show dyserythropoiesis with an increased number of ring sideroblasts (≥ 15%). The WBC count and BM cellularity may also be increased. Proliferation of large megakaryocytes, a feature commonly seen in ET or PMF, is required for the diagnosis.

Mutations in genes encoding for components of the RNA-splicing machinery have been discovered to be prevalent in MDS patients, particularly those with increased ring sideroblasts. *SF3B1* mutations have been discovered in up to 90% of patients with MDS with ring sideroblasts. Due to the strong association between *MDS-RS* and *SF3B1* mutations, MDS-RS can be diagnosed with only 5% ring sideroblasts instead of the 15% typically required for this diagnosis. TET2 mutations were found in 26% of MDS-RS-T cases.

Approximately one-half of patients with MDS/MPN-*SF3B1*-T will carry the *JAK2V617F* mutation. The likelihood of finding a *JAK2* mutation in patients with MDS-RS increases proportionally with the degree of thrombocytosis. Platelet counts < 400,000/μL are usually enough to exclude the disorder.

Reports to date have shown survival rates for patients with MDS/MPN-RS-T to be intermediate between those of MDS-RS and ET but with a higher propensity of thrombosis compared with MDS-RS and a higher risk of leukemia compared with ET. The prognostic significance and therapeutic implications of a *JAK2* mutation in patients with MDS/MPN-RS-T are currently unclear.

Although conventional cytogenetic analysis to detect chromosomal abnormalities is an invaluable tool in the diagnosis and risk stratification of MDS, it is only helpful in the approximately 40% of cases in which it is abnormal. Over the past two decades, the availability and utilization of MDS FISH probes in bone marrow samples have become increasingly common. Due to its ability to target interphase cells, FISH has an improved yield over metaphase karyotyping in malignancies with a low proliferative rate such as multiple myeloma and chronic lymphocytic leukemia. In MDS, however, the utility of FISH is not supported by our experience or the literature. Pitchford et al. performed FISH for −5/−5q, −7/−7q, +8, and del(20q) on 137 MDS cases. In 102 cases with normal cytogenetics, the FISH was abnormal in only one case (showing +8). In 35 patients with abnormal cytogenetics, only one showed a minor discrepancy. Other reported studies have generally been consistent with these findings. Due to its low yield and minimal added clinical benefit, we do not recommend the routine use of FISH for MDS except in cases of karyotype failure.

Correct Answer: C

Case Study 7

A 46-year-old male was evaluated as a potential allogeneic stem cell donor for his sister, who has poor-risk acute myeloid leukemia. A post-transplant bone marrow biopsy showed the patient's sister to be in complete remission with a 46,XY karyotype consistent with full donor chimerism. NGS testing, however, detected a *DNMT3A* mutation that was not present at the time of her initial diagnosis nor before the allogeneic transplant. The patient himself had peripheral blood NGS testing that detected an identical *DNMT3A* variant at a VAF of 6%. He has no cytopenias and peripheral blood smear showed no abnormality.

11) **What is the next step in management?**
    A) Perform a bone marrow biopsy.
    B) No further workup is needed. The patient has clonal hematopoiesis of indeterminate potential (CHIP).
    C) Refer the patient for genetic counselling and testing to see whether the *DNMT3A* mutation is germline.

Expert Perspective: In this case, the patient has an incidental finding of a somatic muta-tion in the *DNMT3A* gene. CHIP is now a well-described entity and has been included in the WHO classification, fifth edition. The consensus definition of CHIP is based on the presence of a leukemia-associated somatic gene mutation at a VAF ⩾ 2%, in the absence of cytopenia or a WHO-defined hematologic malignancy. The prevalence of CHIP increases with age, particularly above the age of 50. With aging both the number of CHIP mutations and VAF of individual mutations increase. *DNMT3A*, *ASXL1*, and *TET2* are the most common variants found in CHIP. Genes that are less often associated with CHIP include *JAK2*, *GNB1*, *BCORL*, *BCOR*, *U2AF1*, *GNAS*, *PPM1D*, *SF3B1*, *SRSF2*, *CBL*, *IDH1*, *IDH2*, and *TP53*. Aging-related clonal hematopoiesis (ARCH) is another category of clonal hematopoiesis in which the gene mutation VAF is less than 2%.

Germline mutations that predispose to myeloid malignancies are probably more common than previously anticipated and should be explored in patients with a strong family history with referral to a specialist. Example of implicated genes include *DDX41*, *RUNX1*, and *GATA2* (see chapter on familial myeloid neoplasms). Testing of normal skin tissue for dermal fibroblasts is recommended to prevent potential contamination with malignant cells. The VAF in a germline mutation is usually expected to be > 25%; however, this does not automatically imply presence of a germline mutation. The results should be interpreted in the context of complete medical history.

Correct Answer: B

12) **Which of the following statement is true?**
  A) Individuals with CHIP mutations are at increased risk of cardiovascular disease compared to the general population.
  B) CHIP mutations are associated with increased risk of hematological malignancies.
  C) Individuals with CHIP mutations have excess mortality compared to age-matched population.
  D) All of the above are correct.

Expert Perspective: The presence of one or more CHIP mutations is associated with an increased risk of atherosclerosis including ischemic stroke, myocardial infarction, and heart failure. Similarly, population studies have demonstrated an increased risk of hema-tologic malignancies estimated to be about 0.5–1% per year. Overall, patients with CHIP mutations have excess mortality compared to the general population. Pathophysiology of CHIP mutations and its role in cardiovascular disease or malignancy is an evolving area. There are still no consensus recommendations for management, surveillance, or interven-tion in these patients. Interestingly, recent data have shown that the presence of CHIP in allogeneic stem cell transplant donors has no effect on the overall survival of the recipi-ents. Some have still advocated for routine testing for CHIP in potential stem cell donors, but its implications for the transplant recipient are not entirely clear.

Correct Answer: D

Case Study 8

A 72-year-old woman is found to have pancytopenia on a routine primary care visit. Her hemoglobin is 7.7 g/dL, WBC count is 2100/μL, absolute neutrophil count is 1000/μL, and platelet count is 25,000/μL. On review of records, her last CBC five years ago had mild anemia. A bone marrow biopsy is done and shows a hypercellular marrow for age, trilineage dysplasia, and 14% blasts by morphologic assessment. Flow cytometry confirmed these blasts to be myeloid in origin, and conventional cytogenetics revealed an abnormal clone with 5q deletion in 17 out of 20 metaphases. Next-generation sequencing identifies *TP53* and *ASXL1* mutations.

13) What is the diagnosis?
  A) MDS with low blasts and isolated 5q deletion.
  B) MDS with multilineage dysplasia.
  C) MDS with increased blasts.
  D) B and C.

Expert Perspective: MDS with low blasts and isolated 5q deletion (MDS-5q) is a distinct entity in the WHO classification. Patients are more likely to be female and usually present with anemia and normal to high platelet counts. The bone marrow morphology exhibits dysplasia including characteristic micromegakaryocytes with monolobulated and bilobulated nuclei and erythroid hypoplasia. The blast percentage in bone marrow and peripheral blood should be < 5% and < 2%, respectively. By definition, karyotyping identifies an isolated deletion of 5q with or without one other cytogenetic abnormality except monosomy 7 or deletion 7q. MDS-5q is considered a lower-risk MDS with a relatively favorable prognosis.

A proportion of patients with MDS-5q can have additional molecular aberrations such as presence of *TP53* mutation. Concurrent *TP53* mutations are associated with a suboptimal response to lenalidomide and a higher risk of transformation to AML. In fact, acquisition of *TP53* mutations while on treatment is a common mechanism of acquired resistance to lenalidomide.

Another new entity in the updated 2022 WHO classification is MDS with *biallelic TP53* aberration (MDS-*biTP53*) in which two or more *TP53* alterations are identified (mutations by sequencing, structural deletions, or copy-neutral loss of heterozygosity) resulting in the loss of residual TP53 protein. Most patients with this diagnosis will have complex cytogenetics with very high risk disease by IPSS-R and a poor clinical prognosis. MDS-*biTP53* can be considered an AML equivalent for therapeutic purposes.

In this case, the patient's bone marrow shows 14% myeloblasts, so this should be considered MDS with increased blasts (MDS-IB2). Unlike MDS with isolated del(5q), these patients do not respond well to lenalidomide, have a higher likelihood of progression to AML, and much poorer overall prognosis.

Correct Answer: C

Recommended Readings

Bewersdorf, J.P., Xie, Z., Bejar, R. et al. (2023 July). Current landscape of translational and clinical research in myelodysplastic syndromes/neoplasms (MDS): proceedings from the 1st International Workshop on MDS (iwMDS) Of the International Consortium for MDS (icMDS). *Blood Rev* 60: 101072. doi: 10.1016/j.blre.2023.101072. Epub 2023 Mar 11. PMID: 36934059.

DeZern, A.E., Malcovati, L., and Ebert, B.L. (2019 January). CHIP, CCUS, and other acronyms: definition implications, and impact on practice. *Am Soc Clin Oncol Educ Book* 39: 400–410. doi: 10.1200/EDBK_239083. Epub 2019 May 17. PMID: 31099654.

Estey, E., Hasserjian, R.P., and Döhner, H. (2022 January 20). Distinguishing AML from MDS: A fixed blast percentage may no longer be optimal. *Blood* 139 (3): 323–332. doi: 10.1182/blood.2021011304. PMID: 34111285.

Halfdanarson, T.R., Kumar, N., Li, C.Y., Phyliky, R.L., and Hogan, W.J. (2008 June). Hematological manifestations of copper deficiency: a retrospective review. *Eur J Haematol* 80 (6): 523–531. doi: 10.1111/j.1600-0609.2008.01050.x. Epub 2008 Feb 12. PMID: 18284630.

Jaiswal, S., Fontanillas, P., Flannick, J., Manning, A., Grauman, P.V., Mar, B.G. et al. (2014 December 25). Age-related clonal hematopoiesis associated with adverse outcomes. *N Engl J Med* 371 (26): 2488–2498. doi: 10.1056/NEJMoa1408617. Epub 2014 Nov 26. PMID: 25426837; PMCID: PMC4306669.

Khoury JD, Solary E, Abla O, et al. The 5th edition of the World Health Organization Classification of Haematolymphoid Tumours: Myeloid and Histiocytic/Dendritic Neoplasms. *Leukemia*. 2022 Jul;36(7):1703–1719. doi: 10.1038/s41375-022-01613-1. Epub 2022 Jun 22. PMID: 35732831; PMCID: PMC9252913.

Kim, P.G., Niroula, A., Shkolnik, V., McConkey, M., Lin, A.E., Słabicki, M. et al. (2021 December 6). Dnmt3a-mutated clonal hematopoiesis promotes osteoporosis. *J Exp Med* 218 (12): e20211872.

List, A., Ebert, B.L., and Fenaux, P. (2018 July). A decade of progress in myelodysplastic syndrome with chromosome 5q deletion. *Leukemia* 32 (7): 1493–1499. doi: 10.1038/s41375-018-0029-9. Epub 2018 Jan 30. PMID: 29445113.

Malcovati, L., Gallì, A., Travaglino, E., Ambaglio, I., Rizzo, E., Molteni, E. et al. (2017 June 22). Clinical significance of somatic mutation in unexplained blood cytopenia. *Blood* 129 (25): 3371–3378. doi: 10.1182/blood-2017-01-763425. Epub 2017 Apr 19. PMID: 28424163; PMCID: PMC5542849.

Malcovati, L., Karimi, M., Papaemmanuil, E., Ambaglio, I., Jädersten, M., Jansson, M. et al. (2015 July 9). SF3B1 mutation identifies a distinct subset of myelodysplastic syndrome with ring sideroblasts. *Blood* 126 (2): 233–241. doi: 10.1182/blood-2015-03-633537. Epub 2015 May 8. PMID: 25957392; PMCID: PMC4528082.

Marnell, C.S., Bick, A., and Natarajan, P. (2021 December). Clonal hematopoiesis of indeterminate potential (CHIP): linking somatic mutations, hematopoiesis, chronic inflammation and cardiovascular disease. *J Mol Cell Cardiol* 161: 98–105. doi: 10.1016/j.yjmcc.2021.07.004. Epub 2021 Jul 21. PMID: 34298011; PMCID: PMC8629838.

Pitchford CW, Hettinga AC, Reichard KK. Fluorescence In Situ Hybridization Testing for −5/5q, −7/7q, +8, and del(20q) in Primary Myelodysplastic Syndrome Correlates With

Conventional Cytogenetics in the Setting of an Adequate Study. *Am Journal of Clin Path.* 2010 Feb; 133(2);260–264.

Venugopal, S., Mascarenhas, J., and Steensma, D.P. (2021 March). Loss of 5q in myeloid malignancies - a gain in understanding of biological and clinical consequences. *Blood Rev* 46: 100735. doi: 10.1016/j.blre.2020.100735. Epub 2020 Jul 23. PMID: 32736878.

13

Treatment of Myelodysplastic Syndromes

Rami S. Komrokji

H. Lee Moffitt Cancer Center, Tampa, FL

Introduction

Myelodysplastic syndromes (MDS) represent a spectrum of neoplastic stem cell diseases characterized by bone marrow failure with resultant cytopenias and their complications. The first step is always assuring correct and accurate diagnosis (previous chapter), and appropriate risk stratification incorporating clinical and molecular data. The management is individualized and tailored based on disease risk. In patients with higher-risk MDS, allogeneic stem cell transplantation should be considered early in the disease course. In lower-risk disease, treatment is geared to alleviate cytopenias where anemia is the major indication to treat; isolated thrombocytopenia or neutropenia is less often encountered in lower-risk disease but can dictate choice of therapy. After more than a decade, a couple of new drugs were recently approved for treating MDS.

1) **What is the general approach to the treatment of newly diagnosed myelodysplastic syndrome (MDS)?**

Therapy should be tailored to each patient according to the specific risk profile, and whenever possible, patients should be treated on a clinical trial.

2) **Which patients are good candidates for treatment with erythropoiesis-stimulating agents (ESAs), such as epoetin α or darbepoietin?**

Expert Perspective: ESAs are an appropriate initial treatment for anemia in lower-risk MDS patients. A simple, validated decision model was developed by the Nordic MDS Group (2005/2008) for the use of epoetin alpha and granulocyte colony-stimulating factor (G-CSF) in patients with lower-risk MDS based on their pretreatment serum erythropoietin (EPO) level and the number of red blood cell (RBC) transfusions administered each month. Patients are assigned +2, +1, and −3 points for EPO levels of < 100, 100–500, or > 500 U/L, respectively. Similarly, patients who require fewer than two units of packed RBCs (pRBCs) each month are assigned +2 points, and those who require at least two units each month are assigned −2 points. Patients with a combined score that was greater than +1 had a 74% probability of response, compared to 23% for those with a score between −1 and +1 and 7% for those with scores less than −1. Darbepoetin (150 to 300 mcg once weekly or 500 mcg once every two to three weeks) appears to be equivalent to epoietin α (150 to 300 units/kg once daily or 450 units/kg [up to 40,000 units/dose] once weekly; based on erythroid response after eight weeks may increase to 1,050 units/kg [up to 80,000 units/dose] once weekly), and the use of either agent is reasonable. We typically recommend a 6–8-week trial of ESAs followed by continuation of treatment in responders (the median duration of response is 12–18 months). We reserve the addition of G-CSF (1–2 mcg/kg every 1–2 weeks) for patients who do not respond after a 6–8-week trial of an ESA, a method that has been employed with modest success in multiple prospective trials. In real-world experience roughly 60% of patients clinically benefit from ESA for treating anemia in lower-risk MDS. Primary failure is associated with worse outcomes, and no clear association between somatic mutations landscape and response to ESA had been demonstrated.

3) Which patients are good candidates for treatment with immunosuppressive therapy (IST)?

Expert Perspective: In the phase III trial of anti-thymocyte globulin and cyclosporine versus best supportive care in patients primarily with lower-risk MDS, IST was shown to increase hematologic response rates significantly by six months (29% vs 9%, respectively), but neither two-year progression-free survival (46% vs 55%) nor overall survival (49% vs 63%) was significantly improved. Based on their previous experiences with IST, the National Institutes of Health (NIH 2003) developed and validated a predictive score for response model, which included patient's age, the presence of a human leukocyte antigen (HLA)-DR15 class II phenotype, and the duration of RBC transfusion dependence. The patient's age in years is added to the duration of RBC transfusion dependence in months. A sum ≤ 57 predicts a high probability of response for patients in whom HLA-DR15 is absent, while a sum ≤ 71 predicts higher responses for patients in whom HLA-DR15 is present. Not all studies validated this model. In addition to the above factors, other studies have reported additional predictive factors such as bone marrow hypocellularity, the presence of a parox-ysmal nocturnal hemoglobinuria clone, LGL clones, STAT-3 mutant cytotoxic T-cell clones, and a low or reverse CD4:CD8 ratio correlate with improved response rates. SF3B1 somatic mutation has been reported to be associated with inferior response to IST.

In a recent international study by Stahl et al. (2018), IST demonstrated objective responses in nearly half the lower-risk MDS patients with the highest rate of RBC transfusion independence achieved in patients with hypocellular bone marrows. Hypocellularity of bone marrow (< 20%) and the use of horse ATG plus cyclosporine were associated with increased rates of transfusion independence. In this larger retrospective study, age, prior transfusion dependence, MDS risk assessment scores, presence of PNH or LGL clones, HLA DR15 positivity, and gene mutations did not appear to predict response to IST.

We consider treatment for younger (age < 60 years) low-risk (non 5q and blast < 5%) patients with hypoplastic MDS after ESA failure. We wait 4–6 months after start of horse ATG with cyclosporin to assess response and closely observe for treatment-related toxicity such as infections and cyclosporine toxicity.

4) What is the role of luspatercept in treatment of MDS?

Expert Perspective: Luspatercept, a novel fusion TGFβ ligands trap protein, was approved for treatment of lower-risk MDS patients with ring sideroblasts and MDS/MPN RS-T patients who are transfusion dependent. TGFβ ligands play a role in terminal erythroid differentiation blockage, and so luspatercept is considered first-in-class "erythroid maturation agent" contrary to ESAs, which stimulate early erythropoiesis. The MEDALIST study was a randomized clinical trial 2:1 luspatercept:placebo study demonstrating significantly higher rate of red blood cell transfusion independency with luspatercept. The magnitude of benefit was higher among patients with lower red blood cell transfusion burden suggesting earlier treatment could yield higher responses. Luspatercept is given as subcutaneous injection every three weeks, starting dose is 1 mg/kg escalated after two doses to 1.33 mg/kg and to 1.75 mg/kg after other two doses if no response. Main adverse events included fatigue, musculoskeletal symptoms, diarrhea, and peripheral edema. Most of adverse events subsided after first 2–3 treatments and did not lead to study drug discontinuation. Blood pressure should be monitored and relatively controlled while using luspatercept. Trilineage responses have been reported with luspatercept. Ongoing studies are exploring the role of luspatercept among all MDS patients regardless of *SF3B1* mutation or ring sideroblasts presence comparing it to up-front ESA in the COMMANDS study. The interim analysis of this phase 3, open-label, randomised controlled trial showed that luspatercept improved the rate at which RBC transfusion independence and increased hemoglobin were achieved compared with epoetin alfa in ESA-naive patients with lower-risk MDS. Long-term follow-up and additional data will be needed to confirm these results and further refine findings in other subgroups of patients with lower-risk MDS, including non mutated SF3B1 or ring sideroblast-negative subgroups. Additionally, luspatercept is currently being studied in a Phase IIIB clinical trial assessing its effectiveness and safety of LR-MDS post ESA/ineligible for ESA therapy (LUSPLUS). Other novel TGFβ inhibitors are entering clinical trials.

5) What is the best starting dose for lenalidomide in lower-risk patients with RBC transfusion dependence and a chromosome 5q deletion [del(5q)]?

Expert Perspective: The US Food and Drug Administration (FDA)–approved starting dose for lenalidomide in MDS is 10 mg daily continuously or for 21 days every four weeks based on the MDS-003 phase II registration trial conducted exclusively in transfusion-dependent patients with del(5q). A subsequent phase III trial randomized patients to placebo or two different doses of lenalidomide: 5 mg daily on days 1–28 and 10 mg daily on days 1–21 of a 28-day cycle. This trial was not designed to detect differences in the two lenalidomide arms, but higher rates of transfusion independence and cytogenetic response were seen in the 10 mg arm. In the phase II MDS-003 trial in patients with del(5q), patients were also originally treated with 10 mg on days 1–21, but shortly after activation, the schedule was amended to 10 mg continuous daily dosing in light of the faster times to response observed in the pilot trial. Forty-six patients received the day 1–21 schedule, and 102 received continuous daily dosing, which resulted in a slight trend toward higher erythroid response rates (72% vs 77%, respectively; $P = 0.26$) and faster median time to response (4.7 weeks vs 4.3 weeks). The 10 mg continuous dosing is associated with more frequent neutropenia and thrombocytopenia, but the development of these events is also associated with a higher probability of transfusion independence. Based on the available data, we initiate patients on the 10 mg continuous daily dosing schedule with weekly blood counts for the first eight weeks. Approximately 80% of patients will require a drug holiday after a

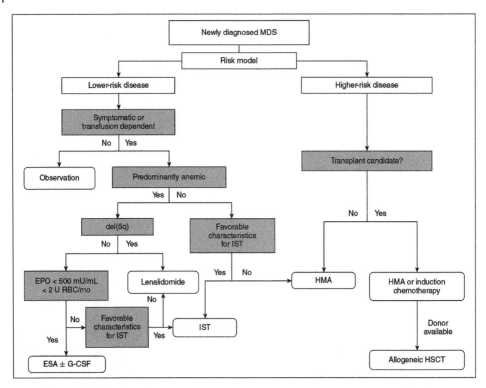

Figure 13.1 General approach to the treatment of newly diagnosed myelodysplastic syndrome. Del(5q), chromosome 5q deletion; EPO, erythropoietin; ESA, erythropoiesis-stimulating agent; G-CSF, granulocyte colony-stimulating factor; HMA, hypomethylating agent; HSCT, hematopoietic stem cell transplantation; IST, immunosuppressive therapy; MDS, myelodysplastic syndrome; RBC, red blood cell. **Newer therapies in MDS are emerging**; these include luspatercept in LR-MDS with symptomatic anemia esp. with high EPO levels (COMMAND study), and imetelstat in patients with heavily transfusion dependent non-del(5q) LR-MDS after failure to ESA (IMerge Study).

median duration of three weeks for myelosuppression. Treatment is held for an average of three weeks, and then the dose is reduced to 5 mg daily. G-CSF can be used to accelerate neutrophil recovery and preempt neutropenia. The median time to response is four weeks, and the median duration of response is approximately three years.

Recent promising data from SINTRA-REV trial were presented introducing lenalidomide at a lower dose (5 mg po daily for two years total duration of therapy), earlier during del(5q) MDS disease course in patients who were not RBC transfusion dependent. The studies suggested longer time to transfusion dependency and higher cytogenetic responses.

6) Can lenalidomide be used in lower-risk patients with anemia and karyotypes other than del(5q)?

Expert Perspective: Yes. The use of lenalidomide in MDS without the del(5q) abnormality is considered off-label; however, a multicenter phase II trial (MDS-002) demonstrated some activity of this agent in lower-risk, transfusion-dependent MDS patients without this specific cytogenetic abnormality. In that trial, 26% of patients achieved RBC transfusion independence that lasted a median of 41 weeks. An additional 17% of patients had at least a 50% reduction in transfusion requirement, for an overall response rate of 43%.

The median time to response (4.8 weeks) in this trial appears similar to the results in patients with del(5q). Unlike the MDS-003 study, however, there were very few cytogenetic responses. Further comparisons between the MDS-002 and MDS-003 trials show a shorter median duration of transfusion independence and a less robust median increase in hemoglobin in patients without the del(5q) abnormality. We consider this a treatment alternative in lower-risk non del(5q) MDS patients requiring frequent transfusions of RBCs who have failed ESAs and have adequate platelet and neutrophil counts. The National Comprehensive Cancer Center Network (NCCN) guidelines for management of MDS list lenalidomide as an option for treatment of anemia in non-del(5q) lower-risk MDS. The USA Intergroup study demonstrated higher and more durable response combining lenalidomide with ESA in non-del(5q) patients. Retrospective study suggests higher response rate if used before hypomethylating agents in lower-risk MDS.

7) Can patients with higher-risk disease and del(5q) be treated with lenalidomide rather than hypomethylating agents (HMAs)?

Expert Perspective: Lenalidomide treatment of higher-risk MDS with del(5q) should be considered investigational, and in our practice, we use lenalidomide exclusively in lower-risk patients. A phase II study of daily lenalidomide in 47 higher-risk MDS patients with del(5q) reported a 27% response rate, including seven complete remissions (CRs). Most responses were rapid, but the duration of response was only 6.5 months. Patients with an isolated del(5q) were more likely to respond compared with those with additional chromosomal abnormalities. While this study utilized lenalidomide at the currently approved dose of 10 mg daily, dose escalation may improve response rates.

8) Does lenalidomide increase the risk of progression to acute myeloid leukemia (AML)? Should patients be monitored for clonal evolution while on lenalidomide therapy?

Expert Perspective: As seen in the long-term follow-up of 42 European patients treated in the MDS-003 trial, 15 patients (36%) progressed to AML and 17 (40%) had karyotypic evolution. Patients who failed to achieve a response to lenalidomide appeared to have a higher rate of AML progression compared to those who responded. These rates of AML progression in this isolated subset of patients may seem higher than historical controls, but patients in the MDS-003 trial were all transfusion dependent, which is a known poor prognostic factor for disease progression. In addition, recent studies indicate that *TP53* gene mutations are demonstrable in approximately 20% of del(5q) MDS patients, expand over time, and are associated with higher risk of disease progression and lower frequency of cytogenetic response to lenalidomide. The rate of AML progression can be as high as 80% in patients with del(5q) and more than 5% blasts; thus, the apparent tendency toward leukemic transformation may actually reflect the natural history of disease in this subset of patients with greater AML potential. A study from the International Working Group on MDS with del(5q) evaluated 295 lenalidomide treated patients on the MDS-003 and -004 studies along with 125 untreated, lower-risk, RBC-transfusion-dependent patients with del(5q) from a registry. The median follow-up was over four years in each cohort. Despite a higher RBC transfusion burden in the lenalidomide cohort, the two-year cumulative AML progression risk was similar between cohorts (hazard ratio [HR] 0.969), but lenalidomide-treated patients had a significant improvement in survival (HR 0.597). In the phase III trial of lenalidomide versus placebo in del(5q) MDS, almost all patients who were randomized to placebo crossed over to the lenalidomide arm; thus, truly randomized prospective data with long-term follow-up are lacking, and the issue of whether lenalidomide truly increases the risk of AML progression remains unclear. Nonetheless, responding patients have a lower frequency of AML than nonresponders, suggesting that a drug effect is unlikely. No formal guidelines currently exist for monitoring cytogenetics in patients on lenalidomide, and we do not routinely perform karyotyping or fluorescent in situ hybridization on our responding patients.

9) How does one manage MDS patients with isolated thrombocytopenia? Are romiplostim or eltrombopag reasonable options?

Expert Perspective: Currently, the only available treatment modalities that can potentially improve platelet counts are IST and the HMAs. The use of the thrombopoietin receptor agonists romiplostim and eltrombopag in patients with MDS can be considered an option. Romiplostim decreased the rate of clinically significant bleeding events and platelet transfusions compared to placebo in a randomized trial of patients with lower-risk MDS and thrombocytopenia. Despite these promising results, the trial was halted prematurely when data emerged showing an apparent increase in peripheral blasts and AML transformation in the romiplostim arm. Longer follow-up showed a lower hazard ratio for progression to AML than was originally reported. Eltrombopag is a noncompetitive thrombopoietin receptor agonist that was shown to be cytotoxic to leukemic myeloblasts in preclinical studies, and it is currently being studied in several early phase trials in patients with MDS. The results of the lower-risk MDS study showed significantly increased platelet counts and decreased bleeding or transfusion events in patients treated with eltrombopag compared to placebo, with no patients progressing to AML in the treatment arm.

10) In lower-risk patients, what schedule of azacitidine should be given?

Expert Perspective: In our practice, we administer five days of azacitidine at 75 mg/m^2 every 28 days in patients with lower-risk disease. A multicenter community-based study randomized patients (most of whom had lower-risk MDS) to three different schedules of azacitidine: (i) a 5–2–2 schedule (75 mg/m^2 subcutaneously for five days, followed by two days of no treatment, then 75 mg/m^2 for two days), (ii) a 5–2–5 schedule (50 mg/m^2 subcutaneously for five days, followed by two days of no treatment, then 50 mg/m^2 for five days), or (iii) a five-day schedule (75 mg/m^2 subcutaneously for five days). Differences in response rates were not statistically significant, but there was a trend toward a higher rate of hematologic improvement and RBC transfusion independence in patients treated on the five-day schedule, with comparable (and perhaps even reduced) hematologic toxicity. It should be noted that 75 mg/m^2 for seven days, which showed survival benefit in higher-risk patients, was not one of the arms in this study. The first randomized phase III study from the Cancer and Leukemia Group B (CALGB), however, used the seven-day schedule and allowed patients with lower-risk disease to be enrolled. Analysis of the whole study population showed only a trend toward survival benefit over best supportive care. Although it can be argued that the crossover design of the study may have confounded the results, definitive survival benefit from azacitidine using the current FDA-approved schedule has never been shown in lower-risk patients. A phase II study from US MDS consortium reported similar efficacy with three days regimen of azacitidine or decitabine compared to historical five days regimen; the phase III clinical study results are pending.

11) How does one manage intermediate-risk patients by the Revised International Prognostic Scoring System (IPSS-R)?

Expert Perspective: Most clinical trials in MDS have risk-stratified patients based on the original IPSS score, dividing patients into lower-risk (low and intermediate-1) and higher-risk (intermediate-2 and high) categories. The development of the Revised IPSS (IPSS-R) resulted in five risk categories (very low, low, intermediate, high, and very high), leaving uncertainty regarding the treatment of patients in the intermediate category. Patients in this risk category had a median survival of 3.0 years and a median time to 25% AML evolution of 3.2 years. Although cohorts from differing eras were used to develop the two risk models, these data appear to be closer to those for IPSS intermediate-1 patients (3.5 years and 3.3 years, respectively) than those for IPSS intermediate-2 patients (1.8 years and 1.1 years, respectively). At this point, therapy must be individualized to the patient by considering additional factors such as age, the presence of specific gene mutations, the presence of bone marrow fibrosis, circulating myeloblasts, transfusion dependency, and disease tempo.

12) Which HMA should be used for higher-risk MDS patients?

Expert Perspective: Both azacitidine and decitabine are approved by the FDA for management of MDS, but they have not been directly compared in a prospective, randomized study. Only azacitidine, however, has been shown to confer overall survival benefit over conventional care regimens in patients with higher-risk disease, including those with refractory anemia with excess blasts in transformation (RAEB-t). In the AZA-001 trial, patients with higher-risk MDS by IPSS treated with azacitidine had a median survival of 24.5 months compared to 15.0 months in patients treated with intensive chemotherapy, low-dose cytarabine, or best supportive care. In contrast, in two phase III trials of decitabine versus best supportive care, only a trend toward overall survival benefit was seen despite the lack of active treatment in the control arm. In both trials of decitabine, however, treatment was not continued until disease progression, which likely affected survival outcomes. In addition, the highest complete response rate ever reported for an HMA (39%) was in patients receiving the five-day 20 mg/m^2/d intravenous decitabine regimen. While both agents have clinical activity, we favor azacitidine in our practice given its documented overall survival benefit, a practice that is supported by current NCCN guidelines. However, decitabine maybe preferred in patients with end-stage renal disease given hepatic metabolism, and some retrospective studies suggested higher response rates among CMML patients and those who harbor TP53 somatic mutation.

13) What are the optimal schedules and routes of administration of azacitidine and decitabine in higher-risk MDS patients?

Expert Perspective: In contrast to patients with lower-risk disease, we administer 75 mg/m^2 of azacitidine subcutaneously on days 1–7 of a 28-day cycle in higher-risk patients whenever possible, as this is the only dose, route of administration, and schedule combination ever shown to improve overall survival. When weekend dosing is not feasible in the community, we generally recommend the 5–2–2 (total of seven days with two days' rest on the weekend) schedule. Although pharmacokinetic data are available showing similar bioavailability between intravenous and subcutaneous administration, only one prospective study has been published evaluating the efficacy of intravenous azacitidine. When given for five consecutive days every 28 days, the overall response rate was 27%, and the median survival was only 14.8 months. The initial FDA-approved schedule for decitabine, based on the phase III trial, was 15 mg/m^2/dose given intravenously every 8 h for three consecutive days every 28 days. This schedule is often inconvenient for patients and requires inpatient hospitalization; thus, many clinicians, including our group, use the alternative FDA-approved schedule of a 20 mg/m^2 dose given intravenously once daily for five consecutive days. As stated in question 11, this schedule is associated with a high CR rate, and it may be less toxic than the three-day schedule due to the lower cumulative dose.

More recently the FDA approved oral decitabine/cedazuridine for treatment of intermediate- and higher-risk MDS and CMML (ASTX727-01-B and ASTX727-02 studies). The ASCERTAIN study demonstrated 99% similar bioavailability and comparable response rates to IV decitabine. Oral azacitidine (QUAZAR AML-001) was approved by the FDA for maintenance therapy in AML after intensive chemotherapy for patients not candidates for allogeneic hematopoietic stem cell transplant; however, the pharmacokinetics are not similar to IV/SC azacitidine and these drugs should not be used interchangeably until further studies configure appropriate dosing in MDS patients.

14) When treating higher-risk patients with HMAs, how should doses be modified for cytopenias?

Expert Perspective: Preferably, doses should not be modified. Cytopenias are the most frequent adverse event associated with HMA therapy, and clinical practice varies widely. The package insert for azacitidine recommends dose reductions of up to 67% of the initial dose depending on nadir absolute neutrophil, white blood cell, and platelet counts. However, dose reductions or delays to allow recovery of counts may be associated with lower efficacy. A consensus panel of experts recommends against dose modifications during the first three cycles even in the presence of severe cytopenias, except in cases of life-threatening infections. Eighty-six percent of patients in the AZA-001 trial did not require dose modifications, and despite the higher incidence of grade 3 or 4 neutropenia and thrombocytopenia compared to best supportive care, there was no increase in the incidence of infections or bleeding. In addition, improvement in cytopenias may occur with subsequent cycles, in particular anemia and thrombocytopenia. The use of G-CSF to improve neutropenia has not been studied systematically and was not allowed on the AZA-001 trial; thus, we do not routinely use this agent to hasten neutrophil recovery after treatment with HMAs. If dose adjustments are needed after the first three cycles, we generally dose-delay rather than dose-reduce therapy.

15) In patients who have had a sustained response to HMA therapy, can cycles be given less frequently than every four weeks or even stopped?

Expert Perspective: Preferably, no. In the absence of toxicities, we attempt to stay on schedule with the administration of HMAs, and we do not stop therapy in responders unless there is evidence of loss of response or disease progression. In circumstances when patients are adamant about prolonging the interval between cycles for quality-of-life purposes, we have a frank discussion regarding the risks of this approach, and we almost never increase the dosing interval beyond six weeks. In the AZA-001 trial, the median duration of therapy for responders was 14 months, and continued treatment with azacitidine after first response led to higher-quality responses in 48% of patients, suggesting that the benefits of HMAs are greater with prolonged exposure. Loss of response after discontinuation can be rapid, and retreatment results in inferior quality and duration of responses compared to initial treatment.

16) Should induction chemotherapy (with an anthracycline and cytarabine) ever be used for higher-risk patients?

Expert Perspective: Compared to AML, induction chemotherapy for MDS generally results in lower CR rates and shorter responses, but it was one of the few options available to higher-risk patients before the age of HMAs. In particular, younger patients with favorable karyotypes appeared to derive the most benefit. Although azacitidine was shown to be superior to conventional care regimens that included induction chemotherapy in the AZA-001 trial, fit patients in whom allogeneic stem cell transplantation was planned were excluded from the trial. As expected, only 14% of patients in the control arm underwent induction chemotherapy, but this resulted in slightly higher remission rates compared to azacitidine (40% vs 29%, respectively), although this was not statistically significant. Although achievement of a complete response is prerequisite to extension in survival with induction chemotherapy, this is not the case for azacitidine. Thus, its role has clearly diminished in the last decade, but induction chemotherapy may still have value only in a highly select group of MDS patients. Ongoing studies are exploring the role of CPX-351, which is approved by the FDA for secondary AML in patients with higher-risk MDS.

17) Some patients develop therapy-related MDS, but they have lower-risk disease by various prognostic scores. How should these patients be managed?

Expert Perspective: The World Health Organization collectively considers therapy-related MDS, therapy-related AML, and therapy-related myelodysplastic/myeloproliferative neoplasms as a distinct clinical entity. This group of diseases generally has a worse prognosis than their *de novo* counterparts. It should be noted that the IPSS, WHO classification–based Prognostic Scoring System (WPSS), and IPSS-R (but not the global MD Anderson MDS risk model) excluded patients with therapy-related MDS; thus, risk scores calculated within these systems must be interpreted with caution. In all phase III trials of both azacitidine and decitabine, therapy-related MDS patients either were excluded or accounted for a very small fraction of the study population; thus, it is unclear whether the benefits of therapy extend to this group of patients. Several retrospective studies, however, have demonstrated response rates of approximately 40% using these agents; thus, we feel their use is justified, and we routinely use azacitidine in this population. Radiation-induced myeloid neoplasms behave more like *de novo* MDS and should be treated accordingly. The outcome of therapy-related myeloid neoplasms is predominantly driven by disease karyotype; thus, we tailor therapy based on karyotype where we may apply a stepwise approach in those with a more favorable karyotype but pursue allogeneic stem cell transplantation in those with poor-risk disease.

18) **What treatment options are available for patients who have failed or progressed on HMAs?**

Expert Perspective: Patients who have initial failure, progress on therapy, or lose initial response to HMAs have a very poor prognosis, with a median survival measured in months. One small trial evaluated the utility of switching to decitabine after azacitidine failure, demonstrating a response in 4 out of 14 patients (28%), but the duration of response was very short. Whenever possible, these patients should be referred for treatment on a clinical trial. It is important to reevaluate disease post HMA failure including molecular profile and somatic mutations. Targeted therapy such as *IDH* and *FLT-3* inhibitors may have therapeutic value, if detected especially in patients with excess blast counts. Intensive chemotherapy can be considered in a small subset of patients for whom there is no adverse cytogenetics or somatic mutations and for whom allogeneic stem cell transplantation is an option. Recent studies suggest also potential responses with addition of venetoclax to HMA.

19) **What is the role of HMAs before allogeneic hematopoietic stem cell transplantation?**

Expert Perspective: Allogeneic stem cell transplant (see next chapter) remains the only curative option for MDS and should be entertained among fit patients with no major comorbidities. A recent study confirmed the benefit of transplant in higher-risk MDS patients when randomized based on donor availability. The screening process before allogeneic stem cell transplantation can often span several months; thus, HMAs are commonly used as bridging therapy, a practice that is supported by NCCN guidelines. This strategy may be helpful in halting disease progression with limited toxicity, allowing more patients to proceed to transplant, but no prospective studies are available. A large retrospective study comparing azacitidine to induction chemotherapy or both before transplant suggests that overall survival, event-free survival, relapse rate, and non-relapse mortality are similar between azacitidine and induction chemotherapy. There was a trend toward poorer overall survival in patients who received both therapies, but this may be a reflection of aggressive disease requiring multiple therapies. The optimal timing of transplantation during HMA therapy is also controversial and is further complicated by the long duration of therapy before the best response is attained. Although patients with lower blast counts at the time of transplantation have better outcomes than those with higher disease burden, the value of cytoreduction before transplant remains unclear. From a practical standpoint, most patients receive at least two or three cycles of azacitidine before a donor is available and the pre-transplant workup is complete. In our practice we attempt achieving best response possible before transplant. Among patients with the *TP53* somatic mutation we attempt to clear the mutation before transplant given the dismal outcome if patients proceed to transplant with detectable high allele burden of this particular mutation. The role of post-transplant azacitidine maintenance remains investigational.

20) **What is the value of iron chelation therapy, and when should it be used?**

Expert Perspective: Although transfusion dependence and elevated ferritin levels are known to correlate with poorer outcomes in patients with MDS, to date no randomized trial has shown a definitive benefit for iron chelation therapy in patients with MDS. Two large phase II studies have shown that deferasirox decreases serum ferritin levels as well as labile plasma iron in lower-risk MDS patients, but both studies also had high rates of discontinuation, mainly due to gastrointestinal, renal, or hepatic toxicities. The potential benefit on the morbidity and mortality of higher-risk patients is uncertain and likely minimal given the overall poor prognosis of these patients. A large, multicenter, placebo-controlled phase III study evaluating deferasirox in IPSS-defined low-risk or intermediate-1-risk MDS patients with a baseline serum ferritin > 1000 mcg/L (TELESTO) demonstrated benefit mainly preventing end organ damage and a trend to better overall survival. We generally consider iron chelation therapy in patients with lower-risk disease, long life expectancy, and serum ferritin > 1000 mcg/L or other clinical evidence of iron overload. There are also considerations about the use of iron chelation for patients who will proceed to allogeneic stem cell transplantation.

21) What is the role of prophylactic antimicrobial, antifungal, and antiviral agents in patients treated with HMAs?

Expert Perspective: Routine infectious prophylaxis in patients with MDS has not been studied extensively. A single retrospective study of patients receiving decitabine reported a lower incidence of febrile episodes in patients who were treated with prophylactic oral antimicrobial agents compared to those who were not. Randomized studies evaluating antibacterial and antifungal prophylaxis in leukemia patients rarely included patients with MDS, and those who were included underwent induction chemotherapy rather than treatment with HMAs. In our practice, we give quinolone, posaconazole, and aciclovir prophylaxis to patients with MDS undergoing induction chemotherapy in accordance with current guidelines. In patients treated with HMAs, we reserve quinolone and aciclovir prophylaxis for patients who have severe baseline neutropenia and other risk factors for infection. We also give secondary prophylaxis to patients who have previously had neutropenic fevers or documented infections while on therapy.

22) What are promising new agents in MDS?

Expert Perspective: Several ongoing trials are exploring novel agents in MDS. In lower-risk MDS, imetelstat, a telomerase inhibitor, demonstrated promising activity in a phase II clinical study with durable red blood cell transfusion independency. The phase III randomized clinical trial is ongoing. In higher-risk MDS, several agents are being tested in combination with HMA. HMA/venetoclax combination yielded promising activity with high response rates and we are currently awaiting data from phase III VERONA study with overall survival as primary endpoint. Magrolimab, anti-CD47 monoclonal antibody targeting the "don't eat meat signal" and engaging macrophages, showed promising activity in phase I/II clinical studies with more than 90% overall response rate and 50% complete response rate agnostic of somatic mutations. Sabatolimab, a TIM-3 inhibitor targeting leukemia stem cell and engaging immune system, showed promising activity with durable responses when combined with HMA. The role of *IDH* inhibitors is being further explored as single agent or in combination with HMA. Early clinical trials with CAR-T therapy for myeloid diseases including MDS are being explored.

Recommended Readings

Ball S., Komrokji R.S., Sallman D.A (2022 June). Prognostic scoring systems and risk stratification in myelodysplastic syndrome: focus on integration of molecular profile. *Leuk Lymphoma* 63 (6):1281–1291. doi: 10.1080/10428194.2021.2018579. Epub 2021 Dec 21. PMID:34933652.

Fenaux, P., Mufti, G.J., Hellstrom-Lindberg, E. et al. (2009). Efficacy of azacitidine compared with that of conventional care regimens in the treatment of higher-risk myelodysplastic syndromes: a randomised, open-label, phase III study. *Lancet Oncol* 10: 223–232.

Fenaux, P., Platzbecker, U., Mufti, G.J. et al. (2020). Luspatercept in patients with lower-risk myelodysplastic syndromes. *N Engl J Med* 382 (2): 140–151.

Garcia-Manero, G., McCloskey, J., Griffiths, E.A. et al. (2019). Pharmacokinetic exposure equivalence and preliminary efficacy and safety from a randomized cross over phase 3 study (ASCERTAIN study) of an Oral Hypomethylating Agent ASTX727 (cedazuridine/decitabine) compared to IV decitabine. *Blood* 134 (Supplement_1): 846–846.

Greenberg PL, Attar E, Bennett JM, et al.; National Comprehensive Cancer Network. NCCN Clinical Practice Guidelines in Oncology: myelodysplastic syndromes. *J Natl Compr Canc Netw.* 2011 Jan;9(1):30–56. doi: 10.6004/jnccn.2011.0005. PMID: 21233243; PMCID: PMC3768131.

Hellstrom-Lindberg, E., Gulbrandsen, N., Lindberg, G. et al. (2003). A validated decision model for treating the anaemia of myelodysplastic syndromes with erythropoietin + granulocyte colony-stimulating factor: Significant effects on quality of life. *Br J Haematol* 120: 1037–1046.

Jabbour, E., Short, N.J., Montalban-Bravo, G. et al. (2017). Randomized phase 2 study of low-dose decitabine vs low-dose azacitidine in lower-risk MDS and MDS/MPN. *Blood* 130 (13): 1514–1522.

Jädersten, M., Malcovati, L., Dybedal, I., Della Porta, M.G., Invernizzi, R., Montgomery, S.M., Pascutto, C., Porwit, A., Cazzola, M., and Hellström-Lindberg, E. (2008 July 20). Erythropoietin and granulocyte-colony stimulating factor treatment associated with improved survival in myelodysplastic syndrome. *J Clin Oncol* 26 (21): 3607–3613. doi: 10.1200/JCO.2007.15.4906. Epub 2008 Jun 16. PMID: 18559873.

Jädersten, M., Montgomery, S.M., Dybedal, I., Porwit-macdonald, A., and Hellström-Lindberg, E. (2005 August 1). Long-term outcome of treatment of anemia in MDS with erythropoietin and G-CSF. *Blood* 106 (3): 803–811.

List, A., Dewald, G., Bennett, J. et al. (2006). Lenalidomide in the myelodysplastic syndrome with chromosome 5q deletion. *N Engl J Med* 355: 1456–1465.

Lyons, R.M., Cosgriff, T.M., Modi, S.S. et al. (2009). Hematologic response to three alternative dosing schedules of azacitidine in patients with myelodysplastic syndromes. *J Clin Oncol* 27 (11): 1850-1856.

Nakamura, R., Saber, W., Martens, M.J. et al. (2021). Biologic assignment trial of reduced-intensity hematopoietic cell transplantation based on donor availability in patients 50-75 years of age with Advanced Myelodysplastic Syndrome. *J Clin Oncol* 39 (30): 3328–3339.

Oliva, E.N., Riva, M., and Niscola, P. (2023 June 9). Eltrombopag for low-risk myelodysplastic syndromes with thrombocytopenia: interim results of a phase-II, randomized, placebo-controlled clinical trial (EQOL-MDS). *J Clin Oncol* JCO2202699. doi: 10.1200/JCO.22.02699. Epub ahead of print. PMID: 37294914.

Platzbecker, U., Della Porta, M.G., Santini, V. et al. (2023 June 9). Efficacy and safety of luspatercept versus epoetin alfa in erythropoiesis-stimulating agent-naive, transfusion-dependent, lower-risk myelodysplastic syndromes (COMMANDS): interim analysis of a phase 3, open-label, randomised controlled trial. *Lancet* S0140-6736(23)00874-7. doi: 10.1016/S0140-6736(23)00874-7. Epub ahead of print. PMID: 37311468.

Santini, V., Almeida, A., Giagounidis, A. et al. (2016). Randomized phase III study of lenalidomide versus placebo in rbc transfusion-dependent patients with lower-risk non-del(5q) Myelodysplastic Syndromes and ineligible for or refractory to Erythropoiesis-Stimulating Agents. *J Clin Oncol* 34 (25): 2988–2996.

Saunthararajah, Y., Nakamura, R., Wesley, R., Wang, Q.J., and Barrett, A.J. (2003 October 15). A simple method to predict response to immunosuppressive therapy in patients with myelodysplastic syndrome. *Blood* 102 (8): 3025–3027. doi: 10.1182/blood-2002-11-3325. Epub 2003 Jun 26. PMID: 12829603.

Stahl, M., Bewersdorf, J.P., Giri, S., Wang, R., and Zeidan, A.M. (2020 January). Use of immunosuppressive therapy for management of myelodysplastic syndromes: a systematic review and meta-analysis. *Haematologica* 105 (1): 102–111.

Stahl, M., DeVeaux, M., de Witte, T. et al. (2018). The use of immunosuppressive therapy in MDS: clinical outcomes and their predictors in a large international patient cohort. *Blood Adv* 2 (14): 1765–1772.

Volpe VO, Garcia-Manero G, Komrokji RS. Myelodysplastic Syndromes: A New Decade. *Clin Lymphoma Myeloma Leuk*. 2022 Jan;22(1):1–16. 10.1016/j.clml.2021.07.031. Epub 2021 Aug 2. PMID: 34544674.

14

Hematopoietic Cell Transplantation and Cellular Therapy in Myelodysplastic Syndromes

Ibrahim Yakoub-Agha

Lille University Hospital, Lille University, Lille, France

Introduction

Allogeneic hematopoietic cell transplantation (allo-HCT) is still the best therapeutic option for patients with higher-risk myelodysplastic syndrome (MDS). The number of allo-HCT for MDS has been increasing over the two last decades and tends to be the second indication after acute myeloid leukemia accounting for almost 1800 transplants/year in the USA and the third indication in Europe with 12% of allo-HCT patients being transplanted for MDS. Through three clinical cases, we tried to address the main questions regarding the management of MDS patients in patients who are suitable candidate for allo-HCT.

Case Study 1

The patient is a 63-year-old male, in good health, who came to our clinic complaining of chronic fatigue. He reports a surgery for discal hernia 10 years ago, no known prior exposure to toxins. His clinical examination was normal except dyspnea at effort. Blood cell count (CBC) showed neutropenia [absolute neutrophil count (ANC): 0.7 G/L], macrocytic anemia [hemoglobin (Hgb): 9.1 g/dL; mean corpuscular volume (MCV) 103 fL], thrombocytopenia [platelet count (PLT) 33 G/L], and reticulocyte count 20 g/L. His other laboratory parameters, including inflammatory markers and chemistry were all unremarkable. Bone marrow smear showed hypocellular marrow with a few megakaryocytes, several morphological abnormalities affecting all three myeloid lineages (hypogranularity with abnormal nuclear lobulation of granulocytes, megaloblastoid erythropoiesis, and nuclear karyorrhexis and micromegakaryocytes), and 3% of marrow blasts. Bone marrow biopsy revealed a bone marrow with low cellularity for age (20%), with no blasts, normal iron stores, and reticulin fibrosis grade 2. His karyotype did not reveal any cytogenetic abnormalities. No

Cancer Consult: Expertise in Clinical Practice, Volume 2: Neoplastic Hematology & Cellular Therapy,
Second Edition. Edited by Syed A. Abutalib, Maurie Markman, James O. Armitage, and Kenneth C. Anderson.
© 2024 John Wiley & Sons Ltd. Published 2024 by John Wiley & Sons Ltd.

gene mutations were found on NGS. Final diagnosis is myelodysplastic syndrome (MDS) with multilineage dysplasia. His R-IPSS is 4.3 corresponding to intermediate risk level.

1) Should this patient receive up-front allogeneic hematopoietic cell transplantation?

Expert Perspective: Allo-HCT cannot be a standard treatment for all MDS patients. Indeed, several factors must be considered in the decision-making process (Figure 14.1).

Those factors are, on one hand, patient-related, such as age and comorbidities that affect the transplantation feasibility. The European Society for Blood and Marrow Transplantation (EBMT) proposed an optimized transplant-specific risk score for MDS patients (Gagelmann et al. 2019). This scoring system along with the comorbidity index (HCT-CI) developed by Sorror et al. are usually used to judge the feasibility of allo-HCT and to predict post-transplant outcomes in an MDS patient.

On the other hand, the disease characteristics that affect the risk of transformation into acute myeloid leukemia (AML) and survival have to be considered. The revised international prognosis scoring system (IPSS-R) has been recognized internationally as the most relevant system to assess disease prognosis (de Witte et al. 2017). This revised scoring system is based on marrow blast percentage, modified cytogenetic risk groups, and the severity of cytopenias. In addition, it is an age-adjusted risk score. The IPSS-R risk categories can function as the platform for disease-related factors with five categories: very

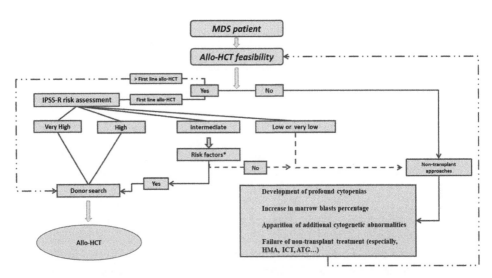

Figure 14.1 Indication of allogeneic hematopoietic cell transplantation (allo-HCT) in myelodysplastic (MDS).
> first line allo-HCT means patients who were not candidate for allo-HCT at first place but who further experience one of the following deteriorations in the disease characteristics: development of profound cytopenia, increase in marrow blasts, having additional cytogenetic abnormalities, and failure with non-transplant approaches.
* Risk factors include more than 5% marrow blasts, poor karyotype, profound cytopenias (i.e. Hb < 8 g/dL, absolute neutrophil count < 0.8 G/L, platelets < 50 G/L), severe bone marrow fibrosis, or poor gene mutations on NGS.
Abbreviations: HMA: hypomethylating agents; ICT: induction-type chemotherapy; ATG: antithymocyte globulin.

low (score ≤ 1.5), low (1.5 < score ≤ 3.0), intermediate (3 < score ≤ 4.5), high (4.5 < score ≤ 6), and very high (score > 6). The 25% AML progression/median survival in the absence of therapy were (not reached/8.8), (10.8/5.3), (3.2/3), (1.4/1.6), and (0.7/0.8) years for patients with very low, low, intermediate, high, and very high risk, respectively. To simplify its clinical use, patients can be categorized into three risk groups when considering allo-HCT: lower risk (LR-MDS), including low and very low risk groups; intermediate risk; and higher risk (HR-MDS), including high- and very high-risk groups.

While allo-HCT is a standard of care in fit patients with higher-risk MDS, the decision becomes more difficult for patients belonging to the intermediate IPSS-R group. In fact, these patients have a median survival of three years without treatment and 25% AML progression at 3.2 years. Patients in the intermediate IPSS-R risk group who present at diagnosis more than 5% marrow blasts, poor karyotype, profound cytopenias (i.e. Hgb < 8 g/dL, ANC < 0.8 g/L, PLT < 50 g/L), or severe marrow fibrosis can be referred for frontline allo-HCT. All the remaining patients in this risk group should be offered non-transplant options as first line of therapy (Della Porta et al. 2009, de Witte et al. 2017).

Case Study continued: In the present case, up-front allo-HCT is the best option for this 63-year-old male with no comorbidities and intermediate IPSS-R score suffering from severe cytopenias and myelofibrosis.

2) Is "debulking" therapy indicated before transplant? And if so, what is the optimal induction regimen?

Expert Perspective: Large studies have shown that the percentage of bone marrow blasts at transplant significantly affect post-transplant outcome for MDS patients, thus justifying the use of pre-transplant cytoreduction treatment. However, debulking treatment before allo-HCT, which aims to reduce the incidence of post-transplant relapse in patients with MDS, is still debated. The achievement of complete remission (CR) before transplant has been shown to improve outcome, although one might question whether this better outcome reflects the selection of responsive patients or is related to a reduction in disease burden. A large retrospective study from the chronic malignancies working party (CMWP) of EBMT failed to demonstrate any impact of changing IPPS-R score between diagnosis and allo-HCT in MDS patients. Therefore, similar survival and disease-free survival were observed in patients who improved, worsened, or maintained their IPSS-R scores between diagnosis and transplant. These results lead to the conclusion that disease biology is the main driver of outcome rather than the disease status at transplant.

Patients with MDS who are candidates for allo-HCT could be offered three pre-transplant strategies including induction-type chemotherapy, hypomethylating agents (HMA), and new drugs (targeted therapies such as *IDH1* and *IDH2* inhibitors, reactivating compound of mutant p53 protein, or venetoclax) alone or associated with HMA.

Although, there are no solid data to support pre-transplant debulking treatment, intensive chemotherapy has been the preferred pre-transplant treatment in patients with more than 10% marrow blasts and an absence of poor cytogenetic abnormalities, and HMA has been offered to older patients who have less than 10% marrow blasts. In a retrospective comparison of intensive chemotherapy and HMA, Damaj et al. observed similar post-transplant outcome with both strategies when patients received either intensive chemotherapy or HMA alone (Damaj et al. 2012). Patients who received intensive chemotherapy and HMA before transplant had higher non-relapse mortality rate and similar incidence of post-transplant relapse compared to patients who received only intensive chemotherapy or HMA, reflecting an additional toxicity rather than a selection of poor prognostic patients (Damaj et al. 2012).

Mutations of *IDH1* and *IDH2* genes are present in 5–10% of MDS. IDH 1 (ivosidenib) and *IDH2* (enasidenib) inhibitors have been approved by the FDA for the treatment of refractory/relapsed (R/R) acute myeloid leukemia (AML) with these mutations. Enasidenib and ivosidenib, as a single oral agent in patients with R/R AML, induced approximately 35% response rate. Data are more limited for patients with *IDH1/2*-mutated MDS with response rate of 53% in 16 R/R high-risk *IDH2*-mutated MDS treated with enasidenib. The potential therapeutic role of *IDH* inhibitors in MDS is currently under investigation, either as a single agent or in combination with HMA.

The *TP53* mutation is present in about 10% of HR-MDS and in 50% of those with complex karyotype. It is associated with lower response rates but, more importantly, much shorter responses to HMA than in patients with wild-type *TP53* gene. A randomized phase III (NCT03745716) is currently evaluating safety and efficacy of APR-246 (eprenetapopt) a first-in-class small molecule that restores wild-type p53 protein functions in TP53-mutant cells is being tested in combination with azacitidine in patients with TP53-mutated MDS and AML.

The preliminary results of a phase Ib study that investigated the safety and efficacy of the association venetoclax-azacitadine showed a high toxicity incidence with this combination in 78 patients with HR-MDS. Venetoclax was initially given at a dose of 400 and 800 mg/d for 28 days but was later amended to an escalating dose regimen (100, 200, and 400 mg) for only 14 of 28 days every cycle due to excessive toxicity.

The overall response rate (ORR) was 77%, including complete remission (CR) and marrow CR (mCR) achieved by 42% and 35% of patients, respectively. Of note, Adverse events ⩾ grade 3 were common with neutropenia (51%) and thrombocytopenia (30%). Febrile neutropenia was observed in 42%, and the 30-day mortality rate was 2%. Two-thirds of patients required a cycle delay for a median of 15 days. Half of patients experienced two or more venetoclax dose interruptions while dose reduction of azacitidine was also necessary in 30% of patients.

This illustrates, once again, that HR-MDS patients constitute a vulnerable patient population in terms of toxicities. In general, pre-transplant debulking treatment can be responsible for morbidities and mortality that can prevent some patients to undergo allo-HCT. Indeed, in a prospective study comparing donor versus no donor in patients with HR-MDS, Robin et al. observed up to 25% of patients died before transplantation mainly because of pre-transplant treatment toxicity. In a large retrospective comparison, Damaj et al. observed no difference in terms of overall survival, relapse-free survival, relapse, and non-relapse mortality between patients who received HMA before allo-HCT for MDS and those who did not (Damaj et al. 2014).

Given the absence of prospective data demonstrating a definite benefit of pre-transplant treatment for post-transplant outcome, another approach would be to simply proceed to transplantation right away after the diagnosis of HR-MDS. Indeed, with the increased number of donors (unrelated or haploidentical), the time to transplant is becoming shorter in most transplant centers worldwide.

Case Study continued: In this 63-year-old male patient with no comorbidities, up-front allo-HCT seems to be the most appropriate strategy.

3) What is the most appropriate donor?

Expert Perspective: Approximately 30% of patients have a human leukocyte antigen (HLA)–identical sibling donor that has been established as the gold standard for malignant and nonmalignant diseases. In addition, outcomes after transplantation from high-resolution HLA-matched unrelated donors (so-called 10/10) were similar to outcomes observed with HLA-identical sibling donors (Yakoub-Agha et al. 2006). Therefore, both HLA-identical sibling and 10/10 HLA-matched unrelated donor are equal and should be considered as a first choice.

Although, allo-HCT from syngeneic donors are reputed to lack graft-versus-leukemia effect, results of such transplantations have similarly shown that they are responsible for lower post-transplant toxicity leading to similar or even better outcomes when compared to HLA-matched related or unrelated donors (Deeg et al. 2000). Indeed, in an EBMT study, a trend for better overall survival was observed in the twin group probably because of lower non-relapse mortality with comparable relapse incidence (Kroger et al. 2005).

In the absence of an HLA-matched donor, allo-HCT from an alternative donor including haploidentical donor, HLA-mismatched related or unrelated donor, and unrelated cord blood can be considered. Of note, in a study that included 3,857 patients, Lee et al. reported that mismatching at a single HLA-A, -B, -C, or -DRB1 locus (7/8) was associated with lower survival and disease-free survival and higher treatment-related mortality compared with 8/8 HLA-matched pairs. Therefore, alternative donor transplants may be considered for young fit patients with HR-MDS for whom no HLA-matched donor can be identified within 2–3 months (de Witte et al. 2017).

Overall, in the absence of an HLA-matched donor for a given patient, a prolonged search in order to identify a fully HLA-matched donor must be balanced against the risk of disease progression and the occurrence of cytopenia-related complications while the search is underway. Depending on the stage of the disease, rapid transplantation with the best available donor, even if allele- or antigen-level mismatched, may offer the best chance for survival.

4) Which hematopoietic CD34+ cell source (PB vs BM) would be most desirable?

Expert Perspective: A large number of studies have compared mobilized peripheral blood stem cells (PBSC) with bone marrow for allo-HCT. Although PBSC has become a preferred graft source in many centers around the world for several reasons, the potential benefits with this source are still unclear. In fact, PBSC has been associated with a high rate of extensive chronic GvHD.

In a prospective multicenter randomized trial that enrolled 551 unrelated transplantations, Anasetti et al. showed a two-year incidence of chronic GvHD of 53% (95% CI 45–61) in PBSC group as compared with 41% (95% CI 34–48) in the BM group ($P = 0.01$) (Anasetti et al. 2012). The absence of the use of ATG as a GvHD prophylaxis in PBSC patients could be an explanation of these results since 72% of the patients had not received ATG within the conditioning. Indeed, the quantity of donor-derived lymphocytes in PBSC grafts could be up to 30-fold greater than in bone marrow grafts. In addition, the absence of ATG was observed to be an independent risk factor for both acute and chronic GvHD in a prospective randomized study that included 201 patients, of whom 164 had received PBSC (Finke et al. 2009). In other studies, incorporating ATG into conditioning regimens for unrelated transplantations has decreased the incidence of GvHD without compromising survival or increasing post-transplant relapse rates (Dulery et al. 2014). The same study by Anasetti et al. also showed that the overall survival rate at two years using PBSC was 51% (95% CI 45–57), compared to 46% (95% CI 40–52) in the BM group (*P* = 0.29), with an absolute difference of 5% points (95% CI –3–14). Results were similar among HLA-mismatched pairs, recipients with advanced disease, and recipients older than 40 years of age, although this trial was not designed to detect potential differences within these subsets. The overall incidence of graft failure in the PBSC group was 3% (95% CI 1–5), versus 9% (95% CI 6–13) in the BM group (*P* = 0.002). In addition, graft failure was more common after marrow transplantation from an HLA-mismatched donor than after marrow transplantation from an HLA-matched donor (16% versus 7%, *P* = 0.04). Graft failure was rarely observed after transplantation from PBSC source from HLA-mismatched donors (2%) or HLA-matched unrelated donors (3%). Among patients randomly assigned to receive peripheral blood grafts, as compared with those randomly assigned to receive marrow grafts, the median time to neutrophil engraftment was five days shorter (*P* < 0.001), and the median time to platelet engraftment was seven days shorter (*P* < 0.001).

In a retrospective study that included 234 MDS patients and compared PBSC with bone marrow using HLA-identical sibling donors, survival was significantly better among recipients of PBSC, except for patients with either refractory anemia or high-risk cytogenetics. Although, there is no international consensus regarding the preferred source of hematopoietic cells between PBSC and bone marrow, in our practice we incorporate ATG at 2.5 mg/kg/day for two consecutive days within the conditioning regimen whenever PBSC graft is used. It is important to note that the paradigm of GvHD prophylaxis is favorably evolving especially with the advent of post-transplantation cyclophosphamide.

Unrelated cord blood, whose use has dramatically decreased nowadays, can be chosen in the absence of an HLA-matched donor in certain centers with expertise.

In summary, it might be reasonable to conclude that for patients with high-risk disease who have already been neutropenic for a prolonged period of time, evidence supports the use of peripheral blood stem cells despite higher risk of chronic GvHD, and for all other situations, BM is the preferred source in hematologic malignancies including MDS.

5) What is the most appropriate intensity of the transplant conditioning regimen?

Expert Perspective: The impact of conditioning intensity on patient outcome after allo-HCT for MDS is still controversial. However, some retrospective studies comparing myeloablative with reduced-intensity conditioning regimens did not show a difference in survival when patients were transplanted in CR1, while none of the patients transplanted with active disease survived after reduced-intensity regimens (Shimoni et al. 2006). Likewise, the results of a prospective randomized study that compared myeloablative versus reduced-intensity conditioning regimens in patients with AML or MDS were clearly in favor of an myeloablative regimen (Scott et al. 2017). In contrary, the EBMT's CMWP study has investigated the impact of conditioning intensity on post-transplant outcome in different scenarios of MDS patients but failed to find any differences (unpublished data).

For the time being, myeloablative conditioning should be the preferred regimen whenever possible. However, age-adjusted HCT-CI as well as disease characteristics should be considered before making the decision regarding conditioning intensity for a given patient (Gagelmann et al. 2019).

Case Study 2

A 56-year-old female is referred to the cellular therapy unit to undergo allo-HCT for MDS, which was diagnosed two weeks ago. At the admission, her CBC showed pancytopenias with neutropenia (ANC: 0.9 G/L), anemia (Hgb: 8.2 g/dL; MCV: 96 fL), and thrombocytopenia (PLT: 77 G/L). Her other laboratory parameters, including inflammatory markers and chemistry, were all unremarkable. A bone marrow smear showed a hypercellular marrow with increased red cell precursors and 7% of blasts consistent with EB1/MDS diagnosis. Bone marrow biopsy was consistent with this diagnosis with no fibrosis. Her karyotype revealed +8 in 16 of 20 assessed metaphases. Her IPSS-R score is 5.18 (high). The ferritin level was found to be elevated at > 2500 ng/mL. Karnofsky index = 100, age-adjusted HCT/CI = 1, and EBMT optimized score = 3 (age, CMV, and unrelated donor) (Gagelmann et al. 2019). An up-front allo-HCT with PBSC from an HLA-matched (10/10) unrelated donor is scheduled in two months. Only supportive care has been recommended before allo-HCT. Conditioning is myeloablative with IV busulfan (130 mg/m^2/day, four days) and fludarabine (30 mg/m^2/day, four days).

6) What is the most appropriate post-transplant disease monitoring?

Expert Perspective: New techniques based on PCR using whole bone marrow or sorted subpopulations have been used to monitor post-transplant chimerism. Declining donor chimerism after allo-HCT are usually considered as a marker of imminent relapse (Platzbecker et al. 2012). In some patients with MDS, the expression of *Wilms' tumor 1* (*WT1*) can be a good quantitative marker for monitoring minimal residual disease after allo-HCT (Dulery et al. 2017). Molecular abnormalities play a significant role in the prognosis of MDS (Nikoloski et al. 2010) and in patient response to allo-HCT. Some genetic abnormalities such as *SF3B1* mutation generally have a favorable prognosis in contrast to SRSF2-mutated cases. In addition, multilineage dysplasias are associated with *DNMT3A*, *TET2*, *IDH1*, and *IDH2* mutations. Furthermore, *RUNX1-*, *U2AF1-*, *ASXL-*, and *TP53*-mutated cases appear to be associated with poor prognosis. Except for the combination of complex karyotype and *TP53* mutations being associated with extremely poor outcome after allo-HCT, to date there is no international consensus that incorporates molecular abnormalities as factors into the treatment decision-making process. Furthermore, there are no robust data to support NGS as biomarkers for minimal residual disease post-transplant monitoring in MDS patients with molecular abnormalities.

7) What is the best prevention of post-transplant relapse?

Expert Perspective: Relapse remains the main cause of transplant failure, especially following reduced-intensity conditioning regimens. Although, there are no solid prospective data to support post-transplant prophylaxis, many phase II studies have reported promising results with the use of HMA alone or associated with donor lymphocyte infusion (DLI) after allo-HCT (Itzykson et al. 2011, Krishnamurthy et al. 2013). On the other hand, a prospective randomized study demonstrated no effect of post-transplant azacitidine in 187 patients with high-risk AML or MDS who underwent allo-HCT following myeloablative and non-myeloablative conditioning regimens (Oran et al. 2020). Oral azacitidine has been assessed as a maintenance therapy in a prospective study with encouraging results, but only seven MDS patients received the drug in this study (de Lima et al. 2017). New drugs are being investigated especially the association of low-dose venetoclax and azacitidine (NCT04128501). Rapid tapering of immunosuppressive treatment with/without prophylactic DLI can be a strategy to reduce post-transplant relapse. However, this latter strategy should be limited to patients at substantial risk of post-transplant relapse (i.e. complex karyotype) since it may be responsible for an increase in GvHD incidence and severity leading to an increase in non-relapse mortality. In this 56-year-old female, we decide not to give her maintenance therapy since there are no strong data to support this strategy so far.

8) How best to manage iron overload in patients with MDS?

Expert Perspective: Iron overload is an important concern after allo-HCT especially in MDS patients because of accumulation of iron mainly as a result of ineffective hematopoiesis and frequent red blood cell transfusion. Iron overload can be responsible for several post-transplant complications (Alessandrino et al. 2010).

Assessment of serum ferritin level is the easiest test to perform in this setting. However, new MRI seems to be the most appropriate test to confirm IOL in the liver and the heart. Myocardial T2* values < 20 ms indicate increased myocardial iron and values < 10 ms are associated with high risk of heart failure within 12 months after allo-HCT.

Iron overload after allo-HCT may be treated by phlebotomies or by iron chelation (de Witte et al. 2017). In this patient with high serum ferritin level, we decide to start iron chelation after 6–12 months post transplant in the absence of concurrent complications.

Case Study 3

A 66-year-old male underwent an allo-HCT from a haploidentical donor for high-risk MDS three years ago. He is just being admitted for post-transplant relapse. CBC showed neutropenia (ANC: 1.6 × G/L), macrocytic anemia (Hgb: 10.1 g/dL; MCV: 106 fL), and thrombocytopenia (PLT: 110 G/L). His other laboratory parameters, including inflammatory markers and chemistry, were all unremarkable. Bone marrow smear showed hypocellular marrow with a few megakaryocytes, and 9% of marrow blasts. His karyotype is complex with three abnormalities, which were observed before allo-HCT. Chimerism revealed 73% of recipient-origin cells.

9) How best to manage post-transplant relapse?

Expert Perspective: The treatment is individualized based on patient desire and performance status at the time of relapse. The options include (i) palliative approaches and best supportive care; (ii) cytoreduction treatment with intensive chemotherapy, HMA, or targeted therapies; and (iii) adoptive immunotherapy (i.e. DLI and/or second transplant). In a retrospective study on 147 MDS patients who relapsed after allo-HCTreported that early (before six months) post-transplant relapse, history of GvHD, platelet count < 50,000, and progression to AML at the time of relapse were the most important factors determining poor outcome (Guieze et al. 2015). Furthermore, longer survival was observed in patients who received immunotherapy (DLI or second allo-HCT) with or without cytoreduction treatment compared with patients who received best supportive care or cytoreduction treatment alone.

An international panel of MDS and transplantation experts recommended immune modulation (DLI or second allo-HCT) in MDS patients who relapse after six months from transplant (de Witte et al. 2017).

Case Study continued: For this patient, who relapsed after six months after allo-HCT with 12% of marrow blasts or more (arbitrary blast number), we recommend a cytoreduction (intensive chemotherapy or venetoclax-azacitidine) treatment followed by DLI in case of full or mixed donor-type chimerism or second allo-HCT preferably from a different donor.

Authors' disclosure: The clinical cases in this chapter do not refer to actual patients. All of the recommendations are in accordance with the international guidelines.

Recommended Readings

Alessandrino, E.P., la Porta, M.G., Bacigalupo, A., Malcovati, L., Angelucci, E., Van Lint, M.T., Falda, M., Onida, F., Bernardi, M., Guidi, S., Lucarelli, B., Rambaldi, A., Cerretti, R., Marenco, P., Pioltelli, P., Pascutto, C., Oneto, R., Pirolini, L., Fanin, R., and Bosi, A. (2010 March). Prognostic impact of pre-transplantation transfusion history and secondary iron overload in patients with myelodysplastic syndrome undergoing allogeneic stem cell transplantation: a GITMO study. *Haematologica* 95: 476–484.

Anasetti, C., Logan, B.R., Lee, S.J., Waller, E.K., Weisdorf, D.J., Wingard, J.R., Cutler, C.S., Westervelt, P., Woolfrey, A., Couban, S., Ehninger, G., Johnston, L., Maziarz, R.T., Pulsipher, M.A., Porter, D.L., Mineishi, S., McCarty, J.M., Khan, S.P., Anderlini, P., Bensinger, W.I., Leitman, S.F., Rowley, S.D., Bredeson, C., Carter, S.L., Horowitz, M.M., and Confer, D.L. (2012). Peripheral-blood stem cells versus bone marrow from unrelated donors. *N Engl J Med* 367: 1487–1496.

Damaj, G., Duhamel, A., Robin, M., Beguin, Y., Michallet, M., Mohty, M., Vigouroux, S., Bories, P., Garnier, A., El Cheikh, J., Bulabois, C.E., Huynh, A., Bay, J.O., Legrand, F., Deconinck, E., Fegueux, N., Clement, L., Dauriac, C., Maillard, N., Cornillon, J., Ades, L., Guillerm, G., Schmidt-Tanguy, A., Marjanovic, Z., Park, S., Rubio, M.T., Marolleau, J.P., Garnier, F., Fenaux, P., and Yakoub-Agha, I. (2012). Impact of azacitidine before allogeneic stem-cell transplantation for myelodysplastic syndromes: a study by the Societe Francaise de Greffe de Moelle et de Therapie-Cellulaire and the Groupe-Francophone des Myelodysplasies. *J Clin Oncol* 36:4533-40

Damaj, G., Mohty, M., Robin, M., Michallet, M., Chevallier, P., Beguin, Y., Nguyen, S., Bories, P., Blaise, D., Maillard, N., Rubio, M.T., Fegueux, N., Cornillon, J., Clavert, A., Huynh, A., Adès, L., Thiébaut-Bertrand, A., Hermine, O., Vigouroux, S., Fenaux, P., Duhamel, A., and Yakoub-Agha, I. (2014). Up-front allogeneic stem cell transplantation following reduced intensity/nonmyeloablative for patients with myelodysplastic syndrome. a study by the Société Française de Greffe de Moelle et de Thérapie Cellulaire (SFGM-TC). *Biol Blood Marrow Transplant* 9:1349-55

de Lima, M., Oran, B., Champlin, R.E., Papadopoulos, E.B., Giralt, S.A., Scott, B.L., William, B.M., Hetzer, J., Laille, E., Hubbell, B., Skikne, B.S., and Craddock, C. (2017). CC-486 maintenance after stem cell transplantation in patients with acute myeloid leukemia or myelodysplastic syndromes. *Biol Blood Marrow Transplant* 24: 2017–2024.

de Witte, T., Hermans, J., Vossen, J., Bacigalupo, A., Meloni, G., Jacobsen, N., Ruutu, T., Ljungman, P., Gratwohl, A., Runde, V., Niederwieser, D., van, B.A., Devergie, A., Cornelissen, J., Jouet, J.P., Arnold, R., and Apperley, J. (2000 September). Haematopoietic stem cell transplantation for patients with myelo-dysplastic syndromes and secondary acute myeloid leukaemias: a report on behalf of the Chronic Leukaemia Working Party of the European Group for Blood and Marrow Transplantation (EBMT). *Br J Haematol* 110: 620–630.

Deeg, H.J., Shulman, H.M., Anderson, J.E., Bryant, E.M., Gooley, T.A., Slattery, J.T., Anasetti, C., Fefer, A., Storb, R., and Appelbaum, F.R. (2000 February 15). Allogeneic and syngeneic marrow transplantation for myelodysplastic syndrome in patients 55 to 66 years of age. *Blood* 95: 1188–1194.

Della Porta, M.G., Malcovati, L., Boveri, E., Travaglino, E., Pietra, D., Pascutto, C., Passamonti, F., Invernizzi, R., Castello, A., Magrini, U., Lazzarino, M., and Cazzola, M. (2009). Clinical relevance of bone marrow fibrosis and CD34-positive cell clusters in primary myelodysplastic syndromes. *J Clin Oncol* 27: 754–762.

Dulery, R., Mohty, M., Duhamel, A., Robin, M., Beguin, Y., Michallet, M., Vigouroux, S., Lioure, B., Garnier, A., El Cheikh, J., Bulabois, C.E., Huynh, A., Bay, J.O., Daguindau, E., Ceballos, P., Clement, L., Dauriac, C., Maillard, N., Legrand, F., Cornillon, J., Guillerm, G., Francois, S., Lapusan, S., Chevallier, P., Damaj, G., and Yakoub-Agha, I. (2014). Antithymocyte globulin before allogeneic stem cell transplantation for progressive myelodysplastic syndrome: a study from the French Society of Bone Marrow Transplantation and Cellular Therapy. *Biol Blood Marrow Transplant* 20: 646–654.

Dulery, R., Nibourel, O., Gauthier, J., Elsermans, V., Behal, H., Coiteux, V., Magro, L., Renneville, A., Marceau, A., Boyer, T., Quesnel, B., Preudhomme, C., Duhamel, A., and Yakoub-Agha, I. (2017). Impact of Wilms' tumor 1 expression on outcome of patients undergoing allogeneic stem cell transplantation for AML. *Bone Marrow Transplant* 52: 539–543.

Finke, J., Bethge, W.A., Schmoor, C., Ottinger, H.D., Stelljes, M., Zander, A.R., Volin, L., Ruutu, T., Heim, D.A., Schwerdtfeger, R., Kolbe, K., Mayer, J., Maertens, J.A., Linkesch, W., Holler, E., Koza, V., Bornhauser, M., Einsele, H., Kolb, H.J., Bertz, H., Egger, M., Grishina, O., and Socie, G. (2009). Standard graft-versus-host disease prophylaxis with or without anti-T-cell globulin in haematopoietic cell transplantation from matched unrelated donors: a randomised, open-label, multicentre phase 3 trial. *Lancet Oncol* 10: 855–864.

Gagelmann, N., Eikema, D.J., Stelljes, M., Beelen, D., de Wreede, L., Mufti, G., Knelange, N.S., Niederwieser, D., Friis, L.S., Ehninger, G., Nagler, A., Yakoub-Agha, I., Meijer, E.,

Ljungman, P., Maertens, J., Kanz, L., Lopez-Corral, L., Brecht, A., Craddock, C., Finke, J., Cornelissen, J.J., Bernasconi, P., Chevallier, P., Sierra, J., Robin, M., and Kroger, N. (2019). Optimized EBMT transplant-specific risk score in myelodysplastic syndromes after allogeneic stem-cell transplantation. *Haematologica* 104: 929–936.

Guieze, R., Damaj, G., Pereira, B., Robin, M., Chevallier, P., Michallet, M., Vigouroux, S., Beguin, Y., Blaise, D., El Cheikh, J., Roos-Weil, D., Thiebaut, A., Rohrlich, P.S., Huynh, A., Cornillon, J., Contentin, N., Suarez, F., Lioure, B., Mohty, M., Maillard, N., Clement, L., Francois, S., Guillerm, G., and Yakoub-Agha, I. (2015). Management of myelodysplastic syndrome relapsing after allogeneic hematopoietic stem cell transplantation: a study by the French Society of Bone Marrow Transplantation and Cell Therapies. *Biol Blood Marrow Transplant* 22: 240–247.

Itzykson, R., Thepot, S., Eclache, V., Quesnel, B., Dreyfus, F., Beyne-Rauzy, O., Turlure, P., Vey, N., Recher, C., Boehrer, S., Gardin, C., Ades, L., Fenaux, P., and Groupe Francophone des Myélodysplasie (GFM). (2011). Prognostic significance of monosomal karyotype in higher risk myelodysplastic syndrome treated with azacitidine. *Leukemia* 25: 1207–1209.

Krishnamurthy, P., Potter, V.T., Barber, L.D., Kulasekararaj, A.G., Lim, Z.Y., Pearce, R.M., de Lavallade, H., Kenyon, M., Ireland, R.M., Marsh, J.C., Devereux, S., Pagliuca, A., and Mufti, G.J. (2013). Outcome of donor lymphocyte infusion after T cell-depleted allogeneic hematopoietic stem cell transplantation for acute myelogenous leukemia and myelodysplastic syndromes. *Biol Blood Marrow Transplant* 19: 562–568.

Kroger, N., Brand, R., van Biezen, A., Bron, D., Blaise, D., Hellstrom-Lindberg, E., Gahrton, G., Powles, R., Littlewood, T., Chapuis, B., Zander, A., Koza, V., Niederwieser, D., de Witte, T., and Myelodysplastic Syndromes Subcommittee of the Chronic Leukaemia Working Party, European Blood and Marrow Transplantation Group. (2005). Stem cell transplantation from identical twins in patients with myelodysplastic syndromes. *Bone Marrow Transplant* 35: 37–43.

Nikoloski, G., Langemeijer, S.M., Kuiper, R.P., Knops, R., Massop, M., Tonnissen, E.R., van der, H.A., Scheele, T.N., Vandenberghe, P., de, W.T., van der Reijden, B.A., and Jansen, J.H. (2010 August). Somatic mutations of the histone methyltransferase gene EZH2 in myelodysplastic syndromes. *Nat Genet* 42: 665–667.

Oran, B., de Lima, M., Garcia-Manero, G., Thall, P.F., Lin, R., Popat, U., Alousi, A.M., Hosing, C., Giralt, S., Rondon, G., Woodworth, G., and Champlin, R.E. (2020). A phase 3 randomized study of 5-azacitidine maintenance vs observation after transplant in high-risk AML and MDS patients. *Blood Adv* 4: 5580–5588.

Platzbecker, U., Wermke, M., Radke, J., Oelschlaegel, U., Seltmann, F., Kiani, A., Klut, I.M., Knoth, H., Rollig, C., Schetelig, J., Mohr, B., Graehlert, X., Ehninger, G., Bornhauser, M., and Thiede, C. (2012). Azacitidine for treatment of imminent relapse in MDS or AML patients after allogeneic HSCT: results of the RELAZA trial. *Leukemia* 26: 381–389.

Scott, B.L., Pasquini, M.C., Logan, B.R., Wu, J., Devine, S.M., Porter, D.L., Maziarz, R.T., Warlick, E.D., Fernandez, H.F., Alyea, E.P., Hamadani, M., Bashey, A., Giralt, S., Geller, N.L., Leifer, E., Le-Rademacher, J., Mendizabal, A.M., Horowitz, M.M., Deeg, H.J., and Horwitz, M.E. (2017). Myeloablative versus reduced-intensity hematopoietic cell transplantation for acute myeloid leukemia and myelodysplastic syndromes. *J Clin Oncol* 35: 1154–1161.

Shimoni, A., Hardan, I., Shem-Tov, N., Yeshurun, M., Yerushalmi, R., Avigdor, A., Ben-Bassat, I., and Nagler, A. (2006 February). Allogeneic hematopoietic stem-cell transplantation in AML and MDS using myeloablative versus reduced-intensity conditioning: the role of dose intensity. *Leukemia* 20: 322–328.

Vittayawacharin, P., Kongtim, P., and Ciurea, S.O. (2023 February). Allogeneic stem cell transplantation for patients with myelodysplastic syndromes. *Am J Hematol* 98 (2): 322–337. doi: 10.1002/ajh.26763. Epub 2022 Oct 28. PMID: 36251347.

Yakoub-Agha, I., Mesnil, F., Kuentz, M., Boiron, J.M., Ifrah, N., Milpied, N., Chehata, S., Esperou, H., Vernant, J.P., Michallet, M., Buzyn, A., Gratecos, N., Cahn, J.Y., Bourhis, J.H., Chir, Z., Raffoux, C., Socie, G., Golmard, J.L., and Jouet, J.P. (2006). Allogeneic marrow stem-cell transplantation from human leukocyte antigen-identical siblings versus human leukocyte antigen-allelic-matched unrelated donors (10/10) in patients with standard-risk hematologic malignancy: a prospective study from the French Society of Bone Marrow Transplantation and Cell Therapy. *J Clin Oncol* 24: 5695–5702.

15

Familial Myeloid Neoplasms—When to Suspect and What to Do?

Ryan J. Stubbins[1,2,5], Amy M. Trottier[3], Simone Feurstein[4], and Lucy A. Godley[1]

[1] Northwestern University Feinberg School of Medicine, Chicago, IL
[2] Leukemia/BMT Program of BC, BC Cancer, Provincial Health Services Authority, Vancouver, BC, Canada
[3] Division of Hematology, Department of Medicine, QEII Health Sciences Centre/Dalhousie University, Halifax, NS, Canada
[4] Section of Hematology, Oncology and Rheumatology, Department of Medicine, Heidelberg University Hospital, Heidelberg, Germany
[5] Leukemia/BMT Program of BC, BC Cancer, Provincial Health Services Authority, Vancouver, BC, Canada

Introduction

Familial myeloid neoplasms are a heterogeneous group of disorders wherein the presence of a germline gene variant leads to a heritable risk of developing myelodysplastic syndromes (MDS), acute myeloid leukemia (AML), or myeloproliferative neoplasms (MPNs). Once thought to be rare, germline disorders are now recognized to be identified in 10% or more of patients with myeloid malignancies and can occur across the entire age spectrum. These findings have implications for patient management, cascade testing of family members, and selection of appropriate donors for allogeneic hematopoietic stem cell transplantation (allo-HSCT). It is important for any clinician who treats patients with myeloid malignancies to understand these disorders. Herein, we outline the approach to identifying patients with germline predisposition syndromes and identify the key components to managing the unique needs of these patients.

Case Study

A 65-year-old woman is referred to you with a presumptive new diagnosis of myelodysplastic syndrome with excess blasts (MDS-EB). She presented with cytopenias on routine bloodwork (neutrophil count 0.9×10^9/L, hemoglobin 8.8 g/dL, platelets 55×10^9/L). She is asymptomatic and previously healthy. Her blood film showed dysplastic neutrophils. A bone marrow biopsy showed hypocellularity (20%), erythroid precursor dysplasia, and 9%

blasts. Cytogenetic analysis was normal. A next-generation sequencing panel is pending. She has one brother (age 58) and one sister (age 55). Upon further questioning, she notes her father and paternal aunt died of acute myeloid leukemia at ages 71 and 73, respectively. She has two children (ages 25 and 28) and is asking whether they are at risk of developing a malignancy.

1) What are familial myeloid neoplasms?

Expert Perspective: Familial myeloid neoplasms are defined by the presence of a pathogenic or likely pathogenic germline gene variant that predisposes an individual to myeloid malignancies, most commonly MDS or AML. Familial predispositions to MPNs also exist but are less common. It is important to define what is meant by a genetic variant: a variant refers to an alteration in the DNA sequence relative to the reference genome that is not found at a high frequency in the general population and can include single nucleotide variants (SNVs), copy number variants (CNVs), insertions/deletions (indels), and truncating variants. Germline SNVs found at a frequency > 1% in the general population are considered common and are generally referred to as single nucleotide polymorphisms (SNPs). The American College of Medical Genetics and Genomics classifies germline variants into five categories: pathogenic (P); likely pathogenic (LP); variant of uncertain significance (VUS); likely benign (LB); and benign (B). Assignment of a detected variant to one of these categories is based on numerous factors, including previously reported clinical phenotype(s), population frequency, segregation data, frequency of detection in large population databases, and the predicted or experimentally established effect of the variant on the protein product. This information is aggregated into databases such as ClinVar (www.ncbi.nlm.nih.gov/clinvar), where the variant classification is reported publicly. The term "gene mutation" is synonymous with a P/LP variant, although the former nomenclature is falling out of favor as individuals can be offended if called mutant.

A germline variant can either be inherited (i.e. the variant was present in a parent's germline tissue) or can occur *de novo* in the early stages after oocyte fertilization. In some disorders, *de novo* germline variants account for a significant fraction of cases (e.g. *GATA2*-related disease). It is important to recognize that germline variants will be present in all cells throughout the body, and this can cause non-hematopoietic manifestations of these disorders. There are also implications that arise from the presence of germline variants that extend beyond the patient to their family members. Somatic variants are acquired later in life and are isolated to a subset of an individual's cells. In the context of MDS/AML, these somatic variants will be found exclusively within the hematopoietic system.

Although familial myeloid neoplasms were once thought to be rare, we now know that they are more common than previously realized. Studies suggest that germline variants can be implicated in up to 50% of childhood MDS/AML and 10% or more of adult cases. The detection of familial myeloid neoplasms and the identification of germline variants can influence familial screening, allo-HSCT donor selection and conditioning, treatment approaches, detection of extra-hematopoietic manifestations, and surveillance strategies for hematopoietic and non-hematopoietic malignancies. Due to increased awareness of familial myeloid neoplasms, there are now established guidelines around screening and management for these disorders, such as those from the National Comprehensive Cancer

Network (NCCN) and the European LeukemiaNet (ELN) and also specific diagnostic categories for these diseases, such as those from the World Health Organization (WHO) and the International Consensus Classification (ICC).

2) When should I consider evaluating a patient with a myeloid neoplasm for a familial syndrome, and how should I approach the initial clinical assessment?

Expert Perspective: A familial syndrome should be considered and assessed for in all patients presenting with a myeloid malignancy. The prevalence of familial predisposition syndromes is high in pediatric and young adult MDS/AML patients. One study examined a cohort of MDS/aplastic anemia (AA) patients diagnosed between 18–40 years of age and identified that 19% carried P/LP germline variants. Any patient diagnosed with MDS or AA under age 40 should undergo clinical testing to identify possible germline variants. It is also important to recognize that familial predisposition syndromes occur across the entire age spectrum. A recent study of MDS patients including patients of all ages demonstrated that at least 7% carry a germline variant, with 6% or more having a germline variant in each age decile. Germline variants in *DDX41* have a median age at MDS/AML onset of 68 years, which approaches the median age for a *de novo* diagnosis.

A critical component of the assessment for hereditary cancer syndromes is a comprehensive and detailed family history. Questions that should be asked for both immediate and extended family members within at least two generations include:

A) Have any family members been diagnosed with a hereditary cancer syndrome?
B) Have any family members been diagnosed with a hematologic malignancy, including MDS, AML, lymphoid malignancies, or AA?
C) Have any family members been diagnosed with non-hematologic cancers?
D) Have any family members had unexplained hematologic abnormalities (i.e. "low blood counts") or bleeding disorders?
E) Have any family members had issues with recurrent, atypical infections (e.g. human papillomavirus [HPV]-related or mycobacterial infections) or immunodeficiency?
F) Have any family members developed non-hematopoietic organ complications that may signal a germline disorder (e.g. pulmonary fibrosis, premature hair graying, nail abnormalities, or lymphedema)?

A patient is generally considered to be at higher risk if within two generations of the patient there is (i) another case of a hematologic malignancy, (ii) another person with hematopoietic abnormalities, or (iii) an individual with a solid tumor diagnosed at age 50 or younger. The presence of these findings should prompt additional testing to identify a germline variant. However, a negative family history does not rule out the possibility of a familial predisposition. As previously noted, *de novo* germline variants can arise, and there are several other factors such as incomplete penetrance, genetic anticipation, smaller family size, genetic heterogeneity, adoption, and unreported parentage that may confound a reported family history.

Another aspect to consider is the patient's own cancer history. Any patient diagnosed with two or more cancers, one of which is a hematopoietic malignancy, should be prioritized for germline testing. A common misconception is that hereditary cancer syndromes that predispose to solid organ malignancies (e.g. *BRCA1/2*) and those that predispose to hematologic malignancies are independent entities. One study demonstrated that, among breast cancer patients that subsequently developed a therapy-related leukemia, 21% harbored a germline variant that predisposes to both breast cancer and leukemia. The most common were *BRCA1* (6%), *BRCA2* (4%), and *TP53* (6%). Another example are *GATA2*-related diseases. In addition to predisposing to MDS/AML, patients carrying germline *GATA2* variants are at high risk of HPV-related squamous cell carcinomas of the skin and aerodigestive tract. As such, it is important to consider a hereditary cancer syndrome in patients who have a personal history of multiple cancers, including therapy-related myeloid neoplasms.

In addition to the history, there are findings on physical examination that may guide one to evaluate for a hereditary cancer syndrome, outlined in Figure 15.1.

3) What types of additional testing should be pursued in patients suspected of having a familial predisposition to myeloid malignancies, and what are the optimal tissue sources for these tests?

Expert Perspective: The selection of appropriate confirmatory germline genetic testing for patients with a suspected familial syndrome is a crucial aspect of patient management. It is important to understand the strengths and limitations of different testing approaches and to select a test capable of identifying possible germline variants of interest. Providers should consider referring patients who require genetic testing for germline variants to a center experienced with these disorders that can provide the appropriate pre- and post-test genetic counseling. The involvement of a certified genetic counselor is highly recommended during the testing process. It is important that the patient fully understands the potential legal, ethical, and financial consequences of identifying a germline variant in order to provide informed consent for testing.

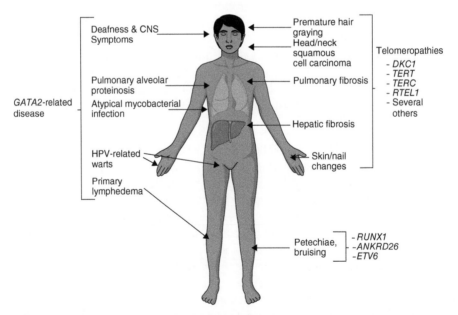

Figure 15.1 Physical exam features of familial myeloid disorders. Physical exam features that are associated with familial myeloid disorders are outlined. It is important to recognize that, although these features may suggest a diagnosis of a particular syndrome, individual phenotypes can be highly variable, and these findings are not always present.

Obtaining appropriate germline (i.e. non-hematopoietic) tissue is critical to establishing the diagnosis of a familial predisposition syndrome. A variant is deemed germline if its presence is confirmed in a non-hematopoietic tissue at an allele frequency > 30% or if it is present in other family members. In some cases, germline tissue may be obtained as a confirmatory measure after a suspected germline variant has already been identified from tumor-directed sequencing or suspected based on the clinical history. However, a sequential testing approach may lead to delays in diagnostic confirmation, particularly given that the turnaround times for sequencing can be several weeks. We suggest collecting germline tissue as early in the diagnostic process as possible. Ideally all MDS/AML patients would have germline tissue collected at the time of diagnosis. This can be done simultaneously with a bone marrow biopsy, although we recognize that most centers are not routinely testing all patients. Delays in establishing the presence of a germline variant can negatively affect patient outcomes in several ways. Although this is an active area of investigation, the presence of undetected germline variants may result in delayed identification of non-hematologic manifestations, use of treatment approaches not optimized for germline variant carriers (e.g., for older patients with deleterious *DDX41* variants or patients with a deleterious *CEBPA* germline variant without a matched related donor etc.), and not having sibling donors properly screened for a germline variant before allo-HSCT.

The gold standard source of non-hematopoietic tissue for germline testing is cultured skin fibroblasts. To obtain fibroblasts, a skin biopsy is collected from the patient. The fibroblasts are expanded and passaged in culture to ensure high purity and a sufficient number of cells for DNA extraction. The benefits of this technique are that a high yield of quality DNA is usually obtained; the DNA is from non-hematopoietic tissue and is a reasonable approximation of the germline; and the cells can be expanded in the future if more DNA is needed and/or the patient has consented to research. Use of samples with blood contamination is a significant concern when testing for germline variants in myeloid malignancies, given that even minimal levels of hematopoietic cells can lead to the detection of tumor- or clonal-hematopoiesis associated variants. The use of cultured skin fibroblasts has some disadvantages: culture failure occurs in approximately 5% of cases, and the time from culture initiation to DNA extraction is relatively long, with a median of 27 days. Other tissue sources that have been investigated include bone marrow-derived mesenchymal stromal cells hair follicles, and nail clippings, although the latter two sources may provide low DNA yields and the latter is subject to hematopoietic contamination. Similarly, buccal swabs are not preferred due to the level of hematopoietic cell contamination. Some have suggested that fluorescence or magnetic cell sorted mature blood lymphocytes can serve as a source of germline tissue, but they are not an ideal DNA source as somatic variants that lead to myeloid malignancies, particularly the clonal hematopoiesis of indeterminate potential ("CHIP") variants in *DNMT3A*, *TET2*, and *ASXL1*, often occur in earlier hematopoietic progenitor cells. As such, the presence of clonal blood lymphocytes descending from an early progenitor carrying somatic variants may confound the diagnosis of a germline variant.

It is important to choose a test that is sufficiently comprehensive to identify germline variants. Although most centers routinely utilize next-generation sequencing (NGS)–based target capture panels for newly diagnosed MDS/AML patients, it is important to realize that most of these panels are insufficient to detect all germline variants. Many do not have a target space that is comprehensive enough (i.e. includes enough genes) to assess for a range of germline variants. In addition, although most NGS panels perform well for the detection of SNVs, they are often incapable of detecting CNVs without specialized design and bioinformatic approaches. This is important, as CNVs have been shown to account for up to 10% of germline variants in a series of MDS/AA patients under the age of 40. Similarly, it is important to capture non-protein coding regions where predisposition alleles can be located. In this same study, 20% of the germline variants were in non-protein coding loci. In the future, it is possible that whole-genome-based sequencing will be used for both diagnostic hematopoietic and germline tissues, since it will allow the identification of structural variants, SNVs, indels, CNVs, and non-coding regions with a single assay and could facilitate the identification of novel candidate germline variants. Currently, the cost and increased interpretation burden preclude its widespread use.

4) What are the most common familial myeloid neoplasms, and how do they present?

Expert Perspective: It can be useful to group the familial myeloid neoplasms into three broad categories: (i) syndromes presenting primarily with MDS/AML, (ii) syndromes associated with thrombocytopenia and platelet abnormalities, and (iii) syndromes associated with marrow failure and extra-hematopoietic manifestations. A more extensive list of these syndromes, including the genes involved, further studies are needed to determine if there is an association between *DDX41* germline variants and these features, is outlined in Table 15.1; here *we* discuss only the most common disorders.

Syndromes presenting primarily with MDS/AML

- *DDX41:* One of the most common familial syndromes that presents primarily with MDS/AML are P/LP variants in DEAD-box helicase 41 (*DDX41*; OMIM 608170). DDX41 is a member of the DEAD box proteins, which bind DNA, are involved in RNA secondary structure, regulate cellular growth and maintenance, and are part of the innate STING immunity pathway. Deleterious germline *DDX41* variants have been reported as causative variants in up to 2.4% of MDS/AML cases. The types of variants that can occur include missense (e.g. p.Y259C) and truncating variants, such as frameshift mutations (e.g. p.D140fs), which are almost exclusively germline. Inheritance is autosomal dominant, and penetrance is high, being at least 40–50%. Somatic *DDX41* variants also occur, and approximately 50% of detected variants are somatic on tumor-focused testing. Often patients carrying a germline *DDX41* variant will have an acquired *DDX41* variant occur on the second allele in the malignant hematopoietic cells, the most common being the p.R525H somatic variant. The median age of disease onset for individuals with germline *DDX41* variants is 68 years. These patients will generally develop high-grade myeloid neoplasms (MDS, AML, or chronic myelomonocytic leukemia [CMML]) and have minimal antecedent manifestations. The bone marrow is often mildly hypocellular, and the karyotype is typically normal or with del(5q). Deleterious germline *DDX41* variants may be associated with solid-organ tumors and/or autoimmune disorders and appear to confer chemosensitivity, at least in hematopoietic *malignancies*. However, the leukemia-predisposing germline variant will persist with chemotherapy alone, and therefore, patients in first remission may benefit from allo-HSCT.
- *CEBPA:* Another described syndrome is familial AML with mutated CCAT/enhancer-binding protein alpha (*CEBPA*; OMIM 116897), which encodes an important transcription factor

Table 15.1 List of described genes for which deleterious germline variants lead to a familial myeloid malignancy predisposition.

Gene	Location	Syndrome Association(s)	Inheritance	Hematologic Disease Manifestations	Non-Hematopoietic Malignancy Risks	Non-Hematopoietic Disease Manifestations	Comments	OMIM
Syndromes Presenting Primarily with Myeloid Malignancy								
CEBPA	19q13.11	Familial AML with mutated *CEBPA*	AD	AML	ND	ND	Inherited as a single-allele, somatic variants on second allele common. About 7–11% of variants are germline in patients with bi-allelic CEBPA variants.	116897
DDX41	5q35.3	Familial AML with mutated *DDX41*	AD	MDS, AML, CMML	Possibly solid organ tumors, lymphoid malignancies	ND	Approximately 50% of *DDX41* variants are germline. Somatic variants can occur often on the second allele	608170
CHEK2	22q12.1	Li-Fraumeni Syndrome 2	AD	CLL, myeloid malignancies	Sarcoma, breast cancer, CNS tumors	ND	Associated with the Fanconi-BRCA1/2 pathway.	604373
MBD4	3q21.3	Familial AML with mutated *MBD4*	AR	AML	Possibly colorectal cancer	Colonic polyps	Rare syndrome, causes an AML with a high mutational rate/burden	603574
SAMD9/9L	7q21.2	MIRAGE syndrome, ataxia-pancytopenia syndrome and myelodysplasia and leukemia with monosomy 7 syndrome	AD	Pancytopenia, myeloid malignancy	Transient monosomy 7 and pancytopenia	Normophosphatemic familial tumoral calcinosis, MIRAGE, adrenal hypoplasia, enteropathy, ataxia	Strongly associated with monosomy 7, up to 20% of pediatric MDS with –7	610456 617053 159550

(Continued)

Table 15.1 (Continued)

Gene	Location	Syndrome Association(s)	Inheritance	Hematologic Disease Manifestations	Non-Hematopoietic Malignancy Risks	Non-Hematopoietic Disease Manifestations	Comments	OMIM
TP53	17p13.1	Li-Fraumeni Syndrome	AD	Myeloid malignancy, hypodiploid ALL	Breast cancer, sarcomas, CNS tumors, adrenocortical carcinoma	ND	Germline *TP53* can occur without classic features of Li Fraumeni syndrome	151623
BRCA1/2	17q21.31 13q13.1	Hereditary breast and ovarian cancer	AD	Myeloid and lymphoid malignancies	Breast, ovarian, prostate, pancreatic cancer	ND	One study suggested 21% of therapy-related MDS/AML in breast cancer patients was related to germline BRCA1/2 & TP53	113705 600185
CSF3R	1p34.3	Severe Congenital Neutropenia	AR	Myeloid and lymphoid malignancies	ND	Hereditary neutrophilia, severe congenital neutropenia	Monoallelic germline *CSF3R* predisposes to myeloid and lymphoid malignances	138971
14q32 duplications	14q32	Myeloid neoplasms with germline predisposition to 14q32 region duplications	AD	AML, MDS, ET, PV, PMF, CMML	ND	ND	Results in a duplication of ATG2B-GSKIP	616604
BLM	15q26.1	Bloom syndrome	AR	Myeloid and lymphoid leukemias	Colon, skin, breast carcinoma	Telangiectasias, café-au-lait spots, immunodeficiency, endocrine abnormalities	Rare disorder, will typically be identified in childhood	210900

Gene	Locus	Disorder	Inheritance	Malignancy				OMIM
PTPN11	12q24.13	Leopold/Noonan syndrome	AD	JMML, AML	Congenital heart disease, bleeding, skeletal malformation, lentigines	Neuroblastoma, melanoma, breast cancer, lung cancer, colorectal cancer	Rare, usually pediatric age at diagnosis	163950
NF1	17q11.2	Neurofibromatosis Type 1	AD	MDS, AML, JMML	CNS tumors, nerve sheath tumors, sarcomas	Café-au-lait macules, lisch nodules, bone abnormalities, neurologic abnormalities	Somatic NF1 variants also occur not uncommonly in MDS/AML	613113 607785
Familial Myeloid Malignancies with Platelet Abnormalities								
RUNX1	21q22.12	Familial platelet disorder with propensity to myeloid malignancies	AD	MDS, AML, T-ALL	ND	Eczema	Variable degree of thrombocytopenia and bleeding propensity, usually mild to moderate.	151385 601399
ANKRD26	10p12.1	Thrombocytopenia 2	AD	MDS, AML	ND	ND	Platelets typically 40,000–50,000 × 10^9/L, also a qualitative defect. Mild bleeding phenotype.	188000 610855
ETV6	12p13.2	Thrombocytopenia 5	AD	MDS, AML, CMML	ND	ND	Typically moderate thrombocytopenia with mild or no bleeding symptoms	600618 616216

(Continued)

Table 15.1 (Continued)

Gene	Location	Syndrome Association(s)	Inheritance	Hematologic Disease Manifestations	Non-Hematopoietic Malignancy Risks	Non-Hematopoietic Disease Manifestations	Comments	OMIM
JAK2	9p24.1	NA	AD	Thrombocytopenia, familial MPN	ND	ND	A very rare syndrome, almost all *JAK2* V617F are somatic. V617I reported once as germline.	147796 614521
MPL	1p34.2	NA	AR or AD	Amegakaryocytic thrombocytopenia, essential thrombocytosis	ND	ND	Germline *MPL* mutations can rarely be a cause of familial thrombocytosis	159530
WAS	Xp11.23	Wiskott-Aldrich syndrome	X-linked	Neutropenia, thrombocytopenia, lymphoid, myeloid malignancies	ND	Thrombocytopenia, bleeding, immunodeficiency, eczema, autoimmune disease	Rare, usually pediatric age at diagnosis	301000

Syndromes Associated with Inherited Marrow Failure Syndromes and Extra-Hematopoietic Manifestations

Gene	Location	Syndrome Association(s)	Inheritance	Hematologic Disease Manifestations	Non-Hematopoietic Malignancy Risks	Non-Hematopoietic Disease Manifestations	Comments	OMIM
GATA2	3q21.3	*GATA2* deficiency syndrome	AD	Marrow failure, MDS, AML, immunodeficiency	HPV-related squamous cell carcinomas of the skin, genitals, aerodigestive tract	Immunodeficiency (mycobacterial infection, HPV-related warts), deafness, CNS symptoms, pulmonary alveolar proteinosis, primary lymphedema, monocytopenia	Early hematologic presentation is often with marrow failure, later progression to MDS/AML	many

Gene(s)	Location	Disorder	Inheritance	Marrow failure/malignancy	Solid tumors	Clinical features	Notes	OMIM
DKC1 TERT TERC RTEL1 others	Xq28 5p15.33 3q26.2 20q13.33	Telomere disorders dyskeratosis congenital (outdated term)	AD AR (TERT)	Marrow failure, MDS, AML	Squamous cell carcinoma (aerodigestive, stomach, rectal), gastrointestinal cancer, lung cancer, liver cancer	Skin hyperpigmentation, nail dystrophy, oral leukoplakia, premature hair graying, hyperhidrosis, cognitive delay, pulmonary fibrosis, endocrine abnormalities, esophageal strictures	Early hematologic presentation is often with marrow failure, later progression to MDS/AML. Reduced-intensity conditions to TBD.	many
FANCA FANCC FANCG others	16q24.3 9q22.32 9p13.3	Fanconi anemia	AR	Marrow failure, MDS, AML	Squamous cell carcinomas, liver cancer, CNS tumors, breast cancers	Congenital abnormalities, renal disease, endocrine abnormalities	High sensitivity to DNA toxic agents, requires special consideration with conditioning chemotherapy	many
SBDS DNAJC21 EFL1 others	7q11.21 15q25.2 5p13.2	Schwachman-Diamond syndrome	AR	Marrow failure, MDS, AML or comp het	ND	Exocrine pancreatic insufficiency, skeletal abnormalities and malformation, growth delay, liver dysfunction, cardiac abnormalities, neurocognitive abnormalities	Classically presents in childhood but can be found in adulthood. Chromosome 7 abnormalities are common at progression.	607444 260400 617538 617048 617052

(Continued)

Table 15.1 (Continued)

Gene	Location	Syndrome Association(s)	Inheritance	Hematologic Disease Manifestations	Non-Hematopoietic Malignancy Risks	Non-Hematopoietic Disease Manifestations	Comments	OMIM
MECOM	3q26.2	MECOM-associated syndrome	AD	Marrow failure, MDS	ND	Radioulnar synostosis, clinodactyly, cardiac and renal malformations, immunodeficiency, hearing loss	Rare, usually pediatric age at diagnosis	165215 616738
SRP72	4q12	Familial aplastic anemia/MDS with SRP72 mutation	AD	Marrow failure, MDS	ND	Deafness	Very rare syndrome, few families reported	602122 614675
ERCC6L2	9q22.32	NA	AR	Marrow failure, AML	ND	ND	Very rare syndrome, few families reported	615667 615715
NBN	8q21.3	Nijmegen breakage syndrome	AR	Marrow failure, ALL	Ovarian cancer	Microcephaly, clinodactyly, syndactyly, GI stenosis, cleft lip/palate, endocrine abnormalities, café-au-lait, immunodeficiency	Rare syndrome, mutations cause chromosomal instability	602667 609135 613065
RECQL4	8q24.3	NA	AR	Marrow failure, myeloid, lymphoid malignancies	ND	Microcephaly, developmental abnormalities	Very rare syndrome	603780
TET2	4q24	NA	AR (homozygous)	Myeloid malignancies and lymphoma	ND	Immunodeficiency	Nearly all *TET2* variants in myeloid malignancies are somatic, but extremely rare germline occurrences have been reported	603780

for hematopoietic differentiation. Deleterious germline variants in *CEBPA* typically are frameshift or nonsense (truncating) variants involving the 5'-end of the gene and therefore affect the protein's N-terminus. These variants are nearly completely penetrant, and carriers develop AML at a median age of 24.5 years in one study, with a range between 1.75 and 46 years. Typically, patients with a germline *CEBPA* variant will sustain a somatic variant on the second allele, usually at the 3'-end of the gene, at the time of leukemic transformation. In AMLs with biallelic *CEBPA* mutations, approximately 7–11% of patients carry a germline variant on one allele. Acquired *GATA2* variants can also be detected. The AML typically has a normal karyotype with aberrant CD7 expression. There are no extra-hematopoietic manifestations. Whether patients harboring a germline *CEBPA* variant should undergo allo-HSCT in first remission is controversial. If chemotherapy-only is used initially, it is important to recognize that there will be a persistent risk due to the ongoing presence of the germline *CEBPA* variant in the hematopoietic cells, and subsequent AMLs are typically independent malignancies, as evidenced by distinct acquired *CEBPA* variants.

Syndromes associated with thrombocytopenia and platelet abnormalities: Familial myeloid malignancies with platelet abnormalities are frequently diagnosed with an acquired platelet disorder (e.g. immune thrombocytopenia) or a bleeding disorder before their diagnosis of a myeloid malignancy. As such, it is important to elicit a history of platelet disorders or bleeding symptoms when assessing patients with a possible familial myeloid malignancy.

- **Familial platelet disorder with propensity to myeloid malignancies (FPD/MM)** (OMIM 601399) was the first such disorder described; it is caused by deleterious germline variants in *RUNX1*, which encodes the α chain of the *RUNX1* transcription factor. There is heterogeneity in the degree and character of the platelet defects in these patients, with both quantitative and qualitative defects. The platelet counts are usually mildly to moderately decreased, although they can also be normal and can fluctuate over time. In addition, patients typically have a mild bleeding propensity. The average age of malignancy onset is in the early 30s, although there is a wide range described. Penetrance is incomplete, with 40% of patients developing a hematologic malignancy in some reports, while almost all individuals will suffer from some degree of thrombocytopenia and/or platelet dysfunction. The disease manifestations are typically MDS/AML, but cases of acute T-cell lymphoblastic leukemia and other hematopoietic malignancies have also been described. The second *RUNX1* allele is sometimes also mutated at disease onset.
- **Thrombocytopenia 2 (THC2)** (OMIM 188000) is caused by deleterious germline variants in *ANKRD26*, typically in the gene promoter. The average platelet count pre-diagnosis is 40,000–50,000 × 10^9/L, and the platelets are qualitatively abnormal, with decreased α-granules and GPIa. Of the patients that develop malignancy, most develop MDS/AML, but chronic myeloid leukemia has also been described. The age of malignancy onset is broad and has been reported between 30 and 70 years.
- **Thrombocytopenia 5 (THC5)** (OMIM 616216) is caused by P/LP germline variants in *ETV6*, which encodes an important hematopoietic transcription factor. These patients usually present with a moderate thrombocytopenia and either mild or no bleeding symptoms. These variants are autosomal dominant and include both missense and truncating variants. A wide range of malignancies has been reported in association with

germline *ETV6* variants, most commonly B-cell ALL but also MDS, AML, CMML, skin, and colorectal cancer. The penetrance of thrombocytopenia is high and is usually mild (typically > 75 × 10^9/L). Bleeding tendency is highly variable, and many have no significant bleeding symptoms. The outcomes of patients with P/LP germline *ETV6* variants who develop MDS/AML are not well described in the literature, but allo-HSCT should be considered in most patients carrying a germline variant that predisposes to leukemia (see Chapters 6 and 12).

Syndromes associated with marrow failure and extra-hematopoietic manifestations: The syndromes associated with inherited marrow failure syndromes and extra-hematopoietic manifestations are a broad and diverse category of disorders.

- The *GATA2*-related syndromes (OMIM 137295), historically designated as MonoMAC or Emberger's syndrome, were eventually discovered to all be caused by germline variants in *GATA2*, which encodes a zinc finger-containing transcription factor important for hematopoietic development. The *GATA2*-related diseases are heterogeneous, and the hematologic manifestations can include MDS, AML, AA and severe immunodeficiency. The penetrance of this disorder is relatively high, with approximately 70% of patients developing MDS/AML, with a median onset age of 29 years. Monosomy 7 or trisomy 8 and *ASXL1* variants are frequently seen at the time of progression. Allo-HSCT is an important consideration in these disorders, and preemptive HSCT should be considered for known carriers of a P/LP germline *GATA2* variant, especially those suffering from severe HPV-linked diseases.
- Fanconi anemia is caused by germline variants in members of the *FANC* gene family; 90% of cases are due to variants in *FANCA, FANCC, and FANCG*. Members of the *FANC* family are important for maintenance of genomic stability. Patients can develop bone marrow failure or MDS/AML. Up to 40% of Fanconi patients will develop MDS and 15% AML, and this can be the initial presenting feature. Clonal evolution is common, with gains of 1q, 3q, 13q, or loss of chromosome 7 being the most common cytogenetic findings. A wide range of extra-hematopoietic manifestations are observed, including skeletal abnormalities, skin abnormalities, eye malformations, renal and urinary tract malformations, central nervous system and ear abnormalities, and solid organ tumors (particularly squamous cell carcinomas). However, typical extra-hematopoietic manifestations are not present in all patients. It is important to be aware that these patients are highly sensitive to DNA toxic agents and require appropriate dose modifications. Chromosomal breakage studies and appropriate choice of DNA sequencing tests for confirmation are critical.

The telomere disorders are another important syndrome to consider when a patient presents with features that include a personal or family history of early-onset MDS or AA, premature hair graying, skin/nail changes, and pulmonary or liver fibrosis. The most common causative germline variants are found in *DKC1, TERT, TERC, RTEL1, and TINF2*, although there are a number of other culprit genes with less frequent variants described. Patients carrying *DKC1* or *TINF2* P/LP germline variants will typically manifest in childhood, whereas *TERT* and *TERC* variant carriers have a broader age range at presentation. These genes are crucial in maintaining telomere length, and loss of function leads to premature shortening and cellular senescence. These variants have incomplete penetrance and demonstrate significant intra-individual heterogeneity in their manifestations. The hematologic manifestations are typically either AA or hypoplastic MDS, but with time, high-grade MDS or AML often develops. The age of onset varies significantly, both with the type of inherited variant and between individual patients, and genetic anticipation can be seen. It is important to be aware that patients with telomeropathies are at risk for lung and liver fibrosis as well as aggressive squamous cell carcinomas, all of which can be severe and life-limiting. In addition to sequencing studies, it is important to pursue telomere length testing. These tests will assess the patient's telomere length and compare them to the age-adjusted population average. A patient with a telomeropathy will typically have telomere lengths < 1% relative to the population average in lymphocytes. It is important to identify these individuals as early intervention, particularly with reduced-intensity conditioning regimens has the potential to improve outcomes in carefully selected patients.

5) What should I do if I incidentally encounter a potential germline variant on my local routine next-generation sequencing panel for myeloid disorders?

Expert Perspective: Diagnostic NGS panels are standard of care for MDS/AML, but it is important to recognize that there is significant heterogeneity in the target space (i.e. types of genes tested) between panels, and many tumor-focused NGS panels include genes that can be mutated either somatically or in the germline. The origin of a detected gene variant may be difficult to assess from molecular profiling of leukemia cells. For this reason, we prefer the term "tumor-based NGS panel" in contrast to the commonly used phrase "somatic NGS panel." An increasingly common dilemma occurs when a provider encounters a tumor-based NGS result that includes variants in genes known to confer germline risk. Deciding whether a patient requires additional testing for germline variants on the basis of a tumor-based NGS panel requires some understanding of what features make a variant more likely germline versus somatic. Clinicians must look deeper into the specific molecular change present in the report. There are some variants (e.g. frameshift *DDX41* variants such as p.D140fs) that are virtually always germline but also several that can occur as either somatic or germline variants. It can be useful to consult large databases (e.g. ClinVar www.ncbi.nlm.nih.gov/clinvar) or a molecular pathology expert for guidance. One common heuristic is examining the variant allele frequency (VAF), with the assumption that a VAF in the range 40–60% suggests a heterozygous (single-allele) mutation and > 90% a homozygous (dual-allele) mutation, which is not typical of acquired somatic variants. We caution against this practice as structural variants, such as CNVs or loss of heterozygosity, and degree of disease burden can confound the VAF and render it unreliable. One study found that VAF alone could assign germline variants in only 48% of confirmed cases.

Although a positive family history or certain mutational characteristics can help add positive predictive value when assessing for a germline variant, there are no reliable clinical tools to add significant negative predictive value. Thus, it is very difficult to rule out the presence of a germline variant without testing true germline tissue. Therefore, we advise testing all patients with a tumor-based NGS panel positive for a possible germline variant with clinical testing of true germline tissue to determine the nature of the variant(s) detected. We also suggest paired testing of germline tissue with the initial diagnostic bone marrow biopsy samples if possible. As we learn more about the impacts of these germline variants on patient outcomes, and the number of known syndromes increases, a complete and systematic approach to identification of germline variants should be the goal. However, recognizing that many centers may not have the expertise or capacity to implement germline tissue testing on a uniform basis, we present a suggested algorithm for prioritizing incidentally discovered potential germline variants in Figure 15.2.

6) **How should I counsel the patient presented in the clinical case study about the risks of their children or relatives developing a myeloid neoplasm, and what types of referrals and testing should be pursued?**

Expert Perspective: This a common and challenging question with hereditary cancer syndromes. Screening for and preventing complications in family members is one of the

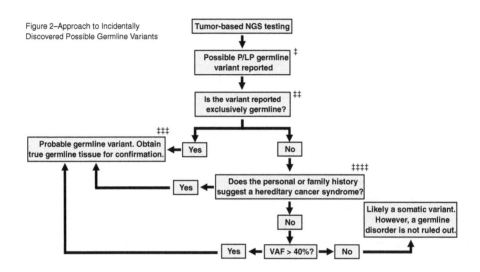

‡ - Examples of genes for which P/LP variants could be germline in origin include:

- DDX41
- CEBPA
- RUNX1
- ETV6
- SAMD9
- SAMD9L
- MBD4
- GATA2
- TERT
- TERC
- RTEL1
- TP53
- ANKRD26
- BRCA1/2
- CHEK2
- CSF3R
- SRP72

‡‡ - Consider consulting large databases (e.g., ClinVar) or a molecular pathology expert for guidance

‡‡‡ - Cultured skin fibroblasts are the preferred source of germline tissue

‡‡‡‡ - Criteria for a strong family history include:

- At least one additional case of a hematologic malignancy within the immediate family
- At least one case of a non-hematologic malignancy within the immediate family diagnosed before age 50 years
- Non-hematopoietic malignancies diagnosed within two or more family members within two generations

Figure 15.2 Approach to incidentally discovered possible germline variants. Although we advocate for universal germline testing in all patients with a myeloid malignancy, we suggest an approach for triaging possible germline variants identified on tumor-focused sequencing panels. Although demonstrating any of these features in this algorithm increases the likelihood of an identified variant being germline, the absence of these features is insufficient to rule out the presence of a germline variant.

primary motivations for individuals seeking germline testing. However, cascade testing is complicated by numerous ethical issues that deserve consideration by clinicians. All patients and family members should be referred to a comprehensive and interdisciplinary program that has experience in managing patients with familial myeloid disorders. The precise risks will depend on the syndrome and variant in question, along with the features of the proband, and often cannot be viewed in a straightforward way. The importance of involving a certified genetic counselor for both pre- and post-test management cannot be overstated. Questions of informed consent become more challenging when discussing family members who may be incapable of informed consent, such as young children. There is no uniform solution to these scenarios, and many factors must be taken into consideration, including the nature and risk of the variant, the presence of useful therapeutic options, and the age at which disease is expected to develop. An optimal approach is one that balances beneficence and identification of potentially actionable variants before complications arise with the autonomy of the future adult that the child represents. We emphasize that counseling around risks should take place in the context of an experienced and multidisciplinary team and that each family requires a tailored approach to counseling, testing, and management.

7) What are the implications for patients needing allogeneic hematopoietic stem cell transplant?

Expert Perspective: Related donors are the most common source for allogeneic hematopoietic stem cells and increasingly haploidentical family members (e.g. parent or child) are being utilized over other alternative donor sources. Given that the affected parent and 50% of first-degree relatives will carry a familial P/LP germline variant in autosomal dominant disorders, there is a significant risk of returning leukemia-predisposing donor cells to an already vulnerable patient. There are likely several risks associated with this, including a higher risk of post-transplant relapse with a donor-derived malignancy and/or delayed or failed engraftment. In addition, exposure of a donor carrying a predisposing germline variant to mobilization with granulocyte colony stimulating factor may accelerate or increase the risk of the donor developing a malignancy.

The questions facing allo-HSCT programs are which and how related donors should be tested for the presence of germline variants. Family members of patients diagnosed with or suspected to harbor a germline variant must undergo further testing before donation should be entertained. This can be challenging, as there are implications for the donor from this testing. Many donors will feel an obligation to undergo testing in order to donate for their loved one, but this raises ethical issues around informed consent, and the risks of the influence of a relative's acute illness in the decision-making process. The testing approach should be individualized for each patient based on the family history and may include a baseline bone marrow biopsy and sequencing studies. The optimal donor selection will depend on the patient, but generally a relative who is proven to lack the familial variant is desirable. However, with the increasing size of unrelated donor registries and the number of patients who can find a well-matched unrelated donor, these may become the preferred option in the future for patients with a suspected or confirmed familial syndrome. However, this does not completely eliminate the risk of re-introducing a germline variant, as asymptomatic unrelated donors may have carry other deleterious germline variants that are not shared with the recipient. We advocate for consideration of universal donor testing as the future standard of care, which has the advantage of providing a global and systematic assessment for deleterious germline variants in donors and may be a means of reducing post-transplant relapse or donor-derived malignancies.

Another important question in the allo-HSCT realm is the role for preemptive transplant for carriers of high-penetrance and high-risk germline variants (e.g. *CEBPA* and *GATA2*). Advantages of this approach include: (i) by replacing the deleterious variant, one can avoid the subsequent development of MDS/AML, for which achieving remission through chemotherapy is not guaranteed; and (ii) transplant outcomes are more favorable in younger age groups, particularly children. There are several factors that one would need to weigh in this scenario, including the variant in question, the penetrance, and the personal and family history of the index case. We suggest that at least a transplant assessment and identification of potential donors should occur early on, ideally shortly after identification of the variant in question. The optimal timing and choice of preemptive transplant should remain an individualized decision (see Chapter 11).

Case Study Conclusion

You refer this patient to a hereditary cancers program, arrange treatment with 5-azacitidine/venetoclax, and initiate an allo-HSCT referral. Shortly after, you receive the NGS-panel results, revealing frameshift *DDX41* (p.D140fs, VAF 48%) and *ASXL1* (Gly646fs, VAF 8%) variants. You recognize the *DDX41* variant is likely germline and expedite cultured fibroblast testing. Four weeks later, it confirms germline status. The patient's WHO classification is revised to "Myeloid neoplasm with germline *DDX41* mutation." Both siblings have been found to be HLA-matched and are seen at the hereditary cancer program. The transplant center recommends testing both siblings for the *DDX41* variant. The sister agrees, but the brother declines. The patient's children defer testing due to insurance concerns. The sister is confirmed as positive for the germline *DDX41* variant and is excluded as a donor. A fully HLA-matched unrelated donor is available, and the patient receives an unrelated donor allo-HSCT in first remission after five cycles of therapy.

Recommended Readings

Ballew, B.J. and Savage, S.A. (2013). Updates on the biology and management of dyskeratosis congenita and related telomere biology disorders. *Expert Rev Hematol* 6 (3): 327–337.

DiNardo, C.D., Bannon, S.A., Routbort, M. et al. (2016). Evaluation of patients and families with concerns for predispositions to hematologic malignancies within the Hereditary Hematologic Malignancy Clinic (HHMC). *Clin Lymphoma Myeloma Leuk* 16 (7): 417.

Feurstein, S., Churpek, J.E., Walsh, T. et al. (2021). Germline variants drive myelodysplastic syndrome in young adults. *Leukemia* 35 (8): 2439.

Feurstein, S., Trottier, A.M., Estrada-Merly, N. et al. (2022). Germ line predisposition variants occur in myelodysplastic syndrome patients of all ages. *Blood* 140 (24): 2533–2548. Hideki's recent Blood paper on DDX41.

Hsu, A.P., Sampairo, E.P., Khan, J. et al. (2011). Mutations in GATA2 are associated with the autosomal dominant and sporadic monocytopenia and mycobacterial infection (MonoMAC) syndrome. *Blood* 118 (10): 2653.

Pabts, T., Eyholzer, M., Haefliger, S., Schardt, J., and Mueller B.U. (2008). Somatic CEBPA mutations are a frequent second event in families with germline CEBPA mutations and familial acute myeloid leukemia. *J Clin Oncol* 26 (31): 5088.

Preudhomme, C., Renneville, A., Bourdon, V. et al. (2009). High frequency of RUNX1 biallelic alterations in acute myeloid leukemia secondary to familial platelet disorder. *Blood* 113 (22): 5583–5587.

Sébert, M., Passet, M., Raimbault, A. et al. (2019). Germline DDX41 mutations define a significant entity within adult MDS/AML patients. *Blood* 134 (17): 1441.

Trottier, A.M. and Godley L.A. (2021). Inherited predisposition to haematopoietic malignancies: overcoming barriers and exploring opportunities. *Br J Haematol* 194 (4): 663–676.

Trottier, A.M., Bannon, S., Bashir, Q. et al. (2019). When should transplant physicians think about familial blood cancers? *Adv Cell Gene Ther* 2: e68.

Trottier, A.M., Cavalcante de Andrade Silva, M., Li, Z., and Godley, L.A. (2019). Somatic mutation panels: time to clear their names. *Cancer Genet* 235–236: 84–92.

Part 4

Myeloproliferative Neoplasms

16

Chronic Myeloid Leukemia: Chronic Phase Disease

Jerald P. Radich

Fred Hutchinson Cancer Center, Seattle, WA

Introduction

Tyrosine kinase inhibitors (TKIs) have irrevocably changed the care of chronic myeloid leukemia (CML) patients, dramatically changing the natural history of this disease. Before TKI therapy, patients without an option of allogeneic transplantation were doomed to a future of progression to advanced-phase disease, with a median life expectancy of about seven years. Now, chronic-phase CML patients who are appropriately treated enjoy life spans comparable to the general population.

There are now three major questions in dealing with a patient with chronic-phase CML. First, at diagnosis, which TKI should you start with? Second, when should you switch TKIs? And lastly, for patients with an excellent response, which patients should consider discontinuation of the TKI, with the prospect of a treatment-free remission (TFR; see Chapter 19)?

Case Study 1

A 55-year-old driftwood sculpter is diagnosed with intermediate-risk (Sokal) chronic-phase CML. He is low risk by both the Sokal and Hasford classification schemes. His peripheral blood BCR-ABL1 level at diagnosis was 64% IS. He is overweight, has a significant smoking history (both cigarettes and marijuana), and has moderately elevated blood pressure and lipid panel, both untreated.

1) **Which tyrosine kinase do you choose for front-line therapy?**
   A) Bosutinib.
   B) Dasatinib.
   C) Imatinib.
   D) Nilotinib.

Expert Perspective: How do we decide which TKI to use? The choices are imatinib and the more potent second-generation TKIs nilotinib and dasatinib. All three second-generation TKIs (dasatinib, nilotinib, and bosutinib) have been compared to imatinib in newly diagnosed chronic-phase CML (Table 16.1). All of these ramdomized trials have shown remarkably consistent results (Table 16.1). Compared to imatinib, second-generation TKIs offer greater complete cytogenetic remissions, greater percentage of cases reaching clinically significant molecular milestones (and faster), less progression to advanced-phase disease, but surprisingly, similar overall survivals. However, the second-generation TKIs have more hematopoietic toxicity compared to imatinib. Most of the second- and third-generation TKIs seem to have more cardiovascular toxicity (hypertension, vascular occlusions) than imatinib (the exception might be bosutinib), and some have serious or bothersome specific side effects (dasatinib, pulmonary effusions; bosutinib, diarrhea). Table 16.2 illustrates some of the attractive and unattractive features of the various TKIs that are available for front-line therapy of CML.

Given these facts and trade-offs, how does one choose a front-line therapy?

Table 16.1 12 month responses in the ENESTnd, DASISION, and US Intergroup trials.

Response	NIL300bid (ENESTnd)	NIL400bid (ENESTnd)	IM 400 (ENESTnd)	DAS 100 (DASISION)	IM 400 (DASISION)	BOS (BFORE)	IM 400 (BFORE)
CCyR	80%	78%	65%	83%	72%	77%	64%
MMR	44%	43%	22%	46%	28%	47%	37%
AP/BC	0.7%	0.4%	4.2%	1.9%	3.5%	1.6%	2.5%

AP/BC: patients progressing to accelerated phase and blast crisis; CCyR: complete cytogenetic remission; MMR: major molecular response.
Source: Data from Saglio G, et al. *N Engl J Med.* 2010;362:2251–9; Kantarjian H, et al. *N Engl J Med.* 2010;362:2260–70; Cortes JE, *J Clin Oncol.* 2017, 36:231–7.

Table 16.2 Front-line and second-line TKI therapy, outcomes, and most common side effects.

Treatment	TKI	CCyR% (yr)	OS% (yr)	Common side effects (%) and comments
Front-line	Imatinib	65 (5)	83 (11)	Muscle spasm (41%), edema (37%). May also see fatigue, rash, hepatotoxicity and diarrhea
	Dasatinib	86 (2)	91 (5)	Neutropenia (29%), pleural effusion (28%), pulmonary arterial HTN ($\leq$5%). May also see prolonged QTc, pericardial effusion (rare), and platelet dysfunction
	Nilotinib	85 (4)	95 (5)	Rash (38%), headache (32%), fatigue (23%), prolong QTc (4%; Hold if >480 msec), increase lipase (28%), avoid strong CYP3A4 inhibitors. May also see hyperglycemia, hepatotoxicity, and vascular disease
	Bosutinib	77 (1)	N/A	Diarrhea (70%), increased ALT (23%). May also see rash and pancreatitis
Second-line				
	Dasatinib	50 (5)	71 (6)	
	Nilotinib	44 (4)	85 (3)	
	Bosutinib	40 (2)	92 (2)	
	Ponatinib	45 (2)	90 (2)	Vascular occlusive events (~30%); hepatotoxicity

There are a few considerations for selection of a front-line therapy: (1) What are the treatment goals? For instance, for a patient diagnosed in their 70s, an appropriate goal is to extend survival without concerns of potential serious toxicities, thus making imatinib a fine choice. For someone much younger, especially those that whish to procreate, it may be appropriate to drive for a deeper response faster, thus a second-gereration TKI. (2) Consider comorbities in the light of each TKIs unique side effect profile. For example, it may not be a good idea to prescribe nilotinib to a patient with cardiac issues or vascular disease or dasatinib to a patient with preexisiting pulmonary problems. (3) Think about their risk score (e.g. Sokal). Patient with high-risk disease (and maybe intermediate) may benefit from starting with a second-generation TKI since the randomized trials showed less transformation with these agents compared to imatinib. (4) All things above being equal, the personal experience of the physician with each of the agents is a relevant factor.

Case Study continued: Given his low-risk status and cardiovascular risk profile, you and the patient decide on starting therapy with imatinib 400 mg a day. Keep in mind necessary dose adjustments required for renal and hepatic impairment(s) and for hematologic toxicity.

Correct Answer: C

2) Without further ado he returns home in his quest for the perfect beached driftwood. He misses several appointments but returns to your office three months later. He has normalized his complete blood count, and his BCR-ABLl is 15% IS. When asked if he is taking his medication, he sheepishly replies, "On most days." As it turns out, he is having some muscle aches with imatinib, and while not debilitating, it does impair his activity on big beach days, so he doesn't take his drug a day or so before planned expeditions.

When do you switch TKI therapy?

Expert Perspective: What does early response mean? Several studies show that early (3–6 months) response, as measured by the peripheral blood BCR-ABL1 level, is an early predictor of longer-term outcomes (Table 16.3). Patients who have a BCR–ABL1 > 10% IS at 3–6 months have an inferior outcome (cytogenetic, molecular, and overall survival) compared to patients with a better response of ⩽ 10% IS. This holds for both up-front CML therapy (no matter which TKI) and those patients who switch to a second-generation TKI after intolerance or resistance. For example, a retrospective study of chronic-phase CML patients treated with imatinib first-line therapy found that patients with three-month BCR-ABL levels of ⩽ 10% IS had OS of 93%, while patients with > 10% had inferior rates of 57%. In addition, cytogenetic and molecular responses also differ based on early molecular response For example, patients treated with dasatnib with a good early response had five-year CCyR, MMR, and MR4.5 rates of 94%, 87%, and 54% while patients with poor early response had rates of 41%, 38%, and 5%, respectively.

This milestone of response is built into NCCN and ELN guidelines. However, poor early response can be from poor adherence, bad biology, or a combination of both. In our case, some experts would advocate switching to an alternative TKI with such a poor three-month *BCR::ABL* PCR result seen in this patient, though the story is complicated here by the knowledge that the patient is not compliant. Thus, for this patient, it is reasonable to continue imatinib, with close follow-up of another *BCR::ABL* at the six-month mark.

Table 16.3 Milestones on TKI therapy and definitions of molecular responses.

BCR/ABL1 (IS)	3 months	6 months	12 months
<10%	Acceptable	Sometime acceptable*	
> 1–10%		Acceptable	
> 0.1–1%		Acceptable	
≤ 0.1%			Acceptable

Definitions of molecular responses (MRs)

MR^2 – $BCR::ABL1 \leq 1\%$; this level roughly corresponds to complete cytogenetic response (CCyR)

MR^3 – $BCR::ABL1 \leq 0.1\%$; this level is equivalent to major molecular remission (MMR)

MR^4 – $BCR::ABL1 \leq 0.01\%$

$MR^{4.5}$ – $BCR::ABL1 \leq 0.0032\%$; this is the current limit of most commercially available assays.

*Sometimes steep decline from start and less than 10% at six months is acceptable.

Back to the case. He stays on imatinib (and promises to be more compliant). His six-, nine-, and 12-month peripheral blood *BCR::ABL* is 9%, 5%, 4%, respectively.

3) Now what?
A) Stay on imatinib.
B) Swith to another TKI.
C) Consider allogeneic transplant.
D) Swith to omaxetaxine.

Expert Perspective: The NCCN and ELN set treatment milestones that are associated with survival outcomes (Table 16.3). They are remarkably similar. The chief takeaways are: (i) the achievement of a CCyR (or its near equivalent, a *BCR::ABL* of ≤ 1% IS) should occur by 12 months of therapy; (ii) thereafter, achievement of an MMR (BCR-ABL1 ≤ 0.1% IS) is desirable, as this level of disease burden is associated with a very low rate of resistance and progression; and (iii) if deeper responses (MR 4.0 and lower) are sustained, it may allow for TKI discontinuation. The failure to reach milestones, or the loss of milestones, should prompt (i) consideration of changing to another TKI, and (ii) mutation testing to inform the decision of which TKI to use as second-line therapy.

The treatment response of CCyR at 12 months of TKI is a prognostic indicator of long-term survival for imatinib or second-generation TKIs. For example, for chronic-phase patients receiving either imatinib or second-generation TKIs, the three-year PFS and OS rates for patients with and without a 12-month CCyR were 98% and 99% vs 67% and 94%, respectively. Achievement of MMR is associated with continued CCyR, less disease progression to advanced phases, and a better OS compared to patients without MMR. For example, in the IRIS study, the 10-year overall survival was 91% with a MMR at 12 months, versus 85% of cases without a MMR. Similar benefits of achieving MMR are seen in patients receiving second-generation TKIs.

Correct Answer: B

4) Again, we get to the question of which second-line therapy to choose?

Expert Perspective: For second-line therapy, the second-generation TKIs dasatinib, nilo-tinib, and bosutinib are joined by the third-generation TKI ponatinib. The first question is why the patient needs to switch. If for pure drug intolerance, the different drug toxicities should allow one to find at least one other potential agent (see the NCCN guidelines for an excellent coverage of TKI toxicities and how to deal with them; also see Table 16.2). In the setting of intolerance, the disease should respond well once adequate drug levels are obtained and maintained.

Changing therapy for resistance (as in our case) is more difficult. Resistance is often associated with single base pair mutations in the *ABL1* tyrosine kinase domain (roughly 30–50% of the cases of resistance), which changes ABL1 protein binding and disturbs TKI binding and inhibition. The strength of this effect depends on the specific mutation and the specific TKI, and there are published tables (refer to CML chapter on transplant) describing which mutations need a particular TKI to maximize efficacy. If there are no mutations, then the same general rules apply as when considering front-line therapy: goals, comorbiditites, and user familiarity.

TKIs have similar efficacy in the second-line therapy. Various studies suggest that these agents in the setting of resistance will yield CCyR in 25–50% of cases. All the second-generation TKIs appear to be equally efficacious for the majority of imatinib resistant/intolerant patients, but importantly at a five-year follow-up of the studies, only a third of patients remain on treatment. The progression-free survival for second-line TKI are > 70%. If/when subsequent relapse occurs, a third-line agent can be used, but in this setting (predictably), responses are unusual. The possible exception is pona-tinib, which in the setting of multiple resistant or *T315I* mutations achieved CCyR > 70%, with two-year PFS rates of ~70%.

There is a worry that "resistance is forever." It is not clear if second-generation TKIs in the resistance setting can effectively "cure" patients like their effect in the front-line setting. Patients who relapse once have a high rate of another relapse and a higher risk of subsequent transformation to advanced-phase disease. Therefore, how long do you follow a patient in this resistance setting to decide that second-line therapy is (or is not) working? And if not, what's next? Studies suggest an evaluation of response after three months of therapy is important in predicting subsequent outcomes. This lines up nicely with the time it generally takes to find an unrelated donor for a transplant (see CML chapter on transplant). Thus, if a patient is a transplant candidate, a formal search can be initiated at the same time as the second-line TKI, and at three months, when a donor is identified, and assessment can be made as to adequacy of TKI response. If the patient has a good response, continue the TKI; if not, proceed with allogeneic trans-plantation.

Case Study 2

Let us assume that string theory is real and there are numerous parallel universes. In another astral plane, the before mentioned 55-year-old driftwood sculpter (his bond with this endeavor is apparently strong!) presents and is treated with imatinib, like before. However, in our new universe he gets a great response: *BCR::ABL* 5% IS by six months, 0.08% by 12 months (MMR), and 0.002% IS (greater than a four-log reduction in *BCR::ABL*) by 18 months. For the next two years, his *BCR::ABL* falls to undetectable. He has been in a deep molecular response (defined as >4 log reduction of *BCR::ABL*) for three years, and he inquires if he can try to get off therapy.

5) **Here's a gentleman with a spectacular result. Do you dare rock the boat? Your options.**
   A) Forbid discontinuation. Just say no!
   B) Allow with appropriate monitoring.
   C) Allow but only if he has two more years of undetectable disease.

Expert Perspective: In in vitro studies, the "CML stem cell" appears practically impervious to TKI therapy, and therefore it was assumed that patients would have to remain on a TKI for life since discontinuation would simply allow the stem cell reservoir to proliferate, assuring certain relapse. However, in a remarkable study, TKI therapy was discontinued in 100 patients who had been without detectable BCR-ABL1 for several years (see chapter by Dr. Larson on cessation of TKI therapy in CML). More than 50% relapsed quickly (generally in three to six months), but remarkably, 40% remained in molecular remission for more than two years. Many discontinuation studies followed and convincingly showed that despite differences in study design (length of time in deep molecular response, depth of deep molecular response, different rules for restarting TKI), roughly 50% of patients remain in a treatment-free remission. The minimum time appears to be at least two years of a deep response, and given that it takes about a year to obtain a deep response, most patients will have had at least three years of therapy. Most (> 90%) of patients who relapse following discontinuation respond well when treatment is reintroduced. Progression to advanced-phase disease after discontinuation appears rare. However, the long-term consequences of discontinuation are unknown, and patients and physicians who wish to try discontinuation are advised to enroll in a clinical trial. Trials examining attempts at a second discontinuation for those patients who failed to achieve a treatment-free remission and who returned to a deep molecular response after restarting therapy are ongoing.

   NCCN guidelines have some ground rules for considering discontinuing a TKI, which include chronic phase without history of advanced disease, at least three years of TKI therapy, at least two years of well-documented deep molecular response (defined as MR4.0 [*BCR::ABL* ≤ 0.01% IS] or below), and availability (and willingness) for frequent testing once discontinuation occurs (every monthly for the first six months following discontinuation and then a less frequent schedule of monitoring). The therapy should be restarted, preferably with the same TKI upon loss of MMR (*BCR::ABL* ≥ 0.1%) with monthly monitoring till MMR is achieved and then every three months.

Correct Answer: B

Back to the case: The patient decides to attempt discontinuation. His peripheral blood BCR-ABL1s for the first three months were all undetectable. However, on months four, five, and six they were 0.005% IS, undetectable, and 0.003% IS, respectively. In addition, around the first month he had a few episodes of increasing muscle fatigue and felt "crummy." He is quite distraught that all this might mean his disease is relapsing.

6) What should you do?

    A) Tell him to chill out and make another sculpture.

    B) Restart his TKI.

    C) Reassure and follow as planned.

Expert Perspective: He has several features that bode well for a successful discontinuation and long treatment-free remission: a long, deep response; a low-risk score; and undetectable *BCR::ABL* before discontinuation and three months beyond. In addition, he appears to have had a brief discontinuation withdrawl syndrome, which occurs in ~30% of discontinuation attempts and is self-limiting usually within weeks. There is some data to suggest that these patients are more likley to have successful treatment-free remission

Correct Answer: C

Back to the case: After your reassurance he returns to providing artistic musings to his devoted collectors, and his *BCR::ABL* hovers between undetectable and 0.004% for the next two years. He continues to have his *BCR::ABL* followed every three months.

Recommended Readings

Attalah, E., Schiffer, C., Radich, J.P. et al. (2020). Assessment of outcomes after stopping tyrosine kinase inhibitors among patients with chronic myeloid leukemia. *JAMA Oncol* 7: 42–50.

Branford, S., Yeung, D.T., Parker, W.T. et al. (2014). Prognosis for patients with CML and >10% BCR-ABL1 after 3 months of imatinib depends on the rate of BCR-ABL1 decline. *Blood* 124: 511–518.

Cortes, J.E., Gambacorti-Passerini, C., Deininger, M.W. et al. (2017). Bosutinib versus imatinib for newly diagnosed chronic myeloid leuekmia: results for the randomized BFORE trial. *J Clin Oncol* 36: 231–237.

Cortes, J.E., Khoury, H.J., Kantarjian, H.M. et al. (2016a). Long-term bosutinib for chronic phase chronic myeloid leukemia after failure of imatinib plus dasatinib and/or nilotinib. *Am J Hematol* 91: 1206–1214.

Cortes, J.E., Saglio, G., Kantarjian, H.M. et al. (2016b). Final 5-year study results of DASISION: The dasatinib versus imatinib study in treatment-naive chronic myeloid leukemia patients trial. *J Clin Oncol* 34: 2333–2340.

Deininger, M.W., Shaw, N.P., Altman, J.K. et al. (2020). NCCN guidelines insights: Chronic myeloid leukemia, version 2.2022. *J Natl Compr Canc Netw* 18: 1385–1415.

Giles, F.J., le Coutre, P.D., Pinilla-Ibarz, J. et al. (2013). Nilotinib in imatinib-resistant or imatinib-intolerant patients with chronic myeloid leukemia in chronic phase: 48-month follow-up results of a phase II study. *Leukemia* 27: 107–112.

Hochhaus, A., Larson, R.A., Guilhot, F. et al. (2017). Long-term outcomes of imatinib treatment for chronic myeloid leukemia. *N Engl J Med* 376: 917–927.

Hochhaus, A., Saglio, G., Hughes, T.P. et al. (2016). Long-term benefits and risks of frontline nilotinib vs imatinib for chronic myeloid leukemia in chronic phase: 5-year update of the randomized ENESTnd trial. *Leukemia* 30: 1044–1054.

Hughes, T., Kaeda, J., Branford, S. et al. (2003). Frequency of major molecular responses to imatinib or interferon alfa plus cytarabine in newly diagnosed chronic myeloid leukemia. *N Engl J Med* 349: 1423–1432.

Mahon, F.X., Rea, D., Guilhot, J. et al. (2010). Discontinuation of imatinib in patients with chronic myeloid leukaemia who have maintained complete molecular remission for at least 2 years: the prospective, multicentre Stop Imatinib (STIM) trial. *Lancet Oncol* 1029–1035.

Nair, A.P., Barnett, M.J., Broady, R.C. et al. (2015). Allogeneic hematopoietic stem cell transplantation is an effective salvage therapy for patients with chronic myeloid leukemia presenting with advanced disease or failing treatment with tyrosine kinase inhibitors. *Biol Blood Marrow Transplant* 21: 1437–1444.

Rousselot, P., Charbonnier, A., Cony-Makhoul, P. et al. (2014). Loss of major molecular response as a trigger for restarting tyrosine kinase inhibitor therapy in patients with chronic-phase chronic myelogenous leukemia who have stopped imatinib after durable undetectable disease. *J Clin Oncol* 32: 424–430.

Senapati, J., Sasaki, K., Issa, G.C., Lipton, J.H., Radich, J.P., Jabbour, E., and Kantarjian, H.M. (2023 April 24). Management of chronic myeloid leukemia in 2023 - common ground and common sense. *Blood Cancer J* 13 (1): 58. doi: 10.1038/s41408-023-00823-9. PMID: 37088793; PMCID: PMC10123066.

Shah, N.P., Rousselot, P., Schiffer, C. et al. (2016). Dasatinib in imatinib-resistant or -intolerant chronic-phase, chronic myeloid leukemia patients: 7-year follow-up of study CA180-034. *Am J Hematol* 91: 869–874.

Soverini, S., Branford, S., Nicolini, F.E. et al. (2014). Implications of BCR-ABL1 kinase domain-mediated resistance in chronic myeloid leukemia. *Leuk Res* 38: 10–20.

17

Chronic Myeloid Leukemia: Advance Phases of the Disease

Michael J. Mauro

Memorial Sloan Kettering Cancer Center, NY

Introduction

While chronic-phase chronic myeloid leukemia (CML) has become markedly more treatable with orally available, rationally designed targeted therapy and has set an example of success in cancer medicine, its evolved and gloomier cousin—advanced-phase CML—remains a challenging endeavor and has not benefitted to the degree seen in earlier phase disease. While chronic phase CML is now viewed as functionally curable with treatment-free-remission as a new target (Chapter 19), blast-phase disease continues to have a poor prognosis along with accelerated-phase disease. Both are oft best managed by subsequent allografting, which brings its own risks (Chapter 20). Understanding the underlying biology of advanced-phase CML, how it evolves from chronic phase, and how to identify the central targets, which may lie beyond *BCR::ABL*, likely hold the promise of greater success. Combination therapy with *ABL* kinase inhibitors and conventional chemotherapy remain as options with a search for better, safer, and novel "nonchemotherapy" agents.

1) How big a problem is advanced-phase CML presently?

Expert Perspective: CML is overwhelmingly a disease diagnosed and managed in the chronic phase. In the era of specific targeted therapy with *ABL* kinase inhibitors, progression of CML to advanced phases of disease (accelerated phase [AP] or blast phase/blast crisis [BP/BC]) has declined dramatically. Given that a diagnosis of CML in chronic phase is most commonly made incidentally, i.e. bloodwork performed for routine health care purpose or for management of another unrelated health issue, access to health care including preventative medicine can impede prompt identification of CML and be permissive of progression to advanced-phase disease; presentation in advanced phase thus remains higher in developing regions or places where health care resources are more limited. While the advent of *ABL* kinase inhibitors has affected advanced disease risk and sharply diminished the prevalence of AP and BC CML, treatment of advanced disease has unfortunately remained less successful. Efficacy of *ABL* inhibitors alone has been limited, and treatment generally necessitates combination therapy with conventional chemotherapy or other agents to gain control or return patients to a chronic phase, with allogeneic stem cell transplant remaining as a key next step, where feasible, to achieve long-term disease control.

Cancer Consult: Expertise in Clinical Practice, Volume 2: Neoplastic Hematology & Cellular Therapy, Second Edition. Edited by Syed A. Abutalib, Maurie Markman, James O. Armitage, and Kenneth C. Anderson. © 2024 John Wiley & Sons Ltd. Published 2024 by John Wiley & Sons Ltd.

2) How exactly is advanced-phase CML defined? And when to suspect "lymphoid blast phase" disease

Expert Perspective: CML staging is divided between three phases, the chronic, accelerated, and blast phases. Chronic phase is characterized by leukocytosis; variable platelet count (thrombocytosis more often than thrombocytopenia); left shifted differential with typically a full spectrum of immature myeloid forms including circulating blasts, basophilia, and possible eosinophilia; and potential splenomegaly. Advanced-phase disease includes accelerated-phase CML and the terminal blast phases, either myeloid or lymphoid blast crisis.

Accelerated-phase: Represents a somewhat heterogenous mix of disease evolution manifestations, recently updated by the World Health Organization (WHO) (Arber et al. 2016). These include clinical findings such as thrombocytopenia independent of therapy, marked basophilia (> 20% in peripheral blood), and blast percentage in the blood or bone marrow increased to between 10% and 19% (although historically up to 15% blasts was considered chronic-phase disease) as well as marked thrombocytosis (> 1000×10^9/L), leukocytosis or increasing WBC (> 10×10^9/L) or increasing splenomegaly unresponsive to therapy. An additional criterion for accelerated phase is the presence at diagnosis, or acquisition during therapy, of additional chromosomal changes in the malignant (Philadelphia chromosome positive) clone especially those identified as "major route" abnormalities (second Ph, trisomy 8, isochromosome 17q, trisomy 19) as well as complex karyotype or abnormalities of 3q26.2, as described by the German CML Study Group (Fabarius et al. 2015). The WHO update formalized broad, provisional "response to TKI" criteria as features of accelerated-phase disease, including: (i) hematologic resistance to the first TKI, (ii) any hematological, cytogenetic, or molecular indications of resistance to two sequential TKIs, (iii) or the occurrence of two or more mutations in *BCR::ABL1* during TKI therapy; these clinical criteria are practical as they are indeed indicative of the need for novel, potent therapies that are able to deal with this higher-risk disease commensurate with a significantly higher risk of poor outcome.

Blast phase: When CML manifests with a high degree of immaturity (20% or greater blast fraction in the blood or bone marrow), i.e. mirroring acute leukemia, or as extramedullary high-grade (myeloid sarcoma, also known as chloroma), it is deemed in a blast phase (BP), also called blast crisis (BC). With the origins of chronic myeloid leukemia in a pluripotent stem cell (Jamieson et al. 2004), acquisition/activation of additional mutations/blocks to differentiation in lineage-specific progenitors leads to blast-phase disease with approximately two-thirds of cases being myeloid blast phase and the remaining third corresponding to lymphoid blast phase. Also noted in the 2016 WHO classification of myeloid neoplasms is the warning (Arber et al. 2016) that since onset of lymphoid blast phase may be quite sudden, the detection of any confirmed lymphoblasts in the blood or marrow should raise concern for a possible impending lymphoid blast phase, warranting timely additional laboratory and genetic studies to exclude the possibility.

Whereas the most common scenario historically was blast-phase disease evolved from incomplete or ineffective treatment of antecedent chronic-phase disease after a highly variable length of time, *de novo* blast-phase disease can occur as well, with growth kinetics of the transformed blast clone overtaking expansion of background indolent CML clones. Neglected or unrecognized CML in chronic phase, with time, can develop increasing disease burden and accumulation of adverse features and can thus shift to a higher risk category within chronic phase by Sokal or other risk modeling; transformation to a defined accelerated- or blast-phase disease may also occur with significant delay or deferral of treatment. In addition to failure of therapy, delay to accessing care, neglect of signs/symptoms of disease, and potentially even lack of routine or symptom-driven blood testing are all potential facilitators of chronic-phase disease evolution to advanced phase.

3) Is it possible to avoid advanced-phase disease?

Expert Perspective: Expectedly, a primary goal of CML treatment is avoidance of blast-phase evolution from within chronic phase. In the management of chronic-phase disease, principles of treatment include several points that may minimize risk of progression to advanced-phase disease, or at least clarify the risk properly to allow appropriate intervention. These include the following:

A) At diagnosis of CML, proper staging is essential. Full and careful blood count assessment coupled with physical exam findings reveal the essential elements needed for risk stratification within current models (Sokal, Eutos Long Term Survival [ELTS; Pfirrmann et al. 2020], and others). Bone marrow assessment continues to be recommended in guidelines and may be essential in revealing the following accelerated phase elements:

   I) Occult morphologic increase in bone marrow blasts heralding AP or BC, including any amount of lymphoblasts prompting concern for emerging/subsequent lymphoid blast phase;

   II) Cytogenetic clonal evolution supporting disease evolution (Fabarius et al. 2015) and potential for AP disease even if seen in isolation;

   III) Unanticipated flow cytometric evidence of higher-risk lymphoid or myeloid blast clones.

B) Achievement of milestones in CP CML minimizes risk of progression to advanced-phase disease, and adherence by providers to guideline-driven response expectations can direct timely dose modification, switch of tyrosine kinase inhibitor, or consideration or reconsideration of alternative pathways for best outcome including referral for allogeneic stem cell transplant. Key elements include proper TKI choice, dosing according to disease phase and risk at diagnosis, correct surveillance for and management of adverse events, and confirming patient adherence to therapy. Examples of higher-risk scenarios in chronic-phase CML include persistent hematologic disease (lack of complete hematologic response to therapy), which is rare, and lack of complete cytogenetic response in the appropriate time frame. Major molecular response (*BCR::ABL1* 0.1% IS or less) is widely viewed as a safe harbor below which progression risk is greatly diminished (Druker et al. 2006) and may be viewed as the best milestone threshold minimizing transformation risk (Chapters 16 and 19).

C) Allogeneic stem cell transplant as a treatment choice for CML has evolved significantly, and referral for consideration as well as decision-making to determine when outcomes may improve by proceeding to allograft are often delayed and opportunities missed. While use of more potent TKI options with activity against specific mutations may be advantageous in chronic-phase disease, transformation to advanced-phase disease is likely best managed with proceeding to allografting if possible and ideally after treatment able to return disease back to a chronic phase or better (Nicolini et al. 2017) (Chapter 20).

4) What is the best approach currently to myeloid blast-phase CML?

Expert Perspective: In the rare case of *de novo* myeloid blast crisis of CML, single-agent TKI therapy preferably with second- or even third-generation agents is reasonable with high rates of hematologic response but risk of early relapse and potential for emergent ABL kinase domain mutations. More common is the scenario of blast phase (myeloid or lymphoid) evolving from treated chronic-phase CML where prior TKI exposure and ABL kinase mutation testing are crucial to advise a best therapy pathway. Given the limited efficacy of single-agent TKI therapy for myeloid blast crisis, efforts to identify an optimal combination therapy approach, incorporating conventional chemotherapy and evolved *ABL* kinase inhibitors, has been ongoing and has been slowed by declining incidence of blast crisis. The MATCHPOINT study (Copland et al. 2022), a seamless phase I/II, multicenter UK trial of oral ponatinib at various doses with intravenous fludarabine (30 mg/m^2 for five days), cytarabine (2 g/m^2 for five days), and idarubicin (8 mg/m^2 for three days), and subcutaneous granulocyte colony-stimulating factor in 16 evaluable patients using EffTox design determined the optimal ponatinib dose of 30 mg daily to combine with FLAG-IDA and demonstrated a 69% return to second chronic phase after one cycle of treatment and 71% rate of proceeding to allogeneic hematopoietic cell transplant (allo-HCT), with acceptable and somewhat expected adverse events, including hepatic and vascular toxicity. Ponatinib–FLAG-IDA thus stands as a preferred salvage therapy for myeloid blast-phase disease and can bridge to allo-HCT.

5) What is the best approach currently to lymphoid blast-phase CML?

Expert Perspective: Similar to myeloid blast phase, the combination of chemotherapy and TKI has emerged as a standard in lymphoid blast-phase disease, with data including imatinib, dasatinib, and more recently ponatinib combined with standard lymphoid induction therapy believed to represent the most active regimen and the current standard of care for the disease (refer to Chapter 2). Such regimens were primarily studied for *de novo* Ph+ acute lymphoblastic leukemia based on incidence and need, and while some studies had combined populations of Ph+ ALL and lymphoid blast-phase disease, much has been extrapolated in clinical use. In the rare case of *de novo* or early emergent lymphoid blast-phase disease, such extrapolation is reasonable. For lymphoid blast phase evolving after prior treatment for chronic-phase CML with TKI therapy, much consideration into TKI choice and investigation into pathogenesis (mutation testing at a minimum) is necessary.

The backbone most studied in Ph+ lymphoid leukemias has been hyperfractionated cyclophosphamide, vincristine, adriamycin, dexamethasone (hyper-CVAD), combined initially with either imatinib or dasatinib (Strati et al. 2014). This regimen yielded hematologic remission in ~90% of patients, cytogenetic remission in ~60%, and minimal residual disease negativity in ~40%; additionally, molecular negativity was observed in ~25% of cases. Bridging to allo-HCT was possible in a subset of patients and led to improved long-term survival, as did the use of dasatinib (CNS penetration as well) rather than imatinib. While hematologic toxicity in all cases and related infections in a majority were observed, discontinuation due to adverse events was rare. With the advent of ponatinib, combination with hyper-CVAD was thus examined in Ph+ ALL (Jabbour et al. 2018) with results as mentioned extrapolated for use in lymphoid blast phase. On study ponatinib dosing evolved, initially 15 mg for 14 days with initial treatment, then 45 mg continuously, then subsequently reduced to 30 mg in subsequent cycles and to 15 mg with complete molecular remission. The three-year event-free survival in a phase II (n = 76) single-center study was 70%, with a predictable adverse event profile including grade 3 or 4 infection (86%), increased transaminases (32%), increased bilirubin and pancreatitis (both 17%), hypertension (16%), bleeding (13%), and skin rash (12%) and two myocardial infarction–related deaths before ponatinib dose revision.

Obviously, a chemotherapy induction may not be suitable for many patients with evolving lymphoid blast-phase CML, as well as for many patients with Ph+ ALL. A chemotherapy-free induction approach was championed by the Italian GIMEMA group in Ph+ ALL, arising initially from the need for lower-risk options for higher-risk, older patients, with over 15+ years of sequential study of imatinib and then dasatinib in combination with steroids and central nervous system (CNS) prophylaxis (Chiaretti et al. 2021). Results have demonstrated very high rates of hematologic response, including 100% response in 53 patients treated with dasatinib + steroid induction. Bridging to allo-HCT was possible even with the original imatinib + steroid regimen, and over time, in a later study, risk-adapted consolidation with dasatinib alone in the case of complete molecular response or chemotherapy/allo-HCT for lesser response led to overall and disease-free survival of ~50%. *ABL* kinase domain mutations were common in relapse, and the incorporation of next-generation TKIs thus followed. Recent publication of ponatinib + steroids for older/unfit patients (n = 44) with Ph+ ALL (Martinelli et al. 2022) demonstrated similarly high rates of hematologic response (86%) and increased rates of complete molecular response (~40%) but was coupled with a 25–30% incidence of treatment emergent cardiac and vascular adverse events suggesting ponatinib dose and risk may need to be reconsidered.

Other TKIs such as bosutinib have been studied in advanced-phase Ph+ disease; a phase I/II study (Jain et al. 2021) of bosutinib at three dose levels (300 mg/d, 400 mg/d, 500 mg/d) in a 3 + 3 design combined with inotuzumab ozogamicin weekly (cycle 1) and then monthly for six cycles in patients with relapsed/refractory Ph+ ALL (n = 16) and lymphoid BC (n = 2) yielded complete response (with and without complete count recovery combined) in 15 of 18 (83%) patients, with 11 of 18 (61%) of cases reverting to negative measurable residual disease by flow cytometry; complete molecular response was noted in 10 of 18 (56%) patients. Importantly the 30-day mortality was 0%, with skin rash and thrombocytopenia (60%) and neutropenia (38%) the main adverse events. No sinusoidal obstructive disease (SOS) was noted, and six patients had a subsequent allo-HCT. Overall, these data point to exploration of other TKI/targeted therapy combinations for such patients. CNS screening and prophylaxis is an integral component of all the anti-ALL systemic therapies (see Chapters 2 and 20).

6) What is the best approach currently for accelerated-phase CML?

Expert Perspective: Accelerated-phase CML should be treated according to its behavior, more like CP or more like BC, based on the spectrum of findings. Early work examining the impact of clonal evolution only as an isolated finding and criteria for AP disease (O'Dwyer et al. 2002) suggested that response to imatinib therapy may be still possible. However, as described below, the specific type of clonal change is very important and may impact disease biology differently. Clinical findings of acceleration akin to blast transformation, namely rising blast counts or other immature forms (excess promyelocytes/"myelocyte bulge") likely suggest impending criteria for blast phase and treatment accordingly.

Aside from single-agent TKI experience in accelerated-phase CML, generally included in reports with chronic-phase disease, combination with a strategy familiar to MDS posing risk of transformation, namely hypomethylating agents, has been explored as well for patients with both AP and BC CML, with the conclusion of both safety and clear activity. In a phase I/II study (Abaza et al. 2020) of decitabine 10 mg/m^2 or 20 mg/m^2 daily for 10 days combined with dasatinib (100 mg increasing to a target dose of 140 mg daily) in 30 patients (7 with AP, 19 with BC CML, and 4 with Ph+ ALL), while high rates of hematologic toxicity were observed, 48% of these patients achieved major hematologic response, 22% minor hematologic response, and in these responding cases, 44% and 33% achieved major cytogenetic and major molecular response, respectively.

7) How can we identify or understand the basis of advanced-phase CML better?

Expert Perspective: In the large German CML IV study (> 1500 patients) predictors of progression were carefully studied (Hehlmann et al. 2020); based on their impact on survival, additional chromosomal abnormalities were considered either high risk (+8, +Ph, i(17q), +17, +19, +21, 3q26.2, 11q23, −7/7q abnormalities; complex) or low risk (all other). From the subset of CP CML patients with additional chromosomal abnormalities (n = 123), 91 were high risk and remarkably, at low (chronic phase) blast levels (1–15%) these additional chromosomal abnormalities posed clear increased risk of progression or death from CML; 63 of those 91 either died or survived treatment or allografting for progression. These data emphasized the importance of cytogenetic testing at diagnosis and when response is lacking in CP CML.

Genomic sequencing clearly has shaped the identification, nature, and behavior of advanced-phase CML. In a comprehensive genetic analysis of a large (n = 216) cohort of patients sampled at CP and/or BC (Ochi et al. 2021), certain genetic lesions were better predictors of survival than clinical parameters, specifically *TP53* mutations, isochromosome 17q, *ASXL1* mutation, trisomy 21, and complex copy number alterations.

The exact totality of genetic lesions that are relevant, however, if noted in screening or at pivotal subsequent points during treatment, likely when response is suboptimal or lost and/ or progression is emerging, is unclear. A recent review (Branford et al. 2019) highlighted *RUNX1*, a master regulator of myeloid and lymphoid differentiation essential for normal hematopoiesis; *ASXL1*, evidenced by its role in chromatin modification and regulation of gene expression; and *IKZF1*, a tumor suppressor encoding the lymphoid transcription factor IKAROS, crucial in hematopoiesis, as well as gene fusions including partners with known impact in other myeloid diseases. Specific modelling of RUNX1-transformed blast-phase disease (Adnan Awad et al. 2021) demonstrated, perhaps logically, disrupted interferon and TNF signaling and stem cell and B-lymphoid factors were upregulated in association with a unique phenotype. Related drug sensitivity and resistance testing pointed to cluster designation antigen 19 positive chimeric antigen receptor (CAR) T cells, glucocorticoids, and therapies inhibiting mTOR, BCL2, and VEGFR pathways; such dissection of blast-phase disease is likely to prove very helpful in sorting highest priority targets and highest yield therapy concepts for study.

Recommended Readings

Abaza, Y., Kantarjian, H., Alwash, Y. et al. (2020 November). Phase I/II study of dasatinib in combination with decitabine in patients with accelerated or blast phase chronic myeloid leukemia. *Am J Hematol* 95 (11): 1288–1295.

Adnan Awad, S., Dufva, O., Ianevski, A. et al. (2021 April). RUNX1 mutations in blast-phase chronic myeloid leukemia associate with distinct phenotypes, transcriptional profiles, and drug responses. *Leukemia* 35 (4): 1087–1099.

Arber, D.A., Orazi, A., Hasserjian, R. et al. (2016 May 19). The 2016 revision to the World Health Organization classification of myeloid neoplasms and acute leukemia. *Blood* 127 (20): 2391–2405.

Branford, S., Kim, D.D.H., Apperley, J.F. et al. (2019 August). International CML Foundation Genomics Alliance. Laying the foundation for genomically-based risk assessment in chronic myeloid leukemia. *Leukemia* 33 (8): 1835–1850.

Chiaretti, S., Ansuinelli, M., Vitale, A. et al. (2021 July 1). A multicenter total therapy strategy for *de novo* adult Philadelphia chromosome positive acute lymphoblastic leukemia patients: final results of the GIMEMA LAL1509 protocol. *Haematologica* 106 (7): 1828–1838.

Copland, M., Slade, D., McIlroy, G. et al. (2022 February). Ponatinib with fludarabine, cytarabine, idarubicin, and granulocyte colony-stimulating factor chemotherapy for patients with blast-phase chronic myeloid leukaemia (MATCHPOINT): a single-arm, multicentre, phase 1/2 trial. *Lancet Haematol* 9 (2): e121–e132.

Druker, B.J., Guilhot, F., O'Brien, S.G. et al. (2006 December 7). IRIS Investigators. Five-year follow-up of patients receiving imatinib for chronic myeloid leukemia. *N Engl J Med* 355 (23): 2408–2417.

Fabarius, A., Kalmanti, L., Dietz, C.T. et al. (2015 December). SAKK and the German CML Study Group. Impact of unbalanced minor route versus major route karyotypes at diagnosis on prognosis of CML. *Ann Hematol* 94 (12): 2015–2024.

Hehlmann, R., Voskanyan, A., Lauseker, M. et al. (2020 August). SAKK and the German CML Study Group. High-risk additional chromosomal abnormalities at low blast counts herald death by CML. *Leukemia* 34 (8): 2074–2086.

Jabbour, E., Short, N.J., Ravandi, F. et al. (2018 December). Combination of hyper-CVAD with ponatinib as first-line therapy for patients with Philadelphia chromosome-positive acute lymphoblastic leukaemia: long-term follow-up of a single-centre, phase 2 study. *Lancet Haematol* 5 (12): e618–e627.

Jain, N., Maiti, A., Ravandi, F. et al. (2021 August 1). Inotuzumab ozogamicin with bosutinib for relapsed or refractory Philadelphia chromosome positive acute lymphoblastic leukemia or lymphoid blast phase of chronic myeloid leukemia. *Am J Hematol* 96 (8): 1000–1007.

Jamieson, C.H., Ailles, L.E., Dylla, S.J. et al. (2004 August 12). Granulocyte-macrophage progenitors as candidate leukemic stem cells in blast-crisis CML. *N Engl J Med* 351 (7): 657–667.

Martinelli, G., Papayannidis, C., Piciocchi, A. et al. (2022 March 22). INCB84344-201: ponatinib and steroids in frontline therapy for unfit patients with Ph+ acute lymphoblastic leukemia. *Blood Adv* 6 (6): 1742–1753.

Nicolini, F.E., Basak, G.W., Kim, D.W. et al. (2017 August 1). Overall survival with ponatinib versus allogeneic stem cell transplantation in Philadelphia chromosome-positive leukemias with the *T315I* mutation. *Cancer* 123 (15): 2875–2880.

O'Dwyer, M.E., Mauro, M.J., Kurilik, G. et al. (2002 September 1). The impact of clonal evolution on response to imatinib mesylate (STI571) in accelerated phase CML. *Blood* 100 (5): 1628–1633.

Ochi, Y., Yoshida, K., Huang, Y.J. et al. (2021 May 14). Clonal evolution and clinical implications of genetic abnormalities in blastic transformation of chronic myeloid leukaemia. *Nat Commun* 12 (1): 2833.

Pfirrmann, M., Clark, R.E., Prejzner, W. et al. (2020 August). The EUTOS long-term survival (ELTS) score is superior to the Sokal score for predicting survival in chronic myeloid leukemia. *Leukemia* 34 (8): 2138–2149.

Strati, P., Kantarjian, H., Thomas, D. et al. (2014 February 1). HCVAD plus imatinib or dasatinib in lymphoid blastic phase chronic myeloid leukemia. *Cancer* 120 (3): 373–380.

18

Chronic Myeloid Leukemia: Treatment Safety During Reproductive Age and Pregnancy

Safety of Therapy during Reproductive Age and Pregnancy

Michael J. Mauro

Memorial Sloan Kettering Cancer Center, NY

Introduction

In considering patients with chronic myeloid leukemia of child-bearing age, desiring the option to plan a family, current tyrosine kinase inhibitor (TKIs) therapy options have created a scenario where optimal leukemia treatment and pregnancy can successfully merge. The average age of patients diagnosed with CML in industrialized countries is 55–65 years of age whereas it is 10–15 years lower in developing countries, where population growth is the greatest (Hoffmann et al. 2015). There is thus a significant population, especially on a global level, for whom preserving the option for pregnancy remains crucial and runs parallel to gaining CML remission, prompting open and active discussion and consideration. While there are reports in the literature regarding strategies to manage the myriad of scenarios related to pregnancy and CML, as well as aggregate data on pregnancy outcomes, organized study of this important area has been elusive; additionally, a call for guidelines has been noted (Pallavee et al. 2019) and is planned to be taken up by various groups. This chapter will focus primarily on the scenario of a female patient with chronic myeloid leukemia and pregnancy. (For more information about CML, see Chapters 16 and 19.)

1) Can pregnancy be considered in the setting of chronic myeloid leukemia (CML)?

Expert Perspective: Unsurprisingly there are many considerations for such an endeavor, including the impact of the CML diagnosis and CML therapy on fertility, pregnancy, and delivery. Importantly and highly relevant to pregnancy considerations, the treatment of CML has evolved to include a focus on the potential for treatment-free remission, whereas in patients with select response characteristics (primarily focused around thresholds of overall TKI duration overall and duration in deep molecular response), treatment can be deliberately stopped, and monitoring increased, to observe for stability and ongoing deep response off therapy.

Currently a significant fraction (majority) but not all CML CP patients are ultimately eligible for treatment-free remission per guidelines (Hochhaus et al. 2020, National Comprehensive Cancer Network 2022), and treatment-free remission is successful roughly 50% of the time. CML research aims to increase the cure fraction—treatment-free remission eligible patients and prediction, success in subsequent (second) treatment-free remission attempts after primary failure, etc. It is logical to combine the agenda of treatment-free remission with a woman's desire to conceive and carry a pregnancy, and with careful planning, optimal outcomes for both CML and pregnancy can be attained. On the opposite spectrum, avoidance of unplanned or unexpected pregnancy, if at all possible, is highly desirable given the incompatibility of active TKI treatment and confirmed pregnancy.

Consideration of pregnancy with a diagnosis of CML and incumbent TKI treatment is a multistep process requiring forethought, involvement of both the patient and their support (spouse/partner/significant other), patience, and flexibility regarding the timing, given compounded uncertainties with CML treatment response kinetics and milestones as well as factors intrinsic to pregnancy including timing and ability to conceive and avoidance of complications leading to miscarriage, among others.

2) What are the important considerations for pregnancy and CML?

Expert Perspective: Not surprisingly, optimal CML management—proper risk stratification of CML diagnosis, thoughtful choice of TKI therapy (potentially favoring rapid, early, and deep molecular remission as a means of facilitating pregnancy at the earliest point possible), toxicity avoidance and treatment adjustments to optimize response and odds of stable deep remission, and guideline-driven milestone monitoring—all constitute the first step toward setting the stage for family planning. Targeting the ideal time to conceive warrants primary focus on the CML remission and treatment status, coupled with as much consideration to the patient's wishes and ideals as possible. Frank discussion of this balance, and emphasis on avoiding unplanned/unexpected pregnancy with the involvement and alliance of patient's support (spouse/partner/significant other, etc.) is crucial.

Additionally, a clear understanding of fertility potential for all parties involved—in particular the female patient desiring to achieve pregnancy and any anatomical, hormonal, or other barriers to conception, successful pregnancy to term, and delivery—is important in all cases. Investigation into male partners of female patients may be warranted as needed for greater certainty of ease of conception when desired. Given the potential uncertainty of pregnancy in CML under certain circumstances, frank discussion with the patient and their spouse/partner/significant other regarding risk and management of CML relapse if it occurs and dual agenda to focus care on the patient and the fetus predelivery or infant/child post delivery; ethical and moral decisions regarding priorities and wishes should the patient's health decline or be in jeopardy should be aired and views shared to minimize stress and anxiety. Last, early involvement, alliance, and effective communication of leukemia specialty physicians with the obstetrics team, and where indicated, higher-risk obstetrics, during pregnancy is very important; as these specialties are quite divergent, each brings vital information and strategy to bear for the success of the endeavor.

3) What is the optimal way to manage pregnancy in someone with newly diagnosed CML?

Expert Perspective: Given the increased risk of both maternal and fetal complications, in accordance with any prior known views, ethics, religious preferences, termination may be discussed and considered in the context of greater maternal than fetal risk due to limitation of treatment options or evolution of the CML. Open discussion of all scenarios is best to ultimately preserve life and manage difficult situations, with no one party oversteering the conversation. In the current era of highly successful TKI options and goal of functional cure, need for intentional delay of treatment initiation and the fact that TKI treatment in the face of confirmed ongoing pregnancy is not recommended are realities making diagnosis during pregnancy particularly challenging.

Despite uncertainty and risk, consideration to allow pregnancy to proceed with observation and close monitoring is feasible based on the oft indolent presentation of CML in chronic phase and historical expectation of several years' time typically in chronic phase before progression to accelerated- or blast-phase disease may manifest. As mentioned, all FDA-approved TKIs fall in pregnancy warning category D (i.e. there is positive evidence of human fetal risk, but the benefits from use in pregnant women may be acceptable despite the risk) and thus are not sanctioned for use. There are variable data on fetal exposure, risks, and outcomes available based on registry and drug safety databases, allowing for provisional judgment of relative harm from TKIs (Abruzzese et al. 2018, Cortes et al. 2015, 2020, Pye et al. 2008). Early data with imatinib cites limited congenital anomalies mostly observed when used in early pregnancy (organogenesis), and clinical experience from its manufacturer and registry data note limited effects resulting from nilotinib exposure during pregnancy. Dasatinib has been associated with fetal harm both early during organogenesis and later in pregnancy, thus relegating it to the TKI with greatest risk to date. There remains a paucity of data regarding impacts of bosutinib and ponatinib, and expectedly, no information is available for asciminib given its recent FDA approval.

Hydroxyurea reliably can provide rapid cytoreduction, but its use in pregnancy is precluded by expectation of teratogenesis; experience is thus limited, and it cannot be recommended. Interferons, both conventional formulations and long acting (pegylated), have been and can be used in CML and other myeloproliferative neoplasms in pregnancy. They are generally considered safe for the fetus, except for a potential concern over polyethylene glycol (PEG), albeit very limited and unlikely to have any consequence.

The woman diagnosed with CML during pregnancy faces the highest likelihood of needing active therapy; goals should include stabilizing/controlling proliferative disease, in particular minimizing risk of leukostasis, thrombosis, and hemorrhage, coupled with preserving healthy maternal fetal placental blood flow and safe delivery assuming proceeding to term is safe. White blood cell count and platelet count goals may be set (for example, $< 50,000$ WBC, avoiding extreme thrombocytosis [$> 1,000,000$]), although each case should be individualized. Kinetics of therapy effect should be considered; while safer, interferon-based therapy may have limited or delayed effect and thus may need to be considered earlier. As previously mentioned, while not sanctioned, TKI use in later stages of pregnancy may be considered necessary for maternal safety, outweighing fetal risk, and generally can provide rapid control of disease.

4) How can you manage ongoing CML treatment with segue into pregnancy?

Expert Perspective: Either resulting from unplanned or unexpected conception or a woman's keen desire to conceive in the setting of CML, a not uncommon scenario is pregnancy despite less-than-optimal CML response. Varying levels of remission may be present—less protective status such as hematologic response only or partial cytogenetic response; expectedly, complete cytogenetic response and molecular response afford more protection and stability. One way to consider this situation would be patient treatment-free remission eligible / not treatment-free remission eligible, meaning that unless the patient meets criteria for treatment-free remission, relapse would be expected during a hiatus for conception and pregnancy. Given this, it is prudent to counsel regarding incremental risk based on CML response at time of potential conception and point at which TKI therapy would be needed to be halted (i.e. risk of relapse/progression: active chronic phase / no hematologic response > hematologic response > cytogenetic response > major molecular response > deep molecular response). Depending on the circumstance, if a patient with less than deep molecular response (not treatment-free remission eligible) decides to conceive or carry a pregnancy, a firm discussion with patient and spouse/partner/significant other regarding potential for adverse leukemia outcome and risk to patient, including risk of progression to advanced phase, is prudent. Ethically it is likely important to prompt couples to develop contingency plans if the mother's health is endangered, or disease progression occurs, in order to ensure proper care for a child brought to term; while such conversations are difficult, transparency and honesty are important elements to managing such circumstances.

When planning conception during CML treatment, whether for patients who are or are not treatment-free remission eligible (see below), facilitating access to rapid pregnancy tests (in-home as well as confirmatory clinic-based assays) is crucial, to allow the quickest identification of pregnancy and to thus guide treatment advice (TKI cessation). As described, TKI use during pregnancy as a general rule is not recommended; in order to avoid long periods entirely off TKI for conception (which could be quite long), it is reasonable to consider continue ongoing CML TKI treatment while actively trying to conceive (with the goal to allow ~50% + of days on treatment per month) while avoiding any TKI exposure immediately after conception, when risk of negative impact may be greatest. Such an approach requires significant commitment and attention to detail by the patient and firm understanding of menstrual cycle length and pattern and fertility indicators. Such a strategy entails administration of TKI therapy before, during, and after menstrual cycle until ovulation; TKI interruption until fertile period has passed / during conception attempts; and resumption of TKI therapy if pregnancy testing is negative or interruption sustained if pregnancy is confirmed.

5) Is it possible to combine treatment-free remission with segue into pregnancy?

Expert Perspective: With the knowledge that a proportion of patients can be treated for a discrete amount of time, and subsequently a fraction may continue in stable deep remission off therapy, the option to marry a treatment-free remission agenda with a subsequent planned pregnancy can offer the safest way for CML and safe pregnancy to coexist. Considering the CML treatment first, monitoring, results, and findings should be according to accepted guidelines (ELN, NCCN), regarding eligibility for treatment-free remission. Aligning the patient with the obstetrics team before treatment-free remission, with agenda to monitor menstrual cycles, fertility indicators, etc., or if needed, to adjust any medications (oral contraceptives, other hormonal manipulation) can avoid unexpected delay or barrier to conception after treatment-free remission. As treatment-free remission is only successful in ~50% of cases, it is prudent to prepare contingency plan if it is unsuccessful (resuming TKI therapy and alternative family planning strategies) to minimize stress on the patient/partner/family.

Ideally, in optimal remission after CML therapy, such cases can proceed with TKI interruption (treatment-free remission) with observation for a recommended minimum six or more months before consideration of attempting to conceive, based on general and patient-specific estimate of kinetics of potential relapse. It is possible thus to counsel the patient regarding odds of ongoing stable treatment-free remission based on available data at time of proceeding to attempt to conceive (PCR at time of TKI cessation, PCR after three months of treatment-free remission, etc.). During treatment-free remission, cases should be monitored according to guidelines; consideration can be given to extend the duration of more frequent early treatment free-remission monitoring (i.e. monthly PCR) if relapse appears more imminent/possible despite proper observation (> six months), or even throughout pregnancy in light of the uncertainty of the effect of concomitant pregnancy on longitudinal treatment-free remission outcomes. Even if the patient remains in deeper remission, ongoing success of treatment-free remission during pregnancy may be estimated based on available data and time elapsed off treatment before pregnancy. A meta-analysis of treatment-free remission data from 3105 patients (Dulucq et al. 2020) noted a probability of molecular recurrence within the first six months after TKI cessation of 35%. After six months the likelihood of relapse decreases significantly, with probability of recurrence in months 7–12 of 8%, in months 13–18, 3%, and in months 19–24, 3% (Abruzzese et al. 2018). This data is agnostic to the individual patient data available leading into treatment-free remission and early into the treatment-free remission endeavor, where further prediction may be made (see Chapter 19).

6) Are there special considerations or risks for men with CML wishing to father children?

Expert Perspective: Early in the development phase of TKIs for CML there was concern over potential effects in men wanting to father children. Animal studies raised questions regarding effects on spermatogenesis and development of reproductive organs, albeit at high exposure. Prescribing information and patient drug information advises against pregnancy and suggests adequate birth control during treatment. Clinical experience has generally concluded minimal effects and inconclusive data on male fertility, with a possibility of decreased sperm counts. A recent review concerning male patients fathering children during or after TKI therapy (Szakács et al. 2020) found no increased incidence of fetal malformations above expected. With this information, there is insufficient information to warrant interruption or pause in therapy (including for "washout", which based on spermatogenesis, would require six to eight weeks of time off therapy) for men with CML on active treatment wishing to father children. It may be prudent to consider any pregnancy involving TKI exposure, whether it is related to a male patient, women with prior exposure, or women with exposure potentially at or after the time of conception, as potentially higher risk and warranting specialized obstetrical investigation or care.

Recommended Readings

Abruzzese, E., Elena, C., Castagnetti, F. et al. (2018). Gimema Registry of conception/pregnancy in adult Italian patients diagnosed with chronic myeloid leukemia (CML): report on 166 outcomes. *Blood* 132 (Suppl. 1): abstract 43.

Cortes, J.E., Abruzzese, E., Chelysheva, E. et al. (2015). The impact of dasatinib on pregnancy outcomes. *Am J Hematol* 90: 1111–1115.

Cortes, J.E., Gambacorti-Passerini, C., Deininger, M. et al. (2020). Pregnancy outcomes in patients treated with bosutinib. *Int J Hematol Oncol* 9: IJH26.

Dulucq, S., Astrugue, C., Etienne, G. et al. (2020 May). Risk of molecular recurrence after tyrosine kinase inhibitor discontinuation in chronic myeloid leukaemia patients: a systematic review of literature with a meta-analysis of studies over the last ten years. *Br J Haematol* 189 (3): 452–468.

Hochhaus, A., Baccarani, M., Silver, R.T. et al. (2020). European LeukemiaNet 2020 recommendations for treating chronic myeloid leukemia. *Leukemia* 34: 966–984.

Hoffmann, V.S., Baccarani, M., Hasford, J. et al. (2015 June). The EUTOS population-based registry: incidence and clinical characteristics of 2904 CML patients in 20 European Countries. *Leukemia* 29 (6): 1336–1343.

National Comprehensive Cancer Network (2022). NCCN clinical practice guidelines in oncology: chronic myeloid leukemia. V3.2022, accessed with permission www.nccn.org.

Pallavee, P., Samal, R., and Ghose, S. (2019 May). Chronic myeloid leukaemia in pregnancy: call for guidelines. *J Obstet Gynaecol* 39 (4): 582–583.

Pye, S.M., Cortes, J., Ault, P. et al. (2008). The effects of Imatinib on pregnancy outcome. *Blood* 111: 5505–5508.

Szakács, Z., Hegyi, P.J., Farkas, N. et al. (2020). Pregnancy outcomes of women whom spouse fathered children after tyrosine kinase inhibitor therapy for chronic myeloid leukemia: a systematic review. *PLoS One* 15 (12): e0243045.

19

Chronic Myeloid Leukemia: Cessation of Therapy

Anand A. Patel and Richard A. Larson

University of Chicago, Chicago, IL

Introduction

In the current era of chronic myeloid leukemia (CML) management, when to consider tyrosine kinase inhibitor (TKI) cessation is a common clinical question that arises. Several prospective trials have established that TKI cessation is both feasible and safe in patients with a sustained deep molecular response. In the current chapter we review chronic adverse effects associated with TKI use and what quality of life improvements patients may expect to see with TKI cessation. We also summarize what factors affect the likelihood of achieving a deep molecular response and parameters that should be met prior to a trial of TKI cessation. Lastly, we discuss frequency of clinical monitoring during a trial of TKI cessation, symptoms that may be seen with TKI cessation, and considerations around when to restart TKI therapy and which TKI to select.

Case Study 1

A 38-year-old man with chronic myeloid leukemia (CML) presented for routine follow-up. He had been diagnosed in chronic phase 18 months earlier, and his EUTOS long-term survival (ELTS) score placed him in the low-risk disease group. He was started on imatinib 400 mg daily, and he has met all optimal disease response mileposts so far. At the one-year mark of treatment, he had no detectable disease by quantitative RT-PCR (qRT-PCR) testing with a sensitivity of 10^{-5}, consistent with a deep molecular remission, and his disease continues to be undetectable in the blood. Before his diagnosis of CML, he was an avid runner. Now, however, he reports persistent fatigue since starting imatinib that has limited his ability to exercise. He would like to discuss stopping imatinib or switching to a different tyrosine kinase inhibitor (TKI) due to the impact on his quality of life.

1) What are the chronic adverse effects of TKIs used for the treatment of CML?

Expert Perspective: The initial choice of TKI in a patient with newly diagnosed CML in chronic phase is influenced by both the presence of high-risk disease characteristics and underlying comorbidities. Common comorbidities of concern include obesity, smoking, hypertension, diabetes mellitus, dyslipidemia, and cardiovascular disease. The Charlson Comorbidity Index is a strong predictor of overall survival in chronic-phase CML patients treated with TKIs, and the presence of multiple comorbidities increases the risk of arterio-occlusive events. As CML patients live longer, they may also develop additional age-related comorbidities. All TKIs used in the treatment of CML have been associated with increased risk of the development of arterio-occlusive events, although the risk is highest with ponatinib and lowest with imatinib.

TKI-specific non-hematologic adverse effects must also be considered in choosing the optimal therapy. Nilotinib is associated with the development of hyperglycemia and dyslipidemia while dasatinib has been associated with the development of pleural and pericardial effusions. Bosutinib has been associated with diarrhea and hepatic toxicity. The incidence of renal dysfunction attributable to TKIs is quite low, although imatinib and bosutinib have been associated with a decrease in GFR in a few reports. A rare but significant complication described with dasatinib, and less commonly with bosutinib, is the development of pulmonary hypertension (see Chapter 16).

Patient-reported outcomes (PROs) have identified adverse effects that have a significant impact on quality of life. An analysis of patients enrolled in the LAST trial found that a proportion of patients reported at least moderately severe symptoms in the following domains: 16% fatigue, 20% depression, 17% diarrhea, 14% sleep disturbance, and 20% interference in daily life due to pain.

2) Which patient-reported outcomes (PROs) typically improve with cessation of TKI?

Expert Perspective: The LAST trial was a prospective discontinuation study that analyzed PROs of 172 patients with CML who met criteria for cessation of TKI. PROs were collected before TKI cessation, monthly for the first six months after cessation, at eight months, at 12 months, and every six months thereafter. A number of symptoms improved significantly after TKI cessation. Twenty-six percent of patients had a meaningful improvement in fatigue at six months after TKI cessation, and 80% of patients had a meaningful improvement at 12 months. Depression symptoms improved in 35% of patients, diarrhea scores improved in 88%, and sleep disturbance scores improved in 21% at the 12-month mark. Interestingly, pain interference scores worsened in 2% of patients at 12 months while 5% of patients had meaningful improvement. PRO scores also worsened in patients who needed to restart a TKI due to molecular recurrence of disease.

3) What clinical and treatment factors are associated with achieving a deep molecular response in CML and subsequently maintaining a treatment-free remission (TFR) after discontinuation of TKI?

Expert Perspective: A deep molecular response is defined as a 4 log or greater reduction in leukemia burden by qRT-PCR on the International Scale (IS) by the European Leukemi-aNet in 2020 and the National Comprehensive Cancer Network (NCCN) Version 2.2022 guidelines. This corresponds to a *BCR::ABL1* transcript level of ≤ 0.01% (IS), also known as MR^4 (a 4 log reduction in mRNA transcripts). In the front-line setting, factors contributing to a higher likelihood of achieving a deep molecular response include the use of a second-generation TKI, a lower CML risk score at diagnosis, and achieving an early molecular response (transcript level < 10% [IS] by three months). Use of a second-generation TKI is associated with higher rates of deep molecular response when compared to imatinib. In the phase III DASISION trial, 33% of patients randomized to imatinib achieved an MR$^{4.5}$ (*BCR::ABL1* ≤0.0032% IS) at five years of treatment compared to 42% of patients on dasatinib. Similarly, in the phase III ENESTnd trial, 35% of patients randomized to imatinib achieved an MR$^{4.5}$ at five years compared to 54% of patients taking nilotinib 300 mg twice daily. In patients treated with imatinib, Sokal score affects the likelihood of achieving a deep molecular response as well. Patients with a low-risk Sokal score treated on imatinib are more likely to achieve a deep molecular response than those with intermediate- or high-risk scores. In contrast, patients treated with either nilotinib or dasatinib achieve similar rates of deep molecular response with low- and intermediate-risk Sokal scores. The early molecular response has been established as a predictor of deep molecular response regardless of TKI generation and CML risk score at diagnosis.

Select TKI discontinuation trials are summarized in Table 19.1. In the STIM1 trial for patients treated with imatinib, Sokal risk score at diagnosis and duration of treatment with imatinib before discontinuation were associated with maintaining molecular remission. In the DESTINY trial, multivariate analyses identified duration of treatment with TKI and achieving MR^4 as being significantly associated with maintaining a molecular remission. A five-year update of the ENESTfreedom study identified the following factors as being favorable for maintaining a treatment-free remission ≥ five years: initial low-risk Sokal score, treatment duration with nilotinib > 44 months, and achieving an MR$^{4.5}$. An interim analysis of patients enrolled on the EURO-SKI study identified treatment duration before TKI discontinuation and duration of deep molecular response before discontinuation as being significantly associated with maintaining a treatment-free remission. Long-term outcomes have recently been reported from the EURO-SKI trial. Of those patients who remained in a treatment-free remission three years after discontinuation, only 1 of the 98 analyzed patients in a MR^4 or better response had a molecular relapse in the following three years. The ENESTop study evaluated treatment-free remission in patients with CML in chronic phase who had received ≥ three years of TKI therapy and achieved sustained deep molecular remission only after switching from imatinib to nilotinib. After one-year nilotinib consolidation, 126 patients attempted treatment-free remission. At 48 weeks (primary analysis), 57.9% (73/126) were in treatment-free remission and at five years 42.9% (54/126) were in treatment-free remission.

4) What criteria are used in considering discontinuation of TKI in patients with CML who achieve a deep molecular response?

Expert Perspective: Criteria for discontinuation have been investigated prospectively, and several variables have been identified as predictors for prolonged molecular remission. Both the European LeukemiaNet (ELN) and the National Comprehensive Cancer Network (NCCN) have designed criteria for discontinuation. These include being in chronic phase (CP) CML without a history of accelerated phase (AP) or blast phase (BP; see Chapters 17 and 20) or resistance to any prior TKI, access to high-quality testing, and duration of deep molecular response ≥ two years. The NCCN specifies a minimum total duration of three years of TKI therapy before discontinuation while the ELN specifies a minimum of four years on a second-generation TKI or five years on imatinib. The full criteria are summarized in Table 19.2. The ELN specifies which criteria are considered mandatory for discontinuation along with differentiating between minimal criteria and optimal criteria for discontinuation. All NCCN criteria should be met before consideration of TKI discontinuation. Data are sparse regarding the treatment-free remission success rate for second attempts or when resistance to the initial TKI was present.

Table 19.1 Select TKI discontinuation trials.

Trial	TKIs investigated	Criteria for discontinuation	Criteria for molecular relapse	Molecular relapse free survival (MRFS)
STIM1	Imatinib	5 log reduction in *BCR::ABL1* levels and undetectable transcripts for ≥ 2 years	Two consecutive positive RT-PCR tests with ≥ 1 log increase or loss of MMR on one RT-PCR test	MRFS at 6 months: 43%. MRFS at 18 months: 40%. MRFS at 60 months: 38%.
DESTINY	Imatinib, nilotinib, dasatinib	TKI therapy for ≥ 3 years and MMR ≥ 1 year	Loss of MMR on two consecutive RT-PCR tests	MMR group: MRFS at 36 months: 36%. MR^4 group: MRFS at 36 months: 72%.
ENEST freedom	Nilotinib	Nilotinib therapy for ≥ 2 years and sustained MR^4 for year during nilotinib consolidation	Loss of MMR on one RT-PCR test	MRFS at 11 months: 52%. MRFS at 60 months: 42%.
EURO-SKI	Imatinib, nilotinib, dasatinib	TKI therapy for ≥ 3 years with MR^4 for ≥ 1 year	Loss of MMR on one RT-PCR test	MRFS at 6 months: 61%. MRFS at 24 months: 51%.

TKI = tyrosine kinase inhibitor; MMR = major molecular remission (*BCR::ABL1* $\leq 0.1\%$ IS).

Table 19.2 Criteria for discontinuation.

ELN	NCCN
Mandatory Criteria	Age ≥ 18 years
CML in first CP	CP-CML without history of AP or BP
Motivated patient	On approved TKI for ≥ 3 years
Access to high-quality qPCR testing using IS with rapid turnaround	Prior evidence of quantifiable *BCR::ABL1* transcript
Minimal criteria	Stable response of MR^4 or deeper for ≥ 2 years documented on 4 tests performed at least 3 months apart
First-line therapy or second-line therapy if intolerance was the reason for switching therapies	Access to qPCR testing with sensitivity of at least $MR^{4.5}$ that provides results within 2 weeks
Typical e13a2 or e14a2 *BCR::ABL1* transcripts	
Duration of TKI therapy > 5 years (or > 4 years if 2nd-generation TKI)	
Duration of DMR > 2 years	
Optimal criteria	
duration of TKI therapy > 5 years	
duration of DMR > 3 years if MR^4	
duration of DMR > 2 years if $MR^{4.5}$	

CML = chronic myeloid leukemia; CP = chronic phase; TKI = tyrosine kinase inhibitor; AP = accelerated phase; BP = blast phase; MR = molecular remission; qPCR = quantitative PCR; IS = International Scale); DMR = deep molecular remission

Case Study 2

A 63-year-old woman was diagnosed with chronic-phase CML five years ago. She was initiated on dasatinib at diagnosis and achieved a major molecular response after one year of therapy. She has had no detectable disease by qRT-PCR-based testing with a sensitivity of 10^{-5} for the past three years. The risks and benefits of TKI discontinuation have been discussed, and a joint decision is made to discontinue dasatinib.

5) How frequently should *BCR::ABL1* testing be performed in patients undergoing cessation of therapy?

Expert Perspective: The large majority of molecular relapses after TKI continuation occur within the first year of discontinuation and most within six months. For example, in the EURO-SKI trial 80% of molecular recurrences of disease occurred within the first six months after TKI discontinuation. Given the high incidence of early molecular relapse, testing is recommended to occur on a more frequent schedule initially. The NCCN recommends monthly testing for the first year of TKI discontinuation, testing every two months for the second year, and testing every three months thereafter. The ELN recommendations are for monthly testing for the first six months, testing every two months for the following six months, and testing every three months thereafter. The goal is to detect a molecular recurrence early enough to prevent a hematologic relapse by restarting TKI therapy quickly.

6) What symptoms may occur in patients that discontinue a TKI?

Expert Perspective: Among the first 50 patients that underwent TKI discontinuation as part the EURO-SKI study, 30% reported musculoskeletal pain ranging from generalized muscle tenderness to symptoms resembling polymyalgia rheumatica. These symptoms were not associated with laboratory abnormalities such as an elevated creatine kinase, and the symptoms gradually resolved one to six weeks after discontinuation of TKI. In patients with severe musculoskeletal symptoms, a short course of corticosteroids was quite effective in controlling the pain and were gradually tapered off. Rates of musculoskeletal symptoms after TKI discontinuation have been reported at 20–30% across TKI discontinuation studies. Interestingly, in an analysis of patient-reported outcomes in patients undergoing TKI discontinuation by Atallah et al., there was no significant increase in pain interference scores after TKI discontinuation.

Case Study 3

A 55-year-old man with chronic-phase CML presented for follow-up. He was originally treated with imatinib and achieved a DMR after 18 months. His DMR was maintained for three years, and his imatinib was then discontinued. He has been getting qRT-PCR monitoring for any recurrence of disease on a monthly basis. Now, six months after cessation of imatinib, his disease has become detectable with a transcript level of 0.05% IS.

7) For patients who have discontinued TKI therapy, when should reinitiation of TKI be considered?

Expert Perspective: A variety of thresholds for reinitiation of TKI therapy have been investigated in the context of TKI discontinuation trials, with the majority specifying loss of MMR.

The STIM1 trial defined molecular relapse as any positivity for *BCR::ABL1* transcripts by qRT-PCR confirmed by a 1 log increase in *BCR::ABL1* transcripts between two successive assessments or loss of MMR at one time point, at which time it was recommended to reinitiate imatinib. On the DESTINY trial protocol, patients were recommended to restart their prior TKI if loss of MMR was documented on two consecutive tests at least one month apart. Both the ENESTfreedom and EURO-SKI trials specified reinitiation of TKI if loss of MMR was documented on a single test. The ELN recommends reinitiation of TKI if loss of MMR is documented on a single test (see Chapter 16).

8) If the decision to reinitiate TKI therapy is made, should the same TKI be restarted?

Expert Perspective: When loss of MMR occurred during one of the TKI discontinuation trials, the great majority of patients regained an MMR within a couple of months after restarting their original TKI. Of the 42 patients enrolled in the STIM1 trial who restarted imatinib due to molecular recurrence, all had disease that had remained sensitive to imatinib, and 62% achieved a complete molecular response after restarting. In the EURO-SKI trial, 86% of patients who restarted their TKI due to molecular recurrence regained an MMR. Ninety-one percent of patients enrolled on the DESTINY trial regained an MMR with reinitiation of TKI due to molecular recurrence while 99% of patients enrolled in the ENESTfreedom regained an MMR with TKI reinitiation. In the ENESTop trial, of the 59 patients who reinitiated nilotinib upon loss of MMR or confirmed loss of MR4, 98.3% regained MMR, 94.9% regained MR^4, and 93.2% regained $MR^{4.5}$. Based on these data, our practice is to restart the same TKI a patient was taking before a discontinuation trial if a molecular relapse occurs. An exception to this strategy would be to switch TKIs at that point if there had been chronic side effects from the initial TKI.

9) If a patient achieves a second DMR lasting several years, can a second trial of TKI discontinuation be considered?

Expert Perspective: The RE-STIM trial, an observational study, evaluated 70 patients who had achieved an $MR^{4.5}$ or better after restarting a TKI after failing an initial discontinuation trial. The median time from TKI resumption to second discontinuation attempt was 32 months, and the median duration in $MR^{4.5}$ before the second discontinuation attempt was 25 months. Treatment-free remission rates at 12, 24, and 36 months were 48%, 42%, and 35%, respectively. In addition, reinitiation of TKI if molecular recurrence again occurred during the second discontinuation attempt was quite effective, and no cases of progression of CML to an accelerated phase were reported. Prospective trials evaluating this question in patients treated with nilotinib and dasatinib are ongoing (NCT02917720, NCT03573596).

Suggested Readings

Atallah, E., Schiffer, C.A., Radich, J.P. et al. (2021). Assessment of outcomes after stopping tyrosine kinase inhibitors among patients with chronic myeloid leukemia: a nonrandomized clinical trial. *JAMA Oncol* 7 (1): 42–50. doi: 10.1001/jamaoncol.2020.5774.

Clark, R.E., Polydoros, F., Apperley, J.F. et al. (2019 July). De-escalation of tyrosine kinase inhibitor therapy before complete treatment discontinuation in patients with chronic myeloid leukaemia (DESTINY): a non-randomised, phase 2 trial. *Lancet Haematol* 6 (7): e375–e383. doi: 10.1016/S2352-3026(19)30094-8. Epub 2019 Jun 12. PMID: 31201085.

Cortes, J. (2020 November 26). How to manage CML patients with comorbidities. *Blood* 136 (22): 2507–2512. doi: 10.1182/blood.2020006911. PMID: 33236757.

Deininger, M.W., Shah, N.P., Altman, J.K. et al. (2020 October 1). Chronic myeloid leukemia, version 2.2021, NCCN clinical practice guidelines in oncology. *J Natl Compr Canc Netw* 18 (10): 1385–1415. doi: 10.6004/jnccn.2020.0047. PMID: 33022644.

Etienne, G., Guilhot, J., Rea, D. et al. (2017 January 20). Long-term follow-up of the French Stop Imatinib (STIM1) study in patients with chronic myeloid leukemia. *J Clin Oncol* 35 (3): 298–305. doi: 10.1200/JCO.2016.68.2914. Epub 2016 Oct 31. PMID: 28095277.

Hochhaus, A., Baccarani, M., Silver, R.T. et al. (2020 April). European LeukemiaNet 2020 recommendations for treating chronic myeloid leukemia. *Leukemia* 34 (4): 966–984. doi: 10.1038/s41375-020-0776-2. Epub 2020 Mar 3. PMID: 32127639; PMCID: PMC7214240.

Hochhaus, A., Masszi, T., Giles, F.J. et al. (2017 July). Treatment-free remission following frontline nilotinib in patients with chronic myeloid leukemia in chronic phase: results from the ENESTfreedom study. *Leukemia* 31 (7): 1525–1531. doi: 10.1038/leu.2017.63. Epub 2017 Feb 20. PMID: 28218239; PMCID: PMC5508077.

Hughes, T.P., Clementino, N.C.D., Fominykh, M. et al. (2021). Long-term treatment-free remission in patients with chronic myeloid leukemia after second-line nilotinib: ENESTop 5-year update. *Leukemia* Epub 12 May. doi: 10.1038/s41375-021-01260-y.

Legros, L., Nicolini, F.E., Etienne, G. et al. (2017 November 15). Second tyrosine kinase inhibitor discontinuation attempt in patients with chronic myeloid leukemia. *Cancer* 123 (22): 4403–4410. doi: 10.1002/cncr.30885. PMID: 28743166.

Radich, J.P., Hochhaus, A., Masszi, T. et al. (2021). Treatment-free remission following frontline nilotinib in patients with chronic phase chronic myeloid leukemia: 5-year update of the ENESTfreedom trial. *Leukemia* doi: 10.1038/s41375-021-01205-5.

Rea, D. (2020 November 10). Handling challenging questions in the management of chronic myeloid leukemia: when is it safe to stop tyrosine kinase inhibitors? *Blood Adv* 4 (21): 5589–5594. doi: 10.1182/bloodadvances.2020002538. PMID: 33170936; PMCID: PMC7656932.

Richter, J., Lübking, A., Söderlund, S. et al. (2021 February 15). Molecular status 36 months after TKI discontinuation in CML is highly predictive for subsequent loss of MMR – Final report from AFTER-SKI. *Leukemia* doi: 10.1038/s41375-021-01173-w. Epub ahead of print. PMID: 33589755.

Saussele, S., Richter, J., Guilhot, J. et al. (2018 June). Discontinuation of tyrosine kinase inhibitor therapy in chronic myeloid leukaemia (EURO-SKI): a prespecified interim analysis of a prospective, multicentre, non-randomised, trial. *Lancet Oncol* 19 (6): 747–757. doi: 10.1016/S1470-2045(18)30192-X. Epub 2018 May 4. PMID: 29735299.

20

Hematopoietic Cell Transplantation in Chronic Myeloid Leukemia

Jerald P. Radich

Fred Hutchinson Cancer Center, Seattle, WA

Introduction

Tyrosine kinase therapy revolutionized the therapy of chronic myeloid leukemia (CML). While hematopoietic cell transplantation (HCT) was the treatment of choice for CML from the 1980s, the advent of imatinib has pushed transplantation to the role of salvage therapy in CML. There are now four TKIs approved for up-front chronic-phase CML (imatinib, dasatinib, nilotinib, and bosutinib), and six approved for cases resistant or intolerant to TKI therapy (dasatinib, nilotinib, bosutinib, ponatinib, omacetaxine, and the new allosteric inhibitor, asciminib). Thus, the question becomes: In what settings should an HCT be considered? The most direct answer is when a TKI can no longer provide long-term survival advantages, such as intolerance to multi-TKIs, resistance to multiple TKIs, or progression to advanced-phase disease (accelerated or blast phase). The cases below outline these clinical settings.

Case Study 1

A 31-year-old male rodeo clown is diagnosed with intermediate risk (Sokal) chronic-phase CML. He is intermediate risk by both the Sokal and Hasford classification schemes. His peripheral blood *BCR::ABL1* level at diagnosis was 73% IS. He has three siblings. He has hypertension, smokes, and has more than occasional alcohol use. He is averse to the idea of taking medicines, and being a risk taker, he is attracted to transplantation since it is "one and done."

1) **All things considered, what do you recommend?**
    A) Tyrosine kinase therapy.
    B) Allogeneic transplantation.
    C) Clinical trial.

Expert Perspective: The question here is whether transplantation should ever be offered as up-front therapy for newly diagnosed chronic-phase CML. In this setting, treatment with any TKI will yield 10-year survival of ~90%, and indeed, several studies have suggested that chronic-phase CML patients on a TKI have a comparable life span to the general

Cancer Consult: Expertise in Clinical Practice, Volume 2: Neoplastic Hematology & Cellular Therapy,
Second Edition. Edited by Syed A. Abutalib, Maurie Markman, James O. Armitage, and Kenneth C. Anderson.
© 2024 John Wiley & Sons Ltd. Published 2024 by John Wiley & Sons Ltd.

(non-CML) population. Compare this to the pre-TKI years, where the median survival for this group would be about six years. Allogeneic transplantation for chronic-phase CML would expect to yield ~85% disease-free survival (with either a matched related or unrelated donor), but it is associated with an up-front risk of morbidity and mortality and potential long-term complications, mostly secondary to chronic graft-versus-host disease (GvHD). Thus, regardless of whether the patient is a risk taker or not, up-front transplant should be strongly discouraged.

After discussion, the patient decides that he will try a TKI after all.

Correct Answer: A

2) Which TKI should you use?
   A) Imatinib.
   B) Dasatinib.
   C) Nilotinib.
   D) Bosutinib.

Expert Perspective: How do we decide which TKI to use? All three second-generation TKIs (dasatinib, nilotinib, and bosutinib) have been compared to imatinib in newly diagnosed chronic-phase CML. All of these ramdomized trials have shown remarkably consistent results (Table 20.1). Compared to imatinib, second-generation TKIs offer greater complete cytogenetic remissions, greater percentage of cases reaching clinically significant molecular milestones, less progression to advanced-phase disease, but surprisingly, similar overall survivals.

Given that this patient presents with intermediate-risk disease by the Sokal and Hasford scores, many physicians would lean toward starting therapy with the more potent second-generation TKI, hoping that the more potent inhibition would better prevent progression to advanced-phase disease. However, the second-generation TKIs have more hematopoietic toxicity, especially grades 3–4 thrombocytopenia (e.g. ~10% grade 3–4 with imatinib versus 20% with dasatinib in the US Intergroup trial). Most of the second- and third-generation TKIs seem to have more cardiovascular toxicity (hypertension, vascular occlusions) than imatinib (the exception might be bosutinib), and some have serious or bothersome specific side effects (dasatinib, pulmonary effusions; bosutinib, diarrhea).

Table 20.1   12-month responses in the ENESTnd, DASISION, and US Intergroup trials.

Response	NIL300bid (ENESTnd)	NIL400bid (ENESTnd)	IM 400 (ENESTnd)	DAS 100 (DASISION)	IM 400 (DASISION)	BOS (BFORE)	IM 400 (BFORE)
CCyR	80%	78%	65%	83%	72%	77%	64%
MMR	44%	43%	22%	46%	28%	47%	37%
AP/BC	0.7%	0.4%	4.2%	1.9%	3.5%	1.6%	2.5%

AP/BC: patients progressing to accelerated phase and blast crisis; CCyR: complete cytogenetic remission; MMR: major molecular response.
Source: Data from Saglio, G, et al. *N Engl J Med.* 2010;362:2251–9; Kantarjian H, et al. *N Engl J Med.* 2010;362:2260–70; Cortes JE, *J Clin Oncol.* 2017, 36:231–7.

Given these considerations, and the patient's occupational propensity to collide with one-ton hoofed animals, you and the patient decide to start therapy with imatinib (A).

Case Study continued: He starts on 400 mg a day and without further ado rejoins the rodeo circuit. He misses several appointments but returns to your office three months later. He has normalized his complete blood count and his *BCR::ABL1* is 25% IS. When asked if he is taking his medication, he replies "mostly."

Correct Answer: A

3) After furrowing your brow, what do you decide?
   A) Continue imatinib.
   B) Switch to a second-generation TKI.
   C) Refer to allogeneic transplantation.

Expert Perspective: What does early response mean? Several studies demonstrate that early (3–6 months) response, as measured by the peripheral blood *BCR::ABL1* level, is an early predictor of longer-term outcomes. Patients who do not have a *BCR::ABL1* < 10% IS at 3–6 months have an inferior outcome (cytogenetic, molecular, and survival) compared to patients with a better response. This relationship seems to hold for both up-front CML and those patients who switch to a second-generation TKI after poor tolerance or efficacy to imatinib. This milestone of response is built into NCCN and ELN guidelines. However, poor early response can be from poor adherence, bad biology, or a combination of both. Some experts would advocate switching to an alternative TKI with such a poor three-month *BCR::ABL1* PCR result seen in this patient, though the story is complicated here by the suspicion that the patient is not compliant. Thus, for this patient, it is reasonable to continue imatinib, with close follow-up of another *BCR::ABL1* at the six-month mark.

He continues imatinib, and while he says he understands your concern and promises to return in three months, he misses his next appointment. After nine months without contact, you receive a postcard from him from the Calgary Stampede rodeo. It states, "Dear Doc. All is going well. Maybe some bruising lately, but it's been a tough week in the pen. Some fevers as well. Guess I caught a bug. See you in a week. Wish you were here." He arrives a week later with a white blood cell count > 50k, with 17% peripheral blood mye-loblasts, an enlarged spleen, and 10 lbs of weight loss.

Correct Answer: A

4) As he is now in accelerated phase, what do you recommend?
   A) Switch to nilotinib, dasatinib, bosutinib, ponatinib, and watch for response.
   B) Start on second-generation TKI, and then move to allogeneic transplant.
   C) AML induction therapy with TKI.

Expert Persepctive: What do you do with the rare patients who progress to aggressive CML? When progression occurs, it really does not make a difference why (compliance or biology). The ship has sailed to deep waters. When TKI fails the patient (not vice versa) and progression occurs, the switch to a more active TKI can sometimes control their disease, but the long-term outcome is likely to be poor. Transplantation is the best alternative. However, a switch to a second- or third-generation TKI should be done while a transplant donor is obtained. An important note—when siblings are available, they should be typed so that the process of finding a donor is done in an urgent setting. Finding a donor can take time (especially if a patient needs to find an unrelated donor), and once progression occurs, time is the enemy.

Correct Answer: C

Case Study 2

You are referred a 45-year-old female clothing inspector ("No. 6") who recently presented in what appeared to be chronic-phase CML. However, her cytogenetic exam showed the Ph in 15/20 metaphases, with five metaphases showing an additional clonal change of del(17p) (the location of the p53 tumor suppressor gene). The bone marrow blast count is 11%, and her peripheral blood *BCR::ABL1* is 81% IS. She started three weeks ago on imatinib 400 mg per day by her local general practitioner, and her counts are responding appropriately. She has no siblings.

5) **Based on this story, what do you recommend?**
   A) Imatinib 400 mg/d.
   B) Imatinib 600–800 mg/d.
   C) Second-generation TKI.
   D) Unrelated donor workup with transplantation without TKI therapy.

Expert Persepctive: What does clonal evolution mean in chronic-phase disease? There is debate about what to do in the case of apparent accelerated phase at diagnosis (as opposed to our previous case, where progression occurred during therapy). A scenario as described above occurs in ~5% or less of chronic-phase cases, and indeed, in some of the TKI clinical trials for chronic-phase patients, those with only additional cytogenetic abnormalities were not excluded. There is limited data on these types of cases. The prognosis seems to be best for cases like this (normal blast count, with clonal evolution only), intermediate for cases with increased blast counts but no clonal evolution, and worst for cases with clonal and blast evolution. Cases with clonal evolution do somewhat worse compared to standard chronic-phase CML, with slower times of response and worse rates of CCyR (71% vs 89%), MMR (67% vs 86%), and failure-free survival (61% vs 76%) but not overall survival by six years of follow-up. Thus, NCCN and ELN guidelines would recommend starting this patient with a TKI.

Thus, it is reasonable to start a TKI, and it would be prudent to use a more potent second-generation variety. High-dose imatinib would provide good kinase inhibition but is generally less well tolerated than the other choices. It would be wise to perform HLA typing on the donor, and at least do a preliminary "world book" search to assess how many donors might be available if needed.

Correct Answer: C

You start her on dasatinib. At three months, her *BCR::ABL1* is 11% IS, and at six months, the level remains steady at 13% IS. She misses her nine-month appointment, and at 12 months, her *BCR::ABL1* is 25%.

6) What should you do?

A) Continue dasatinib for another two weeks and recheck *BCR::ABL1*.

B) Perform mutation testing and switch TKI.

C) Start an official unrelated donor search.

D) B and C.

Expert Persepctive: What do we do with high-risk cases with suboptimal response? While routine cytogenetic testing has been largely abandoned in CML, in this case is called for given her disease state at diagnosis and her lukewarm response to second-generation TKI. What we are looking for is to assess blast counts (by morphology and flow cytometry), cytogenetic state (progression of her clonal abnomality, as well as new abnormalities), and ABL kinase domain test.

It is certainly reasonable to continue dasatinib if you believe you will have the laboratory results back quickly. If not, it is reasonable to presumptively switch to another TKI while you await the results that might guide therapy. In this scenario, the mutaton testing will guide your choice of which TKI to use. The blast count will determine whether you will need chemotherapy in addition to a TKI (e.g. if frank blast crisis). It is essetnial to begin an unrelated donor search since salvage to a complete cytogenetic remission with a durable response seems very unlikely in this scenario, and transplant may be stacking up to be her best curative chance.

She indeed is positive for the *T315I* mutation, her bone marrow blast count is 18%, and her abnormal del(17p) is now in 9/20 metaphases. She is placed on ponatinib while her unrelated search begins. After three months of therapy, her peripheral blood *BCR::ABL1* is 5% IS. She found and then lost a donor because of COVID-related issues and continues ponatinib. A donor is finally secured, and she has a full ablative transplant.

Correct Answer: D

Case Study 3

A 44-year-old male former investment banker now turned BASE jumper was diagnosed two years ago with low-Sokal-risk CML. He has cycled through imatinib, dasatinib, nilotinib, and bosutinib, all with the same story: he has a good treatment response but cannot tolerate the medications due to a series of odd but serious side effects. He no longer has medical insurance, and he is worried that his considerable saved financial resources will be drained by years of TKI therapy. Plus, he has grown weary and despondent over the failure of TKI agents to cure him. Thus, he wants a transplant from his HLA-matched sibling.

He has read up and is curious about pursuing a low-intensity transplant rather than a full ablative, as he suspects the latter approach will sooner return him to his risky and thrilling lifestyle.

7) What should you do?

A) Insist he try a TKI again.

B) Promote an allogeneic transplant.

C) Offer a non-myeloablative transplant.

D) Suggest he go on a clinical trial of a new TKI (there is always a new one).

Expert Persepctive: How intensive a transplant is needed in CML? As opposed to standard "ablative" transplants (so called since the preparative regimen of chemotherapy +/− total body irradiation [TBI] destroys the hematopoiesis so that the patient must be rescued by a donor hematopoietic stem cell infusion), the reduced-intensity conditioning (RIC) transplant uses far less preparative therapy, aiming to cripple rather than destroy the host hematopoietic and immune system. As such, the RIC relies on the graft-versus-leukemia effect to control and destroy the host leukemia.

RIC transplants were first offered for patients unable to receive a full transplant because of advanced age or other medical conditions that would make a full preparative regimen too toxic. However, the regimen proved to be more successful in combating disease and now is used much more routinely. A few things can be said about the RIC compared to the standard ablative transplant in virtually all diseases: (i) the regimen-related toxicity is less, with < 10% at 100 days and < 20% at two years post transplant; (ii) relapse rates tend to be higher; and (iii) graft-versus-host disease (GvHD) rates and severity are similar. As such, for most diseases, survival for RIC is quite comparable to ablative transplants.

Early results using RIC for CML were troubled by high rates of graft rejection (especially with unrelated donors) since in CML the immune system had not been previously exposed to the immunosuppressive effects of chemotherapy. However, with improved protocols, RIC has been used with excellent results with regimen-related mortality, and with ~40% patients achieving a molecular remission. The IBMTR reviewed its extensive database and retrospectively compared the outcomes of > 1,000 CML patients treated with an ablative or RIC regimen. Multivariable analyses revealed no differences in overall survival. RIC transplants were associated with a higher rate of early relapse (HR 1.9) but less chronic GvHD (HR 0.8).

Correct Answer: D

Case Study continued: The patient decides on a RIC transplant. He engrafts by day 28. On his day 10 discharge workup, he has full donor chimerism, normal morhphology and cytogenetics, and a *BCR::ABL1* of 0.008% IS. He had grade II acute GvHD of the skin, which was treated successfully with steroids, and he has no active chronic GvHD.

8) What do you decide to do?
   A) Wait and watch, and repeat PCR in three months.
   B) Immediately discontinue all immunosuppressive medications.
   C) Start a TKI.
   D) Give donor leukocyte infusions (DLIs).

Expert Persepctive: What do you do about "molecular relapse"? Many studies have shown that the presence of *BCR::ABL1* post transplant in chronic-phase CML is associated with subsequent relapse. In general, (i) day + 28 appears to have less consequence than later time points, (ii) disease at 2−12 months is associated with subsequent relapse, and (iii) very low levels of *BCR::ABL1* can occur and persist without subsequent relapse.

BCR::ABL1 molecular relapse has been treated with interferon, DLI, and, more recently, TKI (Table 20.2). The treatment of molecular relapse with TKI is effective. The response to TKI reflects the stage of disease, and complete hematological response was seen in > 90% of chronic-phase cases, > 50% of accelerated-phase cases, and > 20% of cases in blast crisis. A complete cytogenetic remission occurred in > 40% of all cases, with response rates considerably higher in chronic phase. Most of the data are from the use of imatinib. Second-generation TKI appear to have higher toxicity, particularly to the hematopoetic system (especially on platelet counts).

You decide to watch and repeat a PCR in three months. TKI can be held unless the *BCR::ABL1* climbs appreciable (generally, 5–10-fold).

Correct Answer: C

Imagine the same patient as above, but now he is transplanted for accelerated-phase disease. Before transplant, he had no *ABL* mutation. He engrafts at day 28 and has no GvHD.

9) What do you do?
  A) Wait for his day + 28 *BCR::ABL1* to decide what to do.
  B) If his *BCR::ABL1* is negative, watch.
  C) Start prophylactic TKI.
  D) Give TKI or DLI only if his *BCR::ABL1* is highly positive.

Expert Persepctive: Should we give prophylactic TKI? While chronic phase is associated with a low risk of relapse, transplantation for accelerated- or blast-phase CML, or Ph+ ALL, is of sufficient high risk to warrant prophylactic administration of a TKI. Published trials are limited, but they suggest that imatinib can be given safely at engraftment without significant effects on hematological counts. Phase I and II trials of prophylactic TKI suggest no negative effects on GvHD. It does seem to prevent molecular relapse. Twenty-two patients (7 CML and 15 Ph+ ALL) were treated with imatinib after engraftment, and 19 completed the planned course of one year of treatment. At a median follow-up of one and a half years, five of seven of the CML patients and 12 of 15 of the Ph+ ALL cases were in a molecular remission.

One continuing issue is whether the presence of a pre-transplant mutation should influence the selection of a post-transplant TKI. It appears that most of the time if molecular relapse occurs, it does so with the same clone. Thus, if TKI prophylaxis is given for a high-risk patient (that is, even if the *BCR::ABL1* is negative post transplant), using a TKI directed at a known prior mutation is reasonable. However, sometimes a molecular relapse is associated with a different clone—so if you are treating molecular relapse, testing for the TKI kinase domain mutation is important.

Correct Answer: C

He is started on imatinib 400 mg/d. His blood counts tolerate this well. He gets no GvHD. At discharge on day 100, he now has a cytogenetic relapse, with the Ph in 2 of 20 metaphases. The peripheral blood *BCR::ABL1* is 2.5% IS. Mutation analysis shows an *E255V* mutation.

10) What do you do?
  A) Discontinue immunosuppressives.
  B) Change to dasatinib.
  C) Give DLI.
  D) All of the above.

Table 20.2 Post-transplant use of tyrosine kinase inhibitors (TKIs) in patients with chronic myeloid leukemia (CML).

Reference	N pts.	Indication	TKI	Median dose	Significant toxicity	Outcome
Kantarjian et al.[a]	28	Relapse	Imatinib	600 mg	Grade 3–4 hematologic toxicity grade 3–4 liver toxicity	CHR: 74% (CP: 100%, AP: 83%, BP: 43%) CgR: 58% (CP: 63%, AP: 63%, BP: 43%) CCgR: 35%
Olavarria et al.[b]	128	Relapse	Imatinib	400 mg (CP) 600 mg (AP/ BP)	N/A	CCgR: 44% (CP: 58%, AP: 48%, BP: 22%) CMR:26% (CP: 37%, AP: 33%, BP: 11%) CP: 2y OS 100% AP: 2y OS 86% BP: 2y OS 12%
DeAngelo et al.[c]	15	Relapse	Imatinib	600 mg	Grade 3–4 liver toxicity	CCgR: 11/15 (73%) CMR: 7/15 (47%)
Hess et al.[d]	44	Relapse	Imatinib	400 mg	Grade 3–4 hematologic toxicity	CCgR: 73% CMR: 62%
Palandri et al.[e]	16	Relapse	Imatinib	400 mg	Grade 3–4 hematologic toxicity	CCgR:88% CMR:75%
Klyuchnikov et al.[f]	11	Relapse	Dasatinib	50 mg BID	Thrombocytopenia-related gastrointestinal bleeding	Stable response in 4 pts (2 with extramedullary relapse)
Wright et al.[g]	22	Relapse	Imatinib (20), dasatinib (6)	Imatinib 400 mg dasatinib 140 mg	Grade 3–4 hematologic toxicity	CHR: 86% (AP/ BP-79%) CCgR: 77% (AP/BP-71%) CMR: 64% (AP/BP-57%)

Table 20.2 (Continued)

Reference	N pts.	Indication	TKI	Median dose	Significant toxicity	Outcome
Carpenter et al.[h]	22	Prophyl-axis	Imatinib	400 mg	Grade 1–3 nausea, emesis, liver toxicity	CCgR: 5/7 CMR: 5/7
Olavarria et al.[i]	22	Prophyl-axis	Imatinib	400 mg	Not noted	68% relapse at median of 17 month after HCT

CCyR: complete cytogenetic response; CgR: cytogenetic response; CHR: complete hematologic response; CMR: complete molecular response. [a]Kantarjian HM, et al. *Blood*. 2002;100:1590–5. [b]Olavarria E, et al. *Leukemia*. 2003;17:1707–12. [c]DeAngelo DJ, et al. *Clin Cancer Res*. 2004;10:5065–71; and DeAngelo DJ, et al. *Clin Cancer Res*. 2004;10:1–3. [d]Hess G, et al. *J Clin Oncol*. 2005;23:7583–93. [e]Palandri F, et al. *Bone Marrow Transpl*. 2007;39:189–91. [f]Klyuchnikov E, et al. *Acta Haematol*. 2009;122:6–10. [g]Wright MP, et al. *Biol Blood Marrow Transpl*. 2010;16:639–46. [h]Carpenter PA, et al. *Blood*. 2007;109:2791–3. [i]Olavarria E, et al. *Blood*. 2007;110:4614–17.
Source: Bar, M, et al. *J Natl Comp Cancer Network*. 2013;11(3):308–15.

Expert Persepctive: When do we need to give DLI? This patient has a cytogenetic relapse with an imatinib-resistant mutation. A reasonable option would be to taper immunosuppression rapidly, while starting dasatinib (nilotinib is also ineffective with the *E255V* mutation; Table 20.3). The patient's response can be followed by peripheral blood PCR. If the patient gets GvHD, then DLI cannot be given, and one should maintain dasatinib; if no GvHD occurs, gauge the response to dasatinib alone—if his disease is disappearing, maintain dasatinib; and if it is still stable or increasing, DLI is appropriate.

DLI is effective in CML, and many studies demonstrate cytogenetic complete response rates of 50–100% in patients treated for clinically relapsed chronic-phase CML. Response rates are best for patients in early cytogenetic relapse and worst for those who have progressed to advanced-phase disease. The two major complications of DLI are transient marrow failure (seen in cases of frank hematological relapse without adequate residual

Table 20.3 TKI resistance in *BCR::ABL1* leukemias.

TKI	Resistant mutations[†]
Nilotinib	E255V/K; T315I; F359V/C/I; Y253H
Dastatinib	T315I/A; F317L/V/I/C; V299L
Bosutinib	E255V; T315I: V299L; G250E; F317L
Potanatinib	None identified

[†]Asciminib has activity in patients with the T315I mutation and is also approved for patients who are resistant or intolerant to ≥ 2 TKIs Omacetaxine (non-TKI) has also demonstrated activity in some patients with the T315I mutation and in patients who are resistant or intolerant to ≥ 2 TKIs; Mutations in imatinib are too numerous to include. Allo-HCT can overcome all the resistant mutations in CML.

donor hematopoiesis especially if less than 30%) and the development of GvHD, which occurs in ~50% of cases. There is a close correlation between the development of GvHD and the achievement of complete responses to DLI.

Correct Answer: D

Recommended Readings

Chhabra, S., Ahn, K.W., Hu, Z.H. et al. (2018). Myeloablative vs reduced-intensity conditioning allogenic hematopoietic cell transplant for chronic myeloid leukemia. *Blood Adv* 2: 2922–2936.

Cortes, J.E., Jiang, Q., Wang, J., Weng, J., Zhu, H., Liu, X. et al. (2020 August). Dasatinib vs. imatinib in patients with chronic myeloid leukemia in chronic phase (CML-CP) who have not achieved an optimal response to 3 months of imatinib therapy: the DASCERN randomized study. *Leukemia* 34 (8): 2064–2073.

Crawley, C., Szydlo, R., Lalancette, M. et al. (2005). Outcomes of reduced-intensity transplantation for chronic myeloid leukemia: an analysis of prognostic factors from the chronic leukemia working party of the EBMT. *Blood* 106: 2969–2976.

Gratwohl, A. and Heim, D. (2009 September). Current role of stem cell transplantation in chronic myeloid leukaemia. *Best Pract Res Clin Haematol* 22 (3): 431–443.

Gratwohl, A., Pfirrmann, M., Zander, A. et al. (2016). Long-term outcome of patients with newly diagnosed chronic myeloid leukemia: a randomized comparison of stem cell transplant with drug treatment. *Leukemia* 30: 562–569.

Gratwohl, A., Stern, M., Brand, R. et al. (2009). Risk score for outcome after allogeneic hematopoietic stem cell transplantation: a retrospective analysis. *Cancer* 115: 4715–4726.

Guglielmi, C., Arcese, W., Dazzi, F., Brand, R., Bunjes, D., Verdonck, L.F. et al. (2002 July 15). Donor lymphocyte infusion for relapsed chronic myelogenous leukemia: prognostic relevance of the initial cell dose. *Blood* 100 (2): 397–405.

Hochhaus, A., Baccarani, M., Silver, R.T., Schiffer, C., Apperley, J.F., Cervantes, F. et al. (2020 April). European LeukemiaNet 2020 recommendations for treating chronic myeloid leukemia. *Leukemia* 34 (4): 966–984.

Hu, B., Lin, X., Lee, H.C., Huang, X., Tidwell, R.S.S., Ahn, K.W. et al. (2020 December). Timing of allogeneic hematopoietic cell transplantation (alloHCT) for chronic myeloid leukemia (CML) patients. *Leuk Lymphoma* 61 (12): 2811–2820.

Kerbauy, F.R., Storb, R., Hegenbart, U. et al. (2005). Hematopoietic cell transplantation from HLA-identical sibling donors after low-dose radiation-based conditioning for treatment of CML. *Leukemia* 19: 990–997.

Kolb, H.J., Schattenberg, A., Goldman, J.M., Hertenstein, B., Jacobsen, N., Arcese, W. et al. (1995 September 1). European group for blood and marrow transplantation working party chronic leukemia. Graft-versus-leukemia effect of donor lymphocyte transfusions in marrow grafted patients. *Blood* 86 (5): 2041–2050.

Passweg, J.R., Walker, I., Sobocinski, K.A., Klein, J.P., Horowitz, M.M., and Giralt, S.A. (2004 June). Chronic leukemia study writing committee of the international bone marrow transplant registry. Validation and extension of the EBMT risk score for patients with chronic myeloid leukaemia (CML) receiving allogeneic haematopoietic stem cell transplants. *Br J Haematol* 125 (5): 613–620.

Wright, M.P., Shepherd, J.D., Barnett, M.J. et al. (2010). Response to tyrosine kinase inhibitor therapy in patients with chronic myelogenous leukemia relapsing in chronic and advanced phase following allogeneic hematopoietic stem cell transplantation. *Biol Blood Marrow Transplant* 16: 639–646.

21

Polycythemia Vera

Prithviraj Bose and Srdan Verstovsek

The University of Texas MD Anderson Cancer Center, Houston, TX

Introduction

Polycythemia vera (PV) is the most common Philadelphia chromosome–negative myelo-proliferative neoplasm, with a US prevalence estimate of 44 to 57 individuals per 100,000 population. The disease is driven in 99% of cases by an activating mutation in the Janus kinase 2 (*JAK2*) gene and is typically characterized by a pancytosis in the peripheral blood; bone marrow examination classically reveals panmyelosis and pleiomorphic megakaryo-cytes. The disease is slightly more common in males, and the median age of presentation is in the 60s; median survival ranges in different studies from 14 to 19 years. The 2022 WHO diagnostic criteria are displayed in Table 21.1. Younger patients have a much better prog-nosis. The main causes of death in patients with PV are thrombotic events and leukemic transformation. Management focuses on prevention of thrombosis; interventions to reduce or prevent progression to myelofibrosis and transformation to acute leukemia are presently lacking.

1) Is it possible to have polycythemia vera (PV) without a *JAK2* mutation?

Expert Perspective: In the era of widespread *JAK2* mutation testing, it is easy to forget that many laboratories only routinely test for the *JAK2V617F* mutation in exon 14, which is present in approximately 95% of patients with PV. An additional 4% of PV patients will have mutations at various codons within exon 12 of the *JAK2* gene. Rare mutations in other genes are described in patients with unexplained erythrocytosis, including mutations in LNK (SH2B3), a negative regulator of JAK-STAT signaling, and cooperating mutations or promoter hypermethylation in SOCS genes, *TET2*, or *EZH2*; testing for some of these muta-tions is not possible in everyday practice, and therefore, it is possible to encounter a patient with true PV who is *JAK2* mutation–negative in exons 14 and 12.

Cancer Consult: Expertise in Clinical Practice, Volume 2: Neoplastic Hematology & Cellular Therapy, Second Edition. Edited by Syed A. Abutalib, Maurie Markman, James O. Armitage, and Kenneth C. Anderson. © 2024 John Wiley & Sons Ltd. Published 2024 by John Wiley & Sons Ltd.

Table 21.1 2022 World Health Organization (WHO) criteria for the diagnosis of polycythemia vera.

Major criteria

1. Hemoglobin > 16.5 g/dL in men / > 16.0 g/dL in women

or

hematocrit > 49% in men / > 48% in women

or

increased red cell mass (RCM)*

2. BM biopsy showing hypercellularity for age with trilineage growth (panmyelosis) including prominent erythroid, granulocytic, and megakaryocytic proliferation with pleomorphic, mature megakaryocytes (differences in size)

3. Presence of *JAK2V617F* (*exon 14*) or *JAK2 exon 12* mutation

Minor criterion

Subnormal serum erythropoietin level

Diagnosis of PV requires meeting either all three major criteria or the first two major criteria and the minor criterion†. *More than 25% above mean normal predicted value.†Criterion number 2 (BM biopsy) may not be required in cases with sustained absolute erythrocytosis: hemoglobin levels > 18.5 g/dL in men (hematocrit 55.5%) or > 16.5 g/dL in women (hematocrit 49.5%) if major criterion 3 and the minor criterion are present. However, initial myelofibrosis (present in up to 20% of patients) can only be detected by performing a BM biopsy; this finding may predict a more rapid progression to overt myelofibrosis (post-PV MF).

2) What is the optimal therapeutic hematocrit target in patients with PV?

Expert Perspective: There was considerable uncertainty about the importance of "strict" hematocrit control to < 45% as claimed in earlier studies. In the European Collaboration on Low-Dose Aspirin in PV (ECLAP) study, a multinational prospective study of 1638 patients with PV, only 48% of patients were maintained at the recommended hematocrit target of < 0.45, with the remainder maintained at 0.45–0.50 (39% of patients) and > 0.50 (13% patients). Interestingly, in the ECLAP study there was no relationship found between hematocrit level and risk of thrombosis, as had previously been reported, although it can be argued that the entire ECLAP cohort was undertreated as a whole, as reflected by the high event (i.e. thrombosis) rate (3.2% rate of major thrombosis per year). Analysis of the historic PVSG-01 study also failed to show a relationship between thrombosis and hematocrit, albeit at a liberal hematocrit target of < 0.52. These older studies predated the modern practice of routine aspirin prescription and risk stratification by age and prior thrombosis; nevertheless, their results gave plenty of ammunition to proponents of liberal hematocrit targets.

Fortunately, the question of target hematocrit is now definitively answered with the publication of the CYTO-PV study. In this study, 365 patients with PV were randomized to hematocrit targets of < 0.45 (low hematocrit) or 0.45–0.50 (high hematocrit). Notable differences between the CYTO-PV study and previous studies included the use of aspirin in all patients (unless contraindicated), and a recommendation for the use of hydroxyurea in high-risk patients (those age ≥ 65 years and/or with prior thrombosis). After a median follow-up of 31 months, major thrombosis or cardiovascular death occurred in 9.8% of the high-hematocrit group, compared with 2.7% of the low-hematocrit group ($P = 0.007$), a remarkable difference, considering that the median hematocrit differed by only 0.03 between the two groups

(0.44 vs. 0.47). The annual rate of major thrombosis or cardiovascular (CV) death in the high-hematocrit group (4.4% per year) was like that of the ECLAP study (3.2% per year), despite the routine prescription of aspirin and the use of hydroxyurea in high-risk patients in the CYTO-PV study. These observations confirm the critical importance of hematocrit control in PV and highlight the ineffectiveness of aspirin and hydroxyurea in failing to overcome the adverse consequences of poor (> 0.45) hematocrit control.

3) Should the hematocrit target differ between male and female patients with PV?

Expert Perspective: Traditionally, a target of 0.42 is often recommended for female patients. In the CYTO-PV patients, the therapeutic target was identical for male and female patients, and with the caveat of small numbers in subgroup analyses, the event rate in the high-hematocrit group was numerically higher in female (13%) than male (8%) patients. The CYTO-PV trial showed that reduction in hematocrit to physiological levels was important in preventing thrombosis, and if one extrapolates the physiological differences in hemoglobin in healthy state to those in disease state, it will seem reasonable that the target for female patients should be lower than that of male patients. Although there is no prospective evidence at present to support this view, the judicious use of a lower hematocrit target (0.42) in female patients is unlikely to cause harm and represents the practice of some experts.

4) Should extreme thrombocytosis in a patient with well-controlled hematocrit be an indication for cytoreductive therapy in PV?

Expert Perspective: There is a reasonable argument for the use of cytoreduction in extreme thrombocytosis ($\geq 1500 \times 10^9$/L) due to the well-documented association between extreme thrombocytosis and bleeding risk from acquired von Willebrand factor deficiency. Unlike the situation with thrombosis risk, in which there are alternatives to cytoreduction (i.e. control of hematocrit and use of aspirin), the only therapeutic maneuver available to ameliorate the bleeding phenotype in extreme thrombocytosis is by cytoreduction; this practice is supported by expert opinions and consensus guidelines. The preferred choice of cytoreductive agent in this situation for younger patients would be interferon, while in older patients, hydroxyurea is usually the standard of care. While not commonly used in PV because of its selective platelet-lowering action and tolerability concerns, anagrelide can also be a useful agent in this scenario to control isolated extreme thrombocytosis.

5) Should leukocytosis with well-controlled hematocrit be an indication for cytoreductive therapy in PV?

Expert Perspective: The ECLAP study was able to provide insight into the association between white blood cell (WBC) count and thrombosis in PV. About 205 thrombotic events occurred in 1638 patients followed for a mean of 2.7 years in the original ECLAP data set. Of these, 81 were first vascular events. Overall, the effect of leukocytosis was rather weak, being associated mainly with an increased risk of myocardial infarction when the WBC count exceeded 15×10^9/L. Aspirin is highly effective in the secondary prevention of recurrent vascular events in the general population, and data from ECLAP and studies in essential thrombocythemia (ET) suggest that aspirin use is associated with a similar lowering of risk as a reduction in white cell count. However, a multi-variable, time-dependent sub-analysis of the CYTO-PV study, in which the 28 patients who had fatal and nonfatal cardiovascular events were stratified into four approximate quartiles based on their last recorded WBC counts preceding the thrombotic events, showed that the risk of thrombosis was clearly increased in patients with WBC counts $> 7 \times 10^9$/L, becoming statistically significant when the WBC count was $> 11 \times 10^9$/L. This finding is supported by multiple studies in ET that have documented an association between leukocytosis and thrombosis risk. On the other hand, a retrospective study using group-based trajectory modeling of a database of 520 PV patients seen at 10 US academic centers has shown that persistently elevated WBC trajectories were not associated with a thrombosis hazard but rather with increased hazard of disease evolution to myelofibrosis, myelodysplastic syndrome (MDS), or acute myeloid leukemia (AML). Most recently, in an analysis from REVEAL, a large, observational study of 2,510 patients with PV cared for in US community and academic practices, it was demonstrated that elevated WBC counts ($> 12 \times 10^9$/L) were significantly associated with increased risk of thromboembolism when the hematocrit was controlled at $\leq 45\%$. The issue of whether leucocytosis in PV in and of itself represents an indication for cytoreductive therapy, or a change in the same, remains an open one in the field, but it is our practice to try to control progressive increases in WBC counts in PV patients, not just the hematocrit. In the US, consensus guidelines from the National Comprehensive Cancer Network (NCCN) recognize leucocytosis as a potential reason to consider cytoreductive therapy in an otherwise low-risk patients with PV.

6) A patient develops a deep venous thrombosis (VTE) in the context of previously undiagnosed PV. What should be the duration of anticoagulation?

Expert Perspective: PV is a potent provocative factor for venous thromboembolism (VTE). Tight hematocrit control is clearly effective at ameliorating this risk, reducing the rate of major VTE to $< 0.5\%$ per year. The American College of Chest Physicians (ACCP) guidelines state that in VTE provoked by a nonsurgical transient risk factor, treatment with anticoagulation should be continued for three months. Expert opinions in cancer-related thrombosis suggest continuation of anticoagulation while a malignancy is active. As PV is a lifelong condition and almost exclusively a mutant *JAK2*–driven disease (*JAK2* mutation is strongly associated with thrombotic risk in ET, for example), our preference is to continue anticoagulation indefinitely in patients who have had a life-threatening thrombotic event, in addition to low-dose aspirin, which may provide additional protection from arterial thrombosis. This recommendation is, however, tempered by the recognition of excess bleeding events in patients on both aspirin and anticoagulant therapy, as shown in REVEAL, an observational, real-world study of over 2500 patients with PV. These decisions must, therefore, be individualized based on a careful consideration of risks and benefits for each patient.

For thrombosis in less critical sites, the duration of treatment depends on the individual risk-benefit ratio, but for most standard-risk patients we have tended to anticoagulate for three months and until the hematocrit is well controlled and then bridge onto ongoing aspirin therapy. We should not forget that such patients must be on cytoreductve therapy as well.

7) Should reduction in *JAK2V617F* allele burden be a therapeutic goal in PV?

Expert Perspective: The short answer in clinical practice is no because it is unclear how this may translate into clinical benefits for patients. The major cause of morbidity and mortality in PV is thrombosis, which is most clearly related to the intensity of hematocrit control. Most PV-specific therapies (apart from interferons) fail to reduce the *JAK2* mutation allele burden but still result in survival prolongation through reduction of thrombotic risk.

However, as we improve our ability to prevent cardiovascular events through effective control of the hematocrit, the risk of clonal progression to AML and myelofibrosis becomes increasingly relevant. Multiple studies have documented an AML progression rate of approximately 0.8% per year in patients treated with phlebotomy or hydroxyurea. This risk is now relatively important, considering that the risk of cardiovascular death or thrombosis is 1.1% per year in optimally controlled PV. Therefore, contemporary studies are focusing more on reduction of the neoplastic clone as a therapeutic endpoint, based on the premise (established from the treatment of chronic myeloid leukemia) that suppression of the mutant clone during chronic-phase disease may reduce the subsequent risk of transformation. This is perhaps best exemplified by the trials of ropeginterferon alfa-2b, now approved in the US for the treatment of PV patients.

8) How do we interpret the presence of significant bone marrow fibrosis in patients with PV?

Expert Perspective: It is a common misconception that the presence of marrow reticulin fibrosis in patients with PV represents progression to post-PV myelofibrosis. In fact, approximately 20% of marrow specimens in patients with newly diagnosed PV have grade 2 (on a scale 0–3) reticulin fibrosis. Compared with patients without marrow fibrosis, patients with reticulin fibrosis are more likely to have palpable splenomegaly and progress to post-PV myelofibrosis.

Consensus criteria for diagnosis of post-PV myelofibrosis have been published (Figure 21.1; see also Chapter 24). Required criteria are (i) a documented history of PV, and (ii) significant marrow fibrosis (grade 2 to 3 on a 0–3 scale, or grade 3 to 4 on a 0–4 scale). In addition, the patient must have at least two clinical manifestations of myelofibrosis, as defined by (i) anemia or sustained loss of the requirement of treatment for erythrocytosis, (ii) a leucoerythroblastic blood film, (iii) increasing or newly palpable splenomegaly, and (iv) development of constitutional symptoms (≥ 10% weight loss, drenching night sweats, unexplained fever). Thus, post-PV myelofibrosis is a clinicopathological diagnosis and not one based on marrow fibrosis grade alone.

9) Is hydroxyurea therapy truly devoid of leukemia risk?

Expert Perspective: Acute leukemia is a rare but devastating complication of PV. Early reports suggested a relationship between the occurrence of acute leukemia and exposure to mutagenic therapy, but the widespread use of alkylating agents and radiation-based treatment precluded a clear assessment of the underlying leukemia risk. It was not until the PVSG-01 study that the question of acute leukemia in relation to treatment was addressed definitively. This study randomized 431 patients (1:1:1) to treatment with phlebotomy alone, chlorambucil, or radioactive phosphorus. At a median follow-up of

PV May Progress to Post-PV MF or AML

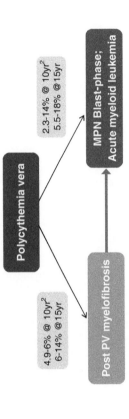

Polycythemia vera

4.9-6% @ 10yr[2]
6-14% @15yr

Post PV myelofibrosis

2.3-14% @ 10yr[2]
5.5-18% @15yr

**MPN Blast-phase;
Acute myeloid leukemia**

IWG-MRT Diagnostic Criteria for Post-PV Myelofibrosis[1]

Required criteria

- Documentation of previous diagnosis of PV as defined by WHO criteria
- **Bone marrow fibrosis grade 2-3 (on 0-3 scale) or grade 3-4 (0-4 scale)**

Additional criteria (2 required)

- Anemia or sustained loss of need for either phlebotomy or cytoreductive therapy
- Leukoerythroblastic peripheral blood picture
- Increase ≥5 cm in palpable splenomegaly or new palpable splenomegaly
- Development of ≥1 of 3 constitutional symptoms (>10% weight loss in 6 mo, night sweats, unexplained fever >37.5°C)

Figure 21.1 IWG-MRT diagnostic criteria for post-PV myelofibrosis[1].
1. Barosi G, et al. *Leukemia.* 2008(2);22:437–438; 2. Cerquozzi S, Tefferi A. *Blood Cancer J.* 2015;5:e366.

6.5 years, acute leukemia occurred in 1 (phlebotomy), 9 (radioactive phosphorus), and 16 (chlorambucil) patients, respectively. PVSG-01 not only demonstrated the mutagenicity of radioactive phosphorus and alkylating agents, but also underscored the low inherent risk of leukemic transformation in non-exposed patients.

The ECLAP study provided further insight into the natural risk of leukemia in patients with PV. Among 1638 patients with PV followed for a median duration of 2.8 years, 22 cases of MDS and AML were diagnosed. Patients were managed according to local practices. Not surprisingly, high rates of MDS and AML were encountered in patients receiving radioactive phosphorus or alkylating agents at registration. The crude MDS and AML rates were 6.4% and 7.3%, respectively. Among patients not receiving treatment, or treated with phlebotomy or interferon, MDS and AML occurred in 5 of 664 (0.8%) over the study period. This rate was the same as that of patients treated with hydroxyurea as the only cytoreductive drug (6 of 736, or 0.8%). Thus, with the caveat of short follow-up, ECLAP provides some degree of assurance that the leukemia risk of hydroxyurea is like that of the natural history of PV.

The French randomized study of pipobroman versus hydroxyurea as first-line therapy of PV provides further evidence for the low risk of acute leukemia in patients receiving long-term hydroxyurea. This study randomized 285 patients younger than 65 years to (1:1) hydroxyurea or pipobroman, with a very mature median follow-up of 16.3 years. The actuarial risk of MDS and AML for patients treated exclusively with hydroxyurea was 7.3% at 10 years, 10.7% at 15 years, and 16.6% at 20 years (i.e. approximately 0.8% per year). Importantly, the MDS and AML risk of pipobroman was approximately double that of hydroxyurea at every time point.

A case/control study of 162 patients who developed MDS and AML in a nationwide myeloproliferative diseases' cohort found that 25% of the AML cases occurred in patients never exposed to cytoreductive therapy and that there was no dose-response effect of hydroxyurea therapy on the subsequent risk of MDS and AML. Finally, a study of 1545 patients with PV defined according to the 2008 WHO criteria found no association between hydroxyurea use and leukemic transformation.

So is hydroxyurea free from leukemia risk? This question cannot be answered definitively based on current evidence, except to note that hydroxyurea is the safest chemotherapeutic drug with respect to leukemogenicity. In a recent propensity score matching analysis of 1042 patients from the ECLAP study who received only phlebotomy or hydroxyurea during the follow-up to keep their hematocrit < 45%, the incidence of fatal or nonfatal CV events was significantly higher in those receiving phlebotomy as compared to those receiving hydroxyurea, testifying to the superiority of hydroxyurea over phlebotomy alone in preventing thrombotic events. Two patients in the phlebotomy group and one in the hydroxurea group developed acute leukemia. Interferons are known to be non-leukemogenic. A head-to-head trial of hydroxyurea and pegylated interferon-alfa failed to show any meaningful differences, but follow-up was short. In the PROUD-CONTINUATION-PV trials that led to the European approval of ropeginterferon alfa-2b, superiority of the latter over hydroxyurea was demonstrated over time. As alluded to above, the ability of this agent to induce clonal remissions may lead to it supplanting hydoxyurea in the first line for high-risk patients with PV. Furthermore, based on its disease-modifying potential as evidenced by the sustained lowering of mutant JAK2 allele burden and its superiority over phlebotomy alone in low-risk patients with PV in the LOW PV trial, it could also lead to a paradigm shift in the management of low-risk PV.

Ropeginterferon alfa-2b is also now approved in the US for the treatment of PV. Additionally, there are no concerns regarding leukemogenicity with the JAK1/2 inhibitor, ruxolitinib, widely used as a second-line treatment for patients with PV who become resistant to or intolerant of hydroxyurea. Both ruxolitinib and hydroxyurea are, however, associated with an increased risk of non-melanoma skin cancers.

10) How do we advise a female with PV who wishes to pursue pregnancy?

Expert Perspective: PV predominantly occurs in older males, and it is relatively rare in females of reproductive age (incidence 0.04–0.25 per 100,000 between the ages of 20 and 39 years). For this reason, there is little information pertaining to pregnancy in patients with PV. Even in healthy individuals, pregnancy itself is a prothrombotic state. Not surprisingly, most complications that occur in patients with myeloproliferative neoplasms relate to thrombosis, whether placental (fetal loss and intrauterine growth retardation) or maternal (venous thromboembolism).

In a recent report of 41 pregnancies occurring in 20 patients with PV, the live birth rate was 51.2%, with 43.9% of the pregnancies ending in spontaneous abortion and 4.9% in stillbirth. The use of PV-specific therapies significantly increased the live birth rate. A systematic review and meta-analysis of 22 studies reporting on 1210 pregancies in patients with MPNs (mostly ET) found the rate of live birth to be 71.3% and the use of aspirin and interferon to be associated with higher odds of the same.

Hence, successful pregnancies can occur in patients with PV, provided that the patient is managed jointly by an experienced team of a hematologist, obstetrician, and ultrasonographer, and meticulous attention is paid to thromboprophylaxis and control of the hematocrit. Patients should cease hydroxyurea prior to conception, and receive aspirin prophylaxis throughout pregnancy, as well as low-molecular-weight heparin for six weeks postpartum. Phlebotomies should aim to maintain the hematocrit in the mid-gestation-appropriate reference range. Patients at especially high risk (e.g. those with previous late-term loss or other severe pregnancy complications, those with platelets $\geq 1500 \times 10^9$/L associated with bleeding risk, or those with VTE within the past six months) should receive cytoreductive therapy with interferon and antenatal coverage with low-molecular-weight heparin when appropriate. Iron supplementation should be avoided. In the postpartum period, women who are breast-feeding can continue to receive aspirin and low-molecular-weight heparin, but they should not take hydroxyurea or interferon.

11) What is the role of ruxolitinib in polycythemia vera?

Expert Perspective: Ruxolitinib is approved by regulatory authorities in the US and Europe for the treatment of patients with polycythemia vera who are resistant to or intolerant of hydroxyurea. Approval was based on the pivotal RESPONSE and RESPONSE-2 trials, which showed sustained haematocrit control, spleen volume reduction (in the RESPONSE study), symptom improvement, and durable complete hematologic responses to ruxolitinib through five years of follow-up. Standard criteria published by the European LeukemiaNet were used to define hydroxyurea resistance and intolerance. Although reduction of thromboembolic events was not an efficacy endpoint, these were captured as adverse events in the trials and were fewer numerically in the patients initially randomized to ruxolitinib as compared to standard or best available therapy. Of note, all patients initially randomized to the latter did cross over to ruxolitinib in both pivotal trials. While hard evidence that ruxolitinib reduces rates of thrombosis in PV is lacking, a systematic review and meta-analysis showed that the number of thrombotic events reported with ruxolitinib was consistently lower than that with best available therapy. Preclinical data supports an anti-thrombotic effect of JAK inhibition via interference with neutrophil extracellular trap formation. Resistance to hydroxyurea in PV is associated with inferior survival and an elevated risk of leukemic transformation, as is the development of cytopenias, especially leukopenia/neutropenia, at the lowest dose of hydroxyurea needed to maintain hematologic response. Ruxolitinib is our second-line drug of choice in PV after failure of hydroxyurea or interferon. Herpes zoster reactivation on ruxolitinib is of some concern in patients with PV, and it is our practice to offer inactivated shingles virus vaccination to older patients when initiating ruxolitinib.

Recommended Readings

Alvarez-Larran, A., Kerguelen, A., Hernandez-Boluda, J.C. et al. (2016 March). Frequency and prognostic value of resistance/intolerance to hydroxycarbamide in 890 patients with polycythaemia vera. *Br J Haematol* 172 (5): 786–793.

Alvarez-Larran, A., Pereira, A., Cervantes, F. et al. (2012 February 9). Assessment and prognostic value of the European LeukemiaNet criteria for clinicohematologic response, resistance, and intolerance to hydroxyurea in polycythemia vera. *Blood* 119 (6): 1363–1369.

Arber DA, Orazi A, Hasserjian RP, et al. (2022 Sept). International Consensus Classification of Myeloid Neoplasms and Acute Leukemias: integrating morphologic, *clinical, and genomic data. Blood* 140 (11):1200–1228.

Barbui, T., Ghirardi, A., Masciulli, A. et al. (2019 August). Second cancer in Philadelphia negative myeloproliferative neoplasms (MPN-K). A nested case-control study. *Leukemia* 33 (8): 1996–2005.

Barbui, T., Masciulli, A., Marfisi, M.R. et al. (2015 July 23). White blood cell counts and thrombosis in polycythemia vera: a subanalysis of the CYTO-PV study. *Blood* 126 (4): 560–561.

Barbui, T., Vannucchi, A.M., De Stefano, V. et al. (2021 March). Ropeginterferon alfa-2b versus phlebotomy in low-risk patients with polycythaemia vera (Low-PV study): a multicentre, randomised phase 2 trial. *Lancet Haematol* 8 (3): e175–e184.

Barbui, T., Vannucchi, A.M., Finazzi, G. et al. (2017 November). A reappraisal of the benefit-risk profile of hydroxyurea in polycythemia vera: a propensity-matched study. *Am J Hematol* 92 (11): 1131–1136.

Barosi, G., Birgegard, G., Finazzi, G. et al. (2010 March). A unified definition of clinical resistance and intolerance to hydroxycarbamide in polycythaemia vera and primary myelofibrosis: results of a European LeukemiaNet (ELN) consensus process. *Br J Haematol* 148 (6): 961–963.

Gerds A.T., Mesa R.A., Burke J.M., et al.(2021Nov). A Real-World Evaluation of the Association between Elevated Blood Counts and Thrombotic Events in Polycythemia Vera (Analysis of Data from the REVEAL Study). *Blood (ASH Annual Meeting abstracts)*138 (Supplement 1): abstract #239.

Gisslinger, H., Klade, C., Georgiev, P. et al. (2020 March). Ropeginterferon alfa-2b versus standard therapy for polycythaemia vera (PROUD-PV and CONTINUATION-PV): a randomised, non-inferiority, phase 3 trial and its extension study. *Lancet Haematol* 7 (3): e196–e208.

Kiladjian, J.-J., Zachee, P., Hino, M. et al. (2020 March). Long-term efficacy and safety of ruxolitinib versus best available therapy in polycythaemia vera (RESPONSE): 5-year follow up of a phase 3 study. *Lancet Haematol* 7 (3): e226–e237.

Kiladjian J-J, Klade C, Georgiev P, et al.(2022 May). Long-term outcomes of polycythemia vera patients treated with ropeginterferon Alfa-2b. *Leukemia* 36 (5):1408–1411.

Landolfi, R., Marchioli, R., Kutti, J. et al. (2004). Efficacy and safety of low-dose aspirin in polycythemia vera. *N Engl J Med* 350 (2): 114–124.

Lasho, T.L., Pardanani, A., and Tefferi, A. (2010). LNK mutations in JAK2 mutation-negative erythrocytosis. *N Engl J Med* 363 (12): 1189–1190.

Marchioli, R., Finazzi, G., Landolfi, R. et al. (2005). Vascular and neoplastic risk in a large cohort of patients with polycythemia vera. *J Clin Oncol* 23 (10): 2224–2232.

Marchioli, R., Vannucchi, A.M., and Barbui, T. (2013). Treatment target in polycythemia vera. *N Engl J Med* 368 (16): 1556.

Masciulli, A., Ferrari, A., Carobbio, A. et al. (2020 January 28). Ruxolitinib for the prevention of thrombosis in polycythemia vera: a systematic review and meta-analysis. *Blood Adv* 4 (2): 380–386.

Maze, D., Kazi, S., Gupta, V. et al. (2019 October 2). Association of treatments for myeloproliferative neoplasms during pregnancy with birth rates and maternal outcomes: a systematic review and meta-analysis. *JAMA Netw Open* 2 (10): e1912666.

Passamonti, F., Griesshammer, M., Palandri, F. et al. (2017 January). Ruxolitinib for the treatment of inadequately controlled polycythaemia vera without splenomegaly (RESPONSE-2): a randomised, open-label, phase 3b study. *Lancet Oncol* 18 (1): 88–99.

Passamonti F, Palandri F, Saydam G, et al.(2022 Jul). Ruxolitinib versus best available therapy in inadequately controlled polycythaemia vera without splenomegaly (RESPONSE-2): 5-year follow up of a randomised, phase 3b study. *Lancet Haematol* 9 (7):e480–e492.

Robinson, S.E. and Harrison, C.N. (2020 May). How we manage Philadelphia-negative myeloproliferative neoplasms in pregnancy. *Br J Haematol* 189 (4): 625–634.

Ronner, L., Podoltsev, N., Gotlib, J. et al. (May 7). Persistent leukocytosis in polycythemia vera is associated with disease evolution but not thrombosis. *Blood* 135 (19): 1696–1703.

Tefferi, A., Rumi, E., Finazzi, G. et al. (2013 September). Survival and prognosis among 1545 patients with contemporary polycythemia vera: an international study. *Leukemia* 27 (9): 1874–1881.

Khoury JD, Solary E, Abla O, et al.The 5th edition of the World Health Organization Classification of Haematolymphoid Tumours: Myeloid and Histiocytic/ Dendritic Neoplasms. *Leukemia*. 2022 Jul;36(7):1703–1719. doi:10.1038/s41375-022-01613-1. Epub 2022 Jun 22. PMID: 35732831; PMCID: PMC9252913.

Vannucchi, A.M., Kiladjian, J.-J., Griesshammer, M. et al. (2015 January 29). Ruxolitinib versus standard therapy for the treatment of polycythemia vera. *N Engl J Med* 372 (5): 426–435.

Wille, K., Bernhardt, J., Sadjadian, P. et al. (2021 July). The management, outcome, and postpartum disease course of 41 pregnancies in 20 women with polycythemia vera. *Eur J Haematol* 107 (1): 122–128.

Wolach, O., Sellar, R.S., Martinod, K. et al. (2018 April 11). Increased neutrophil extracellular trap formation promotes thrombosis in myeloproliferative neoplasms. *Sci Transl Med* 10 (436): eaan8292.

22

Essential Thrombocythemia

Paola Guglielmelli and Alessandro Maria Vannucchi

University of Florence, AOU Careggi, Florence, Italy

Introduction

Essential Thrombocythemia (ET) is one of the Philadelphia chromosome–negative myeloproliferative neoplasms (MPNs), a heterogeneous group of clonal hematopoietic stem disorders that also include polycythemia vera (PV) and primary myelofibrosis (PMF). The incidence varies from 0.38 to 1.7/100.000, according to large epidemiologic studies, while prevalence remains unknown. ETs are usually associated with mutations in *JAK2* (60–65%), *CALR* (20–25%) and *MPL* (5%), collectively defined as "driver" mutations; their characterization is crucial for diagnosis, according to the 2016 WHO criteria, although a minority of patients (10–15%) may lack known mutations (triple-negative ET). With unique mechanisms, all driver mutations lead to constitutive activation of the JAK-STAT signaling, independent of cytokine regulation, which explains many of the pathophysiological traits of ET and MPN in general. Clinically, ET is characterized by an increased rate of thrombosis and risk of hematological progression, which includes transformation to post-ET myelofibrosis and progression to acute myeloid leukemia; it is also associated with a variety of microvascular and systemic symptoms, largely mediated by inflammatory cytokines, which may impair quality of life, and increased risk of other cancers. Treatment is mainly aimed to obtain a reduction of the risk of vascular events, including arterial and venous thrombosis, and major hemorrhage and to improve quality of life by managing symptoms and complications caused by the abnormal myeloproliferation.

1) Should a bone marrow biopsy be performed in all patients suspected to have ET?

Expert Perspective: Yes. According to the 2016 revised WHO diagnostic criteria for ET, there are four major criteria and one minor criterion (Table 22.1).

A bone marrow biopsy is required to make an appropriate morphologic diagnosis of ET and distinguish it from other myeloid neoplasms, in particular prefibrotic primary myelofibrosis (pre-PMF; Chapter 23). However, this distinction—largely based on the isolated proliferation and mature morphology of megakaryocytes and their organization in loose clusters in ET, as opposed to the overall increased myeloproliferation and abnormal megakaryocyte maturation and nuclei abnormalities—together with formation of dense clusters

Cancer Consult: Expertise in Clinical Practice, Volume 2: Neoplastic Hematology & Cellular Therapy,
Second Edition. Edited by Syed A. Abutalib, Maurie Markman, James O. Armitage, and Kenneth C. Anderson.
© 2024 John Wiley & Sons Ltd. Published 2024 by John Wiley & Sons Ltd.

Table 22.1 2016 WHO criteria for the diagnosis of ET.

Major criteria	Minor criterion
1. Platelets $\geq 450 \times 10^9$/L	1. Other clonal marker present or no evidence of reactive thrombocytosis
2. Bone marrow megakaryocyte proliferation and loose megakaryocyte clusters	
3. Not meeting criteria for other myeloid neoplasms	Diagnosis requires all 4 major criteria or the first 3 plus the minor criterion
4. Presence of *JAK2V617F*, *CALR*, or *MPL* mutations	

in pre-PMF may be challenging and requires expertise. Nevertheless, an accurate diagnosis of these disorders has clinical relevance considering the shorter survival and the greater risk to transform to overt primary myelofibrosis of the latter. Bone marrow histopathology may also help to rule out chronic myelogenous leukemia in triple-negative patients (see below), while waiting for *BCR::ABL1* screening results, and other myelodysplastic syndromes / myeloproliferative neoplasms (MDS/MPN), particularly MDS/MPN with ring sideroblasts and thrombocytosis (RS-T), which is often *JAK2V617F-* and *SF3B1*-mutated. Presence of grade 1 fibrosis by no means eliminates the possibility of an ET diagnosis; in fact, up to 10% of patients diagnosed with ET have it. Therefore, unless there are compelling clinical reasons against it, a bone marrow biopsy is always required to firmly establish an ET diagnosis.

2) What genetic tests should be performed in any patients suspected to have ET?

Expert Perspective: It is recommended that genotyping for driver mutations of *JAK2*, *CALR*, and *MPL* is performed in any case of thrombocytosis where ET is suspected. JAK2 is a tyrosine kinase constitutively associated with several growth factor receptors (including erythropoietin [EPO], thrombopoietin [TPO], and granulocyte-colony stimulating factor [G-CSF]) and a variety of immune and inflammatory cytokine receptors; its ligand-dependent activation leads to the recruitment of proteins belonging to STAT family, which are involved in the regulated expression of genes involved in cell proliferation, maturation, and function.

The following facts should be taken into consideration when making decisions about genetic tests for ET:

- The *JAK2V617F* is a valine to phenylalanine substitution at amino acid position 617 (V617F) in exon 14 of *JAK2*; it is found in about 60% of ET cases, as well as in pre- and overt PMF in similar proportion and > 95% of cases of PV (Chapter 21).
- A second type of *JAK2* mutation, comprising in-frame insertions or deletions in exon 12 of the gene, is restricted to a minority of PV patients only (2–4%) and should not be searched for in ET.
- The gene calreticulin (*CALR*) encodes for a 46-kDa chaperone protein, which has a key role in the maintenance of calcium homeostasis and protein folding. There are more than 50 different *CALR* mutations, all in exon 9, known to date; all lead to frameshift and synthesis of a novel protein C-terminus. There are two prototypic CALR mutations that

together account for greater than 80% of all the subtypes; type 1 is a 52-bp deletion (c.1092_1143del p.L367fs*46) and type 2 is a 5-bp insertion (c.1154_1155insTTGTC p.K385fs*47). The other *CALR* mutations are classified either as type 1–like or type 2–like in relation to their structural similarities and effects on C-terminal. *CALR* mutations are found in approximately 20–25% of ET cases, a proportion not dissimilar from patients with PMF; on the other hand, they have not been associated with a PV phenotype.

- *MPL* is the cell surface receptor for TPO, which regulates megakaryocytopoiesis and platelet production and is also expressed on hematopoietic stem cells. Mutations are clustered at *tryptophan 515 (W515)* in exon 10, located in the transmembrane domain of the protein in a region that is essential for protein stability. The most frequent mutations are *W515L* and *W515K*, but other rare mutations at the same position, including *W515R*, *W515A*, and *W515G*, have been reported. Another mutation is *MPLS505N*, which may represent either an inherited mutation in cases of familial thrombocytosis or a somatically acquired abnormality in sporadic cases. MPL mutations in ET patients are found in 3–8%, similar to PMF.

Unless the referring laboratory uses multigene panels, the order in which mutations are usually tested in a patient suspected to have ET is based on their relative frequency.

3) Are these mutations (*JAK2V617F*, *CALR* type 1 and 2, and *MPL*) mutually exclusive in ET?

Expert Perspective: Driver mutations are in general mutually exclusive, but cases of co-occurrence have been reported. Particularly when the *JAK2V617F* variant allele frequency (VAF) (which is a measure of the ratio of mutated versus wild-type *JAK2* alleles in the cell samples used for genotyping—usually peripheral blood, less commonly bone marrow aspirate) is below 1%, it is recommended that mutation of *CALR* is also searched for since co-occurrence may be enriched in these cases and *CALR* represents the prevalent mutation (the one with greater VAF). In double-mutated patients the disease phenotype seems to be dictated by the predominant mutation; however, occurrence of thrombosis or progression to secondary myelofibrosis during follow-up was not different from single-mutated patients. Although there is a growing use of next-generation sequencing (NGS) platforms to approach molecular diagnosis, at present we recommend continuing to adopt conventional tests such as real-time PCR and/or allelic discrimination assays, which have greater sensitivity in the low to very-low VAF range and are cost effective.

4) What percentage of patients have been categorized as triple-negative ET?

Expert Perspective: Patients with a 2016 WHO diagnosis of ET who do not have any one of the above driver mutations are classified as triple-negative. They sum up to 10–15% of all ET patients, a figure not far from PMF (about 10%). According to some recent studies, a minority (less than 20%) of triple-negative ET and PMF patients may have mutations outside of *MPL* exon 10 and *JAK2* exon 14. These noncanonical MPL mutations include T119I, S204F/P, and E230G in the extracellular domain and Y591D/N in the intracellular domain, while in *JAK2* the most common are V625F, F556V, R683G, and E627A. Due to their rarity, the complexity of assays to identify them through sequencing of the entire *JAK2* and *MPL* coding sequence, as well as possible uncertainties about their interpretation (somatic rather than germline variants) and functional role, at present we cannot recommend the search of noncanonical *JAK2* and *MPL* mutations on a routine basis. Finally, it is indicated to perform *BCR::ABL1* rearrangement in any patients with isolated thrombocytosis, and mandatorily in those who are triple negative, to exclude chronic myelogenous leukemia.

5) What are the implications of the additional somatic mutations in triple-negative ET?

Expert Perspective: The identification of a clonal marker highly benefitted from NGS with efficient recognition of additional somatic mutations in ET triple-negative patients, as proposed by the WHO classification. In fact, the extensive use of NGS technologies recently contributed to discover a complex mutational landscape of MPN. Overall, more than 50% of MPN patients harbor other genetic variants in addition to the driver ones, although that figure is approximately halved among ET patients. These mutations, which are collectively called myeloid neoplasm–associated mutations, are not restricted to MPN but are shared with other myeloid malignancies and can also be identified in the context of clonal hematopoiesis of indeterminate potential (CHIP) or age-related clonal hematopoiesis (ARCH). They may affect genes involved in DNA methylation (*TET2, DNMT3A, IDH1, IDH2*), histone modification (*ASXL1, EZH2*), mRNA splicing (*SFRB1, SRSF2, U2AF1, ZRSR2*), signaling (*LNK/SH2B3, CBL, NRAS, KRAS, PTPN11*), and transcription factors (*RUNX1, NFE2, TP53, PPM1D*). A particular mutation profile is considered to impart high-molecular risk features in myelofibrosis, being associated with reduced survival and increased risk of progression to blast phase; its knowledge in a patient contributes to treatment decisions. Also, in ET some mutations are considered to bear adverse significance (discussed later), but currently we cannot recommend their assessment on a routine basis in any patients with ET, unlike we do in most patients with myelofibrosis.

6) Which are the most relevant events associated with progression of ET?

Expert Perspective: Most patients with ET are expected to have normal life span, but others may develop disease progression or life-threatening complications. Median survival is around 20 years for ET. As for the other MPN, there is a risk for ET to transform into secondary acute myeloid leukemia, referred to as MPN blast phase (BP), which is typically refractory to conventional chemotherapy and has a poor prognosis. The 15-year risk of leukemia is estimated at 2.1–5.3% for ET, definitely lower than for other MPNs (5.5–18.7% for PV and greater than 20% for myelofibrosis). Conversely, the rate of fibrotic progression ET and PV are quite similar, estimated at 4–11% and 6–14%, respectively, around 15–20 years after diagnosis. Risk factors for fibrotic transformation in ET include advanced age, male gender, leukocytosis, anemia, reticulin fibrosis, increased LDH, absence of $JAK2^{V617F}$, and presence of *SF3B1* or *U2AF1* mutations for post-essential thrombocythemia myelofibrosis (PET-MF).

7) What are the criteria for post-essential thrombocythemia myelofibrosis?

Expert Perspective: The diagnosis of PET-MF should adhere to criteria published by the International Working Group for MPN Research and Treatment (IWG-MRT), outlined in Table 22.2.

Table 22.2 The IWG-MRT criteria for the diagnosis of post-essential thrombocythemia myelofibrosis.

Required criteria
(both necessary)

	Documentation of a previous diagnosis of ET as defined by the 2016 WHO criteria
	Marrow fibrosis grade 2 to 3 (on 0–3 scale) according to the European classification

Additional criteria
(at least 2 are required)

Anemia (below the reference range for appropriate age, gender, and altitude considerations) and a ≥ 2 g/dL decrease from baseline Hb level

A leukoerythroblastic peripheral blood picture

Increasing splenomegaly defined as either an increase in palpable splenomegaly ≥ 5 cm (distance of the tip of the spleen from the left costal margin) or the appearance of a newly palpable splenomegaly

Increased LDH (above ULN)

Development of ≥ 1 of three constitutional symptoms (> 10% weight loss in 6 months, night sweats, unexplained fever > 37.5°C)

8) Should a patient with ET be risk-stratified for an appropriate treatment?

Expert Perspective: Yes. There is no curative treatment for ET outside of allogeneic transplant. The aim of therapy is to minimize the risk of cardiovascular events, either thrombosis or hemorrhage, and provide best control of symptoms without increasing the risk of progression to post-ET myelofibrosis or acute leukemia. Therefore, treatment is recommended for patients considered at higher risk to develop thrombotic events and/or suffering from disabling symptoms attributable to the underlying hematologic disease. The conventional score for risk-stratifying patients according to their propensity to develop thrombosis is based on age (older than 60 years) and prior history of thrombotic events; presence of either variable qualifies for high-risk condition, hence representing an indication for cytoreduction. More recently, the appreciation of the association of *JAK2V617F* mutation with thrombosis rate, unlike for *CALR* and *MPL* mutations, promoted the development of a novel score, the International Prognostic Score for Essential Thrombocythemia (IPSET) and its revised version, r-IPSET (Table 22.3). It constitutes the basis for current treatment recommendation; presence of generic cardiovascular (CV) risk factors, although not a formal variable in r-IPSET, helps modulating treatment.

Median survival in ET patients is longer than 20 years. A mutation-enhanced international prognostic systems for ET (MIPSS-ET) was recently developed, which incorporates *SF3B1, SRSF2, U2AF1*, and *TP53* mutations, which collectively occur in 10% of ET patients, as negative predictors of survival together with age > 60 years, leukocytosis, and male gender. Three groups were depicted, with median survival of 34 years (low risk), 14 years (intermediate risk), and 8 years (high risk). However, survival prediction has a limited role in tailoring therapy in ET patients, unlike in myelofibrosis; therefore, such score is not

Table 22.3 Revised-IPSET score and risk-based treatment.

Variables	Risk categories	Therapy
☐ Age ≤ 60 years	**Very low:** Age ≤ 60 years, no prior thrombosis *JAK2* wild type	Management of CV risk factors, observation, or low-dose aspirin, unless contraindicated
☐ Prior thrombosis ☐ *JAK2V617F* mutation	DELETE THIS SPACE **Low:** Age ≤ 60 years, no prior thrombosis, mutated *JAK2V617F*	Management of CV risk factors and low-dose aspirin unless contraindicated. Higher-dose aspirin may be used if CV risk factors present
	Intermediate: Age > 60 years, no prior thrombosis, wild-type *JAK2* **High:** Age > 60 years and prior thrombosis or mutated *JAK2V617F*	Management of CV risk factors and cytoreductive therapy plus low-dose aspirin, unless contraindicated. Higher-dose aspirin without cytoreductive therapy if no CV risk factors Management of CV risk factors and cytoreductive therapy plus low-dose aspirin

employed in clinical practice for decision-making but might be useful for selecting defined categories of patients in clinical trials.

9) Should extreme thrombocytosis in a patient with ET be an indication for cytoreductive therapy?

Expert Perspective: Not in a patient with low-risk disease. It is important to underline that no definite correlation exists between the extent of thrombocytosis and the rate of thrombosis; this information should be given at the time of diagnosis to all ET patients since most of them—as expected—are very anxious about their platelet counts based on an assumed count-dependent increase of thrombotic complications rate. Rather, extreme thrombocytosis, conventionally fixed at/above 1.0 million platelets/mm^3, may be encountered in about 20% of patients at diagnosis and/or develop during disease course; it is more common among *CALR*- and *MPL*-mutated than *JAK2V617F* ones and might contribute to the lower rate of arterial thrombosis in the former patients.

Extreme thrombocytosis may rather increase the risk of hemorrhage, mediated by a condition of acquired von Willebrand factor (vWF) deficiency. This phenomenon is attributable to the loss of largest vWF multimers possibly mediated by their increased proteolysis by ADAMST13 protease, promoted by high platelet counts. Assessment of vWF activity (e.g. ristocetin cofactor activity assay, vWF:RCoA), better than quantification of total plasma vWF and FVIII levels, may help to identify patients with extreme thrombocytosis who are at higher risk of hemorrhage, in whom aspirin treatment may be prudently withhold, unless in the presence of other clinical indications. A vWF R:CoA assay lower than 20% activity is generally recommended as the threshold level to stop aspirin. On the other hand, extreme thrombocytosis per se in an otherwise low-risk patient, without microvascular manifestations potentially attributable to thrombocytosis (headache, paraesthesia, tinnitus, scotomas), and in the absence of history or actual hemorrhagic manifestations does not warrant cytoreduction and, according to recent data, does not invariably mandate stop of aspirin. Recent data suggest that myelofibrosis-free survival or thrombosis-free survival were not affected by extreme thrombocytosis, typical of *CALR*-mutated as opposite to *JAK2V617F*-mutated ET.

10) How to manage a raised hematocrit in *JAK2V617F*-mutated ET patients?

Expert Perspective: In patients diagnosed with ET according to the 2016 WHO revised criteria, hemoglobin and hematocrit levels are, by definition, below the threshold required for the diagnosis of PV. However, it is not an infrequent observation that some *JAK2V617F*-mutated ET patients, not receiving cytoreductive therapy, may progressively develop raised hematocrit levels above 45%. Conversely, this is very unlikely to occur in those who are CALR- or MPL-mutated. There is no evidence-based nor consensus recommendations about the need/advantage of normalizing hematocrit in these patients (without PV diagnosis). Our practice is to prescribe phlebotomy when the hematocrit is steadily above 47% in patients who present generic cardiovascular risk factors, beyond recommending fluid intake and strict adherence to the daily aspirin prescription.

Masked polycythemia vera: Sometimes, the increase of hemoglobin/hematocrit may even reach the diagnostic threshold for PV, and in these cases, diagnosis should be shifted; they might be retrospectively interpreted as masked polycythemia vera initially presenting with thrombocytosis only. It is also likely that these cases could have been more correctly diagnosed as PV since initial presentation by means of the measurement of red cell mass by isotope methods, but the test is no longer in use if not in highly specialized centers. In the majority of cases, however, although formal criteria for PV remain not met, the hematocrit remains steadily above 45%, which is considered the optimal target to maintain to reduce the risk of thrombosis in PV patients, as supported by results of the controlled CYTO-PV study.

11) What are first-line cytoreductive drugs and the goal of therapy in ET?

Expert Perspective: IPSET-defined, high-risk patients require cytoreduction, according to current guidelines (Table 22.3). Other reasons for cytoreductive treatment, to address on a case-by-case basis, include (i) progressive and symptomatic splenomegaly (which is a very unusual findings and should rather suggest progression to PET-MF; see Table 22.2), (ii) aspirin-insensitive microvascular disturbances (headaches, erythromelalgia, scotomas), (iii) disease-related symptoms (pruritus, night sweats, fatigue), and (iv) progressive leukocytosis (which is also very rare). Preferred first-line drug is hydroxyurea, as supported by the results of pivotal randomized trials. In the first landmark Bergamo trial, 114 patients, in the majority high-risk patients, were randomized to receive or not hydroxyurea. The rate of thrombotic complications was more than seven-fold lower in the hydroxyurea arm (3.6% versus 24%). Two randomized studies compared hydroxyurea to anagrelide in ET patients. Hydroxyurea resulted superior to anagrelide in reducing arterial thrombosis, major bleeding, and also progression to post-ET PMF, in the Primary Thrombocythemia-1 (PT-1) study, which included 809 ET patients at high risk for vascular events who were randomized to receive hydroxyurea versus anagrelide, on top of low-dose aspirin in both arms. Some advantage was seen for anagrelide regarding venous thrombosis. In the ANAHYDRET study, which included 259 high-risk ET patients strictly diagnosed according to 2016 WHO criteria, no significant difference was seen between the anagrelide and hydroxyurea arm concerning the rates of major arterial and venous thrombosis, severe bleeding events, minor arterial and venous thrombosis, and minor bleeding events. Therefore, all these support hydroxyurea as first-line therapy for the majority of ET patients. Based on an assumed potential leukemogenicity of hydroxyurea—which is not supported by retrospective series and large epidemiologic studies—some physicians prefer to avoid hydroxyurea in younger patients and favor anagrelide or interferon (discussed later). We consider interferon in young women who plan to become pregnant or if there is strong negative position toward hydroxyurea from the patient.

In theory, normalization of platelet count should be the target of therapy. However, since no evidence-based or consensus-generated statement definitely support a precise target level of platelets to maintain with cytoreductive therapy, in practice most patients are dosed to approximate normal platelet counts and/or obtain symptomatic improvements by using the lowest amount of hydroxyurea needed. However, in patients with severe or recurrent thrombotic events or in those who are heavily symptomatic, normalization of blood counts may be a reasonable objective of treatment.

On the other hand, a randomized trial showed there is no advantage in using hydroxyurea in patients with ET age 40–59 years and without high-risk factors or extreme thrombocytosis. After a median follow-up of six years, there was no difference between the two arms in time to arterial or venous thrombosis, serious hemorrhage, or death from vascular cause, which was the study primary endpoint. Also, there were no differences in overall survival, transformation to myelofibrosis, acute myeloid leukemia, or myelodysplasia, or in patient-reported quality of life.

12) How to manage second-line treatment in patients with ET?

Expert Perspective: Resistance or intolerance to hydroxyurea, either hematologic or extra-hematologic, may develop and require shifting to second-line drugs. Criteria for defining resistance/intolerance to hydroxyurea have been developed by the European LeukemiaNet. Second-line alternatives to hydroxyurea are anagrelide and interferon-alpha (IFN-α). Treatment with IFN-α has been associated with high rates of hematologic responses in patients with ET across several studies. In a recent meta-analysis that included 44 studies and 730 ET patients, the overall response rate was 71% with complete hematologic response (i.e. normalization of all blood cell counts) as high as 59.0%. Thrombotic complication rate was low and at least similar to historic controls treated with hydroxyurea. However, interferon was associated with an annual discontinuation rate of almost 9% due to side effects. Importantly, IFN-α induced sustained molecular responses in up to 27% of ET patients, suggesting a disease-modifying effect. However, in a long-term observation report of a phase II prospective study, vascular complications were still observed while on therapy, and the rates of progression to post-ET myelofibrosis and blast phase were similar to a matched control group. The role of IFN-α was further evaluated in a randomized, open-label phase III trial comparing peg-IFN-α-2a with hydroxyurea as front-line treatment in high-risk PV and ET patients. Results showed no difference between the two arms, while interferon was associated with a higher rate of grade 3/4 toxicity. In a phase II trial evaluating single-arm salvage peg-IFN-α-2a for high-risk ET patients resistant or intolerant to HU, overall response rate was 69%, making treatment with IFN-α a valid option in this patient category. Intermittent courses of busulfan, an alkylating agent, may be used in older patients who develop resistance or intolerance to hydroxyurea and are not candidates to interferon.

13) When and how should aspirin be used in ET?

Expert Perspective: While the anti-thrombotic value of low-dose aspirin in preventing vascular events, irrespective of risk categories, has been demonstrated in the randomized ECLAP study in PV patients, no controlled study is available in ET; thus, the indication is largely irrelevant for PV. However, retrospective analyses supported aspirin therapy to be beneficial in *JAK2V617F*-mutated low-risk ET in preventing thrombosis. A recent study, which analyzed the impact of the increased platelet turnover in ET patients in relation to the efficacy of aspirin in reducing platelet activation as measured by serum thromboxane B2 level, supports twice a day aspirin to be more effective, and equally well tolerated, than once daily. In clinical practice, twice daily aspirin may be used in the presence of relevant cardiovascular risk factors or in patients presenting severe microvascular symptoms, after carefully weighting the expected benefits with the risk of gastrointestinal side effects and bleeding. Please refer to Table 22.3 for risk-based indications for aspirin. It is recommended that all *JAK2V617F*-mutated patients are prescribed aspirin, even if low risk; conversely, very low-risk patients, which include CALR- and MPL-mutated patients, may be followed without the use of aspirin, provided they are asymptomatic and have no generic cardiovascular risk factors. A tendency toward bleeding was reported in retrospective series of CALR-mutated ET patients treated with aspirin without overt benefits for thrombosis.

14) What is the role of aspirin therapy during pregnancy in ET?

Expert Perspective: Aspirin therapy may be considered also for the prevention of vascular complications during pregnancy, especially in *JAK2V617F*-mutated women, starting from the very beginning of pregnancy up to two weeks before delivery, when aspirin is substituted with heparin, which is to be maintained for 4–6 weeks after delivery. For the use of aspirin in patients with extreme thrombocytosis see above.

15) What are new drugs in development in ET?

Expert Perspective: The expected long survival in ET, which for most patients may be close to normal life span, on one side, and the overall satisfactory clinical activity and safety of drugs currently used as first-line treatment, on the other side, have largely prevented active therapeutic experimentation in ET, unlike with the other classic forms of MPN such as PV and myelofibrosis (Chapters 21, 23, and 24). While there are a number of potentially active drugs in controlling thrombocytosis in the settings of PMF, with thrombocytopenia eventually representing a dose-limiting toxicity, their use in ET should be carefully weighted against potential toxicities and worsening of quality of life.

The main drugs in this category include:

- **Ruxolitinib:** After promising results of a phase II, single-arm study with the *JAK1* and *JAK2* inhibitor ruxolitinib, in a subsequent phase II controlled trial (MAJIC) ET patients who were resistant/intolerant to hydroxyurea were randomized to receive ruxolitinib versus best available therapy, including hydroxyurea, anagrelide, or interferon. There was no evidence of superiority of the experimental arm over BAT, a part for a slight increase of the proportion of patients who had improvement in some disease-related symptoms. In particular, there was no advantage in major endpoints, including two-year rate of thrombosis, hemorrhage, and transformation to myelofibrosis.

- **Imetelstat,** a competitive inhibitor of telomerase activity known to be dysregulated in most ET patients, which potently inhibits megakaryocyte proliferation in cells from ET patients, was used in a phase II study in a small cohort of ET patients who were refractory or intolerant to prior therapies. Imetelstat produced hematologic responses in the majority of cases and also molecular responses; however, due to side effects, which included neutropenia, anemia, and hepatic abnormalities, and considering its inconvenient route of administration (intravenous) for a chronic disease as is ET, no further studies were conducted.

- **Bomedestat** (previously, IMG-7289) is a small molecule inhibitor of lysine-specific demethylase 1 (LSD1 or KDM1A), an enzyme required for maturation of blood cells, with particular activity on megakaryocytes. It is being investigated in patients with myelofibrosis and received FDA orphan drug and fast-track designation also for ET, with an ongoing phase II study in patients refractory/resistant to hydroxyurea.

Recommended Readings

Barbui, T., Tefferi, A., Vannucchi, A.M. et al. (2018). Philadelphia chromosome-negative classical myeloproliferative neoplasms: revised management recommendations from European LeukemiaNet. *Leukemia.* 32 (5): 1057–1069.

Godfrey, A.L., Campbell, P.J., MacLean, C. et al. (2018). Hydroxycarbamide plus aspirin versus aspirin alone in patients with essential thrombocythemia age 40 to 59 years without high-risk features. *J Clin Oncol.* 36: 3361–3369.

Guglielmelli, P. and Vannucchi, A.M. (2020). Current management strategies for polycythemia vera and essential thrombocythemia. *Blood Rev.* 42: 100714.

Loscocco, G.G., Guglielmelli, P., and Vannucchi, A.M. (2020). Impact of mutational profile on the management of myeloproliferative neoplasms: a short review of the emerging data. *Onco Targets Ther.* 13: 12367–12382.

Tefferi, A. and Barbui, T. (2020). Polycythemia vera and essential thrombocythemia: 2021 update on diagnosis, risk-stratification and management. *Am J Hematol.* 95 (12): 1599–1613.

23

Primary Myelofibrosis

Douglas Tremblay[1], Sangeetha Venugopal[2], John Mascarenhas[3], and Ruben Mesa[4]

[1] *Tisch Cancer Institute, Icahn School of Medicine at Mount Sinai, New York, NY, USA*
[2] *University of Miami, Miami, FL, USA*
[3] *Tisch Cancer Institute, Icahn School of Medicine at Mount Sinai, New York, NY, USA*
[4] *Senior Vice President, Atrium Health Levine Cancer Institute, Charlotte, NC*

Introduction

Primary myelofibrosis (PMF) is a clonal hematologic malignancy clinically characterized by splenomegaly, constitutional symptoms, cytopenias, and evolution to acute myeloid leukemia (AML). PMF is a myeloproliferative neoplasm (MPN), a group of disorders including polycythemia vera (PV), essential thrombocythemia (ET), chronic myeloid leukemia (CML), and several other less well-defined disease entities. MPNs share morphological, pathological, molecular, and clinical features and frequently evolve from one clinical phenotype to another. Specifically, myelofibrosis can be secondary to PV or ET, termed post-PV myelofibrosis (PPV-MF) or post-ET myelofibrosis (PET-MF). While the clinical characteristics do not significantly differ between PMF, PPV-MF, and PET-MF, these diagnoses carry somewhat disparate outcomes. For the purpose of the following discussion, we will discuss PMF, but the concepts covered here will also apply to PPV-MF and PET-MF unless specified.

1) How is PMF diagnosed?

Expert Perspective: The World Health Organization (WHO) has established diagnostic criteria for PMF (Table 23.1). The most common presenting symptom of PMF is severe fatigue although many patients also have complaints related to splenomegaly (early satiety, left upper quadrant fullness), fevers, night sweats, weight loss, and bone pain. Laboratory findings of PMF include anemia, and white blood cell and platelet abnormalities. Peripheral blood smear often demonstrates a leukoerythroblastostic picture with nucleated red cells, immature granulocytes, and dacrocytes (tear drop cells). A bone marrow biopsy is key to establishing the diagnosis of PMF, which must demonstrate fibrosis as visualized on a silver stain for reticulin. Megakaryocytes are tightly clustered with atypical forms including hyperlobation and hypolobation (cloud-like nuclei). In addition, osteosclerosis is frequently observed. The bone marrow biopsy is characteristically difficult to aspirate, resulting in a "dry tap." In order to determine the diagnosis of PMF, it is necessary to exclude other MPNs, in particular chronic myeloid leukemia (CML). At time of bone marrow

Cancer Consult: Expertise in Clinical Practice, Volume 2: Neoplastic Hematology & Cellular Therapy,
Second Edition. Edited by Syed A. Abutalib, Maurie Markman, James O. Armitage, and Kenneth C. Anderson.
© 2024 John Wiley & Sons Ltd. Published 2024 by John Wiley & Sons Ltd.

Table 23.1 Criteria for the diagnosis of overt PMF and pre-PMF (Arber et al. 2016).

Overt PMF criteria	Pre-PMF criteria
Major criteria	
1. Presence of megakaryocytic proliferation and atypia, accompanied by either reticulin and/or collagen fibrosis grades 2 or 3	1. Megakaryocytic proliferation and atypia, without reticulin fibrosis > grade 1, accompanied by increased age-adjusted BM cellularity, granulocytic proliferation, and often decreased erythropoiesis
2. Not meeting WHO criteria for ET, PV, *BCR::ABL1*⁺ CML, myelodysplastic syndromes, or other myeloid neoplasms	2. Not meeting the WHO criteria for *BCR::ABL1*⁺ CML, PV, ET, myelodysplastic syndromes, or other myeloid neoplasms
3. Presence of *JAK2, CALR,* or *MPL* mutation or in the absence of these mutations, presence of another clonal marker,† or absence of reactive myelofibrosis‡	3. Presence of *JAK2, CALR,* or *MPL* mutation or in the absence of these mutations, presence of another clonal marker,† or absence of minor reactive BM reticulin fibrosis‡
Minor criteria	
Presence of at least 1 of the following, confirmed in 2 consecutive determinations:	Presence of at least 1 of the following, confirmed in 2 consecutive determinations:
a. Anemia not attributed to a comorbid condition	a. Anemia not attributed to a comorbid condition
b. Leukocytosis $\geq 11 \times 10^9$/L	b. Leukocytosis $\geq 11 \times 10^9$/L
c. Palpable splenomegaly	c. Palpable splenomegaly
d. LDH increased to above upper normal limit of institutional reference range	d. LDH increased to above upper normal limit of institutional reference range
e. Leukoerythroblastosis	
Diagnosis of overt and pre-PMF requires meeting all 3 major criteria and at least 1 minor criterion	

†In the absence of any of the three major clonal mutations, the search for the most frequent accompanying mutations (e.g. *ASXL1, EZH2, TET2, IDH1/IDH2, SRSF2, SF3B1*) are of help in determining the clonal nature of the disease.
‡BM fibrosis secondary to infection, autoimmune disorder, or other chronic inflammatory conditions, hairy cell leukemia or other lymphoid neoplasm, metastatic malignancy, or toxic (chronic) myelopathies.

biopsy, it is important to also obtain cytogenetic analysis and driver mutational testing (*JAK2, CALR,* and *MPL*), for both diagnostic and prognostic purposes. Next-generation sequencing (NGS) is increasingly employed and incorporated in routine practice for the prognostication and treatment of PMF, as described below.

Diagnosis of PPV-MF and PPV-ET requires development of bone marrow fibrosis in the setting of previously diagnosed PV or ET, accompanied by at least two of the following features: (i) anemia, (ii) leukoerythroblastosis peripheral blood smear, (iii) splenomegaly, and (iv) constitutional symptoms including fevers, night sweats, and weight loss of at least 10% over six months (see Chapters 21 and 22).

2) What is the differential diagnosis of primary myelofibrosis?

Expert Perspective: Bone marrow fibrosis is observed in several hematological (malignant and non-malignant) as well as non-hematological disorders (Table 23.2). Acute panmyelosis with myelofibrosis (APMF) is an aggressive hematological neoplasm classified by the WHO as AML not otherwise specified (AML-NOS). APMF is characterized by fever, cytopenias, and leukoerythroblastosis and differentiated from PMF by its acute presentation, absence of spleno-megaly, and rapidly progressive clinical course. Other long-standing myeloid neoplasms including CML, myelodysplastic syndrome, or related MPNs such as PV and ET may have asso-ciated bone marrow fibrosis but are distinguished from PMF by the presence of t(9;22), dys-plasia or the lack of WHO-defined diagnostic criteria for PMF or secondary MF, respectively. Autoimmune myelofibrosis (AIMF) is a cause of non-malignant bone marrow fibrosis, which frequently occurs in the background of autoimmune disorders such as systemic lupus erythe-matosus. AIMF closely resembles PMF in bone marrow morphology but is often associated with lymphocytic infiltration. AIMF is exquisitely sensitive to corticosteroids and is associated with good prognosis. Other rare conditions that could lead to bone marrow fibrosis include multiple myeloma, lymphoma, metastatic cancers, hyperparathyroidism, or medications. For example, long-term thrombopoietin-receptor agonists (TPO-RA) therapy may cause bone marrow fibrosis due to increased levels of profibrotic cytokines [transforming growth factor-β (TGF-β), basic-fibroblast growth factor, and platelet-derived growth factor] as a result of sustained stimulation of megakaryocytes. These mimics of PMF highlight the need for thor-ough history and expert hematopathological evaluation in the diagnosis of PMF.

3) What is pre-PMF, and how is it managed?

Expert Perspective: In 2016, the WHO defined a new diagnostic entity called pre-PMF pathologically characterized by megakaryocytic atypia reticulin fibrosis of grade 1 or less and a hypercellular marrow (Table 23.1). Clinically, pre-PMF is associated with isolated thrombocytosis, which leads to frequent misdiagnosis as ET. In one review of over 1000 cases of previously diagnosed ET, nearly one in five met criteria for pre-PMF. In comparison

Table 23.2 Differential diagnosis of primary myelofibrosis.

Disease	Distinguishing features from PMF
Acute panmyelosis with myelofibrosis	Acute onset, lack of splenomegaly
Chronic myeloid leukemia	Presence of t(9;22)
Myelodysplastic syndrome	Presence of erythroid, myeloid, megakaryocytic dysplasia
Related myeloproliferative neoplasms	Does not satisfy WHO 2016 criteria for PMF or secondary MF
Autoimmune myelofibrosis	Primary or associated with autoimmune disorders (secondary); sensitive to corticosteroids, good prognosis

PMF: primary myelofibrosis; WHO: World Health Organization.

to overt PMF, pre-PMF is characterized by less frequent splenomegaly and constitutional symptoms with more thrombocytosis, leukocytosis, and lower LDH levels. Regardless, patients with isolated thrombocytosis necessitate a bone marrow biopsy to differentiate ET and pre-PMF given divergent clinical approaches and prognosis. The survival of pre-PMF is significantly improved compared to overt PMF: 14.7 years versus 7.2 years, in one study. However, survival is significantly worse with pre-PMF than ET, as is the propensity to transform to overt PMF and MPN-BP.

There remains controversy on the optimal management of pre-PMF. When applying risk stratification for overt PMF, most patient fall within the low or intermediate-1 scoring system, and observation can be safely recommended. However, in patients with constitutional symptoms or symptomatic splenomegaly, treatment with a JAK inhibitor is appropriate. Additionally, in patients who have a thrombosis, antiplatelet therapy and cytoreductive therapy with hydroxyurea or pegylated interferon should also be considered. In all patients with pre-PMF, close monitoring for progression of splenomegaly, cytopenias, or symptoms is essential. Patients with high-risk features, such as rapidly progressive disease or high molecular risk features, should be referred for consideration of allogeneic hematopoietic stem cell transplantation (HSCT).

4) How do you risk-stratify patients with PMF?

Expert Perspective: Several risk stratification tools utilizing only clinical variables or in combination with cytogenomic variables are in vogue for PMF (Figure 23.1). The Dynamic

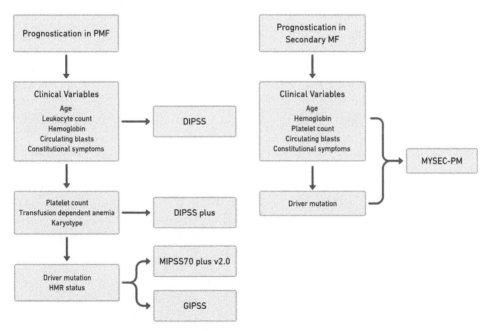

Figure 23.1 Application of prognostic risk models of PMF in clinical practice. PMF: Primary myelofibrosis; DIPSS: Dynamic International Prognostic Scoring System; GIPSS: Genetically Inspired Prognostic Scoring System; HMR: High molecular risk; MIPSS70 + v2.0: mutation-enhanced international prognostic scoring system, version 2.0. MYSEC-PM: Myelofibrosis Secondary to PV and ET-Prognostic Model.

International Prognostic Scoring System (DIPSS) is the most commonly used PMF prognostic model to aid treatment decision-making at any time point in a patient's disease course. Age > 65 years, constitutional symptoms, hemoglobin < 10 g/dL, leukocyte count > 25 × 10^9/L, and circulating blasts ≥ 1% are the prognostic variables included in this model. As disease-related anemia is associated with worse overall survival than that of other variables, hemoglobin < 10 g/dL is assigned two points while the rest are assigned one point each. Based on median overall survival (mOS), this prognostic model categorizes PMF into low-risk (0 points; mOS not reached), intermediate-1 (1–2 points; mOS 14.2 years), intermediate-2 (3–4 points; mOS 4 years), and high-risk (5–6 points; mOS 1.5 years) groups. To refine the prognosis of DIPSS, the DIPSS-plus model was developed. In addition to DIPSS-associated variables, DIPSS-plus also incorporates karyotype, platelet count, and RBC transfusion status assigned one point each for risk stratification. DIPSS-plus also demonstrated that unfavorable karyotype [complex or a single or two abnormalities including + 8, −7/7q−, i(17)q, −5/5q−, 12p−, inv(3), or 11q23 rearrangements] or thrombocytopenia (platelets < 100 × 10^9/L) predicted for inferior leukemia-free survival (LFS). The DIPSS-plus model is used when cytogenetic data is available.

In patients with PPV-MF or PET-MF, the Myelofibrosis Secondary Prognostic Model (MYSEC-PM) is used. In addition to age > 65 years (3 points), MYSEC-PM includes the time to development of MF > 15 years (2 points), history of thrombosis (2 points), constitutional symptoms (2 points), Hgb < 10 g/dL (1 point), and circulating blasts ≥ 1% (2 points). MYSEC-PM categorizes secondary MF into low-risk (mOS not reached), intermediate-risk (mOS 7.9 years), and high-risk (mOS 3.8 years) groups. When applying any of these prognostic models for an individual patient, it should be interpreted with caution as these are medians, and a given patient could be on either end of the survival curve owing to the clinical and biological heterogeneity of PMF.

5) How do you incorporate genomic features into the prognostication of PMF?

Expert Perspective: The prognostic impact of MPN driver mutations, especially the favorable type 1 CALR, and the unfavorable triple-negative (*JAK2/MPL/CALR*-negative) status in PMF prompted the inclusion of genomic data in disease prognostication. Additionally, genomic studies have identified that the presence of *ASXL1, SRSF2, U2AF1 Q157, EZH2, IDH1/2* mutations independently predicted poor outcomes and portended a high molecular risk (HMR) signature in patients with PMF. The Genetically Inspired Prognostic Scoring System (GIPSS) and Mutation-Enhanced International Prognostic Scoring System (MIPSS70 + v2.0) incorporates molecular data in their prognostic models. In terms of genomic variables, absence of type 1–like CALR mutation is included in both models; while GIPSS includes the presence of *ASXL1, SRSF2*, and *U2AF1 Q157, MIPSS70 + v2.0* includes the number of HMR mutations, i.e. *ASXL1, SRSF2, U2AF1 Q157, EZH2, IDH1/2* for prognostication. MIPSS70 + v2.0 is more comprehensive as it incorporates both clinical and cytogenomic variables for risk prognostication. Most recently, targeted sequencing of 69 genes in 2035 patients with MPN, including 309 with myelofibrosis, also identified a prognostic role for *CBL, NRAS, RUNX1, TET2*, and *TP53* mutations among others, in predicting both OS and LFS. This model integrated a number of demographic, clinical, and genomic variables to provide a personalized prognostic prediction in MPNs (a prognostic calculator derived from this model can be accessed at https://cancer.sanger.ac.uk/mpn-multistage). This model compared favorably to the DIPSS model when stratified according to *CALR/ASXL1* mutations and HMR status in patients with PMF.

Undoubtedly, integrating molecular profile with the clinical data vastly improves our cognizance of disease pathogenesis and the biology of leukemic transformation in PMF, although a few caveats are worth mentioning: next-generation sequencing may not be available in all practice settings; testing sample might not be obtainable in some situations (e.g. "dry tap"); most importantly, molecular studies may be less "dynamic" than DIPSS variables, as they cannot be obtained at each visit and may not capture timely clonal evolution. That being said, in the authors' academic clinical practice, we routinely use next-generation sequencing (when possible) to identify the molecular signature of PMF at diagnosis and clinically evident disease progression to guide us in risk-adapted therapy.

6) What are the indications to start a JAK inhibitor in PMF?

Expert Perspective: JAK inhibitors are the mainstay of front-line therapy in patients with PMF independent of *JAK2* mutational status. Ruxolitinib was the first JAK inhibitor approved based on the pivotal COMFORT I and II randomized phase III trials, which compared ruxolitinib to placebo and best available therapy, respectively. Both of these clinical trials demonstrated superiority in terms of spleen reduction and improvement in symptoms. In addition, there are also numerous lines of evidence suggesting improved overall survival with ruxolitinib. However, it is important to note that ruxolitinib does not impact clonal evolution of PMF and has not demonstrated an impact on the rates of progression to acute leukemia, termed MPN blast phase (MPN-BP). Nevertheless, the quality-of-life improvements with ruxolitinib are undeniable. Fedratinib was more recently approved for both previously treated and newly diagnosed myelofibrosis. In clinical practice, fedratinib is rarely given in the front-line setting, although it has been shown to have similar efficacy in patients with platelets 50–100 × 10^9/L as in those with higher platelet counts.

In general, asymptomatic and low-risk patients may be monitored without treatment. Initiation of JAK inhibitor, in particular ruxolitinib, is recommended for patients who have symptomatic splenomegaly or constitutional symptoms such as fevers, night sweats, fatigue, weight loss, pruritus, or bone pain. While the DIPSS prognostic scoring system can be helpful in identifying appropriate patients, we prefer to employ JAK inhibitors based on symptom and spleen-related complaints rather than risk score alone.

It is important to note that ruxolitinib and fedratinib have on-target myelosuppression, given that the erythropoietin and thrombopoietin receptors are JAK-STAT dependent. Therefore, these agents cannot be given to patients with platelet counts < 50 × 10^9/L and should be given with caution in patienst with transfusion-dependent anemia. Importantly, anemia does not affect the response to ruxolitinib, and treatment of emergent anemia with ruxolitinib therapy does not have an adverse impact on overall survival, and thus, anemia should not be the sole reason for discontinuation. In addition, patients with a *JAK2V617F* allele burden less than 50% are less likely to respond to ruxolitinib compared with those who have an allele burden of 50% or greater. Patients with complex genetic disease, as evidenced by three or more non-driver mutations, have a significantly lower rate of spleen response.

Ruxolitinib is generally well tolerated, but there are several adverse effects that are important to recognize. Weight gain is observed almost universally. In the COMFORT I trial, the median weight gain at 24 weeks was 3.9 kg. Although this weight gain is frequently welcomed by cachectic patients, the metabolic impact is unclear and may be detrimental. Ruxolitinib may also increase the risk of infections and secondary malignancies. The most well-established infection that ruxolitinib increase the risk of is herpes zoster. Therefore, vaccination with the recombinant zoster vaccine (Singrex) is recommended. While there is a suggestion that ruxoilitinib may increase the risk of lymphoma, as observed in one study, this relationship has not been validated in multiple other evaluations. However, there is an increase in non-melanomatous skin cancer with ruxolitinib.

7) What are the treatment options for PMF that is relapsed or refractory to a JAK inhibitor?

Expert Perspective: Discontinuation of ruxolitinib is a well-established poor prognostic marker that is associated with a median overall survival of 11–15 months. Ruxolitinib relapse/refractoriness is generally defined as treatment for three or more months with < 10% spleen volume reduction (SVR) or < 30% decrease in spleen length from baseline or regrowth to these parameters. In addition, patients may be intolerant to ruxolitinib because of development of transfusion-dependent anemia or severe thrombocytopenia. Currently, the only United States Food and Drug Administration approved treatment for patients with PMF that are intolerant or refractory to ruxolitinib is the *JAK2/FLT3* inhibitor fedratinib. Data supporting this approval comes from the phase II open-label, single-arm JAKARTA-2 trial. In this trial, 97 MF patients who were either ruxolitinib resistant (67%) or intolerant (33%) were treated with fedratinib 400 mg daily. Of the 83 evaluable at 24 weeks, 46 patients (55%) achieved a spleen reduction of at least 35%. Spleen responses were observed in both ruxolitinib-resistant and -intolerant patients. In the 90 evaluable patients for symptom response, 23 patients (26%) achieved a reduction in the MPN Symptom Assessment Form Total Symptom Score of at least 50%.

Thus, fedratinib is an effective, commercially available treatment option for patients who have continued symptomatic splenomegaly or uncontrolled constitutional symptoms. When transitioning to fedratinib from ruxolitinib, a cross taper is necessary. The authors' current practice is to taper ruxolitinib over five days and start 400 mg fedratinib on day 3 of the taper, therefore overlapping therapy for three days. Similar to ruxolitinib, fedratinib is associated with myelosuppression, although recent data confirms the safety and efficacy at 400 mg daily in patients with a baseline platelet count of $50–100 \times 10^9/L$. Of note, development of fedratinib was temporarily halted as a result of several patients developing Wernicke encephalopathy. Further review of all patients treated with fedratinib suggests that this is an exceedingly rare complication. Regardless, thiamine levels should be checked before starting fedratinib, and any symptoms of encephalopathy should prompt immediate discontinuation of fedratinib and initiation of thiamine supplementation.

Few therapeutic options exist for ruxolitinib relapsed/intolerant patients who are not eligible for fedratinib. In appropriate patients, HSCT should be pursued (Chapter 24). At present, transplant-ineligible patients should be referred for clinical trial. In patients with high-risk features or increasing blast count, hypomethylating agents, most commonly decitabine 20 mg/m^2 for five days in a 28-day cycle, may provide prolongation of survival and reduction in splenomegaly.

8) How do you treat patients with PMF and anemia?

Expert Perspective: Anemia is a common and clinically challenging scenario in the care of patients with PMF. Nearly 40% of patients with PMF have a hemoglobin level less than 10 g/dL at diagnosis, and almost 25% are already transfusion dependent. Anemia has been consistently associated with inferior survival and negatively impacts quality of life. Inadequate erythropoiesis secondary to bone marrow fibrosis, sequestration from spleno-megaly, inflammatory cytokines–mediated increased hepcidin expression, and treatment-related anemia from JAK inhibitors all contribute to anemia in PMF patients.

Several agents have demonstrated efficacy for the treatment of anemia in PMF patients. Erythropoietin stimulating agents (ESAs) may be successfully deployed in patients with low serum erythropoietin levels (less than 125 U/L), although less than half will respond. Patients should be continued for a minimum of three months before discontinuation to evaluate for a response. Danazol, a synthetic attenuated androgen, can induce anemia responses in approxi-mately 40% and 20% of transfusion-dependent and -independent patients, respectively. This agent is well tolerated, although mild transaminitis can occur and prostate-specific antigen must be monitored in men receiving danazol. Of note, a fraction of patients with concomitant thrombocytopenia may also benefit from this treatment. Immunomodulators, namely thalido-mide or lenalidomide, combined with prednisone can also produce an anemia response in approximately 30% of patients with PMF.

Novel agents are also being explored for the treatment of PMF-related anemia. Luspatercept is an activin ligand trap that promotes erythroid differentiation and is approved for the treatment of beta thalassemia and myelodysplastic syndrome. In myelofibrosis clinical trials, this agent was associated with anemia responses in approximately 10% of patients as a single agent and 30% of patients with anemia while being treated with ruxolitinib. This agent is cur-rently being evaluated in a phase III clinical trial (NCT04717414) and may be a treatment option for anemic PMF patients, particularly in the setting of JAK inhibitor treatment.

Next-generation JAK inhibitors are being developed to address anemia in patients with mye-lofibrosis. Momelotinib is a selective inhibitor of *JAK1*, *JAK2*, and *ACVR1*, which is being devel-oped in anemic MF patients. This agent decreases hepcidin production, allowing for increased iron availability and improved erythropoiesis. In the phase III SIMPLIFY trial, momelotinib and ruxolitinib were non-inferior for spleen response but not symptom response. However, transfu-sion requirements and dependence were significantly reduced with momelotinib as compared with ruxolitinib. The FDA approved momelotinib supported by data from the pivotal MOMENTUM study (NCT04173494) and a subpopulation of adults with anemia from the SIMPLIFY-1 phase III trial (NCT01969838). Momelotinib is approved for the treatment of intermediate- or high-risk myelofibrosis, including primary myelofibrosis or secondary myelofi-brosis (post–polycythemia vera and post–essential thrombocythemia), in adults with anemia.

9) How do you treat patients with PMF and thrombocytopenia?

Expert Perspective: Thrombocytopenia has consistently been demonstrated to be a poor prognostic factor in PMF. In a study of 1,269 patients at a large academic setting, platelets less than 50×10^9/L was associated with a survival of 13 months. In addition, thrombocy-topenia is associated with an increased risk of leukemic transformation. Management of thrombocytopenic PMF patients is challenging as currently available JAK inhibitors are associated with thrombocytopenia and cannot be used in patients with a platelet count of less than 50×10^9/L. Eligible patients should be referred for HSCT (Chapter 24). Treatment options for transplant-ineligible patients are limited.

Pacritinib (200 mg twice daily) is a *JAK2/IRAK1* inhibitor that was granted accelerated approval to treat adults who have intermediate or high-risk primary or secondary myelofibrosis and who have platelet levels below 50×10^9/L. This agent has demonstrated effectiveness in patients with myelofibrosis, in particular patients with baseline thrombocytopenia and/or a low *JAK2* allele burden. Pacritinib is contraindicated in patients concomitantly using strong CYP3A4 inhibitors or inducers as these medications can significantly alter exposure to pacritinib, which may increase the risk of adverse reactions or impair efficacy. The drug can also cause prolonged QTc interval. The accelerated approval was based on efficacy results from the pivotal Phase III PERSIST-2 study in patients with myelofibrosis (platelet counts $\leq 100 \times 10^9$/L). Patients were randomized 1:1:1 to receive pacritinib 200 mg twice daily, pacritinib 400 mg once daily, or best available therapy. Prior *JAK2* inhibitor therapy was permitted. In this study, in the cohort of patients with baseline platelet counts below 50×10^9/L who were treated with pacritinib 200 mg twice a day, 29% of patients had a reduction in spleen volume of at least 35% compared to 3% of patients receiving best available therapy, which included ruxolitinib.

Immunomodulatory drugs may improve thrombocytopenia, especially when combined with a corticosteroid. Lenalidomide is the most widely used, but other thalidomide derivatives, including pomalidomide, can improve platelet counts, albeit in a minority of patients. Unfortunately, these agents have an adverse effect profile, which precludes their use in many patients. Surgical splenectomy should also be considered for appropriate patients with refractory thrombocytopenia. However, there is still an urgent need for effective therapies in thrombocytopenic PMF patients.

10) What is the role of allogeneic hematopoietic stem cell transplantation (HSCT) in PMF?

Expert Perspective: Allogeneic HSCT is the only curative intent treatment strategy for myelofibrosis. Both the European and the American Society for Transplantation and Cellular Therapy (ASTCT) guidelines concur that patients aged < 70 years, and with intermediate-2- or high-risk disease per DIPSS/DIPSS-plus should be considered for HSCT (Figure 23.2). Patients aged < 65 years and with intermediate-1-risk disease should be considered if they have refractory, transfusion-dependent anemia, or > 2% circulating blasts, or adverse (per DIPSS-plus score) cytogenetics. But these recommendations were developed before the genomic era of personalized prognosis in PMF, which brings forth the question if transplant-eligible patients with HMR and triple-negative disease should be considered for earlier HSCT. As the risk groups of DIPSS predict only pre-HSCT survival, the Myelofibrosis Transplant Scoring System (MTSS) was developed to predict post-HSCT outcomes in PMF and secondary MF. This model identified pre-HSCT thrombocytopenia ($< 150 \times 10^9$/L), leukocytosis ($> 25 \times 10^9$/L), older age (≥ 57 years), Karnofsky performance status < 90%, a non-*CALR/MPL* or *JAK2V617F* and triple-negative driver mutation genotype, *ASXL1*-mutation, and HLA-mismatched unrelated donor transplant as independent predictors of overall survival. Of note, this model did not include transplant comorbidity index, which significantly affects transplant outcomes; nonetheless, it is a useful tool to

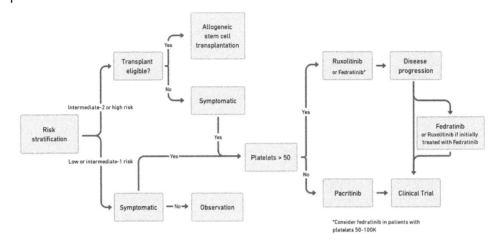

Figure 23.2 Proposed PMF treatment algorithm based on NCCN guidelines. Patients who are intermediate-2 or higher risk by dynamic international prognostic scoring system should be referred for allogeneic transplantation. Symptomatic patients should be treated with ruxolitinib unless they are ineligible because of thrombocytopenia. In patients who are relapsed, refractory, or intolerant to ruxolitinib, fedratinib can be attempted, but early clinical trial evaluation is also appropriate. Momelotinib is the fourth JAK inhibitor approved by FDA (see text).

counsel patients regarding post-HSCT outcomes. The recommendations for younger patients with intermediate-1-risk disease are murkier as the benefit of HSCT must be carefully weighed against the risks of treatment-related morbidity and mortality. In general, the transplant decision is determined by careful comprehensive assessment of the individual patient, guided by a multidisciplinary approach (Chapter 24).

11) Is there a role for ruxolitinib in the peri-transplant setting?

Expert Perspective: In the peri-transplant setting, ruxolitinib by virtue of its *JAK2* inhibition may dampen an inherently pro-inflammatory milieu to improve a patient's performance status, reduce splenomegaly, and potentially shorten the time to engraftment. Studies have demonstrated poor outcomes if ruxolitinib is stopped abruptly leading to cytokine rebound, resulting in occasionally life-threatening "ruxolitinib withdrawal syndrome" characterized by acute symptomatic deterioration, accelerated splenomegaly, worsening of cytopenias, and hemodynamic compromise. Therefore, ruxolitinib should be gradually tapered close to the start of the conditioning regimen, although the optimal tapering schedule varies in different studies. If there is significant concern for withdrawal syndrome, steroids may be added to the taper or ruxolitinib maybe continued throughout, as this strategy has been shown to be well tolerated and does not affect the engraftment. However, there is an increased risk of infections and viral reactivation, especially cytomegalovirus, with ruxolitinib taper closer to the start of conditioning regimen, due to its inhibitory effect on the function of dendritic cells and natural killer cells, warranting close monitoring to prevent graft failure. Ruxolitinib use in the peri-transplant setting does not seem to alter relapse risk, and its role in the prophylaxis of acute graft-versus-host disease needs to be formally evaluated.

12) What are the investigational agents in development?

Expert Perspective: Based on sound mechanistic rationale, there are several agents under clinical investigation in PMF either as stand-alone or combination therapy. These agents exploit several interconnected pathogenetic pathways including epigenetic modifiers, apoptotic pathways, host immunity, tumor microenvironment, and DNA replication. Imetelstat is one such exciting agent, a potent, first-in-class, competitive inhibitor of telomerase enzymatic activity that specifically targets the RNA template of human telomerase. Preclinical studies have shown that patients with MPNs have short telomeres due to enhanced activity of telomerase, independent of *JAK2* mutation status. In 2021, a phase II randomized dose-finding study of imetelstat (9.4 mg/kg or 4.7 mg/kg) in patients with relapsed/refractory (R/R) myelofibrosis reported ≥ 35% spleen volume reduction (SVR35) in 10.2% and ≥ 50% total symptom score reduction (TSS50) in 32.2% of patients in the 9.4 mg/kg arm (0% and 6.3%, respectively, in the 4.7 mg/kg arm). Imetelstat was well tolerated and exhibited on-target activity that correlated with spleen response, symptom response, and OS. Most importantly, patients treated on 9.4 mg/kg imetelstat had a median OS of 29.9 months in addition to the improvement in bone marrow fibrosis (40.5%), which correlated with OS. Based on this encouraging disease-modifying activity, a registration trial of imetelstat in PMF patients relapsed and refractory to JAK inhibitors (NCT04576156) is underway, with overall survival as the primary endpoint, a hitherto unexplored endpoint in the treatment landscape of PMF.

Navitoclax, an oral small-molecule inhibitor of antiapoptotic B-cell lymphoma 2 proteins (BCL-XL, BCL-2, BCL-W) is being evaluated in combination with ruxolitinib in patients with suboptimal response to ruxolitinib. In a phase II study of 34 PMF patients treated with this combination, 27% SVR35 and 30% TSS50 were observed at week 24, and improvement in bone marrow fibrosis was observed in 33% of the cohort. Thrombocytopenia was the common adverse event necessitating dose reduction. Navitoclax and ruxolitinib combination is undergoing phase III evaluation in patients with myelofibrosis in both treatment-naive and relapsed and refractory setting (NCT04472598; NCT04468984).

Phosphatidylinositol 3-kinase (PI3K)/Protein kinase B (Akt) pathway escape has been shown to be a mechanism of suboptimal responses to ruxolitinib. Parsaclisib, a highly selective PI3Kδ inhibitor, is being evaluated as an add-on to ruxolitinib in patients with suboptimal response to ruxolitinib. An elegantly designed dose-finding phase II study identified a daily dose of 5 mg parsaclisib in combination with stable dose of ruxolitinib as the most efficacious and least likely to cause class-specific adverse events of PI3K inhibitors. Parsaclisib and ruxolitinib combination is undergoing phase III evaluation in both treatment naïve (NCT04551066) and those with suboptimal response to ruxolitinib (NCT04551053).

The bromodomain and extra terminal domain (BET) family of proteins regulate gene transcription of several pro-fibrotic cytokines, and BET inhibitor (CPI-0610, pelabresib) has shown preclinical activity in PMF. In a multi-arm phase II study, pelabresib was evaluated as monotherapy in R/R MF, as add-on to ruxolitinib in patients with suboptimal response, and in combination with ruxolitinib in the treatment-naive setting. Pelabresib was generally well tolerated. In the treatment-naive setting, pelabresib in combination with ruxolitinib demonstrated an impressive SVR35 of 67% at week 24, leading to the evaluation of phase III randomized, double-blind study evaluating pelabresib and ruxolitinib combination against ruxolitinib in patients with JAKi-naive myelofibrosis (NCT04603495).

The Murine double minute 2 (MDM2), a key negative regulator of p53, has shown to be overexpressed in CD34 + hematopoietic stem/progenitor cells in MPNs. KRT-232, an oral small molecule inhibitor of MDM2, has shown preliminary efficacy in PMF and is now enrolling on a phase II/III study in the relapsed and refractory setting (NCT03662126).

Additional agents in early phase of clinical development in PMF, include bomedemstat (lysine-specific demethylase 1 inhibitor; NCT03136185), ruxolitinib and pegylated interferon alfa-2a combination (NCT02742324), LCL-161 [second mitochondrial activator of caspases (SMAC) mimetic; NCT02098161], and AVID200 (selective TGFβ1 ligand trap; NCT03895112). Whenever possible, clinicians should strongly consider enrolling PMF patients on a clinical trial as curative intent HSCT is not a feasible option for many, and there is an urgent unmet need for effective therapies in PMF patients with cytopenias, and in the JAKi R/R setting (see Chapter 24).

Recommended Readings

Arber, DA., Orazi, A., Hasserjian, R., Thiele, J., Borowitz, MJ., Le Beau, M.M., Bloomfield, CD., Cazzola, M., Vardiman, J.W. (2016 May 19). The 2016 revision to the World Health Organization classification of myeloid neoplasms and acute leukemia. *Blood* 127 (20): 2391-2405. doi: 10.1182/blood-2016-03-643544. Epub 2016 Apr 11. PMID: 27069254.

Barbui, T., Tefferi, A., Vannucchi, A.M. et al. (2018). Philadelphia chromosome-negative classical myeloproliferative neoplasms: revised management recommendations from European LeukemiaNet. *Leukemia* 32 (5): 1057–1069.

Grinfeld, J., Nangalia, J., Baxter, E.J. et al. (2018). Classification and personalized prognosis in myeloproliferative neoplasms. *N Engl J Med* 379 (15): 1416–1430.

Guglielmelli, P., Pacilli, A., Rotunno, G. et al. (2017). Presentation and outcome of patients with 2016 WHO diagnosis of prefibrotic and overt primary myelofibrosis. *Blood* 129 (24): 3227–3236.

Harrison, C.N., Schaap, N., Vannucchi, A.M. et al. (2017). Janus kinase-2 inhibitor fedratinib in patients with myelofibrosis previously treated with ruxolitinib (JAKARTA-2): a single-arm, open-label, non-randomised, phase 2, multicentre study. *Lancet Haematol* 4 (7): e317–e324.

Kroger, N., Giorgino, T., Scott, B.L. et al. (2015). Impact of allogeneic stem cell transplantation on survival of patients less than 65 years of age with primary myelofibrosis. *Blood* 125 (21): 3347–3350. quiz 3364.

Mascarenhas, J., Hoffman, R., Talpaz, M. et al. (2018). Pacritinib vs best available therapy, including ruxolitinib, in patients with myelofibrosis: a randomized clinical trial. *JAMA Oncol* 4 (5): 652–659.

Newberry, K.J., Patel, K., Masarova, L. et al. (2017). Clonal evolution and outcomes in myelofibrosis after ruxolitinib discontinuation. *Blood* 130 (9): 1125–1131.

Passamonti, F., Cervantes, F., Vannucchi, A.M. et al. (2010). A dynamic prognostic model to predict survival in primary myelofibrosis: a study by the IWG-MRT (International Working Group for Myeloproliferative Neoplasms Research and Treatment). *Blood* 115 (9): 1703–1708.

Vannucchi, A.M., Guglielmelli, P., Lasho, T.L. et al. (2017). MIPSS70: mutation-enhanced prognostic system for transplant age patients with primary myelofibrosis. *Blood* 130 (Suppl 1): 200–200.

Verstovsek, S., Mesa, R.A., Gotlib, J. et al. (2012). A double-blind, placebo-controlled trial of ruxolitinib for myelofibrosis. *N Engl J Med* 366 (9): 799–807.

24

Hematopoietic Cell Transplantation and Cellular Therapy in Primary and Post ET/PV Myelofibrosis

Jerry Luo[1], Irum Khan[2], and Damiano Rondelli[1]

[1] *University of Illinois, Chicago, IL*
[2] *Northwestern University Feinberg School of Medicine, Chicago, IL*

Introduction

Allogeneic stem cell transplantation is currently the only curative therapy for myelofibrosis, and several recent advances have fueled increased utilization in the past decade. Transplant-related mortality remains a significant impediment making this procedure most appropriate in intermediate-1 or higher-risk patients. Refinements in clinical prognostic scoring systems with incorporation of molecular markers have allowed for more judicious selection and monitoring of transplant candidates. The introduction of novel JAK inhibitors such as ruxolitinib has the potential to reduce pre-transplant symptom burden and post-transplant complications such as graft-versus-host disease. The development of reduced-intensity conditioning regimens, liberalization of donor sources, and lower GvHD rates with post-transplant cyclophosphamide have resulted in incremental gains in transplant outcomes in this challenging disease. Future studies will illuminate how best to integrate targeted inhibitors to optimize the outcomes of transplant.

1) Is there a cure for myelofibrosis?

Expert Perspective: Allogeneic hematopoietic stem cell transplantation (allo-HSCT) is currently the only curative therapy for patients with primary myelofibrosis (MF), myelofibrosis secondary to polycythemia vera (PV-MF), or essential thrombocythemia (ET-MF). Advancements in novel therapeutics, resulting in decreased pre-transplant symptom burden and post-transplant acute graft-versus-host disease (GvHD), reduced-intensity conditioning (RIC) regimens, liberalization of donor matching, and improved peri-transplant management have led to incremental utilization of allo-HSCT worldwide. According to the European Society for Blood and Marrow Transplantation (EBMT) database, before 2006, only 389 patients with MF underwent allo-HSCT, compared to nearly 1700 from 2015 to 2018. Due to concerns of transplant-related morbidity and mortality, this therapy remains reserved for intermediate- to high-risk patients. Response criteria in the non-HSCT setting have been established by the International Working Group-Myeloproliferative Neoplasms Research and Treatment (IWG-MRT) and European Leukemia Net (ELN), as well as the MDS/MPN International Working Group (IWG). The criteria for complete remission of myelofibrosis is defined by lasting molecular, pathological, and clinical regression following allogeneic transplantation. This includes the normalization of hematopoiesis, reversal of marrow fibrosis with a reduction in blast cells, reduction of hepatosplenomegaly, and no evidence of extramedullary disease.

Cancer Consult: Expertise in Clinical Practice, Volume 2: Neoplastic Hematology & Cellular Therapy,
Second Edition. Edited by Syed A. Abutalib, Maurie Markman, James O. Armitage, and Kenneth C. Anderson.
© 2024 John Wiley & Sons Ltd. Published 2024 by John Wiley & Sons Ltd.

The effect of transplant relies both on the initial activity of the preparative regimen in reducing disease burden in the marrow and extramedullary sites and on a long-term immunological effect mediated by T lymphocytes in the graft against clonal hematopoietic cells. Complete remission usually occurs over 12–24 months following transplant, and a recent meta-analysis of over 8,000 patients reported five-year overall survival (OS) of 55%. Patients with advanced MF, including accelerated- and blast-phase disease, have inferior outcomes than those in chronic phase; however, transplantation has curative potential in those patients who are eligible for this approach.

Current approved pharmacological treatments are directed toward symptomatology and include several JAK1/2 inhibitors for constitutional symptoms and splenomegaly, while erythropoiesis-stimulating agents, danazol, and recently, activin receptor ligand trap luspatercept are being investigated for anemia. Investigational telomerase inhibitors and recombinant human pentraxin-2 molecule (PRM-151) have demonstrated clinical activity against fibrosis. Interferons have been shown to improve hematologic parameters and induce molecular remission; however, they are also not curative.

2) Who is a candidate for allogeneic HSCT in primary myelofibrosis?

Expert Perspective: Given the marked heterogeneity in the clinical course of myelofibrosis and considerable morbidity and mortality associated with transplantation, it is vital to have a reliable prognostic system to select patients who will benefit most. Studies have shown that long-term survival advantages from allo-HSCT come at the expense of early transplant-related mortality, especially in the first year after transplant, further emphasizing the need to carefully identify suitable candidates for transplant. Furthermore, newer therapies and improved transplant outcomes have led to increasing numbers of transplants in older individuals. An International Prognostic Scoring System (IPSS) was developed in 2009 and encompassed five independent risk factors: age > 65 years, WBC > 25×10^9/L, Hb < 10 g/dL, peripheral blood blasts ≥ 1%, and presence of constitutional symptoms. A subsequent iteration of this prognostic scoring system, called dynamic IPSS (DIPSS), made it applicable at all time points in the disease course and increased weightage for anemia given its disproportionately higher impact on survival. Unfavorable cytogenetic abnormalities were shown to significantly affect post-transplant survival as well as the risk of leukemic transformation in myelofibrosis. DIPSS was modified (DIPSS-plus) to include red cell transfusion dependency, platelet count < 100×10^9/L, and unfavorable karyotype. Based on the presence of 0–4 or more factors, patients at low-, intermediate-1, intermediate-2, and high-risk disease have a median survival of 15.4, 6.5, 2.9, and 1.3 years, respectively. The DIPSS was retrospectively applied to a cohort of transplant patients in two separate analyses with similar results, confirming the prognostic value of this system in a transplant setting.

The newest prognostic scoring systems, the MIPSS70 (mutation-enhanced international prognostic scoring system for transplant-age patients) and GIPSS (genetically inspired prognostic scoring system), integrate mutations and karyotype with clinical risk factors. MIPSS70 applies to patients 70 or younger and includes three genetic (absence of CALR type 1–like mutation, high molecular risk mutations, and presence of ≥ 2 high molecular risk mutations) and six clinical risk factors (hemoglobin < 10 g/dL, WBC > 25×10^9/L, platelet count < 100×10^9/L, circulating blasts ≥ 2%, bone marrow fibrosis grade ≥ 2, and constitutional symptoms). The specific high-risk mutations identified include *ASXL1*,

SRSF2, *EZH2*, and *IDH1/2*. A weighted score of 2 is assigned to leukocytosis, thrombocytopenia, and the presence of ≥ 2 high molecular risk mutations. Total scores in the range 0–5 define low, intermediate, and high-risk disease corresponding to a median survival of 27.7, 7.1, and 2.3 years, respectively. The MIPSS70-plus model only considers three of the aforementioned risk factors (anemia, circulating blasts ≥ 2%, and constitutional symptoms) and adds the presence of an unfavorable karyotype with a weighted score of 3. Total scores can be up to 12 and a very high-risk category was added to scores of ≥ 7. Further revision of the MIPSS in 2018 (MIPSS70+ 2.0) incorporated cytogenic risk stratification and new sex- and severity-adjusted hemoglobin thresholds. It also recognized *U2AF1Q157* as an HMR. When applied retroactively, MIPSS70 and MIPSS70+ 2.0 have been shown to predict transplant outcomes better than DIPSS. The GIPSS is a less complex prognostic score that is exclusively based on karyotype and mutations. In a study of practices across Europe in 2020, the most frequently used scoring system was DIPSS-plus, followed by DIPSS, but many institutions used more than one.

Current consensus guidelines from ELN/EBMT state that patients under 70 years old with intermediate-2 or high-risk disease as determined by IPSS, DIPSS, or DIPSS-plus should be considered potential candidates. Those with intermediate-1-risk disease and age under 65 should be considered if they have either refractory, transfusion-dependent anemia, peripheral blood blasts > 2%, or adverse cytogenetics as defined by DIPSS-plus.

Efforts to develop a model to prognosticate outcomes after HSCT rather than determine who should be referred to transplantation have led to the development of the myelofibrosis transplant scoring system (MTSS). The model incorporates clinical, molecular, and transplantation factors to stratify patients into four risk groups. Factors that differ from existing scoring systems include Karnofsky performance status < 90% and the use of a mismatched unrelated donor. MTSS does not incorporate high-risk mutations, aside from *ASXL1*, or cytogenetic risk factors, as univariable analysis did not show an effect on survival.

Leukemic transformation: One major goal of transplant is to prevent leukemic transformation, which can be a catastrophic terminal event in myelofibrosis. Chances of success with chemotherapy are dismal, with a median survival of 2.7 months. Recent research demonstrated downregulation of liver-inducible kinase (LKB1)/serine/threonine kinase 11 (STK11) appears to be a critical driving event in leukemic transformation, suggesting that LKB1/STK11 acts as a tumor suppressor. This process occurs via stabilization of the transcription factor hypoxia-inducible factor 1-alpha (HIF1α), and thereby presents novel therapeutic targets to prevent leukemic transformation and allow more patients to proceed to transplant. While limited in numbers, in a small series of 13 patients transplanted in the blast phase, 49% of patients were alive after a median follow-up of 31 months.

3) What factors are associated with transplant outcomes?

Expert Perspective: Progress in allo-HSCT over the past two decades was mostly related to the development of novel conditioning regimens using reduced intensity, improved antimicrobial prophylaxis, and improved GvHD prophylaxis. Several non-disease factors such as age, donor type, and comorbidities affect outcome following allo-HSCT in myelofibrosis.

In earlier studies with myeloablative conditioning (MAC) regimens, patient age at the time of transplantation represented an important prognostic factor, with a five-year survival of only 14% in patients older than 45 years compared with 62% in younger patients. Transplant-related mortality significantly decreased upon the introduction of reduced-intensity conditioning (RIC). However, multiple factors have been suggested as independent prognostic factors for toxicity in RIC transplants. A large EBMT retrospective study of 2,224 patients undergoing MAC or RIC transplant between 2000 and 2014 demonstrated similar overall survival (OS) regardless of MAC or RIC regimens overall, but for the younger, fitter patients, MAC resulted in superior relapse and GvHD-free survival while RIC had a significant advantage for patients > 50 years old, those who received transplantation from an unrelated donor, and patients with lower performance status.

The *calreticulin (CALR)* mutation seen in 30% of MF cases has demonstrated predictive potential in transplant outcomes. Patients with mutated CALR had a better OS after allo-HSCT than those with wild-type *CALR* (four-year OS 82% vs 56%, respectively, P = 0.043). More specifically, patients with mutated *CALR* had the best prognosis, patients with *JAK2* or MPL mutations had an intermediate prognosis, and triple-negative patients had the worst prognosis. Kroger et al. similarly demonstrated that *CALR* mutation was associated with lower non-relapse mortality and improved OS. *ASXL1* and *IDH2* mutations were associated with worse progression-free survival.

Another single-center study demonstrated that spleen size > 22 cm, transfusion history > 20 units, and any donor other than a matched sibling donor (MSD) (e.g. a matched or mismatched unrelated donor, or a mismatched related donor) predicted an adverse outcome. Analysis of the French stem cell transplantation registry showed that factors favorably affecting engraftment were splenectomy before allo-HSCT, a human leukocyte antigen (HLA)-matched sibling donor, peripheral stem cell use as a source of stem cells, and the absence of pre-transplant thrombocytopenia. In the GITMO experience, a longer interval between diagnosis and transplant negatively affected survival after allo-HSCT. A recent CIBMTR/EBMT report examined the data of 623 patients undergoing allo-HCT between 2000 and 2016 in the United States (the CIBMTR cohort). A Cox multivariable model was used to identify factors prognostic of mortality. A weighted score using these factors was assigned to patients who received transplantation in Europe (the EBMT cohort; n = 623). Patient age >50 years (HR, 1.39; 95% CI, 0.98-1.96), and HLA-matched unrelated donor (HR, 1.29; 95% CI, 0.98-1.7) were associated with an increased hazard of death and were assigned 1 point. Hemoglobin levels <10 g/dL at time of transplantation (HR, 1.63; 95% CI, 1.2-2.19) and a mismatched unrelated donor (HR, 1.78; 95% CI, 1.25-2.52) were assigned 2 points. The 3-year OS in patients with a low (1-2 points), intermediate (3-4 points), and high score (5 points) were 69% (95% CI, 61-76), 51% (95% CI, 46-56.4), and 34% (95% CI, 21-49), respectively (P < .001). Increasing score was predictive of increased TRM (P = .0017) but not of relapse (P = .12). The derived score was predictive of OS (P < .001) and TRM (P = .002) but not of relapse (P = .17) in the EBMT cohort as well. The proposed system was prognostic of survival in 2 large cohorts, CIBMTR and EBMT, and can easily be applied by clinicians consulting patients with MF about the transplantation outcomes.

With the introduction of JAK1/2 inhibitors, it has been hypothesized that the use of these agents before transplantation may improve performance status, splenomegaly, and reduce cytokine levels, leading to better post-transplant outcomes. A retrospective study from Shanavas et al. (2015) of 100 patients who received JAK1/2 inhibitor therapy revealed a two-year OS of 61% overall and 91% for patients who experienced clinical improvement after therapy. However, response to JAK inhibitors may indicate a more favorable disease phenotype, leading to better outcomes. A German study of 46 patients who received pre-transplant ruxolitinib, compared to 113 patients who did not, showed lower relapse rates in the ruxolitinib group (9% vs 17%) with no difference in OS. Kroger et al. (2021) recently demonstrated similar findings in patients who were responsive to ruxolitinib and had ongoing spleen response at the time of transplant. These patients had significantly higher leukocyte engraftment at day 45 (94% vs 85%) without differences in non-relapse mortality. Those with active spleen response had a lower risk of relapse (8.1% vs 19%) and improved two-year event-free survival (68.9% vs 53.7%).

4) Is there a difference in outcome of allogeneic HSCT based on type of donor?

Expert Perspective: Yes. Several studies, including a large prospective trial, have reported similar outcomes in patients undergoing matched-related (MRD) and matched-unrelated donor (MUD) transplants, while outcomes of mismatched donors were significantly inferior. Contrary to this, using myelofibrosis retrospective data from the Center for International Blood and Marrow Transplant Research (CIBMTR) showed a one-year non-relapse mortality rate of 27% for an HLA-identical allo-HSCT and 43% for an HLA-matched unrelated HCT. Data from GITMO also revealed a reduction in non-relapse mortality associated with the choice of a matched sibling donor. The SFGM-TC registry, including patients with myelofibrosis transplanted between 1997 and 2008, showed engraftment probability and OS to be significantly inferior in non-sibling donors compared to MSDs. An Italian study also indicated that having a donor other than a matched sibling was an independent poor prognostic factor. The ambivalent results from these different studies could be attributable to small sample sizes, retrospective design, patient heterogeneity, and the different chemotherapy regimens utilized. In a prospective study of RIC allo-HSCT in 66 patients, with a median follow-up of 24 months, 78% in the related group are alive compared to 44% in the unrelated group at 12-month follow-up. Possible interpretations of these different results could be the conditioning regimen utilized, the combination of older age and more advanced disease in the unrelated group, or the degree of HLA compatibility. At this time, for patients < 65 years of age, in good overall condition, and with intermediate-2 or high-risk disease, a transplant from an MRD or MUD is indicated.

The use of mismatched related/haploidentical donors has been scarce given the risk of graft failure and GvHD. A significant improvement in the outcome of transplant from mismatched related (haploidentical) donors has been achieved by using post-transplant high-dose cyclophosphamide (PTCy) as GvHD prophylaxis. A retrospective analysis of 56 MMRD transplants from the EBMT database between 2009 and 2015 showed an acceptable 1- and 2-year OS of 61% and 58%, respectively. Neutrophil engraftment occurred in 82% of patients by 28 days, and the cumulative incidence of chronic GvHD at one year was 45%. However, non-relapse mortality at two years was higher at 38%. Another single-center study from Italy experienced an increase in alternative donors from 2011 to 2014 (n = 20) compared to 2000 to 2010 (n = 3) and improved survival in those patients (69% vs 21%), attributed to a reduction in total relapse mortality and relapse. The survival was similar to patients receiving matched sibling grafts (72%). Further studies investigating haploidenti-cal transplantation in the RIC setting are ongoing (NCT04370301).

A handful of studies have examined the feasibility and benefit of umbilical cord blood transplantation (UCBT) in myelofibrosis, but utilization remains rare. Small studies have demonstrated the feasibility of UCBT in patients with primary and secondary MF and further low-power studies demonstrated non-inferior OS when compared to other donor sources. Japanese national registry data (Murata et al. (2019)) showed significantly higher non-relapse mortality and lower incidence of neutrophil recovery with UCBT.

5) Is splenectomy or splenic irradiation indicated before a transplant?

Expert Perspective: Significant splenomegaly at the time of transplant may adversely affect time to engraftment, so the question of whether splenectomy should be offered to these patients has been addressed. A previous analysis at Mayo Clinic showed a 27.7% risk of peri-operative complications and a 6.7% mortality rate for splenectomy in myelofibrosis patients. Conflicting results have been reported on the survival benefit of pre-transplant splenectomy. An EBMT study reported a threefold increased risk of relapse after splenectomy, although it is argued that this may have been a reflection of more advanced disease. In contrast, an Italian study reported a reduced risk of relapse in patients who were splenectomized before allo-HSCT. Pre-transplant splenectomy has also been associated with a higher risk of blast trans-formation, with one study showing a cumulative incidence of 55% in splenectomized patients within 12 years after diagnosis versus 27% in nontransplant patients. A review of the data from the Fred Hutchinson Cancer Center showed that after adjustment for DIPSS score and the Hematopoietic Cell Transplant Comorbidity Index (HCT-CI), patients who had a splenectomy were at lower risk for mortality compared with patients who had not (HR = 0.44). Similarly, a French study demonstrated improved disease-free survival and OS in 39 splenectomized patients who underwent HSCT. However, larger studies examining retrospective data from the EBMT registry and Center for International Blood and Bone Marrow Transplant Research (CIBMTR) and two other studies failed to show an effect of splenectomy on disease-free survival or OS. Analysis of the EBMT registry also showed no difference among those who received MAC versus RIC. Postulated setbacks of splenectomy in the setting of allo-HSCT include a worsened severity of GvHD due to altered immunomodulation and an excess risk of acute myeloid leukemia transformation.

Few studies have examined the role of splenectomy in combination with JAK inhibitor therapy and it is typically reserved for patients that are unresponsive to drug therapy as a bridge to allo-HSCT. A Russian study of 12 patients with primary or secondary MF who had splenomegaly after receiving 3 months of ruxolitinib showed no mortality in the early post-operative period and all patients achieved complete remission with a two-year OS of 90%.

In the absence of any intervention for splenomegaly, successful engraftment can still occur. In a study of 10 patients with extensive splenomegaly, a progressive reduction of splenomegaly within 12 months post-RIC transplant was demonstrated, and it paralleled the reduction of marrow fibrosis. Given the absence of strong favorable evidence and inherent operating risks, at this time, routine splenectomy is not advocated before transplant. Recently, position paper on behalf of the Chronic Malignancies Working Party of the EBMT concluded that myelofibrosis patients with splenomegaly measuring 5 cm and larger, particularly when exceeding 15 cm below the left costal margin, or with splenomegaly-related symptoms, could benefit from treatment with the aim of reducing the spleen size before HSCT. In the absence of, or loss of, response, patients with increasing spleen size should be evaluated for second-line options, depending on availability, patient fitness, and center experience.

Splenic irradiation: Research examining the role of splenic irradiation before allo-HSCT has shown inconsistent evidence in support of the practice. Low-dose splenic irradiation was found to reduce spleen size by a median of 10 cm in a study of eight patients with splenomegaly before transplant without adverse effects. However, a study by Helbig et al. of 44 patients showed no benefit from splenic irradiation on post-transplant outcomes.

6) Myeloablative or reduced-intensity conditioning?

Expert Perspective: Early studies using conventional myeloablative conditioning (MAC) regimens for primary or secondary MF demonstrated prohibitive non-relapse mortality of 27–48%. This led to the introduction of RIC regimens, with the potential reduction in non-relapse mortality making allogeneic transplantation accessible to older patients and those with more advanced disease. In the early 2000s, several retrospective studies showed successful engraftment with stable full-donor hematopoietic chimerism and reversal of marrow fibrosis with RIC transplants in older patients. These studies used MSDs as well as MUDs. Conditioning regimens included mostly fludarabine-based regimens. A retrospective study of 21 patients by the Myeloproliferative Disorders-Research Consortium (MPD-RC) observed an OS of 85% and event-free survival of 76% with a median follow-up of 31 months, despite a median patient age of 54 years and all patients having intermediate- or high-risk disease according to the Lille score system. These encouraging findings suggested that myelofibrosis is highly responsive to donor T-cell alloantigen recognition eliciting a graft-versus-tumor effect.

This data led to a pilot study using RIC with busulfan (10 mg/kg), fludarabine (180 mg/m^2), and anti-thymocyte globulin (ATG) followed by allogeneic stem cell transplantation from related (n = 8) and unrelated donors (n = 13) in 21 myelofibrosis patients with hematological responses in 100%, and after a median follow-up of 22 months, the three-year estimated OS and disease-free survival were 84%. This was followed by an EBMT phase II multicenter prospective trial using a busulfan-fludarabine-based RIC regimen followed by allo-HSCT from related (n = 33) or unrelated donors (n = 70). Acute GvHD occurred in 27% of the patients and chronic GvHD in 43%. The estimated five-year event-free survival and OS rates were 51% and 67%, respectively. However, the prospective multicenter trial of the MPD-RC done in the United States and Europe using a RIC with fludarabine and melphalan (140 mg/m^2) showed better results in MSD vs MUD transplants. Of 66 patients with PMF or MF secondary to polycythemia vera (PV-MF) or essential thrombocythemia (ET-MF), 63 were at intermediate or high risk according to the Lille scoring system, and three were at low risk with thrombocytopenia. After a median follow-up of 24 months, non-relapse mortality was 18% in MSD and 53% in the MUD group, primarily due to a high rate of graft failure in this group. Median survival time has not been reached in the related transplant group and was seven months in the unrelated group.

There have been several retrospective comparisons of myeloablative conditioning versus RIC in myelofibrosis. Ninety-two patients with myelofibrosis in chronic phase underwent allo-HSCT in nine Nordic transplant centers from 1982 to 2009. A MAC regimen was given to 40 patients, and a RIC regimen was used in 52 patients. When adjustment for age differences was made, the survival of the patients in the RIC group was significantly better (*P* = 0.003). These patients, in fact, experienced significantly less acute GvHD. The Swedish experience comparing MAC with RIC at six transplant centers (n = 27) showed that NRM was 10% in the RIC and 30% in the MAC group after a median follow-up of 55 months. In a review of 46 patients who underwent MAC or RIC over a seven-year period, Gupta et al. (2009) reported a reduced risk of GvHD, more rapid engraftment, and reduced hospitalization within the first 100 days with a RIC regimen. Importantly, no difference in relapse rate or rate of histologic regression was noted. Retrospective studies from the GITMO and four major French transplant centers failed to demonstrate any improvement in survival or NRM using RIC over MAC. The largest retrospective study to date examined 2,224 patients from the EBMT database and showed no significant difference in five-year OS between patients who received MAC (n = 781) and RIC (n = 1443). A composite endpoint of five-year GvHD-free/relapse-free survival (GFRS) was lower in the RIC cohort (26.1%) when compared to the MAC group (32.4%). This study also showed advanced age, poor performance status, and use of an unrelated donor were associated with worse OS and non-relapse mortality. A MAC regimen may be a valid therapeutic option for young patients (< 45 years). However, non-relapse mortality after allo-HSCT with RIC regimens, especially in an MRD setting, is in the range of 10–20%, and the risk of relapse in most studies does not exceed that seen with myeloablative conditioning. It appears, therefore, that the majority of patients with myelofibrosis should be conditioned with RIC regimens.

The most common MAC regimens currently are fludarabine and myeloablative dosages of busulfan (Bu4/Flu), and busulfan and cyclophosphamide (Bu/Cy). The most common RIC regimens are fludarabine and dose-reduced busulfan (Bu2/Flu), fludarabine, and melphalan. Overall, based on the EBMT data, the fludarabine/ busulfan RIC regimen with the use of ATG has become the standard in allo-HSCT in many European transplant centers. Myeloablative regimens including two alkylating agents (busulfan and thiotepa) induced a significantly high rate of complete donor chimerism on day +30 and may represent a valid option especially in younger patients. The combination of thiotepa with fludarabine and busulfan has also become more common in conditioning regimens for hematologic malignancies, and a recent EBMT study of 187 patients showed its feasibility. Three-year OS was 55% and non-relapse mortality was 33% with no statistically significant differences based on conditioning intensity or donor type. The use of PTCy in matched as well as in mismatched transplant has shown a reduced risk of GvHD in MAC and RIC transplants for hematologic malignancies, without increasing the risk of relapse. Although at this time there is not yet enough data in MF, it could be hypothesized that future trials will address whether the use of MAC regimens with post-transplant cyclophosphamide (PTCy) improve the outcome of transplant from matched or mismatched donors in high-risk MF, without high rates of non-relapse mortality across different age groups.

7) How is response to allogeneic transplantation defined?

Expert Perspective: As previously mentioned, complete remission in the non-transplant setting has been defined by several groups. In 2013, IWG-MRT also developed criteria defining progressive and relapsed disease. Progressive disease is defined as new palpable splenomegaly at least 5 cm below the left costal margin, 100% increase in palpable distance below left costal margin for baseline splenomegaly of 5–10 cm, 50% increase in palpable distance below left costal margin for baseline splenomegaly of > 10 cm, leukemic transformation (confirmed by bone marrow blast count ≥ 20%), or peripheral blood blast count of

≥ 20% associated with an absolute blast count of 1×10^9/L that lasts for at least two weeks. Relapse is defined as no longer meeting criteria for clinical improvement having achieved complete response, partial response, or clinical improvement, or loss of anemia or spleen response persisting for at least one month.

The EBMT Chronic Malignancies Working Party has proposed definitions for relapse after allo-HSCT distinguished by categories: molecular relapse, cytogenetic relapse, molecular and cytogenetic relapse, and morphological/clinical relapse. Molecular relapse is defined as detectable MRD markers on two consecutive peripheral blood samples obtained at least 28 days apart after previously confirmed clearance by two prior blood samples collected 28 days apart. The possibility of relapse should also be considered when patients have increased mixed myeloid chimerism, defined as < 95% donor myeloid chimerism after day 30. A study by Srour et al. showed that out of 21 patients who developed mixed myeloid chimerism, all but one had concomitant molecular relapse. Cytogenetic relapse is defined as the detection of an informative, previously detected chromosomal abnormality on karyotyping, FISH, or SNP array in patients not meeting criteria for morphological relapse. The group defined morphological relapse as two separate scenarios: relapsed disease and progressive/accelerated disease. Criteria for relapsed disease include increased grade of reticulin/collagen fibrosis, increased age-adjusted cellularity and abnormal M:E ratio, and megakaryocytic abnormalities typically seen in MF. These features must occur after previously confirmed normalization of marrow morphology and reduction in fibrosis after transplant. In progressive or accelerated disease, there must be evidence of myelodysplastic features, increased blast counts in blood or marrow, AML, or persistent monocytosis.

8) Is there a molecular predictor of post-transplant relapse?

Expert Perspective: In addition to its prognostic role, the *JAK2V617F* mutation can also be used as a marker for MRD. A study monitoring patients after transplantation with a quantitative polymerase chain reaction assay for *JAK2V617F* demonstrated that of 15 *JAK2*-positive patients analyzed, three relapsed clinically shortly after the *JAK2* gene mutation was detected in the peripheral blood. A German study demonstrated that 78% of patients with the *JAK2* mutation undergoing a RIC allo-SCT achieved a molecular response after a median of 89 days following transplantation. This achievement of molecular response six months after allo-HSCT predicted a reduced risk of relapse (5% vs 35%). There is controversy surrounding the prognostic value of the *JAK2* allele burden in PMF. In non-transplant patients, low levels of the mutation seemed to predict a worse survival with a higher risk for bone marrow failure. However, in the setting of an allo-HSCT, the allele burden on day 28 post transplantation discriminated against two prognostic groups, with patients having > 1% being at significantly higher risk for relapse and having an inferior overall survival.

Other molecular markers that have been studied in primary and secondary myelofibrosis include the MPL W515L/K mutation and calreticulin (CALR) mutations and Wolschke et al. (2017) demonstrated that molecular clearance was higher in CALR-mutated patients at 100 days post transplant. However, similar to prior studies, the risk of clinical relapse at five years was significantly higher in patients with detectable mutations at days 100 and 180 irrespective of the mutation (62% vs 10% and 70% vs 10%). Importantly for triple-negative patients, chimerism remains an important surveillance strategy.

While these studies demonstrate a potential future role for MRD surveillance, in practice many centers only evaluate for molecular markers when prompted by clinical or hematological signs of relapse.

9) What are the current strategies for the management of transplant complications and relapse?

Relapse rates after allo-HSCT remain significant, ranging from 10 to 40% in various studies, with a median relapse time of around 7.1 months and median survival of less than two years. It is the most common cause of death after transplantation, and management strategies vary but primarily consist of donor lymphocyte infusion (DLI), second allo-HSCT, and targeted palliative therapies such as ruxolitinib. Complications such as poor graft function, graft failure, and GvHD also remain problematic, as there exists a pro-inflammatory, fibrotic milieu within the marrow and often bulky splenomegaly. The EBMT has recently developed definitions for these complications in an effort to create standardized management guidelines for each.

Hepatotoxicity

The most common etiologies of abnormal liver function tests after allo-HSCT are hepatic GvHD, drug-induced hepatitis, and iron overload, whereas severe hepatotoxicity (aminotransferase > 1500 U/L) is mediated mainly by veno-occlusive disease (VOD; now referred to as sinusoidal obstructive syndrome [SOS]) and hypoxia. Patients with myelofibrosis are at a significantly higher risk of early hepatoxicity after allo-HSCT compared to matched controls (n = 53) undergoing transplant for other indications. A history of portal hypertension, biopsy-proven hepatic iron overload, or splanchnic vein thrombosis strongly predicted for this complication. Importantly, moderate or severe hyperbilirubinemia or transaminitis was associated with inferior survival at 12 months (P = 0.02) in myelofibrosis. In light of these risk factors and their impact on survival, some groups are screening for portal hypertension prior to transplantation, and risk stratification for SOS is recommended prior to transplantation.

Graft-versus-Host Disease

The incidence of GvHD must be interpreted in the context of the conditioning regimen, T cell depletion, donor type, and source of stem cells. Rates of acute GvHD (aGvHD) differ with MAC or RIC regimens, and they depend on the use of T-cell immune-modifying agents. The Fred Hutchinson Cancer Center MAC experience revealed a 68% incidence of aGvHD. Use of RIC with ATG appeared to lower the rate of acute grade II–IV GvHD to 27%. Several retrospective comparisons provided conflicting results about the role of RIC in reducing aGvHD. Gupta et al. (2009) reported a day 100 cumulative incidence of aGvHD of 78% in the MAC allo-HSCT group versus 18% in the RIC allo-HSCT recipients, most likely because 70% of the RIC patients received ATG or alemtuzumab. The Nordic data showed 72% of patients undergoing RIC to be free of aGvHD compared to 24% of those undergoing MAC allo-HSCT. This was not confirmed by the British transplant data, in which acute GvHD occurred in 29% and 38% of patients in the myeloablative and RIC groups, respectively, even though 70% of RIC patients received an in vivo T-cell depletion. Chronic GvHD was reported in 40–59% of cases and predicted for improved OS, underscoring the importance of the graft-versus-tumor effect of allogeneic transplantation. In a retrospective study of 73 patients, relapse incidence was significantly higher in the absence of chronic GvHD ($P = 0.006$).

Regarding GvHD prophylaxis, prospective experience at the City of Hope has shown that tacrolimus–sirolimus +/− methotrexate is superior to cyclosporine–mycophenolate mofetil (CsA–MMF) +/− methotrexate. The estimated two-year OS for the CsA–MMF cohort was 55.6%, and for the tacrolimus–sirolimus cohort it was 92.9% ($P = 0.047$). The probability of grade III or IV acute GvHD was 60% for the CsA–MMF patients, and 10% for the tacrolimus-sirolimus group ($P = 0.0102$).

The incidence of GvHD in some studies of myelofibrosis exceeds that in other hematologic malignancies. This has been postulated to be due to elevated proinflammatory cytokines enhancing dendritic cell activation of T cells. An interesting observation in this regard is that the *JAK2* inhibitor CP-690550 abrogated acute GvHD-related mortality in murine models; this effect was largely related to the suppression of donor CD4 T-cell-mediated interferon (IFN) gamma production. Moreover, ruxolitinib has also been shown to reduce the levels of proinflammatory cytokines in PMF. Its superior efficacy in treating glucocorticoid-refractory GvHD in the REACH trials has now led to its approval by the FDA in treating such patients. In myelofibrosis patients, peritransplant use of ruxolitinib has shown to reduce the incidence of acute GvHD, and treatment of acute and chronic GvHD was effective at a dose of 5–10 mg/day. With the increasing rates of allo-HSCT in myelofibrosis, GvHD will continue to be an area of great interest in the era of newer targeted therapies (see Chapters 60 and 61).

Graft Failure

Primary graft failure is defined as pancytopenia (ANC $< 0.5 \times 10^9$/L, Hgb < 80g/L, platelets $< 20 \times 10^9$/L) at day 28 and mixed or lack of donor chimerism in patients undergoing RIC allo-HSCT. Concern about graft failure caused initial reluctance to carry out transplants in patients with myelofibrosis. Previous data showed that graft failure was a problem in only 5–25% of patients, particularly those who received transplants from "alternative" donors (i.e. other than MSD). The MPD-RC 101 prospective study reported a high rate of rejection in patients transplanted with unrelated donors and conditioned with fludarabine-melphalan and ATG. More recent large retrospective studies have shown a cumulative incidence of failure around 7% at one year, with a five-year survival rate of 14%. The use of ruxolitinib before allo-HSCT has also not been shown to affect graft failure rates, but conditioning regimen, including a benefit for two alkylators (Bregante et al. BBMT 2016) and CMV seronegativity appear to be protective against failure. Recommendations for the treatment of graft failure include early and prompt recognition, changes in immunosuppressive therapy, second allo-HSCT if indicated and feasible, and minimizing other post-transplant complications such as GvHD and infection. Minimization of risk factors before transplantation is also essential in preventing graft failure.

Poor Graft Function

The suggested definition for poor graft function includes the persistent presence of cytopenias in at least two hematopoietic lines (neutrophil count $\leq 1.5 \times 109/L$, platelet count $\leq 30 \times 10^9/L$, Hb ≤ 8.5 g/dL) for at least two consecutive weeks following engraftment and in the presence of full donor chimerism. This must occur in the absence of infection, GvHD, and drug-related myelosuppression. Poor graft function was reported in 17% of a cohort of 100 MF patients who underwent reduced-intensity HSCT. Risk factors for poor graft function included older age, male gender, and persistence of splenomegaly at or beyond day 30. While there is no consensus on the prevention treatment of poor graft function, the use of stem cell boost has been shown to be effective in several limited studies. Recently, thrombopoietin receptor agonists such as eltrombopag have been studied as a treatment for poor graft function, and results are encouraging. Expert consensus recommendations from the EBMT currently recommend consideration of growth factor support, post-HSCT splenectomy, stem cell boost, and second allo-HSCT for selected patients.

Donor Lymphocyte Infusion

An immunologic graft-versus-tumor effect can be achieved with DLIs in myelofibrosis patients relapsing after allo-HSCT. In a large retrospective study of 202 relapsed patients, 47 underwent DLI alone and had a median OS of 76 months compared to 23 patients who were treated with chemotherapy only and had a median OS of 23 months. The timing of a DLI, whether as a preemptive or salvage therapy, is debatable. In the salvage setting, responses were observed in 10 of 26 patients. Notably, all 10 responders achieved stable remissions and required no additional treatment. In a series of 17 patients where DLI was used preemptively in 8 patients and as salvage in 9, complete molecular response rate was superior in the preemptive group (68% vs 44%). The use of preemptive DLI was triggered by the detection of *JAK2 V617F*, emphasizing the need for monitoring of donor chimerism and MRD post transplant. The role of lymphodepleting chemotherapy before DLI has been explored. In preclinical models, lymphodepletion potentiates T-cell expansion and function by decreasing competition for cytokines and growth, elimination of regulatory T cells, and enhancement of antigen-presenting cell function.

Second Allograft

The efficacy of a second allo-HSCT has been demonstrated in several studies, but it remains limited to a select number of patients who are deemed healthy and fit enough to withstand another transplantation. A small study reported on 17 patients who underwent a second HSCT at a median interval of 17 months from the first allograft due to relapse (n = 13), graft rejection (n = 3), and transformation to blast phase (n = 1). Fifteen patients were transplanted with cells from alternative donors, and two patients from the same donor. The response rate was 80%, and one-year OS and progression-free survival were 82% and 70%, respectively. A study from the CMWP of the EBMT showed a median OS of

27 months for 51 patients who underwent second HSCT and 54 months for 26 patients who had DLI followed by second allo-HSCT. The group further recently analyzed 216 patients who received repeat transplantation and found a three-year OS of 42% and relapse-free survival of 39%. Factors that predicted a poorer prognosis include low performance status, a shorter interval between transplants, and graft failure as the reason for transplantation.

Stem Cell Boost

Current recommendations from the EBMT/ELN IWG are that patients with late decline of graft function who have full donor chimerism and no evidence of active GvHD should receive a booster infusion of donor stem cells without the need for conditioning. A study from the Hamburg group involving 32 patients (14 with primary MF) with poor graft function who underwent CD34+-stem cell boost demonstrated efficacy with a two-year OS of 45%. The rate of hematologic improvement was 81% with a median response time of 25 days. The use of related donor grafts increased the rate of recovery by approximately 10 days compared to unrelated donors. Cumulative rates of acute and chronic GvHD were 17% and 26%, respectively. This demonstrates that stem cell boost is a safe and effective option for patients with poor graft function, without the need for a second allo-HSCT.

10) Can current targeted therapies improve the outcomes of allo-HSCT?

Expert Perspective: With the advent of JAK inhibitors into the clinical armamentarium for myelofibrosis, there is increasing debate on whether and when to refer a patient with myelofibrosis to a transplant physician. It is interesting to speculate on whether improvement in the DIPSS score due to cytokine inhibition mediated by JAK inhibitors will allow physicians to modify the transplant strategy. It may be that the DIPSS score will be valid only in the absence of therapy with JAK inhibitors or similar compounds. By improving constitutional symptoms and splenomegaly, JAK inhibitors might turn out to be very useful in the pre-transplant setting and favor a more rapid engraftment, and possibly reduce the rates of rejection and/or GvHD. Concerns include a "withdrawal effect" after stopping ruxolitinib, poor engraftment due to the role of JAK signaling in normal hematopoiesis, risk of infection, and decreased graft-versus-leukemia effect due to immunosuppressive effects. A retrospective experience from Germany demonstrated an improved performance status and spleen size with ruxolitinib therapy for a median duration of 97 days before RIC allo-HSCT. The MPD-RC 114 study demonstrated the feasibility of incorporating pre-transplant ruxolitinib in 19 patients with no evidence of withdrawal when a tapering strategy was implemented. However, graft failure and NRM were significant in spite of JAK inhibition, and the study was prematurely terminated due to low accrual and failures. (NCT01790295). A subsequent phase II prospective trial looked at ruxolitinib only in treatment-naive patients before HSCT and showed good outcomes with related donors but not unrelated donors, where a higher mortality was attributed to hyperacute and grades 3–4 GvHD especially in mismatched unrelated donors. Interestingly, the rate of splenectomy was similar in these patients compared to pre-ruxolitinib data, suggesting it did not obviate the need for this high-risk procedure.

The other FDA approved JAK inhibitor, fedratinib, demonstrated a significant reduction in spleen volume and improvement in symptoms and quality of life in primary and secondary myelofibrosis patients (JAKARTA study). Fedratinib is currently being combined with hypomethylating agents in accelerated/blast-phase myelofibrosis prior to HSCT (NCT04282187), and results are awaited (see Chapter 23).

Several newer JAK inhibitors are under development that may have a safer side effect profile when compared to ruxolitinib and fedratinib, which can cause treatment-related adverse events (TRAE) such as anemia or thrombocytopenia. Momelotinib, a JAK1/2 and activin A receptor type-I (ACVR1) inhibitor, has been shown to reduce transfusion dependence and rate when compared to ruxolitinib but was less effective at reducing symptom burden. Pacritinib, a novel JAK2 and interleukin-1 receptor-associated kinase 1 (IRAK-1) inhibitor, has demonstrated superior symptom reduction and spleen reduction when compared to ruxolitinib in MF patients with severe thrombocytopenia. Preclinical studies with pacritinib suggest that inhibiting JAK2 while sparing JAK1 is able to control alloreactivity without impairing normal T-effector and Treg function. A phase I/II acute GvHD prevention trial combining pacritinib with standard immune suppression after allo-HCT is actively being investigated (NCT02891603).

There are a variety of novel therapies currently under investigation that are being evaluated both in combination with JAK inhibitors and alone. They include BET inhibitor (pelabresib), telomerase inhibitor (imetelstat), lysine-specific demethylase (LSD1) inhibitor (bomedemstat), BCL-XL/BCL-2 inhibitor (navitoclax), PI3K inhibitors (buparlisib, parsaclisib), aurora kinase inhibitor (alisertib), CD123 inhibitor (tagraxofusp) and recombinant human pentraxin-2 (PRM-151). However, while they may play a role in the future therapy for MF, their effect in allo-HSCT is still unknown (see Chapter 23).

Conclusion

The decision to opt for an allo-HSCT for patients with myelofibrosis is currently based on multiple considerations. Controversies continue to surround the timing, type of donor, and conditioning regimen. Some guiding principles to consider include the following:

- Comparisons of myeloablative and reduced-intensity regimens are retrospective and spread over many decades. However, RIC allo-HSCT has been shown to be effective. Conditioning intensity should be given to patients based on disease status and HCT-Cl at the time of transplant.
- Although patients with intermediate-2 and high-risk disease, adverse cytogenetics, or transfusion dependence should unequivocally proceed to transplant, there is controversy about transplanting low-risk patients with high risk molecular aberration(s). Low-risk patients should be monitored and newly developed definitions of progression will help in the early identification of patients who will benefit from transplant.
- Molecular markers have been validated in the transplant setting, and several newer models incorporate clinical and molecular features. These underscore a clinical need for NGS testing for accurate treatment selection and should be routinely employed in the care of MF patients.

- Non-relapse mortality remains a challenge in this disease, and donor selection, choice of conditioning, stem cell dose, and pre-transplant therapies including JAK inhibitors and splenectomy all need to be carefully considered. However, ongoing studies with the use of PTCy as GvHD prophylaxis in matched or mismatched transplant could provide new positive results regardless of the choice of MAC vs RIC conditioning regimen.
- Minimal residual disease may represent a useful tool for early detection of relapse, but this data is based on small retrospective studies, and prospective validation is awaited.

Recommended Readings

Alchalby H, Yunus D, Zabelina T. *et al.* (2012). 'Risk models predicting survival after reduced-intensity transplantation for myelofibrosis', *British Journal of Haematology*, 157(1), pp. 75–85. doi: https://doi.org/10.1111/j.1365-2141.2011.09009.x.

Battipaglia G, Mauff K, Wendel L. *et al.* (2021). 'Thiotepa–busulfan–fludarabine (TBF) conditioning regimen in patients undergoing allogeneic hematopoietic cell transplantation for myelofibrosis: an outcome analysis from the Chronic Malignancies Working Party of the EBMT', *Bone Marrow Transplantation*, 56(7), pp. 1593–1602. doi: 10.1038/s41409-021-01222-z.

Bewersdorf J.P, Sheth AH, Vetsa S. *et al* (2021). 'Outcomes of Allogeneic Hematopoietic Cell Transplantation in Patients With Myelofibrosis—A Systematic Review and Meta-Analysis', Transplant Cell Ther, May 28;S2666-6367(21)00935-0. doi: 10.1016/j.jtct.2021.05.016.

Bose, P. and Verstovsek, S. (2021 June 23). SOHO state of the Art Updates and Next Questions: identifying and treating "progression" in myelofibrosis. *Clinical Lymphoma Myeloma and Leukemia* S2152–2650 (21): doi: 10.1016/J.CLML.2021.06.008.

Bregante S, Dominietto A, Ghiso A, *et al.* (2016). 'Improved Outcome of Alternative Donor Transplantations in Patients with Myelofibrosis: From Unrelated to Haploidentical Family Donors', *Biology of Blood and Marrow Transplantation*, 22(2), pp. 324–329. doi: https://doi.org/10.1016/j.bbmt.2015.09.028.

Chiusolo P, Bregante S, Giammarco S, Lamparelli T, Casarino L, Dominietto A, Raiola AM, Metafuni E, Di Grazia C, Gualandi F, Sora F, Laurenti L, Sica S, Barosi G, Guolo F, Rossi M, Rossi E, Vannucchi A, Signori A, De Stefano V, Bacigalupo A, Angelucci E. Full donor chimerism after allogeneic hematopoietic stem cells transplant for myelofibrosis: The role of the conditioning regimen. *Am J Hematol.* 2021 Feb 1;96(2):234–240.

Gagelmann N, Ditschkowski M, Bogdanov R. *et al.* (2019). 'Comprehensive clinical-molecular transplant scoring system for myelofibrosis undergoing stem cell transplantation', *Blood*, 133(20), pp. 2233–2242. doi: 10.1182/BLOOD-2018-12-890889.

Gupta V, Kosiorek HE, Mead A. *et al.* (2019). 'Ruxolitinib Therapy Followed by Reduced-Intensity Conditioning for Hematopoietic Cell Transplantation for Myelofibrosis: Myeloproliferative Disorders Research Consortium 114 Study', *Biology of Blood and Marrow Transplantation*, 25(2), pp. 256–264. doi: 10.1016/j.bbmt.2018.09.001.

Kroger N, Holler E, Kobbe G. *et al.* (2015). 'Impact of allogeneic stem cell transplantation on survival of patients less than 65 years of age with primary myelofibrosis', *Blood*, 125(21), pp. 3347–3350. doi: 10.1182/BLOOD-2014-10-608315.

Kröger N, Panagiota V, Badbaran A. *et al.* (2017). 'Impact of Molecular Genetics on Outcome in Myelofibrosis Patients after Allogeneic Stem Cell Transplantation', *Biology of Blood and Marrow Transplantation*, 23(7), pp. 1095–1101. doi: 10.1016/j.bbmt.2017.03.034.

Kröger, N., Sbianchi, G., Sirait, T. *et al.* (2021). Impact of prior JAK-inhibitor therapy with ruxolitinib on outcome after allogeneic hematopoietic stem cell transplantation for myelofibrosis: a study of the CMWP of EBMT. *Leukemia* 35, 3551–3560 https://doi.org/10.1038/s41375-021-01276-4

Marinaccio C, Suraneni P, Celik H, et al. (2021). 'Lkb1/stk11 is a tumor suppressor in the progression of myeloproliferative neoplasms', *Cancer Discovery*. doi: 10.1158/2159-8290.CD-20-1353.

McLornan D, Szydlo R, Koster L. *et al.* (2019). 'Myeloablative and Reduced-Intensity Conditioned Allogeneic Hematopoietic Stem Cell Transplantation in Myelofibrosis: A Retrospective Study by the Chronic Malignancies Working Party of the European Society for Blood and Marrow Transplantation', *Biology of Blood and Marrow Transplantation*, 25(11), pp. 2167–2171. doi: 10.1016/j.bbmt.2019.06.034.

McLornan DP, Hernandez-Boluda JC, Czerw T, *et al.* (2021). 'Allogeneic haematopoietic cell transplantation for myelofibrosis: proposed definitions and management strategies for graft failure, poor graft function and relapse: best practice recommendations of the EBMT Chronic Malignancies Working Party', *Leukemia*. doi: 10.1038/s41375-021-01294-2.

Murata M, Takenaka K, Uchida N, Ozawa Y, Ohashi K, Kim SW, Ikegame K, Kanda Y, Kobayashi H, Ishikawa J, Ago H, Hirokawa M, Fukuda T, Atsuta Y, Kondo T. Comparison of Outcomes of Allogeneic Transplantation for Primary Myelofibrosis among Hematopoietic Stem Cell Source Groups. Biol Blood Marrow Transplant. 2019 Aug;25(8):1536–1543. doi: 10.1016/j.bbmt.2019.02.019. Epub 2019 Mar 1. PMID: 30826464.

Polverelli, N., Hernández-Boluda, J.C., Czerw, T. et al. (2023 January). Splenomegaly in patients with primary or secondary myelofibrosis who are candidates for allogeneic hematopoietic cell transplantation: a position paper on behalf of the chronic malignancies working party of the EBMT. *Lancet Haematol* 10 (1): e59–e70. doi: 10.1016/S2352-3026(22)00330-1. Epub 2022 Dec 6. PMID: 36493799.

Robin M, de Wreede LC, Wolschke C. et al. 'Long-term outcome after allogeneic hematopoietic cell transplantation for myelofibrosis', *Haematologica*, 104(9), pp. 1782–1788. doi: 10.3324/HAEMATOL.2018.205211.

Robin M, Porcher R, Orvain C, et al. (2021). 'Ruxolitinib before allogeneic hematopoietic transplantation in patients with myelofibrosis on behalf SFGM-TC and FIM groups', *Bone Marrow Transplantation*, 56(8), pp. 1888–1899. doi: 10.1038/s41409-021-01252-7.

Rondelli D, Goldberg JD, Marchioli R. *et al.* (2012). 'Results of Phase II Clinical Trial MPD-RC 101: Allogeneic Hematopoietic Stem Cell Transplantation Conditioned with Fludarabine/Melphalan in Patients with Myelofibrosis', *Biology of Blood and Marrow Transplantation*, 18(2). doi: 10.1016/j.bbmt.2011.12.039.

Scott BL, Gooley TA, Sorror ML. *et al.* (2012). 'The Dynamic International Prognostic Scoring System for myelofibrosis predicts outcomes after hematopoietic cell transplantation', *Blood*, 119(11), pp. 2657–2664. doi: 10.1182/blood-2011-08-372904.

Shanavas M, Popat U, Michaelis LC, Fauble V, McLornan D, Klisovic R, Mascarenhas J, Tamari R, Arcasoy MO, Davies J, Gergis U, Ukaegbu OC, Kamble RT, Storring JM, Majhail NS, Romee R, Verstovsek S, Pagliuca A, Vasu S, Ernst B, Atenafu EG, Hanif A, Champlin R, Hari P, Gupta V. 2016 Mar;Outcomes of Allogeneic Hematopoietic Cell Transplantation in Patients with Myelofibrosis with Prior Exposure to Janus Kinase 1/2 Inhibitors. *Biol Blood Marrow Transplant.* 22(3):432–40.

Tamari, R., McLornan, D.P., Ahn, K.W. et al. (2023 August 8). A simple prognostic system in patients with myelofibrosis undergoing allogeneic stem cell transplantation: a CIBMTR/EBMT analysis. *Blood Adv* 7 (15): 3993–4002. doi: 10.1182/bloodadvances.2023009886. PMID: 37134306; PMCID: PMC10410129.

Wolschke C, Badbaran A, Zabelina T. et al. (2017). 'Impact of molecular residual disease post allografting in myelofibrosis patients', *Bone Marrow Transplantation*, 52(11), pp. 1526–1529. doi: 10.1038/bmt.2017.157.

25

Chronic Myelomonocytic Leukemia

Mrinal M. Patnaik

Mayo Clinic, Rochester, MN

Introduction

Chronic myelomonocytic leukemia (CMML) is a myeloid neoplasm best classified as a myelodysplastic syndrome/myeloproliferative neoplasm overlap syndrome and is characterized by sustained peripheral blood monocytosis. CMML is a disease of aging, with a median age at diagnosis of 73–75 years, with a male preponderance. CMML is a rare disease with an estimated incidence rate of 4 cases per 1,000,000 of the population. CMML tends to occur on a background of clonal hematopoiesis defined by biallelic *TET2* mutations or *TET2* and *SRSF2* mutations, with the subsequent acquisition and expansion of epigentic mutations and signaling mutations giving rise to dysplastic and proliferative phenotypes, respectively. Mutational signatures commonly seen in CMML include *TET2* (60%), *SRSF2* (50%), *ASXL1* (40%), and *RAS* pathway mutations (*NRAS, KRAS, CBL, PTPN11, NF1−*, cumulatively 30%), with *ASXL1* mutations consistently predicting inferior survival rates. The median survival for CMML patients is < 36 months, with 15–30% undergoing AML transformation over 3–5 years.

Case Study 1

A 55-year-old male presented with a one-year history of progressive effort intolerance, 10-pound weight loss, early satiety, and left upper abdominal quadrant fullness. On a physical examination, he was found to have moderate splenomegaly. His bloodwork revealed hemoglobin of 8.0 gm/dL, a mean corpuscular volume of 96 fL, a white blood cell (WBC) count of 19.2×10^9/L, and a platelet count of 100,000/mL. His absolute neutrophil count (ANC) was 3.4×10^9/L, while the absolute monocyte count was 12.6×10^9/L. A peripheral blood smear was remarkable for monocytosis with occasional hypogranular neutrophils.

On reviewing a prior complete blood count (CBC) from a year ago, his hemoglobin was 9.2 g/dL, his WBC count was 7.8×10^9/L, and his absolute monocyte count was 1.8×10^9/L.

A bone marrow biopsy revealed a cellularity of 70% with trilineage hyperplasia and associated trilineage dysplasia. The megakaryocytes were markedly abnormal with hypolobated forms. There were increased butyrate esterase–positive monocytes and dual esterase–positive cells. The myeloblasts were estimated at 5% by morphology and

Cancer Consult: Expertise in Clinical Practice, Volume 2: Neoplastic Hematology & Cellular Therapy, Second Edition. Edited by Syed A. Abutalib, Maurie Markman, James O. Armitage, and Kenneth C. Anderson.

immunohistochemistry. The cytogenetics were diploid: 46XY. Fluorescent in situ hybrid-ization (FISH) studies for *BCR::ABL1*, *PDGFRA*, and *PDGFRB* abnormalities were negative. Next-generation sequencing analysis identifieid mutations involving *ASXL1* (variant allele frequency, or VAF: 45%), *SRSF2* (VAF: 40%), *NRAS* (VAF: 40%), and *TET2* (VAF: 40%).

1) What are the definition and the differential diagnosis for peripheral blood monocytosis?

Expert Perspective: Absolute monocytosis is defined by a peripheral blood AMC $\geq 1 \times 10^9$ cells/L, with monocytes $\geq$ 10% of the white blood count differential. The differential diag-nosis is categorized into clonal versus reactive. Reactive monocytosis is common and is most often seen in association with viral infections and autoimmune diseases. Chronic infections and inflammatory conditions such as tuberculosis, brucellosis, leishmaniasis, sarcoidosis, and connective tissue disorders can be associated with monocytosis. Mono-cytosis is also one of the early signs of a recovering bone marrow (BM) following myelo-suppression, either from chemotherapy, toxins, or viral infections. Clonal monocytosis is often persistent and is associated with hematopoietic stem cell disorders such as chronic myelomonocytic leukemia (CMML), juvenile myelomonocytic leukemia (JMML), myelopro-liferative neoplasms (MPNs), and myeloid disorders, with overlapping features between myelodysplastic syndromes (MDSs) and MPNs (see Chapters 12, 13, 23, and 26). Recently, experts have defined a new entity callled "oligomonocytic CMML," where patients have a sustained peripheral blood monocytosis (AMC $\geq 0.5 \times 10^9$/L and $\geq$ 10% of the white blood cell count differential), without any associated reactive cause for monocytosis and with markers for clonality (including cytogenetic changes and somatic mutations or flow cyto-metric evidence for monocyte repartitioning). Recent updates to the classification schema for CMML have now included oligomonocytic CMML as bona fide CMML.

2) What are the 2016 World Health Organization (WHO) definition and subcategorization criteria for CMML?

CMML is a clonal hematopoietic stem cell disorder with overlapping features of MDS and MPN. It is characterized by:

i) Persistent peripheral blood monocytosis $\geq 1 \times 10^9$/L, with monocytes constituting $\geq$ 10% of the total white blood cell count;
ii) Absence of the Philadelphia chromosome and the *BCR::ABL1* fusion oncogene;
iii) Absence of the *PDGFRA* or *PDGFRB* gene rearrangements;
iv) Less than 20% blasts and promonocytes in the peripheral blood and bone marrow;
v) Dysplasia involving one or more myeloid lineages.

Expert Perspective: If myelodysplasia is absent or minimal, the diagnosis of CMML can still be made if the other requirements are met and one of the following applies: an acquired, clonal, or molecular genetic abnormality is present in the hematopoietic cells, or the monocytosis has persisted for at least three months and other causes of monocy-tosis have been excluded. Molecular abnormalities that can be seen in CMML but are not specific to CMML include somatic mutations involving *ASXL1*, *TET2*, *SRSF2*, and *SETBP1*.

CMML is further subclassified into CMML-0 (< 2% circulating blasts and < 5% BM blasts), CMML-1 (2–4% circulating blasts and 5–9% BM blasts) and CMML-2 (5–19% circulating blasts and 10–19% BM blasts, or when Auer rods are present irrespective of the blast count). CMML can phenotypically also be classified as proliferative and dysplastic CMML subtpyes, with a white blood cell count ⩾ 13×10^9/L being diagnostic of the former. Recent studies have shown that proliferative and dysplastic CMML subtpyes have unique genetic and epigenetic landscapes, with the former being enriched in oncogenic RAS pathway mutations (*NRAS*, *CBL*, *PTPN11*, *KRAS*, and *NF1*). Recent updates to the classification schema for CMML have eliminated the CMML-0 category and now stratify CMML as CMML-1 (< 10% BM blasts and < 5% PB blasts) and CMML-2 (10–19% BM blasts and 5–19% PB blasts), respectively.[1, 2]

3) What are the epidemiology, clinical features, and presenting symptoms of patients with CMML?

Expert Perspective: The incidence of CMML has been approximated at 12.8 cases per 100,000 people per year, with the median age of presentation being 73–75 years. Patients with CMML have features overlapping between those of MDS and MPN. Those with an MDS phenotype present with or develop peripheral blood cytopenias, effort intolerance, easy bruisability, and transfusion dependence. Those with a MPN phenotype present with or develop leukocytosis, monocytosis, hepatomegaly, splenomegaly, and features of myeloproliferation.

4) What are the typical bone marrow morphological findings in patients with CMML?

Expert Perspective: The bone marrows are often hypercellular with granulocytic hyperplasia and dysplasia. Monocytic proliferation can be present but is often difficult to appreciate, and immunohistochemical studies that aid in the identification of monocytes and their precursors are recommended. Almost 80% of patients will demonstrate micromegakaryocytes with abnormal nuclear contours and lobations, and 30% of patients can have an increase in BM reticulin fibrosis. About 20 to 30% of patients can demonstrate nodules composed of mature plasmacytoid dendritic cells. These plasmacytoid dendritic cells are clonal, often have RAS pathway mutations, are CD123 and CD303 positive, and portend an inferior acute luekemia–free survival in CMML.

5) What are the typical immunophenotypic and cytochemical bone marrow findings in patients with CMML?

Expert Perspective: On immunophenotyping, the abnormal bone marrow cells often express myelomonocytic antigens such as CD13 and CD33, with variable expression of CD14, CD68, and CD64. Markers of aberrant expression include CD2, CD15, and CD56 or decreased expression of CD14, CD13, HLA-DR, CD64, or CD36. The presence of myeloblasts can be detected by expression of CD34. The most reliable markers on immunohistochemistry include CD68R and CD163. The monocytic cells are often positive for nonspecific esterases and lysozyme, while the granulocytic precursors are often positive for lysozyme and chloroacetate esterase.

6) Discuss cutaneous findings in CMML.

Expert Perspective: CMML being a monocytic neoplasm and given the plasticity between monocytes and macrophages, cutaneous findings are common. Skin biopsies with immunophenotyping is strongly reommended. Monocytic infiltrates into the epidermis and dermis are the most common finding, whereas the detection of CD34+ blastic forms (leukemia cutis) is suggestive of AML transformation. Occasionally, infiltrating plasmacytoid dendritic cells can be seen in the skin and can be identified by staining for CD123+ and CD303+. Since CMML is one of the most common associated non–mast cell disorders with systemic mastocytosis, urticaria pigmentosa and cutanous mastocytomas can be seen and should be identified by CD117+ and tryptase expression, with aberrant flow markers, CD2+ and CD25+. Finally, CMML can coexist with histocytic neoplasms, and appropriate immunostains for Langerhans and non-Langerhans histocytosis should be assessed for, when clinically suspected.

7) What are the cytogenetic abnormalities seen in patients with CMML?

Expert Perspective: Cytogenetic abnormalities in CMML can be detected by conventional karyotyping or FISH studies. Clonal cytogenetic abnormalities are seen in approximately 20–40% of patients with CMML. Frequent aberrations include +8, monosomy 7, del(7q), and recurring abnormalities of chromosome 12p. In a large Spanish cytogenetic study (n = 304), the karyotype was normal in 73% of patients. The most frequent abnormalities included +8, del(5q), +10, del(11q), del(12p), add(17p), +19, +21, abnormalities of chromosome 7, and complex karyotypes. Cytogenetic abnormalities were more frequent in patients with increased peripheral blood and BM blasts, and those who demonstrated dyserythropoiesis and dysgranulopoiesis. Based on these findings, the Spanish cytogenetic risk stratification system was developed, categorizing patients into three groups; high risk (+8, chromosome 7 abnormalities, or complex karyotype), intermediate risk (all chromosomal abnormalities except for those in the high- and low-risk categories), and low risk (normal karyotype or –Y), with five-year OS of 4%, 26%, and 35% respectively. The Mayo-French cytogenetic model better refined this stratification schema by adding sole der(3q) abnormalities to the low-risk group and by moving +8 from the high-risk to the intermediate-risk group.

8) What is the importance of detecting *PDGFRA* and *PDGFRB* gene rearrangements in patients suspected to have a diagnosis of CMML?

Expert Perspective: The platelet-derived growth factor receptors alpha and beta (*PDGFRA* chromosome 4q12 and *PDGFRB* chromosome 5q31–q32) are type III receptor tyrosine kinases. Rearragement of these genes can be associated with myeloid and lymphoid neoplasms associated with tyrosine kinase fusions. The clinical phenotype in both cases involves prominent blood eosinophilia and marked responsiveness to imatinib mesylate. These abnormalities can be detected by karyotyping and/or FISH techniques, and given their unique response to imatinib, are no longer classified as CMML. Patients presenting with a clinical phenotype of CMML, especially with eosinophilia, should be assessed for t(5;12)(q31–q32;p13), giving rise to the *ETV6(TEL)::PDGFRB* fusion oncogene. Gene rearrangements involving *PDGFRA* are less common, but nevertheless due to their imatinib responsiveness should be evaluated. Of note, the *FIP1L1::PDGFRA* fusion secondary to the *CHIC2* deletion is karyotypically occult and can only be detected by FISH or molecular techniques.

9) What is the current understanding about CMML disease biology?

Expert Perspective: The advent of next-generation sequencing technology has led to the identification of molecular aberrations in > 90% of patients with CMML. These can broadly be divided into the following categories:

i) Mutations involving epigenetic regulator genes, such as *EZH2, ASXL1, TET2, DNMT3A, IDH1*, and *IDH2*;

ii) Mutations involving the spliceosome machinery, such as *SF3B1, SRSF2, U2AF1, ZRSR2, SF3A1, PRPF40B, U2AF65*, and *SF1*;

iii) Mutations involving DNA damage response genes, such as *TP53*;

iv) Mutations involving genes regulating cellular and receptor tyrosine kinases, such as *JAK2, KRAS, NRAS, CBL, NF1*, and *PTPN11*;

v) Mutations involving transcription factors such as *RUNX1*;

vi) Others such as *SETBP1* and cohesin mutations.

TET2 (60%), *SRSF2* (50%), and *ASXL1* (40%) are the three most frequent somatic mutations seen in CMML, with oncogenic RAS pathway mutations being seen in 30%. Among these mutations, nonsense, and frameshift *ASXL1* mutations have consistently been shown to negatively impact overall survival (OS) and have been incorporated into all three contemporary prognostic models—Mayo Molecular Model, GFM CMML model, and the CPSS-Molecular model.

10) Discuss the role of RAS gene mutations in CMML.

Expert Perspective: Mutations involving *NRAS, KRAS, CBL, PTPN11*, and *NF1* are common in patients with CMML (~30%), and they are often associated with a myeloproliferative phenotype with monocytosis (70% of proliferative CMML). The expression of mutated RAS in mice has been associated with an MPN phenotype with monocytosis. Although univariate analysis studies have demonstrated inferior outcomes in CMML patients with RAS mutations, these observations have not held consistently in multivariate models. Approximately 10% of CMML patients do have a proliferative phenotype due to *JAK2V617F* mutations.

11) What are the clinical relevance and prognostic impact of spliceosome mutations in CMML?

Expert Perspective: Mutations in genes of the splicing machinery are common in patients with myeloid malignancies, including CMML. *SF3B1* mutations have a high prevalence (~80%) in MDS and ring sideroblasts, can be seen in patients with CMML and ring sideroblasts (< 10%), and in CMML are associated with lower AML transformation rates. *SRSF2* is the most mutated spliceosome gene in CMML (28–47%) and has been associated with increased age, less pronounced anemia, and a diploid karyotype. Thus far, *SRSF2* mutations have not demonstrated an independent prognostic impact. *U2AF1* mutations are seen in ~10% of patients with CMML and have not been associated either with inferior OS or leukemia-free survival. With the advent of clinical-grade spliceosome complex inhibitors, the recognition of splicing mutations in CMML patients has become important from a therapeutic standpoint.

12) What are the currently available prognostic scoring systems for CMML? Also describe their advantages and disadvantages.

Expert Perspective: Numerous prognostic systems have attempted to better define and stratify the natural history of CMML. The Bournemouth system, Lille system, and International Prognostic Scoring System (IPSS) are limited by the fact that they were mainly designed for patients with MDS and excluded patients with CMML who had a proliferative phenotype (WBC > 12 × 10^9/L).

The MD Anderson Prognostic Scoring System (MDAPS) was developed on a cohort of 213 CMML patients and identified a hemoglobin level < 12 g/dL, the presence of circulating immature myeloid cells, an absolute lymphocyte count > 2.5 × 10^9/L, and ⩾ 10% marrow blasts as independent predictors for inferior survival. This model identified four subgroups of patients with median survivals of 24, 15, 8, and 5 months for low-risk, intermediate-1 risk, intermediate-2 risk, and high-risk disease, respectively.

The MDAPS was then analyzed in 212 CMML patients in the Dusseldorf registry. In a univariate analysis, circulating immature myeloid cells had no prognostic impact, while in a multivariate analysis, elevated LDH, marrow blast count > 10%, male gender, hemoglobin < 12 g/dL, and absolute lymphocyte count > 2.5 × 10^9/L were independently prognostic. The Dusseldorf score classified patients into three risk categories, with a median survival of 93 (low), 26 (intermediate), and 11 (high) months, respectively.

The Spanish cytogenetic risk stratification system analyzed the role of karyotype abnormalities in patients with CMML. This stratification system did not, however, predict for the long-term outcomes.

In 2008, the global prognostic model for patients with *de novo* MDS, secondary MDS, and CMML was proposed. On multivariate analysis, independent factors included older age, poor performance status, thrombocytopenia, anemia, increased marrow blasts, leukocytosis (> 20 × 10^9/L), chromosome 7 or complex cytogenetic abnormalities, and a prior history of red blood cell transfusions. Four prognostic groups were identified with median survivals of 54 (low risk), 25 (intermediate-1 risk), 14 (intermediate-2 risk), and 6 months (high risk), respectively. This model was validated in 176 patients with CMML and leukocytosis (> 12 × 10^9/L).

Some, but not all, studies have demonstrated a negative prognostic impact for *ASXL1* mutations in patients with CMML. Notably, a Mayo Clinic study analyzed several clinical and laboratory parameters, including *ASXL1* mutations, in 226 patients with CMML; on multivariable analysis, risk factors for survival included hemoglobin < 10 g/dL, platelet count < 100 × 10(9)/L, absolute monocyte count > 10 × 10^9/L and the presence of immature myeloid cells. In this study *ASXL1* mutations were detected in 49% of patients and did not impact either overall ($P = 0.08$) or leukemia-free ($P = 0.4$) survival. The study resulted in the development of the Mayo prognostic model, with three risk categories: low (0 risk factors), intermediate (1 risk factor) and high (⩾ 2 risk factors), with median survivals of 32, 18.5, and 10 months, respectively.

In contrast to the findings from the above-discussed Mayo Clinic study, a GFM (Groupe Francais des Myelodysplasies) study demonstrated an adverse prognostic effect for *ASXL1* mutations in 312 patients with CMML; additional risk factors on multivariable analysis included age > 65 years, white blood count (WBC) > 15 × 10^9/L, platelet count < 100 × 10^9/L and hemoglobin level < 10 g/dL in females and < 11 g/dL in males. The GFM prognostic model assigns three adverse points for WBC > 15 × 10^9/L and two adverse points for each one of the remaining risk factors, resulting in a three-tiered risk stratification: low (0–4 points), intermediate (5–7 points), and high (8–12 points), with respective median survivals of 56, 27.4, and 9.2 months, respectively. It should be noted that all nucleotide variations (missense, nonsense, and frameshift) were regarded as *ASXL1* mutations in the

Mayo study, whereas only nonsense and frameshift *ASXL1* mutations were considered in the French study. To further clarify the prognostic relevance of *ASXL1* mutations, an international collaborative cohort of 466 CMML patients was analyzed.(3) In univariate analysis, survival was adversely affected by *ASXL1* (nonsense and frameshift) mutations. In multivariable analysis, *ASXL1* mutations, AMC > 10 × 10^9/L, HB < 10 gm/dL, platelets < 100 × 10^9/L, and circulating IMC were independently predictive of shortened OS. A regression coefficient–based prognostic model based on these five risk factors delineated high (≥ 3 risk factors; HR 6.2; 95% CI 3.7–10.4), intermediate-2 (two risk factors; HR 3.4; 95% CI 2.0–5.6), intermediate-1 (one risk factor; HR 1.9; 95% CI 1.1–3.3), and low (no risk factors) risk categories with median survivals of 16, 31, 59, and 97 months, respectively.(4) This model is referred to as the Mayo Molecular Model.

The CPSS-Mol is a recently developed prognostic model that first computes a genetic score based on cytogenetic abnormalities and mutations involving *ASXL1, RUNX1, NRAS,* and *SETBP1*. This is then computed with clinical variables such as red blood cell transfusion dependency, bone marrow blasts, and white blood cell count and stratifies patients into four categories; low, intermediate-1, intermediate-2, and high risk, with median OS of not reached, 64, 27, and 18 months, respectively. This model was also effective for leukemia free-survival stratification.

13) Discuss the management strategies for a patient with CMML.

Expert Perspective: The treatment for CMML can be broadly divided into two categories: supportive care and directed, or targeted, therapy.

Supportive care: Supportive care focuses on symptom management and palliation, and it comes into play when patients are ineligible for, or have failed, directed therapy. Hydroxyurea, a myelosuppressive agent, is very helpful in palliating symptoms related to massive splenomegaly and in controlling elevated blood counts. Other agents that have been used with less efficacy and tolerability include etoposide, low-dose cytarabine, topotecan, and 9-nitro-campothecin. Erythropoietin analogs can be used in patients with anemia; however, granulocyte colony-stimulating factor should be used with caution, given the risk for splenic rupture in patients with proliferative disease. Recommendations for supportive transfusional care, infectious disease prophylaxis, and iron chelation therapy are like those for patients with MDS, and data for their specific use in CMML do not exist.

Directed and targeted therapy: The hypomethylating agents 5-azacitidine, decitabine, and oral decitabine with cedazuridine (cytidine deaminase inhibitor) have been approved by the US Food and Drug Administration (FDA) for use in patients with MDS and CMML. Given the overlapping MDS–MPN phenotype and the presence of similar genetic and methylation abnormalities in CMML, these agents have been used in CMML with varying success. There currently are no phase III randomized clinical trial data to support their use in CMML. A recent randomized prospective phase III clinical trial randomized patients with high-risk proliferative CMML to decitabine versus hydroxyurea and demonstrated no benefit of decitabine over hydroxyurea in terms of overall survival and event-free survival (DACOTA trial). Based on phase II studies, the overall response rates vary between 40% and 50%, with true CR rates of < 20%. Like MDS, these medications generally take a minimum of four cycles before response assessment can be made. On starting these medications, the worsening of preexisting cytopenias and transfusion dependence is very likely. While hypomethylating agents epigenetically improve cytopenias in a subet of CMML patients, they do not alter mutational allele burdens, and disease progression to AML remains inevitable. While there remain no biomarkers predicting response to hypomethylating agents in CMML, the *TET2* mutant / *ASXL1* wild-type genotype is most likely to respond (based on retrospective data). In addition, proliferative CMML subtypes are least likely to respond to hypomethylating agens (DACOTA trial).

In 2015, the International Working Group for MDS/MPN overlap neoplasms outlined proposed consensus response criteria for CMML, which have been retrospectively validated. There currently exist several CMML-specific clinical trials targeting several aspects of the disease including GM-CSF hypersensitivity, RAS mutations, and CD123 expressing plasmacytoid dendritic cell nodules.

14) Discuss the role for allogeneic hematopoietic stem cell transplantation (allo-HCT) in CMML.

Expert Perspective: Allo-HCT remains the only curative option for patients with CMML. This technique is, however, fraught with complications, such as graft rejection, non-relapse mortality, acute and chronic graft-versus-host disease (GVHD), organ injury, and disease relapse in the post-transplant period. There are no randomized studies comparing allo-HCT with other modalities of care. The advent of reduced-intensity conditioning allo-HCT and the greater availability of matched unrelated donors and alternative donor stem cell sources (umbilical cord blood and haploidentical donors) have made allo-HCT available to more people. Eissa et al. reported outcomes on 85 patients with CMML who underwent allo-HCT (32% reduced-intensity conditioning allo-HCT, 62% peripheral blood stem cell grafts). After a median follow-up of 5.2 years, 49 (58%) had died, 20 from disease relapse and 29 from non-relapse causes; 26% developed grade II–IV acute GVHD; and 40% developed chronic GVHD. A multivariate model identified increasing age, a high allo-HCT comorbidity index, and poor-risk cytogenetics as independent prognosticators for poor survival. A recent European study evaluated allo-HCT in 73 patients with CMML (61% CMML-1 and 43 reduced-intensity conditioning allo-HCT). The three-year OS was 32%, the non-relapse mortality was 36%, and the cumulative incidence of relapse was 35%. OS was not influenced by the CR status, BM blast percentage at allo-HCT, prior treatments, and chronic GVHD. Twenty-eight percent and 34% of patients developed acute grade II–IV and chronic GVHD, respectively. In one of the largest retrospective cohorts involving 513 CMML patients (median age 53 years), the European Group for Blood and Marrow Transplantation reported a four-year RFS rate of 27% and an OS rate of 33%. Engraftment was successfully documented in 95% of patients, while acute (grade 2–4) and chronic GvHD occurred in 33% and 24% of patients, respectively. The achievement of CR at the time of HCT was independently associated with improved RFS and OS. For young patients with high-risk disease, poor prognostic scores, high-risk karyotypes, and increased BM blasts, early allogenenic transplantation strategies should be pursued. For the elderly, the transplant ineligible, and patients with limited donor options, clinical trials, or off-label use of hypomethylating agents can be considered.

Treatment Algorithm for CMML
Based on Risk Stratification According to the *Mayo Molecular Model

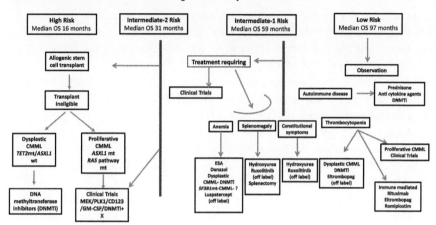

Figure 25.1 Prognostication and management of CMML in the era of precision genomics and clinical trials. OS: overall survival, wt: wild type, mt: mutant, HMA: hypomethylating agents.

Concluding remarks about the case study

Expert Perspective: The patient in the clinical vignette meets the 2016 WHO diagnostic criteria for CMML-1 and has presented with a proliferative phenotype with a high-risk mutational profile (*ASXL1* and *NRAS* mutations). He is symptomatic from his disease and has developed anemia, which is very likely to necessitate red blood cell transfusions. He is considered to be in the higher-risk category by most molecularly integrated CMML prognostic models. Given his younger age, I would HLA-type the patient and his siblings. If there are no sibling matches, unrelated and alternate donor sources should be investigated. If we can identify a suitable stem cell source, and if his pre-transplantation evaluation, including the SCT comorbidity index, is satisfactory, I would give him the option of proceeding with an allo-SCT. If he does not have a stem cell source, or if he is transplant ineligible, I would look to enroll him in clinical trials. Please refer to Figure 25.1 for my therapeutic approach to CMML (1–10).

Recommended Readings

Arber, D.A., Orazi, A., Hasserjian, R.P., Borowitz, MJ., Calvo, K.R., Kvasnicka, H.M. et al. (2022). International consensus classification of myeloid neoplasms and acute leukemia: integrating morphological, clinical, and genomic data. *Blood* 2016 May 19;127 (20): 2391–405. doi: 10.1182/blood-2016-03-643544. Epub 2016 Apr 11.

Arber, D.A., Orazi, A., Hasserjian, R., Thiele, J., Borowitz, M.J., Le Beau, M.M. et al. (2016). The 2016 revision to the World Health Organization classification of myeloid neoplasms and acute leukemia. *Blood* 127 (20): 2391–2405.

Carr, R.M., Vorobyev, D., Lasho, T., Marks, D.L., Tolosa, E.J., Vedder, A. et al. (2021). RAS mutations drive proliferative chronic myelomonocytic leukemia via a KMT2A-PLK1 axis. *Nat Commun* 12 (1): 2901.

Coston, T., Pophali, P., Vallapureddy, R., Lasho, T.L., Finke, C.M., Ketterling, R.P. et al. (2019). Suboptimal response rates to hypomethylating agent therapy in chronic myelomonocytic leukemia; a single institutional study of 121 patients. *Am J Hematol*. 2019 Jul;94 (7): 767–779. doi: 10.1002/ajh.25488. Epub 2019 May 3.

Elena, C., Galli, A., Such, E., Meggendorfer, M., Germing, U., Rizzo, E. et al. (2016). Integrating clinical features and genetic lesions in the risk assessment of patients with chronic myelomonocytic leukemia. *Blood* 128 (10): 1408–1417.

Itzykson, R., Santini, V., Thepot, S. et al. (2023 April 1). Decitabine versus hydroxyurea for advanced proliferative chronic myelomonocytic leukemia: results of a randomized phase III trial within the EMSCO network. *J Clin Oncol* 41 (10): 1888–1897. doi: 10.1200/ JCO.22.00437. Epub 2022 Dec 1. PMID: 36455187.

Hoversten, K., Vallapureddy, R., Lasho, T., Finke, C., Ketterling, R., Hanson, C. et al. (2018). Nonhepatosplenic extramedullary manifestations of chronic myelomonocytic leukemia: clinical, molecular and prognostic correlates. *Leuk Lymphoma* 59 (12): 2998–3001.

Khoury, J.D., Solary, E., Abla, O., Akkari, Y., Alaggio, R., Apperley, JF et al. (2022). The 5th edition of the world health organization classification of haematolymphoid tumours: myeloid and histiocytic/dendritic neoplasms. *Leukemia* 36 (7): 1703–19.

Merlevede, J., Droin, N., Qin, T., Meldi, K., Yoshida, K., Morabito, M. et al. (2016). Mutation allele burden remains unchanged in chronic myelomonocytic leukaemia responding to hypomethylating agents. *Nat Commun* 7: 10767.

Patnaik, M.M., Itzykson, R., Lasho, T.L., Kosmider, O., Finke, C.M., Hanson, C.A. et al. (2014). ASXL1 and SETBP1 mutations and their prognostic contribution in chronic myelomonocytic leukemia: a two-center study of 466 patients. *Leukemia* 28 (11): 2206–2212.

Patnaik, M.M. and Lasho, T. (2020). Myelodysplastic syndrome/myeloproliferative neoplasm overlap syndromes: a focused review. *Hematology Am Soc Hematol Educ Program* 2020 (1): 460–464.

Patnaik, M.M., Padron, E., LaBorde, R.R., Lasho, T.L., Finke, C.M., Hanson, C.A. et al. (2013). Mayo prognostic model for WHO-defined chronic myelomonocytic leukemia: ASXL1 and spliceosome component mutations and outcomes. *Leukemia* 27 (7): 1504–1510.

Patnaik, M.M. and Tefferi, A. (2020). Chronic Myelomonocytic leukemia: 2020 update on diagnosis, risk stratification and management. *Am J Hematol* 95 (1): 97–115.

Wassie, E.A., Itzykson, R., Lasho, T.L., Kosmider, O., Finke, C.M., Hanson, C.A. et al. (2014). Molecular and prognostic correlates of cytogenetic abnormalities in chronic myelomonocytic leukemia: a Mayo Clinic-French consortium study. *Am J Hematol* 89 (12): 1111–5.

26

Eosinophilic Myeloproliferative Disorders

Jason Gotlib

Stanford Cancer Institute, Stanford, CA

Introduction

The internal medicine workup of patients with eosinophilia should first acknowledge that most cases will be attributable to secondary (reactive) causes that stimulate an otherwise normal bone marrow to produce excess numbers of eosinophils that subsequently egress to the blood and other tissue compartments. If an initial diagnostic evaluation does not reveal a secondary cause, a referral to a hematologist should be undertaken to rule out a primary (clonal) basis for eosinophilia, or if no diagnosis is found, idiopathic hypereosinophilia (HE) or hypereosinophilic syndrome (HES) may be considered as a provisional diagnosis.

The incidence and prevalence of HES is not well characterized. Using the International Classification of Disease for Oncology (version 3), and code 9964/3 relating to the term "chronic eosinophilic leukemia", the Surveillance, Epidemiology and End Results (SEER) database from 2004 to 2015 revealed that the age-adjusted incidence rate was approximately 0.4 cases per 1,000,000. Eosinophilias with recurrent genetic abnormalities (e.g. gene fusions involving *PDGFRA, PDGFRB, FGFR1, JAK2, FLT3*, or *ETV6::ABL1*) occur only in a minority of these patients, with the *FIP1L1::PDGFRA* fusion being the most common molecular abnormality in this subgroup. Thus, primary eosinophilias are very rare entities, and patients with a confirmed or suspected diagnosis of one of these entities should be referred to a specialty center with expertise in treating these neoplasms.

Case Study 1

A 54-year-old man with no significant medical history reports a three-month history of mild fatigue during his annual routine checkup with his internist. The physical examination is unremarkable. A complete blood count (CBC) reveals a white blood cell (WBC) count of 9.6×10^9/L, with the manual differential revealing 45% neutrophils, 20% lymphocytes, 5% monocytes, and 25% eosinophils (absolute eosinophil count: 2.5×10^9/L). The hemoglobin and platelet count are normal.

Cancer Consult: Expertise in Clinical Practice, Volume 2: Neoplastic Hematology & Cellular Therapy,
Second Edition. Edited by Syed A. Abutalib, Maurie Markman, James O. Armitage, and Kenneth C. Anderson.
© 2024 John Wiley & Sons Ltd. Published 2024 by John Wiley & Sons Ltd.

1) Should this patient be referred to a hematol ogist for a bone marrow biopsy?

Expert Perspective: No. A systematic approach to the differential diagnosis of eosinophilia should be undertaken before assuming a bone marrow biopsy is immediately necessary to make a diagnosis in this case. The starting point is to recognize the cutoff for a normal eosinophil count. The upper limit of normal for the range of percentage of eosinophils in the peripheral blood is generally 3–5%, with a corresponding absolute eosinophil count (AEC) of $0.35-0.5 \times 10^9$/L. The severity of eosinophilia has been partitioned into mild (AEC from the upper limit of normal to 1.5×10^9/L), moderate (AEC: $1.5-5.0 \times 10^9$/L), and severe (AEC: $> 5 \times 10^9$/L). In the 2011 and, more recently, 2022 Working Conference on Eosinophil Disorders and Syndromes, the term "hypereosinophilia" (HE) is used to denote persistent and marked eosinophilia ($\geq 1.5 \times 10^9$/L).

The first step in the workup of eosinophilia is to rule out reactive (secondary) causes. This requires a thorough history and physical examination to evaluate patient travel and exposures, new medications, and a review of prior blood counts to evaluate the temporality and severity of eosinophilia. In developing countries, eosinophilia most commonly derives from infections, particularly tissue-invasive parasites. In developed countries, allergy/atopy conditions, hypersensitivity conditions, and drug reactions are the most common causes of eosinophilia. Other secondary causes of eosinophilia to consider include collagen-vascular diseases (e.g. Churg-Strauss syndrome and systemic lupus erythematosus), pulmonary eosinophilic diseases (e.g. idiopathic acute or chronic eosinophilic pneumonia, tropical pulmonary eosinophilia, allergic bronchopulmonary aspergillosis), allergic gastroenteritis (with associated peripheral eosinophilia), and metabolic conditions such as adrenal insufficiency. Malignancies may be associated with secondary eosinophilia, which usually results from elaboration of eosinophilopoietic cytokines such as IL3, IL5, and GM-CSF from the tumor. Such cytokine-driven eosinophilia has been associated with various solid malignancies, Hodgkin and non-Hodgkin lymphomas, and acute lymphoblastic leukemia/lymphoma.

Routine testing for secondary causes of eosinophilia typically involves ova and parasite testing, and sometimes stool culture and antibody testing for specific parasites (e.g. strongyloides and other helminth infections). The type and frequency of laboratory and imaging tests (e.g. chest X-ray, electrocardiogram and echocardiography, or computed tomography scan of the chest, abdomen, and pelvis) are guided by the patient's travel history, symptoms, and findings on physical examination. For patients with eosinophilia and signs or symptoms referable to lung disease, pulmonary function testing, bronchoscopy with bronchoalveolar lavage or biopsy, and serologic tests (e.g. aspergillus immunoglobulin E [IgE] to evaluate for allergic bronchopulmonary aspergillosis [ABPA]) may be considered.

The internist finds no reactive causes for eosinophilia. Although a referral is placed to hematology, the patient does not follow up with this consultation. The patient returns six months later complaining of increasing shortness of breath with exertion. On physical examination, an S3 murmur is auscultated, the spleen is palpated 5 cm below the left costal margin, and 2 + lower extremity edema is present. The current CBC reveals a WBC count of 23×10^9/L with 32% eosinophils (absolute eosinophil count: $\sim 7.4 \times 10^9$/L). Myeloid immaturity is not present. An echocardiogram reveals a decreased ejection fraction of 45%. Endomyocardial biopsy reveals an extensive eosinophilic infiltrate. No new reactive causes of eosinophilia have emerged.

2) Does the patient meet the criteria for idiopathic hypereosinophilic syndrome (HES)?

Expert Perspective: No. Historically, idiopathic HES is a diagnosis of exclusion whose criteria are: (i) an absolute eosinophil count > 1.5×10^9/L lasting for more than six months, (ii) signs of organ damage, (iii) and lack of evidence of other causes of eosinophilia. Note, however, that the first criterion is no longer universally accepted, as discussed below. The Working Conference on Eosinophil Disorders and Syndromes uses the term "HES" to indicate HE + organ damage, irrespective of underlying cause of eosinophil-mediated organ damage. Therefore, in addition to idiopathic HES, it may be associated with reactive causes (HES$_R$) or neoplastic cases (HES$_N$).

The recent 2022 5th edition of the World Health Organization classification (WHO) and the International Consensus Classification (ICC) include the category of "myeloid/lymphoid neoplasms with eosinophilia and tyrosine kinase gene fusions." This includes fusions involving platelet-derived growth factor receptor alpha (*PDGFRA*), platelet-derived growth factor receptor beta (PDGFRB), fibroblast growth factor receptor 1 (*FGFR1*), *JAK2*, *FLT3*, and *ETV6::ABL1* (Table 26.1).

"Chronic eosinophilic leukemia (CEL)" is another bone marrow–derived eosinophilic neoplasm, one of seven diseases within the World Health Organization (WHO) category of myeloproliferative neoplasms (MPNs). In the WHO classification, the qualifier "not otherwise specified (NOS)" is dropped but remains part of the disease nomenclature in the ICC, i.e. "CEL-NOS." ICC diagnostic criteria for CEL (NOS) are shown in Table 26.2 and are very similar to WHO criteria. For CEL, the emphasis is on demonstration of both dysplastic bone marrow morphology and evidence of clonality in order to distinguish it from idiopathic HE (also referred to as HE uncertain significance [HE$_{US}$]). If primary and secondary causes of HE are excluded (including lymphocyte-variant hypereosinophilia, discussed further in this chapter), then the diagnosis of idiopathic HE / HE$_{US}$ (organ damage absent) or idiopathic HES (organ damage present) can be considered. The ICC diagnostic criteria for idiopathic HES are shown in Table 26.3.

Duration of eosinophilia: A time window of sustained eosinophilia for six or more months is no longer universally accepted as necessary criterion for HES. Similarly, for the WHO definition of CEL, the time interval to define sustained eosinophilia is decreased to four weeks from six months. This shortening of required duration relates to the fact that modern evaluation of eosinophilia can usually proceed rapidly, and some patients may require immediate treatment. It is difficult to predict what duration and severity of eosinophilia will precipitate tissue damage in individual patients. HES diagnosis requires sustained overproduction of eosinophils, associated with damage to one or more organs due to eosinophilic infiltration and mediator release. Nonetheless, HES is considered a provisional entity that may change to a specific diagnosis if a defined basis for eosinophilia emerges over time.

3) Which of the following genetic markers should be obtained from the peripheral blood as part of the initial workup of primary eosinophilia?
A) *JAK2 V617F*.
B) *BCR::ABL1*.
C) Fluorescent in situ hybridization (FISH) for *CHIC2* deletion.
D) *FLT3 ITD* or D835 mutation.

Table 26.1   Myeloid/Lymphoid Neoplasms with Eosinophilia and Tyrosine Kinase Gene Fusions.

Tyrosine kinase	Rearranged chromosome band	Known partner genes (at least)	Most frequent partner protein	Phenotype	Risk for progression/ death	TKIs	Clinical Outcomes On TKI
PDGFRA	4q12	8	FIP1L1	MPN, rarely AML or ALL	Very low	Imatinib (FDA approved)	Outstanding long-term survival; treatment-free remission possible in some patients
PDGFRB	5q31~33	~35	ETV6	MPN or MDS/MPN	Very low	Imatinib (FDA approved)	
FGFR1	8p11	16	ZNF198	MPN; AML T>B cell lymphoma; MPAL	high	Pemigatibib (FDA after prior therapy)	• In CP, complete remission on TKIs achievable, but durability variable and relapses may occur
JAK2	9p24	4	PCM1	MPN;MDS/MPN; AML; CEL; PH- like ALL	high	Ruxolitinib	• In BP, Limited complete and durable remissions on intensive chemo alone. Use of intensive chemo+/- TKIs or TKIs alone for specific TK fusions followed by allogeneic stem cell transplantation
FLT3	13q12	7	ETV6	MPN; AML; CEL; T-cell ALL/lymphoma	high	Sunitinib sorafenib Midostaurin Gilteritinib	
ETV6::ABL1	9q34	-	-	MPN; AML; Ph-like ALL	Variable	Imatinib Nilotinib Dasatinib	

BP: blast phase; CP: chronic phase; FDA: Food and Drug Administration; MPAL: mixed phenotype acute leukemia; TKI: tyrosine kinase inhibitor.

Table 26.2 International consensus classification diagnostic criteria for chronic eosinophilic leukemia, not otherwise specified (CEL-NOS).

1. Peripheral blood hypereosinophilia (eosinophil count $\geq 1.5 \times 10^9$/L and eosinophils $\geq 10\%$ of white blood cells);

2. Blasts constitute $< 20\%$ of cells in peripheral blood and bone marrow, not meeting other diagnostic criteria for AML[a];

3. No tyrosine kinase gene fusion including *BCR::ABL1*, other *ABL1*, *PDGFRA*, *PDGFRB*, *FGFR1*, *JAK2*, or *FLT3* fusions;

4. Not meeting criteria for other well-defined MPN, chronic myelomonocytic leukemia, or systemic mastocytosis[b];

5. (i) Bone marrow shows increased cellularity with dysplastic megakaryocytes with or without dysplastic features in other lineages and often significant fibrosis, associated with an eosinophilic infiltrate, or (ii) increased blasts $\geq 5\%$ in the bone marrow and/or $\geq 2\%$ in the peripheral blood;

6. Demonstration of a clonal cytogenetic abnormality and/or somatic mutation(s)[c].

The diagnosis of CEL requires all 6 criteria
[a] AML with recurrent genetic abnormalities with $< 20\%$ blasts is excluded.
[b] Eosinophila can be seen in association with SM. However, "true" CEL-NOS may occur as SM-AMN (systemic mastocytosis with associated myeloid malignancies).
[c] In the absence of a clonal cytogenetic abnormality and/or somatic mutation(s) or increased blasts, bone marrow findings supportive of the diagnosis will suffice in the presence of persistent eosinophilia, provided other causes of eosinophilia have been excluded.
Source: Permission required for: From Arber et al., *Blood* 2022;140:1200–1228.

Table 26.3 International consensus classification diagnostic criteria for idiopathic hypereosinophilic syndrome (HES).

1. Persistent peripheral blood hypereosinophilia (eosinophil count $\geq 1.5 \times 10^9$/L and $\geq 10\%$ eosinophils)[a];

2. Organ damage and/or dysfunction attributable to tissue eosinophilic infiltrate[b];

3. No evidence of a reactive, well-defined autoimmune disease or neoplastic condition/disorder underlying the hypereosinophilia;

4. Exclusion of lymphocyte variant hypereosinophilic syndrome[c];

5. Bone marrow morphologically within normal limits except for increased eosinophils;

6. No molecular genetic clonal abnormality, with the caveat of clonal hematopoiesis of indeterminate potential (CHIP).

The diagnosis of idiopathic HES requires all six criteria.
[a] Preferably a minimal duration of six months if documentation is available.
[b] Hypereosinophilia of uncertain significance has no tissue damage but otherwise fulfills the same diagnostic criteria.
[c] An abnormal T-cell population must be detected immunophenotypically with or without T-cell receptor clonality by molecular analysis.
Permission required for: From Arber et al, Blood 2022;140:1200-1228

Expert Perspective: Clues to the presence of a primary eosinophilia may emerge from the evaluation of the blood smear. Review of the peripheral smear for circulating blasts, dysplastic cellular morphology, monocytosis, and elevated serum B_{12} or serum tryptase level(s) in conjunction with bone marrow morphologic, cytogenetic, and immunopheno-typic analyses will help identify whether a WHO-defined eosinophilia-associated myeloid neoplasm is present: acute myeloid leukemia (AML) (esp. inv(16)(p13q22) or t(16;16) (p13;q22)), myelodysplastic syndrome (MDS), systemic mastocytosis (SM), the classic MPNs (chronic myeloid leukemia, polycythemia vera, essential thrombocythemia, and primary myelofibrosis), and MDS/MPN overlap disorders (e.g. chronic myelomonocytic leukemia [CMML]) (Table 26.2).

Laboratory evaluation of primary eosinophilia should begin with screening of the peripheral blood for the *FIP1L1::PDGFRA* gene fusion by reverse transcription polymerase chain reaction (RT-PCR) or interphase or metaphase FISH (Figure 26.1). Probes are available that hybridize to the region between the *FIP1L1* and *PDGFRA* genes where the CHIC2 gene is located; its deletion is a surrogate for the cytogenetically occult 800 Kb deletion on chromosome 4q12 that results in the *FIP1L1::PDGFRA* fusion. If testing for *FIP1L1::PDGFRA* is not available, evaluation of the serum tryptase level may be a useful ancillary test since increased levels have been associated with the presence of the *FIP1L1::PDGFRA* fusion or other myeloproliferative neoplasms with hypereosinophilia. Genetic rearrangement of *PDGFRA* (fusion partners besides *FIP1L1*), *PDGFRB*, *FGFR1*, and *JAK2* can usually be inferred by their abnormal karyotype equivalent: rearrangement of 4q12 (*PDGFRA*), 5q31–33 (*PDGFRB*), 8p11–13 (*FGFR1*), 9p24 (*JAK2*), or 13q12 (*FLT3*). The *ETV6::ABL1* is represented by the t(9;12)(q34;p13). Over 30 gene fusion partners of *PDGFRB* have been described. Eosinophilic myeloid neoplasms related to fusions involving the *FGFR1* gene are similarly rare. In these cases, the association of the t(8p11) breakpoint with lymphoblastic lymphoma with eosinophilia and myeloid hyperplasia was first described in 1995. Sixteen fusion partners of *FGFR1* have been reported, with *ZMYM2::FGFR1* and *BCR::FGFR1* being the most common.

Although eosinophilia can accompany *BCR::ABL1*-positive chronic myeloid leukemia (and acute lymphoblastic leukemia [ALL]), as well as *JAK2 V617F*–positive MPNs, and these mutation tests can be drawn simultaneously with FISH for the *CHIC2* deletion, there are no other clinicopathologic findings in this case to steer the physician to these diagnoses. FLT3 mutations (*ITD* or *D835*) are found primarily in AML and confer a worse prognosis. MPN cases of primary eosinophilia associated with gene fusions involving *FLT3* (e.g. *ETV6::FLT3* and *ETV6::ABL1*) have been published and are now included in the category of myeloid/lymphoid neoplasms with tyrosine kinase gene fusions. It should be noted that eosinophilia is not an invariable finding in these diseases, but if present, it can be a useful prediagnostic checkpoint to think about them.

Correct Answer: C

The patient undergoes peripheral blood testing with FISH for the *CHIC2* deletion, which is positive in 96/200 cells (48%).

4) What treatment should be initiated?
- A) Hydroxyurea.
- B) Corticosteroids (prednisone 1 mg/kg).
- C) Imatinib.
- D) Imatinib + an initial course of prednisone 1 mg/kg.

Expert Perspective: Imatinib is first-line therapy in patients with *FIP1L1::PDGFRA*-positive disease and the rare patients with alternate *PDGFRA* fusions or rearranged *PDGFRB*. The

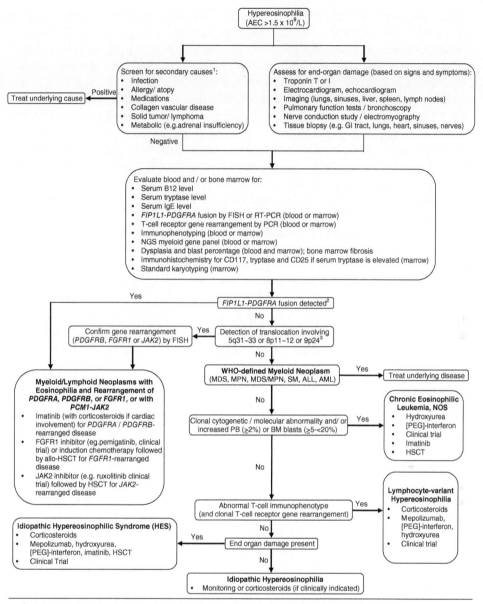

Figure 26.1 Diagnostic algorithm for evaluation of hypereosinophilia. FISH, fluorescent in situ hybridization; MDS, myelodysplastic syndrome; MPN, myeloproliferative neoplasm; NOS, not otherwise specified; RT-PCR, reverse transcription polymerase chain reaction; WHO, World Health Organization.

hematologic benefit of empiric imatinib in myeloid neoplasms associated with eosinophilia was identified in several early studies before the therapeutic target *FIP1L1::PDGFRA* was identified. Molecular remissions were first reported by the NIH group by PCR testing of the peripheral blood in 5 of 6 *FIP1L1::PDGFRA*-positive patients after 1–12 months of imatinib therapy. Several reports have now described rapid induction of molecular remission in imatinib-treated *FIP1L1::PDGFRA*-positive patients. Although 100 mg daily may be sufficient to achieve a molecular remission in some patients, others may require higher maintenance doses in the range of 300–400 mg daily. Maintenance dosing of 100–200 mg weekly may be sufficient to achieve a molecular remission in some patients. The optimal maintenance dose of imatinib that sustains a molecular remission has not been defined, but its clear that this disorder is exquisitively sensitive to TKI inhibition.

The natural history of imatinib-treated *FIP1L1::PDGFRA*-positive myeloid neoplasms was evaluated in an Italian prospective cohort of 27 patients with a median follow-up period of 25 months (range: 15–60 months). Patients were dose-escalated from an initial dose of 100 mg daily to a final dose of 400 mg daily. Complete hematologic remission was achieved in all patients within one month, and all patients became PCR negative for *FIP1L1::PDGFRA* after a median of three months of treatment (range: 1 to 10 months). Patients continuing imatinib remained PCR negative during a median follow-up period of 19 months (range: 6–56+ months). Another European study prospectively assessed the natural history of molecular responses to imatinib doses of 100–400 mg daily. Among 11 patients with high pretreatment transcript levels, all achieved a 3 log reduction in transcript levels by one year of therapy, and 9 of 11 patients achieved a molecular remission.

In patients with rearrangements of *PDGFRB* or *PDGFRA* variants other than *FIP1L1::PDGFRA*, case reports and series indicate that imatinib, usually at doses of 400 mg daily, can produce durable hematologic and cytogenetic remissions. Like *FIP1L1::PDGFRA*, FISH (most commonly) or PCR can be used to assess response to imatinib in *PDGFRB*-rearranged cases.

Caution with TKI therapy: Cardiogenic shock has been reported in a few *FIP1L1–PDGFRA*-positive patients after initiation of imatinib. Steroids during the first 7–10 days of imatinib treatment is recommended for patients with known cardiac disease and/or elevated serum troponin levels, which may be related to eosinophil-mediated heart damage or other cardiac comorbidities. In this patient with a biopsy-proven cardiac eosinophilic infiltrate and signs of heart failure, it would be prudent to begin this individual on a combination of imatinib and prednisone, with tapering of the latter if there is less concern for cardiac decompensation.

Correct Answer: D

The patient commences imatinib 100 mg daily and achieves a complete hematologic remission within one month. Splenomegaly has resolved, but he is maintained on heart failure medications with a repeat echocardiogram (echo) showing an ejection fraction of 50%. After three months, FISH testing for the *CHIC2* deletion from the peripheral blood is negative.

The patient is lost to follow-up and comes back to clinic one year later with complaints of night sweats, a 20-pound weight loss, and progressive dyspnea on exertion. The patient reports having stopped imatinib six months ago because he "felt well." On exam, splenomegaly 15 cm below the left costal margin is noted. A repeat echo shows a restrictive cardiomyopathy with an ejection fraction of 35%. The CBC now reveals a WBC count of 47 × 10^9/L, hemoglobin 8.5 g/dL, and platelet count 94 × 10^9/L. The differential reveals 15% neutrophils, 5% bands, 10% lymphocytes, 52% eosinophils, 12% immature myeloids (myelocytes and metamyelocytes), and 6% blasts. The smear reveals occasional teardrop and nucleated red blood cells. A bone marrow biopsy shows marked hypercellularity and eosinophilia, 8% myeloblasts, and MF-2 reticulin fibrosis. Cytogenetics reveals trisomy 8 and del (20q).

5) What is the next step in management?

A) Switch to prednisone.

B) Multi-agent AML-type (idarubicin–cytarabine) chemotherapy.

C) *JAK2 V617F* mutation testing.

D) Sequence analysis of *PDGFRA* to evaluate for resistance mutation(s).

Expert Perspective: Despite in-depth and durable molecular remissions, discontinuation of imatinib can lead to disease relapse. In a dose de-escalation trial of imatinib in five patients who had achieved a stable hematologic and molecular remission at 300–400 mg daily for at least one year, molecular relapse was observed in all patients after 2–5 months of either imatinib dose reduction or discontinuation. Molecular remissions were reestablished with reinitiation of imatinib in all patients at a dose range of 100–400 mg daily. In a cohort of patients evaluated by the Mayo Clinic, hematologic relapse occurred only several weeks after discontinuation of imatinib in four patients. Recent cohorts reported relapse rate (molecular or hematologic) of 33–57% in patients who discontinued imatinib, within a median of 10 months. Time to imatinib initiation and duration of imatinib treatment were independent factors of relapse after discontinuation of imatinib. Molecular remissions could be reestablished with re-induction of imatinib in most cases at a dose range of 100–400 mg daily. These data indicate that imatinib does not cure *FIP1L1::PDGFRA*-positive disease and argue for ongoing imatinib therapy to suppress the abnormal clone. In the largest cohort to date of 148 imatinib-treated patients, 1-, 5-, and 10-year overall survival rates were 99%, 98%, and 89%, respectively.

FIP1L1::PDGFRA-positive patients can develop resistance to imatinib, mostly involving the T674I mutation within the ATP-binding domain of *PDGFRA*. *T674I PDGFRA* is analogous to the *T315I ABL1* mutation in CML, which confers pan-resistance to the tyrosine kinase inhibitors imatinib, dasatinib, and nilotinib. However, unlike CML, secondary resistance is much less common (less than 10 cases are reported in the literature) and is almost exclusively observed during advanced phases of the disease.

Options for second-line treatment for T674I imatinib resistance are limited. One patient with the *FIP1L1::PDGFRA T674I* mutation in blast crisis responded briefly to sorafenib, but this was followed by rapid emergence of a pan-resistant *FIP1L1::PDGFRA D842V* mutant. Other reports have demonstrated either in vitro or in vivo activity of sorafenib, midostaurin, or nilotinib against the *T674I* mutant. The ability of alternative tyrosine kinase inhibitors to elicit durable clinical remissions (despite *in vitro* data demonstrating inhibitory activity against mutated fusions) has been disappointing. Because the agent avapritinib has activity against the *PDGFRA D842V* mutant in gastrointestinal stromal tumors (GIST), for which the drug is approved, it would be of interest to evaluate this agent in patients with relapsed disease carrying the *FIP1L1::PDGFRA D842V* mutation.

Correct Answer: D

Our patient

In this case, it would be premature to use induction chemotherapy since the patient does not have a diagnosis of AML; however, the patient is demonstrating signs of disease progression and may soon require higher intensity therapy such as induction chemotherapy followed by allogeneic transplantation if a suitable donor can be identified. Nevertheless, his cardiac function may preclude such options. Although the patient has marked splenomegaly and marrow fibrosis, his diagnosis is not myelofibrosis, and the *JAK2 V617F* mutation is unlikely to be present except in rare cases as a tandem mutation. Steroids would not be helpful in this clonal myeloid neoplasm showing evolution toward AML.

Case Study 2

A 46-year-old man reports a four-month history of fevers, night sweats, weight loss, and progressive swelling of lymph nodes in the bilateral cervical, axillary, and inguinal areas. An excisional left inguinal lymph node biopsy reveals T-cell lymphoblastic lymphoma. A CBC reveals a WBC count of 33×10^9/L, with 49% neutrophils; 5% bands; 13% metamyelocytes, myelocytes, and promyelocytes; 4% lymphocytes; 10% monocytes; and 19% eosinophils. A bone marrow biopsy reveals myeloid hyperplasia, no dysplasia or fibrosis, and moderate eosinophilia, consistent with a chronic-phase myeloid neoplasm (specifically a chronic eosinophilic leukemia). Testing for *BCR::ABL1* and *JAK2 V617F* is negative. Marrow cytogenetics reveal t(8;13)(p11;q12), and FISH reveals that the *FGFR1* gene is rearranged. PCR reveals a *ZMYM2–FGFR1* fusion gene.

1) What is the treatment recommendation?
   A) Imatinib.
   B) Selective FGFR tyrosine kinase inhibitor; bridge to allogeneic transplant.
   C) AML or ALL-type induction chemotherapy; bridge to allogeneic transplant.
   D) Hydroxyurea.

Expert Perspective: This patient has a myeloid/lymphoid neoplasm associated with eosinophilia with rearrangement of *FGFR1* according to the WHO and ICC classifications. This entity can present in the marrow as either chronic-phase disease (usually MDS, MPN, mixed MDS/MPN, or CEL), or blast-phase disease (myeloid [AML], lymphoid [ALL]), or mixed phenotype acute leukemia (MPAL). *FGFR1*-rearranged disease can also present with extramedullary disease (EMD), which by definition is a blast disease component. The lineage of the EMD can be AML, or B- or T-cell ALL or mixed phenotype disease and can be of the same or different lineage of the disease involving the bone marrow.

This condition has been historically referred to as 8p11 myeloproliferative syndrome or stem cell leukemia/lymphoma. The natural history of patients with myeloid or lymphoid disease with rearranged *FGFR1* follows an aggressive course, usually terminating in AML in 1–2 years. In chronic phrase, the cumulative incidence of transformation to blast phase at 12 months is almost 50%. The median survival from diagnosis has been reported as low as nine months in patients not receiving transplantation, but long-term remissions have been reported in patients transplanted before transformation. In blast-phase disease, one-year overall survival was 30%. Achievment of a complete remission from intensive induction chemotherapy has been associated with improved survival, and long-term remissions have been reported in patients undergoing allogeneic transplantation.

For chronic-phase patients, hydroxyurea or multikinase inhibitors with anti-FGFR1 activity, including midostaurin and ponatinib, have been used. For blast-phase disease, lineage-specific induction chemotherapy +/− tyrosine kinase inhibitors have been employed with the goal of inducing a complete clinical and cytogenetic remission with the goal of bridging to allogeneic transplantation. However, these treatments for chronic- and blast-phase disease typically result in partial or short-lived complete responses, and complete cytogenetic responses are rare.

Pemigatinib is a potent and selective inhibitor of FGFR1-3, which is being evaluated in an ongoing trial of patients with *FGFR1*-rearranged myeloid neoplasms. An ongoing trial of 31 evaluable chronic- and blast-phase patients (most of whom had progressed on prior therapy including transplant) revealed an overall complete clinical response rate of 77.4% and a complete cytogenetic response rate of 75.8% by central review. Clinical and cytogenetic responses were less frequent and durable compared to chronic-phase disease, but 23% of the blast-phase patients were bridged to transplant. The safety profile was consistent with FGFR inhibition with no unexpected toxicities. The most common toxicities were hyperphosphatemia, alopecia, diarrhea, and stomatitis. These interim trial results suggest that pemigatinib may offer a long-term treatment option for patients with myeloid/lymphoid neoplasms with *FGFR1* fusions and may facilitate bridging to transplant in eligible patients. In summary, in patients with myeloid or lymphoid neoplasms with FGFR1 rearrangements, pemigatinib produced high and durable response rates, despite patients' extensive use of prior treatments or hematopoietic stem cell transplantation, according to the early results of the multicenter phase II FIGHT-203 trial. Pemigatinib was approved by the Food and Drug Administration (FDA) in August 2022 for patients with myeloid/ lymphoid neoplasms with FGFR1 rearrangement after one line of prior systemic therapy.

Correct Answer: B

Our patient

In this case with both chronic-phase and blast-phase components, imatinib would not be expected to have any activity since it does exhibit anti-FGFR1 activity. Hydroxyurea may elicit transient control of blood counts but would not be expected to produce durable clinical responses or cytogenetic responses. Intensive AML- or ALL-type induction chemotherapy may produce clinical and cytogenetic responses but are variable and often short-lived. Although not directly compared to chemotherapy, emerging data suggests that the use of a selective FGFR1 inhibitor such as pemigatinib, now FDA approved, should be considered as a key component of therapy. Futibatinib is another FGFR inhibitor currently under investigation for myeloid/lymphoid neoplasms with FGFR rearrangement. In FGFR1-rearranged cases, if a suitable donor is identified, bridging to allogeneic transplant should be considered as it is the only treatment modality that provides a chance for cure. The safety and efficacy of the combination of lineage-specific induction chemotherapy plus a selective FGFR inhibitor has not been evaluated.

Case Study 3

A 61-year-old woman presents with progressive fatigue and crampy abdominal pain with moderate diarrhea. Mild splenomegaly is present on examination. A CBC reveals a WBC count of 28 × 10^9/L, hemoglobin 8.4 g/dL, and platelet count 82 × 10^9/L. The differential shows 57% eosinophils without increased blasts or myeloid immaturity. Endoscopy reveals a moderate eosinophil infiltrate on gastric and small duodenal biopsies. No causes for reactive eosinophilia are found. A bone marrow biopsy shows a cellularity of 60% with marked eosinophilia and minimal fibrosis without evidence for dysplasia. Cytogenetics is normal. Testing is negative for *BCR::ABL1* and *JAK2 V617F*, and there is no evidence for rearrangement of *PDGFRA/B*, *FGFR1*, or *JAK2*. T-cell receptor gene rearrangement is negative, and immunophenotyping of the bone marrow aspirate reveals a heterogeneous B- and T-lymphocyte population without aberrant markers. A diagnosis of idiopathic HES is made.

1) **Which first-line treatment do you recommend?**
   A) Prednisone.
   B) Hydroxyurea.
   C) Interferon-alfa.
   D) A or B.

Expert Perspective: Corticosteroids (e.g. prednisone 1 mg/kg) are recommended as first-line treatment for HES. Steroids have potent anti-eosinophil activity and can produce rapid reductions in eosinophil count. In a retrospective analysis of 188 patients, 141 HES patients on corticosteroids as first-line monotherapy achieved a complete remission (CR) or partial remission (PR) after one month, with duration of therapy ranging from 2 to 20 years and a median maintenance dose of 10 mg/day. As symptoms improve and eosinophil counts normalize, a steroid taper can be instituted, particularly given the long-term treatment side effects of steroids.

Hydroxyurea at 500–1000 mg daily is also an effective first-line option for HES, with the understanding that, like corticosteroids, hydroxyurea is palliative and does not change the natural course of the disease. Hydroxyurea can be used as monotherapy or in combination with corticosteroids. In the same retrospective study, 64 HES patients (34%) received hydroxyurea monotherapy, with 13 (72%) achieving CR or PR. One should note that for CEL and steroid-refractory idiopathic HES, hydroxyurea has been used as a first-line treatment.

Interferon alpha (IFN-α) has been used effectively to induce hematologic and cytogenetic remissions in patients with HES and CEL-NOS who are refractory to either steroids or hydroxyurea or administered in addition to corticosteroids as a steroid-sparing agent. Of the 188 patients in a retrospective study, 46 were treated with IFN-α in combination with steroids, with response rates ranging from 50% to 75%, respectively. IFN-α remissions have been associated with improvement in clinical symptoms as well as occasional improvement or reversion of end-organ injury, including hepatosplenomegaly and cardiac and thromboembolic complications. The optimal starting or maintenance dose of IFN-α has not been well defined, but the initial dose required to control eosinophil counts often exceeds the doses required to sustain a remission. Initiation of therapy at 1 million units by subcutaneous injection three times weekly (tiw) and gradual escalation of the dose to 3–4 million units or higher tiw may be required to control the eosinophil count. Treatment of four HES patients with pegylated interferon alpha 2b (PEG-IFNα-2b) among a larger cohort of *BCR::ABL1*-negative MPN patients resulted in one CR and one PR, but side effects required that the initial study dose be reduced from 3 to 2 mcg/kg/week. A lower starting dose of 90 mcg/kg/week (e.g., 1–1.5 mcg/kg/week) is better tolerated based on the experience of PEG-IFNα-2a (Pegasys) in PV and ET. Side effects of short- and longer-acting formulations of IFN-α are usually dose dependent and can include fatigue and flu-like symptoms, transaminitis, cytopenias, depression, hypothyroidism, and peripheral neuropathy. IFN-α is considered safe for use in pregnancy.

Second- and third-line agents for the treatment of HES have included vincristine, cyclophosphamide, etoposide, 2-chlorodeoxyadenosine alone or in combination with cytarabine, and cyclosporin-A. Imatinib has been used empirically in *PDGFRA/B*-rearrangement-negative patients (e.g. with HES or CEL). At doses of 400 mg or higher, partial hematologic responses are sometimes observed but are more often transient and may reflect drug-related myelosuppression.

Other treatment options for HES have included the anti-CD52 monoclonal antibody alemtuzumab, based on the expression of the CD52 antigen on eosinophils. In patients with HES who were refractory to other therapies, infusion of alemtuzumab one to three times weekly produced a hematologic remission in 10 of 11 patients (91%), but responses were not sustained when alemtuzumab was discontinued. Longer-term follow-up of patients receiving maintenance therapy on this study was recently reported.

Other antibody treatment approaches to HES include the use of mepolizumab, an anti-IL5 humanized monoclonal antibody that inhibits binding of IL5 to the alpha chain of the IL5 receptor found on eosinophils. Mepolizumab has been evaluated in a large, randomized, double-blind, placebo-controlled trial of 85 HES patients (e.g. *FIP1L1::PDGFRA*-negative patients). Patients were randomized to intravenous mepolizumab 750 mg or placebo every 4 weeks for 36 weeks. No adverse events were significantly more frequent with mepolizumab compared to placebo. A significantly higher proportion of mepolizumab-treated HES patients versus placebo were able to achieve the primary efficacy endpoint of a daily prednisone dose of ≤ 10 mg daily for at least eight consecutive weeks. In a long-term follow-up of 78 patients treated for a mean exposure of 251 weeks (range: 4–302 weeks), the median daily prednisone dose decreased from 20 to 0 mg in the first 24 weeks, and 62% of patients were prednisone-free without other HES medications for ≥ 12 consecutive weeks.

Most recently, a registrational randomized, placebo-controlled clinical trial in HES was reported. In this trial, a total of 108 patients (aged 12 years and older) with uncontrolled idiopathic HES (defined as at least two flares in the past 12 months and AEC ≥ 1×10^9/L) were randomized (1:1) to receive mepolizumab (300 mg subcutaneous) or placebo every four weeks, in addition to their existing therapy, for 32 weeks. Mepolizumab significantly reduced the occurrence of flares (28% in mepolizumab group vs 53% in the placebo group had a flare or withdrew from the trial). In addition, the time to first flare was 66% lower in the mepolizumab group. Both groups had a similar rate of adverse events. This study led to the approval of mepolizumab (300 mg subcutaneous once every four weeks) in idiopathic HES in 2020.

Benralizumab is an anti-IL5 receptor antibody that has been shown to reduce the annual asthma exacerbation rate in two phase III trials of patients with severe, uncontrolled eosinophilic asthma. It was also effective as an oral glucocorticoid-sparing therapy in adults with severe asthma in a randomized phase III trial and is currently FDA approved for adults with severe eosinophilic asthma. Benralizumab has been evaluated in 20 patients with *PDGFRA*-negative HES in a small randomized, double-blind, placebo-controlled, phase II trial. In all, 9 of 10 patients in the benralizumab arm met the primary endpoint of at least 50% reduction in the absolute eosinophil count at 12 weeks, in comparison to 3 of 10 patients who received placebo during the randomized phase ($P = 0.02$). Clinical and hematological responses were sustained for 48 weeks in 14 of 19 patients (74%) during the open phase of the trial, and the median duration of response was 84 weeks. A phase III, randomized, placebo-controlled, registrational trial of benralizumab is currently in progress.

Correct Answer: D

Case Study 4

A 45-year-old man reports a recurrent macular skin rash. A biopsy reveals lymphocytes and increased eosinophils in the dermis, but a specific diagnosis is not rendered. A CBC reveals a WBC count of 18×10^9/L with 45% eosinophils. Primary and secondary causes of eosinophilia are carefully ruled out. T-cell receptor gene rearrangement of the peripheral blood is positive. Immunophenotyping of the peripheral blood reveals a population of CD3 – CD4 + T-lymphocytes.

1) **Does this patient meet the diagnostic criteria for lymphocyte-variant hypereosino-philia?**
   A) Yes, proceed with therapy.
   B) Additional information is required.
   C) None of the above.

Expert Perspective: If both secondary and primary causes of eosinophilias are excluded, lymphocyte-variant hypereosinophilia should be considered next in the diagnostic algorithm before making a diagnosis of idiopathic HES. Patients with lymphocyte-variant hypereosinophilia often have cutaneous signs and symptoms as the primary disease manifestation. Although patients' skin disease can by symptomatic, the natural history of this condition is typically indolent, with rare patients progressing to T cell lymphoma or Sézary syndrome. A clonal T-cell receptor gene rearrangement and/or T cells with an aberrant immunophenotype are characteristic of lymphocyte-variant hypereosinophilia. Abnormal cell populations that have been described by flow immunophenotyping include double-negative immature T-lymphocytes (CD3 +, CD4 –, and CD8 –), an absence of CD3 (CD3 – and CD4 +), elevated expression of CD5 on CD3 – CD4 + cells, and loss of surface CD7 and/or expression of CD27. Elevated serum IgE levels are also commonly described. Research-based analyses have reported T cell production of cytokines (e.g. IL5, IL4, and IL13) consistent with a T-cell helper type 2 (Th2) cytokine profile, and production of TARC (thymus- and activation-regulated chemokine), a chemokine in Th2-mediated diseases.

This syndrome represents a mixture of clonal and reactive processes resulting in the expansion of a clone of T lymphocytes that produce cytokines that drive eosinophilia. Although these laboratory findings constitute basic elements of this syndrome, neither the WHO nor other consensus panels have established specific diagnostic criteria for this condition. The finding of isolated T-cell clonality by PCR without T cell immunophenotypic abnormalities or demonstration of Th2 cytokine production is not adequate to make a diagnosis of this variant. In an analysis of patients diagnosed with HES, 18 of 42 (43%) subjects exhibited a clonal T-cell receptor gene rearrangement by PCR. However, the biologic relevance of such clonal T cell populations to eosinophilia was not established. Therefore, whether such patients should still be referred to as idiopathic HES or as lymphocyte-variant hypereosinophilia remains a matter of debate.

Correct Answer: B

2) **All of the following are associated with relatively worse outcomes in eosinophilic diseases and MPNs, except for which one?**
   A) Cardiac disease.
   B) Corticosteroid refractoriness.
   C) Height of eosinophilia.
   D) Presence of *FIP1L1::PDGFRA*.

Expert Perspective: Older case series identify cardiac disease as the primary etiology of premature death. A review of 57 HES cases published through 1973 reported a median survival of nine months, and the three-year survival was only 12%. Patients usually presented with advanced disease, with congestive heart failure accounting for 65% of deaths at autopsy.

In addition to cardiac involvement, peripheral blood blasts and a WBC count greater than 100×10^9/L were poor prognostic factors. A later report of 40 HES patients cited a five-year survival rate of 80%, which decreased to 42% at 15 years. Factors predictive of a worse outcome included the presence of a myeloproliferative neoplasm, corticosteroid-refractory hypereosinophilia, cardiac disease, male gender, and the height of eosinophilia. It is possible that male gender was identified as a poor prognostic factor because we have learned that almost all patients diagnosed with *FIP1L1::PDGFRA*-positive eosinophilic neoplasms are male. The basis for this gender predominance is unknown. Before the availability of imatinib for such patients, it is quite likely that these individuals experienced poor outcome because their myeloid neoplasms were unsuccessfully treated.

In WHO-defined myeloid malignancies, the prognostic importance of associated eosinophilia has been studied in only a few diseases. In a series of 123 patients with systemic mastocytosis, eosinophilia was prevalent in 34% of cases, but it was prognostically neutral and was not affected by exclusion of *FIP1L1::PDGFRA*-positive cases. However, in a more recent analysis of 2,350 patients from the European Competence Network on Mastocytosis (ECNM) registry, eosinophilia/hypereosinophilia was more common in advanced systemic mastocytosis and was associated with a worse outcome. In a study of 1,008 patients with *de novo* MDS, eosinophilia (and basophilia) predicted a significantly reduced survival without having a significant impact on leukemia-free survival. A retrospective analysis of 288 individuals with newly diagnosed

MDS revealed that significantly higher numbers of patients with eosinophilia or baso-philia (compared to patients with neither) had chromosomal abnormalities carrying an intermediate or poor prognosis. In addition, the overall survival rate was significantly lower and a higher rate of evolution to AML was observed.

Correct Answer: D

Recommended Readings

Khoury, J.D., Solary, E., Abla, O. et al. (2022). The 5th edition of the world health organization classification of haematolymphoid tumours: myeloid and histiocytic/dendritic neoplasms. *Leukemia* 36 (7): 1703–1719.

Arber, D.A., Orazi, A., Hasserjian, R.P. et al. (2022). International consensus classification of myeloid neoplasms and acute leukemias: integrating morphologic, clinical, and genomic data. *Blood* 140 (11): 1200–1228.

Reiter, A. and Gotlib, J. (2017). Myeloid neoplasms with eosinophilia. *Blood* 129: 704–714.

Roufosse, F., Kahn, J.E., Rothenberg, M.E. et al. (2020). Efficacy and safety of mepolizumab in hypereosinophilic syndrome: a phase III, randomized, placebo-controlled trial. *J Allergy Clin Immunol* 146: 1397–1405.

Shomali, W. and Gotlib, J. (2022). World health organization-defined eosinophilic disorders: 2022 update on diagnosis, risk stratification, and management. *Am J Hematol* 97: 129–148.

Valent, P., Klion, D., Horny, H.P. et al. (2012). Contemporary consensus proposal on criteria and classification of eosinophilic disorders and related syndromes. *J Allergy Clin Immunol* e9 130: 607–612.

Valent, P., Klion, A., Roufosse, R. et al. (in press). Proposed refined diagnostic criteria and classification of eosinophil disorders and related syndromes. *Allergy*.

Part 5

Chronic Lymphocytic and Other Leukemias

27

Chronic Lymphocytic Leukemia/Small Lymphocytic Lymphoma

Jayastu Senapati, Nitin Jain[1], and Susan O'Brien[2]

[1] *MDACC, Houston, TX*
[2] *University of California, Irvine, CA*

Introduction

Chronic lymphocytic leukemia / small lymphocytic leukemia (CLL/SLL) is the most common leukemia in the Western Hemisphere. In the most recent update of the SEER database, the age-adjusted incidence of CLL was 4.9 per 100,000 inhabitants per year. By 2021, SEER estimates 21,250 new CLL cases in the United States, which represents 1.1% of all new cancer cases. In 2018, there was an estimated 195,129 people living with CLL in the United States. While the incidence of CLL has been stable over the last two decades, the mortality has been declining. CLL is estimated to have caused contextualized 4,320 deaths in 2021, representing 0.7% of all cancer deaths. It typically occurs in elderly patients with a median age at diagnosis of 70 years. More male than female patients (1.9:1) are affected.

The diagnosis of CLL requires the presence of $\geq 5 \times 10^9$/L clonal B lymphocytes in the peripheral blood, sustained for at least three months. The clonality of these B lymphocytes needs to be confirmed by demonstrating immunoglobulin light chain restriction using flow cytometry. The definition of SLL requires the presence of lymphadenopathy and the absence of cytopenias caused by a clonal marrow infiltrate. Additionally, the number of B lymphocytes in the peripheral blood should be $< 5 \times 10^9$/L. CLL or SLL might be suspected in otherwise healthy adults who have an absolute increase in clonal B lymphocytes but who have $< 5 \times 10^9$/L B lymphocytes in the blood. However, in the absence of lymphadenopathy or organomegaly (as detected by physical examination or imaging studies) or of disease-related cytopenias or symptoms, the presence of $< 5 \times 10^9$/L B lymphocytes is defined as monoclonal B lymphocytosis (MBL). The presence of a cytopenia caused by a typical marrow infiltrate establishes the diagnosis of CLL regardless of the number of peripheral blood B lymphocytes or of the lymph node involvement. MBL has been observed to progress to CLL, requiring treatment at a rate of 1–2% per year. Subjects with MBL appear to share an increased risk of secondary cancers of the skin with CLL patients and should be encouraged to participate in the appropriate screening programs (e.g. for carcinomas of the skin or colon).

Cancer Consult: Expertise in Clinical Practice, Volume 2: Neoplastic Hematology & Cellular Therapy,
Second Edition. Edited by Syed A. Abutalib, Maurie Markman, James O. Armitage, and Kenneth C. Anderson.
© 2024 John Wiley & Sons Ltd. Published 2024 by John Wiley & Sons Ltd.

Case Study 1

A 65-year-old schoolteacher presents to the clinic after being incidentally diagnosed with leukocytosis with lymphocytosis during a yearly routine blood test. CBC showed hemoglobin 15.3 g/dL, WBC count 28 × 10^9/L (lymphocytes 80%), and platelet count 415 × 10^9/L. He had no symptoms attributable to the disease. Physical examination did not reveal any lymphadenopathy or organomegaly. A diagnosis of CLL was established based on peripheral blood flow cytometry. CLL FISH panel showed presence of del(17p). Next-generation sequencing panel showed presence of *TP53* and *NOTCH1* mutations. Testing for IGHV showed unmutated IGHV.

1) **What is the next step in the management of this patient?**
   A) Clinical observation.
   B) Start chemoimmunotherapy.
   C) Start therapy with a targeted agent.
   D) Consider up-front allogeneic SCT or CAR T cell therapy given young age and high-risk disease features.

Expert Perspective: Despite the advent of multiple newer treatment options in CLL over the last decade including immunotherapy such as obinutuzumab, targeted therapies such as Bruton tyrosine inhibitors (BTKi), and BCL2 antagonist, therapy in the absence of iwCLL (International Workshop on CLL) treatment indications has not been shown to be beneficial. The recommendation for this patient should be observation. Patients with CLL should be counseled for adequate vaccination, risk of infection, and age-appropriate cancer screening, including dermatological evaluation for skin cancer screening (Muchtar et al. 2021).

Ongoing clinical trials are trying to study the effect of early therapy initiation in asymptomatic/early-stage high-risk CLL patients. The CLL 12 study by the German CLL study group (GCLLSG) evaluated the effect of ibrutinib therapy in patients with newly diagnosed CLL who did not fulfill the iwCLL treatment criteria for therapy initiation. Patients were randomized to up-front ibrutinib monotherapy versus placebo with the primary endpoint of event-free survival defined as time from randomization until occurrence of active disease according to iwCLL guidelines, new CLL treatment, or death. Patient on the ibrutinib arm had longer event-free survival and time to next treatment as would be expected (since the control arm had received a placebo drug) but had higher incidence of bleeding, hypertension, and arrhythmia episodes. The study will report on overall survival (OS), but at this time the data is immature with no indication of improvement in the treatment arm. The EVOLVE SLL/CLL trial (NCT04269902) is aiming to study the effect on OS of early initiation of venetoclax and obinutuzumab combination therapy in patients with CLL IPI > 4 or with complex karyotype compared to patients who are started when they fulfill iwCLL 2018 recommendations for therapy initiation. The PreVent-ACaLL study (NCT03868722) by the HOVON and NORDIC CLL groups is using a novel machine learning algorithm to identify patients with early-stage CLL who have an increased risk of severe infection (> 65% over two years) and investigate the effect of a three-month combination of venetoclax with acalabrutinib in reducing these grade 3 infections. Data from such trials are needed to better understand the benefit of therapy initiation in early-stage CLL; presently observation alone is standard of care.

Correct Answer: A

2) Do BTK inhibitors such as ibrutinib, zanubrutinib and acalabrutinib and BCL2 antago-nist such as venetoclax act uniformly throughout all disease compartments in CLL?

Expert Perspective: No. BTKi and venetoclax are targeted therapies that have significantly improved the treatment outcomes in CLL. CLL is a multi-compartmental disease involving the peripheral blood, bone marrow, lymph nodes, and other lymphoid organs. The effect of the targeted therapies is not universal throughout all disease compartments. BTKi, through inhibition of chemotaxis and adhesion, result in rapid reduction of lymph nodes / spleen, leading to reactive lymphocytosis. Unlike BTKi, venetoclax affects all compartments (including bone marrow) rapidly and leads to marrow undetectable–measurable residual disease (MRD) remission in the majority of patients when used as initial therapy with obinutuzumab (Senapati and Jain 2021).

3) Among the prognostic markers relevant in the setting of chemoimmunotherapy, which marker has maintained prognostic significance with the use of targeted therapies?
   A) CD38.
   B) IGHV mutation status.
   C) Deletion 17p / *TP53* mutation.
   D) ZAP-70.

Expert Perspective: With the use of chemoimmunotherapy, several risk factors that were established for prognosis including deletion 17p, deletion 11q, unmutated IGHV, TP53 mutation, ZAP-70 positivity, CD38 positivity, elevated β2 microglobulin are losing clinical relevance.

The CLL International Prognostic Index (CLL-IPI) was established in 2016 and included the following factors: TP53 status (TP53 mutation / deletion 17p), IGHV mutation status (mutated or unmutated), β2 microglobulin levels (≤ 3.5 mg/L vs > 3.5 mg/L), clinical stage (Binet A or Rai 0 vs Binet B–C or Rai I–IV), and age (≤ 65 years vs > 65 years); it defined four risk groups with progressively worse survival. In the FCR (fludarabine, cyclophosphamide, rituximab) trial in CLL from MD Anderson Cancer Center (MDACC), patients with an IGHV mutation (IGHV-M) had a significantly better progression-free survival at over 12 years of follow-up (53.9% vs 8.7%) compared to that seen in IGHV-unmutated (IGHV-UM) patients. However, with targeted therapies the prognostic utility of IGHV has reduced significantly. The RESONATE and RESONATE 2 trials did not show an effect of IGHV mutation status on progression-free survival at 6–7 years of follow-up in patients treated with ibrutinib, while del(17p)/TP53 mutation affected progression-free survival in the RESONATE trial. With PI3K inhibitors such as idelalisib and duvelisib, IGHV status also does not affect response rates or survival in the relapsed setting. In the context of venetoclax-based therapy, the CLL14 trial showed inferior progression-free survival for patients with deletion 17p / *TP53* mutated on the venetoclax-obinutuzumab arm. In a recent update of the CLL data, there also appears to be a difference of progression-free survival between mutated and unmutated IGHV.

ZAP-70 and CD38 positivity tend to be present in patients with IGHV-unmutated CLL and have lost their prognostic value in the era of targeted agents. Thus, with refinements in CLL therapy, other than 17p deletion / *TP53* mutation, the majority of the other traditional risk factors have lost their prognostic relevance.

Correct Answer: C

Case Study 2

A 55-year-old tennis coach with hypertension and diabetes presented with lymphocytosis, generalized lymphadenopathy, and mild splenomegaly. She had significant symptom burden. CBC showed hemoglobin 9.6 g/dL, WBC 220 × 10^9/L (ALC 198 × 10^9/L), and platelet 76 × 10^9/L. Workup confirmed CLL. She was initiated on ibrutinib at 420 mg once daily. She achieved a partial response to therapy with normalization of her blood counts, resolution of disease-related symptoms, and resolution of palpable adenopathy. However, she noticed progressive arthralgias affecting her work and worsening hypertension requiring additional anti-hypertensives.

4) What are the potential next lines of treatment? (Choose one or more, as appropriate.)
   A) Switch ibrutinib to acalabrutinib.
   B) Discontinue ibrutinib and change to another class of drug (BCL2 antagonists).
   C) Reduce dose of ibrutinib to 280 mg daily.
   D) Continue ibrutinib at the same dose.

Expert Perspective: Ibrutinib was the first oral targeted therapy approved for CLL. Despite its benefits, ibrutinib can have side effects warranting therapy alteration or discontinuation, especially in data emanating from real-world practices. Data from clinical trials have shown rates of atrial fibrillation at 6–10% in the first year after ibrutinib initiation, and a cumulative rate of about 10–15%. Hypertension (new onset hypertension or worsening of known hypertension with requirement of additional anti-hypertensives) is another side effect of ibrutinib, whose incidence can increase with ongoing therapy. Arthralgia is another common side effect with ibrutinib; most of the time it is grade 1–2 but can be a problem with long-term therapy, necessitating dose reduction/discontinuation. In a patient with worsening hypertension and arthralgia, an appropriate first option will be to reduce the dose of ibrutinib. For many patients, lowering the dose of ibrutinib from 420 mg daily to 280 mg daily and sometimes to 140 mg daily can improve the tolerability of the drug. With the approval of acalabrutinib, a second-generation BTK inhibitor, switching therapy to acalabrutinib in patients who are intolerant to ibrutinib is an appropriate choice as well. Acalabrutinib has greater specificity for BTK than ibrutinib; however, a head-to-head trial has not shown a significant difference in response and progression-free survival, but acalabrutinib resulted in lower rates of atrial fibrillation and hypertension.

Correct Answers: A, C

Case Study 3

A 67-year-old patient was diagnosed with CLL four years ago and initiated on ibrutinib two years ago when he developed progressive lymphadenopathy, anemia, and thrombocytopenia. Molecular characterization of the disease at the time of therapy initiation reported del(13q) on FISH and unmutated IGHV. He presents to the clinic now without any significant symptoms, normal blood counts (Hb 13.8 g/dL, platelet 310 × 10^9/L, WBC 4.6 × 10^9/L with 32% lymphocytes). CT imaging reported no lymphadenopathy larger than 1.5 cm. A bone marrow evaluation reported about 40% abnormal lymphoid infiltrate on morphology. Patient is tolerating ibrutinib well.

5) What is the next best therapeutic option?

A) Ibrutinib should be continued as the patient has attained partial remission and is tolerating ibrutinib well.

B) Presence of persistent disease in bone marrow is indicative of ibrutinib resistance, and the patient should be switched to a second-generation BTK inhibitor such as acalabrutinib.

C) Presence of persistent disease in bone marrow is indicative of BTKi resistance, and the patient should be switched to venetoclax-based regimen.

D) CD20 monoclonal antibody such as rituximab or obinutuzumab should be added to ibrutinib to clear the marrow disease.

Expert Perspective: The iwCLL 2018 response criteria requires the absence of CLL cells or lymphoid nodules in the bone marrow together with a normal CBC, absence of any lymphadenopathy $\geq$ 1.5 cm, and no hepatosplenomegaly to deem the response to therapy as complete (CR) (Hallek et al. 2018). In the above patient, the presence of a 40% lymphoid infiltrate in the bone marrow indicates attainment of a partial remission (PR). BTKi tend to have higher rates of PR compared to those seen with CIT and venetoclax-based therapies. The rate of CR with ibrutinib is low but increases with therapy duration (about 30% at five years in the front-line ibrutinib trials). However, this does not necessarily portend poorly on survival outcomes. In the ECOG1912 trial comparing ibrutinib-rituximab to fludarabine-cyclophosphamide-rituximab CIT in patients with treatment-naive CLL, the CIT arm produced a higher rate of CR (30.3%) compared to that seen in the ibrutinib arm, even though both progression-free survival and OS were superior for the ibrutinib arm at around three years of follow-up (Shanafelt et al. 2019). In the ALLIANCE trial, which compared chemoimmunotherapy (bendamustine with rituximab) versus ibrutinib or ibrutinib and rituximab as front-line therapy in older adults with CLL, the BR arm had higher rates of CR and undetectable-MRD remission than did the two ibrutinib arms but had significantly lower progression-free survival than that seen in ibrutinib arms (Woyach et al. 2018).

With BTKi monotherapy, the majority of patients achieve PR, and this is an acceptable therapy outcome. Therefore, ibrutinib should be continued in this patient as the persistent marrow involvement does not imply failure of BTKi.

Switching to a second-generation BTKi such as acalabrutinib is not indicated as the patient has not failed ibrutinib and is tolerating ibrutinib well. Similarly, use of monoclonal antibodies is not indicated at this time.

Venetoclax-based regimens lead to higher rates of CR and undetectable MRD in both front-line and R/R CLL (Fischer et al. 2019; Seymour et al. 2018). The group from MDACC reported outcomes of venetoclax consolidation in patients who were on prior ibrutinib for a minimum of one year with persistent disease and reported MRD conversion rates of 33% at six months and 67% at 12 months of combination therapy (Thompson et al. 2019). Based on this data, it is likely that this patient can achieve deeper marrow response with the addition of venetoclax; however, this approach is not FDA approved and long-term benefit is not clear at this time.

Correct Answer: A

Case Study 4

A 67-year-old woman was diagnosed with CLL four years ago and initiated on therapy with bendamustine-rituximab (BR) in view of anemia and significant lymphadenopathy. She had features of disease progression after one year of completion of BR (six cycles) with worsening anemia, lymphadenopathy, and fatigue. Genetic and molecular character-ization showed complex karyotype with a TP53 mutation. She was initiated on ibrutinib monotherapy. She attained a PR with ibrutinib but presents now with fever; progressive lymphadenopathy in the cervical, axillary, and intra-abdominal region with a mesenteric nodal mass measuring 3 × 3 × 2 cm and an SUVmax of 10.1 on PET-CT. Serum LDH is 610 IU (normal range: 120–220 IU). CBC is normal. Her ECOG PS is 1. She has no major comor-bidities, except for well-controlled type 2 diabetes mellitus.

6) **Which of the following are correct options in her management plan? (Choose one or more, as appropriate.)**
    A) She has features of CLL progression and needs change in therapy to a BCL2 antagonist.
    B) High SUV on the PET scan and high LDH are suggestive of a likely Richter transfor-mation, so you should biopsy the node with the highest SUV.
    C) Histopathological examination might show presence of CLL/SLL (small cells) and large cell (Richter's transformation) in the same specimen.
    D) As the most recent therapy was ibrutinib and not chemotherapy, the possibility of Richter transformation is low.

Expert Perspective: Disease progression in a patient with CLL on therapy usually indicates progressive CLL, but less commonly, this may represent Richter transformation. Richter trans-formation is a large cell transformation of CLL, usually to diffuse large B cell lymphoma (DLBCL) and rarely Hodgkin's lymphoma. The frequency of transformation is variable, around 1–10%. The gold standard of diagnosis is a PET guided-biopsy (excisional [preferred] or inci-sional) with assessment of the tissue architecture in detail and quantifying the involvement by large (transformed cells) and small cells with CLL/SLL morphology. Fine needle aspira-tion (FNA) is insufficient for RT diagnosis. Rarely infections can mimic RT, and it is important to rule them out. Despite high uptake on PET being considered a marker for RT, a biopsy is warranted to confirm the diagnosis. An SUVmax of > 10 is usually specific and has a good positive predictive value for RT in the correct clinical context but has low sensitivity.

Biopsy is imperative to diagnose Richter transformation as it helps in morphological and molecular characterization of RT. Most RT are DLBCL of the non-GCB subtype. They are usually associated with *TP53* and *MYC* aberrations. Understanding the origin of the DLBCL is impor-tant; those that are heterogeneous from the CLL clone may represent a new lymphoma (rather than transformation) and respond to traditional *de novo* DLBCL therapies (such as R-CHOP) while those similar to the CLL clone have poor response rates and survival outcomes. Nota-bly, expression of the Programmed cell death 1 (PD1) on the transformed tissue can be used as a surrogate to understand the origin of the DLBCL; transformed cells from CLL are usually positive while *de novo* DLBCL are negative (Ding 2018). Novel therapies incorporating PD1 and PDL1 inhibitors in early studies have shown responses in Richter transformation. Additional studies are looking at the BCL2 inhibitor venetoclax, non-covalent BTK inhibitors, and CART therapy for this group of patients Pirtobrutinib, a highly selective, non-covalent (reversible)

BTKi, inhibits both wildtype and C481-mutant BTK. In the phase I/II BRUIN trial, pirtobrutinib exhibited strong activity in patients with relapsed or refractory CLL who had received prior treatment with a covalent BTK inhibitor. About 100 patients (40.5%) had also received prior BCL2 inhibitor such as venetoclax. The percentage of patients with an overall response to pirtobrutinib was 73.3% (95% confidence interval [CI], 67.3 to 78.7), and the percentage was 82.2% (95% CI, 76.8 to 86.7) when partial response with lymphocytosis was included. The median PFS was 19.6 months (95% CI, 16.9 to 22.1). The most common adverse events were infections, bleeding, and neutropenia. Only 9 of 317 patients (2.8%) discontinued pirtobrutinib owing to a treatment-related adverse event.. Patients with Richter transformation should be considered for allogeneic stem cell transplantation when in remission (see Chapters 28 and 43).

Correct Answers: B, C

7) **Which of the following statements is/are correct in the context of CLL treatment?**
   A) Hemoglobin < 10 g/dL or platelet count < 100×10^9/L always indicate disease progression in a patient with CLL on observation and requires initiation of CLL-directed therapy.
   B) BTKi treatment initiation is associated with transient lymphocytosis due to lymphocyte redistribution.
   C) Ibrutinib and venetoclax combination have a synergistic effect in CLL.
   D) Venetoclax treatment initiation should be gradual with a ramp-up to the maximum dose over one week to prevent TLS.

Expert Perspective: The indications for treatment in CLL have been highlighted before (Question 1). An important sign of CLL progression warranting therapy is cytopenia. However, not all cytopenia in CLL is secondary to CLL involvement of the bone marrow. Around 5–10% patients can develop autoimmune hemolytic anemia (AIHA), and a smaller percentage can develop immune thrombocytopenia (ITP), pure red cell aplasia (PRCA), or immune-mediated neutropenia (Visco et al. 2014). Other conditions unrelated to the CLL can cause anemia such as iron or vitamin B_{12} deficiency secondary to malabsorption and anemia of chronic kidney disease; thrombocytopenia can be caused by chronic liver disease related to chronic splenomegaly. For the consideration of AIHA, elevated LDH, indirect hyperbilirubinemia, low serum haptoglobin, positive Coombs test, and elevated reticulocyte counts are important markers. Cytopenia secondary to autoimmune phenomenon in CLL should be treated initially with steroids with or without rituximab.

BTKi such as ibrutinib/acalabrutinib/zanubrutinib lead to post-treatment lymphocytosis considered secondary to redistribution of the lymphocytes from CLL-involved lymph nodes and secondary lymphoid organs, usually within the first month of therapy. The mechanism for this is the reduction in CLL cell adhesion molecules by BTKi in the lymph node, leading to their migration into peripheral blood. Redistribution lymphocytosis is very common in patients with CLL who start BTKi and does not affect long-term outcomes. Importantly, BTKi treatment should not be interrupted. Redistribution lymphocytosis generally resolves over the course of 3–9 months with ongoing BTKi therapy.

BTKi and venetoclax have a synergistic action that might improve disease control. Several preclinical studies have shown their synergistic effect (Patel et al. 2018). Both in the relapsed setting (CLARITY trial) and in the front-line trial (MDACC, CAPTIVATE), ibrutinib plus venetoclax combination regimen showed high rates of MRD-negative remissions. Several combinations of BTKi and venetoclax, with or without CD20 mono-clonal antibodies, are being studied in phase II and phase III clinical trials.

Venetoclax can be associated with a high risk of tumor lysis syndrome in patients with CLL and needs a slow ramp-up over five weeks to the maximum dose (400 mg daily) with close monitoring for TLS. It is important to consider interactions with other concomitant medications (like azole antifungals) that require dose reduction of venetoclax.

Correct Answers: B, C

8) **Which of the following is/are FDA approved non-chemotherapeutic time-limited combination regimen in treatment-naive CLL?**
   A) Ibrutinib with rituximab.
   B) Ibrutinib with obinutuzumab.
   C) Venetoclax with rituximab.
   D) Venetoclax with obinutuzumab.
   E) Venetoclax with ibrutinib.
   F) Acalabrutinib with obinutuzumab.

Expert Perspective: Currently, the only FDA approved time-limited targeted therapy for patients with treatment-naive CLL is venetoclax + obinutuzumab (based on the CLL14 trial). The combination of ibrutinib with venetoclax is being studied in several phase II and phase III studies (CLL GLOW trial); it is currently not yet FDA approved In GLOW, fixed-duration ibrutinib + venetoclax showed superior PFS versus chlorambucil + obinutuzumab in older/comorbid patients with previously untreated CLL. Interestingly, PFS rates at EOT+12 were high among patients treated with ibrutinib + venetoclax regardless of MRD status at end of therapy plus 3 months, 96.3% and 93.3% in patients with undetectable MRD ($<10^{-4}$) and detectable MRD ($\geq 10^{-4}$) in BM, respectively, versus 83.3% and 58.7% for patients receiving chlorambucil + obinutuzumab. PFS rates at end of therapy plus 12 months also remained high in patients with unmutated IGHV receiving ibrutinib + venetoclax, independent of MRD status in BM. All the other combination regimens have a BTKi that needs to be adminis-tered indefinitely, while the time-limited venetoclax + rituximab combination is approved in R/R CLL. Recently, the results of GAIA-CLL13 and Alliance A041702 were reported. GAIA-CLL13 is a phase 3, open-label trial, which randomly assigned, in a 1:1:1:1 ratio, fit patients with CLL who did not have TP53 aberrations to receive six cycles of chemoimmunotherapy (fludarabine-cyclophosphamide-rituximab or bendamustine-rituximab) or 12 cycles of venetoclax-rituximab, venetoclax-obinutuzumab, or venetoclax-obinutuzumab-ibrutinib. Ibrutinib was discontinued after two consecutive measurements of undetectable minimal residual disease or could be extended. The primary end points were undetectable MRD as assessed by flow cytometry in peripheral blood at month 15 and PFS. At month 15 (short fol-low-up), the percentage of patients with undetectable MRD was significantly higher in the venetoclax-obinutuzumab group (86.5%; 97.5% CI, 80.6 to 91.1) and the venetoclax-obinu-tuzumab-ibrutinib group (92.2%; 97.5% CI, 87.3 to 95.7) than in the chemoimmunotherapy group (52.0%; 97.5% CI, 44.4 to 59.5; P<0.001 for both comparisons), but it was not signif-icantly higher in the venetoclax-rituximab group (57.0%; 97.5% CI, 49.5 to 64.2; P = 0.32). PFS at 3 years was also higher with venetoclax-obinutuzumab (87.7%; HR for disease progression or death, 0.42; 97.5% CI, 0.26 to 0.68; P<0.001), but not with venetoclax-rituximab (80.8%; HR, 0.79; 97.5% CI, 0.53 to 1.18; P = 0.18). Grade 3 and grade 4 infections were more common with chemoimmunotherapy (18.5%) and venetoclax-obinutuzumab-ibrutinib (21.2%) than with venetoclax-rituximab (10.5%) or venetoclax-obinutuzumab (13.2%). The study need longer follow-up to see whether the PFS curves start to show a difference between the three and two chemotherapy free regimens. The Alliance A041702 trial is an NCTN phase III clinical trial looking at initial therapy for older patients with previously untreated CLL. The study did not show benefit of triplet over doublets however at a relatively short follow up of 14 months. The study investigated regimen of ibrutinib and venetoclax plus obinutuzumab with the doublet of ibrutinib plus obinutuzumab. The purpose of this study was to see whether adding venetoclax to this doublet might allow more patients to have undetectable MRD and complete responses and thus be able to discontinue therapy. After a year of treatment, and this included just six months of the antibody, all patients underwent a response evaluation. Those patients that were on the doublet arm all then continued ibrutinib indefinitely, and the patients on the triplet arm underwent a response-adapted either discontinuation of ibrutinib or continuation of therapy. However, the results of this study may have been confounded somewhat by the COVID-19 pandemic, where the death rate from COVID-19 was higher in patients treated on the triplet arm than those treated on the doublet arm. Outside of this, the toxicity profile between the two regimens was actually relatively similar. Like GAIA-CLL13 long-term results of study would be of interest.

Correct Answer: D

Table 27.1 FDA Approved combination targeted therapies in patients with newly diagnosed and relapsed and refractory CLL.

Drug combination	FDA approval	Indication	Duration	Approval comments
Ibrutinib with rituximab	April 2020	Treatment naive	Ibrutinib continuously till progression Rituximab for 6 cycles	**ECOG 1912** Phase III trial (Shanafelt et al. 2019): I and R vs FCR in CLL patients ≤ 70 years [del(17p13) excluded]
Ibrutinib with obinutuzumab	Jan 2019	Treatment naive	Ibrutinib continuously till progression Obinutuzumab for 6 cycles (total 8, 1000 mg infusions)	**iLLUMINATE** phase III trial (Moreno et al. 2019): I and G vs. chlorambucil and G in CLL [≥ 65 years or < 65 years with comorbidities or del(17p)/TP53 mutated]
Venetoclax with rituximab	June 2018	After 1 prior therapy (± 17p del)	Venetoclax for 24 months Rituximab for 6 cycles	**MURANO** phase 3 trial (Seymour et al. 2018): V and R vs. bendamustine and R in ≥ 18 years after 1–3 prior therapy

(Continued)

Table 27.1 (Continued)

Drug combination	FDA approval	Indication	Duration	Approval comments
Venetoclax with obinutuzumab	May 2019	Treatment naive	Venetoclax for 12 months Obinutuzumab for 6 cycles (total 8, 1000 mg infusions)	**CLL 14** phase III trial (Fischer et al. 2019): V and G vs. chlorambucil and G in CLL (> 6 cumulative illness rating scale or CrCl < 70 mL/min)
Acalabrutinib with obinutuzumab	November 2019	Treatment naive	Acalabrutinib continuously till progression Obinutuzumab for 6 cycles (total 8, 1000 mg infusions)	**ELEVATE TN** Phase III trial (Hallek and Al-Sawaf 2021; Sharman et al. 2020): A or A-G vs chlorambucil and G in CLL (≥ 65 years or < 65 years with CrCl 30–69 mL/min or CIRS > 6)

Recommended Readings

Ding, W. (2018). Richter transformation in the era of novel agents. *Hematology Am Soc of Hematol Educ Program* 2018 (1): 256–263.

Eichhorst, B., Niemann, C.U., and Kater, A.P. (2023 May 11). GCLLSG, the HOVON and Nordic CLL study groups, the SAKK, the Israeli CLL association, and cancer trials Ireland. First line venetoclax combinations in chronic lymphocytic leukemia. *N Engl J Med* 388 (19): 1739–1754. doi: 10.1056/NEJMoa2213093. PMID: 37163621.

Fischer, K., Al-Sawaf, O., Bahlo, J. et al. (2019). Venetoclax and obinutuzumab in patients with CLL and coexisting conditions. *New England Journal of Medicine* 380 (23): 2225–2236.

Hallek, M. and Al-Sawaf, O. (2021 December 1). Chronic lymphocytic leukemia: 2022 update on diagnostic and therapeutic procedures. *Am J Hematol* 96 (12): 1679–1705. doi: 10.1002/ajh.26367. PMID: 34625994.

Hallek, M., Cheson, B.D., Catovsky, D. et al. (2018). iwCLL guidelines for diagnosis, indications for treatment, response assessment, and supportive management of CLL. *Blood* 131 (25): 2745–2760.

Huber, H., Tausch, E., Schneider, C. et al. (2023 September 14). Final analysis of the CLL2-GIVe trial: obinutuzumab, ibrutinib, and venetoclax for untreated CLL with del(17p)/TP53mut. *Blood* 142 (11): 961–972. doi: 10.1182/blood.2023020013. PMID: 37363867.

Mato, A.R., Woyach, J.A., and Brown, J.R. (2023 July 6). Pirtobrutinib after a co valent BTK inhibitor in chronic lymphocytic leukemia. *N Engl J Med* 389 (1): 33–44. doi: 10.1056/NEJMoa2300696. PMID: 37407001.

Moreno, C., Greil, R., Demirkan, F. et al. (2019). Ibrutinib plus obinutuzumab versus chlorambucil plus obinutuzumab in first-line treatment of chronic lymphocytic leukaemia (iLLUMINATE): A multicentre, randomised, open-label, phase 3 trial. *The Lancet Oncol* 20 (1): 43–56.

Muchtar, E., Kay, N.E., and Parikh, S.A. (2021). Early intervention in asymptomatic chronic lymphocytic leukemia. *Clin Adv Hematol Oncol* 19 (2): 92–103.

Munir, T., Moreno, C., Owen, C. (2023 July 20). Impact of minimal residual disease on progression-free survival outcomes after fixed-duration Ibrutinib-Venetoclax versus Chlorambucil-Obinutuzumab in the GLOW Study. *J Clin Oncol* 41 (21): 3689–3699. doi: 10.1200/JCO.22.02283. Epub 2023 Jun 6. PMID: 37279408; PMCID: PMC10351955.

Patel, V.K., Lamothe, B., Ayres, M.L. et al. (2018). Pharmacodynamics and proteomic analysis of acalabrutinib therapy: similarity of on-target effects to ibrutinib and rationale for combination therapy. *Leukemia* 32 (4): 920–930.

Senapati, J. and Jain, N. (2021). Eradicating minimal residual disease in chronic lymphocytic leukemia. *Adv Oncol* 1: 249–262.

Seymour, J.F., Kipps, T.J., Eichhorst, B. et al. (2018). Venetoclax–Rituximab in relapsed or refractory chronic lymphocytic leukemia. *N Engl J Med* 378 (12): 1107–1120.

Shanafelt, T.D., Wang, X.V., Kay, N.E. et al. (2019). Ibrutinib–Rituximab or Chemoimmunotherapy for chronic lymphocytic leukemia. *N Engl J Med* 381 (5): 432–443.

Sharman, J.P., Egyed, M., Jurczak, W. et al. (2020). Acalabrutinib with or without obinutuzumab versus chlorambucil and obinutuzumab for treatment-naive chronic lymphocytic leukaemia (ELEVATE-TN): a randomised, controlled, phase 3 trial. *The Lancet* 395 (10232): 1278–1291.

Thompson, P.A., Keating, M.J., Jain, N. et al. (2019). Venetoclax added to Ibrutinib in high-risk CLL achieves a high rate of undetectable minimal residual disease. [RTS1]. *Blood* 134 (Supplement_1): 358–358.

Visco, C., Barcellini, W., Maura, F., Neri, A., Cortelezzi, A., and Rodeghiero, F. (2014). Autoimmune cytopenias in chronic lymphocytic leukemia. *Am J Hematol* 89 (11): 1055–1062.

Woyach, J.A., Ruppert, A.S., Heerema, N.A. et al. (2018). Ibrutinib regimens versus Chemoimmunotherapy in older patients with untreated CLL. *N Engl J Med* 379 (26): 2517–2528.

28

Hematopoietic Cell Transplantation and Cellular Therapy in Chronic Lymphocytic Leukemia

Ajay Major, Michael R. Bishop, and Peter A. Riedell

The University of Chicago, Chicago, IL, USA

Introduction

Chronic lymphocytic leukemia / small lymphocytic leukemia (CLL/SLL) is the most common leukemia diagnosed in the United States with an estimated 20,160 new cases in 2022 and approximately 4,410 patients succumbing to the disease (Siddiqi et al. 2023). In the past several years, there has been a shift in the CLL treatment paradigm toward greater utilization of targeted agents over traditional chemoimmunotherapy approaches based on improved efficacy and greater tolerability. Commonly, Bruton tyrosine kinase inhibitors (BTKi) or B-cell lymphoma 2 (BCL2) inhibitors in combination with an anti-CD20 monoclonal antibody are utilized in the front-line setting with encouraging long-term data (see Chapter 27). This paradigm shift has also translated into a steady decline in the utilization of allogeneic hematopoietic stem cell transplantation (HSCT) since 2013 based on data from Phelan and colleagues from the Center for International Blood and Marrow Transplant Research (CIBMTR) registry (2020). In CLL, a variety of novel therapeutic approaches are being explored, including the use of cellular therapy. While chimeric antigen receptor (CAR) T cell therapy is currently investigational in CLL, preliminary studies have shown impressive activity and a tolerable safety profile. These seminal works have provided the foundation for further exploration of cellular therapy in this disease, and researchers predict that cellular therapy will likely be rapidly incorporated into the CLL treatment paradigm in the years to come. Herein, we discuss the role of allogeneic HSCT and other cellular therapy in patients with CLL/SLL.

Case Study 1

A 62-year-old woman with a history of atrial fibrillation sought medical attention from her primary care physician for the recent development of lumps above her left axilla and right supraclavicular region. Upon questioning, she acknowledged progressive fatigue over the preceding two months and occasional fevers and night sweats over the past two weeks. She palpated the masses approximately a week ago and called at her spouse's insistence. On physical examination, she had palpable bilateral cervical, right supraclavicular, bilateral axillary (left greater than right), and bilateral inguinal adenopathy. The spleen tip was palpable 2 cm below the left costal margin with deep inspiration; the liver edge was not palpable. A complete blood count (CBC) demonstrated a white blood cell (WBC) count of 42,700 with 90% mature lymphocytes with occasional prolymphocytes, a hemoglobin (Hb) of 10.8 g/dL, and platelets of 103,000. She was referred to a hematologist, who sent her blood for flow cytometric analysis, which demonstrated a monoclonal B cell population that expressed CD5, CD19, CD20(dim), CD22(dim), CD23, CD38, and CD79(dim); they were negative for CD10 and SmIg. The cells were also positive for ZAP70, and IGHV (immunoglobulin heavy-chain variable region) was unmutated. A bone marrow examination demonstrated a hypercellular marrow with 70–80% replacement by lymphocytes; 10% were prolymphocytes. Cytogenetic analysis demonstrated a deletion of the short arm of chromosome 17 in 19/20 metaphases analyzed, which was further corroborated by fluorescence in situ hybridization (FISH) studies. A CT scan of the chest, abdomen, and pelvis demonstrated diffuse adenopathy and splenomegaly.

The decision was made to initiate treatment with obinutuzumab and venetoclax per the CLL14 study, as the patient preferred time-limited therapy. At the completion of one year of therapy, her adenopathy had completely resolved, and a CBC demonstrated a WBC of 6,700 with 13% lymphocytes on peripheral smear, a Hb level of 14.3 g/dL, and a platelet count of 303,000. The patient was then transitioned to active surveillance.

Approximately 20 months following conclusion of therapy, the patient re-presented with palpable cervical adenopathy. CT imaging confirmed significant cervical adenopathy (3–4 cm) as well as diffuse adenopathy in the chest, abdomen, and pelvis. A CBC demonstrated a WBC of 59,000 with 89% mature lymphocytes, a Hb of 9.0 g/dL, and platelets of 97,000. The patient subsequently initiated treatment with acalabrutinib and had adequate disease control for 14 months, after which time she developed groin pain and was found on CT imaging to have progressive bilateral inguinal lymphadenopathy. An excisional lymph node biopsy demonstrated small lymphocytic lymphoma and no evidence of Richter's transformation (RT). The patient was referred to a tertiary center for treatment options, including cellular therapies and hematopoietic stem cell transplantation (HSCT). The patient has three living siblings who are in good health. A decision is made to treat the patient, outside of a clinical trial, with bendamustine and rituximab (BR).

1) Is it appropriate to consider allogeneic HSCT for the patient at this time?

Expert Perspective: The patient has progressive disease after treatment with both the BCL2 inhibitor venetoclax and a BTK inhibitor. She is relatively young and has high-risk features, including a 17p deletion and relatively short response durations to two prior lines of therapy. Taken together, it is appropriate to consider allogeneic transplantation as a treatment option even if she were to respond to next line of therapy. Whether the patient is an appropriate transplantation candidate is dependent on a number of factors, including the patient's response to third-line therapy, the availability of a donor, and ultimately whether the patient is willing to accept the toxicities associated with allogeneic HSCT.

2) If the patient does not have chemotherapy-sensitive disease, is transplantation contraindicated?

Expert Perspective: Chemotherapy sensitivity is known to be an important prognostic factor; however, there are patients who lack chemotherapy sensitivity, generally defined as at least a partial response (PR), who can achieve long-term remissions and survival with allogeneic HSCT. Pavletic and colleagues (2000) reported on 23 CLL/SLL patients who underwent allogeneic HSCT, including 14 patients with chemotherapy-refractory disease, 12 of which were refractory to fludarabine. Fourteen patients (61%) were alive without disease at follow-up, including eight patients with chemotherapy-refractory disease. Additionally, pre-transplant chemosensitivity was not found to be a predictor of overall survival in a univariate analysis. The literature has demonstrated mixed findings regarding the prognostic significance of chemosensitivity, with an analysis by Khouri and colleagues (2011) at MD Anderson Cancer Center finding that disease status at the time of HSCT had no effect on survival in a multivariable analysis. However, the prospective multicenter phase II German CLL Study Group CLL3X trial by Dreger and colleagues (2010) found that neither the time interval from diagnosis to allogeneic HSCT nor the number of previous regimens correlated with overall survival, but chemotherapy-refractory disease did adversely correlate with overall survival in multivariate analysis. As such, lack of chemotherapy sensitivity is not an absolute contraindication to allogeneic HSCT, but it appears that outcomes may be improved in patients who have chemotherapy-sensitive disease. In our practice, we have found that patients with truly progressive disease at the time of transplant rarely, if ever, benefit from HSCT, and we advise against transplantation for these patients. However, we will offer patients with stable disease the option of allogeneic HSCT, explaining that the risk of relapse is increased.

3) What if the patient does not have an HLA-matched (HLA: human leukocyte antigen) sibling? Are the results significantly worse with a HLA-matched, HLA-mismatched unrelated donor, or even with a related haploidentical donor?

Expert Perspective: Given that only a minority of patients have matched related donors, there has been increasing interest over the past decade in utilizing matched unrelated donors (MUDs) or HLA-haploidentical donors for allogeneic HSCT in various hematologic malignancies. Although transplantation from MUDs were historically considered to have worse outcomes than matched related donors, even with haploidentical donors, several studies within the CLL literature have challenged this notion. In the aforementioned German CLL Study Group CLL3X trial by Dreger and colleagues (2010), which predominantly included poor-risk CLL, donor source (HLA-matched siblings, well-matched unrelated donors, or partially matched unrelated donors) did not adversely affect survival in a multivariable analysis. The use of haploidentical donors in CLL has comparable outcomes to HLA-matched donors, with a retrospective European Society for Blood and Marrow Transplantation (EBMT) analysis by van Gorkom and colleagues (2017) finding a five-year overall survival of 38% with haploidentical HSCT, though the five-year non-relapse mortality (NRM) was 44%, higher than rates seen with HLA-matched donors. It is well known in the transplant literature that transplantation using a haploidentical donor may be associated with higher rates of graft-versus-host disease (GvHD) and NRM, though the adoption of the post-transplant cyclophosphamide (PTCy) platform may mitigate these complications. In a 2018 EBMT study, 38% of patients received PTCy for GvHD prophylaxis, and no difference in the cumulative incidence of NRM was observed between patients who did and did not receive PTCy. A retrospective study by Paul and colleagues (2020) at Johns Hopkins found that, of 64 consecutive CLL patients who underwent reduced-intensity conditioning (RIC) haploidentical HSCT with PTCy, four-year overall survival was 52%, three-year NRM was 24%, and the two-year incidence of chronic GvHD was 17%.

A meta-analysis by Gagelmann and colleagues (2019) confirmed this observation. In summary, although matched related donors are preferred in allogeneic HSCT, the use of MUDs as well as related haploidentical donors with a PTCy platform may result in comparable survival rates for those patients who do not have a suitable related donor.

4) What is the quality of life like for CLL patients who undergo allogeneic HSCT?

Expert Perspective: Given the availability of novel agents in relapsed and refractory CLL, health-related quality of life (HRQoL) must be considered in counseling patients about allogeneic HSCT for CLL. Although there is a tremendous amount of literature on HRQoL in long-term survivors following allogeneic HSCT, particularly the effects of chronic GvHD, there is only a limited data on the HRQoL of CLL patients who have undergone allogeneic HSCT. Malhotra and colleagues (2008) at the Mayo Clinic retrospectively reviewed the outcomes of 12 consecutive CLL patients who had undergone allogeneic HSCT for CLL at their institution. Of the six patients who were alive five years after HSCT, all were reported as having an excellent performance status without ongoing chronic GvHD. Gill and colleagues (2008) evaluated HRQoL of 13 CLL patients treated at the Royal Melbourne Hospital and noted that three out of five patients who were still alive at last follow-up had resumed part- or full-time employment. However, a more recent EBMT registry study involving over 2,500 patients with CLL who had underwent allogeneic HSCT by van Gelder and colleagues (2017) reported a NRM of 40% in the 10 years after HSCT, with 42% of deaths attributed to GvHD. In counseling patients, it is important to emphasize possible long-term complications from allogeneic HSCT, such as GvHD, with a return to a relatively normal quality of life seen largely in patients who achieve long-term remissions.

5) What if the patient had Richter's transformation? Is there any role for HSCT?

Expert Perspective: Both autologous and allogeneic HSCT have historically been used for RT, as they both present opportunities for durable remissions. Cwynarski and colleagues (2012) at the EBMT conducted a retrospective analysis of both autologous and allogeneic HSCT in patients with RT. Of the 59 total patients identified among EBMT centers, 34 had received autologous HSCT and 25 had received allogeneic HSCT. The overwhelming majority of autologous recipients had chemotherapy-sensitive disease, and 36% of allogeneic recipients had chemotherapy-refractory disease. Three-year overall survival (OS) and relapse-free survival (RFS) were 36% and 27%, respectively, for allogeneic HSCT and 59% and 45%, respectively, for autologous HSCT. In a multivariable analysis, chemotherapy-sensitive disease and use of a reduced-intensity conditioning regimen were found to be associated with superior RFS after allogeneic HSCT. A more recent retrospective study by Herrera and colleagues (2021) through the CIBMTR identified 171 patients with RT who underwent autologous (n = 53) and allogeneic (n = 118) HSCT. Three-year OS and RFS were 52% and 30%, respectively, for allogeneic HSCT and 57% and 37%, respectively, for autologous HSCT. As previously demonstrated by the EBMT study, deeper response before allogeneic HSCT was associated with significantly better survival. Additionally, this study found that cytogenetic abnormalities, including 17p deletion, and receipt of previous novel therapies were not significantly associated with outcomes. Both studies concluded that patients with RT who have chemotherapy-sensitive disease appear to benefit from consolidation with either autologous and allogeneic transplantation. The choice between autologous and allogeneic transplantation in this setting requires multidisciplinary discussion and consideration of a patient's comorbidities and preferences surrounding transplant-related morbidity and toxicities (also see chapter 43).

6) What is the upper age limit for allogeneic HSCT in CLL patients?

Expert Perspective: Considering that the average age of CLL patients at diagnosis is older than 60 years, the question of upper-age eligibility for allogeneic transplantation is highly relevant. The utilization of reduced-intensity and nonmyeloablative conditioning regimens has broadened the applicability of allogeneic HSCT to older patients. Additionally, the development of comorbidities indices has aided our ability to assess who are appropriate transplant candidates. Sorror and collaborators within the Seattle Transplantation Consortium (2011) reported on the outcomes of 372 patients with a variety of hematologic malignancies, 60 years or older, who underwent nonmyeloablative allogeneic HSCT while enrolled in prospective clinical HSCT trials. The median patient age was 64.1 years (range: 60.1–75.1 years). Overall, the five-year cumulative incidences of NRM and relapse were 27% (95% CI 22–32%) and 41% (95% CI 36–46%), respectively. The five-year OS and progression-free survival (PFS) rates were 35% (95% CI 30–40%) and 32% (95% CI 27–37%), respectively. These outcomes were not statistically significantly different ($P = 0.18$) when stratified by age groups (60–64 vs 65–69 vs 70 or older). Furthermore, increasing age was not associated with increases in acute or chronic GvHD or organ toxicities. In multivariate models, HCT-specific comorbidity index scores of 1 to 2 (hazard ratio, HR, 1.58; 95% CI 1.08–2.31) and 3 or greater (HR 1.97; 95% CI: 1.38–2.80) were associated with worse survival compared with an HCT-specific comorbidity index score of 0 ($P = 0.003$ overall).

At most transplant centers, the upper age limit is 75 years. This is a relatively arbitrary upper limit, and there are several anecdotal reports of transplantation being performed for even older adults. The most important determination of transplant eligibility involves the assessment of several parameters related to comorbidities, performance status, disease status, and, ultimately, the decision by a well-informed patient relative to risks and benefits (Derman et al. 2019).

Case Study continued: Our 62-year-old patient went on to achieve a partial response from bendamustine and rituximab (BR) and subsequently underwent a nonmyeloablative allogeneic HSCT from a 10-of-10 HLA-matched unrelated donor. She developed late-onset grade II acute GvHD with tapering of her immunosuppression and subsequently limited chronic GvHD of the skin. She achieved a morphologic CR but had persistent evidence of minimal residual disease by polymerase chain reaction monitoring. She eventually had clinical evidence of relapse 27 months after HSCT, and she is currently being evaluated for a clinical trial with CAR T cell therapy.

Case Study 2

A 68-year-old male with no significant past medical history presented for his annual physical examination. Over the past year, he had noted slight fatigue, which he attributed to increased stress at work; he was otherwise asymptomatic. A CBC demonstrated a WBC count of 33,000 with 87% mature-appearing lymphocytes on peripheral smear, a Hb level of 13.7 g/dL, and a platelet count of 278,000. On physical examination, he was noted to have mildly enlarged bilateral (1–2 cm) cervical and axillary adenopathy without hepatosplenomegaly. A peripheral blood sample was sent for flow cytometric analysis and demonstrated a monoclonal B-lymphocyte population expressing CD5, CD19, CD20, CD22(dim), CD23, CD79(dim), and SmIg(dim); they were negative for CD38 and FMC7. A bone marrow examination demonstrated 40% lymphocytes with a diffuse histopathologic pattern. Cytogenetic analysis revealed a normal 46XY karyotype; however, FISH studies demonstrated an 11q deletion, 13q deletion, and IGHV was unmutated. The patient was diagnosed as having B-cell CLL and staged as Rai stage 1. It was recommended that the patient be closely observed with follow-up every three months.

At a follow-up visit six months later, the patient reported increased fatigue and drenching night sweats. On physical examination, his adenopathy had increased in both size and extent, with new palpable adenopathy (2–3 cm) in the bilateral inguinal regions. A CBC demonstrated a WBC of 78,000 with 92% mature-appearing lymphocytes on peripheral smear, a Hb of 10.3 g/dL, and a platelet count of 156,000. Given evidence of clinical progression and symptomatology, the decision was made to begin treatment with front-line chemoimmunotherapy, and he was started on BR. He tolerated therapy well and completed six cycles resulting in a PR based on iwCLL response criteria. Active surveillance was recommended.

The patient was monitored with active surveillance for one year, at which time a progressive increase in his WBC count was noted. Approximately two years after completion of BR therapy, the patient began experiencing night sweats again, at which time a CBC demonstrated a WBC of 49,000 with progressive anemia and thrombocytopenia. A bone marrow biopsy revealed 50% involvement by CLL without any evidence of RT. Repeat cytogenetics revealed an 11q deletion, 13q deletion, along with a 17p deletion. He had widespread lymphadenopathy on CT scan though non-bulky accompanied with an elevated lactate dehydrogenase (LDH). Given his relapsed disease and new 17p deletion, the decision was made to initiate therapy with the BTK inhibitor, ibrutinib. He tolerated ibrutinib well without any clinically significant adverse events. He achieved a partial response to therapy and maintained this response for approximately 24 months before demonstrating signs of progressive disease with lymphocytosis, worsening cytopenias, increased lymphadenopathy, early satiety, and drenching night sweats.

He was then initiated on a combination of venetoclax and rituximab as third-line treatment. He tolerated the venetoclax ramp-up without evidence of tumor lysis syndrome, and after completing six cycles of rituximab, he continued on venetoclax for 24 months, achieving a PR to therapy. Following the conclusion of treatment, active surveillance was again recommended. Unfortunately, 14 months after concluding venetoclax he developed drenching night sweats, lymphocytosis, thrombocytopenia, and increased lymphadenopathy in his right inguinal region. A right inguinal excisional lymph node biopsy was performed and consistent with CLL without evidence of histologic transformation. His FISH studies again revealed an 11q deletion, 13q deletion, and 17p deletion, and cytogenetics revealed a complex karyotype with > five cytogenetic abnormalities. Given his failure of three prior lines of treatment, including chemoimmunotherapy, along with BTK and BCL2 inhibitor therapy, the decision was made to refer him to a tertiary cancer center to discuss allogeneic HSCT or cellular therapies, including CAR T cell therapy. The patient has one living sibling who has metastatic colon cancer and one MUD in the registry, though he is reticent to incur the risks associated with an allogeneic HSCT.

7) What is the current state of CAR T cell therapy in CLL/SLL?

Expert Perspective: Although targeted agents such as BTK inhibitors and venetoclax have significantly improved outcomes for the front-line treatment of CLL as compared to traditional chemoimmunotherapy, most patients will eventually relapse or develop progressive disease while on these therapies (see Chapter 27). There is a scarcity of effective agents for the salvage treatment of CLL after BTK inhibitors and venetoclax therapy, largely limited to phosphatidylinositol 3-kinase (PI3K) inhibitors and allogeneic HSCT, both of which have considerable toxicities. As such, there have been recent investigations of the efficacy of CAR T cell therapy in relapsed or refractory CLL, with promising activity.

At the time of this publication, CAR T cell therapy has not received regulatory approval for CLL, though CAR T cell therapy has a well-established role in the treatment of relapsed and refractory non-Hodgkin lymphomas, with the potential for durable remissions in aggressive large B-cell lymphomas. Currently, there are four autologous CAR T cell products approved by the FDA for use in a variety of lymphoma subtypes, including patients with aggressive large B-cell lymphomas, mantle cell lymphoma, and follicular lymphoma. Additional indications are expected in the near future as cellular therapy is explored in earlier lines of therapy and in more disease subtypes.

Currently enrolling studies evaluating the role of CAR T cell therapy in CLL are largely limited to subjects who are relapsed, refractory, or intolerant to both a BTK and a BCL2 inhibitor. Even with investigational non-covalent BTK inhibitors, risk of mutations that cause resistance to these therapies are emerging. Thus, it is likely that CAR T cell therapy may initially surface as a treatment option in the third-line setting or beyond in CLL. In our patient's case, he harbors high-risk disease features, including a 17p deletion, and therefore experimental therapeutic options such as CAR T cell therapies should be considered.

8) What is the evidence behind CAR T cell therapy in CLL/SLL?

Expert Perspective: Initial small studies on CD19-targeted CAR T cells in relapsed CLL by Porter and colleagues (2015) demonstrated an overall response rate (ORR) of 57% among 14 treated patients, including four patients (29%) who achieved a complete response (CR). These findings were redemonstrated by Geyer and colleagues (2019) with 3 of 12 patients (25%) achieving CR, as well as in a larger cohort of 32 patients by Frey and colleagues (2020) in which nine patients (28%) achieved a CR. Findings from these studies suggest that patients who achieve a CR had persistently detectable CAR T cells after their initial infusion along with no evidence of minimal residual disease (MRD). Cumulatively, these data fostered interest in utilizing CAR T cell therapy to achieve durable long-term responses in patients with relapsed and refractory CLL and led to the further exploration in a variety of clinical trials.

9) Which CAR T cell products are in late stage of clinical development for the treatment of relapsed or refractory CLL/SLL?

Expert Perspective: The results of the TRANSCEND CLL 004 study are expected to lead to regulatory approval of lisocabtagene maraleucel (liso-cel) for patients with relapsed or refractory CLL. In the multicenter phase I study by Siddiqi and colleagues (2023), 24 patients with relapsed or refractory CLL after previous BTK inhibitor treatment failure were treated with liso-cel CAR T cell therapy at two different dose levels. Of 22 efficacy-evaluable patients, the ORR was 82% (45% CR rate), with 45% of patients still in response at 18 months of follow-up. Importantly, patients who achieved undetectable MRD in their peripheral blood or bone marrow had superior median PFS than those with detectable disease, suggesting MRD may serve as a novel prognostic biomarker after CAR T cell therapy in CLL. There were five patients (23%) who developed RT after liso-cel, with three of those patients initially achieving a response to liso-cel. Most recently, primary analysis of phase 1/2 TRANSCEND CLL 004 were reported. Patients (n=117) had at least two previous lines of therapy, including a BTK inhibitor, received an intravenous infusion of liso-cel at one of two target dose levels. A subset of patients had also experienced venetoclax failure (n=70). In the primary efficacy analysis set at dose level 2 (100×10^6 CAR + T cells; n=49), the rate of CR (including with incomplete marrow recovery) was statistically significant at 18% (n=9; 95% CI 9–32; p=0·0006). Toxicities of CAR T-cell therapy from this trial are discussed below and in further detail in Chapter 59.

10) Does the number of lines of prior therapy or disease-risk features affect outcomes of CAR T cell therapy in CLL/SLL?

Expert Perspective: Given the small number of patients with CLL treated with CAR T cell therapy, there are limited data regarding patient- or disease-related characteristics that may predict better outcomes. Turtle and colleagues (2017) treated 24 patients with relapsed CLL who had received a median of five prior therapies including prior ibrutinib with CD19-directed CAR T cells. The ORR was 71% with a high proportion of patients with undetectable disease in their bone marrow after treatment, suggesting that CAR T cell therapy is also effective in ibrutinib-refractory patients. In the aforementioned TRANSCEND CLL 004 study, the median number of prior lines of treatment was four, and 100% of patients had previously received ibrutinib and 65% had previously received venetoclax, suggesting efficacy of CAR T cell therapy in heavily pretreated patients. In relation to disease risk features, the study by Turtle et al. (2017), enrolled patients with high-risk disease, including 67% with complex cytogenetics, 58% with deletion 17p, and 96% who were refractory to or relapsed after a fludarabine and rituximab containing regimen. Similarly, in the TRANSCEND CLL 004 study, 83% of recipients had high-risk features, including deletion 17p (35%), mutated *TP53* (61%), complex karyotype (48%), and/or unmutated IGHV (35%). In summary, CAR T-cell therapy appears to be highly effective in heavily pretreated patients, though longer-term follow-up is needed to better determine if responses in these high-risk subsets translate into durable remissions.

11) What toxicities are associated with CAR T cell therapy in CLL/SLL, and how are they managed?

Expert Perspective: CAR T cell therapy is universally associated with two primary acute toxicities after infusion: cytokine release syndrome (CRS) and neurologic toxicity, both of which are the result of upregulation of inflammatory cytokines that occur during in vivo expansion of the CAR T cell product (see Chapter 59). These toxicities are typically managed with close daily monitoring, supportive care measures, and frequently may require inpatient hospitalization. In general, more serious grades of CRS and neurologic toxicity are managed with anti-cytokine therapies; the IL-6 receptor antagonist, tocilizumab, is the mainstay for management of CRS, and corticosteroids serve as the cornerstone of management of neurologic toxicity. The incidence of CRS and neurologic toxicity may vary depending on the CAR T cell product and the patient population being treated; in the aforementioned CLL studies, CRS rates were 64–100%, with grade ≥ 3 CRS of 8–24% and grade ≥ 3 neurologic toxicity in 6–25% of patients. Importantly, in the TRANSCEND CLL 004 study with liso-cel, grade 3 CRS was reported in ten (9%) of 117 (with no grade 4 or 5 events) and grade 3 neurological events were reported in 21 (18%; one [1%] grade 4, no grade 5 events). Among 51 deaths on the study, 43 occurred after liso-cel infusion, of which five were due to treatment-emergent adverse events (within 90 days of liso-cel infusion). One death was related to liso-cel (macrophage activation syndrome-haemophagocytic lymphohistiocytosis).

Additionally, prolonged cytopenias were reported in 63 (54%) patients, most recovered to grade 2 or lower within 3 months after liso-cel infusion. Grade 3 or higher infections occurred in 20 (17%) patients; the majority were manageable with standard treatments. Management of these toxicities required close monitoring and institution of intravenous immunoglobulins, transfusions of blood products, and growth factor support. In counseling CLL patients about CAR T cell therapy, it is important to discuss that side effects may be delayed and require close monitoring and potentially repeat hospitalizations.

As with the currently FDA approved CAR T cell products in lymphoma, patients should have a designated caregiver to assist during their treatment period and beyond. Additionally, it is expected that all approved cellular therapy products will require treating centers to comply with the risk evaluation and mitigation strategy program, which requires patients to stay in the proximity of the treatment center for approximately four weeks following the CAR T cell infusion to closely monitor toxicity. In the case of patients traveling from afar, local lodging and accommodations should be strongly considered. In instances where adequate social support or access to such accommodations isn't feasible, it is important to collaborate with case managers and social workers to negotiate financial coverage, lodging, and other considerations.

12) What if the patient had Richter's transformation? Is there any role for CAR T cell therapy?

Expert Perspective: Despite advances in novel therapeutics for CLL, RT continues to confer a dismal prognosis and represents a major cause of mortality in relapsed and refractory CLL. CAR T cell therapy for RT remains investigational and is not FDA approved, although several studies have included a small number of patients with RT. For example, in the study by Turtle and colleagues (2017), antitumor activity of the CAR T cell product was evaluated in five patients with RT, with CR in two patients and PR in one patient. In a single-center experience by Kittai and colleagues (2020), nine patients with RT were treated with off-label axicabtagene ciloleucel. Of the eight patients who underwent formal response assessment, all of them (100%) achieved an objective response, with five patients (63%) achieving a CR and seven patients remaining in remission at a median of six months of follow-up. Other small studies have confirmed the activity of CAR T cell therapy in RT, including two out of three patients with CR in a trial by Batlevi and colleagues (2019) and five out of eight patients with CR in a trial by Benjamini and colleagues (2020). Although results are preliminary and longer follow-up is required, there appears to be promising activity of CAR T cell therapy in a disease that is very difficult to treat.

Case Study continued: As for our patient, he enrolled on a clinical trial of CAR T cell ther-apy and successfully received an infusion of liso-cel. His post-treatment course was com-plicated by grade 2 CRS requiring steroids and tocilizumab, as well as grade 3 anemia, which resolved. He achieved a complete response to therapy and has been in a sustained remission for 12 months after CAR T cell treatment.

Recommended Readings

Batlevi, C.L., Palomba, M.L., Park, J., Mead, E., Santomasso, B., Riviere, I., Wang, X., Senechal, B., Furman, R., Yang, J., Kane, P., Hall, M., Bernal, Y., Lund, N., Diamonte, C., Pineda, J., Halton, E., Moskowitz, C., Younes, A., and Sadelain, M. (2019). Phase I clinical trial of CD19-targeted 19-28Z/4-1BBL "armored" car T cells in patients with relapsed or refractory nhl and cll including richter transformation. *Hematol Oncol* 37: 166–167. https://doi.org/10.1002/hon.124_2629.

Benjamini, O., Shimoni, A., Besser, M., Shem-Tov, N., Danylesko, I., Yerushalmi, R., Merkel, D.G., Tadmor, T., Lavie, D., Fineman, R., Jacobi, E., Nagler, A., and Avigdor, A. (2020). Safety and efficacy of CD19-CAR T cells in Richter's transformation after targeted therapy for chronic lymphocytic leukemia. *Blood* 136 (Supplement 1): 40–40. https://doi.org/10.1182/blood-2020-138904.

Blombery, P., Thompson, E.R., and Lew, T.E. (2022 October 25). Enrichment of BTK Leu528Trp mutations in patients with CLL on zan ubrutinib: potential for pirtobrutinib cross resistance. *Blood Adv* 6 (20): 5589–5592. doi: 10.1182/bloodadvances.2022008325. PMID: 35901282; PMCID: PMC9647719.

Cwynarski, K., van Biezen, A., de Wreede, L., Stilgenbauer, S., Bunjes, D., Metzner, B., Koza, V., Mohty, M., Remes, K., Russell, N., Nagler, A., Scholten, M., de Witte, T., Sureda, A., and Dreger, P. (2012). Autologous and allogeneic stem-cell transplantation for transformed chronic lymphocytic leukemia (Richter's syndrome): a retrospective analysis from the chronic lymphocytic leukemia subcommittee of the chronic leukemia working party and lymphoma working party of the European Group for Blood and Marrow Transplantation. *J Clin Oncol* 30 (18): 2211–2217. https://doi.org/10.1200/jco.2011.37.4108.

Derman, B.A., Kordas, K., Ridgeway, J., Chow, S., Dale, W., Lee, S.M., Aguada, E., Jakubowiak, A.J., Jasielec, J., Kline, J., Kosuri, S., Larson, R.A., Liu, H., Mortel, M., Odenike, O., Pisano, J., Riedell, P., Stock, W., Bishop, M.R., and Artz, A.S. (2019). Results from a multidisciplinary clinic guided by geriatric assessment before stem cell transplantation in older adults. *Blood Adv* 3 (22): 3488–3498. https://doi.org/10.1182/bloodadvances.2019000790.

van Gorkom, G., van Gelder, M., Eikema, D.-J., Blok, H.-J., van Lint, M.T., Koc, Y., Ciceri, F., Beelen, D., Chevallier, P., Selleslag, D., Blaise, D., Foá, R., Corradini, P., Castagna, L., Moreno, C., Solano, C., Müller, L.P., Tischer, J., Hilgendorf, I., and Hallek, M. (2017). Outcomes of haploidentical stem cell transplantation for chronic lymphocytic leukemia: a retrospective study on behalf of the chronic malignancies working party of the EBMT. *Bone Marrow Transplant* 53 (3): 255–263. https://doi.org/10.1038/s41409-017-0023-2.

Dreger, P., Döhner, H., Ritgen, M., Böttcher, S., Busch, R., Dietrich, S., Bunjes, D., Cohen, S., Schubert, J., Hegenbart, U., Beelen, D., Zeis, M., Stadler, M., Hasenkamp, J., Uharek, L.,

Scheid, C., Humpe, A., Zenz, T., Winkler, D., and Hallek, M. (2010). Allogeneic stem cell transplantation provides durable disease control in poor-risk chronic lymphocytic leukemia: long-term clinical and MRD results of the German CLL Study Group CLL3X trial. *Blood* 116 (14): 2438–2447. https://doi.org/10.1182/blood-2010-03-275420.

Frey, N.V., Gill, S., Hexner, E.O., Schuster, S., Nasta, S., Loren, A., Svoboda, J., Stadtmauer, E., Landsburg, D.J., Mato, A., Levine, B.L., Lacey, S.F., Melenhorst, J.J., Veloso, E., Gaymon, A., Pequignot, E., Shan, X., Hwang, W.-T., June, C.H., and Porter, D.L. (2020). Long-term outcomes from a randomized dose optimization study of chimeric antigen receptor modified T cells in relapsed chronic lymphocytic leukemia. *J Clin Oncol* 38 (25): 2862–2871. https://doi.org/10.1200/jco.19.03237.

Gagelmann, N., Bacigalupo, A., Rambaldi, A., Hoelzer, D., Halter, J., Sanz, J., Bonifazi, F., Meijer, E., Itälä-Remes, M., Marková, M., Solano, C., and Kröger, N. (2019). Haploidentical stem cell transplantation with posttransplant cyclophosphamide therapy vs other donor transplantations in adults with hematologic cancers: a systematic review and meta-analysis. *JAMA Oncol* 5 (12): 1739–1748. https://doi.org/10.1001/jamaoncol.2019.3541.

Geyer, M.B., Rivière, I., Sénéchal, B., Wang, X., Wang, Y., Purdon, T.J., Hsu, M., Devlin, S.M., Palomba, M.L., Halton, E., Bernal, Y., van Leeuwen, D.G., Sadelain, M., Park, J.H., and Brentjens, R.J. (2019). Safety and tolerability of conditioning chemotherapy followed by CD19-targeted CAR T cells for relapsed/refractory CLL. *JCI Insight* 4 (9): https://doi.org/10.1172/jci.insight.122627.

Gill, S., Grigg, A., Szer, J., and Ritchie, D. (2008). Long-term toxicity of allogeneic stem cell transplantation in fludarabine-refractory chronic lymphocytic leukemia. *Leukemia & Lymphoma* 49 (5): 896–901. https://doi.org/10.1080/10428190801975550.

Herrera, A.F., Ahn, K.W., Litovich, C., Chen, Y., Assal, A., Bashir, Q., Bayer, R.-L., Coleman, M., DeFilipp, Z., Farhadfar, N., Greenwood, M., Hahn, T., Horwitz, M., Jacobson, C., Jaglowski, S., Lachance, S., Langston, A., Mattar, B., Maziarz, R.T., and McGuirk, J. (2021 September 28). Autologous and allogeneic hematopoietic cell transplantation for diffuse large B-cell lymphoma–type Richter syndrome. *Blood Advances* 5 (18): 3528–3539. https://doi.org/10.1182/bloodadvances.2021004865.

Khouri, I.F., Bassett, R., Poindexter, N., O'Brien, S., Bueso-Ramos, C.E., Hsu, Y., Ferrajoli, A., Keating, M.J., Champlin, R., and Fernandez-Vina, M. (2011). Nonmyeloablative allogeneic stem cell transplantation in relapsed/refractory chronic lymphocytic leukemia. *Cancer* 117 (20): 4679–4688. https://doi.org/10.1002/cncr.26091.

Kittai, A.S., Bond, D.A., William, B., Saad, A., Penza, S., Efebera, Y., Larkin, K., Wall, S.A., Choe, H.K., Bhatnagar, B., Vasu, S., Brammer, J., Shindiapina, P., Long, M., Mims, A., O'Donnell, L., Bhat, S.A., Rogers, K.A., Woyach, J.A., and Byrd, J.C. (2020). Clinical activity of axicabtagene ciloleucel in adult patients with Richter syndrome. *Blood Adv* 4 (19): 4648–4652. https://doi.org/10.1182/bloodadvances.2020002783.

Malhotra, P., Hogan, W.J., Litzow, M.R., Elliott, M.A., Gastineau, D.A., Ansell, S.M., Dispenzieri, A., Gertz, M.A., Hayman, S.R., Inwards, D.J., Lacy, M.Q., Micallef, I.N., Porrata, L.F., and Tefferi, A. (2008). Long-term outcome of allogeneic stem cell transplantation in chronic lymphocytic leukemia: analysis after a minimum follow-up of 5 years. *Leukemia & Lymphoma* 49 (9): 1724–1730. https://doi.org/10.1080/10428190802263535.

Naeem, A., Utro, F., Wang, Q., and Cha, J. (2023 May 9). Pirtobrutinib targets BTK C481S in ibrutinib resistant CLL but second site BTK mutations lead to resistance. *Blood Adv* 7 (9): 1929–1943. doi:10.1182/bloodadvances.2022008447. PMID: 36287227; PMCID: PMC10202739.

Paul, S., Tsai, H.-L., Lowery, P., Fuchs, E.J., Luznik, L., Bolaños-Meade, J., Swinnen, L.J., Shanbhag, S., Wagner-Johnston, N., Varadhan, R., Ambinder, R.F., Jones, R.J., and Gladstone, D.E. (2020 March). Allogeneic haploidentical blood or marrow transplantation with post-transplantation cyclophosphamide in chronic lymphocytic leukemia. *Biol Blood Marrow Transplant* 26 (3): 502–508. https://doi.org/10.1016/j.bbmt.2019.11.008.

Pavletic, Z.S., Arrowsmith, E.R., Bierman, P.J., Goodman, S.A., Vose, J.M., Tarantolo, S.R., Stein, R.S., Bociek, G., Greer, J.P., Wu, C.D., Kollath, J.P., Weisenburger, D.D., Kessinger, A., Wolff, S.N., Armitage, J.O., and Bishop, M.R. (2000). Outcome of allogeneic stem cell transplantation for B cell chronic lymphocytic leukemia. *Bone Marrow Transplant* 25 (7): 717–722.

Porter, D.L., Hwang, W.-T., Frey, N.V., Lacey, S.F., Shaw, P.A., Loren, A.W., Bagg, A., Marcucci, K.T., Shen, A., Gonzalez, V., Ambrose, D., Grupp, S.A., Chew, A., Zheng, Z., Milone, M.C., Levine, B.L., Melenhorst, J.J., and June, C.H. (2015). Chimeric antigen receptor T cells persist and induce sustained remissions in relapsed refractory chronic lymphocytic leukemia. *Sci Transl Med* 7 (303): 303ra139–303ra139. https://doi.org/10.1126/scitranslmed. aac5415.

Siddiqi, T., Maloney, D.G., and Kenderian, S.S. (2023 June 5). Lisocabtagene maraleucel in chronic lymphocytic leukaemia and small lymphocytic lymphoma (TRANSCEND CLL 004): a multicentre, open-label, single-arm, phase 1-2 study. *Lancet*. S0140-6736(23)01052-8. doi: 10.1016/S0140-6736(23)01052-8. Epub ahead of print. PMID: 37295445.

Sorror, M.L., Sandmaier, B.M., Storer, B.E., Franke, G.N., Laport, G.G., Chauncey, T.R., Agura, E., Maziarz, R.T., Langston, A., Hari, P., Pulsipher, M.A., Bethge, W., Sahebi, F., Bruno, B., Maris, M.B., Yeager, A., Petersen, F.B., Vindeløv, L., McSweeney, P.A., and Hübel, K. (2011). Long-term outcomes among older patients following nonmyeloablative conditioning and allogeneic hematopoietic cell transplantation for advanced hematologic malignancies. *JAMA* 306 (17): 1874. https://doi.org/10.1001/jama.2011.1558.

Turtle, C.J., Hay, K.A., Hanafi, L.-A., Li, D., Cherian, S., Chen, X., Wood, B., Lozanski, A., Byrd, J.C., Heimfeld, S., Riddell, S.R., and Maloney, D.G. (2017). Durable molecular remissions in chronic lymphocytic leukemia treated with CD19-specific chimeric antigen receptor–modified T cells after failure of ibrutinib. *J Clin Oncol* 35 (26): 3010–3020. https://doi. org/10.1200/JCO.2017.72.8519.

van Gelder, M., de Wreede, L.C., Bornhäuser, M., Niederwieser, D., Karas, M., Anderson, N.S., Gramatzki, M., Dreger, P., Michallet, M., Petersen, E., Bunjes, D., Potter, M., Beelen, D., Cornelissen, J.J., Yakoub-Agha, I., Russell, N.H., Finke, J., Schoemans, H., Vitek, A., and Urbano-Ispízua, Á. (2017). Long-term survival of patients with CLL after allogeneic transplantation: a report from the European Society for Blood and Marrow Transplantation. *Bone Marrow Transplant* 52 (3): 372–380. https://doi.org/10.1038/bmt.2016.282.

29

Prolymphocytic Leukemia

Dima El-Sharkawi and Claire Dearden

The Royal Marsden NHS Foundation Trust, Sutton and Institute of Cancer Research, London, UK

Introduction

Prolymphocytic leukemias (PLLs) are rare, aggressive mature lymphoproliferative disorders. While B-cell PLL (B-PLL) and T-cell PLL (T-PLL) can be readily distinguishable from one another with basic immunophenotyping panels, differentiating them from other mature leukemias can prove challenging. Both can present with an indolent phase that may not require treatment immediately; however, when they progress, patients can be quite symptomatic. Given their rarity and aggressive clinical course, there are comparatively few clinical trials specifically for these diseases, and so evidence for current treatment relies on retrospective case series and basket trials. Chemoimmunotherapy is standard first-line treatment for B-PLL unless there is TP53 disruption and alemtuzumab for T-PLL. Relapsed or refractory disease is associated with short survival rates with current therapies, and so investigations using novel targeted agents are badly needed. Given the poor outcomes with relapsed disease, consideration should be given to allogeneic stem cell transplant in suitable patients during first complete remission.

While B-PLL and T-PLL have often been considered together due to the overlapping clinical and morphological features, with increased availability of flow cytometry worldwide, differentiating between these two entities is much simpler than had been previously. However, both can prove to be challenging from a diagnostic and management perspective. In this chapter we shall thus examine these two diseases separately.

B-Cell Prolymphocytic Leukemia

B-PLL is a neoplasm of B-cell prolymphocytes affecting the peripheral blood, bone marrow, and spleen. Prolymphocytes must constitute > 55% of lymphoid cells in peripheral blood. Cases of chronic lymphocytic leukemia (CLL) with increased prolymphocytes and lymphoid proliferations with relatively similar morphology but with a t(11;14)(q13;q32)

Cancer Consult: Expertise in Clinical Practice, Volume 2: Neoplastic Hematology & Cellular Therapy,
Second Edition. Edited by Syed A. Abutalib, Maurie Markman, James O. Armitage, and Kenneth C. Anderson.
© 2024 John Wiley & Sons Ltd. Published 2024 by John Wiley & Sons Ltd.

(*IGH::CCND1*) translocation or SOX11 expression are excluded; they instead constitute mantle cell lymphoma with leukemic expression. While B-PLL was recognized as an entity in previous versions of the WHO classification, the most recent, 5th WHO classification has removed this diagnostic entity arguing the majority of cases represent either CLL or blastoid variants of MCL and that the remainder of cases should now be classified as splenic B-cell lymphoma/leukemia with prominent nucleoli. This is in contrast to the international classification of mature lymphoid and histiocytic/dendritic neoplasms, which has kept this entity as a defined diagnosis.

Case Study 1

A 65-year-old man presented with a two-month history of sweats and abdominal discomfort. He has massive splenomegaly, a white blood cell count (WBC) of 250 × 10^9/L, and a peripheral blood film showing a homogeneous population of medium-sized lymphoid cells with a prominent nucleolus and basophilic cytoplasm. Twelve months earlier, he had been noted to have a mild lymphocytosis of 20 × 10^9/L, which was unchanged when rechecked six months later.

Quick analysis: The clinical picture and appearance of the abnormal cells in the peripheral blood suggest the possibility of prolymphocytic leukemia (PLL), either B- or T-cell, but further specialist diagnostic investigations are essential to clearly establish the diagnosis. An accurate diagnosis requires a systematic approach and careful integration of the results of morphology (particularly of peripheral blood) with specialist diagnostic tests, including immunophenotyping, cytogenetics, and molecular genetics.

1) What are the characteristic clinical features of B-PLL?

Expert Perspective: B-PLL mainly affects older adults with a mean age at presentation between 65 and 70 years. It is a rare leukemia accounting for < 1% of lymphocytic leukemias. It usually presents in the sixth decade with an equal preponderance in males and females. Most patients will present with symptomatic disease such as B symptoms, lymphocytosis > 100 × 10^9/L, and splenomegaly. While lymphadenopathy is common, it is usually non-bulky. CNS involvement can be a rare feature (Pamuk et al. 2009). The authors have also seen rare paraneoplastic complications with B-PLL such as capillary leak syndrome (Williams et al. 2020).

2) What does the peripheral blood look like in B-PLL?

Expert Perspective: Prolymphocytes are medium-sized lymphoid cells with round nucleus, moderately condensed nuclear chromatin, and a prominent central nucleolus with a relatively small amount of basophilic cytoplasm (Table 29.1). By new definition, for a diagnosis of B-PLL, > 15% of the circulating (and/or bone marrow) lymphoid cells are prolymphocytes, but in practice often > 90% of cells are prolymphocytes. No cytoplasmic hairy projections, or villi, are seen in B-PLL in contrast to hairy cell leukemia variant (HCL-v) and splenic marginal zone lymphoma (SMZL) (Figure 29.1).

3) How can B-PLL be differentiated from other mature B-cell neoplasms?

Expert Perspective: B-PLL can be difficult to distinguish from other mature B-cell neoplasms by morphology and flow cytometry alone and given the lack of specific markers, it

Table 29.1 Clinical and laboratory characteristics of B- and T-cell prolymphocytic leukemias.

Characteristic findings	B-PLL	T-PLL
Clinical features	Median age: 69 M:F ratio: 1.6:1 B-symptoms splenomegaly Minimal lymphadenopathy high WBC	Median age: 61 M:F ratio: 2:1 splenomegaly, lymphadenopathy, skin rash, Edema, and pleuro-peritoneal effusions very high WBC
Morphology	> 55% prolymphocytes (usually > 90%) prolymphocyte is 2 × size of CLL lymphocyte	Basophilic prolymphocytes with cytoplasmic blebs; small-cell (20%) and SS (5%) variants
Immunophenotype	SmIG strong, CD19 +, CD20 +, CD22 +, CD79a +, CD23 −, CD5 −/ + FMC7 +	CD2 +, CD3 +, CD5 +, CD7++ CD4/8 variable CD1a −, TdT −, CD25 −/ +
Cytogenetics	13q del, 11q del, 17p del, 6qdel No t(11;14)	t(14;14); inversion 14; t(X;14); iso8q; complex
Oncogenes	*TP53, C-MYC*	*TCL1, MTCP1, ATM*
Differential diagnosis	T-PLL, CLL/PL, MCL (leukemic phase), SMZL, HCL-v	B-PLL, T-LGL leukemia, A-TLL, SS
Prognosis	Median survival: 3 years	Median survival: 7 months with conventional therapy; 20 months with alemtuzumab; 37 months with alemtuzumab + allogeneic HSCT

A-TLL, adult T-cell leukemia lymphoma; B-PLL, B-cell prolymphocytic leukemia; CLL/PL, chronic lymphocytic leukemia with increased prolymphocytes (< 14%); HCL-v, hairy cell leukemia variant; HSCT, hematopoietic stem cell transplant; MCL, mantle cell lymphoma; SMZL, splenic marginal zone lymphoma; SS, Sézary syndrome; T-LGL, T large granular lymphocytic leukemia; T-PLL, T-cell prolymphocytic leukemia; WBC, white blood cell count.

can be a diagnosis of exclusion. Immunophenotype is of a mature B-cell clone, with strong surface Ig IgM ± IgD with light chain restriction, bright CD20, CD19, CD22, FMC7, and CD79b expression and usually CD5 and CD23 negative, ruling out CLL from the differential diagnosis. Mantle cell lymphoma is excluded by examining for t(11;14) by FISH, or cyclin D1 or SOX11 expression. Classical hairy cell markers are typically negative (CD11c, CD25, CD103, CD123). The phenotype is most similar to hairy cell variant and marginal zone lymphoma; however, morphology can help distinguish B-PLL from either of these, with HCLv also tending to express CD103 and MZL tending to have a more indolent clinical picture.

4) Is bone marrow examination necessary for diagnosis of B-PLL?

Expert Perspective: Given the lack of specific defining features that characterize B-PLL, a bone marrow, nodal, or splenic histology can be useful to aid in diagnosis both for

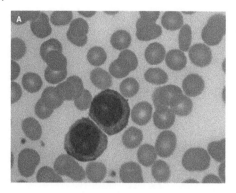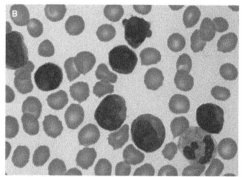

Figure 29.1 Peripheral blood morphology of PLL. (A) B-PLL, showing monomorphic prolymphocytes (PL) with condensed chromatin, prominent nucleolus, and scanty basophilic cytoplasm. (B) T-PLL showing medium-sized lymphoid cells with a regular nuclear outline, single nucleolus, and intense basophilic cytoplasm. An occasional cell shows a cytoplasmic protrusion.

cytogenetic analysis and to also help differentiate B-PLL from other lymphoprolifera-tive disorders. In the largest series reported to date examining the genetic character-ization of B-PLL, most patients had a complex karyotype (73%) with the most common translocation involving the *MYC* gene in 62% (Chapiro et al. 2019). This finding has also been seen by other groups (Flatley et al. 2014). Other frequent cytogenetic aberrations included deletion 17p, trisomy 18, deletion 13q, trisomy 3, trisomy 12, and deletion 8p. The most frequent mutation detected by whole exome sequencing was in *TP53* and, similar to CLL (see Chapter 27), was seen in conjunction with 17p deletion (Chapiro et al. 2019).

5) What are prognostic markers in B-PLL?

Expert Perspective: While there is variable expression of ZAP70, CD38, and variability in IgHV mutation status, in contrast to CLL, these markers are not prognostic in B-PLL (Del Giudice et al. 2006). Despite there being small numbers of patients, Chapiro et al. were able to show that there was a separation in outcomes of patients based on the presence or absence of *MYC* aberration and 17p deletion, with the median overall survival of only 11 months for those who had both aberrations, 125 months for those with a *MYC* aberration alone, and the median of those who did not have a *MYC* aberration was not reached with a survival of 80% at five years (Chapiro et al. 2019).

6) When should treatment be started in patients with B-PLL?

Expert Perspective: As with all mature B-cell neoplasms, should patients be asymptomatic and present during an indolent phase, then it is reasonable to watch and wait, although most patients will require therapy fairly soon after diagnosis. In the largest series reported to date, 29 of the 33 patients had been treated with a median time of first treatment of 3.2 months following diagnosis (range 0–106 months) (Chapiro et al. 2019).

7) What is the best front-line therapy for B-PLL?

Expert Perspective: The treatment of B-PLL has been extrapolated from other lymphoid malignancies, very few trials have included those with B-PLL specifically. Overall survival is reported to be between three and five years (Chapiro et al. 2019; Del Giudice et al. 2006). Given the aggressive nature, in those who are of suitable fitness, consolidation with allogeneic stem cell transplant should be considered with some case reports confirming prolonged remission, although one series of 11 patients had a median PFS of less than 4 months (Arima et al. 2014; Castagna et al. 2005; Kalaycio et al. 2010).

Single-agent purine analogs such as fludarabine, cladribine, and pentostatin may achieve response in 50% of patients including a minority of complete remissions, but with few lasting more than 12 months. A phase II trial using fludarabine and cyclo-phosphomide (FC) showed an overall response rate of 50% with a median survival of 32 months. Combinations of rituximab with fludarabine or bendamustine together with an anthracycline (mitoxantrone [FMR or BMR] or epirubicin [FER]) have also been reported to have activity in B-PLL. Given the excellent responses seen in CLL and MCL (see Chapters 27 and 36) with the combination of fludarabine, cyclophosphamide, and rituximab (FCR), this is a suitable first-line therapy for fit patients without TP53 abnormalities. In our experience this has induced durable complete remissions in two out of four patients lasting for more than five years. Since bendamustine plus rituximab has been shown to have efficacy in CLL and other B-cell malignancies, this could also be an appropriate therapy, and it may be associated with less hematological toxicity. Patients with B-PLL tend to experience higher infusion-related reactions to rituximab and bendamustine.

If there is access to novel therapies (BTKi and BCL2 inhibitors), and patients have complex cytogenetics or *TP53* disruption, then it would be reasonable to consider these as first-line therapy, again as per other lymphoid malignancies there is concern about refractoriness to chemoimmunotherapy in this context.

8) Which treatment options are best suited for relapsed or refractory B-PLL?

Expert Perspective: Given the efficacy of targeted agents in the BCR pathway for other mature B-cell neoplasms, there are unsurprisingly several case reports and small case series of patients with B-PLL who have had responses with ibrutinib in the front-line and relapsed setting (Bindra et al. 2019; Gordon et al. 2017; Oka et al. 2020). Second-generation BTK inhibitors such as zanubrutinib in combination with rituximab and lenalidomide have also been reported with a CR lasting for 12 months at time of publication. Similarly, there have been responses reported with idelalisib-ritxuimab combination (Coelho et al. 2017; Eyre et al. 2019). While responses have been seen in all these reports with some lasting up to two years, median follow-up in all these reports is short. Similarly, venetoclax has been used with success in two case reports but with lack of efficacy seen in a third.

A retrospective study investigating the use of alemtuzumab in CLL did include six patients with B-PLL, with two of these patients showing response; however, the remaining four died primarily related to infection (Fiegl et al. 2014).

If there is access to targeted therapies known to have therapeutic benefit in other B lymphomproliferative disorders, despite the lack of formal investigation in B-PLL, it would be reasonable to consider these treatment options for patients with relapsed/refractory B-PLL.

T-cell prolymphocytic leukemia

T-cell prolymphocytic leukemia (T-PLL) is an aggressive T-cell leukemia characterized by the proliferation of small to medium-sized prolymphocytes with a mature post-thymic T-cell phenotype, involving the peripheral blood, bone marrow, lymph nodes, liver, spleen, and skin. In contrast to B-PLL, T-PLL is a more defined entity with specific diagnostic features. Consensus guidelines from an international expert group have recently been published and outline diagnostic criteria as well as treatment options and response criteria to aid trial development in this condition (Staber et al. 2019).

Case Study 2

A 37-year-old male had been investigated by a pediatrician in childhood for ataxia, dysarthria, intermittent skin erythema, and conjunctival hemorrhages. Genetic studies revealed bi-allelic inactivation of the ATM gene at the 11q23 locus, and ataxia telangiectasia was diagnosed. At the age of 35, he was first noted to have a peripheral blood lymphocytosis (18×10^9/L) on a routine clinic visit and was referred to hematology. He was clinically well with no lymphadenopathy or hepatosplenomegaly. He had a faint erythematous rash across his chest. His peripheral blood film showed a population of small, pleomorphic lymphocytes with hyperchromatic nuclei and basophilic cytoplasm with blebs. His LDH was slightly raised, and other liver function tests were mildly abnormal (ALT: 91; ALP: 117; GGT: 127; Bili: 27). Immunophenotyping of peripheral blood confirmed a clonal T-cell population; and CD4, CD7, CD25, CD2, CD5 positive, with TCR αβ 99%. Cytogenetics showed a complex karyotype, including inversion (14) (q11q32). A diagnosis of T-PLL was made. He remained well for 18 months without treatment and with stable disease. He then progressed with B-symptoms, worsening rash, periorbital edema, and rising WBC (150) and ALT. The bone marrow (BM) showed heavy infiltration with small, mature T-lymphocytes with cytoplasmic blebbing. CT confirmed widespread small-volume lymphadenopathy in the axillary, mediastinal, retroperitoneal, and inguinal regions.

He achieved a complete remission (CR) following alemtuzumab treatment, was not considered a candidate for transplant, and remained in remission for 2½ years. At relapse, he had a short-lived response to alemtuzumab retreatment before losing CD52 expression on T-PLL cells. He failed to respond to other treatment and died 4½ years after the initial diagnosis.

9) How does T-PLL present?

Expert Perspective: Patients typically present with B symptoms, splenomegaly, edema, and serous effusions (~20%). Peri-orbital or conjunctival edema is characteristic of T-PLL (Matutes et al. 1991). Skin involvement is seen in many patients and CNS involvement in rare cases (Hsi et al. 2014; Malkan et al. 2015). White count is often high and tends to rise rapidly. However, an indolent T-PLL clone can be identified in a third of patients (Garand et al. 1998).

10) Any predisposing factors to T-PLL?

Expert Perspective: Ataxia telangiectasia, an autosomal recessive condition caused by mutated *ATM* has been reported to confer a 100-fold higher risk than the general population of T-PLL. Furthermore, in these cases, presenting age is a lot younger (Brito-babapulle and Catovsky 1991; Suarez et al. 2015; Taylor et al. 1996). Nimijen breakage syndrome has also been reported to be a risk factor (Michallet et al. 2003).

11) What does the peripheral blood look like in T-PLL?

Expert Perspective: Medium-sized lymphocytes with a high nuclear-to-cytoplasmic ratio. The nuclei range from round or oval to irregular contours with Sezary-like morphology or small forms with condensed chromatin and a single visible nucleolus. The cytoplasm typically is basophilic with characteristic blebbing in many cases (Figure 29.1).

Case Study 3

A 73-year-old man was referred with a diagnosis of refractory peripheral T-cell lymphoma, not otherwise specified (PTCL-NOS). He had initially presented with a lymphocytosis detected on a routine full blood count (FBC). Mild splenomegaly was detected on computed tomography (CT). Lymphocytes had a CD3, CD4, and CD5 positive (CD7 not done) and CD8 and CD25 negative phenotype, and cytogenetics showed a complex karyotype with inversion 14. However, the BM trephine biopsy was reported as PTCL-NOS. Based on this diagnosis, he was treated with CHOP (cyclophosphamide, doxorubicin, vincristine, and prednisolone), on which he progressed.

- **What mistake was made here?**
  The mistake was to rely on the BM histology, which is nonspecific, rather than a careful examination of the peripheral blood morphology and a failure to integrate the results from all the other investigations, particularly the cytogenetics, which was characteristic for T-PLL.
- **What treatment should he have received?**
  After referral, we confirmed a diagnosis of T-PLL, and he commenced treatment with alemtuzumab. He remains in complete remission four years later.

12) How can T-PLL be distinguished from other T-cell neoplasms?

Expert Perspective: Flow cytometry confirms the T-PLL cells are post-thymic expressing CD2 and CD3 (although membrane expression is often weak or can be absent), as well as CD5, strong CD7 and CD52 and are also exclusively TCR αβ subtype (Figure 29.2). The neoplasm can be either CD4 or CD8 expressing, with double positive cases being fairly specific for T-PLL. The cells are negative for TdT and CD1a. The clinical features, morphology, and immunophenotype can be sufficient in characteristic cases to differentiate T-PLL from other T lymphoproliferative disorders. However, one should be cautious to rely on these alone, as we have had patients referred to us with presumed T-PLL that have been reclassified to PTCL NOS, Sezary syndrome, and LGL. HTLV serology (negative in T-PLL) is important to exclude a potential diagnosis of ATLL. The consensus guidelines have based diagnostic criteria on these features and cytogenetic assessment. T-PLL are positive for CD2, CD5, CD3, and CD7;

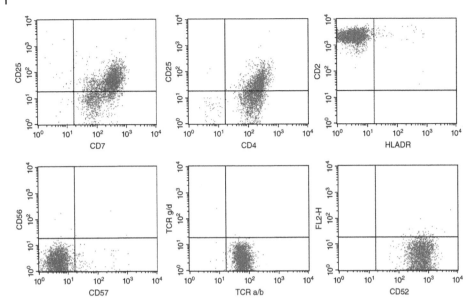

Figure 29.2 Flow cytometry in T-cell prolymphocytic leukemia (T-PLL) showing strong expression of CD2, CD7, CD4, and CD52. Natural killer (NK)-cell markers are negative (*Source:* Ricardo Morilla, The Royal Marsden Hospital, Surrey, UK. Reproduced with permission of Ricardo Morilla).

the membrane expression of CD3 may be weak. CD52 is usually expressed at high density and can be used as a target of therapy.

Cytogenetic aberrations in chromosome 14 are seen in over 90% of cases, typically inv(14) (q11q32) and t(14;14)(q11;q32) (Figure 29.3). This translocation can be identified by FISH, and the aberrant TCL1 protein expression can also be detected by flow cytometry or immunohistochemistry. Translocation t(X;14) is the next most common aberration (Brito-Babapulle et al. 1987; Sun et al. 2018). Like B-PLL, complex karyotype is a common finding.

Recurrent mutations have been identified in T-PLL in genes including *ATM* and *TP53*, but none are specific to T-PLL, and none have been shown thus far to be prognostic (Hu et al. 2017; Kiel et al. 2014; Stengel et al. 2016).

13) Is alemtuzumab still the standard front-line therapy for T-PLL?

Expert Perspective: In the few patients who present with indolent disease, it is reasonable to monitor them initially, but it is important to keep these patients under close surveillance due to the speed of progression when it occurs.

Alemtuzumab is still the recommended first-line treatment of choice, given intravenously three times a week. It is associated with an overall response rate of over 80% (Jain et al. 2017; Krishnan et al. 2010). There is no evidence that adding in chemotherapy routinely to alemtuzumab leads to an improvement (Hopfinger et al. 2013; Pflug et al. 2019). Despite encouraging response rates, relapse in inevitable, and so in those suitable, a stem cell transplant should be considered in first remission. Median progression-free survival post allogeneic stem cell transplant is poor at 12–18 months, with a high non-relapse mortality; however, there is a plateau in the survival curves post allograft, suggesting that

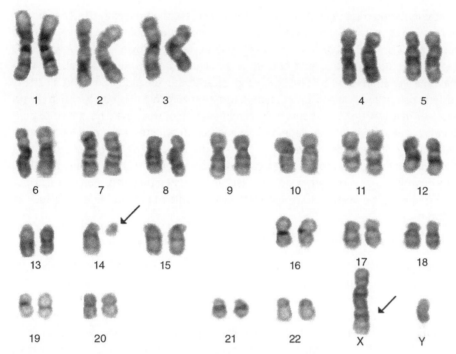

Figure 29.3 Cytogenetics in T-cell prolymphocytic leukemia (T-PLL): complex karyotype from a case of T-PLL showing the characteristic abnormality of t(X,14) (q28,q11), involving the oncogene MTCP1 (*Source:* John Swansbury, The Royal Marsden Hospital, Surrey, UK. Reproduced with permission of John Swansbury).

a proportion of patients will achieve a long-term response (Krishnan et al. 2010). Autologous stem cell transplants have also been reported with some prolonged responses and could be considered if there is concern regarding fitness for allogeneic stem cell transplant or lack of a suitable donor.

14) What are the side effects of alemtuzumab, and how can they be managed?

Expert Perspective: We have found alemtuzumab to be well tolerated in patients with PLL, especially when given as first-line therapy, with fewer infectious complications than when it is used in the relapsed CLL patient group (approximately 10% in T-PLL vs 40% in CLL in our institution). Careful attention to infection prophylaxis for Pneumocystis jirovecii and herpes viruses together with regular monitoring for CMV reactivation have minimized serious infections. Infusion reactions are common on initiating IV therapy but can be readily controlled with the use of premedication and rarely last beyond the first week of treatment. None of our patients has developed tumor lysis.

15) How should patients with an initial slow or poor response to alemtuzumab be managed?

Expert Perspective: In T-PLL, treatment failures with alemtuzumab are in a minority. In those patients where there is a high tumor bulk and WBC remains elevated three weeks or more after initiating treatment, it is reasonable to increase the frequency of alemtuzumab administration to daily (in order to more quickly saturate the binding sites) and/or to add pentostatin at a dose of 4 mg/m^2 once a week for four weeks, followed by every two weeks in responding patients until best response or a maximum of 12 weeks in patients with normal renal function (Dearden 2012; Ravandi et al. 2009; Renaudon-Smith et al. 2014). Pentostatin causes more myelosuppression than alemtuzumab and is also associated with nausea that may last up to 72 hours after administration of the dose. The choice of pentostatin is based on our prior experience The addition of an alternative purine analog or a novel therapy may provide equivalent or superior disease control, but currently the data on combination regimens are limited. Extramedullary disease such as serous effusions and liver involvement more often predict resistance to alemtuzumab monotherapy, but this can frequently be overcome, as discussed by the addition of a purine analog such as pentostatin.

16) What treatment should be used in the relapsed or refractory setting?

Expert Perspective: For those patients who fail or are unsuitable for alemtuzumab re-treatment, a purine analog–based therapy (e.g. FCM) may be used, but response rates are not high. Nelarabine, with or without fludarabine, is an alternative for which there is some evidence of activity in T-PLL. In a phase I study in 11 T-PLL patients, ORR was 20% for nelarabine alone, rising to 63% (13% CR) when given in combination with fludarabine (Gandhi et al. 2008). If the patient is a suitable candidate for an allogeneic transplant, then it is sometimes possible to induce a remission with an intensive combination regimen and proceed directly to HSCT. For those who had a prolonged response to alemtuzumab in the front-line setting, it is reasonable to consider re-treatment if the T-PLL cells are still expressing CD52, although response duration is likely to be shorter (Dearden et al. 2001).

With current treatment options, very few patients will have a successful outcome after relapse. Most patients with T-PLL will still die from their disease, and new therapies are urgently needed. Investigations using whole exome screening and drug screens have been published suggesting possible targeted agents that may have an effect on T-PLL such as agents that target the JAK-STAT pathway (tofacitinib ± ruxolitinib), epigenetic modulators, BCL2 inhibition (e.g. venetoclax ± ibrutinib [VIT-trial] or pentostatin), and PARP inhibitor (e.g. olaparib) and CDK9 inhibition (Alfayez et al. 2020; Andersson et al. 2018; Boidol et al. 2017; Borate et al. 2017; He et al. 2018; Kiel et al. 2014; Pratt et al. 2017; Schrader et al. 2018). Occasional cases and series have been reported of patients responding to some of these agents such as venetoclax and the JAK3 inhibitor tofacitinib; however, there is no convincing evidence to date of durable responses to targeted agents (Boidol et al. 2017; Gomez-Arteaga et al. 2019; Hampel et al. 2021; Li et al. 2017).

Summary

B-PLL and T-PLL are two rare, clinically aggressive but distinct disease entities with characteristic morphological, immunophenotypic, and molecular features. Rituximab-based chemo-immunotherapy combinations should be considered as first-line therapy for

B-PLL, with targeted agents or alemtuzumab used for those presenting with abnormalities of *TP53* or complex cytogenetics. Splenectomy or splenic irradiation may still have a role, especially as palliation. The majority of patients with T-PLL will achieve durable remissions with the use of intravenous alemtuzumab; however, this treatment is not curative, and remission should be consolidated with allogeneic stem cell transplant in suitable patients. Eligible patients with high-risk B-PLL should also be considered for transplant. It is possible that transplant may provide benefit for selected patients with PLL, with some achieving long-term survival (> 5 years). The advent of new targeted therapies may change the treatment landscape in the future.

Recommended Readings

Alaggio, R., Amador, C., Anagnostopoulos, I. et al. (2022). The 5th edition of the World Health Organization classification of haematolymphoid tumours: Lymphoid neoplasms. *Leukemia* 36: 1720–1748.

Arima, H., Ono, Y., Tabata, S., Matsushita, A., Hashimoto, H., Ishikawa, T., and Takahashi, T. (2014). Successful allogeneic hematopoietic stem cell transplantation with reduced-intensity conditioning for B-cell prolymphocytic leukemia in partial remission. *Int J Hematol* 99: 519–522.

Boidol, B., Kornauth, C., Van Der Kouwe, E., Prutsch, N., Kazianka, L., Gültekin, S. et al. (2017). First-in-human response of BCL-2 inhibitor venetoclax in T-cell prolymphocytic leukemia. *Blood* 130: 2499–2503.

Borate, U., Norris, B.A., Lo, P., Tognon, C., Tyner, J., and Spurgeon, S. (2017). Identification of targeted therapies for rare adult mature T -cell leukemia using functional ex vivo screening of primary patient samples. *Am J Hematol* 92: E64–E66.

Castagna, L., Sarina, B., Todisco, E., Mazza, R., and Santoro, A. (2005). Allogeneic peripheral stem-cell transplantation with reduced-intensity conditioning regimen in refractory primary B-cell prolymphocytic leukemia: a long-term follow-up. *Bone Marrow Transplant* 35: 1225–1225.

Chapiro, E., Pramil, E., Diop, M.B., Roos-weil, D., Dillard, C., Gabillaud, C. et al. (2019). Genetic characterization of B-cell prolymphocytic leukemia: a prognostic model involving MYC and TP53. *Blood* blood.201900118 Nov 21;134(21):1821-1831.

Coelho, H., Badior, M., and Melo, T. (2017). Sequential Kinase inhibition (Idelalisib/Ibrutinib) induces clinical remission in B-cell prolymphocytic leukemia harboring a 17p deletion. *Case Rep Hematol* 2017: 1–4.

Dearden, C. (2012). How I treat prolymphocytic leukemia. *Blood* 120: 538–551.

Dearden, C.E., Matutes, E., Cazin, B., Tjonnfjord, G.E., Parreira, A., Nomdedeu, B. et al. (2001). High remission rate in T-cell prolymphocytic leukemia with CAMPATH-1H. *Blood* 98: 1721–1726.

El Hussein, S., Khoury, J.D., and Medeiros, L.J. (2021). B-prolymphocytic leukemia: Is it time to retire this entity? *Ann Diagn Pathol* 54: 151790.

Eyre, T.A., Fox, C.P., Boden, A., Bloor, A., Dungawalla, M., Shankara, P., Went, R., and Schuh, A.H. (2019). Idelalisib-rituximab induces durable remissions inTP53disrupted B-PLL but results in significant toxicity: updated results of the UK-wide compassionate use programme. *Br J Haematol* 184: 667–671.

Gandhi, V., Tam, C., O'Brien, S., Jewell, R.C., Rodriguez, C.O., Lerner, S., Plunkett, W., and Keating, M.J. (2008). Phase I trial of nelarabine in indolent leukemias. *J Clin Oncol* 26: 1098–1105.

Garand, R., Goasguen, J., Brizard, A., Buisine, J., Charpentier, A., Francois Claisse, J., Duchayne, E., Lagrange, M., Segonds, C., Troussard, X., and Flandrin, G. (1998). Indolent course as a relatively frequent presentation in T-prolymphocytic leukaemia. *Br J Haematol* 103: 488–494.

Gomez-Arteaga, A., Margolskee, E., Wei, M.T., Van Besien, K., Inghirami, G., and Horwitz, S. (2019). Combined use of tofacitinib (pan-JAK inhibitor) and ruxolitinib (a JAK1/2 inhibitor) for refractory T-cell prolymphocytic leukemia (T-PLL) with a JAK3 mutation. *Leuk Lymphoma* 60: 1626–1631.

Gordon, M.J., Raess, P.W., Young, K., Spurgeon, S.E.F., and Danilov, A.V. (2017). Ibrutinib is an effective treatment for B-cell prolymphocytic leukaemia. *Br J Haematol* 179: 501–503.

Hampel, P.J., Parikh, S.A., Call, T.G., Shah, M.V., Bennani, N.N., Al-kali, A., et al. (2021). Venetoclax treatment of patients with relapsed T-cell prolymphocytic leukemia. *Blood Cancer J* 11.

He, L., Tang, J., Andersson, E.I., Timonen, S., Koschmieder, S., Wennerberg, K. et al. (2018). Patient-customized drug combination prediction and testing for T-cell prolymphocytic leukemia patients. *Cancer Res* 78: 2407–2418.

Hu, Z., Medeiros, L.J., Fang, L., Sun, Y., Tang, Z., Tang, G. et al. (2017). Prognostic significance of cytogenetic abnormalities in T-cell prolymphocytic leukemia. *Am J Hematol* 92: 441–447.

Jain, P., Aoki, E., Keating, M., Wierda, W.G., O'brien, S., Gonzalez, G.N. et al. (2017). Characteristics, outcomes, prognostic factors and treatment of patients with T-cell prolymphocytic leukemia (T-PLL). *Ann Oncol* 28: 1554–1559.

Kalaycio, M.E., Kukreja, M., Woolfrey, A.E., Szer, J., Cortes, J., Maziarz, R.T. et al. (2010). Allogeneic hematopoietic cell transplant for prolymphocytic leukemia. *Biol Blood and Marrow Transplant* 16: 543–547.

Krishnan, B., Else, M., Tjonnfjord, G.E., Cazin, B., Carney, D., Carter, J. et al. (2010). Stem cell transplantation after alemtuzumab in T-cell prolymphocytic leukaemia results in longer survival than after alemtuzumab alone: A multicentre retrospective study. *Br J Haematol* 149: 907–910.

Malkan, U.Y., Gunes, G., Yayar, O., Demiroglu, H., Yesilirmak, A., and Uner, A. (2015). A T-cell prolymphocytic leukemia case with central nervous system involvement. *Int J Clin Exp Med* 8: 14207–14209.

Oka, S., Ono, K., and Nohgawa, M. (2020). Effective upfront treatment with low-dose ibrutinib for a patient with B cell prolymphocytic leukemia. *Invest New Drugs* 38: 1598–1600.

Pflug, N., Cramer, P., Robrecht, S., Bahlo, J., Westermann, A., Fink, A.M. et al. (2019). New lessons learned in T-PLL: results from a prospective phase-II trial with fludarabine-mitoxantrone-cyclophosphamide-alemtuzumab induction followed by alemtuzumab maintenance. *Leuk Lymphoma* 60: 649–657.

Renaudon-Smith, E., Gribben, J.G., and Agrawal, S.G. (2014). Primary refractory T-cell prolymphocytic leukaemia treated with daily administration of Alemtuzumab plus high-dose methylprednisolone. *Eur J Haematol* 92: 360–361.

Schrader, A., Crispatzu, G., Oberbeck, S., Mayer, P., Pützer, S., Von Jan, J. et al. (2018). Actionable perturbations of damage responses by TCL1/ATM and epigenetic lesions form the basis of T-PLL. *Nature Communications* 9.

Staber, P.B., Herling, M., Bellido, M., Jacobsen, E.D., Davids, M.S., Kadia, T.M. et al. (2019). Consensus criteria for diagnosis, staging, and treatment response assessment of T-cell prolymphocytic leukemia. *Blood* 134: 1132–1143.

Stengel, A., Kern, W., Zenger, M., Perglerova, K., Schnittger, S., Haferlach, T., and Haferlach, C. (2016). Genetic characterization of T-PLL reveals two major biologic subgroups and JAK3 mutations as prognostic marker. *Genes Chromosomes Cancer* 55: 82–94.

Sun, Y., Tang, G., Hu, Z., Thakral, B., Miranda, R.N., Medeiros, L.J., and Wang, S.A. (2018). Comparison of karyotyping, TCL1 fluorescence in situ hybridisation and TCL1 immunohistochemistry in T cell prolymphocytic leukaemia. *J Clin Pathol* 71: 309–315.

30

Hairy Cell Leukemia

Justin M. Watts[1] and Martin S. Tallman[2]

[1] *Memorial Sloan Kettering Cancer Center, New York, NY*
[2] *Northwestern University Feinberg School of Medicine, Chicago, IL*

Introduction

Since 2014, there has been an explosion of new discoveries for the management of hairy cell leukemia (HCL). We have seen the approval of moxetumomab pasudotox, an anti-CD22 immunotoxin, for relapsed/refractory HCL. We have also seen the *BRAF* inhibitor vemurafenib emerge as a viable single-agent oral therapy for relapsed/refractory disease, although resistance can emerge. Recent data suggest that this may be overcome by combining vemurafenib with rituximab in the relapsed/refractory setting, with an 87% CR rate and 78% progression-free survival at median follow-up of 37 months in one study. There have been significant advances in the front-line setting as well, with concurrent or sequential administration of rituximab with cladribine resulting in very high MRD-negative CR rates (≥ 95%) compared to cladribine monotherapy. All of these updates are reviewed in the updated chapter that follows.

Classical hairy cell leukemia (HCL) is a rare mature B-cell hematologic malignancy affecting ~6,000 total people in the United States with an incidence of 600–800 cases per year (Maitre, Cornet, and Troussard, 2020). This represents 2% of all lymphoid malignancies. Most patients are male and over the age of 50. The disease typically presents with pancytopenia, which may be an incidental finding. Untreated, the disease will typically progress over time until patients become symptomatic, usually with fatigue and increased susceptibility to infection. HCL is characterized by the canonical *BRAF-V600E* mutation. Histologically, the marrow is usually hypercellular with infiltration by small- to medium-sized lymphocytic cells with circumferential cytoplasmic projections. At presentation, hairy cells can be rare in the peripheral blood. Monocytopenia is usually present along with neutropenia. Immunohistochemical stains on the trephine biopsy are useful to clarify the extent of leukemic involvement. The typical immunophenotype by flow cytometry includes CD20 (bright), CD22 (bright), CD11c (bright), CD25, CD103, and CD123. Most patients achieve a durable remission (years) with purine analog–based therapy, with or without rituximab. First relapse is often treated by repeating purine analog–based therapy. Multiply relapsed or refractory disease can be treated with *BRAF* inhibitors and immunotoxins. Given the typical long duration of first and second remission, most patients with HCL have a near-normal life expectancy. Hairy cell leukemia variant and splenic marginal zone

Cancer Consult: Expertise in Clinical Practice, Volume 2: Neoplastic Hematology & Cellular Therapy,
Second Edition. Edited by Syed A. Abutalib, Maurie Markman, James O. Armitage, and Kenneth C. Anderson.
© 2024 John Wiley & Sons Ltd. Published 2024 by John Wiley & Sons Ltd.

lymphoma are biologically different diseases that can mimic classical HCL and have a worse prognosis, are treated differently, and should be excluded at diagnosis. Optimizing front-line therapy to lengthen remission duration and improve survival is an area of active investigation, as is the treatment of relapsed/refractory disease.

Case Study 1

A 52-year-old Caucasian man is referred to you with abnormal blood counts. The white blood cell (WBC) count is 3000/μL, absolute neutrophil count (ANC) 1800/μL, hemoglobin 11 g/dL, and platelet count 130,000/μL. Further workup reveals an enlarged spleen of 14.5 cm. The patient continues to work full time as a bank manager. He denies B-symptoms or recurrent infections.

1) **All the following statements about the diagnosis of hairy cell leukemia (HCL) are true EXCEPT:**
   A) Bone marrow examination usually shows a hypercellular marrow with increased reticulin fibrosis, mast cells, and absence of blasts.
   B) Monocytopenia is seen in almost all cases.
   C) Flow cytometry is negative for CD25 and CD22.
   D) There is no specific immunophenotypic marker for the diagnosis of HCL.
   E) Immunohistochemistry (IHC) is positive for DBA.44, TRAP, and ANXA1.

Expert Perspective: HCL is a rare B-cell lymphoproliferative neoplasm that represents approximately 2% of all lymphoid leukemias and affects 600–800 individuals annually in the United States. HCL is more common in Caucasians than African Americans and is more common in males by a ratio of 4:1. The median age at disease onset is 52 years. HCL is characterized by clonal proliferation of small, mature lymphocytes with classic hair-like cytoplasmic projections that accumulate in the peripheral blood, bone marrow, and spleen (Figure 30.1). This leads to decreased production of normal hematopoietic elements, causing anemia, thrombocytopenia, and neutropenia and monocytopenia. Splenomegaly is usually present and may be massive; however, lymphadenopathy is rare except in relapsed disease. Patients typically present with either incidental or symptomatic cytopenias or abdominal symptoms from splenomegaly. Leukocytosis is unusual, and most patients (60–80%) are pancytopenic at diagnosis. On bone marrow examination, the marrow is typically hypercellular with diffusely infiltrating hairy cells and abundant cytoplasm surrounding nuclei may give cells a fried-egg appearance. There is often increased reticulin fibrosis (due to hairy cell infiltration), and there may also be an increased number of bone marrow mast cells. Blasts are not increased. Immunophenotyping by flow cytometry is an important confirmatory test for the diagnosis of HCL, which has a characteristic immunophenotypic profile consisting of both mature B-cell markers (CD19, CD20, and CD22) and aberrant expression of non-B-cell markers (CD11c, CD25, CD103, and CD123). However, there is no one marker or combination of markers that is 100% specific for the disease. Immunohistochemical stains for DBA.44, TRAP, and ANXA1 are typically positive in HCL but have been largely replaced by flow cytometry.

Correct Answer: C

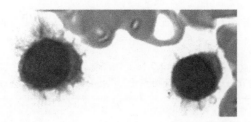

Figure 30.1 Hairy cells with classic circumferential, hairlike cytoplasmic projections. (Color plate 34.1 in previous edition).

2) **All of the following neoplasms are considered in the differential diagnosis of patients presenting with splenomegaly and B-cell lymphoid aggregates in the bone marrow except:**
   A) Splenic marginal zone lymphoma (SMZL).
   B) Transformed prolymphocytic leukemia (PLL).
   C) Chronic lymphocytic leukemia (CLL).
   D) HCL variant (HCL-v)/splenic B-cell lymphoma/leukemia with prominent nucleoli (SBLPN).
   E) Primary myelofibrosis (PMF).

Expert Perspective: Primary myelofibrosis is a myeloid malignancy, and while it may cause splenomegaly it would not result in lymphoid aggregates in the bone marrow. See Table 30.1 for characteristics of A–D in relation to HCL.

Correct Answer: E

3) **The bone marrow biopsy of the patient presented in Question 1 shows a hypercellular marrow, but the marrow was not aspirable (a "dry tap"). Reticulin stain shows grade 2+ fibrosis surrounding hairy cells. Both flow cytometry on the peripheral blood and IHC on the marrow are consistent with the diagnosis of HCL.**

Should this patient be treated or observed?
Expert Perspective: This patient should be observed. Many patients with HCL are asymptomatic and can be observed for months to years before requiring treatment. HCL is typically indolent and slowly progressive, and there is no clear benefit to early treatment. Patients should be treated only when they become symptomatic or develop significant cytopenias. Typical indications for the treatment of HCL include an ANC < 1000/μL, symptomatic anemia with hemoglobin < 11 g/dL, and platelet count < 100,000/μL. Symptomatic splenomegaly — early satiety, abdominal fullness and discomfort, and weight loss — is also an indication for treatment. Bulky lymphadenopathy at initial presentation is rare, and other diagnostic possibilities should be considered if present. Constitutional symptoms, such as fever and night sweats, should also prompt consideration of treatment after infection is ruled out. Infection should always be suspected and treated appropriately in a febrile patient with HCL; bacterial infections are most common, but opportunistic infections can occur as well.

Table 30.1 Characteristics of various neoplasms in relation to hairy cell leukemia (HCL).

Disease	Total white blood cell (WBC) count	Bone marrow involvement	Morphology	Flow cytometry	Splenic involvement
HCL	Typically low or normal	Diffuse	Small cells; long cytoplasmic projections	(+) CD19, 20, 22, 25, 11c, 103, 123; (−) CD5, 23	Yes; red pulp
Splenic marginal zone lymphoma (SMZL)	Usually normal	Nodular	Small cells; short, polar villi	(+) CD19, 20, 22; (−) CD5, 23, 25, 103	Yes; red and white pulp
B-prolymphocytic leukemia (PLL)	High	Variable (nodular, interstitial pattern)	Medium cells; prominent nucleoli	(+) CD19, bright 20, 22, bright surface Ig; (−) CD5, 23, 25, 103	Yes; red and white pulp
Chronic lymphocytic leukemia (CLL)	Variable, can be normal to very high	Varies, in late stages may be diffuse	Small cells; smooth cytoplasmic outline	(+) CD5, 23, 19, weak 20; (−) CD25, 103	Yes; red and white pulp
HCL variant (HCL-v)	High	Variable	Medium cells; projections and prominent nucleoli	(+) CD20, 22, 11c, 103; (−) CD25, 123	Yes; red pulp

Case Study 2

A 65-year-old woman with a history of COPD and recurrent pneumonia is diagnosed with HCL based on incidental pancytopenia detected on routine evaluation. She has been observed without therapy since initial diagnosis about 18 months ago. Now, she reports new onset of fatigue, worsening dyspnea on exertion, and early satiety. The most recent complete blood count shows a WBC of 1300/μL, ANC of 800/μL, hemoglobin of 8.5 g/dL, and platelet count of 80,000/μL. Further workup reveals an enlarged spleen of 18.0 cm. The diagnostic bone marrow biopsy, performed 18 months ago, was consistent with HCL.

4) Should the bone marrow examination be repeated before the initiation of therapy?

Expert Perspective: This patient's clinical course is consistent with the natural history of HCL, and the bone marrow biopsy does not necessarily need to be repeated before treatment unless the initial diagnosis was in question or there is suspicion of another hematologic problem. However, given the time lapse of 18 months, before initiating therapy, it would be prudent to repeat a bone marrow examination to rule out another hematologic disorder or concomitant hematologic malignancy such as chronic lymphocytic leukemia or myelodysplastic syndrome.

5) What is the best therapeutic strategy for this patient with symptomatic HCL?

A) Single-agent purine analog (e.g. cladribine or pentostatin).
B) Cladribine plus rituximab.
C) Cladribine plus granulocyte colony-stimulating factor (G-CSF).
D) Interferon-alpha.
E) Splenectomy and transfusion support.
F) A or B.

Expert Perspective: Single-agent therapy with a purine analog, either cladribine (2-CdA) or pentostatin, has been the standard front-line therapy for patients with symptomatic HCL for the past 25 years. Cladribine and pentostatin are purine analogs that interfere with normal purine metabolism. Typically, cladribine is preferred given the shorter duration of therapy, and it is the most used agent in combination approaches. Mechanistically, cladribine is resistant to adenosine deaminase (ADA), and pentostatin directly inhibits ADA. The mechanism of action of both agents is the accumulation of toxic deoxynucleotides inducing DNA double-strand breaks, which disrupts DNA synthesis and repair and leads to apoptosis. Both agents are highly effective in HCL, but cladribine is usually preferred given its safety profile and tolerability as well as the convenience of administration (given over a single cycle) compared to pentostatin (which is given repeatedly over several cycles). Both agents induce a durable complete remission (CR) in almost all patients with classical HCL, regardless of the extent or bulk of disease, and have similar long-term survival rates (approaching 90% or higher). Clinical trials showing the remarkable effectiveness of a single cycle of cladribine were first reported in the early 1990s. Several large studies have shown CR rates of at least 80–90% (with most other patients achieving a partial response) and four-year progression-free survival (PFS) and overall survival (OS) of approximately 70–80% and 85–95%, respectively. Furthermore, some of these studies had very long follow-up and demonstrated 12-year OS rates of 80–90% (Figure 30.2). Pentostatin has similar response rates and is an acceptable alternative to cladribine. The dosing schedule of pentostatin has varied across clinical trials, but it is commonly given at 4 mg/kg intravenously every two weeks until maximal response (usually around six to eight cycles of treatment). Rituximab has been successfully combined with cladribine in clinical trials, and it may play an important role in relapsed disease. However, it is not currently indicated as part of front-line therapy. A phase II study by Ravandi and coworkers evaluated cladribine followed one month later by eight weekly doses of rituximab in newly diagnosed patients, and while the regimen was well tolerated, remission rates with cladribine alone were excellent, and it is not known if the sequential addition of rituximab improves OS (endpoint not yet reached). Coadministration of G-CSF with cladribine decreases the length of neutropenia but does not affect the incidence or duration of febrile neutropenia or rates of hospitalization and thus is not routinely recommended. Interferon-alpha (IFN-α) is active in HCL and can improve the peripheral blood counts, although achievement of CR is uncommon and there is usually residual splenic and marrow involvement even if it is continued indefinitely. IFN-α is rarely used in the up-front setting given the side effects (e.g. flulike symptoms and depression) and the superiority of purine analog therapy. While splenectomy

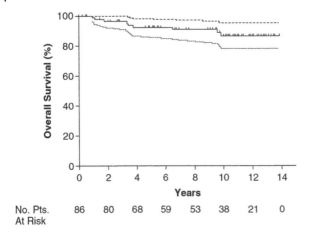

Figure 30.2 Overall survival curve for 86 patients treated with cladribine (26 patients were previously treated). Dotted lines represent the 95% confidence interval. (*Source:* Chadha P, Rademaker AW, Mendiratta P, et al. *Blood* 2005;106:241–246. Reproduced with permission of the American Society of Hematology).

was the first known treatment for HCL and can temporarily improve the peripheral blood counts in most patients for about 1–2 years, it is no longer indicated except for splenic rupture or as salvage in patients with multiply relapsed or refractory disease and no other treatment options.

Recent reports have studied the front-line use of cladribine plus the anti-CD20 B-cell monoclonal antibody rituximab with encouraging results (Chihara et al. 2020). In a 68-patient randomized (1:1) study of concurrent versus delayed (by six months or more and after the detection of MRD in the blood) rituximab, patients who received cladribine with concurrent rituximab had a dramatically higher MRD-negative CR rate (97% vs 24%, $P < 0.0001$) compared to those who received single-agent cladribine (Figure 30.3). Patients who were MRD-positive six months or more after cladribine monotherapy had a lower chance (67%) of achieving MRD negativity with delayed rituximab. Side effects profiles were similar between the groups, except those patients who received concurrent therapy had transiently higher rates of grade 3/4 thrombocytopenia and 35% required platelet transfusions (compared to 0% with single-agent cladribine). While there are no OS data to support the use of concurrent rituximab in the front-line setting (and may never be given practical considerations and the length of follow-up required), the impressive 97% MRD-negative CR rate and good tolerability make it a viable option in appropriate patients and may limit the need for re-treatment or multiple re-treatments in the future. Consideration should be given to the transiently increased risk of bleeding (check CBC 2–3 times/week) and the theoretical risk of increased infection/immunosuppression with concurrent therapy.

Correct Answer: F

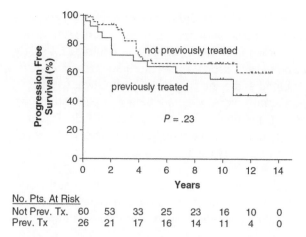

Figure 30.3   Kreitman et al. showed significant improvement in MRD-free survival (bone marrow) and blood MRD–free survival with combined cladribine and rituximab (CDAR) vs cladribine alone (CLA) for first-line therapy of HCL (panels A and B). Also, giving rituximab concurrently with cladribine resulted in improved MRD-negative survival compared to delayed rituximab for patients who were MRD-positive six months or more after initial cladribine therapy (panel C). Long-term follow-up of this study for survival will be important if this is to become the new standard of care, but it is now a reasonable front-line approach, especially in younger patients. There is increased risk of thrombocytopenia in the first month of therapy. It is not known if concurrent cladribine and rituximab is superior to sequential (~one month later) cladribine and rituximab, and the MRD-negative CR rates of 97% and 95% on the two studies, respectively, would suggest that they are equivalent.

6) **Given the patient's older age, pulmonary comorbidities, and concern for infection, particularly COVID-19, a decision to treat with cladribine monotherapy was made after discussing the risks and benefits with the patient.**

- **What is the optimal route and schedule for the administration of cladribine?**
- **How do you manage the fever that commonly occurs after cladribine?**

Expert Perspective: Cladribine is administered intravenously (IV) when treating symptomatic HCL, although there are oral and subcutaneous formulations available. Two recommended dosing schedules exist that are thought to be equivalent: (i) cladribine 0.1 mg/kg per day for seven days by continuous IV infusion, and (ii) cladribine 0.14 mg/kg by two-hour IV infusion daily for five days ("bolus dosing"). The seven-day infusional program was the first to be studied and was the regimen used in many of the large clinical trials leading to the drug's approval. It is generally considered the standard regimen, and it may be more convenient for the patient as there are less outpatient visits required. However, if there are logistical issues with an outpatient seven-day continuous infusion, which requires a peripherally inserted venous catheter (PICC) and portable pump, then the five-day bolus schedule is an acceptable and equivalent alternative regimen.

Approximately 40% of patients will become febrile during treatment with cladribine. This fever is usually non-infectious and coincides with decreasing peripheral neutrophil and hairy cell counts, and it may be related to cytokine release from apoptotic hairy cells. However, given that these patients are often neutropenic, blood cultures should be obtained, and a broad-spectrum oral antibiotic initiated. Usually, patients do not need to be admitted to the hospital for a cladribine-associated fever unless they are systemically ill. If blood and urine cultures are negative at 24 hours, naproxen can be effective for persistent fever. Both cladribine and pentostatin can cause prolonged immunosuppression, and prophylaxis with acyclovir is indicated to prevent herpes zoster. Opportunistic infections are rare, but Pneumocystis jirovecii prophylaxis is advisable if the patient is otherwise immunosuppressed (e.g. on corticosteroids).

In terms of long-term side effects, cladribine has been associated with hypocellularity and foci of aplasia on post-treatment bone marrow biopsies. These findings can be seen in patients with durable remissions and normal blood counts, and they are of uncertain significance.

7) **The patient is successfully treated with a single cycle of cladribine (0.14 mg/kg by two-hour IV infusion daily for days days). What would be the best time for restaging scans and bone marrow examination? How are partial and complete responses defined in hairy cell leukemia?**

Expert Perspective: Approximately 80–90% of patients with newly diagnosed HCL achieve CR after one cycle of cladribine. CR is defined as normalization of peripheral blood counts, resolution of organomegaly, and morphologic remission (absent hairy cells) in the blood and bone marrow (although measurable residual disease [MRD] may still be detectable). A partial response, achieved in 10–15% of patients after cladribine, is defined as normalization of the peripheral blood counts, $\geq$ 50% reduction in organomegaly and bone marrow hairy cells, and < 5% circulating hairy cells. Computed tomography (CT) or other scans are usually not necessary either at initial diagnosis or after treatment. Splenomegaly, which occurs in approximately 80% of patients with HCL, is the most common and often only physical and radiographic finding, and it can be followed by physical examination. In fact, massive splenomegaly (extending into the pelvis) should always prompt consideration of the following limited differential diagnosis: HCL, chronic myeloid leukemia, myelofibrosis, non-Hodgkin's lymphoma, Gaucher disease, and Kala-Azar infection. In the past, restaging bone marrow examinations were typically performed three to six months after treatment. However, our current practice in the purine analog era, when we know that most patients will achieve CR, is to observe patients expectantly without restaging if the blood counts return to normal and splenomegaly resolves. Patients with MRD on post-treatment bone marrow examinations often have durable hematologic remissions, and the detection of MRD in these patients is of unclear significance and would not currently change management (see Question 1).

8) **A 40-year-old male develops increased fatigue and is diagnosed with classic HCL. His WBC is 1.5, Hgb 9.5, and platelets 60,000. BM biopsy shows 90% hairy cells in a hypercellular marrow. He has been vaccinated against COVID-19 and is anxious to start treatment as soon as possible. After a long discussion with the patient, a decision to**

start cladribine with rituximab is made. How should the rituximab be administered in this patient?
A) Concurrently.
B) Sequentially (one month after).
C) Delayed for six months and only given if MRD-positive.
D) A or B.

Expert Perspective: Chihara et al. published on sequential cladribine and rituximab in 2016 (Chihara et al. BJH 2016). This regimen consisted of five days of bolus dose cladribine followed by eight doses of weekly rituximab starting ~one month later. With this regimen, 100% of untreated patients (n = 59) achieved CR, 95% MRD-negative CR, and there was 95% failure-free survival (FFS) at five years. This regimen was also active in relapsed HCL and HCLv (CR rate 100% and 86%, respectively). Across all cohorts, the MRD-negative CR rate was 94%. No safety signals were reported. More recently, Chihara et al. compared concurrent rituximab vs delayed rituximab (68 total patients), to exploit the synergy of cladribine and rituximab when given together, as cladribine is rapidly excreted (within 48 hours of the last dose). On this regimen, cladribine is given days 1–5 (bolus dosing) and rituximab starts weekly for eight doses on day 1. The MRD-negative CR rate with this approach was 97% for untreated HCL. There was a higher rate of thrombocytopenia with concurrent therapy. Either concurrent or sequential administration would be appropriate in this patient. Choice C would be the least desirable option for this young patient, as delayed administration (by six months) had the lowest rates and durability of MRD-negative CR.

Correct Answer: D

9) How is MRD defined, and does it portend relapse in HCL?

Expert Perspective: Measurable residual disease (MRD) can be detected by IHC for markers such as CD20 or DBA.44. Depending on the criteria used, anywhere from 15% to 50% of patients in morphologic CR will have evidence of MRD after one cycle of cladribine; however, it has not been proven that MRD positivity correlates with early relapse. Immunophenotyping by flow cytometry is another useful, and perhaps more sensitive, method for evaluating MRD. Additionally, polymerase chain reaction (PCR) testing for clonal IGH may identify some residual disease even in patients who are MRD-negative by flow cytometry. Post-remission rituximab therapy has been used to successfully eradicate MRD (as detectable by PCR and flow cytometry) in patients with MRD after initial treatment with cladribine, but there is no current evidence that this strategy improves DFS or OS, and it is generally not recommended. Moreover, one study by Sigal and colleagues, which examined 19 patients in continuous hematologic CR for a median of 16 years after a single cycle of cladribine, showed that nine patients had no detectable MRD, seven were MRD-positive, and three had morphologically overt disease (despite having normal blood counts). This highlights the fact that very long-term CRs can occur with a single cycle of cladribine, and that even in the case of MRD or overt bone marrow relapse, patients may have clinically quiescent disease for many years. The clinical significance of MRD in HCL and the role of rituximab to eradicate MRD remain unclear, and we do not recommend routine testing for MRD post cladribine if complete hematologic remission is achieved.

10) If a patient relapses after a single cycle of cladribine, what is the best therapeutic approach?

Expert Perspective: Repeat a single cycle of cladribine with or without rituximab. If the patient did not receive rituximab front-line, then at first relapse we would recommend adding sequential rituximab based on the Chihara 2016 paper cited above (concurrent rituximab is also a consideration in the relapsed setting, but it may cause more toxicity). Relapse of HCL is common but responds very well to repeat courses of purine analog therapy. Several smaller studies have shown that rituximab monotherapy for relapsed HCL after treatment with cladribine can have high response rates, but a larger phase II study showed an overall response rate of only about 25%; therefore, at first relapse a purine analog plus rituximab is advised for most patients. Multiply repeated courses of cladribine or pentostatin are generally not advised due to decreasing effectiveness, increased risk of infection, and risk of bone marrow hypoplasia and secondary myeloid leukemias. In the rare case (< 5%) that a patient is refractory to up-front treatment with cladribine or pentostatin, then the other purine analog should be tried, with rituximab. Treatment options for multiply relapsed or refractory HCL include vemurafenib +/− rituximab, moxetumomab pasudotox, or a clinical trial (see Question 4). Lastly, splenectomy re-treatment. One series showed that at 10 years, 48% of patients treated with cladribine and 42% of those treated with pentostatin had relapsed. However, multiple studies have shown that retreatment with a purine analog leads to a second CR in as many as 70% of patients, and there appears to be no difference in outcome if re-treatment is with the same purine analog used for first-line therapy (e.g. cladribine). Moreover, once a second CR (CR2) is achieved, the CR2 duration may be nearly as long as the duration of first CR (CR1) (Figure 30.4). However, DFS does appear to shorten after multiply repeated courses of purine analog therapy (i.e. after third- or fourth-line treatment).

11) What is the best treatment for patients with multiply relapsed HCL, and is there a role for hematopoietic cell transplantation (HCT)?

Expert Perspective: There are multiple effective treatment options in patients with multiply relapsed or refractory HCL, including many encouraging new clinical trials and recently approved new agents. Vemurafenib plus rituximab had an 87% CR rate (65% of those MRD-negative) in 30 patients with relapsed/refractory HCL (median number of prior therapies was three) (Tiacci et al. NEJM 2021). Progression-free survival (PFS) at 37 months was 78% and RFS at 34 months was 85%, making this a promising new approach for relapsed/refractory HCL, significantly improving on the CR rate and median RFS with vemurafenib alone (35% and nine months, respectively). Moxetumomab pasudotox was also recently approved for relapsed/refractory HCL based on durable CRs. In the pivotal study (n = 80 patients, median number of prior therapies = three), the CR rate was 41% (82% MRD-negative) and the durable CR rate (hematologic recovery > 180 and > 360 days) was 36% and 33%, respectively. Capillary leak syndrome and hemolytic uremic syndrome were seen in up to 10% of patients, some of which were severe, but generally manageable. Patients may require hospitalization. The response rates and durability were not as impressive with single-agent moxetumomab compared to vemurafenib plus rituximab, but nevertheless it remains a viable third- or fourth-line option. We note that the duration

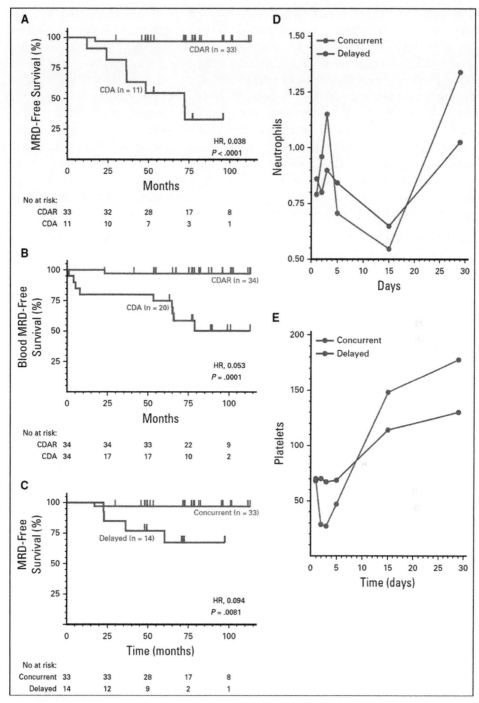

Figure 30.4 Demonstrates the similar progression-free survival (PFS) curves for newly diagnosed patients and those previously treated with one cycle of cladribine. (*Source:* Chadha P, Rademaker AW, Mendiratta P, et al. *Blood* 2005;106:241–246. Reproduced with permission of the American Society of Hematology).

of response shortens after each subsequent line of therapy in multiply relapsed patients, and this remains an area of high unmet need. Given the advent of highly effective new therapies and existing palliative treatment options such as splenectomy and IFN-α, allogeneic HCT is rarely, if ever, indicated. IFN-α can be effective for maintaining adequate blood counts in some patients with relapsed/refractory HCL who have failed all other approved therapies, although IFN-α usually has to be given continuously for an ongoing response. Splenectomy can also be performed for palliation in patients with refractory disease or significant symptoms from massive splenomegaly, although the response typically wanes with time. For early relapse or primary refractory disease, one should consider a different diagnosis, such as HCL variant, which is classically resistant to both purine analogs and splenectomy (and more aggressive in course). Antibody-directed therapies, such as rituximab or an ADC, may be more effective in patients with HCL-v, and sequential or concurrent cladribine plus rituximab is a reasonable first approach.

12) **Which of the following potential therapeutic targets in HCL <u>does not</u> have a corresponding FDA approved agent?**
   A) CD20.
   B) CD22.
   C) CD25.
   D) CD52.
   E) *BRAF* mutation.
   F) All of the above.

Expert Perspective: Rituximab is relatively nontoxic anti-CD20 monoclonal antibody, and multiple clinical trials have shown single-agent efficacy in relapsed or refractory disease, although response rates have varied considerably. More recently, it has been shown to improve MRD-negative CR rates when given concurrently with cladribine as front-line therapy and to have significant activity when combined with vemurafenib in relaped/ refractory disease. Moxetumomab pasudotox is an immunotoxin consisting of an anti-CD22 antibody joined to pseudomonas exotoxin. It is approved for patients who have failed at least two prior lines of systemic therapy and in the pivotal clinical trial had a CR rate of 41% and durable CR rate of 30%. LMB-2, another ADC employing a truncated pseudomonas exotoxin linked to a recombinant anti-CD25 antibody, showed clinical activity in relapsed or refractory HCL in phase I studies but was not further pursued. Alemtuzumab (Campath), an unconjugated anti-CD52 antibody that is highly immunosuppressive, is used more commonly for PLL and HCL-v (now referred as splenic B-cell lymphoma/leukemia with prominent nucleoli [SBLPN]). Given the availability of other effective agents, it is rarely used for classical HCL. Vemurafenib is an FDA approved small-molecule *BRAF* inhibitor for the treatment of stage IV melanoma. The *BRAF V600E* mutation leads to constitutive activation of the MEK–ERK pathway, thereby driving cellular proliferation; has been implicated in almost all cases of classical HCL; and appears to be a driver mutation. Studies have shown that 79–100% of patients with HCL have an activating *BRAF V600E* mutation, and patients with HCL-v appear to be universally wild-type *BRAF*. Dietrich and coworkers (2012) first described a patient with *BRAF*-mutant refractory HCL who had a remarkable response to vemurafenib, achieving CR. In 2015, two single-center studies showed a CR rate of ~40% with single-agent vemurafenib, and more recently the vemurafenib-rituximab combination was shown to be even more active. As in melanoma, mechanisms of resistance to *BRAF* inhibition such as bypass reactivation of MEK and ERK may arise, requiring successive interventions. Rash is common, and frequent skin exams should be done to monitor for skin cancers. In another recent report 6 patients with HCL and progressive disease after vemurafenib plus rituximab, 5 had a response to venetoclax alone or with the addition of rituximab, including 3 complete responses.

Correct Answer: C

13) What is the best front-line therapy in a symptomatic pregnant patient with HCL?

Expert Perspective: Interferon-α. Purine analogs are contraindicated in pregnancy. If treatment is required, then IFN-α can be effective, especially for improving the blood counts, and it has been shown to be safe in pregnancy. If IFN-α is ineffective and cytopenias or symptoms from splenomegaly are severe, then the relative risk and benefits of splenectomy should be carefully considered.

Recommended Readings

Chadha, P., Rademaker, A.W., Mendiratta, P. et al. (2005). Treatment of hairy cell leukemia with 2-chlorodeoxyadenosine (2-CdA): long-term follow-up of the Northwestern University experience. *Blood* 106: 241–246.

Chihara, D., Arons, E., Stetler-Stevenson, M. et al. (2020). Randomized phase II study of first-line cladribine with concurrent or delayed rituximab in patients with hairy cell leukemia. *J Clin Oncol* 38 (14): 1527–1538. doi: 10.1200/JCO.19.02250.

Chihara, D., Kantarjian, H., O'Brien, S. et al. (2016). Long-term durable remission by cladribine followed by rituximab in patients with hairy cell leukaemia: update of a phase II trial. *Br J Haematol* 174 (5): 760–766. doi: 10.1111/bjh.14129.

Dietrich, S., Glimm, H., Andrulis, M., von Kalle, C., Ho, AD., Zenz T. 2012 May 24 BRAF inhibition in refractory hairy-cell leukemia. *N Engl J Med* 366 (21): 2038–2040. doi: 10.1056/NEJMc1202124. PMID: 22621641.

Else, M., Dearden, C.E., Matutes, E. et al. (2009). Long-term follow-up of 233 patients with hairy cell leukaemia, treated initially with pentostatin or cladribine, at a median of 16 years from diagnosis. *Br J Haematol* 145: 733–740.

Grever, M.R. (2010). How I treat hairy cell leukemia. *Blood* 115: 21–38.

Grever, M.R., Abdel-Wahab, O., Andritsos, L.A. et al. (2017). Consensus guidelines for the diagnosis and management of patients with classic hairy cell leukemia. *Blood* 129 (5): 553–560. doi: 10.1182/blood-2016-01-689422.

Kreitman, R.J., Dearden, C., Zinzani, P.L. et al. (2018). Moxetumomab pasudotox in relapsed/refractory hairy cell leukemia. *Leukemia* 32 (8): 1768–1777. doi: 10.1038/s41375-018-0210-1.

Kreitman, R.J., Dearden, C., Zinzani, P.L. et al. (2021). Moxetumomab pasudotox in heavily pre-treated patients with relapsed/refractory hairy cell leukemia (HCL): long-term follow-up from the pivotal trial. *J Hematol Oncol* 14 (1): 35. doi: 10.1186/s13045-020-01004-y. Published 2021 February 24.

Maitre, E., Cornet, E., Troussard, X. 2019 Dec Hairy cell leukemia: 2020 update on diagnosis, risk stratification, and treatment. *Am J Hematol* 94 (12): 1413–1422. doi: 10.1002/ajh.25653. Epub 2019 Oct 31. PMID: 31591741.

Mehta, J., Powles, R., Singhal, S. et al. (1996 March). Clinical and hematologic response of chronic lymphocytic and prolymphocytic leukemia persisting after allogeneic bone marrow transplantation with the onset of acute graft versus host disease: possible role of graft versus leukemia. *Bone Marrow Transplant* 17 (3): 371–375. PMID: 8704689.

Ravandi, F., O'Brien, S., Jorgensen, J. et al. (2011). Phase 2 study of cladribine followed by rituximab in patients with hairy cell leukemia. *Blood* 118: 3818–3823.

Tallman, M.S. (2011). Implications of minimal residual disease in hairy cell leukemia after cladribine using immunohistochemistry and immunophenotyping. *Leuk Lymphoma* 52: 65–68.

Tiacci, E., De Carolis, L., Simonetti, E. et al. (2021). Vemurafenib plus rituximab in refractory or relapsed hairy-cell leukemia. *N Engl J Med* 384 (19): 1810–1823. doi: 10.1056/NEJMoa2031298.

Tiacci, E., Park, J.H., De Carolis, L. et al. (2015). Targeting mutant BRAF in relapsed or refractory hairy-cell leukemia. *N Engl J Med* 373 (18): 1733–1747. doi: 10.1056/NEJMoa1506583.

Tiacci, E., De Carolis, L., Santi, A., and Falini, B. (2023 March 9). Venetoclax in relapsed or refractory hairy-cell leukemia. *N Engl J Med* 388 (10): 952–954. doi: 10.1056/NEJMc2216135. PMID: 36884329.

Tiacci, E., Pettirossi, V., Schiavoni, G., and Falini, B. (2017). Genomics of hairy cell leukemia. *J Clin Oncol* 35 (9): 1002–1010. doi: 10.1200/JCO.2016.71.1556.

Part 6

Hodgkin Lymphoma

31

Classic Hodgkin Lymphoma

Christopher R. D'Angelo[1], James O. Armitage[1], and Nancy L. Bartlett[2]

[1] *University of Nebraska Medical Center, Omaha, NE, USA*
[2] *Washington University School of Medicine, St. Louis, MO, USA*

Introduction

Hodgkin lymphoma (HL) is a unique lymphoid malignancy featuring characteristic Reed-Sternberg cancer cells distributed among a background of inflammatory cells in the tumor microenvironment. HL represents ~10% of all lymphoma cases in developed countries and is separated into classic Hodgkin lymphoma (cHL; 90% of HL cases) and nodular lymphocyte-predominant Hodgkin lymphoma (10% of HL cases; discussed in Chapter 32). The incidence of cHL features a bimodal age distribution with cases peaking in the second and seventh decade of life for a median age at diagnosis in the mid 30s. With current management approaches, over 88% of patients are alive at five years post diagnosis, and most of these patients will be cured of the disease. Given the relatively young age at diagnosis and high rates of cure with current therapy, special attention for late toxicities must be provided. In this chapter, we will present a series of clinical cases designed to highlight common scenarios in the management of patients with cHL. The objective of these cases is to identify optimal management options, recognize toxicities, discuss advances in research, and highlight ongoing controversies in caring for patients with cHL.

Case Study 1

A 19-year-old man presents with a six-week history of an enlarging neck mass, pruritis, and drenching night sweats. A 3.0 × 2.0 cm neck mass and multiple surrounding enlarged cervical lymph nodes are noted by computed tomography (CT). You suspect Hodgkin lymphoma.

1) **What is the best method to biopsy this lesion?**
   A) Bronchosocopy with fine needle aspiration (FNA).
   B) Needle biopsy by interventional radiology.
   C) Surgical consultation for excisional/surgical biopsy.
   D) Any of the above choices are reasonable.

Expert Perspective: Generally, a surgical or excisional biopsy is preferred whenever possible for several reasons. cHL is a unique neoplastic disease where the implicated cancer cell, the Reed-Sternberg cell, is relatively rare within the tumor microenvironment.

Cancer Consult: Expertise in Clinical Practice, Volume 2: Neoplastic Hematology & Cellular Therapy,
Second Edition. Edited by Syed A. Abutalib, Maurie Markman, James O. Armitage, and Kenneth C. Anderson.
© 2024 John Wiley & Sons Ltd. Published 2024 by John Wiley & Sons Ltd.

Reed-Sternberg cells often account for approximately 1% of the cells constituting the tumor tissue. The tumor is instead populated by a dense infiltrate of immune cells with Reed-Sternberg cells scattered within a fibrotic microenvironment. For this reason, obtaining a larger specimen is likely to be more representative of the underlying lymphoma being sampled by both increasing the yield and preserving the underlying architecture. Both features will allow the hematopathologist to make the correct diagnosis. Although a needle biopsy or FNA may possibly be obtained more rapidly, the sample is likely to be nondiagnostic and lead to further diagnosis and treatment delays. A surgical biopsy shows cHL.

Correct Answer: C

2) **What additional study would be most reasonable to complete the staging workup for cHL?**
   A) Whole-body positron emission tomography–computed tomography (PET-CT).
   B) Bilateral bone marrow biopsy with aspirate.
   C) CT of the abdomen and pelvis.
   D) A and B.

Expert Perspective: PET-CT is the preferred imaging modality for initial staging of cHL given its improved sensitivity of 94% compared to 77% with CT. PET-CT upstages approximately 10–20% of patients, resulting in a change in treatment recommendations. If a PET-CT is performed at initial staging, the utility of a bone marrow biopsy appears limited. In a series of 454 HL patients staged with both PET and bone marrow biopsy, no patient with stage I or II disease by PET had bone marrow involvement. Of those with stage III disease, 5 of 106 patients were upstaged by a bone marrow biopsy, but none had a change in treatment plan. A negative PET-CT for focal skeletal lesions has a 99% negative predictive value for marrow involvement (Lugano criteria). Importantly, we do advocate for a PET-CT scan prior to diagnostic mediastinoscopy in case there is easily accessible peripheral adenopathy for biopsy.

Correct Answer: A

Case Study 2

A 26-year-old woman presents with left supraclavicular swelling. CT confirms a conglomerate of enlarged nodes measuring 3.0 × 2.9 cm and a 4.3 × 2.3 cm anterior mediastinal mass. An excisional lymph node biopsy reveals cHL. A PET-CT scan shows no other sites of disease. Initial labs were unremarkable, including an erythrocyte sedimentation rate (ESR) of 10 mm/h. She receives two cycles of ABVD. An interim PET-CT after two cycles demonstrates a Deauville 2 response.

3) **What is the best course of management for this patient?**
   A) Two additional cycles of ABVD (four total).
   B) 20 Gy involved field radiation therapy (IFRT) (total two cycles ABVD + 20 Gy IFRT).
   C) Six cycles of ABVD.
   D) Choices A and B are reasonable.

Expert Perspective: This patient has non-bulky, stage II HL with favorable features. In general, stage I–II HL is stratified according to the presence of unfavorable risk factors. Patients who do not have any of these factors are considered to have favorable disease and may be candidates for less intensive therapy. The definition of unfavorable risk factors differs according to society guidelines used in clinical trials, which limits the comparison and generalizability of study results and can occasionally lead to mismanagement of patients.

- The National Comprehensive Cancer Network (NCCN) includes an ESR ⩾ 50 mm/h, presence of bulky disease (> 10cm), number of nodal sites > 3, and a mediastinal mass ratio (maximum width of mass/ maximum intrathoracic diameter) > 0.33 as unfavorable risk factors.
- The German Hodgkin Study Group (GHSG) defines unfavorable disease as a mediastinal mass ratio greater than one-third, ESR ⩾ 50 mm/h in the absence of B-symptoms or ⩾ 30 mm/h with B-symptoms, extranodal disease, or ⩾ 3 involved lymph node sites.
- The definition of a nodal site may also differ according to GHSG or NCCN criteria.

Although therapy for early-stage HL continues to evolve, current evidence-based options include combined modality therapy (chemotherapy and radiation) versus chemotherapy alone (Table 31.1). Cure rates approximate 90% with either approach. When choosing a therapeutic approach informed by clinical trial results, it is important to understand what definitions were used to define favorable or unfavorable risk, and often the most important factor to guide treatment decision is the presence of bulky disease.

Currently, most experts and guidelines support the use of interim PET/CT to direct therapy. The summary of three important randomized studies in this particular area are highlighted as follows (Table 31.1):

- The largest study of PET-adapted therapy, H10, was conducted by the European Organization for Research and Treatment of Cancer. Patients with favorable cHL were randomized to three cycles of ABVD and involved nodal radiotherapy or to an experimental PET-adapted approach, where PET-negative (Deauville score 1–2) patients after two cycles of ABVD went on to receive two more cycles of ABVD but no radiation. Five-year progression-free survival was 99% versus 87% (hazard ratio, HR, 15.8; 95% CI 3.8–66.1) for the three ABVD and radiation group versus the four cycles of ABVD alone

Table 31.1 PET-guided PET-negative early-stage Hodgkin lymphoma studies.

Study	N	Treatment	PFS	OS
H10	1,950	ABVD × 3 + INRT vs ABVD × 2 → PET → ABVD × 2	5-year 99% vs 87%	5-year 100% vs 99.6%
RAPID	602	ABVD × 3 → PET− → 30 Gy IFRT vs Obs	3-year 95% vs 91%	3-year 97% vs 99%
HD16	1,150	ABVD × 2 + 20 Gy IFRT vs ABVD × 2 → PET− → Obs	5-year 93% vs 86%	5-year 98% vs 98%

PFS: progression-free survival; OS: overall survival; ABVD: doxorubicin, bleomycin, vinblastine, dacarbazine; INRT: involved nodal radiation therapy; IFRT: involved field radiation therapy; Obs: observation.

group. There was no difference in five-year overall survival (100% vs 99.6%) in radiation versus no radiation groups, respectively.

- The United Kingdom National Cancer Research Institute RAPID trial treated non-bulky, stage I–IIA HL patients with three cycles of ABVD followed by interim PET. Those with a negative interim PET (PET−), defined as a Deauville score ≤ 2, were randomized to observation versus IFRT, whereas those with a positive interim PET (PET+) received one additional cycle of ABVD followed by IFRT. At a median follow-up of 60 months, the PET− patients on observation had a three-year progression-free survival of 90.8% compared to 94.6% with IFRT (HR 1.57; 95% CI 0.84–2.97) while PET+ patients had an 87.6% three-year PFS. There was no difference in three-year OS.
- The GSHG conducted the HD16 trial comparing two cycles of ABVD + 20 Gy involved field radiation therapy versus two cycles of ABVD alone if PET− (Deauville 1–2). Five-year progression-free survival was 86.1% in the ABVD group versus 93.4 in the chemotherapy and radiation group (HR 1.78; 95% CI 1.02–3.12). There was no difference in five-year OS (98.1% vs 98.4%) in the chemotherapy and radiation versus chemotherapy alone groups, respectively.

In summary, treatment using chemotherapy and radiation, or chemotherapy alone are effective strategies for managing patients with early-stage, favorable HL. The results of H10, RAPID, and HD16 consistently demonstrate improved progression-free survival but not OS with the addition of radiation to ABVD chemotherapy in patients with interim PET-negative disease. Given the concern for late toxicities with radiation therapy including an increased risk of secondary malignancies and excellent survival outcomes for chemotherapy-alone approaches, we recommend four cycles of ABVD chemotherapy for interim PET-negative (Deauville score 1–2) cHL. We note that chemotherapy and radiation remains a reasonable and evidence-based option. Patients with Deauville 3 responses from interim PET may benefit from the addition of radiation therapy as all Deauville 3 early-stage patients on these trials received radiation.

Correct Answer: D

Case Study 3

A 28-year-old woman presents with generalized pruritis and bilateral cervical lymphadenopathy. A cervical lymph node biopsy shows cHL. The PET-CT reveals a 10 cm anterior mediastinal mass and bilateral cervical adenopathy.

4) **Which of the following is (are) the most appropriate therapy (therapies)? (Choose one or more, if appropriate.)**
   A) Four to six cycles of ABVD followed by 30 Gy of IFRT.
   B) Four to six cycles of ABVD.
   C) Two cycles of ABVD followed by 20 Gy of IFRT.
   D) Two cycles of ABVD followed by an interim PET; if PET negative, then four more cycles of AVD (omitting bleomycin).

Expert Perspective: This patient presents with unfavorable, bulky, early-stage HL. Patients with bulky, early-stage disease have been included in both advanced-stage and early-stage unfavorable trials. Similar to the HD10 trial, the GHSG conducted a parallel HD11 trial for patients with early-stage, unfavorable HL based on the GHSG criteria. Patients treated with four cycles of ABVD + 30 Gy IFRT had a superior five-year freedom from treatment failure (87.2% vs 82.1%) compared to those treated with four cycles of ABVD + 20 Gy IFRT. While no subgroup analysis was done, approximately 20% of patients had bulky mediastinal disease.

The UK RATHL study included stage IIB, stage IIA with either bulky disease (> 10cm or MMR > 0.33 features) or > 2 involved sites and advanced-stage HL patients. Patients received two cycles of ABVD followed by interim PET-CT. Those with a Deauville score 1–3 were considered PET negative and were randomized to four additional cycles of ABVD versus four cycles of AVD with the omission of bleomycin. The three-year progression-free survival rate was 85.7% versus 84.4% in the ABVD versus AVD group, respectively There was no difference in three-year OS rates (97.2% and 97.6%, ABVD vs AVD, respectively). For stage II bulky disease with negative interim PET-CT, three-year PFS was 91.5%.

Based on these data, either a chemotherapy and radiation or chemotherapy-alone approach could be considered for unfavorable early-stage cHL. When determining which approach is ideal, we consider what fields would be included in radiation therapy as well as the age and sex of the patient to aid in consideration of late toxicities as well as fitness for six cycles of multi-agent chemotherapy. Patients with bulky mediastinal disease will likely have RT fields that encompass the heart and significant portions of the breasts, which would increase the future risk for breast cancer and heart disease. Discussion in a multidisciplinary meeting of medical oncology and radiation oncology is also recommended. Most recently, the 3-year follow-up analysis of safety and survival safety data from the NIVAHL trial were reported. Patients (age <60 years) were randomly assigned to receive either concomitant therapy with 4 cycles of nivolumab + AVD or sequential therapy with 4 cycles of nivolumab followed by 2 cycles of nivolumab + AVD and subsequently 2 cycles of AVD. Both groups underwent consolidation by 30 Gy IFRT. There were no PFS or OS events over a median follow-up period of 41 months after treatment completion. Overall, the 3-year PFS estimate was 99%, and the 3-year OS estimate was 100%.

Correct Answers: A or D

Case Study 4

A 45-year-old man presents with cervical and supraclavicular lymphadenopathy. Biopsy of a cervical node reveals cHL. Routine blood tests show a white blood cell (WBC) count of 17,000/mm^3, an absolute lymphocyte count of 300/mm^3, hemoglobin (Hgb) 9.8 mg/dL, albumin 3.2 mg/dL, and an ESR of 52 mm/h. A PET-CT reveals multiple enlarged supraclavicular, cervical, mediastinal, and retroperitoneal lymph nodes and splenomegaly. Bone marrow biopsy and aspirate examination is positive for cHL.

5) What is this patient's five-year progression-free survival with ABVD chemotherapy?
   A) 25%.
   B) 42%.
   C) 66%.
   D) 50%.

Expert Perspective: This patient presents with high-risk disease based on the Hasenclever International Prognostic Score (IPS) for advanced cHL, which assigns one point to each of the following adverse features: age ⩾ 45 years, albumin < 4.0 mg/dL, Hgb < 10.5 g/dL, stage IV disease, WBC ⩾ 15,000/mm³, ALC < 600/mm³, and male gender. The initial publication of the IPS predicted the following five-year freedom from disease progression rates based on the number of risk factors: 0 = 84%, 1 = 77%, 2 = 67%, 3 = 60%, 4 = 51%, and ⩾ 5 = 42%. More modern series have shown improved cure rates with standard ABVD, with five-year progression-free survival rates of 66% for IPS ⩾ 5, which are perhaps related to better supportive care and greater efforts to administer chemotherapy at full dose on schedule.

Correct Answer: C

6) **What is the best treatment option for this patient with advanced cHL?**
   A) Escalated BEACOPP × 4–6 cycles.
   B) Brentuximab vedotin plus AVD (BV-AVD).
   C) ABVD × two cycles → interim PET and if negative → four cycles of AVD.
   D) Nivolumab-AVD × six cycles on a clinical trial.
   E) All of the above are correct.

Expert Perspective: The optimal treatment for stage III–IV HL varies by country. The ECHELON-1 study compared six cycles of ABVD to six cycles of BV-AVD. Recently, the ECHELON-1 trial results were updated and identified an overall survival advantage for the BV-AVD arm versus the ABVD arm. The 6-year overall survival estimates were 93.9% vs 89.4% in the BV-AVD versus ABVD arms, respectively (HR 0.59, 95% CI 0.40-0.88). BV-AVD was associated with increased rates of neuropathy, neutropenic fever, and sepsis requiring administration of prophylactic growth factor. The Germans have adopted the escalated BEACOPP (escBEACOPP) regimen based on the results of a randomized trial showing an improved freedom from treatment failure when compared to COPP and ABVD. Toxicity was significantly higher in the escBEACOPP group, including hematologic toxicity, secondary leukemias, and nearly universal infertility. Follow-up studies of escBEACOPP compared to ABVD confirmed the advantage of escBEACOPP in terms of progression-free survival but showed no difference in OS. Based on these additional studies and the significant toxicity of escBEACOPP compared to ABVD, most oncologists outside of Germany continue to use ABVD as first-line therapy, understanding that more patients will relapse and require autologous stem cell transplantation (see Chapter 33). Based on the updated OS results from ECHELON-1, though there is some room for debate, we consider BV-AVD to be a new standard of care for front-line management of advanced stage cHL. Importantly, there may still be a role for ABVD in areas lacking access to brentuximab, for patients with significant baseline neuropathy, or those where the risk of neuropathy may have a significant impact on quality of life or ability to work, where shared decision making between patient and physician is encouraged. For these situations, we will administer ABVD and perform an interim PET after two cycles and if negative (Deauville 1–3) will omit bleomycin and complete four more cycles of AVD per RATHL.

The remarkable efficacy of programmed death-1 (PD-1) inhibitors in relapsed/refractory cHL has prompted novel clinical trials examining the impact of PD-1 inhibition in combination with chemotherapy for front-line management of cHL. Currently a large multicenter trial led by the Southwestern Oncology Group (SWOG) S1826 is evaluating the combination of nivolumab + AVD versus BV-AVD in newly diagnosed advanced-stage cHL. The results were presented during ASCO 2023 meetings. Nivolumab + AVD significantly prolonged PFS and was better tolerated when compared with BV-AVD in patients with advanced-stage Hodgkin lymphoma ⩾ 12 years of age. Results from the second planned interim analysis, based on 50% of the total expected PFS events among 976 evaluable patients, revealed a 52% reduction in the risk of disease progression or death with the use of nivolumab + AVD versus BV-AVD (HR 0.48, 99% CI [0.27, 0.87]; P = .0005). G-CSF was received by 54% and 95% of patients in the nivolumab +AVD and BV+AVD arms, respectively. Radiotherapy was given to 0.4% and 0.8% of patients, respectively. Based on these data, investigators believe that nivolumab + AVD is poised to become a new standard therapy for advanced stage Hodgkin lymphoma.

Correct Answer: E

Case study 4 continued: This patient receives two cycles of ABVD and has an interim PET-CT done to evaluate response. He has had marked improvement in disease but has residual fluorodeoxyglucose (FDG) avidity in a residual mediastinal node with uptake slightly greater than the liver consistent with Deauville score of 4.

7) Which of the following statements is correct?
- A) Alter the therapy.
- B) Continue with same therapy.
- C) Both choices A and B are acceptable options.

Expert Perspective: The optimal management approach for PET+ advanced-stage cHL remains to be determined, and the limited number of patients preclude definitive analysis in a large randomized controlled trial. Patients with PET+ disease after two cycles of ABVD on the RATHL study proceeded to BEACOPP therapy. The three-year progression-free survival and OS data were 67.5% and 87.8%, respectively, suggesting encouraging responses can be obtained with this approach. Similar results were noted for the Southwest Oncology Group (SWOG) S0816 trial. BEACOPP cannot be recommended for elderly patients with PET+ disease for toxicity concerns. In our practice, patients with Deauville 5 responses on interim PET, regardless of initial regimen, should be biopsied to confirm refractory cHL. Those with confirmed disease who received ABVD who are fit and young may be eligible to proceed with BEACOPP therapy. Patients receiving BV-AVD should be switched to salvage treatment regimens with a plan for autologous stem cell transplantation. Transplant-ineligible patients with progression on BV-AVD should receive individualized approaches, and we suggest PD-1 inhibitors. Elderly patients receiving ABVD, given the lack of trial data to guide therapy decisions, may be considered to switch to BV-AVD to complete six cycles or consider salvage regimens based on fitness as discussed above. For patients with Deauville 4 responses on interim PET, we recommend either two additional cycles of ABVD and repeat PET-CT or switching to BV-AVD with repeat PET-CT testing. Patients who remain PET positive should have biopsies to confirm the presence of disease and proceed to salvage chemotherapy regimens with a plan for autologous stem cell transplantation in eligible patients or relapsed/refractory cHL regimens if unfit.

Correct Answer: C

Case Study 5

A 65-year-old man presents with relapsed cHL now one year post autologous stem cell transplantation using carmustine, etoposide, cytarabine, and melphalan (BEAM) conditioning. He originally received six cycles of BV-AVD with a relapse one year later and received two cycles of ifosfamide, carboplatin, and etoposide salvage therapy with remission prior to transplant. Now he has diffuse disease. He remains thrombocytopenic post therapy, and a bone marrow biopsy demonstrates hypocellularity without evidence of myelodysplasia.

8) What therapy would you recommend next?
   A) Gemcitabine/vinolrelbine/liposomal doxorubicin.
   B) CD30 chimeric antigen receptor T cell (CAR-T) therapy.
   C) PD-1 inhibition with pembrolizumab or nivolumab.
   D) Single-agent brentuximab vedotin.
   E) Lenalidomide.

Expert Perspective: The unique biology of cHL renders it far more susceptible to immunotherapy approaches involving PD-1 inhibitors compared to other lymphomas. cHL has been demonstrated to overexpress PD-1 ligands. This relates to the genetic amplification of chromosome 9p24.1 in HRS cells commonly observed in patients with cHL. The unique, predominant immune infiltrate present in cHL tumors is a further opportunity for activation by PD-1 inhibition. Pembrolizumab and nivolumab have both received FDA approval for treatment of relapsed cHL after multiple lines of therapy. Phase II studies of both drugs have demonstrated high overall response rates in approximately 70% of patients, with up to a quarter experiencing a complete response (CR). The median duration of response extends beyond one year, suggesting the potential to achieve durable benefit. KEYNOTE-204 compared pembrolizumab to BV in the relapsed setting with improvements in median PFS (13.2 vs 8.3 months, HR 0.65; 95% CI 0.48–0.88). The results of KEYNOTE-204 provide further support to the use of PD-1 inhibitors relapsing following autologous stem cell transplantation, and we reserve BV for relapses after PD-1 inhibitors in this scenario based on this data.

Recently, combination therapy of pembrolizumab, gemcitabine, vinorelbine, and liposomal doxorubicin as salvage therapy was reported to produce a CR rate of 95% with 36/39 patients proceeding to autologous stem cell transplantation and 100% of those alive and progression-free after one year of median follow-up. These impressive results are supported by recent publication of nivolumab alone or in combination with ifosfamide, carboplatin, and etoposide as salvage therapy ahead of auto transplant. In this study, CR rates were over 90% and the two-year progression-free survival rate was 72%, suggesting this approach may also produce durable benefit and even avoid salvage chemotherapy ahead of stem cell transplantation.

Multi-agent chemotherapy is unlikely to be safe given this patient's prior exposures and ongoing hematologic toxicities. Lenalidomide has some activity in relapsed/refractory disease but far less and with the potential for greater toxicity compared to PD-1 inhibitors. We recommend proceeding with single-agent checkpoint inhibition using pembrolizumab or nivolumab based on its efficacy and manageable toxicity profile.

CD30 is universally expressed by HRS and CD30 CAR-T therapy has been studied in phase I/II studies involving limited population of heavily pretreated patients with relapsed/refractory cHL. While the overall response rate is encouraging (62%, 51% CR), these responses do not appear durable, and most patients will relapse within two years of therapy. Nevertheless, this therapeutic approach holds great promise as distinct novel therapy in the management of relapsed/refractory cHL. The ongoing multicenter phase II CHARIOT study is being conducted to continue to investigate the safety and efficacy of CD30 CAR-T therapy in cHL, and we highly suggest participation when applicable.

Correct Answer: C

Case Study 6

A 77-year-old woman is diagnosed with cHL presenting as fatigue and pruritis. Staging PET-CT demonstrates PET-avid lymph nodes above and below the diaphragm. Her medical history is notable for hypertension and diabetes mellitus managed with metformin. She lives with her husband and participates in regular household chores. She continues to volunteer at her local church.

9) What additional testing would you recommend?
   A) Bone marrow biopsy.
   B) Geriatric assessment.
   C) Lumbar puncture with cerebral spinal fluid analysis for cHL cells.

Expert Perspective: Elderly patients, defined as age $\geq$ 60 years, are poorly represented in the large, randomized trials that guide general medical recommendations. Older cHL patients are more at risk for inferior outcomes due in part to different disease biology compared to younger patients as well as an increased rate of comorbidity and frailty. Special considerations need to be taken in the care of the elderly patient with cHL and should begin with a comprehensive frailty assessment. Geriatric assessments provide a robust measure of functional performance and comorbidity and are effective at identifying subtle degrees of frailty that may contribute to increased risks of toxicity and inferior outcomes. For situations where a geriatrician cannot be reliably or timely referred to, we suggest evaluating for comorbidity, activities of daily living, and screening for falls, malnutrition, depression, and cognitive dysfunction. Use of geriatric asessment before initiation of therapy can help identify fit versus frail patients to help guide initial treatment decision-making. Finally, we consider the patient's prior functional baseline in making initial treatment recommendations. Situations where a clear deterioration in functional status can be attributable to HL may suggest they will experience improvements with initial therapy, potentially with a dose reduction to account for a poor performance status.

Correct Answer: B

10) She undergoes a geriatric assessment and is determined to be fit to receive definitive therapy. You recommend the following:
   A) Six cycles of ABVD.
   B) Two cycles of BV → six cycles of AVD → four cycles of BV.
   C) Two cycles of ABVD and then PET/CT with four additional cycles of AVD for PET-negative disease or six cycles of AVD.
   D) B or C are reasonable.

Expert Perspective: The incidence of bleomycin toxicity increases dramatically with age and cumulative dose exposure, reaching upwards of 30% with a high rate of mortality once diagnosed. Efforts to avoid bleomycin and resulting toxicity are highly recommended, and a full course of ABVD should be avoided, with some experts recommending completely avoiding bleomycin in patients 60 years or older. Although the RATHL study only featured a limited set of patients aged ≥ 60 years (115/1203, 9.6%), the advantage of a PET-adapted approach and early omission of bleomycin suggests that this approach would be reasonable. Alternatively, a sequential approach incorporating BV followed by AVD chemotherapy and a subsequent BV course has been studied specifically in a geriatric population in a phase II study of 48 patients. Proceeding to single-agent BV therapy is also likely to avoid the risks of neutropenia and sepsis observed with BV-AVD combined therapy and allow for potential improvements in performance status with better disease control before using multi-agent chemotherapy. This approach appeared to be well tolerated with grade 3 or 4 events largely related to hematologic toxicities but low rates of febrile neutropenia (8% patients). The two-year progression-free survival and OS rates were 84% and 93%, respectively, suggesting this regimen is effective as well. Alternatively, BV alone or in combination with dacarbazine can achieve good responses but is limited by high rates of neuropathy and modest PFS (~10 and ~18 months, BV vs BV + dacarbazine). Front-line use of single-agent PD-1 inhibitors such as nivolumab or pembrolizumab have not been evaluated in a clinical trial but based on their efficacy in the relapsed setting are likely to be active and well tolerated in the elderly population.

Correct Answer: D

Case Study 7

A 23-year-old woman with stage IV cHL is currently receiving ABVD. She presents for cycle 2 of treatment and has an absolute neutrophil count (ANC) of 100. She is afebrile and feels well.

11) **How should you manage her?**
    A) Administer full-dose ABVD chemotherapy today.
    B) Hold treatment and recheck counts in a week.
    C) Administer ABVD with a 35% dose reduction today.
    D) Administer full-dose ABVD and start prophylactic peg filgrastim.

Expert Perspective: In several large series, the incidence of febrile neutropenia with ABVD was < 5% despite high rates of neutropenia. Prophylactic growth factors are not indicated with ABVD and should not be instituted for asymptomatic neutropenia. Retrospective studies have shown a possible increase in serious bleomycin lung toxicity in patients receiving granulocyte colony-stimulating factor with ABVD, providing another reason to avoid growth factors with this regimen.

Correct Answer: A

Case Study 8

A 44-year-old man has received two cycles of ABVD for bulky, stage II cHL. He presents for cycle 3 of treatment and has pulmonary function tests (PFTs) performed before therapy. He denies shortness of breath, fever, or other associated symptoms. His oxygen saturation is 95% on room air. A chest X-ray shows no pulmonary infiltrates. You observe on his PFTs that his diffusion capacity for carbon monoxide (DLCO) has declined by 40% compared to his baseline. When you probe him further, he states he has started to notice a dry cough.

12) You recommend:

    A) Continue ABVD and repeat PFTs next cycle.
    B) Omit bleomycin and continue AVD.
    C) Hold therapy and repeat PFTs in one week.

Expert Perspective: Bleomycin lung toxicity commonly presents as a dry cough without associated symptoms. One of the earliest findings to suggest bleomycin lung toxicity is a drop in the DLCO, and patients are often asymptomatic. In a large retrospective study of patients receiving bleomycin for treatment of cHL, lung toxicity occurred in 18% of patients and was fatal in 24% of patients. When fevers, pulmonary infiltrates, shortness of breath, or hypoxia develop, the prognosis is more guarded. Thus, bleomycin toxicity should be considered in all patients on ABVD presenting with a decrease in the DLCO or new cough. In our practice, we obtain PFTs as a baseline and before every cycle of ABVD. We omit bleomycin for patients with new pulmonary symptoms (excluding clear unrelated causes) or with a decline in their DLCO ⩾ 25%. Data from the RATHL study demonstrate that bleomycin can be safely omitted following two cycles of ABVD in PET-negative patients. Additional retrospective data show no difference in outcome when bleomycin is discontinued prematurely.

Correct Answer: B

Case Study 9

A 26-year-old woman completed six cycles of ABVD chemotherapy four weeks ago for stage IIIB cHL. Her post-treatment PET-CT reveals a complete metabolic response to therapy with no FDG-avid disease. She has a 2 cm residual mediastinal mass that has decreased by 75% compared to pretreatment.

13) What follow-up imaging should she receive?
    A) No surveillance imaging.
    B) PET-CT every 6–12 months for five years.
    C) PET-CT every 6–12 months for two years.
    D) CT chest abdomen pelvis every 6–12 months for five years.
    E) CT chest abdomen pelvis every 6–12 months for two years.
    F) A and E.

Expert Perspective: In a prospective surveillance trial in which cHL patients in remission underwent a PET-CT scan every six months for four years, 85% of relapses occurred in the first 18 months following treatment. Despite lacking supportive data, the National Comprehensive Cancer Network (NCCN) guidelines recommend obtaining imaging studies of the chest (X-ray or CT) and abdomen and pelvis (CT) every 6–12 months for the first 2–3 years following completion of therapy. Importantly, there is no evidence that routine surveillance scans improve the outcome of patients with relapsed HL. In retrospective studies, 65–80% of relapses are detected by patient symptoms or physical exam findings, not by surveillance imaging, and these studies show no difference in patient outcomes based on method of relapse detection. In addition, there is a risk of false-positive results when obtaining surveillance PET-CT and CT scans. The largest trial looking at the predictive value of surveillance scans was published by the Dana-Farber Cancer Institute and revealed a positive predictive value for detecting recurrent cHL of 22.9% and 28.6% in PET–CT and CT, respectively. In our practice, we recommend against routine surveillance imaging but employ a shared decision-making approach. For these reasons, a choice of no surveillance imaging or surveillance per NCCN guidelines is reasonable on case-by-case basis.

Correct Answer: F

Case Study 10

A 38-year-old woman presents to establish care with a new primary care physician. Her past medical history is significant only for cHL diagnosed at the age of 15, which was treated with ABVD followed by IFRT to the mediastinum. Her physician calls you to discuss screening and preventative care. She has not been followed by a physician for the past 10 years.

14) Which of the following should you recommend?
    A) Screening colonoscopy.
    B) Pneumococcal and meningococcal vaccination.
    C) Screening mammogram and breast magnetic resonance imaging (MRI).

Expert Perspective: Successful improvements in treatment of patients with HL have led to an increasing number of long-term survivors of the disease. Long-term follow-up studies have noted a marked increased risk for competing causes of death from treatment-related complications, including secondary malignancies, heart, and lung disease, in addition to thyroid dysfunction and infertility. The most common second cancers following treatment of HL are breast and lung cancer. This patient's risk of developing breast cancer is five-fold that of the normal population, with an absolute risk approaching 25% at 30 years of age and 35% at 40 years. Annual mammograms and breast MRIs are recommended for all women treated for HL with mediastinal or axillary RT between ages 10 and 30.

Correct Answer: C

Case Study 11

A 40-year-old man was treated with ABVD and mediastinal RT 10 years ago. He has a family history of coronary artery disease and was recently found to have a low-density lipoprotein (LDL) level of 130 and a high-density lipoprotein (HDL) level of 35.

15) What would you recommend to the patient's internist?

    A) Dietary consult and recheck in 12 months.

    B) Start a statin.

    C) Start a statin and consider cardiology referral +/– echocardiography.

Expert Perspective: Patients treated with mediastinal RT are at high risk of developing cardiovascular disease following treatment, and this includes a threefold increased risk of fatal myocardial infarction. By 10 years, 4.5% of patients have evidence of clinically significant cardiac disease, a number that increases to 23.2% by 25 years following completion of therapy. Additionally, radiation exposure increases the risk for valvular heart disease. Given this elevated risk, all patients who have had mediastinal RT should be considered high risk for cardiovascular disease. These patients should undergo counselling on risk factor reduction, including the use of statin therapy for cholesterol management. Echocardiography to screen for heart failure following radiation and anthracycline exposure should also be considered. Finally, referral to cardiology for a more complete discussion of risk factor management and coronary artery disease screening is encouraged.

Correct Answer: C

Recommended Readings

Ansell, S.M., Radford, J., Connors, J.M. et al. (2022). ECHELON-1 Study Group. Overall survival with brentuximab vedotin in stage III or IV Hodgkin's lymphoma. *N Engl J Med* 387 (4): 310–320.

Bröckelmann, P.J., Bühnen, I., Meissner, J., et al. (2022). Nivolumab and AVD in early-stage unfavorable hodgkin lymphoma: final 1 analysis of the randomized GHSG phase II NIVAHL trial. *J Clin Oncol* JCO.22.02355.

Herrera, A.F., LeBlanc, M.L., Castellino, S.M. et al. (2023). SWOG S1826, a randomized study of nivolumab(N)-AVD versus brentuximab vedotin(BV)-AVD in advanced stage (AS) classic Hodgkin lymphoma (HL). *J Clin Oncol* 41 (suppl 17): LBA4. doi:10.1200/JCO.2023.41.16_suppl.LBA4

Connors, J.M., Jurczak, W., Straus, D.J. et al. (2018 January 25). Brentuximab vedotin with chemotherapy for stage III or IV Hodgkin's Lymphoma. *N Engl J Med* 378 (4): 331–344. doi: 10.1056/NEJMoa1708984. Epub 2017 Dec 10. Erratum in: N Engl J Med. 2018 Mar 1;378(9):878. PMID: 29224502; PMCID: PMC5819601.

Eich, H.T., Diehl, V., Gorgen, H. et al. (2010). Intensified chemotherapy and dose-reduced involved-field radiotherapy in patients with early unfavorable Hodgkin's lymphoma: Final analysis of the German hodgkin study group HD11 trial. *J Clin Oncol* 28: 4199–4206.

Evens, A.M., Advani, R.H., Helenowski, I.B. et al. (2018 October 20). Multicenter phase II study of sequential brentuximab vedotin and doxorubicin, vinblastine, and dacarbazine chemotherapy for older patients with untreated classical hodgkin lymphoma. *J Clin Oncol* 36 (30): 3015–3022. doi: 10.1200/JCO.2018.79.0139. Epub 2018 Sep 4. PMID: 30179569.

Johnson, P., Federico, M., Kirkwood, A. et al. (2016 June 23). Adapted treatment guided by interim PET-CT scan in advanced Hodgkin's Lymphoma. *N Engl J Med* 374 (25): 2419–2429. doi: 10.1056/NEJMoa1510093. PMID: 27332902; PMCID: PMC4961236.

Kuruvilla, J., Ramchandren, R., Santoro, A. et al. (2021 April). Pembrolizumab versus brentuximab vedotin in relapsed or refractory classical Hodgkin lymphoma (KEYNOTE-204): an interim analysis of a multicentre, randomised, open-label, phase 3 study. *Lancet Oncol* 22 (4): 512–524. doi: 10.1016/S1470-2045(21)00005-X. Epub 2021 Mar 12. Erratum in: Lancet Oncol. 2021 May;22(5):e184. PMID: 33721562).

André, M.P.E., Girinsky, T., Federico, M. et al. (2017 June 1). Early positron emission tomography response-adapted treatment in stage I and II hodgkin lymphoma: final results of the randomized EORTC/LYSA/FIL H10 trial. *J Clin Oncol* 35 (16): 1786–1794. doi: 10.1200/JCO.2016.68.6394. Epub 2017 Mar 14. PMID: 28291393.

Radford, J., Illidge, T., Counsell, N. et al. (2015 April 23). Results of a trial of PET-directed therapy for early-stage Hodgkin's lymphoma. *N Engl J Med* 372 (17): 1598–1607. doi: 10.1056/NEJMoa1408648. PMID: 25901426.

Swerdlow, A.J., Cooke, R., Bates, A. et al. (2012). Breast cancer risk after supradiaphragmatic radiotherapy for hodgkin's lymphoma in England and wales: a national cohort study. *J Clin Oncol* 30: 2745–2752.

32

Nodular Lymphocyte-Predominant Hodgkin Lymphoma

Dennis A. Eichenauer

University Hospital Cologne, Cologne, Germany, and German Hodgkin Study Group (GHSG), Cologne, Germany

Introduction

Nodular lymphocyte-predominant Hodgkin lymphoma (NLPHL) is a rare entity accounting for about 5% of all Hodgkin lymphoma (HL) cases. Hence, its incidence is approximately 1–2/1,000,000 per year. The disease is characterized by a male predominance since men account for roughly 75% of cases. The clinical course is usually indolent despite a tendency toward late relapses and histologic transformation into aggressive B-NHL. Most patients present with early-stage disease at the initial diagnosis.

1) **Nodular lymphocyte-predominant Hodgkin lymphoma (NLPHL) and classic Hodgkin lymphoma (cHL) are usually treated similarly. However, there are significant differences. With respect to which features do NLPHL and cHL differ?**
   A) Immunohistology.
   B) Clinical presentation.
   C) Course of the disease.
   D) All of the above.

Expert Perspective: NLPHL substantially differs from the histological subtypes of cHL in terms of immunohistology, clinical presentation, and disease course. The consistent expression of the B-cell marker CD20 represents a hallmark of the disease-defining lymphocyte predominant (LP) cells in NLPHL. In contrast, CD20 is only infrequently found on Hodgkin and Reed-Sternberg (H-RS) cells in cHL. Additional immunohistological differences between the malignant cells in NLPHL and cHL include the lack of the antigens CD15 and CD30 on LP cells; these surface antigens are typically expressed on H-RS cells. These and other markers that can be used to distinguish LP cells from H-RS cells are summarized in Table 32.1.

The most comprehensive data addressing the differences between NLPHL and cHL in terms of clinical presentation and course came from the German Hodgkin Study Group (GHSG). In a retrospective analysis, Nogova and coworkers compared the characteristics and outcomes of 394 NLPHL and 7,904 cHL patients treated within GHSG trials between 1988 and 2002. Sixty-three percent of patients with NLPHL were diagnosed in early, 16% in

Cancer Consult: Expertise in Clinical Practice, Volume 2: Neoplastic Hematology & Cellular Therapy,
Second Edition. Edited by Syed A. Abutalib, Maurie Markman, James O. Armitage, and Kenneth C. Anderson.
© 2024 John Wiley & Sons Ltd. Published 2024 by John Wiley & Sons Ltd.

Table 32.1 Staining characteristics of nodular lymphocyte-predominant Hodgkin lymphoma (NLPHL) and classic Hodgkin lymphoma (cHL).

	NLPHL	cHL
CD20	+	−/+
CD30	−	+
CD15	−	+
CD45	+	−
CD79A	+	−/+
EBER	−	−/+
EMA	+/−	−
OCT-2	+	−/+
BOB.1	+	−/+
PU.1	+	−

EBER: Epstein-Barr encoding region in situ hybridization for EBV; EMA: epithelial membrane antigen; +: positive; −: negative; +/ −: usually positive, may be negative; −/ +: usually negative, may be positive. *Source:* Adapted and modified from Smith LB. *Arch Pathol Lab Med.* 2010;134(10):1434 – 9.

intermediate, and 21% in advanced stages. In contrast, 22%, 39%, and 39% of patients with cHL were diagnosed with early, intermediate, and advanced stages, respectively. Patients with NLPHL had B-symptoms less frequently (9% in NLPHL vs 40% in cHL; $P < 0.0001$). The presence of clinical risk factors such as elevated erythrocyte sedimentation rate (ESR) (4% in NLPHL vs 45% in cHL; $P < 0.0001$), the involvement of three or more nodal areas (28% in NLPHL vs 55% in cHL; $P < 0.0001$), extranodal disease (6% in NLPHL vs 14% in cHL; $P < 0.0001$), mediastinal bulk of more than one-third of the maximum thoracic width (31% in NLPHL vs 55% in cHL; $P < 0.0001$), and elevated lactate dehydrogenase (LDH) (16% in NLPHL vs 32% in cHL; $P < 0.0001$) was also less common in NLPHL (Table 32.2).

In summary, NLPHL is characterized by pathological and clinical features that differ significantly from those of cHL.

Correct Answer: D

2) **In cHL, combined-modality treatment was shown to result in a superior clinical outcome as compared with RT alone and is thus considered one of the standards of care for early stages. In NLPHL, RT alone represents the widely accepted standard of care for stage IA disease without clinical risk factors.**

Is this recommendation based on randomized clinical trials?

Expert Perspective: No. Randomized clinical trials exclusively including patients with NLPHL have not been conducted to date due to the low incidence of the disease. Thus, recommendations in NLPHL are based on results from smaller prospective phase II studies and retrospective analyses (Table 32.3).

Table 32.2 Characteristics of nodular lymphocyte-predominant Hodgkin lymphoma (NLPHL) and classic Hodgkin lymphoma (cHL) patients.

	NLPHL (n = 394)	cHL (n = 7904)
Age (median)	37	33
Male gender (%)	75	56
B-symptoms (%)	9	40
Elevated ESR (%)	4	45
Three or more nodal areas involved (%)	28	55
Extranodal disease (%)	6	14
Large mediastinal mass (> 1/3 of the max. thoracic width) (%)	31	55
Elevated LDH (%)	16	32
Early favorable stages (%)	63	22
Intermediate (%)	16	39
Advanced stages (%)	21	39

ESR: erythrocyte sedimentation rate; LDH: lactate dehydrogenase.
Source: Adapted and modified from Nogova, L., et al. *J Clin Oncol.* 2008;26(3):434–9. Reproduced with permission of the American Society of Clinical Oncology.

Table 32.3 Risk group allocation applied by the GHSG.

Risk group	Stage
Early stage	Stage I/II with no risk factors (see below)
Intermediate stage	Stage I/IIA with ≥ 1 risk factor(s) Stage IIB with risk factors C/D but not A/B
Advance stage	Stage IIB with risk factors A/B Stage III/IV

Risk factors

(A) Large mediastinal mass: > 1/3 of the maximum horizontal chest diameter

(B) Extranodal disease

(C) Elevated ESR: > 50 mm/h without B-symptoms, > 30 mm/h with B-symptoms.

(D) ≥ 3 nodal areas

Stage I disease: The largest analysis investigating patients with stage IA NLPHL without clinical risk factors came from the GHSG. Patients had received involved-field radiotherapy (IF-RT) alone (n = 108), extended-field RT (EF-RT) alone (n = 49), or combined-modality treatment consisting of a brief chemotherapy followed by consolidation RT (n = 72). There were no differences in terms of progression-free survival (PFS) and overall survival (OS) between the treatment groups. At eight years, the PFS was more than 85% and the OS was close to 100%. Similar results were obtained in an analysis including 113 patients with stage I/II NLPHL treated at academic hospitals in the United States. Outcomes of patients who had RT alone for stage I NLPHL could not be improved by the addition of chemotherapy. The 10-year PFS after RT alone was 89%, 10-year OS was 96%. Limited-field RT alone was therefore adopted as standard treatment for most patients with stage IA NLPHL without clinical risk factors.

The question of whether radiation can be safely reduced from IF-RT to involved-site RT (IS-RT) is an ongoing matter of debate. A recent retrospective single-center analysis included 71 patients with stage I/II NLPHL of whom 36 patients received RT alone consisting of EF-RT (n = 9), IF-RT (n = 13), or IS-RT (n = 14). Short-term disease control did not differ between the three RT approaches so that a reduction from IF-RT to IS-RT is likely possible. However, follow-up analyses are necessary to draw final conclusions since the median observation time of patients who had IS-RT alone was only 2.6 years.

Stage II disease: In comparison with stage I NLPHL, patients with stage II disease have an inferior PFS after RT alone. Thus, this approach may not be optimal in this patient group. This impression is supported by the results from a retrospective study from Canada. The outcome of 32 patients treated with RT alone between 1966 and 1993 was compared with the outcome of 56 patients treated with combined-modality treatment between 1993 and 2009. The analysis revealed a significantly better PFS for patients who had combined-modality treatment. Although this analysis has some limitations and results must be interpreted with caution because patients were treated over a period of more than four decades, the improved tumor control with combined-modality treatment should be kept in mind when choosing treatment for patients with NLPHL in early stages other than stage IA.

3) The minority of NLPHL patients are diagnosed in intermediate or advanced stages.

What are treatment differences between NLPHL and cHL in these stages?

Expert Perspective: Only a minority of NLPHL patients are diagnosed in intermediate and advanced stages (Table 32.3). According to a large retrospective analysis performed by the GHSG, intermediate and advanced stages accounted for 37% of NLPHL cases (16% intermediate stages and 21% advanced stages). It is important to acknowledge that there is no consensus regarding a preferred chemotherapy regimen for NLPHL.

Intermediate-stage disease: Treatment of patients with intermediate-stage NLPHL is usually very similar to that for cHL. A retrospective analysis by the GHSG including 76 intermediate-stage NLPHL patients indicated a 10-year PFS of 72.1% and a 10-year OS of 96.2% after stage-adapted HL-directed therapy within randomized studies. In all, four cycles of ABVD-based chemotherapy followed by limited-field RT thus appears to be a highly active treatment for patients with NLPHL in intermediate stages (Table 32.3) and should therefore be considered in this patient group.

Advanced-stage disease: The optimal treatment for patients with advanced NLPHL has not been defined either. The 10-year PFS and OS rates among 144 patients who mostly had treatment with BEACOPP-based chemotherapy within randomized GHSG studies were 69.8% and 87.4%, respectively. However, given the rather indolent course of NLPHL and the often low lymphoma burden, it is unclear whether all patients with advanced NLPHL benefit from intensive treatment with BEACOPP. Promising results were also obtained with the R-CHOP protocol as used in DLBCL. A single-center retrospective analysis included 14 patients with stage III/IV NLPHL who had treatment with R-CHOP. The five-year PFS was 85.7%. A smaller case series comprising nine patients of which eight had advanced disease evaluated the BR protocol. All patients responded to treatment. After a median observation time of 34 months, none of the patients had relapsed. The ABVD regimen that represents the standard of care in advanced cHL in many countries seems to be associated with inferior outcomes in this group of patients. According to a Canadian analysis, approximately 40% of patients with advanced NLPHL experienced lymphoma recurrence either with NLPHL histology or histological transformation into aggressive B-NHL after first-line treatment with ABVD or ABVD-like protocols. The question of whether outcomes with ABVD can be impoved by the addition of an anti-CD20 antibody is not answered until now as larger analyses addressing this issue are pending.

4) **In NLPHL, the consistent expression of the B-cell marker CD20 represents a hallmark of the disease-defining LP cells. Therefore, it is tempting to treat NLPHL with approaches including anti-CD20 antibodies as a single agent.**

Are there prospective data on the value of anti-CD20 antibodies in this entity?
   A) Yes, for all stages.
   B) Yes, but only for some stages.
   C) No, there are no data at all.

Expert Perspective: Several phase II trials evaluating anti-CD20 antibodies in NLPHL have been conducted. A study from the United States included a total of 39 patients; 21 patients had newly diagnosed NLPHL, while 18 patients had relapsed disease. Patients received either four weekly standard doses of rituximab alone or four weekly standard doses followed by rituximab maintenance every six months for two years. All patients responded to treatment. However, the five-year PFS estimates were only 39.1% for patients receiving four doses of rituximab alone and 58.9% for patients receiving rituximab induction with four weekly doses followed by rituximab maintenance. The GHSG conducted a phase II study comprising 28 patients with newly diagnosed stage IA NLPHL who were treated with four weekly doses of rituximab. The response rate was 100%. However, similarly to the study from the United States, the excellent response rate did not translate into a high rate of individuals with long-term disease control. After a median follow-up of 9.7 years, the 10-year PFS was only 51.1% and thus clearly worse than with RT alone.

Prospective studies from the GHSG also investigated rituximab and the second-generation anti-CD20 antibody ofatumumab in patients with relapsed NLPHL. Rituximab was evaluated in 15 patients. Among those, 94% responded to four weekly standard doses. After a median follow-up of 63 months, the median time to progession was 33 months. A total of 28 patients with relapsed NLPHL were included in a phase II study investigating ofatumumab. The antibody was given once weekly for eight consecutive weeks. The response rate was 96%. After a median observation time of 26 months, the one- and two-year PFS estimates were 93% and 80%, respectively.

Based on these data, single-agent anti-CD20 antibody treatment is usually not used in the first-line treatment of NLPHL, although there are a few exceptions. In contrast, patients with disease recurrence are often candidates for salvage treatment with an anti-CD20 antibody given as single agent. These patients do not seem to require aggressive second-line treatment with high-dose chemotherapy and autologous stem cell transplantation in many cases as demonstrated by different retrospective analyses.

Correct Answer: B

5) **A 45-year-old male patient was diagnosed with stage IIIA NLPHL eight years ago. He achieved continuous remission after six cycles of escalated BEACOPP. The patient now presents with cervical and mediastinal lymphadenopathy, B-symptoms are not reported, and the LDH is slightly elevated.**

What is the next diagnostic or therapeutic step?

A) Start treatment with rituximab.

B) Plan high-dose chemotherapy and autologous stem cell transplantation after salvage treatment and stem cell harvest.

C) Obtain a lymph node biopsy.

D) Start treatment with steroids.

Expert Perspective: In NLPHL patients presenting with clinical signs of relapse, a lymph biopsy should be obtained whenever possible. This is due to an increased risk of transformation from NLPHL into aggressive B-NHL, in particular T-cell and histiocyte-rich B-NHL (TCRBNHL; see Chapters 34 and 43). Some analyses addressing this issue have been performed to date. A registry-based analysis comprising 164 patients initially diagnosed with NLPHL between 1973 and 2003 came from France. At a median follow-up of 9.5 years for survivors, 66 patients had recurrence of lymphoma, of which 19 presented with histological transformation into aggressive B-NHL. The median time from the initial NLPHL diagnosis to the occurrence of transformation was 4.7 years; the cumulative 10-year transformation rate was 12%. Patients with transformation were treated with either conventional chemotherapy (10 of 19) or high-dose chemotherapy followed by autologous stem cell transplantation (9 of 19) and thus received more aggressive treatment than most patients who relapse with NLPHL histology.

A second report from Canada using the British Columbia Cancer Agency (BCCA) database included a total of 95 patients initially diagnosed with NLPHL. Transformation into aggressive B-NHL occurred in 13 of them; the median time to transformation was 8.1 years. The actuarial risks for the development of transformed lymphoma after initial diagnosis of NLPHL were 5%, 7%, 15%, 31%, and 36% after 5, 10, 15, 20, and 25 years, respectively. Interestingly, two clusters of transformation were seen. One cluster of early transformation occurred less than three years after the initial lymphoma diagnosis (5 of 13), while a cluster of late transformation occurred 10–25 years after the initial lymphoma diagnosis (7 of 13). Transformation was more likely in patients with initial splenic involvement ($P = 0.006$). In agreement with the French report, the prognosis after diagnosis of aggressive B-NHL was worse than expected after NLPHL relapse. Although patients with transformed lymphoma were being treated with multi-agent chemotherapy mostly followed by high-dose chemotherapy and autologous stem cell transplantation, 10-year estimates for PFS and OS were only 52% and 62%, respectively.

An analysis from the United Kingdom included 26 patients who had developed histological transformation into aggressive B-NHL. At transformation, patients were either treated with R-CHOP or high-dose chemotherapy and autologous stem cell transplantation. The five-year PFS was 64.1%, and the five-year OS was 70%.

Given the risk for the development of histological transformation, a rebiopsy should be obtained whenever possible if clinical signs of relapse occur in patients initially treated for NLPHL. The most appropriate treatment can be chosen only based on a correct histological diagnosis. Treatment options range from anti-CD20 antibody treatment for patients with NLPHL histology and low tumor burden to aggressive treatment approaches including high-dose chemotherapy and autologous stem cell transplantation for patients relapsing with transformation into aggressive B-NHL.

Correct Answer: C

6) **Which group of patients with NLPHL could be potential candidates for active surveillance at diagnosis?**

Expert Perspective: In some patients with advanced NLPHL, i.e. those with a low lymphoma burden and an indolent course of disease, an active surveillance strategy comparable to advanced indolent B-NHL can be considered. The largest analysis on this approach came from the Memorial Sloan Kettering Cancer Center. A total of 37 NLPHL patients who did not undergo systemic treatment or radiation at initial diagnosis were considered. After a median observation time of 69 months, patients who were only followed had an impaired PFS but a similar OS in comparison with 126 patients who had any first-line treatment. Unlike individuals with advanced NLPHL, only a small minority of patients with early-stage NLPHL may be candidates for an active surveillance approach since this strategy bears the risk of relevant disease progression during observation requiring more intensive treatment than it would have been necessary at initial diagnosis.

Recommended Readings

Binkley, M.S., Rauf, M.S., Milgrom, S.A., Pinnix, C.C., Tsang, R., Dickinson, M. et al. (2020 June 25). Stage I-II nodular lymphocyte-predominant Hodgkin lymphoma: a multi-institutional study of adult patients by ILROG. *Blood* 135 (26): 2365–2374. doi: 10.1182/blood.2019003877. PMID: 32211877.

Eichenauer, D.A., Plütschow, A., Fuchs, M., Sasse, S., Baues, C. et al. (2020 Mar 1). Long-term follow-up of patients with nodular lymphocyte-predominant hodgkin lymphoma treated in the HD7 to HD15 trials: a report from the german hodgkin study group. *J Clin Oncol* 38 (7): 698–705. doi: 10.1200/JCO.19.00986. Epub 2019 Oct 18. PMID: 31626571.

Eichenauer, D.A., Plütschow, A., Fuchs, M., von Treschow, B., Böll, B., Behringer, K. et al. (2015 September 10). Long-term course of patients with stage IA nodular lymphocyte-predominant hodgkin lymphoma: a report from the German hodgkin study group. *J Clin Oncol* 33 (26): 2857–2862. doi: 10.1200/JCO.2014.60.4363. Epub 2015 Aug 3. PMID: 26240235.

Eichenauer, D.A., Plütschow, A., Schröder, L., Fuchs, M., Böll, B., von Treschow, B., Diehl, V., Borchmann, P., and Engert, A. (2018 October 4). Relapsed and refractory nodular lymphocyte-predominant Hodgkin lymphoma: an analysis from the German hodgkin study group. *Blood* 132 (14): 1519–1525. doi: 10.1182/blood-2018-02-836437. Epub 2018 Jul 31. PMID: 30064977.

Eichenauer, D.A., Bühnen, I., Plütschow, A., Kobe, C., Dietlein, M., Wendtner, C.M., Thorspecken, S., Topp, M.S., Mauser, M., von Tresckow, B., Fuchs, M., Borchmann, P., and Engert, A. (2022 March 21). IPhase II study of fixed-duration single-agent ibrutinib in relapsed nodular lymphocyte-predominant Hodgkin lymphoma: a report from the German Hodgkin Study Group. *Hematol Oncol.* doi: 10.1002/hon.2986. Epub ahead of print. PMID: 35313381.

Fanale, M.A., Cheah, C.Y., Rich, A., Medeiros, L.J., Lai, C.M., Oki, Y. et al. (2017 July 27). Encouraging activity for R-CHOP in advanced stage nodular lymphocyte-predominant Hodgkin lymphoma. *Blood* 130 (4): 472–477. doi: 10.1182/blood-2017-02-766121. Epub 2017 May 18. PMID: 28522441; PMCID: PMC5578726.

Hartmann, S., Soltani, A.S., Bankov, K. et al. (2022 November). Tumour cell characteristics and microenvironment composition correspond to clinical presentation in newly diagnosed nodular lymphocyte predominant Hodgkin lymphoma. Br J Haematol 199 (3): 382–391. doi: 10.1111/bjh.18376. Epub 2022 Jul 26. PMID: 35880396.

Hartmann, S. and Eichenauer, D.A. (2020 January). Nodular lymphocyte predominant Hodgkin lymphoma: pathology, clinical course and relation to T-cell/histiocyte rich large B-cell lymphoma. *Pathology.* 52(1):142–153. doi: 10.1016/j.pathol.2019.10.003. Epub 2019 Nov 28. PMID: 31785822.

33

Hematopoietic Cell Transplantation and Cellular Therapy in Hodgkin Lymphoma

Narendranath Epperla[1], Alex F. Herrera[2], and Matthew Mei[2]

[1] *Ohio State University, Columbus, OH*
[2] *City of Hope, Duarte, CA,*

Introduction

Autologous hematopoietic cell transplantation (auto-HCT) is the standard treatment for patients with relapsed/refractory classic Hodgkin lymphoma (cHL) and cures most patients with chemosensitive disease. Allogeneic hematopoietic cell transplantation (allo-HCT) is also an option in relapsed/refractory cHL and provides a potentially curative approach, including patients who have progressed after auto-HCT. The non-transplant management of cHL and nodular lymphocyte-predominant Hodgkin lymphoma (NLPHL) are discussed in the preceding chapters (Chapters 31 and 32, respectively). In this chapter we will focus on practical management questions regarding cellular therapies in cHL including auto-HCT and allo-HCT with a focus on novel therapies.

Autologous HCT in cHL

1) Is there an optimal second-line therapy?

Expert Perspective: With the introduction of brentuximab vedotin and PD-1 blockade (nivolumab and pembrolizumab), the selection of second-line therapy in cHL has become an increasingly complex decision. Platinum- or gemcitabine-based combination chemotherapy has historically been the mainstay of second-line cHL therapy, and about half of patients will achieve complete remission (CR). No single regimen has been shown to be superior to another, and commonly used combinations include ICE (ifosfamide, carboplatin, etoposide) and GVD (gemcitabine, vinorelbine, liposomal doxorubicin).

Novel agents that are highly effective for the treatment of relapsed/refractory HL have been incorporated into earlier lines of therapy, including the second-line salvage setting.

Cancer Consult: Expertise in Clinical Practice, Volume 2: Neoplastic Hematology & Cellular Therapy,
Second Edition. Edited by Syed A. Abutalib, Maurie Markman, James O. Armitage, and Kenneth C. Anderson.
© 2024 John Wiley & Sons Ltd. Published 2024 by John Wiley & Sons Ltd.

Brentuximab vedotin is an anti-CD30 antibody conjugated to monomethyl auristatin E (MMAE), an antitubulin agent, and is highly effective for the treatment of relapsed/refractory cHL. Sequential and combination brentuximab vedotin–based salvage regimens have been studied (Table 1), and CR rates are in excess of 70% with this approach. Notably, although a minority of patients will achieve CR with brentuximab vedotin alone as initial salvage therapy, these patients have excellent long-term outcomes after auto-HCT, similar to patients who achieve CR after sequential brentuximab vedotin followed by chemotherapy.

In addition to brentuximab vedotin, nivolumab or pembrolizumab have become standard therapy for multiply relapsed/refractory cHL. A study that used combination brentuximab vedotin (1.8 mg/kg) and nivolumab (3 mg/kg) given every three weeks for four cycles (n = 91) demonstrated a CR rate of 67% and a three-year progression-free survival of 77%. Patients with primary refractory disease had only a 61% three-year progression-free survival as opposed to 90% in patients with relapsed disease, and the estimated three-year progression-free survival was 91% among patients who proceeded directly to auto-HCT after brentuximab vedotin and nivolumab. The combination was well tolerated with 18% of patients requiring systemic steroids for immune-related adverse events and no treatment discontinuation due to immune-related adverse events. Infusion-related reactions were common (43%), but most were grade 1–2.

Checkpoint inhibitors have also been tested independent of brentuximab vedotin in the second-line setting. In a study of 38 patients receiving second-line pembrolizumab with gemcitabine, vinorelbine, and liposomal doxorubicin, 95% achieved CR with 36 patients proceeding to auto-HCT, all of whom remain in ongoing remission at a median follow-up of 13.5 months post transplant. In another study with pembrolizumab and ICE, the CR rate

Table 33.1 Brentuximab vedotin–based salvage therapies in cHL.

	Patients	Primary refractory patients	Relapsed patients	CMR (%)	PFS(%)	Reference
BV → augmented ICE	45	25	20	76	82 at 3 yr	Moskowitz
BV → salvage therapy	57	35	22	74	71 at 2 yr	Herrera
BV + ICE						
BV-ICE × 2	16	11	5	69	Not reported	Cassaday
BV-ICE × 2–3	42	12	30	69	69 at 1 yr	Stamatoullas
BV + ESHAP	66	40	26	70	71 at 30 mo	Garcia-Sanz
BV + DHAP	61	23	38	79	76 at 2 yr	Hagenbeek
BV + Gemcitabine	45	29	16	67	Not reached	Cole
BV + Bendamustine	55	28	27	74	62.6 at 2 yr	LaCasce
BV + Nivolumab	91	38	53	67	78 at 2 yr	Herrera, Moskowitz

Abbreviations: BV: brentuximab vedotin; ICE: ifosfamide, carboplatin, etoposide; ESHAP: etoposide, cytarabine, cisplatin, methylprednisolone; DHAP: dexamethasone, cytarabine, cisplatin; N ±ICE: nivolumablumab with or without ICE; yrs: years; mo: months; CMR: complete metabolic response by PET.

was 86.5% following two cycles with 35 of the 37 evaluable patients proceeding to auto-HCT with a median progression-free survival of 26.9 months at a median follow-up of 27 months. No difference in outcomes was observed in patients with primary refractory or early relapsed disease vs patients with later relapse. Finally, patients who received sequential nivolumab followed either by auto-HCT (if CR) or nivolumab with ICE (other patients) found that the CR rate for nivolumab alone was 70% and nivolumab plus ICE was 86% suggesting that nivolumab monotherapy may be sufficient for many patients in the 2L setting.

Ultimately the choice of second-line therapy remains unanswered, and further studies are planned to clarify this issue further. In the meantime, decision-making should be driven by patient characteristics (for instance, brentuximab vedotin–based salvage is a poor choice in patients who were refractory to front-line brentuximab vedotin) and physician comfort level.

2) Is chemosensitivity required for successful auto-HCT?

Expert Perspective: It has long been taken as dogma that chemosensitivity is required for successful auto-HCT in lymphoma. This notion has been upended in recent years in cHL given that brentuximab vedotin monotherapy, brentuximab vedotin and nivolumab, and PD-1 blockade alone are all able to bridge patients successfully to auto-HCT without concurrent cytotoxic chemotherapy. The use of anti-PD1 monotherapy as a bridge to auto-HCT especially challenges the traditional paradigm of chemosensitivity being necessary for successful auto-HCT since brentuximab vedotin is a drug that provided targeted delivery of chemotherapy. For instance, second-line brentuximab vedotin monotherapy allows over a third of patients to proceed to auto-HCT without further chemotherapy, and probably about two-thirds of patients are likely cured with second-line brentuximab vedotin and nivolumab followed by auto-HCT. More provocatively, there has been evidence demonstrating a striking synergy between PD-1 blockade and auto-HCT: Herrera et al. found that most patients could proceed to auto-HCT after second-line nivolumab alone, and a large multicenter analysis found that auto-HCT performed in chemo-refractory patients who received subsequent PD-1 blockade was associated with an 81% two-year progression-free survival (78% in patients that were refractory to two consecutive therapies prior to PD-1 blockade). Hence, it may be more important to have treatment-sensitive disease than chemosensitive disease, although a longer follow-up will be needed to confirm these preliminary results.

3) Who should receive consolidation therapy post auto-HCT?

Expert Perspective: The AETHERA study, a phase III double-blind randomized study that evaluated brentuximab vedotin as consolidation therapy following auto-HCT in patients with high-risk features, demonstrated significant improvement in progression-free survival in those receiving maintenance brentuximab vedotin (median progression-free survival of 42.9 months) compared to those who received placebo (median progression-free survival of 24.1 months) with sustained progression-free survival benefit on long-term follow-up data (five-year progression-free survival 59% vs 41%, respectively). The high-risk features in the study included primary refractory disease, relapse within 12 months of initial therapy, or extranodal involvement at relapse. Of note, patients with ≥ 2 adverse risk factors (primary refractory disease or relapse within 12 months of initial therapy, extranodal involvement at relapse, B-symptoms at relapse, less than a CR at auto-HCT, or requiring two or more salvage therapies before auto-HCT) seemed to derive the most benefit from post-auto-HCT brentuximab vedotin consolidation. Brentuximab vedotin consolidation is not recommended in patients who have demonstrated brentuximab vedotin resistance (e.g. best response stable disease or progressive disease < 3 months after brentuximab vedotin) before auto-HCT. Brentuximab vedotin BV consolidation could be considered in high-risk patients who remain brentuximab vedotin–sensitive after a short course of brentuximab vedotin before auto-HCT (e.g. CR to brentuximab vedotin–based salvage), especially as recent data from the AMAHRELIS study suggest that such patients may still potentially benefit from brentuximab vedotin consolidation.

PD-1 blockade is also being evaluated as post-auto-HCT consolidation/maintenance therapy to improve rates of durable remission. In a phase II study, pembrolizumab was administered (200 mg IV every three weeks for up to eight cycles) as consolidation therapy to relapsed/refractory cHL patients following auto-HCT. In the 28 evaluable patients, the progression-free survival was 82% at 18 months. Similarly, nivolumab consolidation following auto-HCT in patients with relapsed/refractory cHL is currently ongoing (NCT03436862). Another study that evaluated the combination of nivolumab with brentuximab vedotin (1.8 mg/kg of brentuximab vedotin and 3 mg/kg nivolumab every 21 days for eight cycles) as post-auto-HCT consolidation therapy showed durable remission (estimated 18-month progression-free survival was 95%). Of note, the study not only included high-risk relapsed/refractory cHL patients but also patients with prior treatment with brentuximab vedotin and/or anti PD-1 antibodies. However, given the lack of randomized data, consolidation therapy with PD-1 blockade is not recommended outside of a clinical trial setting.

4) What is the value of peri-transplant radiation therapy?

Expert Perspective: High-energy radiation therapy was the first curative therapy for cHL and continues to be a part of many successful treatment strategies. Occasional patients with late localized relapse can be cured with involved-field radiation therapy and can avoid auto-HCT. But what about the patient who presents with extensive recurrent disease and is to undergo auto-HCT? Does the patient benefit from additional radiation treatment to the involved region? This is one of the most enduring unresolved questions in this area.

Most studies of involved-field radiation therapy as a component of auto-HCT in cHL have been retrospective, small studies, and the results are controversial. Most studies show an improvement in local disease control, but none have convincingly demonstrated a benefit in overall long-term survival. In a study from the University of Rochester (n = 62), among the patients who underwent auto-HCT for relapsed/refractory cHL, although the rate of loco-regional and distant relapses was strikingly different between those who received post-auto-HCT involved-field radiation therapy (n = 32) versus those who did not (n = 30), the multivariate analysis failed to show an advantage for those receiving involved-field radiation therapy. In a more recent study from MD Anderson Cancer Center (n = 189), peri-transplant radiation therapy (n = 22) was associated with improved local control of the high-risk localized disease.

In patients with disseminated relapses or with multifocal progression, radiation therapy may be useful to select sites where local disease control has been a dominant clinical problem. More specifically, patients who might benefit from radiation therapy include those who have persistent FDG-avid disease after conventional-dose salvage chemotherapy or after auto-HCT and/or have a primary refractory disease with a distribution that allows for radiation therapy administration with acceptable risks of morbidity. In addition, radiation therapy is appropriate to address involvement at sites where local control is especially critical, such as disease compressing the spinal cord or nerve roots, obstructing the superior vena cava, airways, ureters, or lymphatics with problematic lymphedema. Of note, the timing of peri-transplant radiation therapy for relapsed/refractory cHL is not clearly defined and is dependent on several factors including the response to salvage therapy and sites of involvement. In addition, one needs to weigh the pros and cons of pre- versus post-auto-HCT involved-field radiation therapy which is determined on a case-by-case basis.

Allogeneic HCT in cHL

There has been a growing body of literature establishing the role of allogeneic hematopoietic cell transplantation (allo-HCT) as curative therapy in relapsed/refractory cHL, particularly for those who relapse after a prior auto-HCT. In the past decade, the advent of novel agents (brentuximab vedotin and checkpoint inhibitor) has revolutionized the therapeutic landscape and reinvigorated the discussion on the relevance and timing of allo-HCT. In this section, we will address some questions regarding allo-HCT in the era of novel agents.

5) What is the best conditioning regimen?

Expert Perspective: One of the important factors that determine the long-term outcomes following allo-HCT in relapsed/refractory cHL is the type of conditioning regimen / conditioning intensity. Several high-quality retrospective studies demonstrated a lack of superiority of myeloablative conditioning over reduced-intensity conditioning leading to increased utilization of reduced-intensity conditioning regimens over the past decade. A recent CIBMTR analysis examined three different reduced-intensity conditioning regimens: fludarabine/intravenous busulfan, fludarabine/melphalan, and fludarabine/cyclophosphamide. A total of 492 adult patients with cHL, who underwent a first allo-HCT using either a matched sibling or matched unrelated donor between 2008 and 2016, were included in the study. There was no significant difference in four-year overall survival, progression-free survival, nonrelapse mortality, and GvHD between the three regimens; however, fludarabine and cyclophosphamide had worse long-term overall survival driven by increased late non-relapse mortality. Nonetheless, the applicability of this study to present-day practice is limited by the exclusion of post-transplant cyclophosphamide-based graft versus host disease (GvHD) prophylaxis, which appears to be important in patients who have been exposed to prior PD-1 blockade.

6) What is the optimal graft?

Expert Perspective: Multiple single-arm studies have shown promising results for haploidentical transplants in relapsed/refractory cHL with chronic GvHD rates far lower than historical controls as well as lower relapse rates. These data have spurred interest in optimal donor selection in cHL given the widespread availability of haploidentical donors compared to matched unrelated donors. The EBMT group evaluated the outcomes of patients undergoing haplo-HCT that used post-transplant cyclophosphamide-based GvHD prophylaxis (n = 98) with those of matched sibling donor (n = 338) and matched unrelated donor (n = 273). In the study, haploidentical transplant with post-transplant cyclophosphamide prophylaxis was associated with a lower risk of chronic GvHD (26%) compared with matched unrelated donors (41%; $P = 0.04$). On multivariable analysis, relative to matched sibling donor, non-relapse mortality was similar in haploidentical transplant ($P = 0.26$) and higher in matched unrelated donor ($P = 0.003$), and the risk of relapse was lower in both haploidentical transplant ($P = 0.047$) and matched unrelated donor ($P < 0.001$). Two-year overall survival for HLA-haploidentical, matched sibling donor, and matched unrelated donor were 67%, 71%, and 62%, respectively, while two-year progression-free survival were 43%, 38%, and 45%, respectively. There were no significant differences in overall survival or progression-free survival between haploidentical, matched sibling donor, and matched unrelated donor. Similarly, in a study by CIBMTR that compared haploidentical with post-transplant cyclophosphamide strategy and matched sibling donor, haploidentical donor transplants were associated with both lower incidences of chronic GvHD and relapse, with progression-free survival and overall survival outcomes comparable with matched sibling donor. Umbilical cord blood transplantation has also been shown to be inferior to haplo-HCT and is not recommended.

At present, there are insufficient data to specifically recommend haplo-HCT over conventional donors (i.e. matched sibling donor, matched unrelated donor). Although the preliminary data have pointed to strong outcomes with haploidentical transplants, more recent data have suggested that these may be due to the universal use of post-transplant cyclophosphamide-based GvHD prophylaxis as opposed to matched sibling donor / matched unrelated donor transplantation where calcineurin inhibitor–based prophylaxis had long been the norm. Nonetheless, we consider haploidentical transplants to be a viable and non-inferior mode of allo-HCT compared to a conventional donor allo-HCT.

7) Who should be considered for allo-HCT in cHL?

Expert Perspective: The overall response rate and CR rates to checkpoint inhibitor in relapsed/refractory cHL are around 70% and 20–30%, respectively. In patients who achieve CR, checkpoint inhibitor is continued until progression, with consideration of discontinuation after six months (at the earliest) and usually after two years; most patients who have responded before will respond to retreatment as well at the time of disease progression. Although the overall response rate to brentuximab vedotin or checkpoint inhibitor monotherapy is high, the CR rate and ultimate curative potential with either type of agent is relatively low. Although allo-HCT is typically delayed until patients have progressed after both brentuximab vedotin and checkpoint inhibitor, both brentuximab vedotin and PD-1 blockade have been studied as a bridge to allo-HCT with favorable outcomes. For instance, in the case of the occasional patient who only received treatment with prior chemotherapy and auto-HCT and achieved a CR with brentuximab vedotin for post-auto-HCT relapse, we would not typically proceed to allo-HCT directly given the lack of prior PD-1 blockade, which can maintain disease control for several years.

An increasingly common scenario in modern hematology practice is the patient with relapsed/refractory cHL who has been through auto-HCT and prior brentuximab vedotin who is now responding well to checkpoint inhibitor—what should the timing of allo-HCT be for such a patient? The concern in such a case is that early allo-HCT (i.e. directly while in CR) may not be needed given the usual long remission duration, whereas waiting until the disease relapses or becomes refractory may result in missing a window to optimize allo-HCT outcomes.

While there is no absolute answer to this question, there are a couple of considerations that can help with decision-making in this difficult scenario. There are ample data to suggest that the duration of response to checkpoint inhibitor is long, especially in the case of CR, and the response rate to retreatment (in the case of prior treatment interruption) is also very high. As such, a common practice is to not proceed directly to allo-HCT for patients in first response while on checkpoint inhibitor. Moreover, checkpoint inhibitors tend to sensitize patients to cytotoxic chemotherapy, so typically there is some provision to bridge to allo-HCT with either combination checkpoint inhibitor plus GVD or even brentuximab vedotin plus chemo-therapy. Nonetheless, proceeding to allo-HCT earlier is also reasonable and ultimate deci-sion-making should take patient preference and physician experience level into account as well. If allo-HCT is done directly after checkpoint inhibitor therapy, an interval of > 80 days from checkpoint inhibitor to allo-HCT was associated with lower rates of grades 2–4 and 3–4 acute GvHD in a large retrospective analysis. We typically wait until after the patients have failed both brentuximab vedotin and checkpoint inhibitor before considering allo-HCT.

8) Is there an optimal GvHD prophylaxis regimen?

Expert Perspective: This question has become relevant ever since the first reports of relapsed/refractory cHL patients undergoing allo-HCT after prior checkpoint inhibitor demonstrated lower than expected rates of relapse but with a few cases of unusually severe cases of fatal acute GvHD. A consensus statement in 2018 had suggested the use of GvHD prophylaxis utilizing post-transplant cyclophosphamide as opposed to standard calcineurin inhibitor–based regimens as well as consideration of the use of bone marrow as opposed to peripheral blood grafts. A larger retrospective cohort was published in 2021 with the finding that the two-year composite endpoint of GvHD-free, relapse-free survival strongly favored post-transplant cyclophosphamide prophylaxis with no real difference in outcomes for haploidentical vs non-haploidentical donors. Therefore, we strongly recommend post-transplant cyclophosphamide-based GvHD prophylaxis for all patients with cHL and consider this imperative for patients with recent exposure to checkpoint inhibitor (see Chapters 60 and 61).

Recommended Readings

Advani, R., Moskowitz, A.J., Bartlett, N.L. et al. (2021). Brentuximab vedotin in combination with nivolumablumab in relapsed or refractory Hodgkin lymphoma: 3-year study results. *Blood, The Journal of the American Society of Hematology,* 138 (6): 427–438.

Armand, P., Chen, Y.B., Redd, R.A. et al. (2019). PD-1 blockade with pembrolizumab for classical Hodgkin lymphoma after autologous stem cell transplantation. *Blood* 134 (1): 22–29.

Bolaños-Meade J, Hamadani M, Wu J, et al. (2023 Jun 22) BMT CTN 1703 Investigators. Post-Transplantation Cyclophosphamide-Based Graft-versus-Host Disease Prophylaxis. *N Engl J Med* 388 (25): 2338–2348. doi: 10.1056/NEJMoa2215943. PMID: 37342922.

Constine, L.S., Yahalom, J., Ng, A.K., Hodgson, D.C., Wirth, A., Milgrom, S.A. et al. (2018). The role of radiation therapy in patients with relapsed or refractory Hodgkin lymphoma: guidelines from the international lymphoma radiation oncology group. *Int J Radiat Oncol Biol Phys* 100 (5): 1100–1118.

Merryman, R.W., Castagna, L., Giordano, L. et al. (2021 September). Allogeneic transplantation after PD-1 blockade for classic Hodgkin lymphoma. *Leukemia* 35 (9): 2672–2683. doi: 10.1038/s41375-021-01193-6. Epub 2021 Mar 3. PMID: 33658659.

Moskowitz, C.H., Nademanee, A., Masszi, T. et al. (2015). Brentuximab vedotin as consolidation therapy after autologous stem-cell transplantation in patients with Hodgkin's lymphoma at risk of relapse or progression (AETHERA): A randomized, double-blind, placebo-controlled, phase 3 trial. *Lancet* 385 (9980): 1853–1862.

Part 7

Non-Hodgkin's Lymphomas

34

Pitfalls in the Diagnosis of Non-Hodgkin's Lymphomas

Carmen Barcena[1] and Laurence de Leval[2]

[1] Hospital Universitario 12 de Octubre, Department of Pathology, Madrid, Spain
[2] Lausanne University Hospital and Lausanne University, Switzerland

Introduction

The proper management of patients with a lymphoma relies on an accurate and precise pathologic diagnosis, since the biology of the tumors, natural history of the diseases, and ultimately optimal treatment of the patients markedly vary according to the many types of lymphoma histotypes. After an era of confusion with multiple competing classification systems, lymphoma diagnosis has become more standardized since the introduction of the principles of the REAL (Revised European American Lymphoma Classification), adopted by the WHO classification since 2001 (Swerdlow et al. 2017). The approach to a diagnosis relies on a first step of careful morphological assessment, followed by additional ancillary studies. Immunophenotyping (immunohistochemistry and/or flow cytometry) is mandatory in essentially all cases, while clonality testing, fluorescent in situ hybridization (FISH) assays, mutation analyses, and other molecular tests are applied in selected cases. Besides diagnostic utility, several biomarkers may be assessed for their theranostic or prognostic significance. Of utmost importance is that the adequate clinical information is provided to the pathologist because clinical features also represent an important component and criterion of disease definition. Accordingly, infection status (HIV, HTLV1, hepatitis viruses), previous history of lymphoma, immune context (immunosuppression, autoimmune diseases), and disease localization and extension are important factors to take into account in the diagnostic process.

Here, we are providing a few clinical histories and examples of more or less common diagnoses to discuss their differential diagnoses, highlight some of the difficulties that might be encountered, and emphasize the clinical importance of a correct diagnosis.

Cancer Consult: Expertise in Clinical Practice, Volume 2: Neoplastic Hematology & Cellular Therapy,
Second Edition. Edited by Syed A. Abutalib, Maurie Markman, James O. Armitage, and Kenneth C. Anderson.
© 2024 John Wiley & Sons Ltd. Published 2024 by John Wiley & Sons Ltd.

Case Study 1

A 57-year-old woman presented with acute onset of abdominal pain and a 15 cm retroperitoneal mass. A needle biopsy (Figure 34.1) showed a dense diffuse proliferation of pleomorphic medium to large lymphoid cells with irregular nuclei and sometimes prominent nucleoli. Mitotic figures and apoptotic bodies were frequent, focally imparting a "starry sky" appearance. The cells expressed CD20, PAX5, CD10, BCL2, BCL6, c-MYC, and MUM1, with a Ki-67 labeling index up to 80%, and they were negative for cyclin D1 and CD138. Fluorescence in situ hybridization (FISH) analysis using break-apart (BA) probes revealed many split (green or red) signals indicative of *MYC* and *BCL2* gene rearrangements.

What is the diagnosis?

A) Burkitt lymphoma (BL).
B) Diffuse large B-cell lymphoma, not otherwise specified (DLBCL-NOS).
C) High-grade B-cell lymphoma with *MYC* and *BCL2* rearrangements.
D) Mantle cell lymphoma, blastoid.

Expert Perspective: High-grade B-cell lymphoma with *MYC* and *BCL2* rearrangements.

Double-hit lymphomas harboring rearrangements of *MYC* (8q24) and *BCL2* (18q21) or *MYC* and *BCL6* (3q27) and triple-hit lymphomas (harboring rearrangements of *MYC*, *BCL2*, and *BCL6*) constitute a subset of aggressive high-grade B-cell lymphomas that are defined by their genetic features. Morphologically, they may resemble DLBCL, show intermediate features between DLBCL and Burkitt lymphoma (high proliferation fraction and a starry sky appearance with cells larger or more pleomorphic than the spectrum of classical Burkitt lymphoma), or feature blastoid cytology. Intermediate or blastoid

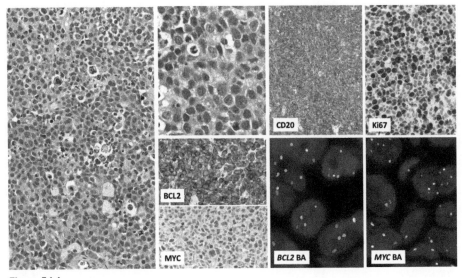

Figure 34.1

morphology imparts an even worse prognosis. Double- or triple-hit high-grade B-cell lymphomas represent about 8% of lymphomas with diffuse large B-cell morphology, and *MYC* plus *BCL2* double hits account for about 60% of these cases. The majority of HGBCL with *MYC* and *BCL2* rearrangements have a germinal center B-cell phenotype with expression of CD10 and BCL6 and are strongly positive for *BCL2*—in contrast to Burkitt lymphoma. They may occur *de novo* or result from transformation of follicular lymphoma. HGBCL with large cell morphology and rearrangements of *MYC* and *BCL2* or *BCL6* have worse outcomes than DLBCL-NOS when treated with standard DLBCL therapies, and the negative prognostic impact is largely observed in patients with *MYC* double-hit / triple-hit disease in which *MYC* is translocated to an IG partner (see Chapter 42) (Scott et al. 2018; Rosenwald et al. 2019).

Burkitt lymphoma

BL comprises endemic, sporadic, and immunodeficiency-associated clinical variants, more commonly seen in children and young adults. BL is a B-cell lymphoma with typical morphology (monomorphic, medium-sized cells with round nuclei, multiple nucleoli, and basophilic cytoplasm containing small lipid vacuoles) and immunophenotypic features (CD10 +, BCL6 +, MYC +, with a Ki-67 proliferation index close to 100%). BCL2 expression is negative or weakly positive. Cytogenetically, nearly all cases harbor a translocation involving the MYC gene at the 8q24 locus, most commonly with the immunoglobulin heavy chain (IGH) on chromosome 14q32. The association with EBV is variable: > 95% of endemic BL, 20–30% of sporadic BL, and 25–40% of immunodeficiency-related cases. Accurate diagnosis and distinction from other aggressive B-cell lymphomas are crucial for proper clinical management, as BL requires more intensive chemotherapy (see Chapter 44).

Diffuse large B-cell lymphoma, not otherwise specified

DLBCL is a diffuse proliferation of large lymphoid cells (centroblastic, immunoblastic, and/or anaplastic) morphologically distinct from BL. The neoplastic cells express B-cell markers, being variably positive for BCL2, CD10, GCET1, LOM2, BCL6, MUM1, FOXP1, c-MYC, and may co-express CD5 and/or CD30. Two molecular subgroups defined by gene expression signatures resembling that of germinal center or activated B cell are delineated, and immunohistochemical algorithms have been developed as surrogates to identify them routinely. DLBCL expressing BCL2 (with a cut-off defined at > 50% tumor cells positive) and MYC (cut-off 40% positive nuclei), so-called "double expressors," have a relatively worse outcome. P53 overexpression can also be found and is associated with a poor prognosis.

The most common genomic alterations consist of rearrangements of *BCL6* or *BCL2*. *MYC* rearrangement, found in 7–14% of *de novo* DLBCLs, has been found to predict a more aggressive behavior (see Chapter 39).

Mantle cell lymphoma, blastoid variant

The blastoid variant of mantle cell lymphoma (bMCL) enters in the differential diagnosis of high-grade B-cell neoplasms. It is both immunophenotypically and genetically similar to classic MCL (cMCL) and is composed of monotonous medium-sized lymphocytes with finely dispersed chromatin and absent or indistinct nucleoli, resembling lymphoblasts. Numerous mitoses and a starry sky pattern may be seen. The immunophenotype is similar to that of cMCL (CD20 +, CD79a +, PAX5 +), usually coexpressing CD5, SOX11, CD43, and negative for CD10, BCL6, and CD23. Most cases show overexpression of cyclin D1. However, aberrant phenotypes and genetics in bMCL exist, including expression of BCL6 and CD10 or overexpression of P53. In addition, CD5 and/or cyclin D1 may be absent, and coexistence of *CCND1* and *MYC* rearrangements has been reported (see Chapter 36).

Correct Answer: C

Case Study 2

A 36-year-old female presented with shortness of breath. Imaging studies revealed a bulky anterior mediastinal mass. The biopsy (Figure 34.2) showed a diffuse infiltrate of large cells with round, oval or lobulated nuclei (long arrows) with abundant clear cytoplasm in a background of compartmentalizing sclerosis. Occasional Hodgkin/ Reed-Sternberg (HRS)–like cells were seen (short arrows). The tumor cells were intense and diffusely positive for B-cell markers (CD20, PAX5, OCT2, BOB1), coexpressed MUM1, BCL6, CD30 (weakly), and CD23. CD10 and CD15 were negative. The Ki-67 index was around 40%. In situ hybridization (ISH) with EBER (Epstein-Barr early RNA) probes produced no signal. By staging, the disease was confined to the mediastinum (stage I).

What is the diagnosis?
A) Nodular sclerosis classical Hodgkin lymphoma.
B) Diffuse large B-cell lymphoma, not otherwise specified.

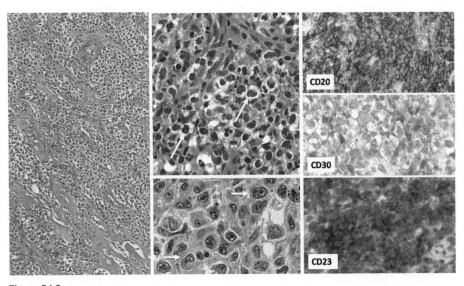

Figure 34.2

C) Primary mediastinal (thymic) large B-cell lymphoma.

D) B-cell lymphoma, unclassifiable, with features intermediate between diffuse large B-cell lymphoma and classical Hodgkin lymphoma.

Expert Perspective: Primary mediastinal (thymic) large B-cell lymphoma.

Clinical, morphological, and immunohistochemical features are consistent with primary mediastinal large B-cell lymphoma (PMBL), a distinct DLBCL entity arising in the mediastinum, thought to be derived from thymic B cells. PMBL tends to occur in young patients (median age 35 years old), affecting women more commonly than men.

Patients often present with a bulky anterior mediastinal mass and symptoms related to impingement of local anatomic structures. The disease is usually localized at diagnosis, but may progress by disseminating to other extranodal sites, including lung, liver, kidneys, adrenals, ovaries, brain, and gastrointestinal tract.

Histologically, PMBL is a diffuse proliferation of medium to large cells. Particular, although not entirely specific, morphologic features include a background of fine compartmentalizing alveolar fibrosis. The atypical cells express B-cell antigens but often lack surface immunoglobulin (Ig), despite expression of the IG-associated transcription factors PAX5, BOB.1, OCT2, and PU.1. They are usually positive for BCL6, MUM1/IRF4, and CD30. A variable proportion of cases expresses BCL2, CD23, p63, MAL, PDL1, and PDL2. By gene expression profiling (GEP), PMBL has a molecular signature distinct from that of both germinal center-like (GCB) and activated (ABC) DLBCL and partly overlapping with that of classic Hodgkin lymphoma, characterized by low levels of expression of multiple B-cell signaling components and co-receptors and high expression of cytokine pathway components, tumor necrosis factor (TNF) family members, and extracellular matrix elements. Altered JAK-STAT signaling, manifested by constitutive activation of STAT5 and STAT6, represents another alteration shared by PMBL and cHL.

The most frequent genetic abnormalities are gains and amplifications at chromosome 9p24, including the *JAK2/PDL1/PDL2* locus in up to 75% of cases and gains of *REL* on chromosome 2p (50% cases). Moreover, CIITA translocations of MHC class II transactivator CIITA, resulting in downregulation of MHC class II molecules, are highly recurrent (about 40% of cases) in PMBL (Mottok et al. 2018) (see Chapter 41).

PBML versus classic Hodgkin lymphoma versus B-cell lymphoma, unclassifiable, with features intermediate between diffuse large B-cell lymphoma and classic Hodgkin lymphoma

PBML and classic Hodgkin lymphoma (cHL), especially nodular sclerosis type (NSHL), have overlapping features. Both frequently present in young patients as mediastinal neoplasms with prominent sclerosis, Reed-Sternberg, or Reed-Sternberg–like cells. Making a correct diagnosis is important due to differences in management and prognosis. In PMBL, large cells are often positive for CD30 but more weakly and heterogenous than in cHL. CD20 and PAX5 are strongly expressed in PMBL while Reed-Sternberg cells are generally CD20-negative and weakly positive for PAX5. *In situ* hybridization for EBV, when positive, strongly favors the diagnosis of cHL. Both PMBL and cHL have a constitutively activated JAK/STAT signaling pathway. There remain cases of B-cell mediastinal lymphomas that have features intermediate between those of PMBL and cHL that cannot be classified despite thorough phenotyping and molecular studies. It is important to recognize these cases designed as "B-cell lymphoma unclassifiable with features intermediate between PMBL and cHL" as they carry a more aggressive clinical course and a worse prognosis than both cHL and PMBL. Cases categorized as such include those morphologically resembling NSHL but immunohistochemically consistent with PMBL (strong and diffuse expression of CD20 and other B-cell antigens) and those morphologically suggestive of PMBL with strong expression of CD15.

PBML versus DLBCL-NOS, involving the mediastinum

This distinction cannot be made based on histopathological grounds only. Although PMBL features distinct morphological and immunohistochemical characteristics, none is entirely specific, and clinical correlation is mandatory. Staging procedures must rule out secondary mediastinal involvement by a systemic DLBCL; extrathoracic lymph node or bone marrow involvement would favor the latter diagnosis. Rearrangements of *MYC*, *BCL2*, and *BCL6* are rare in PMBL. The gene expression signature of PMBL differs from that of DLBCL, and mutations involving the STAT6 DNA-binding domain or *PTPN1*, which may be found in PBML, are mostly absent in DLBCL-NOS.

Correct Answer: D

Case Study 3

A 62-year-old female without prior history presented with abdominal lymph nodes. No B-symptoms. An excisional biopsy (Figure 34.3) showed diffuse polymorphous lymphoid infiltrate comprising many large, atypical lymphoid cells, including occasional Reed-Sternberg–like cells, admixed with histiocytes, small lymphocytes, and occasional eosino-phils. They were positive for CD20, PAX5, OCT-2, BOB-1, BCL6, MUM1, and CD30 and were admixed with numerous small T (CD3 +, CD5 +) cells. CD15 was negative. The large cells were positive for EBER by *in situ* hybridization.

What is the diagnosis?
A) EBV+, diffuse large B-cell lymphoma, not otherwise specified.
B) Classic Hodgkin lymphoma.
C) Angioimmunoblastic T cell lymphoma.
D) T-cell/histiocyte-rich large B-cell lymphoma.

Expert Perspective: EBV+ DLBCL-NOS.

EBV+ DLBCL-NOS, is an aggressive B-cell lymphoma that tends to occur in elderly individuals and is thought to be associated with immunosenescence, but similar cases also occur in younger people. Histologically, this entity encompasses polymorphic and monomorphic variants. The polymorphic cases consist of a spectrum of lymphoid cells of variable size, including centroblasts, immunoblasts, HRS-like cells, lymphoplasmocytoid cells admixed with a reactive background of small lymphocytes, plasma cells, and histiocytes. The monomorphic cases are morphologically alike EBV-negative DLBCL. Geographic necrosis is frequent in both subtypes of EBV+ DLBCLs. Immunohistochemically, the neoplastic cells

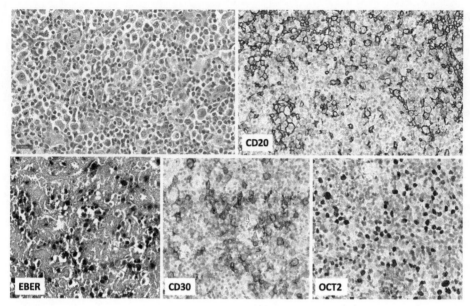

Figure 34.3

usually express B-cell markers (CD19, CD20, PAX5), but we may find CD20– cases, which hinders the diagnosis. In addition, they harbor a non-germinal center-like (non-GC) immunophenotype, being positive for MUM1 and negative for CD10. Expression of NF-kB and pSTAT3 are often seen in EBV+ cases and not in EBV– DLBCL. In contrast to EBV– DLBCLs, EBV+ DLBCLs show activation of JAK/STAT and NFkB pathways, and mutations present in EBV-DLBCL of activated (ABC) type, such as MYD88, CD79B, and CARD11 are absent in EBV+ cases (Beltran et al. 2020).

EBV+, DLBCL-NOS versus EBV+ classic Hodgkin lymphoma (cHL)

Polymorphic EBV+ DLBCL resembles especially the mixed cellularity cHL because both have HRS-like cells or HRS cells in a similar reactive background. Immunohistochemically, both HRS-like cells and HRS may be CD20+ CD30+, instead CD15 is usually negative in EBV+ DLBCL. Besides, in EBV+ DLBCL lesions EBERish highlights HRS-like cells as well as bystander cells of variable sizes whereas EBERish only stains HRS cells in cHL. Furthermore, IGH rearrangements are frequent in EBV+ DLBCL, but not in cHL.

EBV+, DLBCL versus angioimmunoblastic T-cell lymphoma (AITL)

The polymorphic subtype of EBV+ DLBCL and AITL share morphologic features. Both usually exhibit a heterogenous cellularity admixed with EBV+ large cells. Nevertheless, AITL have atypical T cells and numerous eosinophils in contrast to EBV+ DLBCL. TFH (PD1, BCL6, CD10, ICOS, CXCL13) markers expression by the lymphomatous cells together with TR gene rearrangements support the diagnosis of AITL.

EBV+, DLBCL versus T-cell/histiocyte-rich large B-cell lymphoma (THRLBCL)

The polymorphic subtype of EBV+ DLBCL can mimic THRLBCL. In contrast to EBV+ DLB-CLs, THRLBCL is in principle negative for EBV, its background is less heterogenous, being essentially composed of small lymphocytes and histiocytes without eosinophils or plasma cells (see Chapters 39 and 46).

Correct Answer: A

Case Study 4

A 16-year-old boy underwent excision of a persistent 2 cm submandibular adenopathy. Histologically (Figure 34.4), the architecture was partially effaced by numerous large, expansile, coalescent follicles comprising medium-sized centroblasts surrounded by a preserved or focally attenuated mantle zone. The follicular centers showed numerous mitoses, macrophages with apoptotic debris, and a starry sky pattern. CD20 and PAX5 stained the follicles and an interfollicular component of B cells. CD3, CD5, and CD43 only stained small T cells in the background. Follicular B cells were strongly positive for CD10 and BCL6, negative for BCL2, with monotypic IgM + D + kappa expression and a Ki67 proliferation index close to 100%. CD21 stained a follicular dendritic meshwork within the follicles.

What is the diagnosis?
A) Pediatric-type follicular lymphoma.
B) Marginal zone lymphoma.
C) Follicular lymphoma.
D) Reactive follicular hyperplasia.
E) Large B-cell lymphoma with IRF4 rearrangement.

Expert Perspective: Pediatric-type follicular lymphoma.

Pediatric-type follicular lymphoma (PTFL) is a variant of follicular lymphoma (FL) that occurs in children and young adults and rarely in older patients. Typically presents as a clonal follicular proliferation, resulting in a localized adenopathy in the head and neck region. The features that are distinct from those of conventional FL are large expansile or coalescent follicles composed of medium-sized blastoid cells with inconspicuous nucleolus, high Ki67 proliferation index, and lack of BCL2 expression and IGH-BCL2 rearrangement. Similar to FL, PTFL usually expresses BCL6 and CD10 and is negative for IRF4/MUM1. PTFLs are also clinically distinct from FL in that they remain localized and are curable, even after excision alone in some cases. PTFL has a very low genomic complexity and has a unique mutational profile, including *TNFRSF14* and *MAP2K1* mutations.

Pediatric-type follicular lymphoma versus follicular lymphoma

The distinction between both entities is important because follicular lymphoma (FL) is considered an indolent but incurable disease, usually associated with recurrence after systemic chemotherapy. In contrast, although PTFLs are usually grade 3, they usually remain localized and curable. BCL2 immunostaining is often helpful in the differential diagnosis of PTFL and FL, since the neoplastic follicles are typically BCL2-negative in PTFL and usually

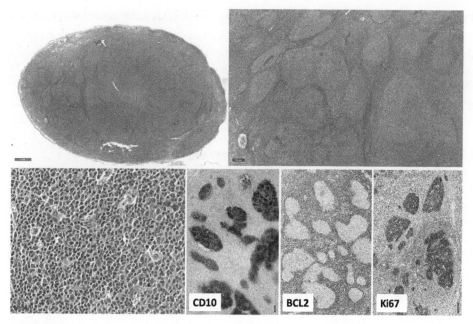

Figure 34.4

BCL2-positive in FL. However, a subset of classical FL, especially grade 3B, lack BCL2 expression and BCL2 gene rearrangement. *TNFRSF14* mutations are common in both PTFL and FL. Nevertheless, mutations of histone-modifying genes (*EZH2, KMT2D, CREBBP*) involved in the pathogenesis of FL are rarely observed in PTFL (Schmidt et al. 2016).

Pediatric-type follicular lymphoma versus reactive follicular hyperplasia

More problematic is the differential diagnosis between PTFL and reactive follicular hyperplasia (RFH) as both are more common in children and young adults, and in both entities the follicle centers lack BCL2 expression. Morphologically, in RFH there is no architectural effacement as seen in PTFL; the lymphoid follicles are large and irregularly shaped, often coalescent, but generally restricted to the cortex. The germinal centers are prominent and polarized and the periphery is sharply demarcated by a mantle of small, mature lymphocytes. The cell population is heterogenous and contains macrophages engulfing nuclear debris. Immunophenotyping is helpful in demonstrating polytypic B cells and plasma cells in benign hyperplasia as well as Ki67. Sometimes the distinction between PTFL and florid follicular hyperplasia with monotypic light-chain expression and clonal IGH gene rearrangement by polymerase chain reaction (PCR) can be extremely difficult. The starry sky appearance characteristically seen in nodal PTFL cases further complicates the matter. In these situations, architectural effacement, recognition of a monotonous blastoid cytology without polarization and scant plasma cells is helpful to make the differential diagnosis. PCR for detection of a clonal B-cell population appears to be a very sensitive test in PTFL.

Pediatric follicular lymphoma versus pediatric nodal marginal zone lymphoma (PNMZL)

The distinction between PFL and PNMZL also can be problematic, due to overlapping features, as both are more frequent in young male patients, who present with localized disease with predilection of the head and neck region. However, characteristics seen in PNMZL, such as expanded interfollicular areas by B cells and progressive transformation of germinal centers, are usually absent in PFL. Immunophenotype and genetics in PNMZL are similar to those of its adult nodal counterpart.

PTFL versus large B-cell lymphoma with IRF4 rearrangement

Large B-cell lymphoma (LBCL) with *IRF4* rearrangement is an uncommon subtype of LBCL (provisional entity in the revised 2017 WHO classification). Similarly, to PTFL it also presents as localized adenopathies mainly involving the head and neck region or Waldeyer's ring. LBCL may present with a diffuse or nodular growth pattern, and nodular forms must be distinguished from PTFL. LBCL with *IRF4* rearrangement comprises medium to large cells, lacks a starry sky pattern, and strongly expresses MUM1. *IRF4/MUM1* rearrangement by FISH studies confirms the diagnosis (see Chapter 35).

Correct Answer: A

Case Study 5

A 79-year-old female presented with a right tonsillar mass. The biopsy (Figure 34.5) showed a lymphoepithelial tissue infiltrated by a vaguely nodular and partially diffuse monomorphic lymphoid proliferation composed of medium-sized cells with slightly irregular nuclear contours, fine chromatin, and inconspicuous nucleolus. The tumor cells were strongly positive for CD20, CD5, SOX11, BCL2, CD30, p53, and p57, weakly expressed CD43, and were monotypic for IgM kappa. They were negative for CD10, BCL6, CD23, cyclin D1, and TdT.

What is the diagnosis?
A) Mantle cell lymphoma (MCL) cyclin D1-negative, blastoid variant.
B) TdT-negative lymphoblastic lymphoma.
C) Small lymphocytic lymphoma with large proliferation centers.
D) CD5-positive DLBCL with blastoid morphology, which requires MYC testing.

Expert Perspective: Cyclin D1-negative mantle cell lymphoma.

The general view of MCL is that of a genetically homogenous B-cell lymphoma characterized by CCND1 rearrangement, usually by the t(11;14) translocation, resulting in cyclin D1 overexpression. Nevertheless, cases of "cyclin D1-negative MCL" have been documented. These cases show morphologic and molecular features indistinguishable from cyclin D1-positive MCL, but they lack *CCDN1* rearrangement and cyclin D1 expression and are otherwise similar to *cyclin D1*-positive MCL in their genetic profile. The identification of *CCND2/D3* translocations with immunoglobulin genes (IGK or IGL) in virtually all cyclin D1-negative MCL together with SOX11 expression help to diagnose these lymphomas (Martín-Garcia et al. 2019).

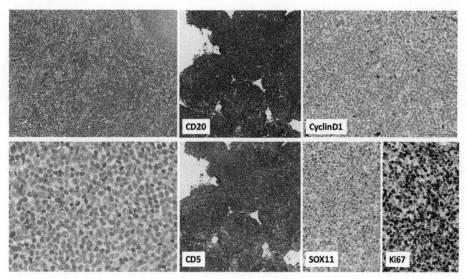

Figure 34.5

The most frequent alternative genetic event in cyclin D1-negative MCL is the occurrence of *CCND2* translocations (55% cases) with consequent cyclin D2 overexpression. The diagnosis of cyclin D1-negative MCL has to be made with caution as many small B-cell lymphomas, such as marginal zone lymphomas, follicular lymphomas, and small lymphocytic lymphomas may coexpress CD5 and/or to some extent may mimic MCL. The transcription factor SOX11 is a specific and highly reliable biomarker of MCL, including for cyclin D1-negative MCL, as it is negative in other types of mature B-cell lymphomas. Clinically, extranodal involvement has been reported more frequently in cyclin D1-negative MCL compared to cyclin D1-positive cases (see Chapter 36).

Correct Answer: A

Case Study 6

A 50-year-old man presented with abdominal pain; clinically there were no peripheral lymphadenopathy, and the spleen was palpable. Thoracoabdominal CT scan disclosed enlarged mesenteric and retroperitoneal lymph nodes, a large lesion in the liver, and several nodules in the spleen. Biopsy of a large mesenteric lymph node was performed (Figure 34.6). The lymph node showed complete architectural effacement by a mostly diffuse lymphoproliferation comprising mainly small lymphocytes and histiocytes admixed with scattered large, atypical cells with irregular contours, multilobated nuclei, pale chromatin, and prominent nucleoli (left panel, circles). Confluent sheets of large, atypical cells were not seen. No significant infiltrate of eosinophils or plasma cells observed. The large, atypical cells were CD20+, BCL6+, IgD−, CD15−, CD30−, and EMA−; the small lymphocytes were mostly (CD3+, CD5+) T cells, including numerous PD1+ cells. EBER was negative. No follicular dendritic cell proliferation was demonstrated by immunohistochemistry in those areas. In one of the sections (lower right panels), the pattern was vaguely nodular as highlighted by the CD20 immunostaining, which also underlined a few admixed small B cells, and CD21+ dendritic cell meshwork was also present in those areas.

What is the diagnosis?
A) Classic Hodgkin lymphoma.
B) T-cell histiocytic rich large B-cell lymphoma.
C) Peripheral T-cell lymphoma.
D) Nodular lymphocytic predominant Hodgkin lymphoma.

Expert Perspective: Nodular lymphocytic predominant Hodgkin lymphoma (NLPHL).

NLPHL is a rare disease and commonly presents with localized lymphadenopathy. The lymph node architecture is altered by a nodular or nodular and/or diffuse proliferation of a few large neoplastic cells called lymphocyte-predominant (LP) cells, or "popcorn" cells, embedded in a background of numerous small lymphocytes, histiocytes, and follicular dendritic cells. LP cells are strongly positive for CD45, CD20, PAX5, OCT2, CD45, BCL6, and sometimes for EMA or IgD. Conversely, they are mostly negative for CD30 and CD15. Six immunoarchitectural patterns with prognostic significance have been described: (i) pattern A is a classic B-cell rich nodular with LP cells within the nodules (the more typical), (ii) pattern B has serpiginous/interconnected nodules, (iii) pattern C has prominent extranodular LP cells, (iv) pattern D is T-cell rich nodular, (v) pattern E diffuse (T-cell/histiocyte-rich large B-cell lymphoma-like), and (vi) pattern F is diffuse moth-eaten, B-cell-rich. Patterns A and B are considered classical patterns, and patterns C–F are considered variant patterns. Variant patterns are observed in about one quarter of the cases, as a major or less commonly minor component of the biopsy. Variant patterns correlate with higher-stage disease at presentation and shorter progression-free survival (but not with reduced overall survival). It is also reported that with subsequent relapses NLPHL tends to progress to more diffuse patterns. Thus, it is recommended that the diagnosis of NLPHL should encompass a description of the disease pattern(s) (Fan et al. 2003).

In this case, the dominant pattern was pattern E, associated to a minor component of pattern D (see Chapter 32).

NLPHL versus classic Hodgkin lymphoma (cHL)

NLPHL must be distinguished from cHL, especially the lymphocyte-rich type. By immunohistochemistry, the neoplastic cells of NLPHL are typically CD45+, CD20+, OCT2+ (strong), and usually negative for CD30 and CD15. Conversely, the Reed-Sternberg cells of cHL are always strongly CD30+, often CD15+, negative for CD45, and when CD20+, they usually express this antigen heterogeneously and express OCT2 moderately to weakly. EMA is often detected in the LP cells and typically negative in cHL. EBV may be detected in HRS cells, while is generally negative in NLPHL (see Chapters 31 and 32).

NLPHL versus T-cell and histiocytic-rich large B-cell lymphoma (THRLBCL)

The distinction between these two entities can be very problematic but is crucial as they have distinct clinical courses. THRLBCL is an aggressive neoplasm, while NLPHL is usually relatively indolent, so they require different therapies.

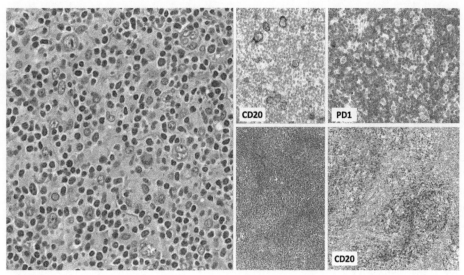

Figure 34.6

In both diseases, the neoplastic cells have large B cells with overlapping morpho-logic, immunophenotypic, and molecular genetic features. The main distinctive fea-tures are (i) the architecture of the lymphoid proliferation and (ii) the nature of the associated background. THRLBCL is diffuse and lacks a follicular dendritic cell mesh-work by CD21 or CD35 staining, whereas NLPHL manifests at least partially a nodular pattern in association with follicular dendritic cells. The difficulty lies in the recog-nition of those rare cases of NLPHL that are diffuse (patterns E and F). Regarding the reactive cellular background, morphology alone is not discriminant as in both entities it comprises mostly small lymphocytes and a variable proportion of histiocytes that may form clusters or microgranulomas. Immunohistochemistry shows a CD8-positive T-cell rich background with few CD57-positive cells and scant small B cells in THRLB-CL, versus an IgD+ B-cell rich background with many CD4+, PD1+, and CD57+ T cells in NLPHL, some of them forming rosettes around LP cells, not seen in THRCL. Important-ly, although the presence of reactive small B cells is a defining feature of NLPHL, the small B-cell population may be obscured by abundant reactive T cells. Regarding the differential between diffuse NLPHL (pattern E) from THRLBL, morphology and immu-nohistochemistry may not be helpful. Therefore, data of biological aggressiveness, such as extensive disease, bone invasion, or elevated LDH may support the diagnosis of THRLBCL.

NLPHL versus peripheral T-cell lymphoma (PTCL), not otherwise specified (NOS)
Unlike NLPHL, PTCL-NOS comprises atypical T cells with frequent loss of T-cell antigens and in the majority of cases shows TR rearrangements (see Chapters 32 and 48).

Correct Answer: D

Case Study 7

A supraclavicular enlarged lymph node was excised in a nine-year-old boy who also had a mediastinal mass.

The lymph node (Figure 34.7) had a thickened fibrotic capsule and disclosed annular sclerosis (upper left panel, trichrome stain). There were sheets of very large, atypical cells showing lobated nuclei, prominent nucleoli, and abundant cytoplasm, with features suggestive of Reed-Sternberg cells. A sinusoidal infiltration by the neoplastic cells was focally seen. By immunohistochemistry, the large cells were strongly and diffusely positive for CD30 with a membrane and paranuclear staining pattern, partially CD15+, faintly PAX-5+, and strongly MUM-1-positive. Several T-cell markers tested stained not only a predominantly T-cell-rich reactive infiltrate but also distinctly highlighted a significant proportion of the neoplastic cells, which were positive for CD3, CD2, CD4, and CD5. ALK was negative, and there was no expression of cytotoxic markers. *In situ* hybridization for *EBV* was negative.

What is the diagnosis?
A) Anaplastic large cell lymphoma, ALK-negative.
B) Peripheral T-cell lymphoma, not otherwise specified.
C) Nodular sclerosis Hodgkin lymphoma.
D) Diffuse large B-cell lymphoma, anaplastic type.

Expert Perspective: Classic Hodgkin lymphoma expressing T-cell markers.

This is an example of classical Hodgkin lymphoma, nodular sclerosis type, expressing T-cell markers. Expression of one or commonly more than one T-cell antigen(s) by the Reed-Sternberg cells is observed in a small proportion of classical Hodgkin lymphoma,

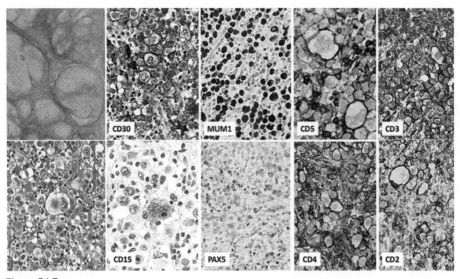

Figure 34.7

more often of the nodular sclerosis type, and more commonly in cases with abundant neoplastic cells (so-called syncitial variant). CD2 and CD4 are the most commonly expressed T-cells antigens, less commonly expressed markers are CD3, CD5, CD7, and CD8. Aberrant T-cell antigen expression in classical Hodgkin lymphoma is associated with decreased event-free survival and overall survival. Because of the usual rosetting of T cells around Reed-Sternberg cells, expression of T-cells antigens at the membrane of the neoplastic cells may be difficult to discern, and an unambiguous positivity in at least 10% of the neoplastic cells must be observed before concluding a T-cell antigen-positive Hodgkin Lymphoma. Two studies have suggested that the expression of T cells or cytotoxic molecules phenotype in classic Hodgkin lymphoma represent a prognostic factor with a predictive of shorter overall and event-free survival.

CD30 positive T-cell lymphomas

Strong and homogeneous expression of CD30 is a constant and basic characteristic of anaplastic large cells lymphomas (either ALK+ or ALK−). In addition, while the characteristic hallmark cells of anaplastic large cells lymphoma are typically large and relatively homogeneous forming cohesive sheets, often with a sinusoidal pattern, there's a subset of ALK+ or ALK− ALCL that has Hodgkin-like features with more pleomorphic, larger, and multilobated nuclei. MUM1 expression is a common characteristic to both ALCL and HRS cells. PAX5 expression, which is typically seen in classic Hodgkin lymphomas, has been reported variably expressed in a subset of ALK− ALCL as well, as a consequence of gene amplification.

At a genomic level, ALCL is a T-cell-derived lymphoma, unlike classical Hodgkin lymphomas, which have a B-cell genotype, even those with expression of T-cell antigens. Expression of CD30, usually more heterogeneous, is also seen in various other mature T-cell lymphoma entities, including peripheral T-cell lymphoma, not otherwise specified (see Chapters 48 and 49).

Diffuse large B-cell lymphoma, anaplastic type

The anaplastic variant of diffuse large B-cell lymphoma, not otherwise specified, is characterized by large to very large cells, with bizarre pleomorphic nuclei that may at least partially resemble Hodgkin Reed-Sternberg cells or may suggest anaplastic large cells lymphoma. In addition, there may be a sinusoidal or cohesive growth pattern and often associated CD30 expression, but this lymphoma of B-cell derivation is ALK-negative and otherwise completely unrelated to anaplastic large cell lymphomas.

Correct Answer: C

Recommended Readings

Alaggio, R., Amador, C., Anagnostopoulos, I., et al. (2022 July). The 5th edition of the World Health Organization classification of haematolymphoid tumours: lymphoi d neoplasms. *Leukemia* 36 (7):1720–1748. doi: 10.1038/s41375 022 01620 2. Epub 2022 Jun 22. Erratum in: (2023 July 19). *Leukemia*. PMID: 35732829; PMCID: PMC9214472.

Beltran, B.E., Castro, D., Paredes, S. et al. (2020). EBV-positive diffuse large B-cell lymphoma, not otherwise specified: 2020 update on diagnosis, risk-stratification and management. *Am J Hematol* 95 (4): 435–445.

Fan, Z., Natkunam, Y., Bair, E. et al. (2003). Characterization of variant patterns of nodular lymphocyte predominant Hodgkin lymphoma with immunohistologic and clinical correlation. *Am J Surg Pathol* 27 (10): 1346–1356.

Mottok, A., Wright, G., Rosenwad, A. et al. (2018). Molecular classification of primary mediastinal large B-cell lymphoma using routinely available tissue specimens. *Blood* 132 (22): 2401–2405.

Martín-Garcia, D., Navarro, A., Valdés, R. et al. (2019). CCND2 and CCND3 hijack immunoglobulin light-chain enhancers in cyclin D1− mantle cell lymphoma. *Blood* 133 (9): 940–951.

Rosenwald, A., Bens, S., Advani, R. et al. (2019). Prognostic significance of *MYC* rearrangement and translocation partner in diffuse large B-cell lymphoma: a study by the lunenburg lymphoma biomarker consortium. *J Clin Oncol* 37 (35): 3359–3368.

Scott, D.W., King, R.L., Staiger, A.M. et al. (2018). High –grade B-cell lymphoma with MYC and BCL2 and/or BCL6 rearrangements with diffuse large B-cell lymphoma morphology. *Blood* 131: 2060–2064.

Schmidt, J., Gong, S., Farafioti, T. et al. (2016). Genome-wide analysis of pediatric-type follicular lymphoma reveals low genetic complexity and recurrent alterations of TNFRSF14 gene. *Blood* 128: 1101–1111.

Venkataraman, G., Song, J.Y., Tzankov, A., Dirnhofer, S. et al. (2013). Aberrant T-cell antigen expression in classical Hodgkin lymphoma is associated with decreased event-free survival and overall survival. *Blood* 121 (10): 1795–1804.AQ1

35

Follicular Lymphoma

Danielle Wallace, Nancy Torres, and Carla Casulo

Wilmot Cancer Institute, University of Rochester, NY

Introduction

Follicular lymphoma (FL) is the most common form of indolent non-Hodgkin lymphoma (NHL). In the United States, it accounts for approximately 15–20% of all new cases of NHLs and has an approximate incidence rate of 2.7 new cases per 100,000 people. It is most frequently diagnosed among people aged 55–64 years, with a median age of 63 years, and it affects men and women equally. In terms of race and ethnicity, the Caucasian population is affected more than twice as much as the African and Asian populations. While it remains incurable in most instances, there are a variety of treatment options. In this chapter, we will discuss the diagnosis, prognosis, and non-transplant management of FL. The role of transplant and other cellular therapies (CAR T and bispecifics) in relapsed and refractory FL are discussed in Chapter 38.

Case Study 1

A 54-year-old retired accountant presented to his primary care physician (PCP) with a history of three months of intermittent drenching night sweats and unintentional weight loss of 10 pounds. Otherwise, he is feeling well. He also noted some nontender cervical lymphadenopathy. Patient does not smoke or drink alcohol. On physical examination, he was found to have enlarged cervical lymph nodes with the largest measuring 2.5 cm. No other lymphadenopathy was found, and he did not have hepatomegaly or splenomegaly. He was given a 10-day course of oral antibiotics without change. His PCP then suspected a low-grade lymphoma and decided to pursue further workup.

1) **What is the best lymph node biopsy technique for a definitive diagnosis of low-grade lymphoma / follicular lymphoma, and what should be included in the initial workup?**
   A) Fine needle aspiration.
   B) Core needle biopsy.
   C) Excisional biopsy.
   D) None of the above.

Expert Perspective: The diagnosis of follicular lymphoma (FL) is best made by excisional tissue biopsy. Adequate tissue sampling is required for morphological assessment,

Cancer Consult: Expertise in Clinical Practice, Volume 2: Neoplastic Hematology & Cellular Therapy,
Second Edition. Edited by Syed A. Abutalib, Maurie Markman, James O. Armitage, and Kenneth C. Anderson.
© 2024 John Wiley & Sons Ltd. Published 2024 by John Wiley & Sons Ltd.

immunophenotyping, and molecular studies. The evaluation of the lymph node architecture is paramount for diagnosis as well as for tumor grading based on centroblast count, which has therapeutic implications. Follicular lymphomas are histologically classified as grade 1–3 according to the number of centroblasts per high power field (grade 1: 0–5; grade 2: 6–15; grade 3: > 15). Grade 3 FL is subclassified into 3a and 3b, with some centrocytes and sheets of centroblasts (or immunoblasts), respectively. The vast majority of the FLs, 80–90% in most unselected series, are of grade 1–2. Small biopsies can miss areas of nodular growth leading to a wrong or missed diagnosis (see Chapter 34).

The initial workup for a patient with newly diagnosed FL includes a complete history and physical examination with attention to node-bearing areas and laboratory studies (complete blood count with differential, full comprehensive metabolic profile including uric acid, lactate dehydrogenase, β-2 microglobulin, and serologic testing for hepatitis B and C virus). A bone marrow aspirate and biopsy is recommended in patients with cytopenias. A PET-CT scan is preferred over CT scans especially to assess for extranodal involvement. Additionally, PET-CT scans are more accurate than CT scans in identifying areas of suspected large cell transformation.

Correct Answer: C

Case Study 2

A 61-year-old man was incidentally found to have mediastinal and bulky para-aortic lymphadenopathy on imaging performed for surveillance of an abdominal aortic aneurysm. He is otherwise asymptomatic. Biopsy revealed follicular lymphoma, grade 2. Laboratory analysis showed normal blood counts, normal comprehensive metabolic profile, and a serum lactate dehydrogenase of 170 U/L (reference range 100–200 U/L).

2) **Which of the following parameters are used to evaluate prognosis in patients with follicular lymphoma?**
   A) Ann Arbor stage.
   B) Serum lactate dehydrogenase.
   C) Hemoglobin.
   D) Age.
   E) All of the above.

Expert Perspective: The Follicular Lymphoma International Prognostic Index (FLIPI) is the most widely used validated tool to establish prognosis and overall survival (OS). However, it is not used to guide therapy. The FLIPI score divide patients into three groups: low, intermediate, and high risk with corresponding OS rates (Table 35.1). The factors included in the FLIPI are age above 60, serum lactate dehydrogenase concentration above normal, hemoglobin level less than 12 g/dL, Ann Arbor stage III or IV, and more than four involved nodal areas. One point is given to each parameter. The patient described in the vignette has a calculated FLIPI of 2 (age above 60 and Ann Arbor stage III) that corresponds with a 5- and 10-year overall survivals of 78 and 51%, respectively.

Correct Answer: E

Table 35.1 Follicular lymphoma international prognostic index (FLIPI) and corresponding estimated OS.

Risk group	Score	5-year OS (%)	10-year OS (%)
Low	0–1	91	71
Intermediate	2	78	51
High	3 or more	52	36

Case Study 3

An asymptomatic 54-year-old woman presented with a 2.5 cm nontender cervical lymph-adenopathy. Biopsy revealed follicular lymphoma grade 1–2. Staging confirms stage I disease. Laboratory analysis was unremarkable.

3) What are the features that aid in the decision to initiate therapy versus active surveillance?

Expert Perspective: The decision to start therapy in patients with newly diagnosed FL is based on criteria established by The Groupe d-Etude des Lymphomes Folliculaires (GELF) to assess for low or high tumor burden (Table 35.2). The presence of any of one of these criteria defines a patient with high tumor burden and in most cases assist in decision to start some sort of therapy in the real-world practice; in clinical trial settings these criteria dictate initiation of therapy in addition to the modified GELF and British National Lymphoma Investigation (BNLI) criteria. In general, patients with high tumor burden are more likely to receive some form of therapy. For patients who are asymptomatic with low tumor burden, active surveillance is a reasonable approach.

4) Which of the following treatment options could potentially cure stage I FL?
   A) Radiation therapy.
   B) Observation (watchful waiting).
   C) Rituxumab monotherapy.
   D) R-CHOP.

Table 35.2 The Groupe d-Etude des Lymphomes Folliculaires (GELF) criteria.

GELF Criteria for treatment in follicular lymphoma
Involvement of 3 or more nodal sites measuring $\geq$ 3 cm
Nodal or extra nodal tumor mass measuring $\geq$ 7 cm in diameter
Presence of B-symptoms
Splenomegaly > 16 cm
Presence of ascites or pleural effusion
Cytopenias (neutrophil count < 1,000 or platelet count < 100 000)
Circulating lymphoma cells (leukemic phase)

Expert Perspective: Approximately 15–25% of cases present with stage I or II at the time of diagnosis. Radiation therapy (total of 24 Gy in 12 fractions not to exceed 30 Gy) is considered a treatment option for patients with non-bulky (~< 7cm) stage I and contiguous stage II disease with potential curative intent resulting in long-term disease control > 86%. A multicenter retrospective study by the International Lymphoma Radiation Oncology Group evaluated RT alone in patients with newly diagnosed stage I–II FL and found a five-year progression-free and overall survival rates of 69% and 96%, respectively. Few studies suggest incorporation of rituximab may prolong progression-free survival but does not appear to improve OS after radiation therapy.

Correct Answer: A

Case Study 4

A 65-year-old woman developed axillary lymphadenopathy. An excisional lymph node biopsy revealed follicular lymphoma grade 2. She is asymptomatic. Her PET-CT scan shows stage II disease with low SUV uptake in axilla bilaterally (left and right axilla 2 cm and 1.9 cm lymph nodes, respectively). Her laboratory analysis was unremarkable. She has no B-symptoms. Patient is uncomfortable with her condition.

5) What are some reasonable options for this patient?
   A) Watchful waiting.
   B) Rituxumab monotherapy.
   C) R-CHOP (cyclophosphamide, doxorubicin, vincristine, and prednisone plus rituximab).
   D) BR (bendamustine and rituximab).
   E) All of the above.
   F) A and B.

Expert Perspective: For patients determined to have low tumor burden disease by GELF criteria, watchful waiting or single-agent rituximab can be considered as therapy options. No difference in OS was observed when comparing observation to chemotherapy. A multicenter randomized trial by the British National Lymphoma Investigation (BNLI) group (Ardeshna et al.) showed no survival advantage to chemotherapy (chlorambucil) when compared to watchful waiting for asymptomatic patients, who were followed for 16 years. Moreover, a study by Ardeshna et al in 2014 compared observation to rituximab alone, followed by rituximab maintenance and found not difference in OS or rates of histological transformation. However, rituximab monotherapy showed a significant delay in disease progression and time until chemotherapy or radiotherapy when compared with a watchful waiting approach. Additionally, this study showed that rituximab induction can be delivered without a reduction in quality of life and patients had an improvement in some aspects of it when compared with watchful waiting (Ardeshna et al. 2014). The RESORT trial evaluated rituximab followed by retreatment at the time of progression versus maintenance and showed that survival is favorable in low tumor burden disease without the additional benefit of maintenance (Kahl et al. 2014).

Based on these data, either observation or single-agent rituximab given for four doses (every eight weeks) are appropriate standard therapies for low tumor burden disease. Therapy with chemoimmunotherapy in this particular patient does not appear to be a good option given that she is asymptomatic with low disease burden.

Correct Answer: F

Case Study 5

A 75-year-old man presented with a palpable lower abdominal mass. Imaging revealed widespread supradiaphragmatic and infradiaphragmatic lymphadenopathy, including multiple sites with lymph nodes greater than 3 cm. A biopsy of the lower abdominal mass showed grade 1–2 follicular lymphoma. A bone marrow biopsy confirms low-level involvement of follicular lymphoma; he has no cytopenias. He denies B-symptoms, but the lower abdominal mass is bothersome. He desires treatment that would be completed in a few months and does not cause alopecia.

6) Given his preferences, what would be the optimal front-line therapy for FL grade I/II high tumor burden disease?

A) R-CHOP (cyclophosphamide, doxorubicin, vincristine, and prednisone plus rituximab).
B) BR (bendamustine and rituximab).
C) Lenalidomide + rituximab.
D) Bendamustine + obinutuzumab with maintenance obinutuzumab.

Correct Answer: B

Expert Perspective: Given his stated preferences, bendamustine in combination with rituximab is likely the best choice for him. The treatment goal is not curative with available chemoimmunotherapy.

Choice of chemoimmunotherapy: Two trials have assessed BR vs R-CHOP in the frontline setting for patients with follicular lymphoma.

- In the phase III non-inferiority (margin of 10%) STIL trial, each regimen was given for six cycles in indolent (including FL) and older mantle cell lymphoma patients. BR had an improved PFS of 69.5 vs 31.2 months (hazard ratio [HR] 0.58; 95% CI 0.44–0.74) without an OS benefit (70% vs 66% at 10 years, respectively). However, BR compared to R-CHOP was associated with lower rates of severe cytopenias and infections. Erythematous skin reactions were more common in patients in the BR group than in those in the R-CHOP group (16% vs 9%; $P = 0.024$).
- The phase III non-inferiority BRIGHT trial also included indolent and mantle cell lymphoma patients. They received BR, R-CHOP, or R-CVP (cyclophosphamide, vincristine, and prednisone) per the investigator's choice for six cycles; two additional cycles were permitted at investigator's discretion. BR was shown to be non-inferior to R-CHOP or R-CVP in terms of complete (31% vs 25%, respectively; $P = .0225$ for non-inferiority [0.88 margin]) and overall response rates (97% and 91%, respectively;

P = 0.0102). BR had higher incidences of vomiting, hypersensitivity reactions, and secondary malignancies with a lower incidence of neuropathy and alopecia. The progression-free survival rates at five years were 65.5% in the BR treatment group and 55.8% in the R-CHOP/R-CVP group. The difference in progression-free survival was considered significant with a hazard ratio of 0.61 (95% CI 0.45–0.85; *P* = 0.0025). The hazard ratio for event-free survival and duration of response (*P* = 0.0020 and 0.0134, respectively) also favored the BR regimen over R-CHOP/R-CVP. However, no significant difference in overall survival was observed. The overall safety profiles of BR, R-CHOP, and R-CVP were as expected; no new safety data were collected during long-term follow-up. A higher number of secondary malignancies was noted in the BR treatment group.

The authors of this chapter favor BR over R-CHOP in patients with FL grade 1–2 disease. Notably, older patients (older than age 70 years) have been shown in other trials to have higher incidence of fatal adverse events when bendamustine is used, so a dose reduction to 70 mg/m^2 instead of the traditional 90 mg/m^2 should be considered. The effect of bendamustine dose reduction on FL outcomes is unknown. The role of maintenance rituximab is discussed in later in the chapter.

Anti-CD20 preference: Obinutuzumab, a novel CD20 monoclonal antibody, is an option to rituximab. The phase III GALLIUM study assessed chemotherapy backbones (CHOP, bendamustine, or CVP) in combination with either rituximab or obinutuzumab, which was continued for up to two years for maintenance therapy in FL patients with stage II–IV. Obinutuzumab-containing regimens showed similar response rate, but an improved three-year PFS (80.0% vs 73.3%); however, this impact on PFS may depend on the chemotherapy backbone (CHOP or bendamustine were superior to CVP). High-grade adverse events were more common with obinutuzumab-based chemotherapy. The overall survival results were similar at last follow-up.

Non-chemotherapy approach: Lenalidomide and rituximab (R^2) has been assessed in the first-line setting in FL patients in the RELEVANCE trial. Patients were randomly assigned to R^2 vs R-chemo (investigators' choice of R-CHOP, BR, or R-CVP) and were given a total of 30 months of therapy—R^2 was given for 18 months followed by a year of rituximab maintenance, and R-chemo was given for approximately six months followed by two years of rituximab maintenance. Patients who received R^2 had similar CR rates and similar PFS and OS compared to R-chemo. They experienced more rash and gastrointestinal toxicity with R^2 but less severe neutropenia and febrile neutropenia. However, they also experienced higher rates of dose reduction, interruption, and treatment consideration, suggesting there is still moderate toxicity associated with this chemotherapy-free regimen.

7) **What would be the recommended therapy if his pathology report showed grade 3b disease?**
   A) R-CHOP (cyclophosphamide, doxorubicin, vincristine, and prednisone plus rituximab).
   B) BR (bendamustine + rituximab).
   C) Lenalidomide + rituximab.
   D) Bendamustine + obinutuzumab with maintenance obinutuzumab.

Expert Perspective: Grade 3b disease is determined on histology by solid sheets of centroblasts, or large noncleaved cells, without centrocytes, which are the small, cleaved cells that constitute most follicular lymphoma. Grade 3b disease is generally clinically aggressive and is therefore treated as a diffuse large-B cell lymphoma with R-CHOP chemotherapy. Patients with GL grade 3 were excluded from the STIL and BRIGHT trial, and therefore BR is not often considered. From the management standpoint, FL grade 3a disease is controversial; some experts prefer treating with BR and others with R-CHOP, based on the clinical presentation of the disease.

Correct Answer: A

Case Study 6

A 56-year-old woman presents with advanced-stage grade 1 follicular lymphoma requiring treatment. She is started on rituximab with cyclophosphamide, vincristine, and prednisone (R-CVP) and at the end of treatment scans show a complete response. She wonders if anything can be done to maximize the duration of her response.

8) **What are the expected results of maintenance rituximab based on the PRIMA study?**
   A) Increased overall survival.
   B) Increased progression-free survival.
   C) Increased rate of infections.
   D) A and C.
   E) B and C.

Expert Perspective: The PRIMA study assessed previously untreated patients with FL who received rituximab combined with CHOP, CVP, or FCM (fludarabine, cyclophosphamide, and mitoxantrone) with or without rituximab maintenance given every eight weeks for two years. This showed an improvement in PFS (three-year PFS of 74.9% vs 57.6%) but no difference in overall survival. Infections were the most common adverse event, occurring in 39% vs 24% of patients with and without maintenance therapy, respectively.

   Maintenance rituximab can be considered in otherwise healthy patients to improve progression-free survival However, consideration must be given to the higher rate of infection, and we generally avoid this approach in elderly patients and during the pandemic. Notably, BR was not included in this study, so there is currently no prospective evidence to suggest that there is benefit to rituximab maintenance after CR from BR, although a retrospective analysis by Hill et al. suggested prolonged progression-free survival akin to PRIMA study (Hill et al. 2019).

Correct Answer: E

9) **Which of the following about maintenance rituximab therapy based on the FOLL12 study results is correct?**
   A) Measurable residual disease (MRD) response–adapted post-induction was superior to standard rituximab maintenance.
   B) PET scan–based response–adapted post-induction was superior to standard rituximab maintenance.

C) Standard rituximab maintenance reduced the risk of disease progression.

D) A and B.

Expert Perspective: Most recently the results of the FOLL12 study were reported. This study was conducted with the hypothesis that a PET and measurable residual disease (MRD) response–adapted post-induction management of patients with high-tumor burden FL responding to standard immunochemotherapy was non-inferior in terms of progression-free survival compared with standard rituximab maintenance. The study demonstrated (i) that standard rituximab maintenance was better than the response-adapted management in terms of progression-free survival, (ii) that standard rituximab maintenance reduced the risk of disease progression also for patients with the best quality of response, and (iii) the lack of any overall survival difference between study arms. The results of the FOLL12 trial do not support a response-adapted post-induction-based maintenance in FL.

Correct Answer: C

Case Study 7

A 54-year-old woman presented with high-tumor burden, stage II, grade 2 follicular lymphoma. She was treated with BR. She relapses with palpable lymphadenopathy and cytopenias approximately 18 months after diagnosis.

10) **What can you tell her about the frequency and prognostic significance of relapsed FL within 24 months ("early relapse")?**

A) Occurs in about 20% of patients, with no change in overall survival.

B) Occurs in about 60% of patients, with no change in overall survival.

C) Occurs in about 20% of patients, with decrease in overall survival.

D) Occurs in about 60% of patients, with decrease in overall survival.

Expert Perspective: A consistent approximately 20% of patients across multiple databases have been shown to have progression of their follicular lymphoma within two years of initial diagnosis. An analysis of the National LymphCare Study by Casulo et al. determined that early progression of disease was significantly associated with decreased overall survival (hazard ratio of 7.17), and this held true whether or not patients received R-CHOP, RCVP, or rituximab-fludarabine. This study helped determine that patients with early relapse with progression of disease within 24 months (POD24) should be separately assessed in future studies and perhaps treated more aggressively at time of relapse, including consideration, outside of a clinical trial, of autologous or allogeneic stem cell transplant.

Correct Answer: C

11) **What are the next steps in the management of her potentially relapsed disease?**

A) PET scan.

B) CT scan.

C) Excisional biopsy.

D) Bone marrow biopsy.

E) Choices A, C, D.

Expert Perspective: At the time of clinical relapse, consideration should be given to obtaining a PET scan. Follicular lymphoma has the potential to progress to more aggressive or transformed large B-cell lymphoma at the rate of approximately 1–2% a year. PET scans have the additional benefit of assessing metabolic activity compared to CT scans, and if there are areas of discordant SUV, biopsy of the area with the highest SUV should be considered. Biopsy should therefore be considered at the time of progression in an attempt to assure relapsed FL as opposed to transformation, and if cytopenias occur, a bone marrow biopsy should also be performed to confirm FL involvement of the marrow. Consideration for transformation (see Chapters 34 and 43) is particularly important especially in patients who have early relapse, as several studies have suggested that there is higher rate of disease transformation in such group of patients. In the retrospective analysis of the PRIMA study (Sarkozy et al.), 37% of biopsies performed during the first year showed histologic transformation (Sarkozy et al. 2016).

Correct Answer: E

12) **She is interested in learning about the various treatment options available to her. Which of the following are treatment options for relapsed follicular lymphoma?**
    A) Bendamustine and obinutuzumab (BO).
    B) Lenalidomide and obinutuzumab.
    C) Lenalidomide and rituximab.
    D) Copanlisib.
    E) All of the above.

Expert Perspective: There are multiple options available for her.

- For patients who are rituximab refractory (defined as patients who failed to respond or progressed within six months of the last rituximab dose), the GADOLIN trial showed that bendamustine and obinutuzumab followed by obinutuzumab maintenance resulted in improvement in progression-free-survival over bendamustine monotherapy.
- For patients who have already received bendamustine or who wish to avoid additional chemotherapy, lenalidomide-containing regimens can be considered. Lenalidomide, an immunomodulatory agent, was combined with obinutuzumab with maintenance in the GALEN trial in patients who had previously received rituximab-containing regimens. This combination showed a 79% overall response rate; 70% of patients had an ongoing response at two years. In regard to the POD24 population, a secondary analysis of the GALEN population showed that the POD24 patients had an overall response rate, progression-free survival, and overall survival that was surprisingly similar to the patients without early progression; we, therefore, consider this regimen as a reasonable second-line choice in patients with early relapsed follicular lymphoma.
- Lenalidomide can also be combined with rituximab (R^2) as shown in the AUGMENT trial, which compared R^2 to rituximab alone. Lenalidomide was continued for 12 28-day cycles in combination with rituximab for the first five cycles. R^2 showed an improvement in PFS and a prolonged duration of response (median 39.4 months vs 14.1 months) vs rituximab monotherapy. Given the relatively limited duration of therapy compared to obinutuzumab-containing regimens, we consider this option for patients with late-progressing relapsed disease who have already received bendamustine.

- PI3K inhibitors target the PI3 kinase pathway that is downstream from the B-cell receptor pathway. Selection of these agents is generally guided by patient preference for infusions (copanlisib) or oral (idelalisib [withdrawn by the company], umbralisib [withdrawn by the FDA], and duvelisib [withdrawn by the company in FL]) therapies, and by their side effect profiles (Table 35.3). In general, they all have a median duration of response of about one year; we usually sequence these agents following lenalidomide- or obinutuzumab-containing regimens.
- Cellular therapies including CAR T cell therapy and bispecifics in relapsed and refractory FL are discussed in Chapter 38.

Correct Answer: E

Table 35.3 Therapeutic options (non-transplant/cellular therapy) for relapsed follicular lymphoma.

Therapy for relapsed disease	Schedule/route	Outcome	Side effects
Bendamustine and obinutuzumab	6 monthly cycles of bendamustine (IV) and obinutuzumab (IV) with 2 years of obinutuzumab maintenance	Median PFS 25.6 months	Infusion reactions, neutropenia, infections
Lenalidomide and obinutuzumab	Induction with lenalidomide (PO) for 3 weeks of each monthly cycle and obinutuzumab (IV) for 6 cycles, maintenance year 1 with lenalidomide and obinutuzumab every other month; maintenance year 2 with obinutuzumab every other month	2-year PFS 65%	Fatigue, neutropenia, diarrhea
Lenalidomide and rituximab	Lenalidomide (PO) for one year with rituximab (IV/subQ) for 5 cycles	Median PFS 39.4 months	Neutropenia, diarrhea, fatigue
Copanlisib	IV 3 of every 4 weeks, continued until disease progression	Median PFS 12.5 months	Hyperglycemia, colitis, hypertension
Idelalisib (withdrawn—see text)	PO, twice daily until disease progression	Median PFS 11 months	Neutropenia, hepatitis, colitis, pneumonia
Duvelisib (withdrawn—see text)	PO, twice daily until disease progression	Median PFS 9.5 months	Neutropenia, colitis, fatigue
Umbralisib (withdrawn—see text)	PO, daily until disease progression	Median DOR of 11.1 months	Colitis, rise in creatinine, infections
Tazemetostat	PO, twice daily until disease progression	Median PFS 13.8 months in EZH2^{mut} patients; 11.1 months in EZH2^{WT}	Thrombocytopenia, neutropenia, anemia

13) The recently approved agent tazemetostat is an inhibitor of which enzyme in patients with follicular lymphoma?

A) FOXO1.

B) MEF2B.

C) EZH2.

D) CREBBP.

E) CARDII.

Expert Perspective: Tazemetostat is a recently approved agent for relapsed follicular lymphoma that inhibits EZH2, a histone methyltransferase that can have gain-of-function mutations in about 20% of FL patients. In a phase II study, patients who progressed following two or more lines of therapy were given tazemetostat and were stratified by *EZH2* mutation status (Morschhauser et al. 2020). Those in the *EZH2* mutated group had a median progression-free survival of 13.8 months compared to 11.1 months in the wild-type *EZH2*; the ORR was also better at 69%, although interestingly the wild-type *EZH2* patients still have a 35% response rate. While not yet universally performed, consideration should be given to assessing *EZH2* mutation status at the time of relapse, especially in the POD24 population as that study showed overall similar response rates to the non-POD24 population (63% and 25%); POD24 patients historically have poorer response rates to agents in the relapsed setting than patients who had late progression, so this suggests tazemetostat is a promising therapy choice for this patient population. It is generally well tolerated, with mostly grade 1 or 2 toxicities including nausea or fatigue.

Correct Answer: C

Recommended Readings

Ardeshna, K.M. Smith P, Norton A, et al. (2003Aug 16). Long-term effect of a watch and wait policy versus immediate systemic treatment for asymptomatic advanced-stage non-Hodgkin lymphoma: a randomised controlled trial. *Lancet* 362 (9383); 516–522. doi: 10.1016/s0140-6736(03)14110-4. PMID: 12932382.

Ardeshna KM, Qian W, Smith P, et al. (2014). Rituximab versus a watch-and-wait approach in patients with advanced-stage, asymptomatic, non-bulky follicular lymphoma: an open-label randomised phase 3 trial. *Lancet Oncol* 15 (4); 424–435.

Bachy E, Houot R, Feugier P, et al. (2022 Apr 14). Obinutuzumab plus lenalidomide in advanced, previously untreated follicular lymphoma in need of systemic therapy: a LYSA study. *Blood.* 139(15):2338–2346. doi: 10.1182/blood.2021013526. PMID: 34936697.

Batlevi CL. (2022 Apr 14; Chemotherapy-free regimens in frontline follicular lymphoma. *Blood.* 139(15):2263–2264. doi: 10.1182/blood.2021015120. PMID: 35420687.

Flinn, I.W. et al. (2019 April 20). First-line treatment of patients with indolent non-Hodgkinlymphoma or mantle-cell lymphoma with bendamustine plus rituximab versus R-CHOP or R-CVP: results of the BRIGHT 5-year follow-up study. *J Clin Oncol.* 37 (12): 984–991. doi: 10.1200/JCO.18.00605. Epub 2019 Feb 27. PMID: 30811293; PMCID: PMC6494265).

Hill BT, Nastoupil L, Winter AM, et al. (2019). Maintenance rituximab or observation after frontline treatment with bendamustine-rituximab for follicular lymphoma. *Br J Haematol* 184 (4); 524–535.

Jacobson CA, Chavez JC, Sehgal AR, et al. (2022 Jan). Axicabtagene ciloleucel in relapsed or refractory indolent non-Hodgkin lymphoma (ZUMA-5): a single-arm, multicentre, phase 2 trial. *Lancet Oncol.* 23(1):91–103. doi: 10.1016/S1470-2045(21)00591-X. Epub 2021 Dec 8. PMID: 34895487.

Kahl BS, Hong F, Williams ME. et al. (2014). Rituximab extended schedule or re-treatment trial for low-tumor burden follicular lymphoma: eastern cooperative oncology group protocol e4402. *J Clin Oncol* 32 (28); 3096–3102.

Luminari S, Manni M, Galimberti S, Versari A, et al. (2022 Mar 1), Fondazione Italiana Linfomi. Response-Adapted Postinduction Strategy in Patients With Advanced-Stage Follicular Lymphoma: The FOLL12 Study. *J Clin Oncol.* 40(7):729–739. doi: 10.1200/JCO.21.01234. Epub 2021 Oct 28. PMID: 34709880.

Morschhauser F, Tilly H, Chaidos A. et al. (2020). Tazemetostat for patients with relapsed or refractory follicular lymphoma: an open-label, single-arm, multicentre, phase 2 trial. *Lancet Oncol* 21 (11); 1433–1442.

Russler Germain, D.A., Krysiak, K., Ramirez, C., et.al. (2023 July 26). Mutations associated with progression in follicular lymphoma predict inferior outcomes at diagnosis (Alliance A151303). *Blood Adv bloodadvances.*2023010779. doi: 10.1182/bloodadvances.2023010779. Epub ahead of print. PMID: 37493986.

Sarkozy C, Trneny M, Xerri L, et al. (2016). Risk factors and outcomes for patients with follicular lymphoma who had histologic transformation after response to first-line immunochemotherapy in the PRIMA trial. *J Clin Oncol* 34 (22); 2575–2582.

Seymour JF, Marcus R, Davies A. et al. (2019 June). Association of early disease progression and very poor survival in the GALLIUM study in follicular lymphoma: Benefit of obinutuzumab in reducing the rate of early progression. *Haematologica* 104 (6): 1202–1208. doi: 10.3324/haematol.2018.209015. Epub 2018 Dec 20. Erratum in: Haematologica. 2020 May;105(5):1465. PMID: 30573503; PMCID: PMC6545851.

Trotman J, Pettitt AR. Is it time for PET-guided therapy in follicular lymphoma? *Blood.* 2022 Mar 17;139(11):1631–1641. doi: 10.1182/blood.2020008243. PMID: 34260714.

36

Mantle Cell Lymphoma

Christina Poh and Stephen D. Smith

University of Washington/Fred Hutchinson Cancer Center, Seattle, WA

Introduction

Mantle cell lymphoma (MCL) is a B-cell lymphoproliferative neoplasm characterized by a variable disease course, with the majority of cases exhibiting an aggressive behavior. It is a relatively uncommon disorder, constituting approximately 7% of adult non-Hodgkin lymphomas. It is generally considered a disease of the elderly, with a median age at diagnosis of 68 years, and affects men three times as often as women with rising incidence in the USA. This chapter will discuss the clinical manifestations, prognostic factors, and management of MCL.

Case Study 1

A previously healthy 59-year-old male presents with adenopathy and night sweats. Lymph node biopsy reveals MCL with a blastoid growth pattern, a Ki-67 proliferation index of 40%. Fluorescence in situ hybridization is normal, but sequencing shows a TP53 mutation. Total white blood cell (WBC) count is $12.5 \times 10^6/\mu L$ and serum lactate dehydrogenase (LDH) is 240 IU/L (normal 100–220).

1) **What favorable prognostic feature does this patient have in MCL?**
   A) Age.
   B) Blastoid variant.
   C) LDH level.
   D) Ki-67 proliferation index.
   E) TP53 mutation status.

Expert Perspective: This patient's only favorable prognostic feature is his relatively younger age of 59 years. Several studies have demonstrated age over 60 (or 70) to be an adverse prognostic feature in MCL, affecting relapse risk and survival.

MCL is categorized into four histologic variants: classic or typical, marginal zone–like, blastoid, and pleomorphic. Blastoid and pleomorphic variants are aggressive and associated with poorer prognosis compared to the other two variants.

Leukemic non-nodal MCL is a clinical variant in which the patients present with peripheral blood, bone marrow, and sometimes splenic involvement but without significant adenopathy (typically defined as peripheral lymph nodes < 1–2 cm and without adenopathy on CT scan, if performed). This entity is often clinically indolent and often show unique features, including kappa light-chain restriction (as opposed to lambda, which is more typical for MCL), hypermutated immunoglobulin heavy-chain genes (seen in a minority of MCL cases), and absent nuclear staining for the transcription factor SOX11. The presentation of patients with leukemic non-nodal variant of MCL often resembles CLL.

The Mantle Cell Lymphoma International Prognostic Index (MIPI) provides disease risk stratification based on age, LDH level, performance status, and total WBC count; this patient falls into the high-risk category. The MIPI has been validated in several data sets and has been proven superior to the International Prognostic Index in some series. A further refinement to the MIPI incorporates the Ki-67 proliferation index; the median Ki-67 index in mantle cell lymphoma is about 20–30%, with values above the median range adversely prognostic.

TP53 mutation, mostly missense mutations in the DNA binding domain, can be found in approximately 10% of all previously untreated MCL patients, and is associated with exceedingly poor outcomes following standard chemoimmunotherapy and autologous transplant (ASCT).

Correct Answer: A

Case Study 2

A previously healthy 53-year-old male is diagnosed with MCL, intermediate-risk by the MIPI score, and with a Ki-67 of 50%. He has a 6 cm adenopathy in the retroperitoneum, has low back pain, and has lost 15% of his weight in the last six months. He has no renal, cardiac, or hepatic comorbidities.

2) **Among the choices listed below, what treatment approach would you recommend for this patient?**
   A) Observation.
   B) FCR (fludarabine, cyclophosphamide, and rituximab).
   C) R-CHOP (rituximab, cyclophosphamide, doxorubicin, vincristine, and prednisone) followed by maintenance rituximab.
   D) Alternating R-CHOP/R-DHAP (rituximab, dexamethasone, cytarabine, and cisplatin) followed by consolidative ASCT and maintenance rituximab.

Expert Perspective: The current treatment approach for newly diagnosed MCL is dependent on several patient-specific factors such as age, functional status, and comorbidities. For younger, fit patients, an intensive chemoimmunotherapy regimen using augmented R-CHOP and cytarabine as a backbone followed by high-dose chemotherapy with ASCT followed by maintenance therapy with rituximab (every two months for three years) is the most appropriate option among those listed.

MCL has historically been associated with poor outcomes with conventional chemotherapy. Although randomized trials are lacking, more intensive induction chemoimmunotherapy approaches—in particular those incorporating high-dose cytarabine, rituximab, and ASCT—

have emerged as the modern standard of care for younger MCL patients based on an array of data. Bendamustine and rituximab (BR) is also a feasible front-line MCL regimen, particularly when combined with cytarabine and rituximab, affording a high complete response (CR) rate, without a negative impact on stem cell collection.

ASCT was previously shown to be superior to interferon maintenance after CHOP-like induction therapy in a randomized clinical trial involving adults younger than 65 years. This study established the role of ASCT for improving disease control in MCL for eligible, young patients after CHOP therapy. However, it is unclear whether ASCT still provides the same benefit with the development of novel agents such as Bruton Tyrosine Kinase (BTK) inhibitors and incorporation of more intensive induction regimens over the past decade.

A phase III trial which randomized advanced stage MCL patients who were eligible for transplant to either induction therapy with RCHOP or RDHAP followed by ASCT and observation, RCHOP or RDHAP induction plus ibrutinib followed by ASCT and 2 years of ibrutinib maintenance, or RCHOP or RDHAP induction plus ibrutinib and 2 years of ibrutinib maintenance (without ASCT) revealed improved failure-free survival (FFS) for patients who received ibrutinib-containing therapy. This study casts uncertainty on the role of ASCT in first-line MCL when BTK inhibitors are used, but key questions regarding durability of responses, toxicity management, optimal choice of BTK inhibitor, and whether some subgroups may still benefit from ASCT. The other answers do not describe optimal first-line therapy for a young, symptomatic MCL patient. Observation is not appropriate for progressing, symptomatic MCL patients. FCR is not used in younger MCL patients due to toxicity, including to the stem cell compartment before potential ASCT. R-CHOP is inferior to bortezomib-containing therapy (VR-CAP) in transplant-ineligible patients and represents inadequate therapy for young, fit MCL patients.

Correct Answer: D

Case Study 3

A 75-year-old male with newly diagnosed MCL, intermediate-risk by the MIPI score, presents to establish care. He endorses progressive inguinal adenopathy, fevers, and weight loss of 20 lbs over the past two months. Comorbidities include hypertension, hyperlipidemia and atrial fibrillation for which he is taking apixaban. On exam, he appears frail with an ECOG of 2. He strongly prefers a chemotherapy-free treatment approach.

3) **Among the choices listed below, what treatment approach would you discuss for this patient, assuming good renal and hepatic function?**
   A) HyperCVAD alternating with high-dose cytarabine and rituximab.
   B) Single-agent rituximab.
   C) Lenalidomide with rituximab.
   D) Venetoclax and Ibrutinib.

Expert Perspective: For older, unfit MCL patients, commonly used induction chemotherapeutic approaches include BR and VR-CAP (bortezomib, rituximab, cyclophosphamide, doxorubicin, and prednisone) with an overall response rate exceeding 85%, and half of patients achieving complete responses. However, for patients who are not eligible for, or decline, chemotherapy, lenalidomide with rituximab is a potential treatment option based on a relatively small phase II trial. This study included 38 previously untreated MCL patients with low- or intermediate-risk disease or unfit patients with high-risk disease per MIPI and demonstrated an overall response rate (ORR) of 92% and a CR rate of 64%. A response to treatment correlated with improvement in quality of life. Long-term follow-up showed a three-year progression-free survival (PFS) and overall survival (OS) of 80% and 90%, respectively, suggesting durable responses. Disadvantages to the lenalidomide with rituximab approach included its off-label (unapproved) use and long-term adminstration of both agents with cumulative toxicity risks.

The other answers do not represent standard first-line therapy for an elderly, intermediate risk MCL patient. HyperCVAD is an inappropriate choice for elderly patients given toxicity and single agent rituximab has limited efficacy in MCL. BTK inhibitors are being combined with chemotherapy, antibodies and other targeted agents including venetoclax (the latter for high-risk *TP53*-mutated MCL). While such combinations are likely to emerge as future standards of care, they are not presently approved. In addition, pre-existing atrial fibrillation and anticoagulation in this case make ibrutinib-containing therapy suboptimal.

Correct Answer: C

Case Study 4

A 74-year-old male with MCL who underwent R-CHOP for six courses and rituximab maintenance for three years is seen for evaluation. Now one year after completion of rituximab maintenance, he has developed progressive pancytopenia. Bone marrow biopsy shows 40% involvement with MCL, a hypocellular marrow, and reduced trilineage hematopoiesis, and imaging reveals 3 cm retroperitoneal adenopathy. Absolute neutrophil count is 600/μL, hemoglobin is 8.6 g/dL without evidence of hemolysis, and platelet count is $92 \times 10^3/\mu L$.

4) What is the next best therapy?
   A) BR with rituximab and cytarabine.
   B) Acalabrutinib.
   C) Bortezomib.
   D) Lenalidomide.

Expert Perspective: Despite multiple effective front-line treatment options for MCL, patients inevitably relapse and require additional therapy. Treatment of R/R MCL requires consideration of an individual's prior therapy, comorbidities, and the nature and timing of their relapse. BTK inhibitors, ibrutinib, acalabrutinib and zanubrutinib, and lenalidomide with rituximab are preferred second-line treatment regimens for MCL.

The efficacy of ibrutinib was evaluated in a pivotal open-label, multi-center, single-arm trial of 111 previously treated MCL patients, which demonstrated an ORR of 67% and a CR rate of 23% with a median duration of response of 17.5 months; this led to its FDA approval in MCL patients who have received at least one prior therapy. The second-generation BTK inhibitor acalabrutinib was also approved for the same patient population based on an open-label, phase II, single-arm trial, which demonstrated an ORR of 81% and a CR rate of 40%. The median duration of response had not been reached after a follow-up of 15.2 months. Although there are no head-to-head studies between BTK inhibitors in MCL, acala-brutinib was associated with less cardiotoxicity and a lower rate of discontinuation due to adverse events compared to ibrutinib in relapsed high-risk chronic lymphocytic leukemia. The efficacy of zanubrutinib was evaluated in two trials, BGB-3111–206 and BGB-3111-AU-003, with both studies demonstrating the same ORR of 84%. However, the CR rate differed at 59% and 22%, respectively, which may partially be due to differences in patient populations and response assessment. None of the BTK inhibitors mentioned above are effective against C481S resistant mutation.

Bortezomib is FDA approved for the treatment of MCL in patients who have received at least one prior treatment based on the results of the multicenter PINNACLE study. However, this approval (2006) was before BTK inhibitors, which have better activity against MCL

Newer-generation BTK inhibitors are in development. Pirtobrutinib, FDA approved, non-covalent BTK inhibitor, has demonstrated promising efficacy in heavily pretreated MCL patients including those who have progressed on a prior BTK inhibitor. Orelabrutinib has recently obtained breakthrough therapy designation by the FDA for the treatment of R/R MCL.

Correct Answer: B

5) **The patient was started on acalabrutinib which he tolerated well. After 1 year on aca-labrutinib, patient was noted to have progressive disease. Among the choices listed below, what treatment approach would you recommend for this patient?**
   A) Ibrutinib.
   B) Zanubrutinib.
   C) Pirtobrutinib.

BTK inhibitors are a growing therapeutic class, including non-covalent agents with a unique mechanism of BTK binding and high specificity. These agents have potential to overcome tumor resistance while exhibiting lower toxicity. Pirtobrutinib, a non-covalent BTK inhibitor, recently received FDA approval for MCL patients who have received at least two prior lines of systemic therapy, including a BTK inhibitor. Efficacy was evaluated in BRUIN, an open-label, multicenter, single-arm trial of pirtobrutinib monotherapy that included 120 patients with MCL previously treated with a BTK inhibitor. The most common prior BTK inhibitors received were ibrutinib (67%), acalabrutinib (30%), and zanubrutinib (8%); 83% had discontinued their last BTK inhibitor due to refractory or progressive disease. The ORR was 50% with a complete response rate of 13%. The estimated median duration of response was 8.3 months and the estimated duration of response rate at 6 months was 65.3%. The most common adverse reactions ($\geq$15%) were fatigue, musculoskeletal pain, diarrhea, edema, dyspnea, pneumonia, and bruising. Grade 3 or 4 laboratory abnormalities in $\geq$10% of patients were decreased neutrophil counts, lymphocyte counts, and platelet counts. Orelabrutinib also received breakthrough therapy designation by the FDA for the treatment of R/R MCL. Further randomized trials are needed to inform optimal sequencing and use of this growing therapeutic class.

Ibrutinib and zanubrutinib, a 1st and 2nd generation BTK inhibitor, are not recommended for those who have progressed on another 2nd generation BTK inhibitior.

Correct Answer: C

Case Study 5

A previously healthy 58-year-old female with MCL who underwent induction therapy with the NORDIC regimen (dose-intensified induction chemoimmunotherapy with R-CHOP [maxi

CHOP] alternating high-dose cytarabine and rituximab) followed by consolidative ASCT four years ago subsequently found to have relapsed disease and has been on acalabrutinib for the past two years. She now presents with progressive lymphadenopathy. Lymph node biopsy reveals MCL with a pleomorphic growth pattern and a Ki-67 proliferation index of 60%.

6) What is the next best therapy?
- A) Zanubrutinib.
- B) BR.
- C) Brexucabtagene autoleucel.
- D) Allogeneic Stem Cell transplantation.

Expert Perspective: Although BTK inhibitors have shown impressive efficacy in patients with R/R MCL, approximately one-third of patients display poor response to BTK inhibitors, and most patients eventually progress; these patients have a poor prognosis. Brexucabtagene autoleucel, a CD19-directed chimeric antigen receptor (CAR) T cell therapy, is approved for the treatment of R/R MCL based on the ZUMA-2 trial. This was a single-arm, open-label study that investigated the efficacy of brexucabtagene autoleucel in 74 R/R MCL patients who had previously received anthracycline- or bendamustine-containing chemotherapy, an anti-CD20 monoclonal antibody therapy, and a BTK inhibitor with either ibrutinib or acalabrutinib. Among the intention-to-treat population, ORR was 85% and CR rate was 59% with a median time to response of one month. Interestingly, patients with poor prognostic factors such as a Ki-67 proliferation index of 50% or higher, blastoid or pleomorphic variants or *TP53* mutation still had objective responses although the sample size in these subgroups were small. This suggests that brexucabtagene autoleucel may be particularly beneficial and should be utilized earlier during the course of treatment for patients with high-risk MCL or those with poor prognostic features. The most common grade 3 or higher adverse events were related to cytopenias and infections, which occurred in 94% and 32% of patients, respectively. Grade 3 or higher cytokine release syndrome and neurotoxicity occurred in 15% and 31% of patients, respectively. A study investigating the addition of ibrutinib to tisagenlecleucel, another CD19-directed CAR T-cell therapy, in patients with R/R MCL preliminarily revealed high rates of durable response.

The other answers do not describe optimal therapy for a young, fit, high-risk MCL patient. Allogeneic stem cell transplantation produces durable remission for 30–40% of heavily pretreated MCL patients but considering its short- and long-term risks, would generally not take precedence over CAR T cell therapy. Bispecific antibodies are under investigation. One such example is glofitamab, a CD20xCD3 T-cell engaging Bispecific antibody, which likely has a favorable toxicity profile compared to CAR-T therapy. However, longer follow-up is needed to determine the durability of response.

Correct Answer: C

Recommended Readings

Chen, R.W., Li, H., Bernstein, S.H. et al. (2017 Mar). RB but not R-HCVAD is a feasible induction regimen prior to auto-HCT in frontline MCL: results of SWOG study S1106. *Br J Haematol* 176 (5): 759–769. doi:10.1111/bjh.14480. Epub 2016 Dec 19. PMID: 27992063. PMCID: PMC5318240.

Cohen, J.B., Shah, N.N., Alencar, A.J. et al. (2022 Oct). MCL-133 pirtobrutinib, a highly selective, non-covalent (reversible) BTK inhibitor in previously treated mantle cell lymphoma: updated results from the phase 1/2 BRUIN study. *Clin Lymphoma Myeloma Leuk* 22 (Suppl 2): S394–S395. doi:10.1016/S2152-2650(22)01569-5. PMID: 36164120.

Dreyling, M., Doorduijin, J.K., Gine, E. et al. (2022). Efficacy and safety of ibrutinib combined with standard first-line treatment or as substitute for autologous stem cell transplantation in younger patients with mantle cell lymphoma: results from the randomized triangle trial by the European MCL network. *Blood* 140 (Suppl 1): 1–3.

Dreyling, M., Goy, A., Hess, G. et al. (2022 Apr 13). Long-term outcomes with ibrutinib treatment for patients with relapsed/refractory mantle cell lymphoma: a pooled analysis of 3 clinical trials with nearly 10 years of follow-up. *Hemasphere* 6 (5): e712.

Eskelund, C.W., Dahl, C., Hansen, J.W. et al. (2017). TP53 mutations identify younger mantle cell lymphoma patients who do not benefit from intensive chemoimmunotherapy. *Blood* 130 (17): 1903–1910.

Jain, et al *Ibrutinib With Rituximab in First-Line Treatment of Older Patients With Mantle Cell Lymphoma*. *JCO*:40, no. 2 (January 10, 2022) 202–212.

Mato, A.R., Shah, N.N., Jurczak, W. et al. (2021). Pirtobrutinib in relapsed or refractory B-cell malignancies (BRUIN): a phase 1/2 study. *Lancet* 397 (10277): 892–901.

Merryman, R.W., Edwin, N., Redd, R. et al. (2020). Rituximab/bendamustine and rituximab/cytarabine induction therapy for transplant-eligible mantle cell lymphoma. *Blood Adv* 4 (5): 858–867.

Minson, A., Hamad, N., Cheah, C.Y. et al. (2022). Time-limited ibrutinib and tisagenlecleucel is highly effective in the treatment of patients with relapsed or refractory mantle cell lymphoma, including those with *TP53* mutated and Btki-refractory disease: first report of the tarmac study. *Blood* 140 (Suppl 1): 181–183.

Ruan, J., Martin, P., Christos, P. et al. (2018). Five-year follow-up of lenalidomide plus rituximab as initial treatment of mantle cell lymphoma. *Blood* 132 (19): 2016–2025.

Wang, M., Munoz, J., Goy, A. et al. (2020). KTE-X19 CAR T-cell therapy in relapsed or refractory mantle-cell lymphoma (Brexucabtagene autoleucel). *N Engl J Med* 382: 1331–1342.

Wang, M., Rule, S., Zinzani, P.L. et al. (2018). Acalabrutinib in relapsed or refractory mantle cell lymphoma (ACE-LY-004): a single-arm, multicentre, phase 2 trial. *Lancet* 391 (10121): 659–667.

Wang, M.L., Jurczak, W., Jerkeman, M. et al. (2022 Jun 30). Ibrutinib plus bendamustine and rituximab in untreated mantle-cell lymphoma. *N Engl J Med* 386 (26): 2482–2494. doi:10.1056/NEJMoa2201817. Epub 2022 Jun 3. PMID: 35657079.

Wang, M.L., Blum, K.A., Martin, P. et al. (2015). Long-term follow-up of MCL patients treated with single-agent ibrutinib: updated safety and efficacy results. *Blood* 126 (6): 739–745.

Wang et al. *Ibrutinib plus Bendamustine and Rituximab in Untreated Mantle-Cell Lymphoma. (The SHINE trial) NEJM* 2022; 386:2482–2494.

37

Marginal Zone Lymphoma

Erin Mulvey, Wayne Tam, and Peter Martin

Weill Cornell Medicine, Department of Medicine, New York, NY
Weill Cornell Medicine, Department of Pathology and Laboratory Medicine, New York, NY

Introduction

Marginal zone lymphomas (MZLs) are a heterogenous group of indolent non-Hodgkin lymphomas (NHLs) comprised of three distinct clinicopathologic entities: nodal MZL (NMZL), extranodal MZL of mucosa-associated lymphoma tissue (MALT lymphoma), and splenic MZL (SMZL). MZLs are frequently associated with chronic immune stimulation and share some common molecular features; however, each entity presents its own specific genotypic findings and clinical manifestations. In the Western world, MZLs accounts for approximately 5–15% of all NHLs, with extranodal MZLs representing approximately 70% of cases, SMZL 20% of cases, and NMZL < 10% of cases. In the United States, it is estimated that there are 1000 to 2300 cases per year of MZL, with a median age of diagnosis of 67 years old and a slight male predominance. The five-year survival rates are estimated at 76.5% for NMZL, 88.7% for MALT lymphoma, and 79.7% for SMZL. While the majority of MZLs have a relatively indolent course, transformation to diffuse large B-cell lymphoma (DLBCL) occurs in 5–10% of cases.

1) How is marginal zone lymphoma (MZL) distinguished from other non-Hodgkin lymphomas (NHLs)?

Expert Perspective: MZLs originate in the marginal zone B-cells of lymph nodes, spleen, or mucosa-associated lymphoid tissue. The marginal zone is particularly prominent in areas of chronic exposure to antigenic stimulation, from either infectious or inflammatory sources. Exactly how chronic inflammation results in tumorigenesis is unclear and may vary among the different MZL subtypes. It is likely that there is a stepwise progression from reactive B-cell, to localized antigendependent tumor, to antigen independence and more aggressive phenotypes. Ultimately, abnormal B-cell clones arise and then proliferate and replace the normal B-cell population.

Cytological features of MZLs are quite variable. They can resemble germinal center centrocytes, with small to medium size, slightly irregular nuclei, moderately clumped chromatin, and inconspicuous nucleoli. Sometimes they have a monocytoid appearance with round or irregular nuclei, more abundant pale cytoplasm, and distinct cytoplasmic membranes. In some cases, they resemble closely small lymphocytes. Plasmacytoid or plasmacytic differentiation can be seen in up to 30–50% of cases. Scattered larger transformed cells resembling centroblasts or immunoblasts are usually present. These large cells should not constitute the majority of the cells present, become confluent, or form diffuse sheets, which would signify disease progression and transformation to large-cell lymphoma. The growth pattern of the lymphoma cells is frequently parafollicular with a marginal zone distribution. Interfollicular and diffuse areas of involvement may also be seen. In nodal MZL (NMZL) and extranodal MZL of mucosa-associated lymphoid tissue (MALT lymphomas), residual reactive follicles are frequently present, which can be hyperplastic, regressed, or sometimes colonized by neoplastic cells. The typical immunophenotype of MZL is CD20+, CD79a+, CD5−, CD10−, and CD23−. CD21 can be positive. Most nodal MZLs and MALT lymphomas are sIgM+ and IgD−, while sIgG+ and sIgA+ are less common. Splenic MZL (SMZL) is typically sIgMD+. Rare cases of MZL are CD5+ and may carry a worse prognosis. Two markers, immune receptor translocation-associated protein 1 (IRTA1) and myeloid nuclear differentiation antigen (MNDA), are clinically useful to help distinguish MZL from other indolent B-cell lymphomas. IRTA1 expression was detected in 42% of 74 MZLs vs 2% of other small B-cell neoplasms ($P < 0.001$). MNDA staining was positive in 64% of MZLs, and its expression was particularly uncommon in follicular lymphoma (21%; $P = 0.003$). Neoplastic B-cells in cases with plasmacytoid or plasmacytic differentiation express MUM1–IRF4 and monocytypic cytoplasmic immunoglobulins. Evidence of plasmacytic differentiation is uncommon in chronic lymphocytic leukemia/small lmphocytic lymphoma (CLL/SLL), mantle cell lymphoma (MCL), and follicular lymphoma (FL). Extranodal MZLs are commonly associated with chromosomal abnormalities including trisomy 3 or 18, and translocations t(11;18)(q21;q21), t(14;18)(q32;q21), and t(1;14) (p22;q32) leading to upregulation and constituative activation of the nuclear factor kappa B (NF-kB) pathway through the BCL10/MALT1 signaling complex, suggesting a vital role in its pathogenesis as well as a potential target for future therapies. Another frequently identified translocation, t(3;14)(p12;q32), fuses the FOXP1 gene on chromosome 3 to the IgH gene, resulting in elevated nuclear levels of the FOXP1 transcription factor. Sequencing efforts have identified distinctive molecular profiles of MZLs. Mutations in NOTCH2 and KLF2, which are genes involved in the differentiation and homeostasis of MZ B cells, are hallmark of MZL, mainly SMZL and NMZL, suggesting that deregulation of MZ B-cell development pathway plays a key role in the pathogenesis of these lymphomas.

Due to limitations in available pathologic material, it can be challenging to differentiate MZL from other subtypes of indolent B-cell lymphomas, and "small B-cell lymphoma" is frequently reported as the diagnosis. The following subquestions discuss diagnoses that can be confused with MZL and tips to differentiate between them. A collaborative effort between clinicians and pathologists is often required to arrive at the correct diagnosis.

- **How is MZL distinguished from chronic lymphocytic leukemia/small lymphocytic lymphoma (CLL/SLL)?**

Expert Perspective: CLL/SLL are characterized by small lymphocytes in the peripheral blood, bone marrow, spleen, and lymph nodes. The typical immunophenotype is CD5 + and CD23 + . Rare cases of CD5 + MZL can be difficult to distinguish from CLL and SLL. For those cases, dim CD20 and surface immunoglobulin expressions, as well as lack of FMC7, favor CLL or SLL. Immunohistochemistry for the lymphocyte enhancer-binding factor 1 (LEF1) can be a useful marker in the differential diagnosis of CLL/SLL in difficult cases. LEF1 is present in about 70% of CLL/SLL and is negative in the vast majority of MZL. A nodal or extranodal clinical presentation with minimal marrow involvement favors a diagnosis of MZL but should not be used as the sole criterion for differentiation. Morphologically, CLL and SLL tend to exhibit more monotony and have a diffuse growth pattern. Proliferation centers (pseudo-follicles) are frequently seen, particularly in the lymph nodes. MZL is characterized by small to medium-sized lymphocytes resembling small lymphocytes, centrocytes or monocytoid cells, with a marginal zone or diffuse growth pattern. In addition, plasmacytic and plasmacytoid differentiation is common in MZL but not CLL or SLL. Except for unusual cases, these diseases do not share common cytogenetic abnormalities, and fluorescent in situ hybridization (FISH) for common genetic anomalies associated with CLL, SLL, and MZL can be helpful in differentiating MZL from CLL/SLL. The commonly observed chromosomal abnormalities in CLL/SLL, including deletions in 13q14.3, trisomy 12 and 11q deletion, are not seen in MZL, while gains in chromosome 3 and 18, as well as the recurrent chromosomosomal translocations seen in MALT, are not present in CLL/SLL. Mutation profile of CLL/SLL is also noticeably different from MZL. The most commonly mutated genes in CLL/SLL, affecting ~ 3–15% of cases, are NOTCH 1, SF3B1, TP53, ATM, BIRC3, POT1 and MYD88.

- **How is follicular lymphoma (FL) distinguished from MZL?**

Expert Perspective: FL is the most common indolent non-Hodgkin lymphoma and can present similarly to MZL. However, the vast majority of FL cases are primary nodal FL, although extranodal dissemination can occur. FL is characterized by a follicular growth pattern, consisting of neoplastic germinal centers with markedly attenuated or absent mantle zones. Nodal MZL and MALT occasionally have a follicular growth pattern mimicking FL when follicular colonization is extensive. Staining for germinal center–associated markers such as BCL6 and CD10, as well as BCL2 and Ki67, may also help to distinguish between FL and MZL with prominent follicular colonization. The residual germinal center B cells are BCL6 and CD10 positive and BCL2 negative, with a very high proliferation rate highlighted by Ki67; the neoplastic MZL cells infiltrating the follicles are BCL6 and CD10 negative and BCL2 positive, with a low proliferation rate. FL with marginal zone differentiation may mimic nodal NZL. In those cases, immunostains with BCL6 and CD10 will help in the diagnostic evaluation. SMZLs usually have a micronodular growth pattern that may be mistaken for FL with splenic infiltration. However, the biphasic appearance of SMZL, coupled with the lack of BCL6 and CD10, differentiates it from FL. CD21 staining to highlight the distribution of follicular dendritic cell (FDC) meshwork is also useful in differentiating between FL and MZL (nodal and MALT types). In FL, FDC meshworks are often expanded and relatively more regular. In MZLs, the FDC meshworks can be expanded and fragmented when follicles are run over or colonized by the neoplastic MZL cells, or they can be small and tight, as seen in regressed follicles. While the majority (about 80%) of FL harbor t(14;18)(q32; 21) involving the *BCL2* gene, t(14;18)(q32; 21) can also be found in a small percentage of MALT lymphomas. However, the *MALT1* gene, not BCL2, is rearranged in t(14:18) in MALT lymphoma. Mutations in *KMT2D* (MLL2), *TNFRSF14*, and *EZH2* are common in FL. *KMT2D* mutations can also be seen in MZL, particularly in NMZL (~34%), but this frequency is much less compared to FL (~85%).

- **How is mantle cell lymphoma (MCL) distinguished from MZL?**

Expert Perspective: MCL typically presents with lymphadenopathy, but bone marrow and gastrointestinal tract involvement are very common. Morphologically, lymph nodes involved by MCL have a nodular or diffuse growth of monotonous small to medium-sized lymphocytes with irregular nuclear contours. MCL is CD5+, CD23−/dim+, FMC7+, and CD43+ and is characterized by overexpression of cyclin D1 and the presence of t(11;14). FISH for t(11;14) is almost always positive, even in CD5− cases, making it relatively easy to distinguish from other types of lymphoma, including MZL. Cyclin D1–negative MCL may be difficult to distinguish from CD5-positive MZL. SOX11 is a useful ancillary stain in those circumstances. SOX11 is frequently positive in MCL, while it is negative in MZL.

- **How is lymphoplasmacytic lymphoma (LPL) distinguished from MZL?**

Expert Perspective: LPL is an indolent lymphoma of small B lymphocytes with plasmacytic differentiation (i.e. plasmacytoid lymphocytes and plasma cells are also present); it tends to involve the bone marrow but can be found in lymph nodes or spleen in 15–30% of cases. A paraprotein, usually immunoglobulin M (IgM), is common but is not diagnostic of LPL and can also occur in cases of MZL with plasmacytoid differentiation. There is considerable morphologic and immunophenotypic overlap between MZL and LPL. Centrocyte-like and monocytoid cells, which can be seen in MZL, are absent in LPL. However, in bone marrow biopsies, neoplastic MZL cells appear often as small lymphocytes, and MZL with plasmacytoid and plasmacytic differentiation can be difficult to distinguish from LPL, especially when the involvement by the former is extensive. Immunohistochemistry is rarely helpful in differentiating between LPL and MZL with evidence of plasmacytic differentiation. CD25 is more commonly positive in LPL, and CD11c is more commonly positive in MZL. The neoplastic B cells and plasma cells in LPL usually express IgM, sometimes IgG, and rarely IgA. IgD is typically negative. This heavy-chain expression pattern may sometimes by useful in differentiating LP from SMZL, as the latter is predominantly IgMD-positive. Comparative genomic hybridization may help to differentiate MZL from LPL. While the two entities may share deletions of 6q23 and gains of 3q13–q28, 6p, and 18q, gains of 4q and 8q are associated with LPL but not MZL. The L256P hotspot mutation of the MYD88 gene may be helpful in establishing the diagnosis of LPL in pathologically challenging cases. MYD88 L256P mutation was present in nearly all cases of LPL (> 90%) but was uncommon in MZL, reported only in ~10% of SMZL, ~6–9% of MALT, and ~10% in NMZL.

- **How are other indolent splenic B-cell lymphomas distinguished from SMZLs?**

Expert Perspective: The differential diagnoses for SMZLs include several small B-cell lymphomas involving the spleen that are recognized by the World Health Organization (WHO) as hairy cell leukemia (HCL) and splenic B-cell lymphoma, unclassifiable. The two best-defined provisional entities with the category of splenic B-cell lymphoma, unclassifiable are splenic diffuse red pulp small B-cell lymphoma (SDRPL) and hairy cell leukemia variant (HCL-v). Differentiation of these entities by peripheral blood cytology can be difficult since they share similarities including the presence of villi. Other morphologic features are more distinct among these entities. In the spleen, SMZL involves the white pulp and also the red pulp in a follicular or micronodular pattern. A biphasic cytological pattern typically observed is characterized by small round lymphocytes in the interior of the follicles surrounded by an outer zone of marginal zone cells with more abundant pale cytoplasm, admixed with scattered larger transformed cells. Splenic diffuse red pulp small B-cell lymphoma involves the red pulp with both cord and sinusoidal patterns. The neoplastic cell population is composed of small to medium-sized lymphocytes with round and regular nuclei and clumped chromatin monotonous with scattered larger cells with more prominent nucleoli. It does not show follicular replacement, biphasic cytology, or marginal zone infiltration. An intrasinusoidal infiltration pattern is consistently seen in the bone marrow. HCL and HCL-v diffusely involve the red pulp, and the white pulp is atrophic. Immunophenotypically, SMZL cells express IgM and almost always IgD, while splenic diffuse red pulp small B-cell lymphoma, HCL, and HCL-v tend to be IgG positive. CD103 and CD11c are more frequently positive in HCL and HCL-v. Contrary to SMZL, HCL is also positive for annexin A1, TRAP, and CD25. About 40% of SMZLs show allelic loss of chromosome 7q22–36, which is not found in splenic diffuse red pulp small B-cell lymphoma. HCL has been found to harbor a V600E mutation in the BRAF gene, leading to constituative activation and ongocenic signlaing throught the MEK-ERK cascade. This may serve as a molecular marker for HCL that could potentially distinguish it from SMZL, although it has not yet been adopted into diagnostic criteria. While HCLv typically exhibits wild-type BRAF, activating mutations in the MAP2K1 gene encoding MEK1 are found in most cases. In the upcoming 5th edition of World Health Organization (WHO) Classification of Haematolymphoid Tumours, HCLv is no longer considered as a separte entity but instead placed in a newly proposed diagnostic category termed splenic B-cell lymphoma/leukemia with prominent nucleoli (SBLPN), along with B-prolymphocytic leukemia (B-PLL). This re-classification of HCLv is proposed because HCLv appears to be biologically distinct from HCL and is morphologically similar to B-PLL with regard to the prominence of the nucleoli. However, this new classificaton is not universally accepted, as HCLv remains as a separate entity in the International Consensus Classification (ICC). Although analysis of both bone marrow and peripheral blood lymphocytes is the primary means of diagnosis, occasionally the only way to acquire sufficient material for pathologic diagnosis is to perform a splenectomy. Under these circumstances, the clinician must weigh the benefits of having a precise diagnosis against the risks of the procedure.

2) How are the types of MZL distinguished?

- **How is SMZL different from nodal MZL and MALT lymphoma?**

Expert Perspective: Although considered an MZL like nodal MZL and MALT lymphoma, SMZL actually is quite distinct from the other two entities in terms of clinical, immunophenotypic, and genetic features. The putative origin of SMZL is a splenic B cell of unknown differentiation stage with variable somatic mutations (present in about 50% of cases) in the Ig heavy-chain variable (IGHV) region. Its relationship to normal marginal zone B cells is controversial, but it is thought that SMZL might develop from a B cell that has been exposed to chronic antigenic stimulation in the germinal center and has the capacity for marginal zone differentiation supported by the splenic environment. Analysis of the B-cell receptors of SMZL revealed stereotypical antigen-binding regions and selective usage of specific immunoglobulin heavy variable alleles, for example VH1-2, implying that stimulation of the B-cell clones is driven by a common antigen. SMZL is frequently associated with hepatitis C infection. The mechanism may involve an interaction between the HCV E2 glycoprotein, with CD81 resulting in B-cell receptor activation and proliferation of B cells.

Although SMZL shares some cytogenetics abnormalities, for example, gains of chromosomes 3 and 18 and loss of 6q23-24, with NMZL and MALT, there are distinct cytogenetics differences among the entities. Deletion 7q is present in about 30% of SMZL and is rarely found in other lymphoma subtypes, including NMZL and MALT lymphoma. In addition, SMZL lacks the recurrent reciprocal translocations frequently present in other B-cell lymphomas, including those associated with MALT lymphomas: t(11;18)(q21;q21) (BIRC3-MALT1), t(14;18)(q32;q21) (IGH-MALT1), t(1;14)(p22;q21) (IGH-BCL10), and t(3;14)(p12;q32) (IGH-FOXP1). Genomic profiling of SMZL revealed KLF2 and NOTCH2 mutations as the most frequent genetic lesions (10–40% and 10–25% of cases, respectively). Other members of the NOTCH pathway are also recurrently targeted by genetic lesions. In addition, mutations in other signaling pathways, including NF-kB, chromatin remodeling/ transcription regulation, B-cell receptor, and TP53 pahtways, can also be seen. Mutations in KLF2 and NOTCH2 are also frequently seen in NMZL (~14% and 20%, respectively), implying a biologic link between SMZL and NMZL. However, there are distinct genetic differences between SMZL and NMZL (see next section), supporting that these are related but different entities and justifying the WHO classification of these tumors.

Patients with SMZL typically present with splenomegaly and associated cytopenias. Lactate dehydrogenase is typically within normal limits, but beta 2-microglobulin is frequently elevated. A monoclonal paraprotein is seen in 10–40% of cases. These patients often have splenomegaly but are not always symptomatic. Autoimmune hemolytic anemia, immune thrombocytopenic purpura, cold agglutinin, acquired von Willebrand disease, lupus anticoagulant, and other autoimmune phenomena are found in 10–15% of SMZL patients. SMZL commonly involves the bone marrow as well as peripheral blood and splenic hilar lymph nodes. Dissemination to other extranodal sites is uncommon, making clinical presentation one of the more important diagnostic factors. The diagnosis of SMZL is typically made from morphologic and immunophenotypic examination of peripheral blood or bone marrow; examination of the spleen pathology is not usually required. SMZLs frequently have peripheral blood involvement, which is rare in nodal MZL and MALT lymphoma. The immunophenotype of SMZL is similar to that of other MZLs, except that IgD is almost always present in SMZL but tends to be absent in MALT lymphoma and NZML.

- ### How is nodal MZL (NMZL) different from SMZL and MALT lymphoma?

Expert Perspective: NMZL was categorized as a distinct type of lymphoma in the 2008 as well as the most recent 2017 WHO classifications. It develops in lymph nodes and is often disseminated at presentation (stage III–IV). Reported five-year OS in NMZL ranges from 55 to 75% as compared to 50–85% in SMZL and 85% in MALT lymphoma. For a primitive diagnosis of NMZL, primary involvement of extranodal sites must be excluded, as one-third of cases with nodal involvement are secondary to extranodal disease. NMZL is less likely to be associated with autoimmune disease than MALT lymphoma, although cases of hemolytic anemia have been reported. SMZL often involves splenic hilar lymph nodes and, infrequently, other peripheral lymph nodes. Dissemination to bone marrow is found more frequently in SMZL than NMZL but occurs in about one-half of patients with NMZL. NMZL may be difficult to distinguish from nodal dissemination of a MALT lymphoma or

SMZL in lymph node biopsies based on morphological grounds. Thus, a thorough clinical history is very important for making this distinction.

Pathologically, in both NMZL and MALT lymphoma, the neoplastic B cells can resemble small lymphocytes or centrocytes or have a monocytoid appearance. Variable number of scattered larger transformed cells are present. They can be seen surrounding reactive germinal centers and infiltrating to the interfollicular area, with occasional follicular colonization, diffuse growth pattern, or plasma cell differentiation. In some cases of NMZL, the growth pattern can mimic that of SMZL, with a micronodular growth pattern and sparing of the sinuses. The presence of IgD favors SMZL, as NMZL is usually IgD negative. Other immunophenotypic markers are not useful in distinguishing NMZL from SMZL or MALT lymphoma. These three MZL entities share overlapping cytogenetic abnormalities, including trisomy 3 or 18 and loss of 6q23–24. However, NMZLs lack the del(7q) commonly seen in SMZL and the reciprocal chromosomal translocations associated with MALT lymphoma. Compared to SMZL, NMZLs harbor similar molecularly deregulated pathways including chromsome remodeling and transcriptional regulation, NF-kB pathway and NOTCH pathway, and share similar mutation signature characterized by mutations in NOTCH2 and KFL2, with the exception of KMT2D (MLL2) and receptor protein tyrosine phosphatase delta (PTPRD) mutations. Mutations in KMT2D are present much more frequently in NMZL than in SMZL (~34% vs ~8%). PTPRD mutations and deletions are enriched in NMZL (~20%), rare in other B-cell lymphomas (< 1%), and absent in SMZL and MALT lymphomas. These lesions are deleterious to the normal functions of PTPRD, which is a tumor suppressor known to be frequently mutated and inactivated in other human cancers. Genetic alterations in PTPRD, though not highly sensitive, can potentially be used as a useful biomarker for the diagnosis of NMZL. In addition, their enrichment in NMZL supports the current lymphoma classification of NMZL as a distinct clinico-pathologic entity.

Treatment Controversies

3) What is the role of splenectomy in SMZL?

Expert Perspective: Splenectomy may serve both diagnostic and therapeutic roles in SMZL. Although the gold standard for diagnosis is evaluation of spleen histology, splenectomy is infrequently worthwhile as a purely diagnostic procedure. The morphology, immunophenotype, and cytogenetics of peripheral blood and bone marrow can be used to make the diagnosis in most cases. Diagnostic splenectomy is absolutely indicated only when more aggressive lymphomas or histologic transformation is suspected, and interventional radiology–guided biopsy is not safe. The degree of fluoro-deoxyglucose uptake seen on positron emission tomography imaging can be associated with indolent versus aggressive histologies and can be helpful in guiding management.

When SMZL is associated with hepatitis C virus (HCV), antiviral treatment should be initiated, as pegylated interferon and ribavirin have been shown to result in a complete remission of SMZL in 75% of cases. Many patients with HCV-indepentent SMZL can be monitored closely without treatment until cytopenias or symptoms secondary to splenomegaly necessitate therapeutic intervention. Therapeutic splenectomy is followed by a median of eight years without treatment despite persistent bone marrow and peripheral blood involvement and is commonly cited as the standard first-line approach in patients who are fit for surgery. Importantly, patients undergoing splenectomy should receive pre-operative immunizations and appropriate lifelong antibacterial prophylaxis. Over the past two decades, the therapeutic splenectomy has declined significantly, largely related to increasing experience with rituximab. In contrast to the morbidity and mortality associated with splenectomy, single-agent rituximab is associated with minimal impact on quality of life, results in a low risk of infection, appears to result in durable remissions in most patients, and may be reused successfully at the time of relapse. A study of 108 patients with SMZL requiring treatment reported that six weekly infusions of rituximab given in the front-line setting followed by optional maintanence therapy resulted in an overall response rate of 92% (98 of 106), with complete response or unconfirmed complete response achieved in 65% (69 of 106) of patients and partial reponse in 27% (29/106). Following a median follow-up of 57 months, the 5- and 10-year freedom-from-progression rates were 71% and 64%, respectively and 5- and 10-year overall survival rates were 93% and 85%.

In the IELSG36 study, 56 patients with SMZL were treated with rituximab plus benda-mustine for up to six cycles. Hematological toxicity, especially neutropenia, was common, and roughly 5% of patients experienced neutropenic fever, while 9% of patients went off study due to toxicity. The overall and complete response rates were 91% and 73%, respectively, with a three-year progression-free survival of 93%. A retrospective review of 43 patients with SMZL reported that 34/43 patients treated with rituximab (either alone or in addition to chemotherapy) achieved a complete response. Disease-free survival at three years was 79% with rituximab and 29% with splenectomy alone. Rituximab monotherapy appeared equally as effective as rituximab combined with chemotherapy (90% vs 79%, $P = 0.7$) with significantly fewer toxicities.

We therefore rarely recommend diagnostic or therapeutic splenectomy. We recommend watchful waiting in asymptomatic patients with SMZL, antiviral therapy for those cases associated with HCV, and a consideration of rituximab for front-line treatment in symptomatic patients who are HCV negative. The addition of chemotherapy to rituximab should be considered depending on patient factors (e.g. age and comorbid conditions) and disease factors (e.g. the extent of disease and acuity of illness).

4) What is the best treatment for localized MALT lymphoma?

Expert Perspective: Here, we review treatment of early-stage MALT lymphomas. While there is evidence to support treatment of localized MALT in particular sites, a review of 44 patients with stage I–II MALT did not find a significant difference in five-year overall survival among those patients treated with curative intent versus those who were not treated with curative intent. Nevertheless, options for treatment of localized MALT include surgical resection, radiation, and various chemoimmunotherapy regimens.

- **What is the role of surgery for pulmonary MZL (or bronchial-associated lymphoid tissue [BALT] lymphoma)?**

Expert Perspective: BALT lymphomas, like other types of MZL, are indolent and often remain solely in the lung(s) for many years. A standard treatment approach has not yet been established. The largest cohort identified was 326 patients from the SEER database. Fifty-one percent were treated with surgery. All the patients who had surgical resection of BALT lymphoma had a complete response. The second most common treatment modality was radiation (7%). Median overall survival was 112 months. This suggests that these patients do well regardless of treatment modality.

In addition to surgical resection, radiation, or watchful waiting, several small studies have reported outcomes following treatment with various chemotherapy regimens. Reponses related to treatment with rituximab were often reported in combination with chemotherapy regimens and rarely as a single agent. In a review of 21 patients, responses to chemotherapy regimens, including (i) cyclophosphamide, vincristine, prednisone (CVP) or (ii) chlorambucil and prednisone were variable: two patients had complete response, two had partial response, two had stable disease, and one had progressive disease. The four untreated patients remained free from progression of the disease after 40.5 months. Second-line treatment with radiation resulted in complete response in all patients who were treated with that modality. A review of 22 patients suggested that surgery is optimal for unilateral disease whereas multifocal disease could be treated with combination chemotherapy or watchful waiting. In that study, six patients were treated with surgery, two were treated with radiation therapy, and 12 were treated with chemotherapy and/or rituximab. Seven of nine patients who received a complete response had unilateral disease. The two treated with single-agent rituximab had a partial response. All patients, including the 2 of 10 patients with bilateral disease, were alive after a median follow-up time of 36 months. A recent retrospective study of 17 patients treated with fludarabine and mitoxantrone, plus or minus rituximab, reported a complete response in over 80% of patients. Patients were treated up front if they had bilateral disease or if they developed progression respiratory symptoms. All patients who received fludarabine and mitoxantrone plus rituximab achieved complete response. At a median follow-up time of five years, 75% of patients were still in complete response. The reported side effects were primarily related to myelosuppression.

Given the indolent nature of the disease, we believe that asymptomatic patients with BALT lymphoma can be followed closely without treatment. Surgical resection is a reasonable first-line option for those who have localized disease, although surgery is not without risks and often causes reduction in lung function. Radiation can be considered but may be associated with similar morbidity. No strong data support the use of rituximab monotherapy in BALT lymphoma but given its role in other B-cell lymphomas we typically add it to other systemic therapies. In symptomatic patients, data for treatment with fludarabine and mitoxantrone are compelling, though potential side effects are serious and should be weighed when considering treatment.

- **Which cases of gastric MALT lymphoma are least likely to respond to eradication of *Helicobacter pylori*? Should they be treated with radiation?**

Expert Perspective: Gastric MALT lymphoma is the sole subtype for which strong evidence of response to antibiotic therapy exists. However, among patients with early-stage gastric MALT lymphoma, the response to *H. pylori* eradication varies from 60 to 100%. First, those patients without evidence of *H. pylori* infection are unlikely to respond to antibiotic therapy. Second, gastric lymphomas with the t(11;18) cytogenetic aberration are unlikely to respond to *H. pylori* eradication and should probably be managed with alternative therapies such as radiation. Finally, those patients with locally advanced disease (i.e. involvement of the muscularis mucosae or local lymph nodes) have a significantly lower complete response rate. Nonetheless, it may be reasonable to attempt antibiotic therapy in patients with locally advanced disease without other indications for more aggressive therapy since the disease is likely to be indolent and *H. pylori* eradication would otherwise be recommended. Patients with localized disease that does not respond to *H. pylori* eradication should be considered for radiotherapy. Despite the potential advantage of therapy with curative intent, there is no evidence that it necessarily prolongs survival, and watchful waiting can be considered in asymptomatic patients. Most of these patients will eventually require radiotherapy or chemotherapy.

- **Should ocular adnexal MALT lymphoma (OAMZL) be treated with antibiotics?**

Expert Perspective: While there is agreement on the value of *H. pylori* eradication in gastric MALT lymphomas, a bacterial etiology in nongastrointestinal MALT lymphomas has been less clearly established. MZL of the ocular adnexae (conjunctiva, lacrimal gland, or orbit soft tissue) has been associated with Chlamydial psittaci infection. Diagnosis of C. psittaci requires a labor-intensive process of PCR from DNA extracted from ocular specimens or conjunctival swabs. The detection of this infection in patients with ocular adnexal MZL varies significantly depending on geographic location even within the same country. The highest incidence has been reported in Italy, Austria, Korea, and Germany. A phase II trial in Italy investigated the use of doxycycline 100 mg daily for three weeks in patients with stage IE MZL of the ocular adnexae. The patients in this study received antibiotic therapy regardless of their chlamydial infection status. Eradication of C. psittaci was documented in 14/34 patients with objective regression of the lymphoma in 12 of those cases (six complete responses and six partial responses). A study of 38 patients reported that OAMZL patients initially unresponsive to a three-week course of doxycycline demonstrated an improved response after a second three-week course of the antibiotic. The use of clarithromycin 500 mg orally twice daily for six months has also been evaluated in a pilot study of 13 patients with relapsed/refractory EMZL who were previously treated with doxycycline. An overall response rate of 38% was reached, with two patients achieving complete response.

Chemotherapy and radiation therapy are alternate treatment options for OAMZL. Chlorambucil was studied in 33 patients with a median total dose of 600 mg over four courses of treatment; 79% had complete response. Mean follow-up time was 32 months, and no major side effects occurred. The TRGO 05.02/ALLG study evaluated 24–30 Gy in early-stage MZL, including 39 patients with OAMZL. With seven years of follow-up, most patient remained free from disease, and none of the OAMZL patients experienced an in-field relapse. Radiation to the ocular adnexae has been associated with conjunctivitis, dry eye, keratitis, and cataracts.

Single-agent rituximab has infrequently been reported in OAMZL patients. In a study of eight patients treated with this agent, five previously untreated patients had a complete response after receiving rituximab, but the median time to relapse was four months. Radioimmunotherapy with ^{90}Y ibritumomab tiuxetan has also been reported as an effective front-line treatment option and is worthy of further evaluation in this setting.

We do not think that antibiotics are sufficient to cure most cases of ocular adnexal MZL, particularly in North America. However, in certain populations and in asymptomatic individuals, it may be worthwhile to start with a trial of doxycycline. Radiotherapy is currently the most accepted front-line treatment for symptomatic patients, although systemic therapy is also a reasonable option. As with other indolent lymphomas, we believe that it is important to avoid overtreatment and frequently observe asymptomatic patients or pursue trials of less aggressive treatment (single-agent rituximab) before initiating radiotherapy or chemotherapy.

● **How should primary cutaneous MZL (PCMZL) be managed?**

Expert Perspective: PCMZL is an uncommon form of MZL in which patients present with unifocal or, more commonly, multifocal cutaneous lesions. Two types of PCMZL have been described on the basis of surface immunoglobulins expression. The "class-switched" group expresses IgG or, more rarely, IgA and IgE, and is characterized by a nodular and scattered distribution of B cells in a T-cell helper 2 environment. The "non-class-switched" group expresses IgM and is characterized by a diffuse distribution of B cells and a less represented T-cell population. IgM-positive cases more frequently show secondary skin involvement of MZL. PCMZL can also show evidence of plasmacytic differentiation, becoming more progressively plasmacytic with cutaneous recurrences over time.

Primary cutaneous marginal zone lymphoma has been associated with Borrelia burgdorferi infection in Europe where the B. afselii strain is endemic; however, such a link has not been established in North America or Asia. The efficacy of antibiotic treatment in B burdorferi–associated PCMZL has not been clearly demonstrated. A retrospective review of several case reports and series found that 6 of 14 patients with B burdorferi–associated PCMZL achieved complete response with various antibiotic regimens.

Rarely does PCMZL develop extracutaneous manifestations in the absence of aggressive transformation. Management is dependent on the extent of the disease. Solitary lesions or regional disease can be treated with curative intent using local radiotherapy and/or surgical resection, but relapse at a distant site is common. We do not believe the data supports the use of antibiotic therapy in North America. Other options for skin-directed therapy include topical treaments such as steroids, imiquimod, nitrogen mustard, and bexarotene, or intralesional steroids, interferon-alpha, or rituximab. Generalized skin disease can often be managed with observation alone in asymptomatic patients. Systemic treatment options include rituximab or chemotherapy. A retrospective analysis of 35 patients with indolent primary cutaneous lymphomas, including 18 patients with MZL treated with intralesional rituximab (often in second- or third-line settings), reported complete response of 71% with a median follow-up of 21 months. Though the complete response rate with intralesional or intravenous rituximab is less than that observed with surgery or radiotherapy, it is a reasonable option for treatment in cases in which there are multiple lesions or lesions located in areas in which it would be difficult to surgically excise or radiate. Chemotherapy should be reserved for cases that fail to respond to these approaches or cases with extracutaneous disease, suggesting a more aggressive biology.

5) What is the optimal first-line treatment for advanced-stage NMZL?

Expert Perspective: There is no standard front-line treatment approach for advanced NMZL. A prognostic scale has not been developed specifically for NMZL, but the International Prognostic Index (IPI) and Follicular Lymphoma International Prognostic Index (FLIPI) scales have been used to stratify patients with NMZL. Overall, patients with NMZL tend to have a poorer prognosis than those with MALT lymphoma even in stage IV disease; they also have a poorer prognosis than patients with FL or CLL. Asymptomatic patients with a low tumor burden can be monitored without treatment. We generally avoid front-line use of purine analogs due to concern over risk of myelodysplasia. Controversy exists regarding the use of regimens containing anthracyclines, with some suggesting that anthracyclines should be considered in NMZL because of a more aggressive course than other MZLs. Based on the reported efficacy of non-anthracycline regimens, we typically reserve anthracyclines for use in patients with known or suspected large cell transformation. The recent phase III study comparing bendamustine–rituximab (BR) with rituximab, cyclophosphamide, doxorubicin, vincristine, and prednisone (R-CHOP) in patients with indolent or mantle cell lymphoma included a small number of patients with NMZL and SMZL. Although this study reported a significant increase in median progression-free survival with BR in the overall study population (69.5 vs 31.2 months; hazard ratio: 0.58; 95% CI 0.44–0.74), this difference was not significant in patients with MZL. To date, there have been no phase III studies that have evaluated the addition of rituximab to chemotherapy in patients with NMZL. The International Extranodal Lymphoma Study Group (IELSG) 19 trial evaluated chlorambucil with or without rituximab in patients with advanced-stage MALT lymphoma and found a superior response rate and event-free survival with no difference in OS at five years. We recommend managing patients with advanced-stage ENMZL similarly to patients with FL. We generally observe asymptomatic cases, consider rituximab as a single agent in low-risk patients, and treat with rituximab plus chemotherapy in patients with more extensive and/or symptomatic disease.

6) What is the role of maintenance rituximab?

Expert Perspective: The RESORT trial reported on the use of maintenance rituximab in patients with previously untreated, low-tumor-burden CLL, SLL, MZL, and FL. All but one of the 137 patients with MZL, CLL, or SLL were at stage III–IV. Each patient was treated with single-agent rituximab 375 mg/m^2 weekly for four weeks. The 57 patients who achieved a complete response or partial response were randomized to receive maintenance rituximab (one treatment every three months) or rituximab at time of progression (four treatments). In contrast to patients with FL, fewer patients with CLL, SLL, and MZL responded to the initial rituximab, but of those who did respond, the time to treatment failure was significantly longer in those treated with maintenance rituximab (3.74 years) versus treatment at time of progression (1.07 years). This suggests that there may be a role for maintenance rituximab in those patients with low-tumor-burden MZL who respond to single-agent rituximab when given as front-line therapy. The use of rituximab maintenance following immunochemotherapy has not been adequately evaluated in MZL. We recommend caution when extrapolating data from phase III trials in other histologies and general avoid maintenance in this setting.

7) What novel agents are available for MZL?

Expert Perspective: While most clinical trials studying targeted therapies in indolent lymphomas are not designed specifically for MZL, there are emering data supporting the use of several novel agents.

The BTK inhibitor ibrutinib is currently approved for MZL based on a single-arm phase II study in 63 patients with MZL with relapsed disease following anti-CD20 antibody therapy. The overall response rate was 48% with two patients achieving complete response. With a median follow-up of 19.4 months, median progression-free survival was 14.2 months. Median progression-free-survival by MZL subtype was 13.8 months for extranodal MZL, 19.4 months for SMZL, and 8.3 months for NMZL. In the MAGNOLIA study, zanu-brutinib was evaluated in 68 patients with relapsed/refractory MZL following prior anti-CD20 therapy. The overall response rate was 56% with a 20% complete response rate and at a median follow-up time of 8.3 months, the median duration of response had not yet been reached, with 85% of responders still in remission at 12 months. These data led to the FDA's approval for zanubrutinib in patients with relapsed or refractory MZL who have received at least one anti-CD20-based regimen.

Lenalidomide has been studied both as a single agent and in combination with rituximab in indolent NHL, including limited numbers of MZL patients, with promising outcomes. A phase II trial combining lenalidomide with rituximab (R^2) in untreated indolent lymphoma reported 18 (67%) complete responses and six (22%) partial reponses among 27 patients with MZL. The phase III AUGMENT trial compared rituximab monotherapy versus R^2 in patients with relapsed/refractory inoldent lymphoma, including 63 patients with MZL. This study demonstrated improved progression-free survival with R^2 vs lenalidomide alone (39.4 months vs 14.1 months); however, in the MZL subgroup there was no statistically significant difference. The ongoing phase III MAGNIFY study is evaluating the optimal duration of lenalidomide therapy in patients with relapsed/refractory FL, MZL, or MCL. Following induction therapy with R^2 for 12 28-day cycles, patients are randomized to con-tinue maintenance with lenalidomide plus rituximab or rituximab alone to complete 30 cycles. After a median follow-up of 23.7 months, the overall response rate to induction R^2 among patients with MZL was 63% with 38% complete response / unconfirmed complete response and median progression-free survival of 41.2 months.

Based on the combined data from these trials, the combination of lenalidomide plus ritux-imab has been approved by the FDA for previously treated marginal zone lymphoma.

PI3K inhibitors have demonstrated activity in several types of NHL, although the data are significantly limited due to small numbers of patients with MZL. Both copanlisib and idelal-isib appear to have activity in relapsed/refractory MZL, with overall response rates of 78% and 53%, respectively; however, these trials included small numbers of MZL patients, and these agents do not have regulatory approval. The FDA withdrew its approval for the oral PI3K inhibitor umbralisib, which had previously been approved for use in patiehts with R/R MZL, due to emerging safety concerns from the phase III UNITY-CLL clinical trial.

Radioimmunotherapy with ^{90}Y ibritumomab tiuxetan, a murine anti-CD20 monoclonal antibody conjugated to the radioisotope yttrium-90, is approved by the FDA for use in patients with relapsed or refractory low-grade B-cell NHL or previously untreated follic-ular lymphoma who achieve a partial or complete response to first-line chemotherapy. In the phase II Zeno trial, 30 patients with relapsed or refractory extranodal MZL received ^{90}Y ibritumomab tiuxetan. The overall response rate was 90%, with 23 patients achieving a complete response (77%), and four patients achieving a partial response (13%) with a median duration of reponse of 81.3 months.

MZL is unique in the requirement for a multidisciplinary approach to diagnosis, staging, and treatment, especially among pathologists and clinicians. Cooperative groups such as the IELSG, and collaborative relationships between academic and community physicians will play an important role in improving the understanding and management of these lymphomas. MZLs are an interesting group of diverse lymphomas, each one rare as a single entity, but all share a common pathogenesis. As we learn more about the biology of the MZLs, we are likely to discover additional features or therapeutic targets that are common to other B-cell lymphomas.

Recommended Readings

Andorsky, D.J., Coleman, M., Abdulraheem, Y. et al. (2020). MAGNIFY phase IIIb interim analysis of induction R2 followed by maintenance in relapsed/ refractory indolent NHL. *J Clini Oncol* 38 (15_suppl): 8046–8046.

Bertoni, F., Coiffier, B., Salles, G. et al. (2011). MALT lymphomas: pathogenesis can drive treatment. *Oncol* 25 (12): 1134–1142.

Falini, B., Agostinelli, C., Bigerna, B. et al. (2012 Nov). IRTA1 is selectively expressed in nodal and extranodal marginal zone lymphomas. *Histopathol* 61 (5): 930–941.

Ferreri, A.J.M., Govi, S., and Pasini, E. (2012). *Chlamydophila psittaci* eradication with doxycycline as first-line targeted therapy for ocular adnexae lymphoma: final results of an international phase II trial. *J Clin Onc* 30 (24): 2988–2994.

Govi, S., Dognini, G., Licata, G. et al. (2010 Jul). Six-month oral clarithromycin regimen is safe and active in extranodal marginal zone B-cell lymphomas: final results of a single-centre phase II trial. *Br J Haematol.* 150 (2): 226–229.

Huh, S.J., Oh, S.Y., Lee, S. et al. (2020). Mutational analysis of extranodal marginal zone lymphoma using next generation sequencing. *Oncol Lett* 20 (5): 205.

Iannitto, E., Bellei, M., Amorim, S. et al. (2018 December). Efficacy of bendamustine and rituximab in splenic marginal zone lymphoma: results from the phase II BRISMA/IELSG36 study. *Br J Haematol* 183 (5): 755–765. doi: 10.1111/bjh.15641. Epub 2018 Nov 8. PMID: 30407629.

Jaffe, E.S. (2020 January). Navigating the cutaneous B-cell lymphomas: avoiding the rocky shoals. *Mod Pathol* 33 (Suppl 1): 96–106. doi: 10.1038/s41379-019-0385-7.

Kalpadakis, C., Pangalis, G., Sachanas, S. et al. (2018). Rituximab monotherapy in splenic marginal zone lymphoma: prolonged responses and potential benefit from maintenance. *Blood* 132 (6): 666–670.

Kang, H.J., Kim, H.J., Kim, S.J. et al. (2012). Phase II trial of rituximab plus CVP combination chemotherapy for advanced stage marginal zone lymphoma as a first-line therapy: consortium for improving survival of lymphoma (CISL) study. *Ann Hematol* 91: 543–551.

Martinez-Lopez, A., Curiel-Olmo, S., Mollejo, M. et al. (2015). MYD88 (L265P) somatic mutation in marginal zone B-cell lymphoma. *Am J Surg Path* 39 (5): 644–651.

Oquendo, C.J., Parker, H., Oscier, D. *et al.* (2019). Systematic review of somatic mutations in splenic marginal zone lymphoma. *Sci Rep* 9: 10444.

Rossi, D., Trifonov, V., Fangazio, M. et al. (2012). The coding genome of splenic marginal zone lymphoma: activation of NOTCH2 and other pathways regulating marginal zone development. *J Exp Med* 209 (9): 1537–1551.

Spina, V., Khiabanian, H., Messina, M. et al. (2016). The genetics of nodal marginal zone lymphoma. *Blood* 128 (10): 1362–1373.

Stoll, J.R., Willner, J., Oh, Y. et al. (2021 November). Primary cutaneous T-cell lymphomas other than mycosis fungoides and Sézary syndrome – Part 1: clinical and histologic features and diagnosis. *J Am Acad Dermatol* 85 (5): 1073–1090. doi: 10.1016/j.jaad.2021.04.080. Epub 2021 Apr 30. PMID: 33940098S0190–9622(211)00926-9 (E-pub ahead of print).

Thieblemont, C., Davi, F., Noguera, M. et al. (2011). Non-MALT marginal zone lymphoma. *Curr Opin Hematol* 18: 273–279.

Veeriah, S., Brennan, C., Meng, S. et al. (2009 June 9). The tyrosine phosphatase PTPRD is a tumor suppressor that is frequently inactivated and mutated in glioblastoma and other human cancers. *Proc Natl Acad Sci U S A* 106 (23): 9435–9440.

Wang, Z. and Cook, J.R. (2019 February 4). IRTA1 and MNDA expression in marginal zone lymphoma: utility in differential diagnosis and implications for classification. *Am J Clin Pathol* 151 (3): 337–343.

Zinzani, P.L., Pellegrini, C., Gandolfi, L. et al. (2013). Extranodal marginal zone B-cell lymphoma of the lung: experience with fludarabine and mitoxantrone-containing regimens. *Hematol Oncol* 31: 183–188.

Alaggio, R., Amador, C., Anagnostopoulos, I. *et al.* The 5th edition of the World Health Organization Classification of Haematolymphoid Tumours: Lymphoid Neoplasms. *Leukemia* **36**, 1720–1748 (2022). https://doi.org/10.1038/s41375-022-01620-2

Campo E, Jaffe E, Cook J, et al. The International Consensus Classification of Mature Lymphoid Neoplasms: a report from the Clinical Advisory Committee. *Blood* 2022; 140 (11): 1229–1253. doi: https://doi.org/10.1182/blood.2022015851

38

Hematopoietic Cell Transplantation and Cellular Therapy in Indolent Non-Hodgkin's Lymphomas

Karthik Nath[1] and Craig S. Sauter[2]

[1] Adult Bone Marrow Transplant Service, Memorial Sloan Kettering Cancer Center, New York, NY, USA
[2] Taussig Cancer Institute, Cleveland Clinic, Cleveland, OH, USA

Introduction

The role of hematopoietic stem cell transplantation in indolent non-Hodgkin's lymphoma is still being defined. Allogeneic stem cell (allo-HCT) transplant offers a possibility for cure with a substantial graft-versus-lymphoma effect, but non-relapse mortality is a concern. Autologous stem cell transplant is a safer option, but post-transplant relapse remains an issue and randomized data are limited. Furthermore, newer treatments such as cell-based therapies are offering promise and likely to change our approach to the management of these patients. Considering follicular lymphoma constitutes 70% of indolent lymphomas in Western countries, it is this histology in which outcomes are most frequently reported. This chapter will primarily cover the role of hematopoietic cell transplantation and cell therapy in follicular lymphoma.

1) **What is the role of autologous hematopoietic stem cell transplantation (auto-HCT) and allo-HCT in follicular lymphoma (FL) patients with early-relapsing/ refractory (R/R) disease as defined by progression of disease within 24 months of initial induction therapy (POD24)?**

Expert Perspective: Follicular lymphoma (FL) is the second most common type of non-Hodgkin lymphoma (NHL) in Western countries. It is characterized by a waxing and waning disease course wherein patients can experience multiple relapses between disease-free periods. Although patients with prolonged responses have an excellent prognosis, those with early relapse after initial chemoimmunotherapy have dismal outcomes. Casulo et al. first demonstrated that 20% of FL patients treated with up-front R-CHOP (rituximab-cyclophosphamide, doxorubicin, vincristine, prednisone) experience progression of disease within 24 months (POD24) of initial therapy (Casulo et al. 2015). The five-year overall survival in POD24 patients was only 50%, compared to 90% in their non-early-relapsing counterparts (Casulo et al. 2015). Inferior outcomes of POD24 patients have also been reported with up-front bendamustine-rituximab (BR) (Freeman et al. 2019). Notably, the majority of POD24 patients had histological transformation in this cohort, and treatment recommendations for transformed FL are provided in responses to questions 6 and 7 of this chapter (also see Chapters 35 and 43) (Freeman et al. 2019). Obinutuzumab-based chemoimmunotherapy was shown to reduce POD24 rates compared to rituximab-based chemoimmunotherapy, but this study also validated previous findings that early disease progression in FL is associated with a poor prognosis irrespective of the initial treatment arm (John et al. 2019). As such, POD24 has emerged as an important endpoint in FL (John et al. 2019), particularly with regard to consideration of risk-adapted consolidation strategies with HCT.

Auto-HCT: Currently, there is no uniformly accepted treatment strategy for patients with early-relapsing FL. Identifying novel therapies in this population has emerged as the most unmet need in lymphoma clinical research by the National Cancer Institute and, resultantly, a clinical trial should be favored (Maddocks et al. 2017). However, in the absence of a clinical trial, there are data supporting auto-HCT in transplant-eligible early-relapsing FL patients. Casulo and colleagues assessed whether high-dose chemotherapy and auto-HCT improved clinical outcomes of POD24 patients; 175 POD24 patients who proceeded to auto-HCT were identified from the Center for International Blood and Marrow Transplant Research (CIBMTR) registry, and 174 POD24 patients who did not proceed to an auto-HCT were identified from the retrospective National LymphoCare Study (Casulo et al. 2018). All patients received an up-front rituximab-containing chemoimmunotherapy regimen, and those with histologic transformation were excluded. Although there was no difference in overall survival between the two cohorts, a subgroup analysis demonstrated that patients who proceeded to an early auto-HCT (i.e. within one year of treatment failure, N = 123) had a significantly higher five-year overall survival compared to their non-auto-HCT counterparts (73% vs 60%, $P = 0.05$). On multivariate analysis, early auto-HCT was the only factor associated with reduced mortality. Indeed, the German Low-Grade Lymphoma Study Group also demonstrated a significantly higher five-year second-line overall survival with auto-HCT compared to no transplant (77% vs 59%, $P = 0.031$) (Jurinovic et al. 2018). Based on these findings, early consolidation with auto-HCT is recommended in transplant-eligible patients experiencing POD24 in their second chemotherapy-sensitive remission. This is supported by the random-assignment CUP Trial (Schouten et al. 2003).

Allo-HCT: In the appropriate patient, there is also limited evidence for allogeneic hematopoietic stem cell transplant (allo-HCT) in early-relapsing FL. An observational study showed similar five-year overall survival rates were between auto-HCT and matched-sibling donor allo-HCT (70% vs 73%, respectively) (Smith et al. 2018). In view of this limited evidence, we recommend consideration of a matched-sibling donor allo-HCT for early-relapsing FL where patients are either chemo-refractory or have extensive bone marrow involvement precluding auto-HCT. In those that are not transplant eligible, consideration should be given to novel therapeutic agents such as lenalidomide and idelalisib (Andorsky et al. 2017, Gopal et al. 2017).

2) What is the role of CAR T cell therapy in R/R FL?

Expert Perspective: Beyond stem cell transplantation, clinical trials of chimeric antigen receptor (CAR) T cell therapy have demonstrated highly promising results in POD24 patients. The anti-CD19 CAR T cell therapy axicabtagene ciloleucel (axi-cel) is now FDA approved for patients with relapsed/refractory (R/R) indolent B-cell NHL after two prior lines of therapy based on results from the pivotal ZUMA-5 trial (Jacobson et al. 2020,

Jacobson et al. 2022). Of the 124 patients with R/R FL in this phase II study, 55% had POD24, and 24% received a prior autologous HCT. The overall response rate was 94% with a complete response (CR) of 79%. Among responding FL patients, approximately 80% had an ongoing response at 12 months, and the safety profile appeared comparable to that previously reported for this product in large B-cell lymphoma. Importantly, the presence of POD24 status was not associated with therapy response. There are also data from an external control cohort in R/R FL (SCHOLAR-5) to provide comparative evidence of clinical outcomes in R/R FL patients meeting ZUMA-5 eligibility criteria (Ghione 2022). Therapeutic regimens were highly heterogeneous in the real-world SCHOLAR-5 cohort of R/R FL, and the overall response rate, progression-free survival, and overall survival were significantly higher in ZUMA-5 compared to SCHOLAR-5. In the absence of a randomized trial, these provocative findings provide additional support that axi-cel, and CAR T cell therapy in general, addresses an important unmet need for the management of R/R FL.

The second anti-CD19 CAR T cell product that is FDA approved in R/R FL is tisagenlecleucel (tisa-cel), which was approved based on the phase II ELARA trial (Schuster et al. 2021, Fowler et al. 2022). Ninety-four patients were evaluated in this study, with a median four lines of prior therapies and 36% having undergone a prior auto-HCT. Most patients were refractory to their last line of therapy, and 63% had experienced POD24. The overall response rate of the entire cohort was 86%, with a CR of 66%. The CR in POD24 patients was 59%, compared to 88% in non-POD24 patients.

Although it is difficult to make cross-trial comparisons, we highlight some key differences between the ELARA and ZUMA-5 trials. Firstly, the median time from enrollment to tisa-cel infusion in the ELARA trial was 46 days, compared to only 17 days from leukapheresis to axi-cel infusion in patients treated on the ZUMA-5 trial. Secondly, the ELARA population had a higher percentage of patients with baseline high-risk Follicular Lymphoma International Prognostic Index (FLIPI), POD24, bulky disease, and number of lines of prior therapy versus ZUMA-5. The tisa-cel product has a 41-BB costimulatory domain within the CAR T cell construct, and axi-cel has a CD28 costimulatory domain. Differences in the patient baseline characteristics, time to infusion, and CAR T cell constructs may account for differences in the safety and efficacy between the two studies.

Nonetheless, the high efficacy from these data inspires cautious optimism regarding the role of CAR T cell therapy in R/R FL in the third line, particularly in those with POD24. Longer follow-up is necessary to determine durability, and a randomized-controlled study is required to determine if CAR T cell therapy is superior to consolidation with auto-HCT in FL patients experiencing POD24.

3) Are there any therapeutic agents that are best avoided in FL patients being considered for future auto-transplant or CAR T cell therapy?

Expert Perspective: Most FL patients considered for future HCT or other cellular therapies are likely to have been exposed to chemotherapeutic agents and targeted therapies.

Therapy preceding auto-HCT: Lenalidomide is an orally active immunomodulatory agent that has an increasing role in the management of up-front and relapsed FL. FDA approval for the rituximab-lenalidomide combination (R^2) in R/R FL was based on the large phase III AUGMENT and MAGNIFY trials. While the R^2 combination has increasing use in the relapsed FL setting, there are limited data on the impact of lenalidomide to collect peripheral blood stem cells for future auto-HCT in FL. Previous studies in multiple myeloma have suggested an adverse impact of lenalidomide exposure on stem cell collection, but this issue been largely overcome with access to effective bone marrow stimulants such as plerixafor. Nonetheless, for R/R FL patients on R^2 and planned for future auto-HCT, it would be reasonable to withhold lenalidomide for a short duration before stem cell collection. The impact of pre-transplant bendamustine exposure should also be considered when planning mobilization strategies given a higher risk of failed stem cell collections with this agent in NHL (Alahwal et al. 2018). Given the above, for clearly physiologically transplant-eligible patients with POD24 to NCCN-recommended first-line chemoimmunotherapy programs (i.e. CHOP-like or bendamustine-based), if the patient is to be considered for auto-HCT consolidation at the time of second induction, we would recommend non-cross resistant chemoimmunotherapy (i.e. CHOP-like or bendamustine-based depending on initial induction). This strategy would ensure demonstrable cytotoxic chemotherapy sensitivity prior to auto-HCT, providing further rationale for consolidation with high-dose cytotoxic therapy associated with auto-HCT. We would then recommend agents such as: lenalidomide, PI3K inhibitors, EZH2 inhibitor, or CAR T cells in the third line (see Chapter 35).

Therapy preceding and after CAR T cell therapy: A more intriguing question is whether exposure to specific targeted therapies may augment the activity of cellular therapies, such as CAR T cell therapy. Indeed, there is promising data in other NHL subtypes regarding this. The ZUMA-2 investigators reported extremely favorable results of a phase II clinical trial with an anti-CD19 chimeric receptor in R/R mantle cell lymphoma, with an overall response rate of 93% (67% CR). At 12 months the progression-free and overall survival were 61% and 83%, respectively, suggestive of potentially durable responses (Wang et al. 2020). Importantly, all patients enrolled onto ZUMA-2 required prior exposure to a Bruton's tyrosine kinase inhibitor (BTKi), and most patients had previous ibrutinib therapy. There are data that prior exposure to BTKi enhances T-cell phenotypes used for the subsequently engineered CAR T cell product. In chronic lymphocytic leukemia, it has been shown that prior BTKi exposure improved the expansion of CD19-directed CAR T cells and reduced the expression of immune checkpoints on T cells (Fraietta et al. 2016). Enhanced CAR T-cell function with BTKi therapy has also been demonstrated in animal models (Geyer et al. 2019). Moving forward, the impact of prior BTKi as a favorable efficacy signal in CAR T cell therapy needs to be studied in a controlled clinical trial (see Chapters 28 and 36).

In addition to BTKi, the role of lenalidomide to augment CAR T cell efficacy requires consideration, especially as this would have a significant impact on sequencing of therapies in R/R iNHL. Lenalidomide is known to prevent defects that cause an impairment of T-cell synapse in B-cell NHL (Ramsay et al. 2012). There is some evidence that early treatment with lenalidomide in patients who relapse post CAR T cell therapy in R/R diffuse large B-cell lymphoma (DLBCL) is associated with high responses rates, suggesting that lenalidomide may enhance CAR T-cell efficacy (Thieblemont et al. 2020). Moreover, there are preclinical data suggesting that phosphoinositide 3-kinase (PI3K) inhibition may improve CAR T function, and this is a class of agents FDA approved in the R/R FL setting (Zheng et al. 2018). Whether to avoid cytotoxic immune-suppressive chemotherapies such as bendamustine before apheresis and instead use potentially synergistic agents such as BTKi, PI3Ki, and lenalidomide before CAR T cell therapy warrants further investigation.

4) Is there a role for bispecifics and autologous transplant in FL beyond two lines of therapy?

Expert Perspective: There is currently no standard of care for FL patients undergoing second-line treatment or beyond. One of the challenges in multi-relapsed FL is determining the optimal sequencing of therapies and the patient population most likely to benefit from auto-HCT. This is particularly relevant in the contemporary era of novel agent development. Most recently, FDA granted accelerated approval to mosunetuzumab, a bispecific CD20-directed CD3 T-cell engager for adult patients with R/R FL after two or more lines of systemic therapy. Mosunetuzumab was evaluated in GO29781 (NCT02500407), an open-label, multicenter, multi-cohort study. The efficacy population consisted of 90 patients with R/R FL who had received at least two prior lines of systemic therapy, including an anti-CD20 monoclonal antibody and an alkylating agent. The ORR was 80% (95% CI: 70, 88), with 60% achieving complete responses. With a median follow-up of 14.9 months among responders, the estimated median duration of response was 22.8 months (95% CI: 10, not reached) and the estimated duration of response rate at 12 months and 18 months was 62% and 57%, respectively. Mosunetuzumab should be administered for 8 cycles unless patients experience unacceptable toxicity or disease progression. After 8 cycles, patients with a complete response should discontinue therapy. Patients with a partial response or stable disease should continue treatment up to 17 cycles unless they experience progressive disease or unacceptable toxicity.

In the absence of POD24, the optimal timing of auto-HCT in R/R FL patients is debated. However, there appears to be no significant benefit to high-dose therapy and auto-HCT as a consolidative strategy in first remission. Sebban et al. studied the role of consolidative auto-HCT in treatment-naive advanced-stage FL patients (Sebban et al. 2006). In this randomized study there was no event-free or overall survival benefit to first-line high-dose therapy with auto-HCT in FL. Similarly, another randomized study was unable to demonstrate an overall survival benefit for auto-HCT in first remission, with significant enrichment of second primary malignancies in the transplant arm (Gyan et al. 2009). The lack of a survival benefit for auto-HCT in first remission was also confirmed in a meta-analysis (Al Khabori et al. 2012).

Auto-HCT has a more defined role in multi-relapsed FL. Initially, the European CUP trial randomized patients with relapsed FL post three cycles of salvage chemotherapy to either further chemotherapy, unpurged auto-HCT, or purged auto-HCT. The study concluded that the incorporation of auto-HCT significantly improved progression-free and overall survival, and importantly no benefit was observed through graft purging (Schouten et al. 2003). Subsequent retrospective studies of patients with relapsed FL who underwent an auto-HCT revealed impressive outcomes, with a median progression-free survival of almost 10 years and overall survival exceeding 20 years (Jiménez-Ubieto et al. 2017). However, such benefits were less robust in patients treated beyond their second complete remission. A single-center experience demonstrated that performing an auto-HCT in second remission resulted in a 20% higher progression-free survival and significantly higher overall survival at 10 years, compared with transplantation in subsequent remissions (Kothari et al. 2014). Other retrospective studies have validated these findings. Vose and colleagues demonstrated that auto-HCT in relapsed FL after three or more lines of therapy predicted a worse overall survival (Vose et al. 2008). Similarly, in another study, the survival

Table 38.1 Major publications of autologous hematopoietic stem cell transplantation in follicular lymphoma.

Reference	Patient Population	Total No. of patients	No. of patients in each arm	Transplant type	EFS	PFS	OS	No. of 2nd malignancies
Casulo et al. 2018	POD24 in FL	297	174	No auto-SCT	-	-	5-yr: 60%	-
			123	early auto-SCT	-	-	5-yr: 73%	-
Jurinovic et al. 2018	POD24 in FL	113	61	No auto-SCT	-	5-yr: 19%	5-yr: 59%	-
			52	auto-SCT	-	5-yr: 51%	5-yr: 77%	-
Sebban et al. 2006	Up-front treatment of FL	401	209	No auto-SCT	7-yr: 28%	-	7-yr: 71%	-
			192	auto-SCT	7-yr: 38%	-	7-yr: 76%	1
Gyan et al. 2009	Up-front treatment of FL	166	80	No auto-SCT	9-yr: 39%	9-yr: 39%	9-yr: 80%	1
			86	auto-SCT	9-yr: 56%	9-yr: 64%	9-yr: 76%	12
Madsen et al. 2015	Up-front treatment of tFL	34	13	No auto-SCT	-	5-yr: 62%	5-yr: 67%	-
			21	auto-SCT	-	5-yr: 71%	5-yr: 76%	-
Madsen et al. 2015	tFL, (with FL previously treated)	51	18	No auto-SCT	-	5-yr: 6%	5-yr: 36%	-
			33	auto-SCT	-	5-yr: 53%	5-yr: 62%	-
Sarkozy et al. 2016	tFL at relapse #1 of FL	40	23	No auto-SCT	-	-	median: 1.7yr	-
			17	auto-SCT	-	-	median: NR	-

POD24: progression of disease at 24 months; FL: follicular lymphoma; tFL: transformed follicular lymphoma; No.: number; auto-SCT: autologous stem cell transplant; EFS: event-free survival; PFS: progression-free survival; OS: overall survival; yr: year; NR: not reached; -: not available.

of patients undergoing auto-HCT in second remission was significantly longer than those treated later in the course of their illness (Rohatiner et al. 2007). Collectively, these data suggest that auto-HCT warrants consideration in FL at the time of second complete remission and is best avoided beyond two lines of therapy. Table 38.1 summarizes the major auto-HCT studies in FL.

5) In an era of cellular and targeted therapies, should allo-HCT still be considered as a treatment option in relapsed FL?

Expert Perspective: Allo-HCT is a potentially curative treatment for patients with FL. In addition to the cytotoxic conditioning regimen, this is in large part contributed by the anti-lymphoma effect from transplantation of immune-competent donor cells. Indeed, there is circumstantial evidence of a substantial graft-versus-lymphoma (GVL) effect in FL as the development graft-versus-host disease (GvHD) is associated with a significantly reduced risk of relapse, including in patients with chemo-resistant disease (Urbano-Ispizua et al. 2015). On the contrary, no such association between GvHD and lower relapse rates were observed in DLBCL, Hodgkin lymphoma, and peripheral T-cell lymphoma (Urbano-Ispizua et al. 2015). Donor lymphocyte infusions also appear to be particularly effective in the treatment of relapsing indolent lymphoma post allo-HCT, again supporting a potent GVL effect (Mandigers et al. 2003).

Registry studies of allo-HCT with reduced-intensity conditioning (RIC) regimens have reported encouraging three-year overall survival rates of approximately 80% (Laport et al. 2016). There is also provocative data from a smaller cohort demonstrating an improved event-free survival with allo-HCT over auto-HCT in R/R FL with at least two lines of prior therapy and a prior remission duration of ≤ 12 months (Lunning et al. 2016). The Blood and Marrow Transplant Clinical Trials Network (BMT CTN) 0202 trial that was launched to prospectively study auto-HCT versus RIC allo-HCT in relapsed FL closed early due to slow accrual. Of the 30 enrolled patients, the three-year overall survival was 73% in the 22 auto-HCT patients versus 100% in the eight patients that underwent allo-HCT (Tomblyn et al. 2011).

However, despite the promising efficacy and potentially curative nature of allo-HCT in FL, its use in FL is gradually reducing, particularly with the recent advancements of less-toxic novel targeted treatment options. Furthermore, both CIBMTR registry data and NCCN have demonstrated that any potential survival benefit of allo-HCT over auto-HCT in R/R FL is offset by its high non-relapse mortality (Evens et al. 2013, Klyuchnikov et al. 2015). Another large retrospective study of RIC allo-HCT in FL patients relapsing after an autologous transplant demonstrated a five-year progression-free and overall survival of 48% and 51%, respectively (Robinson et al. 2016). These findings suggest that RIC allo-HCT can be an effective salvage therapy in relapsing FL after a prior autograft as a subset of patients can achieve durable disease control. It is therefore suggested that allo-HCT be reserved as a salvage option in fit patients with relapsing FL post autograft. Another situation where allo-HCT warrants consideration in R/R FL is in those with incipient myelodysplastic syndrome or where there is failure of autologous stem-cell mobilization. Table 38.2 summarizes the major allo-HCT studies in FL.

Table 38.2 Major publications of allogeneic hematopoietic stem cell transplantation in follicular lymphoma.

Reference	Patient Population	Total No. of patients	Transplant type: No.	Donor type in allo-HCT: No.	Relapse	PFS	OS	NRM	GvHD in Allo-HCT
Laport et al. 2016	R/R FL	62	Allo (RIC)	MSD: 33 MUD: 29	3-yr: 13%	3-yr: 71%	3-yr: 82%	3-yr: 16%	2-yr acute: 37% 2-yr chronic: 61%
Klyuchnikov et al. 2015	R/R FL	518	Auto: 250 Allo (RIC): 268	MSD: 143 MUD: 103 mismatched: 22	5-yr: 54% 5-yr: 20%	5-yr: 41% 5-yr: 58%	5-yr: 74% 5-yr: 66%	5-yr: 5% 5-yr: 26%	100-d acute: 28% 5-yr chronic: 60%
Evens et al. 2013	R/R FL	184	Auto: 136 allo: 48	MSD: 63% MUD: 37%	-	3-yr: 32% 3-yr: 16%	3-yr: 87% 3-yr: 61%	3-yr: 3% 3-yr: 24%	-
Robinson et al. 2016	relapse post-auto in FL	183	Allo (RIC)	MSD: 77 MUD: 87 mismatched:19	5-yr: 16%	5-yr: 48%	5-yr: 51%	2-yr: 27%	180-d acute: 45% 2-yr chronic: 51%
Ghosh et al. 2016	Lymphomas	987	Allo (RIC)	MSD: 807 haplo: 180	3-yr: 40% 3-yr: 37%	3-yr: 48% 3-yr: 48%	3-yr: 62% 3-yr: 61%	3-yr: 13% 3-yr: 15%	1-yr chronic: 45% 1-yr chronic: 12%
Kanate et al. 2016	Lymphomas	917	Allo (RIC + ATG) allo (RIC – ATG) allo (RIC)	MUD: 241 MUD: 491 haplo: 185	3-yr: 36% 3-yr: 28% 3-yr: 36%	3-yr: 38% 3-yr: 49% 3-yr: 47%	3-yr: 50% 3-yr: 62% 3-yr: 60%	1-yr: 20% 1-yr: 13% 1-yr:11%	1-yr chronic: 33% 1-yr chronic: 51% 1-yr chronic: 13%
Tomblyn et al. 2011	Relapsed FL	30	Auto: 22 allo: 8	MSD: 8	3-yr: 15% 3-yr: 14%	3-yr: 63% 3-yr: 86%	3-yr: 73% 3-yr: 100%	- -	- -
Villa et al. 2013	tFL	172	Auto: 97 allo: 22 R-chemo: 53	MSD: 14 MUD: 7 mismatched: 1	- - -	5-yr: 55% 5-yr: 46% 5-yr: 40%	5-yr: 65% 5-yr: 46% 5-yr: 61%	5-yr: 5% 5-yr: 23% -	acute: 50% chronic: 42%
Smith et al. 2018	POD24 in FL	440	Auto: 240 allo (MSD) allo (MUD)	MSD: 105 MUD: 95	5-yr: 58% 5-yr: 31% 5-yr: 23%	5-yr: 38% 5-yr: 52% 5-yr: 43%	5-yr: 70% 5-yr: 73% 5-yr: 49%	5-yr: 5% 5-yr: 17% 5-yr: 33%	2-yr chronic: 54% 2-yr chronic: 58%

R/R: relapsed/refractory; FL: follicular lymphoma; tFL: transformed follicular lymphoma; POD24: progression of disease at 24 months; No.: number; auto: autologous; allo: allogeneic; HCT: hematopoietic cell transplant; RIC: reduced-intensity conditioning; ATG: anti-thymocyte globulin; R-chemo: rituximab-chemotherapy; PFS: progression-free survival; OS: overall survival; NRM non-relapse mortality; GvHD: graft versus host disease; yr: year.

6) Can allogeneic HCT be considered in FL patients in the absence of a HLA-matched sibling or matched unrelated donor?

Expert Perspective: An HLA-matched sibling is the preferred donor for allo-HCT, but only about 30% of individuals would have such a donor available. Therefore, in the United States, the National Marrow Donor Program (NMDP) was established in the 1980s and facilitates identification of matched unrelated donors as an alternative donor source. More than half of allogeneic HCT procedures in the United States have used grafts from unrelated donors. However, optimally matched HLA unrelated donors are not always available, particularly in individuals with diverse ethnic and racial backgrounds. Furthermore, even if a suitable matched unrelated donor is identified there can be logistical challenges and delays in transplantation. However, nearly all patients will have an available related HLA-haploidentical donor (a donor with whom they share a single haplotype) and with contemporary post-transplant cyclophosphamide GvHD prophylaxis, outcomes of haploidentical transplantation have been encouraging.

Ghosh et al. (2016) studied the outcomes of haploidentical allo-HCT to matched sibling donor allo-HCT with RIC. Using the CIBMTR database, 987 patients with non-Hodgkin and Hodgkin lymphoma were identified, of which 807 had an MSD allo-HCT and 180 underwent haploidentical allo-HCT. This analysis demonstrated that survival, risk of relapse, and non-relapse mortality were virtually identical between the two cohorts. Interestingly, those patients undergoing haploidentical allo-HCT had significantly lower rates of chronic GvHD compared to their MSD allo-HCT counterparts. This is likely contributed by the effective depletion of alloreactive donor T cells with post-transplant cyclophosphamide. Kanate et al. evaluated the outcomes in lymphoma patients who underwent haploidentical allo-HCT compared to matched unrelated donor allo-HCT, with and without antithymocyte globulin (ATG) (Kanate et al. 2016). All groups underwent RIC. The study demonstrated that three-year survival was similar between haploidentical and matched unrelated donor transplants, irrespective of ATG use. However, haploidentical allo-HCT was associated with lower rates of chronic GvHD compared to unrelated donor transplants. Together, these data suggest that RIC haploidentical allo-HCT with post-transplant cyclophosphamide should be considered as an acceptable option in FL patients without a matched sibling or matched unrelated donor.

7) Should a consolidative transplantation be performed in patients with transformed FL?

Expert Perspective: FL can undergo biologic transformation to an aggressive histology that mandates urgent clinical intervention. The rate of histologic transformation of FL is approximately 2 to 3% per year, leading to a cumulative risk of transformation of 25–30% at 10 years (Montoto et al. 2007). Furthermore, histologic transformation appears to be enriched within patients with POD24 (Freeman et al. 2019). Although there are several aggressive histological subtypes that may be encountered upon re-biopsy, the most common is DLBCL. Patients with transformed FL can be broadly categorized into those that are treatment-naive at clinical presentation and those who have had previous therapy for their indolent disease.

Auto-HCT in treatment-naive transformed FL: The treatment of transformed FL can be variable and is limited by retrospective studies, but in general terms, treatment-naive patients with disease transformation are typically offered conventional systemic chemoimmunotherapy with R-CHOP. Though there has been limited evidence that incorporating auto-HCT may improve survival outcomes in treatment-naive transformed FL compared to historical controls (Elhassadi et al. 2017), it has been demonstrated that the outcomes of previously untreated transformed FL patients are not significantly different to those with *de novo* DLBCL (Magnano et al. 2017, Wang et al. 2019). Furthermore, another study of composite transformed indolent lymphoma (i.e. coexisting evidence of both an indolent and aggressive histology at time of diagnosis), did not show a benefit for consolidative auto-HCT after initial chemoimmunotherapy (Madsen et al. 2015). Whether this relates to a greater sensitivity of patients to front-line chemoimmunotherapy warrants consideration. More recently, Chin and colleagues used a propensity-score matched cohort to demonstrate an improvement in progression-free survival with a consolidative auto-HCT in previously untreated transformed FL after R-CHOP, and this was attributable to fewer relapses of indolent lymphoma. However, there was no impact on overall survival and patients who relapsed post auto-HCT had significantly inferior outcomes compared to their non-transplanted counterparts (Chin et al. 2020). Taken together, these data suggest that consolidative auto-HCT can be differed in treatment-naive transformed FL patients who achieve a CR after chemoimmunotherapy (see chapter 43).

Auto-HCT in previously treated FL and transformation: Consolidative HCT in patients with transformed FL exposed to prior therapy warrants strong consideration. A retrospective, multicenter analysis demonstrated that patients with transformed FL who received prior treatment for their indolent lymphoma had inferior outcomes to standard chemoimmunotherapy compared to their treatment-naive counterparts (Lerch et al. 2015). Inferior outcomes have also been shown to be more pronounced in patients previously exposed to rituximab pre-transformation, highlighting the challenges of treating lymphoma patients who have progressed after anti-CD20 antibody therapy (Ban-Hoefen et al. 2013, Madsen et al. 2015). An overall survival advantage for auto-HCT was demonstrated in a subset of patients from the PRIMA study who had subsequent histological transformation compared to those who were not transplanted (Sarkozy et al. 2016). Likewise, Madsen and colleagues demonstrated improved progression-free and overall survival in FL patients with subsequent histological transformation receiving auto-HCT compared to a rituximab-containing conventional chemotherapy regimen (five-year OS 62% vs 36%, respectively, $P = 0.07$; progression-free survival 53% vs 6%, $P = 0.002$) (Madsen et al. 2015). Taken together, these studies suggest that there is a demonstrable benefit for auto-HCT in transformed FL patients with prior exposure to chemoimmunotherapy for their indolent lymphoma. Indeed, previously treated patients with transformed indolent lymphoma have similar outcomes to those with relapsed DLBCL. Therefore, like relapsed DLBCL, salvage chemotherapy and auto-HCT require consideration as a standard of care in previously treated transformed FL (Kuruvilla et al. 2015).

Allo-HCT vs auto-HCT vs CAR T cell therapy in previously treated FL and transformation: The role of allo-HCT in transformed FL has also been studied. A retrospective cohort study from the Canadian Blood and Marrow Transplant Group evaluated the efficacy of allo-HCT in FL with subsequent biopsy-proven transformation, with most patients in this study having received rituximab-containing chemotherapy before transformation (Villa et al. 2013). On multivariate analysis patients who underwent auto-HCT for transformed FL had a significantly higher five-year overall survival compared to patients who only received rituximab-containing chemotherapy at transformation, and there was no benefit to allogeneic transplantation (Villa et al. 2013). The five-year OS after transformation was 46% for patients treated with allo-HCT, compared to 65% with auto-HCT (Villa et al. 2013). Any potential improvement in overall survival with allogeneic transplantation was offset by high transplant-related mortality. Similar findings were reported by the CIBMTR (Wirk et al. 2014). Allo-HCT in this setting would need to be carefully considered in the era of CAR T cells with long-term follow-up data pending with FDA approved axi-cel, considering inherent risks of morbidity and mortality with allo-HCT (see Chapters 39, 43, and 40).

8) What is the role of cellular therapies in transformed FL?

Expert Perspective: CAR T cell therapy has led to a transformational advancement in the management of aggressive B-cell malignancies. CAR T cell receptors are composed of an antigen-binding domain, transmembrane domain, co-stimulatory domain, and CD3-zeta intracellular signaling domain. Three anti-CD19 CAR T cell therapies are now US FDA and EMA approved for R/R large B-cell lymphoma, including transformed FL, after at least two prior lines of systemic therapy.

Of the 111 patients in the pivotal phase II trial (ZUMA-1) of axi-cel in refractory large B-cell lymphoma, 16 had transformed FL (Neelapu et al. 2017). The best overall response rate of the entire cohort was 83% (CR: 58%) with a median duration of response of 11.1 months, validating the efficacy of CD19-targeted CAR T cell therapy in this disease (Locke et al. 2019). Response rates and safety assessments within the transformed FL was not reported separately. The JULIET study of tisagenlecleucel (tisa-cel) included 21 patients with R/R DLBCL that had transformed from FL. Within the entire cohort, the best overall response rate was 52% (CR: 40%). Again, outcomes within the transformed FL subtype were not reported separately (Schuster et al. 2018). More recently, Abramson et al. reported findings of lisocabtagene maraleucel (liso-cel), which is formulated at a specified $CD4^+:CD8^+$ composition, in R/R large B-cell lymphoma. The TRANSCEND NHL 001 study had a higher representation of transformed FL with a total of 60 patients (Abramson et al. 2020). The overall response rate was 73% (CR: 53%) in the entire study cohort. Interestingly, the duration of response and progression-free survival in patients with DLBCL transformed from FL (and those with primary mediastinal B-cell lymphoma) were longer than for other subtypes with a median that was not reached at time of publication (Abramson et al. 2020).

The US Lymphoma CAR T Consortium recently reported real-world data of clinical outcomes with axi-cel in the standard of care setting for the approved indication. The safety and efficacy of axi-cel in the real-world setting was comparable to the registrational ZUMA-1 study, and importantly, real-world patients were older and had more comorbidities suggesting that CAR T cell therapy can be more broadly applicable than suggested by the original studies (Nastoupil et al. 2020). Of the 298 patients from this real-world setting, 76 (26%) had transformed FL. There were no differences in toxicity, CR (62% at 12 months), progression-free survival (51% at 12 months), or overall survival (70% at 12 months) in transformed FL compared to other histological subtypes, demonstrating that anti-CD19 CAR T cell therapy is at least as efficacious in transformed FL compared to other DLBCL histological subtypes (Nastoupil et al. 2020). Based on the current data, it would be reasonable to consider anti-CD19 CAR T cell therapy in transformed FL that has relapsed post auto-HCT or in chemo-resistant disease precluding auto-HCT (Smith 2020) (see Chapter 40).

9) **Can the data on HCT and cellular therapies from FL be extrapolated to less common indolent non-Hodgkin's lymphomas such as lymphoplasmacytic lymphoma and marginal zone lymphoma?**

Expert Perspective: Marginal zone lymphoma (MZL) is an indolent disease representing 7% of all mature NHL. Given the rarity of this condition, the role of HCT has not been studied in the prospective setting. Avivi et. al retrospectively analyzed outcomes of 199 MZL patients who underwent auto-HCT. Patients had a median of two lines of prior therapy, and the five-year event-free and overall survival were 53% and 73%, respectively, demonstrating that auto-HCT can provide clinical benefit in R/R MZL (Avivi et al. 2018). Regarding the role of anti-CD19 CAR T cell therapy, 24 of the 146 patients in the ZUMA-5 study had MZL with encouraging overall response rate of 85% (60% CR). Patients were heavily pretreated having received a median of three prior lines of therapy, but only 13% underwent a prior auto-HCT. Although it appears that the response rates were lower for MZL than FL, this is largely due to the finding that 15% of MZL patients were found not to have measurable disease by central review. In the absence of high-quality data for HCT and cellular therapies in MZL, it would be reasonable to extrapolate some of the data reported in FL to make treatment decisions. In the setting of the FDA approval of ibrutinib in the R/R MZL setting, extrapolation of ZUMA-2 toward sequencing BTKi followed immediately by CAR T cell therapy should be strongly considered (see Chapter 37).

Lymphoplasmacytic lymphoma is another rare form of B-cell lymphoma. With few large studies, defining treatments in the relapsed setting has been challenging. However, auto-HCT can be a salvage option in lymphoplasmacytic lymphoma with the European Society for Blood and Marrow Transplantation (EBMT) reporting five-year progression-free and overall survival rates of 40% and 69%, respectively, in a heavily pretreated population (Kyriakou et al. 2010). Similarly, outcomes of previously treated patients who received allo-HCT was reported by the EBMT. Among patients who underwent RIC, the progression-free and overall survival was 49% and 64%, respectively, with a 23% non-relapse mortality at three years (Kyriakou et al. 2010). Therefore, in very select cases, RIC allo-HCT can be considered for R/R lymphoplasmacytic lymphoma. At present, the role of CAR T cell therapy in lymphoplasmacytic lymphoma has not been studied in detail (see Chapter 47).

Recommended Readings

Casulo, C., Friedberg, J.W., Ahn, K.W., Flowers, C., DiGilio, A., Smith, S.M. et al. (2018). Autologous transplantation in follicular lymphoma with early therapy failure: a national lymphocare study and center for international blood and marrow transplant research analysis. *Biol Blood Marrow Transplant: J Am Soc Blood Marrow Transplant* 24 (6): 1163–1171.

Ghosh, N., Karmali, R., Rocha, V., Ahn, K.W., DiGilio, A., Hari, P.N. et al. (2016). Reduced-intensity transplantation for lymphomas using haploidentical related donors versus

HLA-matched sibling donors: a center for international blood and marrow transplant research analysis. *J Clin Oncoly* 34 (26): 3141–3149.

Jacobson, C., Chavez, J.C., Sehgal, A.R., William, B.M., Munoz, J., Salles, G. et al. (2020). Primary analysis of zuma-5: a phase 2 study of axicabtagene ciloleucel (Axi-Cel) in patients with relapsed/refractory (R/R) indolent non-hodgkin lymphoma (iNHL). *Blood* 136 (Supplement 1): 40–41.

Kanate, A.S., Mussetti, A., Kharfan-Dabaja, M.A., Ahn, K.W., DiGilio, A., Beitinjaneh, A. et al. (2016). Reduced-intensity transplantation for lymphomas using haploidentical related donors vs HLA-matched unrelated donors. *Blood* 127 (7): 938–947.

Laport, G.G., Wu, J., Logan, B., Bachanova, V., Hosing, C., Fenske, T. et al. (2016). Reduced-intensity conditioning with fludarabine, cyclophosphamide, and high-dose rituximab for allogeneic hematopoietic cell transplantation for follicular lymphoma: a phase two multicenter trial from the blood and marrow transplant clinical trials network. *Biol Blood Marrow Transplant* 22 (8): 1440–1448.

Madsen, C., Pedersen, M.B., Vase, M., Bendix, K., Møller, M.B., Johansen, P. et al. (2015). Outcome determinants for transformed indolent lymphomas treated with or without autologous stem-cell transplantation. *Ann Oncol* 26 (2): 393–399.

Nastoupil, L.J., Jain, M.D., Feng, L., Spiegel, J.Y., Ghobadi, A., Lin, Y. et al. (2020). Standard-of-care axicabtagene ciloleucel for relapsed or refractory large B-cell lymphoma: results from the US lymphoma CAR T consortium. *J Clin Oncol* 38 (27): 3119–3128.

Schuster, S.J., Dickinson, M., Dreyling, M., Martinez-Lopez, J., Kolstad, A., Butler, J. et al. (2021). Efficacy and safety of tisagenlecleucel (TISA-CEL) in adult patients (PTS) with relapsed/refractory follicular lymphoma (R/R Fl): primary analysis of the phase 2 elara trial. *Hematol Oncol* 39 (S2).

Tomblyn, M.R., Ewell, M., Bredeson, C., Kahl, B.S., Goodman, S.A., Horowitz, M.M. et al. (2011). Autologous versus reduced-intensity allogeneic hematopoietic cell transplantation for patients with chemosensitive follicular non-Hodgkin lymphoma beyond first complete response or first partial response. *Biol Blood Marrow Transplant: J Ame Soc Blood Marrow Transplant* 17 (7): 1051–1057.

Villa, D., Crump, M., Panzarella, T., Savage, K.J., Toze, C.L., Stewart, D.A. et al. (2013). Autologous and allogeneic stem-cell transplantation for transformed follicular lymphoma: a report of the Canadian blood and marrow transplant group. *J Clin Oncol* 31 (9): 1164–1171.

39

Diffuse Large B Cell Lymphoma

Alessia Castellino[1,2] and Grzegorz S. Nowakowski[2]

[1] *Santa Croce and Carle Hospital, Cuneo, Italy*
[2] *Mayo Clinic, Rochester, MN, USA*

Introduction

Diffuse large B-cell lymphoma (DLBCL) represents a clinically and molecularly heterogeneous group of aggressive non-Hodgkin lymphomas (NHL), and it is the most common type of NHL in the United States and in Europe, representing approximately 24% of new cases of NHL each year. The clinical course of the disease is typically aggressive, presenting with rapidly enlarging lymphadenopathy, relatively high rate of extranodal disease involvement, and frequently local or constitutional symptoms, requiring prompt diagnostic assessment and treatment.

Since 1993, the International Prognostic Index (IPI), based on five clinical factors, has been used to characterize prognosis in DLBCL. However, in the past two decades, many efforts have been made to identify different DLBCL subtypes by gene expression profile cell of origin (COO), presence of *BCL2* with and without *MYC* translocation, MYC and BCL2 expression, and more recently molecular clusters, which can be used independently of the IPI to identify high-risk disease and predict poor outcome. On these bases, many attempts for improving the therapeutic approach and the clinical outcome of high-risk patients have been done, but currently, the standard treatment remains chemoimmunotherapy, R-CHOP (rituximab, cyclophosphamide, doxorubicin, vincristine, and prednisone) or R-CHOP-like therapy. With this standard therapeutic approach, over 60–70% of patients are cured, though the remainder relapses or shows a progression and often succumbs to the disease, representing an unmet clinical need. In this chapter, we review the pathobiology of DLBCL and the considerations regarding staging, management, and prognosis.

Cell of Origin and Molecular Characterization

1) How best to determine cell of origin, and how do subtypes influence outcomes with R-CHOP therapy?

Expert Perspective: The 2017 revised WHO classification requires to differentiate DLBCL by COO subtypes. Based on gene expression profile (GEP), DLBCL can be differentiated into two main subgroups: germinal center B cell (GCB; 50–60% of cases) and activated B cell (ABC; 30–40% of cases). However, approximately 10–15% of cases cannot be included in either of these groups and remain unclassified. This subtype along with ABC are grouped as non-GCB DLBCL. These subtypes have distinct oncogenic driver pathways and thus different prognosis

Cancer Consult: Expertise in Clinical Practice, Volume 2: Neoplastic Hematology & Cellular Therapy,
Second Edition. Edited by Syed A. Abutalib, Maurie Markman, James O. Armitage, and Kenneth C. Anderson.
© 2024 John Wiley & Sons Ltd. Published 2024 by John Wiley & Sons Ltd.

with best outcomes for patients with GCB systemic DLBCL. They showed different response if treated with standard R-CHOP: GCB subtypes had cure rates of about 70–80%, while ABC of about 40%. Intriguingly, polatuzumab vedotin-R-CHP appears to be remarkably beneficial for ABC DLBCL. The gold standard method to define COO is GEP using RNA microarray analysis, but, because of logistical difficulties, several studies to identify COO subtype on the bases of protein expression evaluated by immunohistochemistry on tissue microarrays were conducted. Importantly, COO status does not influence the choice of initial treatment for advanced-stage DLBCL. The most widely used algorithm was proposed by Hans et al, which assigns COO based on the expression of three stains, CD10, BCL6, and MUM1 in a stepwise progression (Figure 39.1). Compared to GEP, the Hans algorithm showed a concordance rate of 80%.

Digital expression profiling assays have been developed to identify DLBCL COO on formalin-fixed paraffin-embedded (FFPE) tissue. A pilot study to identify COO using nanostring technology on 93 genes was conducted by Lenz et al. Then 15 genes were selected based on their ability to contribute to accurate replication of the COO assignment. Nanostring technology was then used to determine the expression of 20 genes in FFPE tissues–derived RNA from the training cohort and allowed a model to be built: the Lymphoma/Leukemia Molecular Profiling Project's Lymph2CX assay, performed by Scott et al. It was the first digital gene expression ("NanoString")–based test for COO assignment in FFPE tissues, based on a 20-gene assay, trained using 51 FFPE samples and validated using an independent cohort of 68 FFPE biopsies. The assay showed to be robust, accurate, with only one case with incorrect COO assignment, and with > 95% concordance of COO assignment between two independent laboratories. It is commercially available.

2) How is double expressor DLBCL defined?

Expert Perspective: 2017 WHO classification update recognized co-expression of MYC and BCL2 proteins, defined by IHC, as a new negative prognostic marker. However, the "double expressor lymphoma (DEL)" does not constitute a separate category in WHO. The IHC threshold for MYC is ≥ 40% and > 50% for BCL2 to define DEL. Of note, abnormal MYC protein expression was only associated with worse outcome when accompanied by BCL2 expression. Further studies are needed to clarify the prognosis of lymphomas that overexpress BCL2 and MYC. On the other side, a new entity defined by the 2017 WHO classification included high-grade lymphomas (HGBL) with *MYC* and *BCL2* and/or *BCL6* rearrangements (double- or triple-hit lymphomas [DHL or THL]), for whom, because of their dismal outcome if treated with standard R-CHOP, an intensified approach with high-dose chemotherapy, like the one

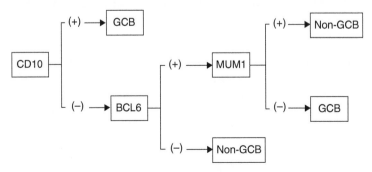

Figure 39.1 Hans Algorithm. (+) if ⩾ 30% on IHC.

used in Burkitt lymphomas, is often recommended, based on case series and phase II studies; however, there are no prospective randomized studies (see Chapters 40, 42, and 44).

3) Can we identify additional molecular signatures in DLBCL?

Expert Perspective: In 2018, a novel approach based on multiplatform analysis of structural genomic abnormalities and gene expression provided a new and evolving understanding of molecular heterogeneity of DLBCL; how this information can influence therapeutic response is briefly discussed below.

Additional Molecular Taxonomy in DLBCL

- In the report by Schmitz et al., the authors identified four prominent genetic subtypes in DLBCL, termed *MCD, N1, BN2, and EZB*. The genetic subtypes *MCD* and *N1* showed mainly an ABC COO phenotype and correlated, as an independent factor, with a worse prognosis if treated with standard R-CHOP, while *BN2* and *EZB* subgroups showed to be predictive of a better outcome. (Table -39.1)
- These interesting findings, which open the way to a new and evolving knowledge in DLBCL complexity, were in accord to what was reported in another manuscript, by Chapuy et al. They described six different "clusters," or signatures (clusters 0–5) that partially overlapped with the genetic subtypes identified by Schmitz et al. Cluster 5 showed uniform 18q gain, increasing expression of BCL2, concordant with frequent $MYD88^{L265P}$ and *CD79B* mutations; they are more likely to have an ABC phenotype for COO and to be associated with extranodal tropism (central nervous system and testicular), like the MCD genetic subgroup described by Schmitz et al. Cluster 1 was characterized by *NOTCH2* mutations, *BCL6* translocations, NF-KB B cell receptor (BCR) pathway alterations, *SPEN* and *BCL10* mutations, and $MYD88^{non-L265P}$ mutations: according to what was described in the analogous *BN2* genetic subgroup, this signature reminds what was observed in marginal zone lymphomas, suggesting a chronic inflammation–driven pathogenesis and the involvement of immune-escape mechanisms. Cluster 3 harbored *BCL2, EZH, PTEN* mutations and alterations in PI3K pathways, while Cluster 4 was characterized by JAK-STAT pathway involvement; they both can be included in the *EZB* genetic subtype and, accordingly, they both showed mainly GCB phenotype. Cluster 2 was characterized by biallelic inactivation of *TP53* and 17p copy loss and seemed to be a cross cluster among the previous ones, including both GCB and ABC subtypes. Cluster 0 was observed to be a less common subtype and included mostly T-cell/histocyte-rich DLBCL, morphologically characterized by high inflammatory/immune infiltrate and the absence of typical detectable driven mutational events, which may reflect a different pathogenetic mechanism.

Deep biological heterogeneity of DLBCL has two main implications: First, highly heterogeneous driven genetic alterations, critical in the initial lymphomagenesis are necessary for activation of key signaling pathways, such as loss-of-function lesions targeting negative regulators of BCR signaling. Second, a temporal order of these genetic events, demonstrated by different subclonal mutation patterns, highlights the role of subsequent alterations in the development of different molecular subtypes and in drug-resistance mechanisms. Moreover, this complexity is compounded by host immune response and its interaction with tumor cells, with the development of a mechanism of immune-surveillance escape. Future efforts should address personalized therapy utilizing novel agents targeting specific molecular subtypes and signaling pathways.

Table 39.1 Genetic subtypes of DLBCL.

Genetic subtypes	Mutations pattern	Other recurrent mutations/ epigenetic attributes	Signature	Prevalent COO	Clinical features	Outcome after R-CHOP (5y-OS %)	Possible target therapy
MCD/ C5	MYD88^{L265P} CD79B	Gain or amplification of SPIB (TR relate to IRF4), PRDMN1 mutation (inhibits plasmacytic differentiation), NF-kB BCR pathway mutations MYC induced genes expression Less TP53 mutations	Proliferation, chronic active BCR	ABC	Extranodal involvement	Unfavorable (26%)	BTK-I (Ibrutinib), PI3K-I, lenalidomide, SYK-I
BN2/ C1	BCL6 fusions, NOTCH2 mutations	SPEN mutation, DTX1 mutation, NF-kB BCR pathway mutations (PRKCB, BCL10), CD70 (immune escape), MYC induced genes expression	Oncogenic, proliferation, fibrotic microenviroment, chronic active BCR	Uncl, ABC, GCB	-	Favorable (65%)	PKCb-I, BTK-I
N1/C2	NOTCH1 mutations	IRF4, ID3, BCOR (contribute to plasmacytic phenotype)	Quiescient, tumor microenviroment signature	ABC	-	Unfavorable (36%)	Lenalidomide, check point inhibitors
EZB/C3 + C4	EZH2 mutations, BCL2 translocation	REI amplification, Jak-STAT pathway, PI3K and MTOR mutations, PTEN	oncogenic, fibrotic microenviroment	GCB	Better PS	Favorable (68%)	PI3K-I, mTOR-I, BCL2-I

PCOO: cell of origin; R-CHOP: rituximab, cyclophosphamide, doxorubicin, vincristine, and prednisone; 5y-OS: five-year overall survival; BCR: B-cell receptor; ABC: activated B-cell; Uncl: unclassified; GCB: germinal center B-cell; MTK-i: Bruton tyrosin kinasse inhibitos; PI3K-I: phosphatidil-inosil 3 kinase inhibitor; SIY-i: spleen inducible kinase inhibitor; PKC-I: protein kinase 3 beta inhibitor; mTOR: mammalian target of rapamycin; PS: performance status; Cluster 0 (not included in the table), less common subtype, included mostly T-cell/histocyte-rich DLBCL, morphologically characterized by high inflammatory/immune infiltrate and the absence of typical detectable driven mutational events, which may reflect a different pathogenetic mechanism.

4) How can we identify high-grade lymphomas with MYC and BCL2 and/or BCL6 rearrangements (double- or triple-hit lymphomas)? In which patients should this analysis be performed?

Expert Perspective: The last revised 2017 WHO Classification of lymphoid neoplasms introduced important changes in the categorization of mature B-aggressive lymphomas defining a new wide entity under the name of high-grade B-cell lymphomas (HGBL), mostly due to the recent understanding of the importance of *MYC, BCL2*, and *BCL6* rearrangements. Therefore, a new category previously known as double-hit/triple-hit lymphoma (DHL/THL) was defined and named high-grade B-cell lymphomas with *MYC* and *BCL2* and/or *BCL6* rearrangements (HGBL,R) which includes all large B-cell lymphomas with *MYC* and *BCL2* and/ or *BCL6* rearrangements, excluding cases of lymphoblastic or follicular lymphomas. On the other hand, all cases with morphologically aggressive features including those that appear like blastoid or Burkitt lymphoma (BL), and lymphomas with features intermediate between diffuse large B-cell lymphomas and Burkitt lymphoma (DLBCL/BL) but that lack an *MYC* and *BCL2* and/ or *BCL6* rearrangement were placed in a unique category under the name of high-grade B-cell lymphomas, not otherwise specified (HGBL-NOS).

These (HGBCL and DLBCL/BL) new entities have a well-known dismal prognosis, representing a diagnostic and therapeutic challenge for pathologists and clinicians. A comprehensive histopathological diagnosis of HGBL should include IHC, FISH, and cytogenetic studies. FISH analysis is considered the gold standard analysis for identification of HGBL with *MYC* and *BCL2* and/or *BCL6* rearrangement (*MYC* rearrangement at chromosome 8q24.2, BCL2 rearrangement at chromosome 18q21.3, BCL6 rearrangement on chromosome 3q27.3). The presence of only copy number increase, amplification, or somatic mutation without the rearrangement is not sufficient for diagnosis of HGBCL. The frequency of HGBL,R cases among tumors with DLBCL morphological features is estimated to range from 1 to 12%. Among HGBCL, most cases have a *BCL2* rearrangement (*MYC/BCL2* or *MYC/BCL2/BCL6*) whereas *MYC/BCL6* DHLs are less common. A clear consensus to provide guidelines to which patients must be investigated with genetic probes has not yet been reached. Some pathologists and clinicians suggest a further investigation only in cases with GCB phenotype, cases with high-grade morphological features, and those with MYC protein overexpression (> 40%). Nevertheless, neither morphology, Ki-67 proliferation index, nor immunohistochemical overexpression of MYC or BCL2 prognosis has sufficient sensitivity and specificity to identify DHL/THLs and cannot be used as surrogate marker. Certainly, this approach could identify most of DHL/THLs, and it should be considered a reasonable strategy in an effort to control costs and save time. However, few considerations are needed: (i) while almost 100% of DHL with *MYC* and *BCL2* rearrangements have a GCB phenotype, 20 to 50% of *MYC/BCL6* DHL are characterized by non-GCB type, if tested by IHC; (ii) not all patients with *MYC* rearrangement overexpress the protein, so MYC as well as BCL2 protein expression, although independently valuable prognostic factors, are not ideal predictors of DHL/THLs; HGBLs typically show high Ki-67 proliferation index, but no clear cut-off value has been defined. Due to the lack of consensus and the clinical impact of *MYC, BCL2*, and *BCL6* aberrations, WHO classification strongly advises that all DLBCL cases should undergo FISH studies. These patients show poor outcome if treated with standard R-CHOP, so an intensified approach with high-dose chemotherapy is often recommended (Figure 39.2). However, standard treatment for HGBL has not yet been defined and represents a therapeutic challenge (see Chapters 34 and 42).

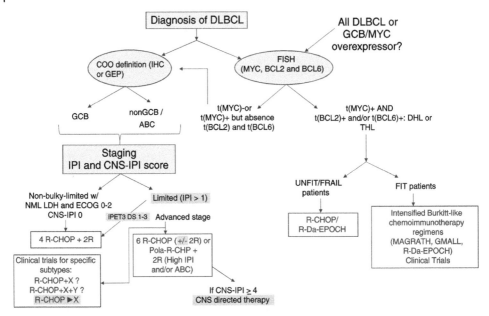

Figure 39.2 Diagnostic and therapeutic algorithm in newly diagnosed DLBCL. COO: Cell of origin; IHC: immunohistochemistry; GEP: gene-expression profiling; FISH: fluorescent *in situ* hybridization; GCB: germinal center B-cell; ABC: activated B-cell; DHL: double-hit lymphoma; THL: triple-hit lymphoma; IPI: International Prognostic Score; CNS-IPI: central nervous system-IPI; R-CHOP: rituximab, cyclophosphamide, doxorubicin, vincristine, and prednisone; Pola-R-CHP: Polatuzumab vedotin, rituximab, cyclophosphamide, doxorubicin, and prednisone R-Da-EPOCH: dose-adjusted EPOCH-R (etoposide, prednisone, vincristine, cyclophosphamide, doxorubicin, and rituximab), MAGRATH: four courses, 2 regimen A: CODOX-M (cyclophosphamide, doxorubicin, adriamycin, vincristine with intrathecal methotrexate and cytarabine followed by high-dose systemic methotrexate) 2 regimen B: IVAC (ifosfamide, cytarabine, etoposide, and intrathecal methotrexate); GMALL protocol for Burkitt lymphoma.

Limited-Stage Disease

5) A 45-year-old male patient with newly diagnosed DLBCL, stage IA, aaIPI 0, no bulky disease, comes to your clinic. He has ECOG performance status of 1.

Which of the following is the best option to cure this patient?

A) High-dose immunochemotherapy plus autologous stem cell transplantation.

B) Six cycles of R-CHOP21 therapy with interim PET scan.

C) Four cycles of R-CHOP21 plus two additional doses of rituximab followed by PET scan.

D) Three cycles of R-CHOP21 followed by PET scan.

Expert Perspective: Two approaches are feasible in patients with and without specific adverse features at diagnosis.

1) **Absence of adverse features at diagnosis:** The results coming from the recently published FLYER trial suggested that a selected group of young DLBCL patients with favorable prognosis and limited-stage disease could benefit from a short chemoimmunotherapy course with four cycles of R-CHOP plus two additional doses of rituximab monotherapy, instead of the standard six cycles of R-CHOP courses. Patients enrolled in the trial

were aged between 18 to 60 years old, mostly had limited stage I–II, age-adjusted IPI (aa-IPI) 0, and non-bulky disease (< 7.5 cm) with ECOG performance status of 0–2. They were randomized to received four vs six R-CHOP courses: the three-year progression-free survival, event-free survival, and overall survival were superimposable in the two groups, with a 30% reduction of adverse events in the cohort randomized to the short course of chemoimmunotherapy.

2) **Risk-adapted approach:** Moreover, the recent results from the S1001 SWOG trial showed that newly diagnosed DLBCL 18 to 60 years old patients with limited-stage I–II, non-bulky (< 10 cm) disease (regardless of performance status and LDH), who achieved complete remission with negative PET scan after three courses of R-CHOP (iPET3-DS1-3) therapy could safely avoid radiotherapy consolidation and complete therapy with an additional R-CHOP cycle (total of four cycles).

The data from these two trials stated a short course of chemoimmunotherapy with four cycles of R-CHOP as a new standard treatment for limited-stage, low-risk, newly diagnosed DLBCL patients up to 60 years of age.

Case Study continued: Our patient does not have any adverse features; therefore, he will follow the treatment algorithm from the FLYER study.

Correct Answer: C

Advanced-Stage Disease

6) **First line treatment of advanced-stage DLBCL: Could we find something better than R-CHOP?**

Expert Perspective: Although R-CHOP21 currently remains the standard backbone of first-line treatment in newly diagnosed DLBCL, this approach can cure only about 60% of patients with advanced disease. The remainder still experiences relapses and often succumbs to the disease (see Chapter 40). In the past two decades, tremendous efforts have been performed with manifold clinical trials aimed to ameliorate this standard therapy. Many attempts to improve R-CHOP21 results with different treatment schedules or with other chemoimmunotherapy regimens have been done, including increasing dose density (R-CHOP14), altering drug delivery methods (Da-EPOCH), using alternative drugs (R-ACVBP), or including a high-dose intensity regimen, such as R-MegaCHOP, high-dose cytarabine, or ASCT consolidation after first-line treatment. However, none of these trials achieved the goal of demonstrating a significant improvement in outcome if compared to standard R-CHOP21. The advances in immunotherapy and the development of novel, more active monoclonal antibodies laid the groundwork for novel combination trials. The studies along with their results are summarized below.

- **POLARIX study (2022):** R-pola-CHP (rituximab, polatuzumab vedotin, doxorubicin, prednisone) was associated with two-year overall survival of 89%, which was similar to R-CHOP; nonetheless, the two-year progression-free survival of 77% and two-year event-free survival of 76% were superior to R-CHOP. Pola-R-CHP appears to be remarkably beneficial for ABC DLBCL. Toxicity of the two regimens was similar; grade ≥ 3 adverse events with R-pola-CHP were primarily cytopenias, febrile neutropenia, and 1.6% grade ≥ 3 peripheral neuropathy. On April 19, 2023, the FDA approved R-pola-CHP for adult patients who have previously untreated DLBCL, not otherwise specified, or high-grade B-cell lymphoma and who have an IPI Index score of 2 or greater.

- **The GOYA study (2017):** randomized previously untreated DLBCL patients to receive standard R-CHOP vs obinutuzumab-CHOP (Ga-CHOP) front-line therapy, on the basis of promising results showed by this novel glycoengineered, type II, anti-CD20 monoclonal antibody in follicular lymphomas. The three-year progression-free survival rates were 70% vs 67%, in Ga vs R arm, respectively. The overall response rates as well were similar between arms. In exploratory subgroup analyses, patients with GCB subtype had a better progression-free survival than did patients with activated B cell–like subtype, irrespective of treatment. The authors concluded that Ga-CHOP did not improve the primary endpoint of progression-free survival compared with R-CHOP in previously untreated DLBCL, even if Ga-CHOP showed a good safety profile.

- **REMoDL-B (2019 and 2023 with 5 year follow-up) and other studies with bortezomib:** Constitutive NF-kB activation is more common, even if not exclusive, in ABC subtype of DLBCL. It has been investigated on ABC cell line *in vitro* and showed a dose-depending growth inhibition traducing in activation of mitochondrial apoptosis pathway. Bortezomib seemed to be able to sensitize patients to chemotherapy but as single agent does not show the same efficacy in DLBCL. In relapsed/refractory setting, it has been investigated in association to Da-EPOCH regimen, showing overall and complete response (CR) rate much higher in ABC vs GCB DLCBL (overall response rate 83% vs 13% and CR 41% vs 6.5% in ABC vs GCB subtype, respectively). Overall survival as well was dramatically superior in ABC vs GCB group (10.8 vs 3.4 months, respectively). These data suggested to evaluate bortezomib also in newly diagnosed non-GCB DLBCL. The phase II study LYM-2034 investigated bortezomib as a replacement for vincristine within the R-CHOP regimen (VR-CAP) in previously untreated non-GCB DLBCL patients, but no significant difference in overall response rate and overall survival were observed compared to R-CHOP. The phase II PYRAMID trial, which also compared R-CHOP vs VR-CHOP in newly diagnosed non-GCB DLBCL patients, was unable to demonstrate any difference between the two regimens. However, both trials stratified patients based on IHC and not GEP. The phase III REMoDL-B study (2019 and 2023) randomized more than a thousand newly diagnosed DLBLC to receive VR-CHOP vs R-CHOP. Patients were stratified in ABC vs GCB subtype defined by central GEP assay, resulting in 27% ABC, 52% GCB, and 22% unclassifiable. Despite the promising preclinical evidence, this trial failed to show significant differences in terms of overall response rate, CR and progression-free survival between the two treatment arms in all three subtypes groups. Clinical trials frequently include multiple end points that mature at different times. The recent 5 year follow-up of the same study using a gene expression-based classifier identified a molecular high-grade (MHG) group with worse outcomes. Eligible patients were age older than 18 years with untreated DLBCL, fit enough for full-dose chemotherapy, and with adequate biopsies for GEP. Of 1,077 patients registered, 801 were identified with ABC, Germinal Center B-cell, or MHG lymphoma. At a median follow-up of 64 months, again, there was no overall benefit of bortezomib on PFS or OS (5-year PFS hazard ratio [HR], 0.81; P = .085; OS HR, 0.86; P = .32). However, improved PFS and OS were seen in ABC lymphomas after RB-CHOP: 5-year OS 67% with R-CHOP versus 80% with VR-CHOP (HR, 0.58; 95% CI, 0.35 to 0.95; P = .032). Five-year PFS was higher in MHG lymphomas: 29% versus 55% (HR, 0.46; 95% CI, 0.26 to 0.84). The study concluded that patients with ABC and MHG DLBCL may benefit from the addition of bortezomib to R-CHOP in initial therapy.

- **PHOENIX (2019) and other studies with ibrutinib:** Ibrutinib is an oral Bruton tyrosine kinase (BTK) inhibitor, which has a key role in B-cell receptor (BCR) pathway, linking BCR with NF-kB signaling. Single-agent ibrutinib was tested in phase I and II studies in relapsed/refractory B-cell malignancies. A phase II study in previously treated DLBCL, administered with single-agent ibrutinib showed an overall response rate of 37% in ABC-DLBCL (CR 16%), while only a small number of responses (5%) in patients with GCB subtype. Median progression-free survival was 2.02 vs 1.31 months and median OS 10.32 vs 3.35 months in ABC vs GCB subtypes, respectively. Response to ibrutinib was particularly evident in ABC lymphoma with BCR mutations, especially those with concomitant myeloid differentiation primary response 88 (MYD88) mutation. On these promising bases, ibrutinib was investigated in association with R-CHOP in untreated DLBCL. A phase I–II trial established as 560 mg/day the maximum tolerated dose of ibrutinib in addition to R-CHOP, with overall response rate of 94% with 71% and 100% of CR in GCB and non-GCB DLBCL, respectively. Consequently, a phase III randomized PHOENIX study comparing R-CHOP versus ibrutinib-R-CHOP (RI-CHOP) in 838 non-GCB DLBCL patients, assessed by central IHC according to Hans algorithm, was conducted. Unluckily, the study did not show an improvement by the addition of ibrutinib, in the intent to improve event-free survival. However, in patients aged younger than 60 years, RI-CHOP improved event-free survival (HR = 0.579), progression-free survival (HR = 0.556), and overall survival (HR = 0.330) and slightly increased serious adverse events (35.7% vs 28.6%). In contrast, in patients older than 60 years, ibrutinib plus R-CHOP worsened survival, increased serious adverse events (63.4% vs 38.2%), and decreased the proportion of patients able to receive at least six cycles of R-CHOP (73.7% vs 88.8%). Despite the advantage in young patients, the study did not meet its primary endpoint. Further subanalysis is ongoing and will try to shed some light on these negative results.

- **ROBUST (2021) and other studies with lenalidomide:** Many preclinical studies suggested a synergism between lenalidomide and rituximab and xenograft model of DLBCL, undercover a major effect on ABC-subtype disease, which was associated with downregulation of NF-kB pathway, through an inhibition of the transcription factor interferon regulatory factor 4 and of cereblon. Lenalidomide has been largely studied in several series of relapsed/refractory DLBCL in monotherapy or in association with rituximab, showing promising efficacy, with good safety profile. A report from Hernandez Ilizaliturri et al, showed the results of a retrospective analysis on 40 patients with relapsed/refractory DLBCL treated with lenalidomide. Tissue samples of these patients were classified by IHC in GCB and non-GCB: the results suggested a significantly improved response (53% vs. 9%, $P = 0.006$) and median progression-free survival (6.2 vs. 1.7 months; $P = 0.004$) in the non-GCB versus GCB subtype, underlined a major activity of lenalidomide in non-GCB DLBCL. Lenalidomide was thus largely investigated in front-line treatment. Three prospective multicenter phase I/II studies analyzed the efficacy and safety the association of lenalidomide with R-CHOP (R2-CHOP) in newly diagnosed DLBCL (REAL07 study by Fondazione Italiana Linfomi, MC078E trial by Mayo Clinic, and R2CHOP study by LYSArc, including also indolent lymphomas). All these studies suggested good safety profile and high efficacy of the combination, especially in non-GCB subtype. The MC078E study compared 64 patients treated with R2-CHOP regimen with a historical control group of 87 patients treated with standard R-CHOP. In the historical control group, as expected, patients with non-GCB subtype experienced inferior two-year progression-free survival (28% vs 64%) and two-year overall survival (46% vs. 74%) than those with the GCB DLBCL. On the other hand, in patients treated with R2-CHOP, two-year progression-free survival and two-year OS were similar for both COO subtypes (60% vs. 59% and 83% vs. 75%, respectively), suggesting improved outcome for non-GCB DLBCL patients if treated with R2-CHOP compared to R-CHOP. On these bases, a randomized multicenter phase III, double-blind trial, the ROBUST trial, was designed only to address previously untreated DLBCL with ABC profile, characterized by GEP on FFPE tissue with NanoString technology. A total of 570 patients were enrolled: median progression-free survival was not reached for either arm (HR = 1.04; *P* = 0.73). The overall response rate was 91% for both arms, with CR 69% vs 65% and two-year OS 79% vs 80% for R2-CHOP vs placebo/R-CHOP, respectively. Despite a positive progression-free survival trend in R2-CHOP over R-CHOP in high IPI score risk and advanced-stage disease, ROBUST trial did not meet the primary endpoint. At the same time, the phase II ECOG 1412 study randomized 280 DLBCL, not differentiated by COO, patients to received R2-CHOP vs placebo/R-CHOP. The schedule of lenalidomide was slightly different than in ROBUST, and the time from enrollment to treatment was very short since centralized pathology review was not necessary. The ECOG 1412 showed improvement in progression-free survival in patients treated with R2-CHOP with statistically significant 34% reduction in risk of death or progression. There was also a positive trend in overall survival and overall response rate toward improved outcome. COO was performed in 234 patients. In the 40% ABC subtype there was a trend toward improved progression-free survival and overall survival for patients treated with R2-CHOP as opposed to R-CHOP alone. However, the ECOG 1412 was a randomized phase II trial in contrast to ROBUST, which was phase III, and hence these encouraging results did not change the practice.

- **CAVALLI study (2021):** Another molecule investigated in R-CHOP + X combination was venetoclax, a BCL2 inhibitor. The phase II CAVALLI trial enrolled 208 DLBCL patients to received R-CHOP in combination with venetoclax: an advantage was observed for patients with BCL2 overexpression or translocation, compared to a matched cohort from GOYA trial. The combinations were affected by high rate of toxicities (cytopenia, infection, febrile neutropenia).

- **Other R-CHOP + X studies:** At the 2020 American Society of Hematology (ASH) Annual Meeting, other trials investigating novel R-CHOP-X combinations have been reported. Selinexor, an oral selective inhibitor of exportin-1, overexpressed in NHL, already studied in relapsed/refractory DLBCL with overall response rate 29% and CR 13%, was investigated in combination to R-CHOP in untreated patients in a phase I trial on 12 cases. Among 10 patients evaluable for response, results were encouraging, with overall response rate 100% and CR 90%, even if many patients discontinued selinexor because of toxicities. A phase II trial is now ongoing in front-line DLBCL and Richter syndrome. Pembrolizumab, a monoclonal antibody anti-programmed death ligand 1(PD-L1), has been investigated in association to R-CHOP in newly diagnosed DLBCL, showing no significant additive results and promising two-year progression-free survival 83%. These results have been confirmed at a long-term follow-up analysis recently reported.

Even if new molecules are under investigation in phase I–II in combination to R-CHOP to improve outcome in frontline treatment of DLBCL, the negative results of the main randomized phase III trials with R-CHOP-single X combinations suggested the need to move toward doublets or triplets to add to the CHOP backbone, on the basis of increasing knowledge on the deep complexity of DLBCL biology.

- **Smart Start study (2023):** Following this new concept, the phase II Smart Start trial evaluated lead-in treatment with rituximab, lenalidomide (25 mg on days 1–10), and ibrutinib (560 mg daily; RLI) in patients with newly diagnosed DLBCL. RLI as lead in for two cycles followed by RLI combined with standard chemotherapy for six cycles in newly diagnosed non-GCB (according to Hans criteria) was administered. A total of 60 patients (age range, 29-83 years)) were enrolled: 42% had high-risk IPI, 65% had advanced stage, 77% had a Ki-67 of ≥ 80%, and 62% of patients with available tissue were double expressor. Adverse events were slightly higher to what is expected with chemotherapy alone, with the exception of rash in 32% (9% grade 3) and CNS aspergillosis (n = 1). Two patients suffered grade 5 events (CNS aspergillosis, clostridium difficile colitis). Overall response rate for two cycles of RLI alone was 86% (n = 50), CR was 36% (n = 21), and patients achieving a partial response had an 81% median tumor reduction from baseline. At the end of therapy overall response rate is 100% (CR: 95%, partial response 5%), with none of the partial response patients having relapsed to date without further therapy, with a median follow-up of 31 months, the progression-free survival and overall survival were at 91.3% and 96.6% at 2 years, respectively. This Smart Start trial demonstrates the RLI combination before and with chemotherapy results in impressive response rates and survival in newly diagnosed non-GCB DLBCL compared with historical outcomes.

FRONT-MIND study: Following this new concept, preliminary results of another trial investigating tafasitamab (MOR208) plus lenalidomide in combinations with R-CHOP have been presented. Tafasitamab is a humanized, Fc-enhanced, anti-CD19 monoclonal antibody, showing an improved antibody-dependent cellular cytotoxicity and phagocytosis, which demonstrated to be effective in relapsed/refractory DLBCL in monotherapy and in combination with lenalidomide. Thus, this doublet was studied in combination with R-CHOP in front-line treatment of DLBCL. Recruitment is ongoing, but safety data from phase Ib were reassuring, and efficacy data are soon expected. On these bases, a phase III trial, the FRONT-MIND study, has been designed to evaluate the efficacy of the combination tafasitamab-lenalidomide-R-CHOP in a large population of intermediate and high-risk newly diagnosed DLBCL.

Central Nervous System (CNS) Prophylaxis

7) Which newly diagnosed patient with DLBCL should be considered for CNS-directed prophylaxis?

Expert Perspective: Central nervous system (CNS) relapse is a rare but potentially fatal event in the natural history of DLBCL, occurring in 2–4% of patients. CNS dissemination usually occurs within less than one year from lymphoma diagnosis with or without systemic recurrence. Patients with CNS progression have a dismal prognosis with a median survival of 4–5 months. Several clinical features at disease diagnosis are used to identify the high-risk patients. Presently, the most common score used to define CNS-relapse risk of aggressive lymphoma is CNS-IPI, which is based on six different clinical variables: age older than 60 years, ECOG performance status (PS) > 2, elevated LDH serum level, advanced III–IV stage disease, presence of two or more extranodal sites, and renal or adrenal involvement. Patients are classified in low risk (0–1 risk factor), intermediate risk (2–3 risk factors), or high risk (4–6 risk factors). Patients have an estimated two-year rate of CNS disease of < 1% vs 2.4% to 4.7% vs > 5% in low- vs intermediate- vs high-risk group, respectively. In particular, high-risk patients with four to six risk factors have rates of 7.4%, 15.0%, and 32.5%, respectively. Actually, the application of this clinical score has been a matter of debate because of its low sensitivity. Integrating biomarkers into clinical CNS-IPI, such as COO subtype or MYC and BCL2 expression, may improve the identification of high-risk patients and should be investigated in a large series of prospective cases. For example, pattern of CNS relapse was analyzed in 1,418 DLBCL patients treated with Ga-CHOP or R-CHOP in the phase III GOYA study. COO assessed using GEP, BCL2, and MYC protein expression in IHC were analyzed in a multivariate Cox regression model: high CNS-IPI score, ABC or unclassified COO subtypes were found independently associated with risk of CNS relapse. BCL2/MYC dual-expression status did not affect CNS relapse risk. Three risk subgroups were identified based on the presence of high CNS-IPI score and/or ABC/unclassified COO (CNS-IPI-C model): low risk (no risk factors), intermediate risk (one factor), and high risk (both factors). Two-year CNS relapse rates were 0.5%, 4.4%, and 15.2%, in the respective risk subgroups. This is an example of how the combinations of biological and clinical features could improve CNS relapse prediction and identify a patient subgroup at high risk for developing CNS relapse. Intrathecal chemotherapy prophylaxis has been largely used in the past decades; however, cumulative data have challenged its efficacy in reducing the incidence of CNS recurrence. In recent years, administration of systemic high-dose methotrexate (HD-MTX) as CNS prophylaxis, in addition to first-line treatment, has been used in patients with high CNS-IPI risk. Nevertheless, two recent reports by real-world retrospective analysis showed a lack of effectiveness even of systemic HD-MTX in preventing CNS relapse in DLBCL, suggesting that optimizing front-line therapy to achieve better systemic disease control may be a more effective strategy to reduce the risk of CNS recurrence than prophylactic HD-MTX alone. Treatment of secondary CNS recurrence in patients with aggressive lymphomas remains an unmet clinical need, and standard therapeutic approach has not been defined yet. Intensified chemoimmunotherapy regimens, including HD-MTX, followed by autologous transplant, have been investigated. Novel drugs could hopefully have a key role in improving the current therapeutic approach (see Chapter 45).

8) Could maintenance treatment with rituximab or other agents, such as lenalidomide, ameliorate the outcome of DLBCL patients?

Expert Perspective: A recent phase III randomized trial, conducted by the Haemato Oncology Foundation for Adults in the Netherlands (HOVON) and the Nordic Groups, compared standard R-CHOP treatment vs a regimen based on an intensified dose of rituximab, showing no advantages from this last intensified scheme. Patients who achieved complete remission were randomized to receive observation vs rituximab maintenance, with standard schedule every eight weeks for two years. The results showed no significative differences in terms of five-year disease-free survival (74% vs 79% in observation vs rituximab maintenance, respectively, HR 0.83) and superimposable OS between the two arms, demonstrating limited role for rituximab maintenance in DLBCL patients responding to first-line treatment.

Different could be the role of maintenance with other agents, such as lenalidomide, in selected groups of DLBCL patients. In the phase III REMARC study (2020) elderly patients, aged between 60 to 80 years old, with DLCBL, who achieved CR or partial response to R-CHOP treatment, were randomized to maintenance with lenalidomide vs placebo. Lenalidomide maintenance was administered with the schedule of 25 mg/day for 21 days of every 28-day cycle for 24 months. A total of 650 patients were enrolled. At a median follow-up of 39 months from random assignment, median progression-free survival was not reached vs 58.9 months for lenalidomide maintenance vs placebo, respectively (HR 0.708; 95% CI 0.537–0.933; $P = 0.01$). Nevertheless, OS were similar among different arms. These results showed that lenalidomide maintenance in elderly patients responding to R-CHOP treatment could prolong progression-free survival. However, the absence of advantages in terms of OS suggested that patients who experienced a relapse after first-line treatment could be saved by salvage therapy, such as lenalidomide, given only to patients who required retreatment. At this time, maintenance therapy cannot be recommended for all patients with DLBCL.

Further Insight

DLBCL is the most common lymphoma worldwide, and it is pathologically and clinically heterogeneous. The increasing possibility to characterize DLBCL through advanced-sequencing techniques in the genomic era ushered large new opportunities but also great challenges. The extensive heterogeneity of mutations among individual patients and within a tumor of a given individual patient made the "one size fits all" approach clearly inappropriate. Although R-CHOP21 remains the standard of care for DLBCL, several new combinations have been investigated, even if with conflicting results, making difficult to draw definitive conclusions regarding the choice of a specific drug or drug combination for specific subgroup of patients. Recently published POLARIX study has added new option in advanced-stage DLBCL with an IPI index score of 2-5 (discussed above). It is becoming increasingly clear that the goal of personalized treatment for lymphomas is ultimately attainable and researchers should keep trying to reach it.

Recommended Readings

Chapuy, B., Stewart, C., Dunford, A.J. et al. (2018). Molecular subtypes od diffuse large B-cell lymphoma are associated with distinct pathogenic mechanism and outcomes. *Nat Med* 24: 679–690.

Coiffier, B., Lepage, E., Briere, J., Herbrecht, R., Tilly, H., Bouabdallah, R. et al. (2002). CHOP chemotherapy plus rituximab compared with CHOPalone in elderly patients with diffuse large-B-cell lymphoma. *N Engl J Med* 346 (4): 235–242.

Davies, A.J., Barrans, S., Stanton, L. et al. (2023 May 20). Differential efficacy from the addition of bortezomib to R-CHOP in diffuse large B-cell lymphoma according to the molecular subgroup in the REMoDL-B study with a 5-Year follow-up. *J Clin Oncol* 41 (15): 2718–2723. doi: 10.1200/JCO.23.00033. Epub 2023 Mar 27. PMID: 36972491.

Dührsen, U., Müller, S., Hertenstein, B. et al. (2018 July 10). PETAL trial investigators. positron emission tomography-guided therapy of aggressive non-hodgkin lymphomas (PETAL): a multicenter, randomized phase III trial. *J Clin Oncol.* 36 (20): 2024–2034. doi: 10.1200/JCO.2017.76.8093. Epub 2018 May 11. PMID: 29750632.

Farooq, U., Maurer, M.J., Thompson, C.A. et al. (2017). Clinical heterogeneity of diffuse large B-cell lymphoma following failure of front-line immunochemotherapy. *Br J Haematol* 179: 50–60.

Habermann, T.M., Weller, E.A., Morrison, V.A. et al. (2006). Rituximab-CHOP versus CHOP alone or with maintenance rituximab in older patients with diffuse large B-cell lymphoma. *J Clin Oncol* 24: 3121–3127.

Lenz, G., Wright, G., and Dave, S.S. (2008). Stromal gene signatures in large-B-cell lymphomas. *N Engl J Med* 359 (22): 2313–2323.

Nowakowski, G.S., Chiappella, A., Gascoyne, R.D. et al. (2021 April 20). ROBUST: A phase III study of lenalidomide plus R-CHOP versus placebo plus R-CHOP in previously untreated patients with ABC-type diffuse large B-cell lymphoma. *J Clin Oncol* 39 (12): 1317–1328.

Persky, D.O., Li, H., Stephens, D.M., Park, S.I. et al. (2020 September 10). Positron emission tomography-directed therapy for patients with limited-stage diffuse large B-cell lymphoma: results of intergroup national clinical trials network study S1001. *J Clin Oncol* 38 (26): 3003–3011. doi: 10.1200/JCO.20.00999. Epub 2020 Jul 13. Erratum in: J Clin Oncol. 2020 Oct 10;38(29):3459. PMID: 32658627; PMCID: PMC7479758.

Poeschel, V., Held, G., Ziepert M. et al. (2019 December 21). Four versus six cycles of CHOP chemotherapy in combination with six applications of rituximab in patients with aggressive B-cell lymphoma with favourable prognosis (FLYER): a randomised, phase 3, non-inferiority trial. *Lancet* 394 (10216): 2271–2281.

Schmitz, N., Zeynalova, S., Nickelsen, M. et al. (2016 September 10). CNS International prognostic index: a risk model for CNS relapse in patients with diffuse large B-cell lymphoma treated with R-CHOP. *J Clin Oncol* 34 (26): 3150–3156. doi: 10.1200/JCO.2015.65.6520. Epub 2016 Jul 5. PMID: 27382100.

Schmitz, R., Wright, G.W., Huang, D.W. et al. (2018). Genetics and pathogenesis of diffuse large B-cell lymphoma. *Nejm* 378: 1396–1407.

Swerdlow, S.H., Campo, E., Pileri, S.A. et al. (2016). The 2016 revision of the World Health Organization classification of lymphoid neoplasms. *Blood* 127: 2375–2390.

Tilly, H., Morschhauser, F., Sehn, L.H. et al. (2022 January 27). Polatuzumab Vedotin in previously untreated diffuse large B-cell lymphoma. *N Engl J Med* 386 (4): 351–363. doi: 10.1056/NEJMoa2115304. Epub 2021 Dec 14. PMID: 34904799.

Tilly, H., Morschhauser, F., Bartlett, N.L. et al. (2019 July). Polatuzumab vedotin in combination with immunochemotherapy in patients with previously untreated diffuse large B-cell lymphoma: An open-label, non-randomised, phase 1b-2 study. *Lancet Oncol* 20 (7): 998–1010. doi: 10.1016/S1470-2045(19)30091-9. Epub 2019 May 14. PMID: 31101489.

Westin, J., Davis, R.E., Feng, L. et al. (2023 February 1). Smart start: rituximab, lenalidomide, and ibrutinib in patients with newly diagnosed large B-cell lymphoma. *J Clin Oncol* 41 (4): 745–755. doi: 10.1200/JCO.22.00597. Epub 2022 Aug 11. PMID: 35952327.

Younes, A., Sehn, L.H., Johnson, P. et al. (2019 May 20). Randomized phase III trial of ibrutinib and rituximab plus cyclophosphamide, doxorubicin, vincristine, and prednisone in non-germinal center B-cell diffuse large B-cell lymphoma. *J Clin Oncol* 37 (15): 1285–1295.

40

Hematopoietic Cell Transplantation and Cellular Therapy in Diffuse Large B Cell Lymphoma

Shreya Desai[1], Syed Maaz Tariq[2], Arjun Patel[3], Istvan Redei[3], and Syed A. Abutalib[4]

[1] Department of Medicine, Rosalind Franklin University of Medicine and Science, North Chicago, IL, USA
Division of Hematology/Oncology, Georgia Cancer Center at Augusta University, Augusta, GA, USA
[2] Jinnah Sind Medical University, Karachi, Sind, Pakistan
[3] City of Hope, Zion, IL
[4] Aurora St. Luke's Medical Center, Milwaukee, WI

Introduction

About 30–40% of patients with newly diagnosed advanced diffuse large B-cell lymphoma (DLBCL) experience relapse, and 10% are refractory to R-CHOP (cyclophosphamide, doxorubicin, vincristine, and prednisone). Most relapses occur during the first two years although late relapses after five years have been observed. At relapse, patients are categorized into one of two therapeutic groups: (i) transplant eligible or (ii) transplant ineligible. Transplant eligible patients who respond (≥ partial response [PR]) to platinum-based immunochemotherapy proceed with curative intent to high-dose chemotherapy and autologous hematopoietic transplantation (auto-HCT). Certain disease characteristics, such as primary refractoriness, early (< 12 months) relapse, a high second-line age-adjusted International Prognostic Index (IPI), and double- or triple-hit genetic lesions in the tumor (rearrangement of *MYC* with *BCL2* or *BCL6* [or both]), have been associated with lower likelihood of response to salvage therapy. Some of these patients are more fit for second-line CAR T cell therapy. It is important to recognize that approximately 50% of transplant-eligible patients will not receive the intended auto-HCT owing to the failure of platinum-based immunochemotherapy; this subgroup of patients are candidates for third-line therapies including three FDA approved CAR T cell therapies (tisagenlecleucel [tisa-cel], axicabtagene ciloleucel [axi-cel], and lisocabtagene maraleucel [liso-cel]). The standard of care second-line therapy for transplant ineligible is undefined and evolving (Table 40.1).

Cancer Consult: Expertise in Clinical Practice, Volume 2: Neoplastic Hematology & Cellular Therapy,
Second Edition. Edited by Syed A. Abutalib, Maurie Markman, James O. Armitage, and Kenneth C. Anderson.
© 2024 John Wiley & Sons Ltd. Published 2024 by John Wiley & Sons Ltd.

Table 40.1 Therapeutic options in relapsed/refractory, transplant-ineligible DLBCL patients.

Lisocabtagene maraleucel (liso-cel)
Gemcitabine, oxaliplatin ± rituximab
Polatuzumab vedotin ± bendamustine ± rituximab
Tafasitamab + lenalidomide
CEOP (cyclophosphamide, etoposide, vincristine, prednisone) ± rituximab
DA-EPOCH ± rituximab
GDP ± rituximab OR gemcitabine, dexamethasone, carboplatin ± rituximab
Gemcitabine, vinorelbine, ± rituximab
Rituximab
Brentuximab vedotin for CD30 + disease
Bendamustine ± rituximab
Ibrutinib (non-GCB DLBCL)
Lenalidomide ± rituximab (non-GCB DLBCL)

Third line and subsequent therapy
Loncastuximab tesirine
Glofitamab
Epcoritamab

Case Study

You are requested to see a 68-year-old very successful hedge fund manager with diffuse large B-cell lymphoma (DLBCL). He comes to you for a third medical oncology opinion with recently diagnosed stage IIIB disease. He has excellent performance status. At the time of diagnosis, the LDH was above the upper limit of normal. His lymphoma does not have C-MYC gene rearrangement or overexpression. The Hans criteria points toward the activated B-cell (ABC) subtype. The gene expression profiling (GEP) analysis confirms the ABC subtype. Approximately eight weeks ago, he completed six cycles of R-CHOP (rituximab plus cyclophosphamide, doxorubicin, vincristine, and prednisone) chemoimmunotherapy with positron-emission tomography (PET) negativity (Deauville score 1). The cycles were given every three weeks. His assistant made an Internet search and told him that he has a "high-risk" lymphoma. He informs you, "I'm a fixer, and I want to be sure that my lymphoma does not come back ever."

1) **What is the next best management strategy?**
    A) High-dose chemotherapy (HDT) and autologous hematopoietic cell transplant (auto-HCT).
    B) Rituximab maintenance for two years.
    C) Surveillance.
    D) Additional two cycles of R-CHOP (total of eight cycles).

This question highlights two important clinical issues in the management of newly diagnosed DLBCL

A) What are the optimal number of R-CHOP cycles (e.g. six versus more than six, especially in HI/HR risk category or ABC DLBCL) in newly diagnosed patients with DLBCL?

Expert Perspective: The RICOVER-60 trial compared six vs eight cycles with and without rituximab in 1,222 patients ages 61–80 years with aggressive NHL; however, the cycles were every two weeks (R-CHOP14). The authors concluded that six cycles should be the standard using R-CHOP-14. Additionally, the results from the exploratory analysis of the international phase III GOYA study, which compared six vs eight cycles of R-CHOP21 in 712 patients with previously untreated DLBCL, also showed no additional benefit in progression-free survival. The authors concluded that six cycles of R-CHOP21 should be considered the standard of care. Population data from Nordic lymphoma group concluded that the outcomes of patients treated with six cycles of R-CHOP21 were non-inferior to the outcomes of those treated with eight cycles of R-CHOP21.

In our opinion, extrapolation of these data with R-CHOP21 in older adults with HR disease is an unsettled issue. The RICOVER-60 trial incorporated histologies other than DLBCL (20% of the patients did not have DLBCL) and < 50% of the patients with aggressive lymphoma (all histologies included) had IPI > 3. In our practice, we prefer R-CHOP21 × 6 cycles in most adults with *de novo* (absence of *c-MYC* gene rearrangement and not transformed from low grade lymphoma) DLBCL. However, European Society of Medical Oncology (ESMO) 2015 guidelines for DLBCL recommend six cycles of R-CHOP21 in patients with low IPI scores and eight cycles of R-CHOP21 in healthy older patients aged > 60–80 years with high IPI scores. Alternatively, the ESMO guidelines recommend six cycles of R-CHOP14 with additional two doses of rituximab (total eight doses of rituximab) for all healthy older patients up to age 80 years. The National Comprehensive Cancer Network (NCCN) guidelines 2023 recommend six cycles of R-CHOP21 with an addition of involved-site radiation therapy (ISRT) in selected bulky cases, which is defined as tumor mass ≥ 10 cm.

B) What is the role of high-dose chemotherapy and auto-HCT in newly diagnosed patients with DLBCL?

Expert Perspective: Most randomized clinical trials have failed to demonstrate OS benefit with front-line auto-HCT in DLBCL. In addition, two meta-analyses (Strehl et al. 2003 and Greb et al. 2007) were unable to show OS benefit. On the contrary, detrimental effects with transplant were observed in low-risk IPI patients. The evidence for or against front-line auto-HCT in patients with high IPI scores continues to be debated especially following the results of the SWOG 9704 study published in the New England Journal of Medicine in 2013. This North American Intergroup study was designed and approved before rituximab; however, the drug was incorporated into the CHOP regimen upon its availability. In this large RCT, patients with high-intermediate risk (HI) and HR IPI received CHOP +/ − rituximab × 5 and then were randomized to either three additional cycles of CHOP +/ − rituximab (n = 128) or one additional cycle of CHOP +/ − rituximab followed by auto-HCT (n = 125). Obviously, the randomization was performed only in patients who achieved greater than or equal to a partial response ("chemosensitive disease"). The study was unable to demonstrate an OS benefit with front-line auto-HCT, not even in patients who received rituximab (n = 72). Subset analysis showed that only patients with high-risk IPI had OS benefit with auto-HCT with two-year OS of 82% versus 64%; however, this was compared between only 44 and 40 patients in the auto-HCT and CHOP +/ – R arms, respectively. In addition, this subset analysis was not specified a priori, and the conditioning regimen used in the study is not the standard of care (BEAM), which reduces generalizability. Therefore, these positive results in favor of auto-HCT for high-risk IPI patients beg caution. In addition, not all patients in this exploratory analysis had DLBCL (22% of all patients had other types of B-cell lymphomas), and rituximab was administered in 48% of patients with B-cell lymphomas.

The GOELAMS 075 study did not demonstrate OS benefit with auto-HCT compared to R-CHOP. In fact, the three-year event-free survival was superior with R-CHOP compared to auto-HCT (56% vs 36%, respectively), with no impact of IPI risk categories on outcomes.

The Italian Lymphoma Foundation (DLCL04) reported a 2 × 2 trial comparing R-CHOP14 with R-MegaCHOP in the first randomization and auto-HCT versus continuation of the original induction regimen in the second randomization, for patients with HR disease. The CR/unconfirmed CR (CR/CRu) rates were 70% for R-CHOP14 and 77% for R-MegaCHOP. With second randomization, there was a two-year progression-free survival in favor of the auto-HCT arm compared with the continuation-of-induction-chemotherapy arm. It was 72% for auto-HCT versus 59% for chemotherapy ($P = 0.008$), with no difference seen in OS.

At present, the American Society for Transplantation and Cellular Therapy (ASTCT) guidelines (updated 2020) and the NCCN guidelines do not advocate front-line auto-HCT in patients with any risk category or molecular classification. In view of the benefit of auto-HCT in the salvage setting, it is likely that certain subgroups of newly diagnosed DLBCL patients may benefit from this or other type of cellular therapy (for example, CAR T) in the front-line setting.

Correct Answer: C

Case Study continued: Unfortunately, approximately 13 months following front-line immunochemotherapy, the patient develops severe B-symptoms; a PET–computed tomography (PET-CT) scan reveals extensive fluoro-deoxyglucose (FDG)-avid lymphadenopathy at original sites (Deauville score 5). Repeat biopsy confirms relapse of ABC DLBCL. Bone marrow examination remains negative for disease.

2) **Which salvage regimen would you recommend for relapsed DLBCL?**
    A) R-DHAP (rituximab, dexamethasone, high-dose cytarabine, and cisplatin).
    B) R-ICE (rituximab, ifosfamide, etoposide, and carboplatin).
    C) R-GDP (rituximab, gemcitabine, dexamethasone, and cisplatin).
    D) Any of the above regimens is a reasonable option.

Expert Perspective: Salvage platinum-based chemotherapy followed by auto-HCT is standard of care for all transplant-eligible patients with chemosensitive disease (⩾ partial response). The choice of a specific salvage regimen should take into consideration patient's comorbidities, physician's comfort level with a particular regimen, and the regimen's ability to reduce disease burden without hampering the stem cell mobilization process. Achievement of complete response is always preferred over partial response, but it is not a prerequisite to proceed with auto-HCT as long as chemosensitivity is demonstrated.

Multiple salvage regimens have been developed, and there remains no standard of care. As such, there is no single best regimen; thus, patients should be encouraged to participate in clinical trials. It must be stated that outcomes are suboptimal even for patients responding and proceeding to auto-HCT. Chemotherapy responders who proceed to autologous transplant have a cure rate of approximately 50%, implying 50% are not cured.

In the rituximab era, the landmark Collaborative Trial in Relapsed Aggressive Lymphoma (CORAL) intergroup study is a randomized controlled trial that compared the two most utilized salvage regimens, R-ICE and R-DHAP, and responding patients received BEAM (carmustine, etoposide, high-dose cytarabine, and melphalan) high-dose therapy and auto-HCT. A second randomization between observation and rituximab maintenance for one year was done after auto-HCT. Several important questions related to relapsed and refractory DLBCL were elegantly addressed in this phase III trial as highlighted in Table 40.2. Noteworthy, only half of the patients were able to receive the intended auto-HCT. This was mainly secondary to progressive disease and highlights the key limitations of currently available salvage regimens and not of auto-HCT.

A larger randomized controlled trial (NCIC CTG LY12) with similar design under National Cancer Information Center (NCIC) sponsorship compared R-GDP (gemcitabine, dexamethasone, and platinum) with R-DHAP regimen in patients with aggressive NHL. The R-GDP was non-inferior to R-DHAP with less toxicity.

In aggregate, it is prudent to effectively incorporate novel agents, preferably early during the disease course especially in patients who are deemed as high risk for refractory or recurrent disease.

Correct Answer: D

3) What is the role of second salvage therapy in relapsed/refractory DLBCL?

Expert Perspective: In the CORAL study, about 30% of the patients who could not proceed to auto-HCT still benefited from a third-line salvage chemotherapy and consolidation autologous transplant, with a significant improvement in long-term survival. In this study, the OS was significantly better in transplanted chemosensitive patients with lower IPI with a one-year OS of 41.6% compared with 16.3% for those not transplanted ($P < 0.0001$).

4) What are the data for CAR T cell therapy as second-line approach in transplant-eligible patients with early (< 12 months) relapsed or primary refractory DLBCL?

Expert Perspective: Early results of three randomized controlled trials have been reported with conflicting results. The primary endpoint of these studies was event-free-survival; however, it was defined differently in these three studies.
The results of the three randomized studies are summarized below.

1) **BELINDA**: Tisa-cel as second-line therapy in aggressive relapsed (early) and refractory NHL patients did not have a higher protocol defined event-free-survival vs standard of care. Interestingly, in the context of this trial, only 32.5% of patients received auto-HCT, a true comparator of CAR T cell therapy. The possible contributing factors for a negative study include study design (primary endpoint, more than one salvage regimen allowed), delay of tisa-cel infusion until after week six assessment, imbalances in relevant patients' characteristics, dose of lymphodepleting chemotherapy, and tisa-cel dose variability. Additional studies are needed to assess which patients may obtain the most benefit.

2) **TRANSFORM**: In the prespecified interim analysis at a median follow-up 6.2 months, liso-cel demonstrated statistically significant and clinically meaningful improvement in protocol-defined event-free-survival compared with standard of care. Of 91 patients in control arm, only 43 patients received auto-HCT, of which 28 achieved CR with second-line chemotherapy. Safety results in the second line setting were consistent with the liso-cel safety profile in third-line or later large B-cell lymphoma. On June 24, 2022,liso-cel was FDA approved for adult patients with large B-cell lymphoma (LBCL) who have refractory disease to first-line chemoimmunotherapy or relapse within 12 months of first-line chemoimmunotherapy; or refractory disease to first-line chemoimmunotherapy **or** relapse after first-line chemoimmunotherapy and are not eligible for auto-HCT due to comorbidities or age.

3) **ZUMA-7**: Axi-cel vs standard of care in relapsed (early) and refractory large B-cell lymphoma demonstrated a statistically significant and clinically meaningful improvement in protocol-defined event-free-survival (HR: 0.398; *P* < 0.0001), with a trend towards OS improvement (HR 0.730; *P* = .027) and expected level of high-grade toxic effects. It is important to recognize the sobering fact that about 80 patients responded to salvage regimen, but only 62 patients received auto-HCT compared to 170 out of 180 axi-cel assigned patients received axi-cel. The investigators noted that in patients who received auto-HCT the outcomes were not as poor. On April 1, 2022, the FDA approved axi-cel for adult patients with large B-cell lymphoma that is refractory to first-line chemoimmunotherapy or relapses within 12 months ("early relapse") of first-line chemoimmunotherapy.

The authors prefer CAR T cell therapy over auto-HCT in patients with early first relapse or primary refractory DLBCL

Case Study continued: Your patient received two cycles of R-DHAP and achieved second remission with a Deauville score of 1 according to the Lugano PET–CT criteria.

5) **What would you recommend for this patient now?**
   A) High-dose chemotherapy and auto-HCT.
   B) Additional three cycles of R-DHAP.
   C) Surveillance.

Expert Perspective: The superiority of auto-HCT over conventional salvage chemotherapy for relapsed and refractory DLBCL was first demonstrated in the PARMA trial (1995) in which 109 patients who had a chemosensitive disease (≥ partial response) were randomly assigned to receive four cycles of DHAP chemotherapy (n = 54) or high-dose chemotherapy with autologous hematopoietic cell rescue (n = 55). Radiotherapy was part of the transplantation protocol and was indicated at the sites of bulky (≥ 5 cm) disease. Patients assigned to transplantation had superior overall survival of 53% versus 32% in the control arm. The overall response rate (84% vs 44%), and event-free survival (46% vs 12%), were also superior in the auto-HCT compared to control arm.

Although widely regarded as the standard approach, the relevance of this study to current management of relapsed DLBCL is uncertain. Eligibility to the PARMA study was restricted to patients younger than 60 years with a previous CR to front-line chemotherapy, and none of the patients had evidence of bone marrow involvement at diagnosis. Moreover, all patients in this study underwent bone marrow harvest, and the study accrued additional histologies other than DLBCL. Another important factor is that this trial was conducted before rituximab was available. With dramatic improvements in supportive care and global use of peripheral blood as the source of hematopoietic stem cells, greater number of auto-HCT are being offered to older adults such as your patient in the case.

Another study on behalf of the European Group for Blood and Marrow Transplantation (EBMT), analyzed the benefit of auto-HCT in relapsed DLBCL patients in second complete remission. The study retrospectively compared disease-free survival after auto-HCT with the duration of CR1 for each patient. Out of 470 patients, 119 patients (25%) received rituximab before auto-HCT whereas 351 patients (75%) were rituximab naive. Overall, the duration of progression-free survival after auto-HCT was significantly increased compared with the duration of first complete remission (median, 51 months vs 11 months; $P < 0.001$). The benefit of auto-HCT was seen regardless of previous exposure to rituximab. The five-year progression-free survival and OS were 48% and 63%, respectively. This EBMT study concluded that even in rituximab era, auto-HCT remains a good therapeutic approach for patients with relapsed and refractory DLBCL who have chemosensitive disease.

In our opinion, patients responding to a salvage regimen should still be considered for auto-HCT. We acknowledge that some patients who relapse early or have a partial response might have inferior outcomes. Such patients should be considered for CAR T cell therapy with T cell apheresis prior to T cell toxic bridging therapy. A recent CIBMTR retrospective study (2021) showed similar progression-free survival and OS following auto-HCT in relapsed patients irrespective of timing to relapse (progression-free survival 41% vs 41%, $P < 0.93$; OS 51% vs 63%, $P < 0.09$).

Correct Answer: A

Case Study continued: From the options given, you recommend high-dose chemotherapy and autologous transplant. The patient is inquisitive about different conditioning regimens. He wants to know which high-dose regimen you would select and why.

6) What do you recommend as high-dose regimen?
   A) TBI and Cy (total body radiation and cyclophosphamide).
   B) BEAM (carmustine, etoposide, cytarabine, melphalan).
   C) 90Y-Ibritumomab tiuxetan with BEAM (Z-BEAM).
   D) 131-Iodine tositumomab with BEAM (I-BEAM).
   E) CBV (cyclophosphamide, carmustine, and etoposide).

Expert Perspective: Commonly used myeloablative conditioning regimens include BEAM, CBV, TBI-Cy, and BuCyVP-16 (busulfan, cyclophosphamide, and etoposide). Although there has been no randomized controlled trial in this setting, comparative studies between TBI-based and non-TBI-based regimens suggest higher rates of secondary hematologic and nonhematologic toxicities without any additional clinical benefit with TBI-based regimens. We recommend BEAM conditioning regimen.

Radioimmunotherapy has been brought forward into the arena of conditioning regimens with hopes of eradicating disease more effectively without added toxicities of TBI. Radioimmunotherapy delivers targeted radiation to lymphoma sites (primarily anti-CD20) while protecting other tissues. Two radiolabeled antibodies, iodine-131 tositumomab (Bexxar) and yttrium-90 ibritumomab (Zevalin), have been approved by the US Food and Drug Administration (FDA) to treat relapsed indolent lymphoma. Press et al. (2006) combined iodine-131 tositumomab (Bexxar) with etoposide and cyclophosphamide in the setting of relapsed NHL. Comparison of this regimen with historical TBI-based conditioning control demonstrated significant improvement in progression-free survival and overall survival. Multiple phase II studies have been published that incorporated radioimmunotherapy to the conditioning regimen, showing lower treatment-related mortality and promising efficacy. These promising phase II data paved the way for radioimmunotherapy to be tested in a randomized controlled trial (CTN 0401) under the supervision of the Bone Marrow Transplant Clinical Trials Network (BMT CTN). The trial enrolled 224 adult patients with persistent or recurrent, chemosensitive DLBCL. Before autologous transplant, patients were randomly assigned to R-BEAM versus BEAM plus conventional-dose iodine-131 tositumomab (I-BEAM). The two-year progression-free survival was 47.9% for I-BEAM and 48.6% for R-BEAM (*P* = 0.94). The two-year overall survival rate was 61% for I-BEAM and 65.6% for R-BEAM (*P* = 0.38). The treatment-related mortality rate was 4.9% in the radioimmunotherapy-BEAM arm and 4.1% in the R-BEAM arm at 2 years (*P* = 0.97). In summary, this phase III study was unable to recapitulate previously reported positive phase II data. In a separate study by Shimoni et al. (2012), standard-dose yttrium-90 ibritumomab tiuxetan (Zevalin) was added to BEAM (Z-BEAM) and was compared with a conventional BEAM regimen in a small, randomized, multicenter study. Forty-three patients with chemosensitive DLBCL were randomized to one of the treatment arms. The progression-free survival with Z-BEAM and BEAM was 59% and 30% at two years, respectively (*P* = 0.20). The overall survival was 91% and 62% at two years, respectively (*P* = 0.05). There was no significant added toxicity with the Z-BEAM regimen. Further large, well-designed, randomized studies are needed to evaluate the exact role of Z-BEAM as a conditioning regimen.

Correct Answer: B

7) What is the role of adding rituximab to BEAM regimen?

Expert Perspective: Although prospective data are lacking, a large CIBMTR registry data of 862 patients with DLBCL from 2013 to 2017 compared BEAM versus R-BEAM in patients who received rituximab during induction and salvage therapy. The study showed no statistically significant difference in progression-free survival (*P* = 0.61) and OS (*P* = 0.83) between the two cohorts; also, there was no significant difference in early infectious complications between the two groups.

Case Study continued: Your patient underwent a successful apheresis CD34 + cell collection followed by BEAM chemotherapy and autologous transplant. A post-transplant PET-CT scan remains negative, and he went back to work two months after auto-HCT.

Now he asks, "Is there anything else that I can do to prevent relapse?"

8) What do you recommend?
   A) Rituximab maintenance therapy for two years.
   B) Surveillance.
   C) Options A and B are reasonable.

Expert Perspective: Maintenance rituximab therapy in relapsed/refractory DLBCL has been evaluated in the context of short treatment courses administered soon after auto-HCT. Prolonged cytopenias and increased incidence of infections have been reported with this strategy.

Haioun et al. (2009) reported no advantage of rituximab maintenance on 269 patients who were randomly assigned to either a control group or four weekly rituximab treatments after auto-HCT.

In the CORAL trial (Table 40.2), there was no difference in EFS, progression-free survival, or overall survival in the maintenance versus observation arm. The four-year post-auto-HCT event-free survival was 52% in the maintenance arm versus 53% in the observation group ($P = 0.07$). A higher incidence of infections was reported in the maintenance arm after day 100. A subset analysis based on gender difference showed that there was a statistically significant difference in progression-free survival favoring females at the time of second randomization ($P = 0.0135$) and after maintenance therapy ($P = 0.0044$). There was

Table 40.2 Data from CORAL study simplified with answers to important questions in relapsed and refractory DLBCL.

Treatment algorithm: R-ICE vs R-DHAP $\rightarrow$ BEAM and auto-HCT $\rightarrow$ rituximab vs observation		
Question	**Answer[†]**	**Comments**
RICE and R-DHAP are comparable salvage regimens	Yes	EFS: 26% vs 35% ($P = 0.6$) at 3 years OS: 47% vs 51% ($P = 0.5$) at 3 years
Did prior (front-line) rituximab-based regimen affect outcomes differently?	Yes	Probability of survival was 34% vs 66% with and without rituximab, respectively
Did relapse greater or less than 12 months affect outcomes differently?	Yes	3-year EFS was 20% vs 45% for relapse > 12 or < 12 months, respectively
Did prior (front-line) rituximab-based regimen affect outcomes differently if relapse was within 12 months of initial therapy?	Yes	3-year EFS was 21% (< 12 months) vs 41% (> 12 months)
Did prior (front-line) rituximab-based regimen affect outcomes differently if relapse was > 12 months following initial therapy?	No	No difference in EFS or OS between the two subgroups with or without rituximab exposure
Did secondary aaIPI had any bearing on prognosis?	Yes	3-year EFS with secondary aaIPI 2–3 was 18% vs 40% for secondary aaIPI 0–1 ($P = 0.0001$)
Did patients with GCB DLBCL respond better to a salvage regimen compared to ABC DLBCL (COO defined by the Hans criteria)?	Yes	Retrospective analysis of the CORAL study showed PFS 70% and OS 74% for GCB DLBCL vs PFS 28%, and OS 40% for ABC DLBCL
Did patients with GCB DLBCL fare better in outcomes with R-DHAP compared to R-ICE (COO defined by the Hans criteria)?	Yes	Retrospective analysis of CORAL study showed PFS at 3 years of 100% with R-DHAP and 27% with R-ICE, but this needs confirmation by a prospective study

(Continued)

Table 40.2 (Continued)

Treatment algorithm: R-ICE vs R-DHAP → BEAM and auto-HCT → rituximab vs observation

Question	Answer[†]	Comments
Did patients with ABC DLBCL fare better in outcomes with R-ICE compared R-DHAP (COO defined by the Hans criteria)?	No	Retrospective analysis of the CORAL study showed equally poor outcomes in ABC DLBCL (via the Hans criteria) with either regimen
Was incidence of C-MYC greater in GCB DLBCL compared to ABC DLBCL by the Hans criteria?	Yes	Retrospective analysis showed that C-MYC by FISH was positive in 17 patients with GCB DLBCL vs 10 patients with ABC DLBCL
Was incidence of C-MYC greater in GCB DLBCL compared to ABC DLBCL by GEP analysis?	Yes	Retrospective analysis showed that C-MYC was more common in GCB DLBCL (n = 3), whereas no cases were associated with ABC DLBCL
Does R-DHAP show OS improvement when compared to R-ICE in patients with C-MYC (genetically defined) positive relapsed or refractory DLBCL?	No	Retrospective analysis showed that the type of salvage regimen, R-DHAP or R-ICE, had no impact on survival, with 4-year PFS rates of 17% vs 19% and 4-year OS rates of 26% vs 31%, respectively
Were most biological characteristics similar between diagnosis and relapse in the 45 matched-pair biopsies studied?	Yes	Retrospective analysis showed this to be true in 87% of the cases
Did maintenance rituximab therapy following auto-HCT improve PFS?	No	The 4-year post–autologous transplant EFS rates were 52% and 53% for the 122 patients with rituximab and the 120 patients in the observation group, respectively ($P = 0.7$)

Abbreviations: aaIPI: age-adjusted International Prognostic Index score; ABC: activated B-cell; auto-HCT: autologous hematopoietic cell transplant; BEAM: carmustine, etoposide, high-dose cytarabine, and melphalan; COO: cell of origin; EFS: event-free survival; FISH: fluorescent in situ hybridization; GCB: germinal B-cell; OS: overall survival; R-DHAP: rituximab, dexamethasone, high-dose cytarabine, and cisplatin; R-ICE: rituximab, ifosfamide, etoposide, and carboplatin.
[†]Applicable to patients between the ages of 18 and 65 as in the CORAL study.

no such gender difference noted in the observation arm ($P = 0.5382$). The authors hypothesized that the lower progression-free survival in males may be a result of hormone-related pharmacokinetic variation that caused higher rituximab clearance, resulting in lower rituximab exposure.

In addition, NCIC CTG LY.12 study studied the role of rituximab as maintenance therapy following auto-HCT. At a median follow-up of 63 months, there was no statistical difference in the two-year event-free survival between rituximab group vs observation group (HR 0.74; 95% CI 0.48–1.14; $P = 0.11$). Additionally, there was no difference in OS at four years among both arms (R 69%, observation 68%, $P = 0.64$).

Newer agents should also be explored following auto-HCT as maintenance therapy. An example for this sort of approach would be the use of CT-011, which is a humanized anti-program death-1 (PD1) antibody. It blocks PD1 function and enhances the activities of natural killer (NK) cells and T cells against PD-L1-positive tumors. Gordon et al. (2011) reported results of 72 chemosensitive relapsed DLBCL patients who received three doses of CT-011 every six weeks, 30–90 days after auto-HCT. Compared with historical data, CT-011 resulted in improved progression-free survival and overall survival in patients with relapsed DLBCL after auto-HCT with acceptable toxicity. Randomized phase III trials are warranted to confirm these intriguing findings. Other agents that are candidates for maintenance therapy include lenalidomide, bortezomib, and vorinostat in selected patients with DLBCL

Correct Answer: B

Case Study continued: The patient came back to see you for one-year post-transplant follow-up. He is very happy because his hedge fund did very well lately. Sadly, the exam and CT scans showed new bulky lymphadenopathy. The biopsy confirmed relapsed DLBCL. He tells you, "Doctor I must live—I have so many things to do." His performance status is excellent.

9) What is the best management strategy following failure after auto-HCT?
- A) Salvage chemotherapy followed by second autologous transplant.
- B) Allogeneic transplant.
- C) CAR T cell therapy.
- D) Hospice.

Expert Perspective: The prognosis of DLBCL patients who relapse after auto-HCT remains poor. In the SCHOLAR-1 study (2017), the median overall survival of patients with relapsed and refractory DLBCL was 6.3 months. The FDA and European Medical Agency (EMS) have approved three CD-19 directed CAR T cell therapies for patients with relapsed and refractory DLBCL after failure of two lines of therapy with one being auto-HCT (Table 40.3).

In the following section we highlight CAR T cell therapy data that led to their approvals in relapsed and refractory DLBCL after at least two lines of therapy including after auto-HCT.

- **Axi-cel** was approved on October 18, 2017. In the ZUMA-1 trial, axicabtagene was administered to patients with DLBCL within one year after auto-HCT; it reported overall response rate of 82% with complete response of 54%. Cytokine release syndrome and neurotoxicity events occurred in 13% and 28% of the patients, respectively. At a follow up of 63 months, response was ongoing in 31% of patients. Median OS was 25.8 months and 5 year OS rate was 43%.
- **Tisa-cel** was approved on May 1, 2018. In the JULIET trial of 165 patients, complete response was achieved in 40% of patients and overall response rate in 52% of the patients. Additionally, relapse-free survival was reported in 65% of patients at a follow-up of 12 months. Grade 3 cytokine release syndrome occurred in 22% of patients, and neurotoxicity events were observed in 12% of patients.
- **Liso-cel** was approved February 5, 2021. The TRANSCEND NHL 001 trial, conducted with 342 patients, showed a favorable overall response rate of 73% and complete response of

Table 40.3 Results of the FDA approved CAR T cell therapy trials in relapsed and refractory DLBCL after failure to two lines of therapy.

	FDA indication	ORR	CR rate	CRS rate (all grades, grade ⩾ 3)	NT rate (all grades, grade ⩾ 3)	Grade ⩾ 3 Cytopenias*
Axicabtagene ciloleucel (ZUMA-1)	Relapsed or refractory LBCL after 2 or more lines of systemic therapy, including DLBCL-NOS, PMLBCL, high-grade LBCL, and DLBCL arising from FL	82%	58%	93%,13%	64%, 28%	Not reported
Tisagenlecleucel (JULIET)	Relapsed or refractory after 2 or more lines of systemic therapy including DLBCL-NOS, high-grade LBCL, and DLBCL arising from FL	52%	40%	58%, 22%	21%,12%	32%
Lisocabtagene maraleucel (TRANSCEND NHL 001)	Relapsed or refractory LBCL after 2 or more lines of systemic therapy, including DLBCL-NOS, high-grade LBCL, PMLBCL, FL grade 3B	73%	53%	42%, 2%	30%, 10%	37%

Abbreviations: ORR: objective response rate; CR: complete response; CRS: cytokine release syndrome; NT: neurologic toxicity; LBCL: large B-cell lymphoma; DLBCL-NOS: diffuse large B-cell lymphoma, not otherwise specified; FL: follicular lymphoma; PMLBCL: primary mediastinal large B-cell lymphoma.
*Grade ⩾ 3 cytopenias not resolved by day 28.

53%. Cytokine release syndrome and neurotoxicity events occurred in 2% and 10% of the patients, respectively. Median PFS was at 6.8 months with median OS at 19.9 months.

Additionally, several real-world registry studies by CIBMTR, US CART consortium, and Dana Farber Institute have showed comparable responses. The use of CAR T-cell therapy is associated with unique immune-mediated toxicities such as cytokine release syndrome and immune effector cell-associated neurotoxicity syndrome (ICANS), which are discussed in more detail in Chapter 59.

Conventional-dose salvage chemotherapy can induce remission in a very small minority of patients. The results of a second auto-HCT are usually disappointing. Allogeneic transplant would be a reasonable consideration in patients after CAR T cell therapy Selected allo-HCT data, after failure to auto-HCT (and without prior CAR T cell therapy) is discussed below.

- **Allo-HCT** using a myeloablative conditioning regimen can achieve durable CRs. However, it has also been associated with exceedingly high non-relapse mortality of approximately 50%. The development of less intensive conditioning regimens that rely more on harnessing on graft-versus-lymphoma (GvL) effect has increased the number of patients who are candidates for this life-saving modality, including patients who relapse after auto-HCT. Two retrospective analyses were published evaluating the results of allo-HCT in patients with DLBCL who relapsed after auto-HCT.

- The analysis of the EBMT database included 101 patients; conditioning regimen was non-myeloablative in 64 patients. The three-year progression-free survival and overall survival were 41% and 53%, respectively. Patients with long remission after auto-HCT and with chemosensitive disease before allo-HCT had the best outcomes.
- Rigacci et al. (2010) analyzed 165 patients whose data were reported to the Gruppo Italiano Trapianto di Midollo Osseo (GITMO) registry; 70% of the patients received non-myeloablative conditioning regimens. The one-, three-, and five-year OS were 55%, 42%, and 39%, respectively. The non-relapse mortality was 28%. Interestingly, the three-year OS was 27% in chemotherapy-refractory patients.

These two retrospective registry studies that include relatively large numbers of patients indicate a role for allo-HCT in patients with DLBCL relapsing after auto-HCT. These data are also suggestive of a possible GvL effect because both progression-free survival and OS curves seem to form a plateau in a heavily pretreated patient population. However, allo-HCT has been largely challenged and replaced by CAR T cell therapy as discussed previously. Nonetheless, once patients relapse after CAR T cell therapy, allo-HCT or clinical trial with bispecific antibodies are reasonable options.

Correct Answer: C

1) Which of the following statements about bispecific antibodies is correct?
- A) They do not require manufacturing of patient's T cells.
- B) They are a form of off-the-shelf immunotherapy.
- C) They do not require lymphodepleting conditioning.
- D) All of the above.

Expert Perspective: Bispecific antibodies are molecules designed to specifically target two different surface antigens, usually one on lymphoma cell (e.g. CD19 or CD20) and a second one ("bispecific") on immune effector T cell such as CD3. This synapse cross links cancer cells with immune cells, resulting in cell-mediated cytotoxicity (immuno-therapy). Subsequently, T cells undergo activation as the result of CD3 cross-linking, which is associated with an increase in T-cell activation markers (CD25 and CD69), cyto-kine release (interferon-gamma, tumor necrosis factor α, interleukin-2, -6, -10), and cyto-toxic granule release (granzyme B). Several CD20/CD3 bispecific antibodies, including blinatumomab, glofitamab, mosunetuzumab, odronextamab, plamotamab, and epcori-tamab, have shown promising activity in B-cell lymphomas with CD19 and CD20 targets. Unlike CAR T cell therapy, bispecfic antibodies do not require lymphodepletion.

Some of the other major advantages of bispecific antibodies over CAR T cell therapy include less severe cytokine release syndrome and neurotoxicity. In relapsed/refractory large B-cell lymphoma, early data has shown overall response and complete response rates from 37 to 80% and 19 to 55%, respectively. In addition, bispecifics may extend excellent activity even after failure to anti-CD19 CAR T cell therapy. Given their remarkable profile, bispecifics are also being investigated in newly diagnosed DLBCL Table (40.4).

Table 40.4 Selected trials of bispecific immunotherapies in relapsed and refractory and previously untreated B-cell non-Hodgkin lymphomas (NHLs).

Antibody	Target	Trial number(s)
Glofitamab	CD20/CD3	NCT04914741
		NCT04657302
		NCT04313608
		NCT04408638
Mosunetuzumab	CD20/CD3	NCT03677154
		NCT04313608
Odronextamab	CD20/CD3	NCT03888105
Epcoritamab	CD20/CD3	NCT04358458
		NCT04628494
		NCT04663347
Blinatumomab	CD19/CD3	NCT02568553
		NCT03023878
		NCT03072771
		NCT03340766

Presently, two bispecific antibodies with similar mechanism of action, are in clinical use. They have not been compared hear-to-head.

(i) Glofitamab (administered every three weeks by intravenous infusion for 12 cycles), a bispecific CD20-directed CD3 T-cell engager, was studied in trial NP30179 (NCT03075696), an open-label, multicenter, single-arm trial that included 132 patients for the evaluation of efficacy. In all, 80% of patients had R/R DLBCL, NOS and 20% had LBCL arising from follicular lymphoma. Patients had received at least two prior lines of systemic therapy (median 3, range 2-7). The trial excluded patients with active or previous central nervous system lymphoma or disease. The overall response rate was 56% (95% CI: 47, 65) with 43% achieving complete responses. With an estimated median follow-up of 11.6 months among responders, the estimated median duration of response was 18.4 months (95% CI: 11.4, not estimable). The 9-month Kaplan-Meier estimate for duration of response was 68.5% (95% CI: 56.7, 80.3). The median time to response was 42 days. Among 145 patients with relapsed or refractory LBCL evaluated for safety, CRS occurred in 70% (Grade 3 or higher CRS, 4.1%), ICANS in 4.8%, serious infections in 16%, and tumor flare in 12%.

(ii) Epcoritamab (administrated subcutaneously every two weeks until disease progression or unacceptable toxicity) is also a bispecific CD20-directed CD3 T-cell engager, was evaluated in EPCORE NHL-1, an open-label, multi-cohort, multicenter, single-arm trial in patients with relapsed or refractory B-cell lymphoma. The efficacy population consisted of 148 patients with R/R DLBCL, NOS, including DLBCL arising from indolent lymphoma, and high-grade B-cell lymphoma after two or more lines of systemic therapy, including at least one anti-CD20 monoclonal antibody-containing therapy. The overall response rate was 61% with 38% of patients achieving complete responses. With a median follow-up of 9.8 months among responders, the estimated median duration of response was 15.6 months. Among the 157 patients with R/R large B-cell lymphoma who received epcoritamab at the recommended dose, CRS occurred in 51% of patients, ICANS in 6%, and serious infections in 15%. For CRS, Grade 1 occurred in 37% of patients, Grade 2 in 17%, and Grade 3 in 2.5%. For ICANS, Grade 1 occurred in 4.5% of patients, Grade 2 in 1.3%, and Grade 5 in 0.6%. As opposed to glofitamab, epcoritamab is administered subcutaneously and is not a time limited therapy.

Correct Answer: D

Recommended Readings

Abramson, J.S., Palomba, M.L., Gordon, L.I. et al. (2020 September 19). Lisocabtagene maraleucel for patients with relapsed or refractory large B-cell lymphomas (TRANSCEND NHL 001): a multicentre seamless design study. *Lancet* 396 (10254): 839–852. doi: 10.1016/S0140-6736(20)31366-0. Epub 2020 Sep 1. PMID: 32888407.

Bishop, M.R., Dickinson, M., Purtill, D. et al. (2022 February 17). Second-line tisagenlecleucel or standard care in aggressive B-cell lymphoma. *N Engl J Med* 386 (7): 629–639. doi: 10.1056/NEJMoa2116596. Epub 2021 Dec 14. PMID: 34904798.

Caimi, P.F., Ai, W., Alderuccio, J.P. et al. (2021 June). Loncastuximab tesirine in relapsed or refractory diffuse large B-cell lymphoma (LOTIS-2): A multicentre, open-label, single-arm, phase 2 trial. *Lancet Oncol* 22 (6): 790–800. doi: 10.1016/S1470-2045(21)00139-X. Epub 2021 May 11. PMID: 33989558.

Crump, M., Kuruvilla, J., Couban, S. et al. (2014 November 1). Randomized comparison of gemcitabine, dexamethasone, and cisplatin versus dexamethasone, cytarabine, and cisplatin chemotherapy before autologous stem-cell transplantation for relapsed and refractory aggressive lymphomas: NCIC-CTG LY.12. *J Clin Oncol* 32 (31): 3490–3496. doi: 10.1200/JCO.2013.53.9593. Epub 2014 Sep 29. PMID: 25267740.

Crump, M., Neelapu, S.S., Farooq, U. et al. (2017). Outcomes in refractory diffuse large B-cell lymphoma: results from the international SCHOLAR-1 study [published correction appears in blood. *Blood* 130 (16): 1800–1808. doi: 10.1182/blood-2017-03-769620. 2018 Feb 1;131(5):587-588].

Del Toro-Mijares, R., Oluwole, O., Jayani, R.V., Kassim, A.A., et al. (2023 April). Relapsed or refractory large B-cell lymphoma after chimeric antigen receptor T-cell therapy: current challenges and therapeutic options. *Br J Haematol* 201 (1): 15–24. doi: 10.1111/bjh.18656. Epub 2023 Jan 29. PMID: 36709623.

Gisselbrecht, C., Glass, B., Mounier, N., Singh Gill, D., Linch, D.C., Trneny, M., Bosly, A., Ketterer, N., Shpilberg, O., Hagberg, H., Ma, D., Brière, J., Moskowitz, C.H., and Schmitz, N. (2010 September 20). Salvage regimens with autologous transplantation for relapsed large B-cell lymphoma in the rituximab era. *J Clin Oncol* 28 (27): 4184–4190. doi: 10.1200/JCO.2010.28.1618. Epub 2010 Jul 26. Erratum in: J Clin Oncol. 2012 May 20;30(15):1896. PMID: 20660832; PMCID: PMC3664033.

Jagadeesh, D., Majhail, N.S., He, Y. et al. (2020). Outcomes of rituximab-BEAM versus BEAM conditioning regimen in patients with diffuse large B cell lymphoma undergoing autologous transplantation. *Cancer* 126 (10): 2279–2287. doi: 10.1002/cncr.32752.

Locke, F.L., Miklos, D.B., Jacobson, C.A. et al. (2022 February 17). Axicabtagene ciloleucel as second-line therapy for large B-cell lymphoma. *N Engl J Med* 386 (7): 640–654. doi: 10.1056/NEJMoa2116133. Epub 2021 Dec 11. PMID: 34891224.

Neelapu S.S., Jacobson C.A., Ghobadi A. et al. (2023). 5-Year Follow-Up Supports Curative Potential of Axicabtagene Ciloleucel in Refractory Large B-Cell Lymphoma (ZUMA-1). *Blood.* 2023 Feb 23:blood.2022018893. doi: 10.1182/blood.2022018893. Epub ahead of print. PMID: 36821768.

Neelapu, S.S., Locke, F.L., Bartlett, N.L. et al. (2017 December 28). Axicabtagene ciloleucel CAR T-cell therapy in refractory large B-cell lymphoma. *N Engl J Med* 377 (26): 2531–2544. doi: 10.1056/NEJMoa1707447. Epub 2017 Dec 10. PMID: 29226797; PMCID: PMC5882485.

Salles, G., Duell, J., González Barca, E. et al. (2020 July). Tafasitamab plus lenalidomide in relapsed or refractory diffuse large B-cell lymphoma (L-MIND): a multicentre, prospective, single-arm, phase 2 study. *Lancet Oncol* 21 (7): 978–988. doi:10.1016/S1470-2045(20)30225-4. Epub 2020 Jun 5. PMID: 32511983.

Schuster, S.J., Tam, C.S., Borchmann, P. et al. (2021 October). Long-term clinical outcomes of tisagenlecleucel in patients with relapsed or refractory aggressive B-cell lymphomas (JULIET): a multicentre, open-label, single-arm, phase 2 study. *Lancet Oncol* 22 (10): 1403–1415. doi:10.1016/S1470-2045(21)00375-2. Epub 2021 Sep 10. PMID: 34516954.

Sehn, L.H., Herrera, A.F., Flowers, C.R. et al. (2020 January 10). Polatuzumab vedotin in relapsed or refractory diffuse large B-cell lymphoma. *J Clin Oncol* 38 (2): 155–165. doi: 10.1200/JCO.19.00172. Epub 2019 Nov 6. PMID: 31693429; PMCID: PMC7032881.

Stiff, P.J., Unger, J.M., Cook, J.R. et al. (2013 October 31). Autologous transplantation as consolidation for aggressive non-Hodgkin's lymphoma. *N Engl J Med* 369 (18): 1681–1690.

Thieblemont, C., Briere, J., Mounier, N. et al. (2011 November 1). The germinal center/activated B-cell subclassification has a prognostic impact for response to salvage therapy in relapsed/refractory diffuse large B-cell lymphoma: A bio-CORAL study. *J Clin Oncol* 29 (31): 4079–4087. doi: 10.1200/JCO.2011.35.4423. Epub 2011 Sep 26. PMID: 21947824.

41

Primary Mediastinal Large B Cell Lymphoma

Alessandro Broccoli and Pier Luigi Zinzani

IRCCS Azienda Ospedaliero-Universitaria di Bologna, Istituto di Ematologia "L. e A. Seràgnoli"; Dipartimento di Medicina Specialistica, Diagnostica e Sperimentale, Università di Bologna; Bologna, Italy

Primary mediastinal large B-cell lymphoma (PMBL) is a subtype of diffuse large B-cell lymphoma (DLBCL) that has distinct clinical and molecular features. First recognized in the 1980s, PMBL was formally established as a distinct subtype of DLBCL in the revised European and American classification of lymphoid neoplasms and, more recently, the World Health Organization classification. It represents 2–3% of all non-Hodgkin's lymphoma cases and 6–10% of all DLBCL, and it has a worldwide distribution. PMBL occurs more often in young women, with a male-to-female ratio of 1:2 and a median age in the fourth decade.

Clinical Features

PMBL is characterized by a locally invasive anterior mediastinal mass. The mass originates in the thymus and frequently produces compressive symptoms early on, compromising the airway or great vessels, and producing a superior vena cava syndrome. As a result, at the time of diagnosis, 80% of cases have stage I–II disease; in 70% of patients, the mediastinal tumor is larger than 10 cm, often directly infiltrating the lung, chest wall, pleura, and pericardium. Pleural or pericardial effusions are present in one-third of cases. Local invasion results in cough, chest pain, dyspnea, or complaints resulting from caval obstruction. Systemic symptoms, mainly fever or weight loss, are present in less than 20% of cases. Spread to peripheral lymph nodes is infrequent; extranodal sites, however, may be involved, particularly at the time of disease recurrence, with a propensity for involvement of the kidneys, adrenals, liver, ovaries, and central nervous system. Bone marrow infiltration at presentation is rare.

Primary Management

Initial therapy is critical in treating PMBL patients. Salvage therapy for recurrence or progressive disease is of limited efficacy; thus, the imperative is to cure at the first attempt when possible. In PMBL, there are several controversial topics that warrant further study, and they are matters of debate, such as the superiority of third-generation regimens (i.e.

Cancer Consult: Expertise in Clinical Practice, Volume 2: Neoplastic Hematology & Cellular Therapy,
Second Edition. Edited by Syed A. Abutalib, Maurie Markman, James O. Armitage, and Kenneth C. Anderson.
© 2024 John Wiley & Sons Ltd. Published 2024 by John Wiley & Sons Ltd.

DA-EPOCH/R [dose-adjusted etoposide, prednisone, vincristine, cyclophosphamide, doxorubicin, rituximab]) over cyclophosphamide, doxorubicin, vincristine, and prednisone (CHOP)-based regimens, the impact of rituximab, the use of involved-field radiotherapy, the assessment of clinical response by PET scan, and the utility of high-dose therapy as front-line consolidation.

1) Front-line therapy: First-generation or third-generation regimens?

Expert Perspective: An optimum chemotherapy regimen option for patients with PMBL has not been clearly established, and the optimal treatment for PMBL patients has always been a matter of debate. This is the consequence of the rarity of the disease and the inability to design adequately powered randomized studies to evaluate different front-line approaches.

The approaches to this entity range from the first-generation CHOP regimen to third-generation chemotherapy regimens, with (or without) the use of radiation therapy. CHOP with or without radiation therapy, however, seems not sufficient, because cure rates do not exceed 50–60%. Whereas the CHOP regimen has been used by American investigators, several European centers have suggested that a combination of methotrexate, doxorubicin, cyclophosphamide, vincristine, bleomycin, and prednisone (MACOP-B), or alternatively a similar regimen, with etoposide instead of methotrexate (VACOP-B), may be superior to CHOP. Two Italian preliminary studies with MACOP-B in 50 and in 89 patients with PMBL, demonstrated complete response (CR) rates of 86% and 88%, respectively, with five-year relapse-free survival (RFS) rates of 93% and 91%, respectively.

In addition, a multinational retrospective study compared the outcomes of 426 patients with PMBL after first-generation (CHOP or CHOP-like regimens; 105 patients), third-generation (MACOP-B or VACOP-B; 277 patients), and high-dose chemotherapy schedules followed by autologous stem cell transplant (ASCT; 44 patients). In all these groups, for the most part, patients underwent radiation therapy after chemotherapy. With chemotherapy, CR rates were 49%, 51%, and 53%, with the first-generation, third generation, and high-dose chemotherapy strategies, respectively. The final CR rates, after radiation therapy on the mediastinum, became 61% for CHOP and CHOP-like regimens, 79% for MACOP-B and VACOP-B regimens, and 75% for high-dose regimens. Projected 10-year overall survival (OS) rates were 44%, 71%, and 77%, respectively, and projected 10-year progression-free survival rates were 35%, 67%, and 78%, respectively. In addition, after radiation therapy, 81% of the patients who had already achieved a partial response (PR) obtained a CR status.

A retrospective analysis of 153 patients from British Columbia reviewed outcomes from a geographical region where treatment choice was mandated by era-specific guidelines. Between 1980 and 1992, MACOP-B or VACOP-B was administered, moving to CHOP between 1992 and 2001 and then to rituximab with CHOP (R-CHOP) thereafter. The OS for the cohort was 75% at five years, with the OS at five years for those treated with MACOP-B or VACOP-B significantly higher at 87% compared with 71% for those patients treated with CHOP ($P = 0.048$).

2) What is the role of rituximab?

Expert Perspective: Although derived from a very limited number of cases, preliminary clinical observations suggested the superiority of R-CHOP with or without radiation therapy over CHOP with or without radiation therapy, with a CR rate > 80%. Those initial findings deserved confirmation in larger series, because the impressive results might have been a result of patient selection, publication bias, or merely chance. The Vassilakopoulos et al. study demonstrated that R-CHOP with radiation therapy, or even alone, may cure most patients with PMBL, based on the analysis of 76 patients with adequate follow-up, demonstrating a five-year progression-free survival rate of 81% and a long-term OS rate of 89%. Anyway, the experience of R-CHOP in PMBL patients remains limited, being mainly derived from small patient series. In a review of the Vancouver series, 18 patients aged < 65 years were treated with R-CHOP and radiation therapy, achieving a three-year OS rate of 82%, which is slightly (but not significantly) inferior to those seen with MACOP-B or VACOP-B.

In the context of the MabThera International Trial (MInT), 87 patients with good-prognosis PMBL (bulky stage I or stage II–IV, and an age-adjusted International Prognostic Index score of 0 or 1) aged < 60 years received six cycles of chemotherapy versus rituximab plus the same chemotherapy. More than 90% of patients received R-CHOP or R-CHOP with etoposide (R-CHOEP). Radiation therapy was routinely administered to patients with bulky disease so that 71% of the patients received 30–40 Gy mediastinal radiation therapy. The addition of rituximab to chemotherapy minimized the development of primary refractory disease (3% vs 24%; $P = 0.006$) and resulted in higher three-year progression-free survival (88% vs 64%; $P = 0.006$) and event-free survival (78% vs 52%; $P = 0.012$) rates, but the OS rate was only slightly greater (89% vs 78%; $P = 0.16$). Although derived from an unplanned subgroup analysis, these data provide the strongest evidence to date for the superiority of R-CHO(E)P over CHO(E)P in the treatment of PMBL patients.

A reasonable question is whether rituximab combined with more intensive third-generation chemotherapy regimens would further improve the impressive results already reported. In an Italian study published in 2009, patients treated with a rituximab plus MACOP-B or VACOP-B regimen plus radiation therapy had a CR rate of 80%. This value overlaps with the one obtained with the combination of third-generation chemotherapy regimens and radiation therapy without rituximab: in fact, literature data showed a mean CR of 83% (range: 79–88%) using MACOP-B or VACOP-B plus radiation therapy. Moreover, in the previously reported Italian experiences with third-generation regimens, the relapse-free survival rates were 93% at 96 months and 91% at nine years, respectively, with all relapses occurring within 10 months. In a retrospective multinational study on 426 PMBL patients, the progression-free survival rate was 67% at 10 years in the 277 patients treated with third-generation regimens plus mediastinal radiation therapy.

Taken together, these studies suggest that: (i) the addition of rituximab can improve outcomes in comparison to chemotherapy alone when CHOP is used as induction therapy, and (ii) the combination of rituximab with third-generation regimens has a less clear benefit, albeit nowadays is considered the standard.

3) What is the role of R-DA-EPOCH as front-line therapy?

Expert Perspective: In 2013, Dunleavy et al. from the National Cancer Institute have demonstrated in a phase II prospective trial involving 51 patients that the dose-adjusted etoposide, prednisone, vincristine, cyclophosphamide, doxorubicin, rituximab (R-DA-EPOCH) regimen yielded five-year event-free survival and OS rates of 93% and 97%, respectively. Importantly, the key message of this study was that the use of R-DA-EPOCH could obviate the need of radiation therapy in 96% of the cases, with no relapsing patients over a median follow-up of more than five years. Following the publication of these encouraging results, the use of R-DA-EPOCH has significantly increased at many institutions worldwide.

Giulino-Roth et al. have reported the outcomes of a large retrospective series of patients affected by PMBL (118 adults and 38 children) treated with R-DA-EPOCH. Nearly 16% of cases were irradiated after chemoimmunotherapy. Three-quarters of patients met complete remission criteria at the end of induction; the event-free survival at three years was 85.9% for the entire cohort of patients and 87.4% for adults; the OS at three years was 95.4%. Shah et al. have compared retrospectively the outcomes of 142 PMBL patients treated with either R-CHOP or R-DA-EPOCH at several American institutions: 56 patients received R-CHOP and 76 R-DA-EPOCH; 59% of patients in the R-CHOP group received radiation therapy, against 13% in the R-DA-EPOCH cohort. The complete remission rates at the end of chemoimmunotherapy were 84% and 70% for R-DA-EPOCH and R-CHOP, respectively, and both median progression-free survival and OS were not reached in either treatment arms at a median follow-up of 40 and 20 months for R-CHOP and R-DA-EPOCH, respectively. The OS was similar in both treatment groups, as 89% of R-CHOP-treated patients and 91% of those who received R-DA-EPOCH were alive at two years.

4) Is high-dose therapy followed by ASCT useful as frontline consolidation?

Expert Perspective: The low frequency of marrow involvement and the relatively young age of the PMBL patient population is the basis of consideration of HDT and ASCT to consolidate first remission. Results from the GELTAMO registry on 35 patients in first complete remission, but considered at high risk of relapse, receiving HDT/ASCT with various preparative regimens, indicated that four-year OS and progression-free survival were 84% and 81%, respectively. In the IELSG analysis, a limited number of patients (n = 44) underwent HDT with ASCT, which resulted in an estimated OS of 77% at 10 years. In the Memorial Sloan Kettering experience, HDT with ASCT at first remission was not superior to dose-dense sequential therapy. Based on the results achieved with third-generation regimens and the likely benefit from the addition of rituximab, there is little at present to recommend an HDT followed by ASCT approach to consolidate first complete remission, even in poor-risk patients.

Radiotherapy as Local Consolidation

The role of mediastinal radiation therapy upon completion of chemotherapy remains a matter of debate. The best reported outcomes in PMBL have been achieved with regimens that have incorporated radiation therapy in their planned primary treatment. Furthermore, it is clear from the IELSG series that many patients completing chemotherapy in partial response may be converted to complete remission following radiation therapy and that radiation therapy may render active residual mediastinal masses negative at PET scan (more on this topic later in Question 5). Univariate and multivariate analysis in two retrospective series have suggested that receiving radiotherapy correlated to better event-free survival or OS.

However, excellent long-term results have been achieved with chemotherapy alone in some series. Following an era-specific shift in British Columbia toward the use of radiation therapy to consolidate response, there was no difference in progression-free survival or OS by year of intervention, i.e. with or without post-chemotherapy irradiation. This was true even with initially bulky tumors, and indeed in the whole population there was a trend toward improved progression-free survival in the era before routine radiation therapy. In the subgroup analysis of the UNFLODER study (with the limitation of a pre-PET-era), the results suggest a benefit of radiotherapy only for patients responding to R-CHOP with PR. In the Memorial Sloan Kettering series, only 7% of patients treated with the NHL-15 regimen (comprising intensified doxoroubicin, vincristine, and cyclophosphamide) received radiation therapy: excellent results with an OS of 84% at a median follow-up of 11 years are reported with this chemotherapy-only approach. Similarly, in an Italian experience with 74 patients, all treated with a rituximab and MACOP-B induction, PET-negative cases were only observed, while PET-positive patients received mediastinal radiation therapy. The OS and progression-free survival rates at 10 years demonstrated no differences between irradiated and not-irradiated patients. Finally, the excellent results reported with R-DA-EPOCH, at least in patients achieving a complete remission after induction, support a radiation therapy–free approach.

The IELSG 37 trial was designed to investigate whether consolidative radiation therapy can be omitted in patients with a negative PET scan after induction treatment based on rituximab combined with an anthracycline-containing regimen. At a median follow-up of 30 months, the number of observed events was considerably lower than expected; evidence from IELSG 37 supports the omission of RT in patients achieving a CMR after immunochemotherapy. The primary endpoint analysis was performed, with ≥80% of patients having a minimum follow-up of 30 months. In all, 545 patients were enrolled. Induction immunochemotherapy was completed and response assessed in 530 patients, 268 of them (50.6%) achieved a complete metabolic response and were randomly allocated to observation (n = 132) or RT (n = 136). The PFS at 30 months was 98.5% (95%CI, 94.3 – 99.6) in the RT arm and 96.2% (95%CI, 91.1-98.4) in the OBS arm (P = 0.278). The estimated relative effect of radiotherapy vs observation in terms of hazard ratio (HR) was 0.47 (0.12-1.89) without adjustments and 0.79 (0.19-3.31) after stratification for the variables used for randomization. At 30 months the absolute risk reduction from RT was 2.3% (-1.5 to 6.2) unadjusted, and 0.8% (-3.0 to 8.3) with stratified HR. The number needed to treat is high (43 patients, unadjusted, and 126 after stratification). The 5-year overall survival was 99% in both arms. Longer follow-up is needed to examine late toxicity.

Toward a PET-guided PMBL Management

5) What is the role of the PET scan?

Expert Perspective: Owing to the prominent fibrotic component of PMBL, a residual mediastinal mass is often present upon completion of therapy. Distinction is needed between those who have residual disease and those who have simple fibrotic tissue. PET scan performed at the end of chemoimmunotherapy may be a useful tool to identify patients who obtain a complete metabolic response, thus being free of residual vital tissue. The high negative-predictive value of PET scan is in fact clearly demonstrated in PMBL; on the contrary, its positive-predictive value is rather poor and highly variable among published series, given that PET-avid inflammatory components within masses otherwise negative for cancer can be frequently detected. End-of-treatment PET-positive cases therefore require a cautious interpretation in terms of disease persistence, and biopsy should be performed whenever possible to solve any doubts.

6) Are PET findings useful to choose wisely?

Expert Perspective: The Deauville five-point scale, when applied in PMBL cases at the end of induction (after 6–8 weeks), may provide guidance for the following management of the patient (Figure 41.1). Patients with a Deauville score of 3 at the end of chemoimmunotherapy do not show worse OS and progression-free survival than patients with a Deauville score of 1 or 2, i.e. displaying a complete metabolic response. These patients can be simply observed, with no need of consolidative radiation therapy, especially if treated with R-DA-EPOCH induction. If consolidative radiation therapy is judged necessary, involved-site irradiation (ISRT) at the dose of 30–36 Gy is recommended.

The management of patients displaying a Deauville score of 4 is much more controversial, given that PET positivity may be secondary to inflammatory processes rather than

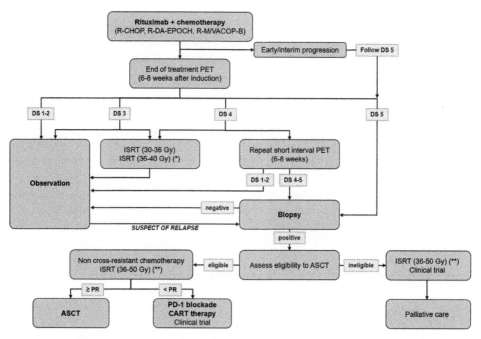

Figure 41.1 Clinical practice flowchart. Rounded rectangles indicate key steps in patients' management. Smaller rectangles indicate decision points. DS: Deauville five-point scale; ISRT: involved-site radiation therapy. (*) 30–36 Gy is intended as consolidation in DS3 cases; 36–40 Gy may be used in DS4 cases. (**) Suitable in DS5 with partial response or stable disease and localized disease only.

residual disease. Some authors recommend a conservative approach with PET repetition after a short interval (6–8 weeks) and close monitoring of fluorodeoxyglucose avidity within the involved tissue. Repeatedly positive PET findings should point physicians to mediastinal biopsy (through mediastinoscopy, anterior mediastinotomy, or thoracoscopy). If the biopsy is negative for disease, the patient requires close monitoring only. On the other hand, radiation therapy may be judged as the option of choice due to the higher incidence of relapse rate of patients with DS of 4 compared to those with a Deauville score of 1–3.

Patients with an end-of-induction Deauville score of 5 are a heterogeneous group that includes those with a partial response, a stable disease, or an over progression, in any case presenting with metabolically active neoplastic tissue. Repeat tissue biopsy is highly recommended in these cases; if positive for disease, the patient should be directed to a second-line approach, which should include non-cross resistant chemotherapy and ASCT if deemed feasible.

Relapsed and Refractory PMBCL

Disease relapse develops early after post-treatment follow-up, generally within the first 18 months, in up to 15–20% of patients. Outcomes for patients with refractory (or relapsed) disease are indeed poor, as the disease often shows chemo-refractoriness. The optimal disease management is represented by the application of a platinum- or ifosfamide-based salvage regimen, followed by ASCT (Figure 41.1). Patients who do not respond adequately to second-line therapies can be directed to programmed death-1 (PD-1) blockers or eventually to chimeric antigen receptor (CAR) T cells.

7) What is the role of anti-PD-1 agents?

Expert Perspective: The blockade of the interaction of PD-1 with its cognate ligand PDL-1 by means of anti-PD-1 monoclonal antibodies helps restore an adequate immunosurveillance against the disease.

In the phase IB KEYNOTE-013 and phase II KEYNOTE-170 trials, adults with relapsed or refractory PMBL received pembrolizumab for up to two years or until disease progression or unacceptable toxicity. The overall response rate was 48% in KEYNOTE-013 and 45% in KEYNOTE-170, with 33% of patients in KEYNOTE-013 and 13% in KEYNOTE-170 achieving a complete remission. After a median follow-up time of 29 months in KEYNOTE-013 and 13 months in KEYNOTE-170, the median duration of response was not reached in either study. None of the patients in complete remission experienced progression. The estimated progression-free survival rates at 12 months were 47% and 38% in each study, respectively. The median OS was 31 months in KEYNOTE-013, while it was not reached in KEYNOTE-170. In KEYNOTE-170 with median duration of follow-up of 48.7 months (range, 41.2-56.2) the ORR was 41.5% (complete response, 20.8%; partial response, 20.8%). The median duration of response was not reached; no patients who achieved a complete response progressed at the data cutoff. The median PFS was 4.3 months; the 4-year PFS rate was 33.0%. The median OS was 22.3 months; the 4-year OS rate was 45.3%. At the data cutoff, 30 patients (56.6%) had any-grade treatment-related adverse events; the most common were neutropenia, asthenia, and hypothyroidism. Grade 3 and 4 treatment-related adverse events occurred in 22.6% of the patients; no grade 5 adverse events occurred. After 4 years of follow-up, pembrolizumab continued to provide durable responses, with promising trends for long-term survival and acceptable safety in R/R PMBCL.

The combination of nivolumab and the anti-CD30 agent brentuximab vedotin in PMBL patients with relapsed or refractory disease after ASCT or two previous lines of systemic therapy was explored in a separate cohort of 30 cases within the phase II portion of the CheckMate 436 study. At a median follow-up of 11 months, the overall response rate was 73%, with 37% of patients obtaining a complete remission and 37% a partial response. The six-month progression-free survival and OS rates were 64% and 86%, respectively, with median progression-free survival and median OS not reached.

8) CAR T cells in PMBL

Expert Perspective: Axicabtagene ciloleucel (axi-cel) is a CAR T cell construct of patients' T-cell lymphocytes engineered to express an anti-CD19 single chain fragment on the extracellular surface. The phase II ZUMA-1 trial with axi-cel involved histologically confirmed large B-cell lymphoma patients, including DLBCL, PMBL, and transformed follicular lymphoma, with refractory or relapsed disease after ASCT, who have received a previous anti-CD20 monoclonal antibody containing–regimen and an anthracycline-containing chemotherapy (see Chapter 48). Within the pooled cohorts of PMBL and transformed follicular lymphoma patients (n = 24), an overall response rate of 83% was obtained, including a complete remission in 71% of the cases. Cytokine release syndrome and neurologic adverse events are a major concern with this treatment, although manageable, with an incidence of grade ≥ 3 complications of 11% and 32%, respectively (see Chapter 59). Lisocabtagene maraleucel (liso-cel) is also approved for R/R PMBCL. the complete indication includes approval in adult patients with large B-cell lymphoma (LBCL; excluding CNS LBCL) who have refractory disease to first-line chemoimmunotherapy or relapse within 12 months of first-line chemoimmunotherapy; or refractory disease to first-line chemoimmunotherapy or relapse after first-line chemoimmunotherapy and are not eligible for ASCT due to comorbidities or age. Approval of liso-cel for the treatment for second-line treatment of R/R LBCL is supported by findings from the phase 3 TRANSFORM trial (NCT03575351) and the phase 2 PILOT trial (NCT03483103).

Recommended Readings

Armand, P., Rodig, S., Melnichenko, V. et al. (2019). Pembrolizumab in relapsed or refractory primary mediastinal large B-cell lymphoma. *J Clin Oncol* 37: 3291–3299.

Broccoli, A. and Zinzani, P.L. (2018). The unique biology and treatment of primary mediastinal B-cell lymphoma. *Best Pract Res Clin Haematol* 31: 241–250.

Dunleavy, K., Pittaluga, S., Maeda, L.S. et al. (2013). Dose adjusted EPOCH-rituximab therapy in primary mediastinal large B-cell lymphoma. *New Engl J Med* 368: 1408–1416.

Held, G., Thurner, L., Poeschel, V., et al. (2023 July 5). Radiation and Dose-densification of R-CHOP in primary mediastinal B-cell Lymphoma: subgroup analysis of the UNFOLDER trial. Hemasphere 7 (7): e917. doi: 10.1097/HS9.0000000000000917. PMID: 37427145; PMCID: PMC10325764.

Hoppe, B.S., Advani, R., Milgrom, S.A. et al. (2021). Primary mediastinal B cell lymphoma in the positron-emission tomography era executive summary of the American Radium Society appropriate use criteria. *Int J Radiat Oncol Biol Phys* 111: 36–44.

Kamdar, M., Solomon, S.R., Arnason, J., et al. (2022 June 18). TRANSFORM Investigators. Lisocabtagene maraleucel versus standard of care with salvage chemotherapy followed by autologous stem cell transplantation as second-line treatment in patients with relapsed or refractory large B-cell lymphoma (TRANSFORM): results from an interim analysis of an open-label, randomised, phase 3 trial. Lancet 399 (10343): 2294–2308. doi: 10.1016/S0140-6736(22)00662-6. Erratum in: (2022 July 16). Lancet 400 (10347): 160. PMID: 35717989.

Locke, F.L., Ghobadi, A., Jacobson, C.A. et al. (2019). Long-term safety and activity of axicabtagene ciloleucel in refractory large B-cell lymphoma (ZUMA-1): a single-arm, multicenter, phase 1-2 trial. *Lancet Oncol* 20: 31–42.

Mohty, R., Moustafa, M.A., Aljurf, M., Murthy, H., and Kharfan-Dabaja, M.A. (2022 November 7). Emerging role of autologous CD19 CAR T-Cell therapies in the second-line setting for large B-cell Lymphoma: a game changer? Hematol Oncol Stem Cell Ther 15 (3): 73–80. doi: 10.56875/2589-0646.1025. PMID: 36395495.

Zinzani, P.L., Broccoli, A., Casadei, B. et al. (2015). The role of rituximab and positron emission tomography in the treatment of primary mediastinal large B-cell lymphoma: experience on 74 patients. *Hematol Oncol* 33: 145–150.

Zinzani, P.L., Martelli, M., Bendandi, M. et al. (2001). Primary mediastinal large B-cell lymphoma with sclerosis: a clinical study of 89 patients treated with MACOP-B chemotherapy and radiation therapy. *Haematologica* 86: 187–191.

Zinzani, P.L., Martelli, M., Bertini, M. et al. (2002). Induction chemotherapy strategies for primary mediastinal large B-cell lymphoma with sclerosis: a retrospective multinational study on 426 previously untreated patients. *Haematologica* 87: 1258–1264.

Zinzani, P.L., Thieblemont, C., Melnichenko, V., et al. (2023 July 13). Pembrolizumab in relapsed or refractory primary mediastinal large B cell lymphoma: final analysis of KEYNOTE 170. *Blood* 142 (2): 141 145. doi: 10.1182/blood. 2022019340. PMID: 37130017.

Zinzani, P.L., Santoro, A., Gritti, G. et al. (2019). Nivolumab combined with brentuximab vedotin for relapsed/refractory primary mediastinal large B-cell lymphoma: efficacy and safety from the phase II CheckMate 436 study. *J Clin Oncol.* 37: 3081–3089.

42

Double-Hit and Double-Expressor Lymphomas

David A. Russler-Germain and Brad S. Kahl

Washington University School of Medicine, St. Louis, MO

Introduction

Diffuse large B-cell lymphoma (DLBCL) is an aggressive non-Hodgkin lymphoma with roughly 20,000 new cases annually in the USA. Even when presenting at an advanced stage, newly diagnosed DLBCL can be cured by front-line R-CHOP chemoimmunotherapy in approximately 60% of patients. However, approximately 5–10% of tumors morphologically consistent with DLBCL possess chromosomal rearrangements involving *MYC* as well as *BCL2* and/or *BCL6*, termed "double-hit lymphoma" (DHL) or "triple-hit lymphoma" (THL), and these patients suffer extremely poor outcomes. Patients with DHL/THL are typically older and more likely to present with worse performance status, elevated lactate dehydrogenase (LDH) levels, and extranodal or central nervous system (CNS) involvement. To date, there are no completed prospective randomized studies to guide the specific treatment of patients with DHL/THL. However, multiple retrospective studies highlight the prognostic importance of achieving a complete response (CR) to induction therapy for DHL/THL, as well as the potential for intensified induction regimens such as DA-EPOCH-R to improve the rate of front-line CR compared to the standard R-CHOP regimen. In turn, DHL is now formally a distinct entity as of the 2016 WHO classifications: high grade B-cell lymphoma, with *MYC* and *BCL2* and/or *BCL6* rearrangements. In contrast, "double-expressor lymphoma" (DEL) is a subclassification of DLBCL with MYC and BCL2 protein overexpression (irrespective of BCL6 expression) but without associated chromosomal rearrangements. DEL is more common than DHL, constituting approximately 30% of DLBCL, and this designation confers modest adverse risk. Nonetheless, standard R-CHOP remains the preferred approach for DEL. Hopefully the results of ongoing clinical trials exploring the addition of novel agents such as venetoclax or acalabrutinib to chemoimmunotherapy or earlier utilization of cellular approaches such as chimeric antigen receptor (CAR) T cell therapy will improve upon the historically poor outcomes in DHL/THL and DEL.

Cancer Consult: Expertise in Clinical Practice, Volume 2: Neoplastic Hematology & Cellular Therapy,
Second Edition. Edited by Syed A. Abutalib, Maurie Markman, James O. Armitage, and Kenneth C. Anderson.
© 2024 John Wiley & Sons Ltd. Published 2024 by John Wiley & Sons Ltd.

1) What is DHL/THL, and how are outcomes different?

Expert Perspective: The classification system for B-cell non-Hodgkin lymphomas (B-NHL) has undergone multiple revisions over the past four decades, reflecting a growing understanding of the pathogenesis and clinical features of these diverse neoplasms. The 2008 World Health Organization (WHO) classification of lymphoid neoplasms introduced the category of "B-cell lymphoma, unclassifiable, with features intermediate between diffuse large B-cell lymphoma (DLBCL) and Burkitt lymphoma (BL)." This was intended to address the subset of very aggressive lymphomas in which the distinction between DLBCL and BL was difficult. However, the utility of this morphologically driven diagnosis was limited due to its vagueness and being nonuniformly implemented in clinical practice. The 2016 update eliminated the B-cell lymphoma, unclassifiable, with features intermediate between DLBCL and BL category, and created a new category not defined by morphology but rather by high-risk combinations of genomic alterations. All large B-cell lymphomas with *MYC* and *BCL2* and/or *BCL6* rearrangements were henceforth included in a single category designated "high-grade B-cell lymphoma, with *MYC* and *BCL2* and/or *BCL6* rearrangements." The simpler alternative labels of "double- / triple-hit" lymphoma (DHL/THL) derive from whether only one or both of *BCL2* and *BCL6* are rearranged in addition to the obligatory *MYC* rearrangement.

Before the 2016 revision of the WHO classification schema, it was noted that tumors categorized as B-cell lymphoma, unclassifiable, with features intermediate between DLBCL and BL category typically had a mixture of medium- to large-sized cells, with a high proliferation rate, and frequent (~35–50%) translocations involving 8q24/*MYC* (a hallmark of classic BL). However, approximately 10–15% of tumors in the DLBCL not otherwise specified (NOS) category were also found to have a *MYC* rearrangement, which appeared to confer a poor prognosis in both the pre- and post-rituximab (R) plus CHOP eras. It was additionally noted that about 50% of *MYC* rearranged tumors also possessed a translocation between chromosomes 14 and 18, the hallmark of follicular lymphoma (FL) that juxtaposes *IGH* and *BCL2*. This led to the adoption of the term DHL, and these patients were noted to have dismal outcomes with either CHOP or R-CHOP treatment. Early, albeit small, cohorts reported median overall survival (OS) intervals in the range of 1–2 years, with very few long-term survivors. Subsequent cohorts of patients with DHL with a *BCL6* rearrangement instead of *BCL2* (or those with THL having all three gene rearrangements) also observed poor outcomes. In general, THL and DHL are viewed as similar entities, and thus most providers evaluate and treat them identically in practice.

With the recognition of DHL/THL as an extremely high-risk subset of B-NHL, several larger retrospective cohorts were assembled in the mid-2010s to better describe these patients' baseline clinical characteristics and responses to treatment. Overall, patients with DHL/THL are more frequently older, suffer from poor performance status, and present with extranodal involvement, elevated lactate dehydrogenase (LDH) levels, central nervous system (CNS) involvement, and higher international prognostic index (IPI) scores. Within DHL, leukocytosis at presentation was also associated with a poor prognosis. The role of intensified induction treatment in classical BL was well-defined, so many providers extrapolated this approach to the treatment of DHL. Pre-2016, the most frequently used induction for DHL was standard R-CHOP (~33%); however, the majority of patients were being treated with intensified induction regimens, most commonly R-HyperCVAD/MA, DA-EPOCH-R, or R-CODOX-M/IVAC (~15–20% each). Retrospective analyses found that patients with DHL receiving intensive induction had significantly higher rates of complete responses (CR) and longer progression-free survival (PFS) intervals, although without a corresponding improvement in OS. Further, a meta-analysis of 11 retrospective studies examining 394 patients with DHL found that front-line treatment with DA-EPOCH-R, specifically, was associated with significantly improved PFS compared with R-CHOP, but again no OS advantage was observed.

To date, there have been no completed prospective randomized clinical trials to guide the treatment of patients specifically with DHL/THL. Nearly all of the large phase III studies of front-line treatment for advanced-stage DLBCL have included patients with DHL/THL, confirming their relative poorer prognoses. However, modern cohorts suggest only ~8% of tumors with DLBCL morphology are found to be DHL/THL. Thus, trial-level subgroup analyses of DHL/THL have lacked statistical power to draw meaningful conclusions regarding any potential benefit of treatment strategies other than R-CHOP due to the low numbers of these patients in each study. As a result, and given the relative rarity of this condition, most providers rely on a combination of expert consensus and institutional prac-tices to shape their approaches to treat DHL/THLs.

2) What is double-expressor lymphoma, and how are outcomes different?

Expert Perspective: During the early investigation of the features of B-NHL with *MYC*, *BCL2*, and/or *BCL6* rearrangements, it was discovered that a subset of DLBCL without rearrangements involving these genes could still demonstrate increased expression of the corresponding proteins. The vast majority of DHLs express both MYC and BCL2. However, several retrospective studies of patients with DLBCL treated with R-CHOP found that patients with expression of both MYC and BCL2 by immunohistochemistry (IHC), without associated translocations, often suffered worse outcomes than other patients with DLBCL whose tumors lacked expression of both proteins. Multiple studies corroborated this trend despite using a variety of dichotomized cutoffs for positive versus negative MYC and BCL2 expression by IHC. The modern consensus is that double (pro-tein)–expressor lymphoma (DEL) is defined by expression of MYC in $\geq 40\%$ and BCL2 in $\geq 50\%$ of neoplastic B cells. BCL6 expression is not involved in the DEL categorization, in contrast to its role in the DHL/THL designations. By these criteria, patients with DEL make up approximately 33% of all DLBCL diagnoses and share many of the high-risk clinical features of DHL including frequently being older age, suffering from poor performance status, and presenting with extranodal involvement, elevated LDH levels, higher IPI scores, and CNS involvement. They also have been shown to have lower response rates to front-line R-CHOP and poorer three-year OS rates compared to patients with non-DEL/DHL. Despite a large portion of DLBCL being DEL, there is scant evi-dence (even retrospective) that alternative front-line treatment approaches to R-CHOP benefit these patients, although this is an area of interest in ongoing clinical trials.

3) How do DHL and DEL relate to cell-of-origin?

Expert Perspective: Given the clinical heterogeneity of DLBCL, gene expression–profiling studies aimed to identify biologically distinct subtypes of this disease. This led to the proposal of the cell-of-origin (COO) concept, based on the ability to segregate DLBCL tumors by simi-larities to the gene expression–profiling signatures of benign germinal center B (GCB) or non-GCB cells (activated B-cells [ABC] or primary mediastinal B-cells). The COO classification

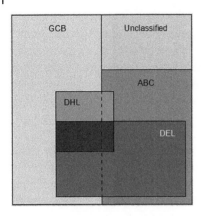

Figure 42.1   Classification of aggressive B-cell lymphomas. Cell-of-origin categories of germinal center B (GCB) cell or activated B-cell (ABC) overlap with double-hit lymphoma (DHL) and double-expressor lymphoma (DEL) designations.

revealed striking differences in clinical outcomes, as patients with GCB-like disease experienced far better outcomes than those with ABC-like disease. This trend was independent of IPI score at diagnosis. In practice, COO is determined not by gene expression profiling but rather using the surrogate Hans algorithm based on IHC of CD10, BCL6, and MUM1. This approach shows about 80% concordance with the gold-standard gene expression–profiling assays, which aren't available for routine clinical application but are incorporated into several clinical trials. Irrespective of the assay used, large cohort studies have found DLBCLs to be approximately 50:50 GCB COO versus non-GCB COO.

The relationship between COO and DHL and DEL is important to consider from a pathobiology perspective as well as in terms of how newly diagnosed lymphomas undergo pretreatment evaluation (Figure 42.1). It has been proposed that many new cases of DHL with a *BCL2* rearrangement are in fact *de novo* presentations of an aggressive transformation of a previously undiagnosed FL, with the *MYC* rearrangement being a transforming event. It is thus fitting that approximately 90% of DHL with *MYC* and *BCL2* rearrangements (which make up about 80% of DHL) are of GCB COO given that FL is a GCB-like disease. While patients with DLBCL of GCB COO tend to have better outcomes, there is a subgroup that suffer markedly worse outcomes, and this subgroup is largely composed of DHL. Therefore, to prognosticate based strictly upon COO is overly simplistic and establishing the DHL status is essential. In contrast, the majority (~66%) of DELs are of non-GCB subtype. This co-association has made it difficult to independently determine the risk conferred by each biologic feature.

4) How do I ensure my hematopathologist correctly identifies these entities, and does type of MYC translocation partner (IG vs. non-IG) predict prognosis in DHL/THL?

Expert Perspective: As of 2021, IHC for COO assessment, as well as for BCL2 and MYC (among other markers), are deemed essential components of the DLBCL workup, per the NCCN guidelines. COO classification by itself does not yet have a role in deciding the treatment of DLBCL in the front-line setting, but it provides important prognostic information for patients and clinicians, as well as informs second-line and beyond treatment strategies due to differences in response rates for selected therapies based on COO. Examples include favorable outcomes with salvage R-DHAP in GCB over non-GCB disease (Chapter 5 – Transplant and cell therapy in DLBCL), as well as favorable (albeit still modest) response rates to immunomodulatory drugs (such as lenalidomide) or Bruton's tyrosine kinase (BTK) inhibitors (such as ibrutinib) in non-GCB over GCB disease.

Fluorescence in situ hybridization (FISH) testing for *MYC* rearrangements should also be performed at baseline. FISH assessment for *MYC* rearrangement is typically done with a break-apart probe targeting 8q24, as the common *MYC* rearrangement partners can include *IGH* (heavy), *IGL* (lambda), or *IGK* (kappa), if not one of several other rarer loci. The advantage to this approach is that it should yield a lower false-negative rate (~4% vs ~22%) due to being agnostic to the rearrangement partner. More recently, though, several shortcomings are being identified including cryptic *MYC* rearrangement events not captured by the break-apart probe strategy, as well as the inability to discern the specific rearrangement partner of *MYC*. In the case of the former dilemma, many DLBCLs with cryptic *MYC* fusions (if also present with either *BCL2* or *BCL6* rearrangements) have gene expression profiles and poor clinical outcomes that align with DHL/THL, despite not being formally assigned this diagnostic designation. Additionally, some studies suggest that only DHL/THL with *MYC* rearrangements specifically involving immunoglobulin gene partners (~50–60% of cases) have the poor prognoses as historically described. As our understanding of these nuances and our clinical laboratory tools continue to improve, so too will our ability to provide better risk-adjusted therapeutic approaches for subsets of patients with DLBCL and DHL/THL.

It is debated whether all B-NHL of DLBCL morphology should also undergo FISH testing for *BCL2* and *BCL6* rearrangements, irrespective of *MYC* FISH results, or whether a reflex approach that only does additional testing on MYC-rearranged tumors is more appropriate. Some have also proposed only testing GCB-DLBCL for these rearrangements by FISH. Our center and many others favor the more comprehensive approach, testing all DLBCL for the three rearrangements despite the modest increase in cost this entails. Limiting FISH testing to GCB COO suffers from the pitfalls of only about 80% concordance between the surrogate Hans algorithm IHC strategy and gold-standard gene expression profiling assays, as well as the fact that ~10–20% of DHL/THL may be non-GCB by the Hans algorithm, which would be missed. Further, excessive use of reflex FISH testing would likely negate the cost savings of running fewer FISH tests by imposing additional burdens on the sample processing, pathology sign-out, and physician results review workflows that may additionally increase the likelihood of errors. At the present time, the NanoString™ gene expression profiling COO classifiers (e.g., Lymph2Cx) and the recently described RNA sequencing assays for determining molecular high-grade (MHG) or double-hit signature (DHsig) gene expression profiles are not yet available for routine clinical use and should be implemented in the context of clinical trials.

5) What is the appropriate staging evaluation for DHL/THL and DEL?

Expert Perspective: The standard workup of DLBCL includes physical examination, assessment of performance status and classic B-symptoms, PET-CT scan, and laboratory testing for complete blood counts, LDH, comprehensive metabolic panel, uric acid, and serostatus for HIV, hepatitis B, and hepatitis C (Figure 42.2). This approach permits calculation of the IPI score. Patients receiving an anthracycline-based regimen should undergo echocardiogram or similar cardiac pretesting. Testing for beta-2-microglobulin is useful in

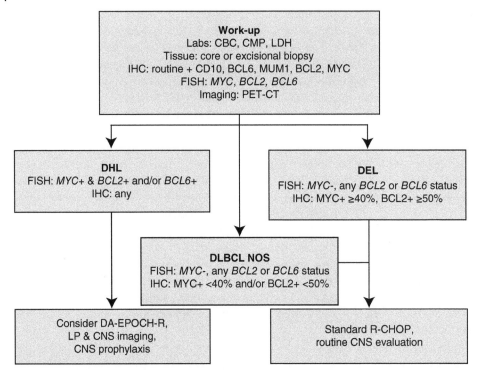

Figure 42.2 Proposed workflow for evaluation and treatment of DHL, DEL, and DLBCL NOS.
*For limited DHL/THL stage (I/II) disease R-CHOP ± RT is preferred over DA-EPOCH unless aggressive presentation or CNS involvement (see text, Question 7).

select cases. The major nuances of the evaluation of DHL/THL and DEL relate to the higher risk of CNS involvement observed in patients with these disease subtypes. Asymptomatic CNS involvement by most lymphomas at the time of diagnosis that would be detectable by preemptive screening imaging is very rare. Thus, radiographic evaluations should largely be reserved for patients with suspicious symptomatic complaints and/or physical examination findings. However, if a clinician determines that intrathecal chemotherapy for CNS prophylaxis is warranted, documentation of negative CSF involvement by lymphoma via cytology and flow cytometry at the time of the first two administrations of intrathecal chemotherapy administration is highly recommended. Occult CNS involvement by lymphoma in pretreatment CSF should trigger completion of a brain MRI to assess for parenchymal disease.

6) Do I need to administer central nervous system prophylaxis in DHL/THL and DEL?

Expert Perspective: Patients with newly diagnosed DHL/THL and DEL typically present without signs or symptoms of CNS involvement at diagnosis, despite their higher risk for occult baseline CNS involvement and CNS relapse. One retrospective study published in 2014 described 311 patients with newly diagnosed DHL, of which 23 (7%) had CNS involvement at time of diagnosis. Whether this was parenchymal and/or leptomeningeal involvement, as well as the motivations for CNS assessment (symptomatic workup versus empiric screening), are not described. However, 102 of the 311 patients (33%) did not have baseline CNS assessment. Patients with either DHL/THL or DEL are more likely to be older, with poor performance status, and elevated LDH level, advanced-stage disease, and extranodal involvement at diagnosis. All of these features are independent risk factors for CNS relapse, as they are components of the CNS-IPI score. Furthermore, there is some evidence that the increased risk of CNS relapse in non-GCB COO DLBCL relative to GCB lymphomas is driven by the DEL subset of non-GCB lymphomas. In general, we discuss CNS prophylaxis with all DHL/THL patients, regardless of CNS-IPI score, and we recommend utilizing the CNS-IPI score to help determine the role for CNS prophylaxis in DEL. At the same time, we acknowledge the limited data regarding the magnitude of benefit associated with either intravenous or intrathecal methotrexate and the lack of certainty regarding the number needed to treat prophylactically in this cohort to prevent CNS relapse.

7) Do we know the best route (intrathecal vs intravenous) of CNS prophylaxis?

Expert Perspective: There has been considerable recent debate regarding the larger role for CNS prophylaxis in DLBCL. The retrospective evidence for and against this practice is significantly confounded by practice variation between providers and centers, evolving criteria used to select patients for CNS prophylaxis, different induction treatment regimens, and comorbidities that could preclude administration of CNS prophylaxis. Overall, the vast majority of lymphoma relapses in the CNS involve the brain parenchyma, with very few isolated leptomeningeal relapses being described. Among patients with any CNS relapse of lymphoma, approximately 50% also have concurrent systemic relapse. In turn, as systemic relapse is the biggest risk factor for CNS relapse, ensuring successful administration of the intended front-line systemic treatment course is paramount if CNS prophylaxis is pursued. Thus, patients who receive intensified induction treatment for DHL/THL, for example with DA-EPOCH-R, are typically paired with intrathecal methotrexate akin to the treatment regimens for Burkitt lymphoma. This was the approach taken in a phase II single-arm study in aggressive DLBCL with *MYC* rearrangements that enrolled high-risk patients including those with baseline leptomeningeal involvement and/or poor performance status. Patients with DHL/THL made up 24 of the 53 enrollees on this study, and an unprecedented 63% OS rate at two years was reported. There is less data to support systemic high-dose methotrexate sequentially or intercalated with DA-EPOCH-R, but this approach has been described in the literature. Patients with DHL/THL or DEL receiving R-CHOP induction therapy are generally first considered for a strategy incorporating intravenous high-dose methotrexate for CNS prophylaxis. For these patients, there is also the decision of whether to intercalate these doses (often given during cycles 2, 4, and 6 on day 15 of 21-day cycles of R-CHOP) or to consolidate these doses at the end of treatment.

Despite the bioplausibility of using intrathecal or intravenous methotrexate for CNS prophylaxis based on the more robust evidence supporting these approaches for the treatment of active leptomeningeal or parenchymal CNS lymphoma, the real-world effectiveness of CNS prophylaxis has been called into question by two large retrospective series from late 2021. In one study (n = 1,384), prophylactic intravenous methotrexate was given to 750 and 634 patients via intercalated or consolidated end-of-treatment strategies, respectively. A total of 78 CNS relapses were observed, with no difference in the 24-month CNS relapse rates between the two strategies. However, intercalated administration was significantly associated with more frequent delays in chemotherapy administration. Surprisingly, patients receiving either strategy had CNS relapse rates very similar to other published comparable high-risk cohorts receiving infrequent CNS prophylaxis, suggestive of a very small benefit from either prophylaxis intravenous methotrexate administration strategy. Furthermore, in the second study (n = 2,300), 410 patients received intravenous methotrexate with or without intrathecal methotrexate, 435 patients received intrathecal methotrexate alone, and 1,455 patients received no CNS prophylaxis. There was no difference in the adjusted five-year risk of secondary CNS relapse between the intravenous methotrexate and no intravenous methotrexate groups (8.4% vs 9.1%; difference not statistically significant). The authors concluded that, despite the limitations of the non-randomized and retrospective design, it appeared unlikely that intravenous methotrexate is associated with a clinically meaningful reduction in CNS relapse rates even in these high-risk patients. In turn, there is likely to be substantial evolution in CNS prophylaxis practice patterns based on these new data, with fewer patients receiving either intrathecal or intravenous methotrexate for prophylaxis. If prophylaxis is pursued, deciding between any of these strategies must be based on numerous patient-specific factors including tolerability of induction therapy, patient preference, logistical hurdles, trends in laboratory parameters, and performance status during treatment.

8) How do I get my patient with limited-stage disease into first complete remission?

Expert Perspective: Because we favor the standard approach of six cycles of R-CHOP for advanced-stage DEL, we similarly recommend the typical strategies of R-CHOP with or without radiotherapy for limited-stage DEL. One recently published retrospective cohort of 33 patients with limited-stage DEL did not find DEL status to be significantly associated with worse PFS or OS compared to 171 patients with limited-stage non-DEL/DHL. In contrast, bulky disease was the single statistically significant adverse risk factor in a multivariate analysis of prognostic factors. Regarding DHL, only about 25% of patients with this already uncommon diagnosis present with limited-stage disease. In turn, the vast majority of the evidence (albeit largely retrospective) that motivates us to consider DA-EPOCH-R for induction treatment in advanced-stage DHL does not apply to patients with limited-stage DHL. In one series of patients with DHL, a multivariate analysis of prognostic factors found advanced stage to be a strong adverse risk factor in newly diagnosed DHL, second only to baseline CNS involvement. Another retrospective series of 40 patients with limited-stage DHL achieved similar PFS and OS compared to an inclusive cohort of 104 patients with limited-stage *MYC*-rearranged DLBCL. Patients with DHL had similar response rates and survival outcomes whether they were treated with R-CHOP or intensive induction regimens. In practice, we factor a patient's burden of disease and aggressiveness of presentation into the decision on whether to recommend standard DLBCL approaches or DA-EPOCH-R for limited-stage DHL. A younger and previously fit patient with widespread intraabdominal/pelvic (stage II) DHL that presents acutely is likely better suited for DA-EPOCH-R, compared to an older patient with small volume cervical and axillary (stage II) DHL that is noted coincidently on a routine physical examination, for whom R-CHOP with radiation would offer less toxicity and reasonable outcomes.

9) How do I get my patient with advanced-stage disease into first complete remission, and then what is the next recommended step?

Expert Perspective: There is general consensus that outcomes are disappointing in DHL/THL treated with R-CHOP induction, but the evidence for alternative front-line treatment strategies is imperfect. One key analysis showed that a cohort of 159 patients with DHL/THL who were in a CR three months after the end of induction therapy achieved remarkably good outcomes, with long-term relapse-free and overall survival rates > 75%. In contrast, multiple smaller cohorts of patients with relapsed or refractory (rel/ref) DHL/THL who went on to intensive salvage chemotherapy and consolidative autologous hematopoietic cell transplantation (auto-HCT) suffered very poor outcomes with few long-term survivors. This was driven largely by high rates of chemotherapy-refractoriness in the salvage setting as well as many patients only achieving partial responses (PR) before auto-HCT. These analyses highlight the particular importance of achieving disease control for DHL/THL with induction therapy, as the likelihood of curing DHL in the rel/ref setting is considerably lower than in non-DHL/THL. Regarding how to accomplish this, several retrospective subgroup analyses showed better CR rates in DHL with intensified induction therapy and/or consolidative auto-HCT in first CR (with or without intensified induction therapy). In the modern era, the most commonly used intensified induction regimen is DA-EPOCH-R given its favorable toxicity profile with comparable outcomes (analyzed retrospectively) relative to R-CODOX-M/IVAC or R-HyperCVAD/MA. Our practice is to use DA-EPOCH-R in fit patients with newly diagnosed advanced-stage DHL, and we do not administer consolidative auto-HCT in first CR for these patients or those in whom R-CHOP may be preferred. If we elect to pursue CNS prophylaxis, we generally pair intrathecal methotrexate with DA-EPOCH-R based on familiarity with and tolerability of this approach.

In our practice, we tend to utilize standard R-CHOP for DEL. Negative results from the recent randomized head-to-head comparison of induction DA-EPOCH-R to R-CHOP in 491 newly diagnosed cases of DLBCL (irrespective of *MYC/BCL2* rearrangement or expression status) are most applicable to the DEL cohort due to this subtype being more common and better represented in this study (compared to the rarer DHL/THL subtype). There is also no specific evidence to support any role for consolidative auto-HCT in first CR for patients based on having DEL, specifically. Thus, we administer six cycles of R-CHOP on 21-day cycles to patients with DEL. In DLBCL-NOS, post-induction maintenance therapies including rituximab or lenalidomide are not indicated due to minimal, if any, PFS benefits and no OS benefits being seen in large phase III clinical trials. No studies to our knowledge have looked at whether a potential benefit from maintenance therapy can be seen specifically in *de novo* DHL/THL or DEL subtypes; thus, we discourage off-label use of these approaches.

10) My patient has relapsed; what are the recommended steps?

Expert Perspective: After induction therapy for either DHL/THL or DEL, we perform routine surveillance with a low threshold for CNS-directed imaging and CSF sampling for concerning symptoms. This applies even if a patient received CNS prophylaxis. Most relapses of DLBCL occur in the first two years after front-line therapy, and this trend is accentuated in DHL/THL (and to a lesser degree DEL), with multiple studies indicating that potentially > 80–90% of DHL/THL relapses occur within the first 12 months after completing induction therapy. While early relapses are highly likely to be a patient's prior DHL/THL or DEL, we prefer to biopsy an accessible site of suspected systemic relapse to exclude the relapse of an underlying low-grade lymphoma, especially in the setting of DHL with a *BCL2* rearrangement or THL.

Patients with confirmed relapse of DHL/THL or DEL unfortunately have very poor prognoses, and there is limited data specific to the DHL/THL or DEL subtypes to guide the choice of a second-line treatment regimen. While outcomes after intensive salvage and auto-HCT are poor in rel/ref DHL/THL, some nuanced decision-making can be applied. First, as many patients with DHL/THL will have been treated with DA-EPOCH-R in the front-line, we often avoid second-line R-ICE due the overlapping agent of etoposide. Additionally, there is some evidence that salvage R-DHAP is preferentially active in the GCB subtype, and this regimen advantageously entails CNS-penetrating doses of cytarabine. Thus, treatment of rel/ref DHL/THL with R-DHAP (or R-DHAX) is one possible strategy that exploits our clinicopathologic understanding of this disease. For patients with rel/ref DHL/THL or DEL who received induction with R-CHOP, salvage with R-ICE is certainly a reasonable option and is commonly used at our institution for fit patients. Options for auto-HCT conditioning include BEAM, BCNU/thiotepa, and busulfan/cyclophosphamide/thiotepa, with the latter two options being considered for fit patients with CNS involvement.

There is no strong evidence to guide the treatment of patients with an initial relapse of DHL/THL who are unfit for intensive salvage therapy. Commonly used approaches including rituximab plus gemcitabine and oxaliplatin (R-GemOx) are reasonable, but there is growing consensus that patients not fit for intensive salvage and auto-HCT may still be good candidates for CAR T cell therapies. In turn, the choice of second- and sometimes third-line treatment regimens to bridge patients with rel/ref DHL/THL to CAR T cell therapy should seek to balance the need for disease debulking, optimization of patient fitness, and protection of the T-cell compartment (e.g., avoiding bendamustine, predominantly) to maximize CAR T production success. It is unknown to what extent prior progression on a FDA approved CD19-directed therapy (such as tafasitamab or loncastuximab tesirine) could affect the subsequent response to an anti-CD19 CAR T cell therapy, but we anticipate the availability of data to help guide sequencing of these treatments in the next few years. Of note, the phase II clinical trial leading to approval of loncastuximab tesirine did include patients with DHL, whereas these patients were not eligible for enrollment in the phase II study of tafasitamab plus lenalidomide.

While DHL is rarely non-GCB in COO, DEL is more likely to be non-GCB and thus agents preferentially active in this subgroup of DLBCL are more often considered for the treatment of rel/ref DEL. Options include ibrutinib and lenalidomide (with or without rituximab). In theory these therapies may have efficacy in patients with CNS involvement and/or help reduce the risk of CNS relapse, but durations of responses to these agents are often limited. As a result, the potentially curative therapy of CAR T cells is just as attractive in rel/ref DEL as in other subtypes of DLBCL.

11) What are promising investigational approaches?

Expert Perspective: The NCCN opinion that the best management of any patient with cancer is a clinical trial is particularly applicable to DHL/THL and DEL. Until the 2019 initiation of the Alliance for Clinical Trials in Oncology A051701 study (NCT03984448), there were no prospective randomized clinical trials exploring the treatment of DHL/THL or DEL, specifically. This ongoing study has two components, one for DHL/THL and one for DEL. Newly diagnosed patients are randomized to receive the oral BCL2 inhibitor venetoclax or placebo in addition to standard-of-care rituximab plus chemotherapy: those with DHL/THL receive DA-EPOCH-R, while those with DEL receive R-CHOP. The rationale to add venetoclax stems from evidence that BCL2 overexpression drives resistance to combination chemotherapy in DLBCL, and the DHL/THL and DEL tumors typically (if not by definition) overexpress BCL2. Initial results from the DEL cohort have not yet been presented. However, despite promising safety and outcomes in the phase I of DA-EPOCH-R plus venetoclax, the DHL cohort of A051701 was prematurely closed in 2021 due to excess treatment-related morbidity and mortality in the experimental arm of DA-EPOCH-R plus venetoclax. The investigators emphasized that this unfortunate outcome highlights both the vital need and potential to conduct randomized trials in DHL. In contrast, the CAVALLI study was a non-randomized phase Ib/II study of R-CHOP plus venetoclax in DLBCL irrespective of BCL2 expressions status. The recently published interim results of the phase II component (with 80 of 179 patients having DEL) demonstrated impressive PFS data relative to the comparable cohort of patients on the GOYA study of front-line R-CHOP versus obinutuzumab plus CHOP (O-CHOP). Whether an OS benefit is observed in CAVALLI remains unknown, and the randomized A051701 study component that exclusively enrolls DEL will provide more formal clarity into the role of adding venetoclax to R-CHOP.

While not selecting for DEL specifically, the ongoing ESCALADE / ACE-LY-312 study (# NCT04529772) is a randomized phase III trial of acalabrutinib versus placebo in combination from front-line R-CHOP for untreated DLBCL of non-GCB COO in patients ≤ 65 years of age. The completed PHOENIX study looking at ibrutinib versus placebo plus R-CHOP in non-GCB DLCBL (irrespective of age) showed a promising OS signal in a subgroup analysis of younger patients. It appeared that older patients receiving ibrutinib plus R-CHOP had more adverse events that limited their ability to receive the intended number of cycles and dose intensity of the R-CHOP backbone, negating the benefits of adding ibrutinib. Given the association between DEL and non-GCB COO, the ESCALADE study (with a prespecified age cutoff) may provide useful insight into the treatment of this higher-risk subset of patients with DLBCL.

Other strategies being explored for the treatment of high-risk patients including DHL/THL and DEL include moving CAR T cell therapies earlier, which is particularly relevant to rel/ref DHL/THL given the frequently inadequate responses seen with intensive second-line salvage chemotherapy-based treatment in this disease. Data from trials comparing second-line CAR T cell therapies to standard-of-care salvage and auto-HCT have been recently published, with some studies showing impressive positive results. Two CAR T cell therapy products have since received FDA approval for DLBCL (irrespective of DEL and DHL status) refractory to or relapsing within 12 months after frontline treatment. These patients should be promptly referred to centers with cellular therapy services given the potentially safe use of CAR T cells in patients upwards of 80 years of age. There are also ongoing studies of early pivoting to CAR T cell therapy in high-risk patients who have inadequate interim responses to induction chemotherapy.

12) What are the takeaways about DHL/THL and DEL?

Expert Perspective: DHL/THL and DEL are subtypes of B-NHL that would otherwise be referred to morphologically as DLBCL. While representing a small portion of DLBCL cases, patients with DHL/THL have among the worst prognosis of any DLBCL subgroup. Patients with DEL are more common and have intermediate outcomes compared to DHL/THL and non-DEL/DHL DLBCL. The majority of patients with DHL/THL present with advanced-stage disease and other high-risk features, and historical data suggest that standard R-CHOP induction therapy is inadequate. Unfortunately, retrospective data with multiple confounding factors provide the foundation for any argument to offer patients alternatives to R-CHOP in the front-line setting. We feel the rationale behind intensified induction treatment, such as with DA-EPOCH-R at our center and many others, should be discussed with patients with newly diagnosed advanced-stage DHL/THL despite the absence of pro-spective randomized data supporting this recommendation. Similarly, the mixed retro-spective data on CNS prophylaxis should be discussed with patients in the context of their predicted individualized risk of CNS relapse. Experienced centers may consider DA-EPOCH-R with intrathecal methotrexate prophylaxis or R-CHOP with intercalated or end-of-therapy high-dose intravenous methotrexate as reasonable options for the treatment of newly diagnosed advanced-stage DHL/THL. For DEL, we still utilize standard R-CHOP induction therapy, with a similar personalized risk assessment for CNS relapse guiding our recommendation for CNS prophylaxis. While the sample sizes are small, two recent studies did not observe poorer outcomes in patients with newly diagnosed limited-stage DHL/THL or DEL. Thus, we also consider standard approaches of R-CHOP with or without radio-therapy for these patients with an exception as described above. In the future, hopefully we will better understand whether novel agents such as the BCL2 inhibitor venetoclax and the BTK inhibitor acalabrutinib should be incorporated into the front-line treatment of DHL/THL and/or DEL. How we diagnose these subtypes of B-NHL is also likely to continue to evolve, as advances in DNA and RNA profiling shed further light into the biology that drives the poor outcomes in these patients. These research tools may also migrate into clinical practice, helping better predict the patients most likely to need novel and/or inten-sified treatment strategies.

Recommended Readings

Alduaij, W., Collinge, B., Ben-Neriah, S., et al. (2023 May 18). Molecular determinants of clinical outcomes in a real-world diffuse large B-cell lymphoma population. *Blood* 141 (20): 2493–2507. doi: 10.1182/blood.2022018248. PMID: 36302166.

Cortese, M.J., Wei, W., Cerdeña, S., Watkins, M.P., et al. (2023 January). A multi-center analysis of the impact of DA-EPOCH-R dose-adjustment on clinical outcomes of patients with double/triple-hit lymphoma. *Leuk Lymphoma* 64 (1): 107–118. doi: 10.1080/10428194.2022.2140281. Epub 2022 Nov 2. PMID: 36323309

Dodero, A., Guidetti, A., Marino, F., et al. (2022 May 1). Dose-adjusted EPOCH and rituximab for the treatment of double expressor and double-hit diffuse large B-cell lymphoma: impact of TP53 mutations on clinical outcome. *Haematologica* 107 (5): 1153–1162. doi: 10.3324/haematol.2021.278638. PMID: 34289655; PMCID: PMC9052894.

Dunleavy, K., Fanale, M.A., Abramson, J.S., et al. (2018). Dose-adjusted EPOCH-R (etoposide, prednisone, vincristine, cyclophosphamide, doxorubicin, and rituximab) in untreated aggressive diffuse large B-cell lymphoma with MYC rearrangement: a prospective, multicentre, single-arm phase 2 study. *Lancet Haematol* 5: e609–e617.

Green, T.M., Young, K.H., Visco, C., et al. (2012). Immunohistochemical double-hit score is a strong predictor of outcome in patients with diffuse large B-cell lymphoma treated with rituximab plus cyclophosphamide, doxorubicin, vincristine, and prednisone. *J Clin Oncol* 30: 3460–3467.

Herrera, A.F., Mei, M., Low, L., et al. (2016). Relapsed or refractory double-expressor and double-hit lymphomas have inferior progression-free survival after autologous stem-cell transplantation. *J Clin Oncol* 35: 24–31.

Johnson, N.A., Slack, G.W., Savage, K.J., et al. (2012). Concurrent expression of MYC and BCL2 in diffuse large B-cell lymphoma treated with rituximab plus cyclophosphamide, doxorubicin, vincristine, and prednisone. *J Clin Oncol* 30: 3452–3459.

Landsburg, D.J., Falkiewicz, M.K., Maly, J., et al. (2017). Outcomes of patients with double-hit lymphoma who achieve first complete remission. *J Clin Oncol* 35: JCO.2017.72.215.

Morschhauser, F., Feugier, P., Flinn, I.W., et al. (2020). A phase 2 study of venetoclax plus R-CHOP as first-line treatment for patients with diffuse large B-cell lymphoma. *Blood* 137: 600–609.

Petrich, A.M., Gandhi, M., Jovanovic, B., et al. (2014). Impact of induction regimen and stem cell transplantation on outcomes in double-hit lymphoma: a multicenter retrospective analysis. *Blood* 124: 2354–2361.

Rosenwald, A., Bens, S., Advani, R., et al. (2019). Prognostic significance of MYC rearrangement and translocation partner in diffuse large B-cell lymphoma: a study by the Lunenburg Lymphoma Biomarker Consortium. *J Clin Oncol Official J Am Soc Clin Oncol* 37: 3359–3368.

Scott, D.W., King, R.L., Staiger, A.M., et al. (2018). High-grade B-cell lymphoma with MYC and BCL2 and/or BCL6 rearrangements with diffuse large B-cell lymphoma morphology. *Blood* 131: 2060–2064.

Torka, P., Kothari, S.K., Sundaram, S., et al. (2020). Outcomes of patients with limited-stage aggressive large B-cell lymphoma with high-risk cytogenetics. *Blood Adv* 4: 253–262.

43

Transformed Lymphoma

Frederique St-Pierre and Jane N. Winter

Robert H. Lurie Comprehensive Cancer Center of Northwestern University, Chicago, IL

Introduction

Any indolent B-cell lymphoma, particularly follicular lymphoma (FL), can transform into a aggressive histology. Histologic transformation from FL is expected to occur at a rate of 2 to 3% each year and is associated with treatment resistance and poor prognosis. Recent modifications to the physiopathologic mechanism of transformed FL have been proposed, including genetic and epigenetic mechanisms as well as a role for the microenvironment. Disease progression of FL and histological transformation exhibit different clonal dynamics that are driven by distinct evolutionary mechanisms. The acquisition of a transformed phenotype through divergent evolution might not be predictable at the time of diagnosis. Deciphering the earliest initiating lesions and identifying the molecular alterations leading to disease progression currently represent important goals; accomplishing these could help identify the most relevant targets for precision therapy. Clinically, suspicion for transformation should arise in patients who exhibit a sudden rise in lactate dehydrogenase (LDH), new hypercalcemia, and discordant growth among other factors that will be discussed in the chapter. The gold standard for diagnosis of transformation is histologic, but this might not be possible in certain situations. The goal of treatment is to achieve a durable remission of FL and potentially cure the high-grade component. Tranformed FL is generally associated with a poor prognosis, with an expected survival of approximately five years. There have been no randomized trials for the treatment of transformed FL, and most data comes from retrospective single-center studies. In patients with double- or triple-hit gene rearrangements at transformation, a more aggressive regimen such as R-DA-EPOCH is preferred over R-CHOP. Autologous stem cell transplant (ASCT) and chimeric antigen receptor (CAR) T cell therapy are options as well and will be discussed in this chapter. Some prospective trials for DLBCL are now including patients with transformed lymphoma, which hopefully will help further define the optimal treatment for these patients.

1) **All of the following constitute transformation except for which one?**
   A) New diagnosis with areas of follicular lymphoma (FL) grade 1–2 and 5% diffuse large B-cell lymphoma (DLBCL).
   B) Long-standing FL, new mass with biopsy showing DLBCL.

Cancer Consult: Expertise in Clinical Practice, Volume 2: Neoplastic Hematology & Cellular Therapy,
Second Edition. Edited by Syed A. Abutalib, Maurie Markman, James O. Armitage, and Kenneth C. Anderson.
© 2024 John Wiley & Sons Ltd. Published 2024 by John Wiley & Sons Ltd.

C) Long-standing FL grade 1–2 with progression in one of the lymph nodes to FL grade 3A.

D) Long-standing chronic lymphocytic leukemia (CLL) previously untreated with a rapidly increasing cervical mass with a biopsy that shows DLBCL.

Expert Perspective: The diagnosis of transformed lymphoma is challenging because there is a lack of consensus regarding the definition of histologic transformation. Most experts agree that grade 1–2 follicular lymphoma that progresses to DLBCL, Burkitt lymphoma, or other high-grade B-cell lymphoma represents histologic transformation (Figure 43.1). Progression of FL grade 1–2 to FL grade 3A (situation C) is not considered histologic transformation but rather progression with a greater number of large cells but not the sheets of large cells required for FL grade 3B or areas of frank DLBCL. Situation A is perhaps the most controversial. Some authors have considered the presence of both FL and DLBCL in the same lymph node to represent a "composite" lymphoma, and some have referred to it as "transformation at diagnosis." Others require a defined interval between the diagnosis of FL and the DLBCL; an interval of six months between the initial FL and the high-grade lymphoma has been proposed by some authors. Regardless, a diagnosis of diffuse large B-cell lymphoma must be made to qualify as a transformation. In all, because transformed FL cannot be morphologically distinguished from *de novo* DLBCL or

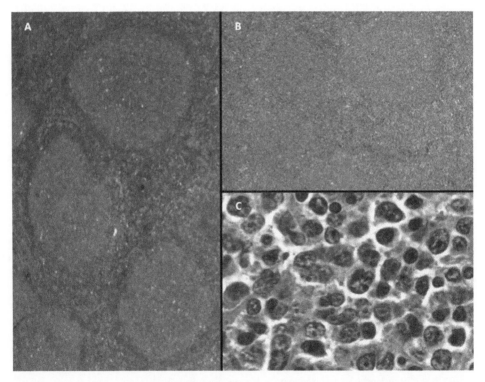

Figure 43.1 (A) Follicular lymphoma at diagnosis of an untreated patient. (B) At transformation: top area with follicles but diffuse architecture in the lower area composed of sheets of large cells. (C) High-power field of the diffuse area of Figure 1B. Large cells, prominent nucleoli, and irregular shape are noted. (also in color plate)

high-grade B-cell lymphoma, the presence of both an indolent and aggressive lymphoma in the same lymph node implies transformation. Rarely, FL may transform to other histologies such as acute B-cell lymphoblastic leukemia or, as recently described elsewhere, to histiocytic or dendritic cell sarcoma.

Although histologic transformation is most described in FL and in CLL (described as Richter's transformation; see Chapters 27 and 28), it may occur in any indolent type of non-Hodgkin lymphoma (NHL) including marginal zone lymphoma (see Chapter 37) and lymphoplasmacytic lymphoma (see Chapter 47). The first description of histologic transformation in CLL/SLL was made in 1928 by Richter and constitutes situation D. Rarely, CLL/SLL can transform to Hodgkin lymphoma or B-cell prolymphocytic leukemia (see Chapter 29).

A scientifically robust definition of "transformation" requires demonstration of a clonal relationship between the original indolent lymphoma and the subsequent aggressive counterpart. Clonal relationship may be best demonstrated by molecular techniques characterizing the immunoglobulin gene. In the daily clinical setting, demonstrating that the two lymphomas have the same light-chain restriction is usually sufficient to suggest a clonal relationship. The immunophenotype of the transformed lymphoma may, however, differ from the original indolent lymphoma. Loss of CD10 expression occurs in 10% of cases, and a gain of MUM1 or CD30 occurs, each in 25% of cases. A change in phenotype does not preclude a clonal relationship between the two lymphomas.

Correct Answer: C

Case Study 1

A 45-year-old male was recently diagnosed with stage IVA FL.

2) What is his chance of histological transformation to DLBCL?
- A) 1% per year.
- B) 2–3% per year.
- C) 10% per year.
- D) 12% per year.

Expert Perspective: Population-based and single-institution studies of FL estimate the overall rate of transformation at approximately 3% per year. The methodology, follow-up period, and definition of transformation vary among case series, which explains the slightly different results. One of the largest series is from the database of the British Columbia Cancer Agency, which included 600 patients with 170 transformations (Al-Tourah et al. 2008). The annual risk of transformation was a continuous 3%. This series included patients diagnosed with transformation based on clinical features alone when biopsy was not considered to be safe. A similar estimated rate of transformation (2%) was reported by investigators from the University of Iowa and Mayo Clinic (Link et al. 2013) in a series in which the majority (85%) were biopsy proven.

More recently, Wagner-Johnston et al. (2015) analyzed the large, prospective National LymphoCare Study (NCLS) database of nearly 2,700 patients in the rituximab era, although fewer than half of all transformations were pathologically confirmed. At median follow-up of 6.8 years, transformation had occurred in 14.3% of patients, which corresponds to approximately 2% per year, similar to earlier studies. Long-term results of the multicenter PRIMA study (2016) of 1,018 patients, show a remarkable transformation rate of only 4.2% at nine years, corresponding to approximately 0.5% per year. All patients in the PRIMA study received immunochemotherapy with or without rituximab maintenance. This very low rate of transformation may reflect improved outcomes in FL treated with rituximab-containing regimens or patient selection biases and higher rates of biopsy confirmation associated with clinical trials. This is further discussed in case Case study 2, Question 3.

The incidence of transformation is lower in the non-follicular lymphoproliferative disorders. For example, in patients with CLL/SLL, the MD Anderson Cancer Center experience from 1975 to 2005 reported a cumulative risk of proven transformation to large-cell lymphoma (Richter's syndrome) of 3.7%, a risk of transformation to Hodgkin lymphoma of 0.4%, and a risk of transformation to prolymphocytic leukemia of 0.1%. In a cohort of 340 patients with MZL, histologic transformation was observed in 3.8% of patients at five years.

Correct Answer: B

Case Study 2

A 56-year-old female with a 10-year history of FL grade 1–2, initially treated with rituximab, cyclophosphamide, vincristine, and prednisone (R-CVP) and two years ago with R-bendamustine for symptomatic recurrence, now presents with rapidly increasing left cervical adenopathy, B-symptoms, and high lactate dehydrogenase (LDH). A biopsy confirms histologic transformation.

3) Do you need a biopsy to prove your suspicion?

Expert Perspective: The obvious answer to this question is yes, or at least whenever possible. What if you suspect transformation in a retroperitoneal lymph node that is difficult to access in a patient with risks or contraindications to biopsy? In the past, biopsies were generally required, but a high clinical suspicion was considered acceptable evidence of transformation. For example, in the British Columbia series (JCO; 2008), 36% of the 170 patients with transformation were diagnosed based on clinical criteria because biopsy was considered not feasible. The presence of at least one of the following was considered indicative of transformation: sudden rise of LDH to more than twice the upper limit of normal, rapid discordant localized nodal growth, new involvement of unusual extranodal sites (liver, bone, muscle, or brain), new B-symptoms (tricky!), or new hypercalcemia. Notably, the median overall survival was not different in the group of patients diagnosed by biopsy compared to those diagnosed based on these clinical or laboratory findings (20 months vs. 16 months; $P = 0.2$). Today, however, a biopsy showing transformation to a high-grade lymphoma B-cell lymphoma, double- or triple-hit (see Chapter 42), or to Burkitt lymphoma (see Chapter 44) would result in a more aggressive treatment strategy than would transformation to diffuse large B-cell lymphoma, NOS, and additionally would require the inclusion of central nervous system (CNS) prophylaxis. Hence, pathologic confirmation of transformation is key to patient management. At times, FL can behave in an aggressive fashion in the absence of transformation and may be better served by strategies specific to follicular lymphoma. Today, a biopsy to confirm the diagnosis of transformation should be performed whenever possible without prohibitive risk. A core biopsy under computed tomography (CT) or ultrasound guidance is usually sufficient in difficult situations, but a fine-needle aspiration is NOT considered adequate. Lastly, FL, which remains incurable, can recur after successful treatment of transformed lymohoma, stressing the importance of biopsy after each progression.

4) What are the molecular or genetic events that underlie the process of histologic transformation?
   A) *p53* mutations.
   B) *c-Myc* alterations.
   C) *BCL-6* mutations or translocations.
   D) Amplification of *c-REL*.
   E) All of the above.

Expert Perspective: Detailed genetic analyses indicate that there is no single molecular or genetic event driving the process of transformation from FL to DLBCL. Rather, the process of transformation is complex and involves genomic, transcriptional, and epigenetic mechanisms. Interaction with the non-neoplastic immune cells in the tumor microenvironment (TME) likely also plays an important role. For an in-depth overview of this subject, the reviews by Fischer et al. (Ann Hematol; 2018) and by Huet S et al. (Nature Rev Cancer; 2018) are excellent resources.

Whole genome sequencing has been performed on paired samples from patients with transformed FL to compare the genetic composition of the clonal populations present at initial diagnosis of FL to those present at time of transformation. Genetic analysis has also been performed in patients with progressed FL (not transformed), for comparison. These studies indicate that FL clones that cause progression of disease without transformation generally have similar genetic composition to the clones from the initial diagnostic specimens, supporting a linear accumulation of oncogenic mutations leading to disease progression. In contrast, transformed specimens are generally composed of clones that were rare or absent in diagnostic specimens. This pattern is independent of treatment modality and time to transformation. This suggests the likely existence of common progenitor cells (CPCs) that have the potential to produce multiple different FL clones, each with a unique genetic profile. When one of these clones acquires the necessary genetic mutation pattern, histologic transformation occurs.

Genetic alterations underlying transformation in FL affect multiple different cell processes. The first is programmed cell death, often through mutated *BCL-2*, facilitated by the presence of t(14;18), which places the antiapoptotic *BCL-2* oncogene under control of the immunoglobulin heavy-chain enhancer. The second is epigenetic regulation of the tumor microenvironment through mutations involving histone and chromatin modification enzymes such as MLL2, EZH2, and CREBBP. Alterations in DNA damage response is another important potential mechanism. One of the most identified genetic lesions in transformed lymphoma is mutation of the tumor suppressor gene *TP53* (on chromosome 17p), present in 20–30% of cases, and leading to impaired DNA damage response and genomic instability. *CDKN2A/B* loss is also associated with inactivation of the *p53* tumor suppressor protein, as well as with low expression of p16 protein, which plays an important role in cell cycle regulation.

Alterations involving *MYC* have also been shown to play an important role in transformation. When arising in patients with FL with t(14;18), MYC rearrangements result in very aggressive transformed lymphomas called "double-hit lymphomas classified as high-grade B-cell lymphomas with *MYC* and *BCL-2* rearrangements by the WHO. Most double-hit lymphomas arise *de novo* and cannot strictly be considered transformations, but approximately 35% of cases arise from a previous FL. This subgroup of transformed lymphoma has a particularly bad prognosis with a two-year overall survival of 50%. *BCL-6* translocation may additionally occur during transformation, characterizing a triple-hit lymphoma *(MYC/BCL-2/BCL-6)*.

A growing list of other contributing genetic events have been identified in transformed lymphoma, including amplification of the proto-oncogene *c-REL* (10%), and mutations in TNF receptor TNFRSF14 (56%), DNA-binding transcription factor STAT6 (23%), and others. Karyotypic abnormalities including del(6q), trisomy 7, and trisomy 12 have also been implicated in histologic transformation.

Correct Answer: E

5) What is the expected survival for this patient?
  A) Less than one year.
  B) 1–3 years.
  C) 3–5 years.
  D) More than 5 years.

Expert Perspective: Historically, the median OS for transformed FL was estimated to be between one and two years, based on several case series. Most patients in these series were treated before 2000 and did not have access to rituximab. The median OS reported in more recent studies is closer to five years and possibly up to 10 years, based on results from several large cohorts. A recent pooled analysis of French and US series of 1,654 patients with FL diagnosed between 2001 and 2013 showed a 10-year cumulative risk of lymphoma-related mortality of 45.9% in patients with histologic transformation (Sarkozy et al. 2019).

Several recent studies have identified variables that may be useful in determining prognosis in patients with histologic transformation. First, the timing of histologic transformation seems to be of importance. Histologic transformation occurring early within 18 to 24 months of initial FL diagnosis is associated with worse overall survival than later relapses in multiple studies. One study indicated a two-year OS of 38% in patients who transformed within 24 months of front-line treatment with bendamustine-rituximab.

How the initial treatment for FL affects prognosis at the time of histologic transformation remains controversial. Several studies have indicated superior OS in patients who were naive to systemic therapy prior to histologic transformation. In the NCCN study of 118 patients with biopsy-proven histologic transformation between 2000 and 2011 (Ban-Hoefen et al. 2013), patients who were untreated had superior two-year OS compared to those who had received prior systemic therapy (chemotherapy and/or immunotherapy) for FL (81% vs 39%, *P* = 0.003). This difference was even more pronounced when comparing prior chemotherapy exposure, with two-year OS of 100% vs 35% ($P = 0.03$), in favor of the chemotherapy-naive group. The NLCS study of 2,700 FL patients enrolled between 2004 and 2007 (Blood; 2015), however, did not find a statistically significant difference in post-transformation OS based on treatment at initial presentation of FL vs observation. Differences between these studies may relate to time period and details of the prior therapy including use of rituximab and anthracycline.

Using rituximab in the treatment of histologic transformation is associated with superior survival outcomes, including PFS and OS, in several studies. One study of 317 patients with DLBCL, 60 of whom had a diagnosis of transformed lymphoma, showed that patients treated with rituximab and chemotherapy following histologic transformation had a five-year OS of 72%, similar to patients with *de novo* DLBCL. Autologous stem cell transplant (ASCT) after histologic transformation also appears to lead to superior survival outcomes compared to patients who do not undergo transplant in some series. Consolidation with ASCT may be of particular benefit in those previously treated with chemoimmunotherapy for FL. In a sub-analysis of the PRIMA study (Sarkozy et al. 2016) of 1,018 patients with FL, treated with R-CHOP with or without maintenance rituximab, patients with HT who were treated with ASCT had an improved OS compared to those who did not undergo ASCT (not reached vs 1.7 years).

Another emerging question is whether outcomes differ between patients who transform to DLBCL and patients who transform to a high-grade lymphoma with double-hit or triple-hit status, i.e. with the presence of *MYC* rearrangement in addition to preexisting BCL-2 and/or BCL-6 translocations characteristic of FL. While patients with transformed FL and those with *de novo* DLBCL have similar outcomes, those who transform to high-grade B-cell lymphoma with *MYC* and *BCL2* and/or *BCL6* rearrangements have poor overall survival.

Correct Answer: D

Case Study 3

A 56-year-old male who was in partial remission two years ago after treatment with R-bendamustine for a stage IVA FL grade 1–2 suddenly presents with drenching night sweats, unexplained fever, and an LDH level of 750 U/L. There is no palpable lymphadenopathy and no splenomegaly on exam.

6) How might a positron emission tomography (PET) scan be useful in the context of histologic transformation?
   A) To adequately stage the suspected histologic transformation.
   B) To identify a site for biopsy.
   C) To confirm your clinical suspicion of transformation.
   D) A and B are correct.

Expert Perspective: The usefulness of PET-CT scan in FL is usually for confirmation of newly diagnosed disease suspected to be of limited stage, when curative radiotherapy is contemplated. However, when HT is suspected, a PET–CT scan may be helpful to identify a site for biopsy.

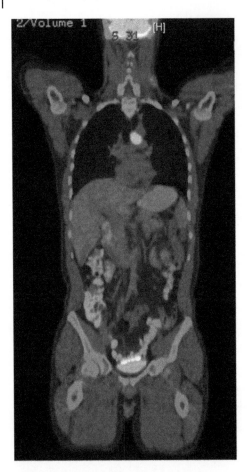

Figure 43.2 PET-CT of a newly diagnosed patient with FL. Aorto-pulmonary node had a standardized uptake value of 21.2 compared to 5.4 for a left inferior cervical node. The pathology of the aorto-pulmonary node showed FL, grade 3a. (also in color plate)

Higher maximum standardized uptake value (SUVmax) has been associated with more aggressive lymphomas. In fact, indolent lymphomas are not always detectable with fluoro-deoxyglucose (FDG) PET. One study showed that a SUVmax of more than 10 excludes indolent lymphoma with 81% specificity, and several single-center studies have established a correlation between SUVmax and FL grade and proliferation levels (Ki-67 expression). Figure 43.2 outlines an example of how PET can be utilized to identify a biopsy site. That being said, there is a considerable degree of overlap in the FDG uptake in lymphoproliferative diseases. Results from the recent GALLIUM study support this discordance. In this large phase III trial of patients with FL, cases with and without subsequent histologic transformation had similar mean baseline SUVmax leading the authors to conclude that baseline SUVmax does not predict histologic transformation. Similarly, a study at Memorial Sloan Kettering Cancer Center retrospectively identified patients with biopsy-confirmed histologic transformation who had baseline PET scans before starting treatment and reported a considerably wide range of SUV of the biopsied site.

A recent study of patients with FL and clinical suspicion of histologic transformation showed that the incidence of biopsy-proven HT was higher in the group where workup included PET-CT, presumably because PET facilitates the selection of the most metabolically active areas.

Therefore, in addition to its utility for staging and evaluation of treatment response, the clinical utility of a PET scan in the context of transformation is possibly, although not definitively so, to guide in the selection of a biopsy site. Functional imaging should not replace biopsy to diagnose transformation.

Correct Answer: D

7) **Which of the following are risk factors for transformation in a patient with FL grade 1–2?**
   A) High Follicular Lymphoma Prognostic Index (FLIPI) score.
   B) Advanced stage.
   C) Elevated LDH.

D) High β2 microglobulin.

E) Failure to achieve complete response (CR) with initial treatment.

F) All of the above.

Expert Perspective: As a rule, factors that are associated with poor outcomes in FL at diagnosis are predictive for transformation. As such, the FLIPI, which was developed specifically for prediction of outcomes of patients with FL, is also a predictor of transformation. Age more than 60 years, Ann Arbor stage III–IV, a hemoglobin level of less than 120 g/L, and four or more nodal areas are factors associated with high-risk FLIPI scores. More recent studies, conducted in the rituximab era, have identified additional independent clinical risk factors for transformation including elevated LDH or β2 microglobulin, Eastern Cooperation Oncology Group (ECOG) performance status > 1, bulky lymphadenopathy, extra-nodal disease, presence of B-symptoms, and failure to achieve a CR with the initial treatment. Pathological and genetic risk factors are emerging as novel predictors of risk, although these biomarkers need to be validated in large prospective cohorts. Potential pathologic findings include histological grade (higher risk of transformation with grade 3A FL), presence of BCL-6 translocation, absence of *BCL-2* translocation, and positive expression of *IRF4*. Potential genetic features include chromosome changes (segmental deletions within 1p and 6p, or gains involving 2, 3q, and 5), somatic gene mutations in the *BCL-6* and *BCL-2* genes, *MYC* rearrangements, mutations in *TP53*, deregulation of *MDM2*, and inactivation of *CDKN2A*.

A more controversial and important issue is whether the initial management of FL changes the risk of transformation. Some studies, including the largest population-based series from the British Columbia Cancer Agency (JCO; 2008), have reported no difference in the risk of transformation among patients initially treated with chemotherapy, radiotherapy, or watchful waiting. Some population-based trials have suggested lower risk of transformation with the "watch and wait" approach, although there is often a significant bias in therapy selection in these studies, as patients with higher-risk disease based on FLIPI tend to be treated up front, while patients who have lower risk disease are more likely to be observed.

On the other hand, several studies found that watchful waiting was associated with the highest risk of transformation when compared with other up-front therapies, including the Iowa/Mayo series (JCO; 2013) and the National LymphoCare series (Blood; 2015). Notably, patients who received rituximab monotherapy as initial treatment had the lowest risk of transformation. A recent multicenter study of 8,116 patients with FL across 11 institutions in Europe showed that the 10-years cumulative risk of histologic transformation was 5.2% in patients who had received systemic therapy, which included rituximab, compared to 8.7% in those who had not received rituximab as part of their treatment regimen (HR 0.73, *P* = 0.004). This newer evidence suggests that when treatment for FL is indicated, treatment with a rituximab-containing regimen decreases risk of transformation. Beyond this, the optimal regimen to prevent transformation is not yet clear, including the role of anthracyclines in prevention of histologic transformation. One recent study of 643 patients did compare R-CVP (rituximab, cyclophosphamide, vincristine, and prednisone) with rituximab and bendamustine for treatment of FL and found no significant difference in risk of transformation between the two regimens. It should still be considered that the data above is from retrospective cohorts, and bias in therapy selection is a significant issue.

It should be noted that the use of purine analogs has been reported to increase the risk of transformation. Al-Tourah et al. (JCO; 2008) compared two cohorts of patients with FL with similar baseline characteristics, treated with either BPVACOP (bleomycin, cisplatin, etoposide, doxorubicin, cyclophosphamide, vincristine, and prednisone) and 25 Gy of radiation to involved nodal sites, or cyclophosphamide and a purine analog (fludarabine or cladribine). The risk of transformation at 10 years was 18% and 30% ($P = 0.01$), respectively. Whether or not purine analogs are indeed associated with higher rates of transformation in indolent lymphomas is unknown. Purine analogues are now rarely used in the treatment of FL due to their limiting toxicities.

Correct Answer: F

Case Study 4

A 57-year-old woman with a previous history of an untreated stage IV FL presents with biopsy-proven transformation to DLBCL.

8) What is the most appropriate treatment?
   A) CHOP plus rituximab (R-CHOP) for six cycles.
   B) CHOP for six cycles followed by mainatence rituximab.
   C) R-CHOP for six cycles followed by high-dose chemotherapy and autologous transplantation.
   D) R-ICE (rituximab, ifosfamide, carboplatin, and etoposide) or R-ESHAP (rituximab, etoposide, methylprednisolone, cytarabine, and cisplatin) followed by high-dose chemotherapy and autologous transplantation.

Expert Perspective: It is important to mention that there have been no randomized trials for the treatment of transformed lymphoma. Most of the information comes from retrospective, often single-center studies. Some of the new prospective trials for DLBCL have now included transformed lymphoma. We hope that the inclusion of transformed lymphoma in these trials will help define the best treatment for this population.

The goal of treatment for the patient described here is a durable remission. In a chemotherapy-naive patient, we would favor an anthracycline-based treatment such as R-CHOP. The Mayo/Iowa series found that patients with transformed FL who were anthracycline-naive had similar outcomes to those with *de novo* DLBCL when treated with rituximab-based chemotherapy. The five-year OS rate following R-chemotherapy was 73% in these patients. Comparison of studies in the pre-rituximab and post-rituximab era show a considerable improvement in outcomes when adding rituximab to the chemotherapy regimen, and therefore answer B is incorrect.

The data for or against maintenance rituximab in transformed FL is weak; an analysis of 311 patients with treatment-naive transformed FL at MDACC, as well as a Canadian registry analysis of 107 patients with discordant or composite lymphomas, showed no benefit to maintenance rituximab.

If a patient with a preexisting indolent lymphoma were to present with a highly aggressive histology such as B-cell lymphoma, unclassifiable, with features intermediate between BL and DLBCL or with a high-grade B-cell lymphoma (*MYC* and *BCL-2* or *BCL-6* rearrangements translocation), we would favor a more aggressive regimen than R-CHOP such as dose-adjusted infusional etoposide, vincristine, and doxorubicin with prednisone, cyclophosphamide, and rituximab (R-DA-EPOCH) because of the poor outcome with conventional anthracycline-based treatments. The role of up-front consolidative transplantation is controversial, but some centers will consider some form of transplantation in patients who achieve remission. A prospective multicenter trial of 53 patients with untreated *MYC* + aggressive B-cell lymphomas showed durable remissions with R-DA-EPOCH without consolidative ASCT, although patients with transformed FL were not included in the study.

ASCT is generally considered for patients who have had prior treatment for their FL at time of transformation and will be discussed in more detail in Case study 5 (see also Chapter 40).

Correct Answer: A

Case Study 5

A 58-year-old male with a long history of recurrent FL grade 1–2 stage IVA has previously been treated with rituximab monotherapy, bendamustine-rituximab, and six cycles of R-CHOP. He now presents with rapid disease progression and biopsy of an FDG avid lymph node is performed. Histology shows transformation to DLBCL, with no *MYC* rearrangement. He has stage IIIB disease and a good performance status.

9) What treatment would you recommend?
   A) Supportive or palliative therapy only.
   B) R-ICE or R-ESHAP or other salvage therapy followed by high-dose therapy and autologous stem cell transplant (ASCT).
   C) Chimeric antigen receptor (CAR) T cell therapy.
   D) Tafasitamab and lenalidomide followed by lenalidomide maintenance.

Expert Perspective: This patient represents an example of a young heavily pretreated patient who presents with a transformed lymphoma. His prognosis is relatively poor, but a durable remission is still possible, so we would advise him against a palliative approach. His prior exposure to anthracycline precludes the use of this class of agents, although a limited number of cycles may be tolerable if given with cardioprotection.

The data to support the role of ASCT after salvage therapy comes from retrospective studies and case series (Table 43.1). There is some variation in survival data between these studies, with studies in the pre-rituximab era (first five studies in Table 46.1) showing 20–35% of patients alive without progression at five years, and studies in the rituximab era showing progression-free survival ranging between 45% and 60% at five years (see Chapter 40). In retrospective studies that compared ASCT to non-ASCT strategies, there appears to be a survival benefit to ASCT. The largest of these, by Villa et al. (JCO; 2013), showed improved OS with ASCT compared to rituximab-based chemotherapy with a hazard ratio (HR) of 0.13 ($P < 0.001$). Transplant-related mortality (TRM) appears to be low for patients treated with ASCT in the rituximab era, ranging from 0 to 5% at five years.

Allogeneic transplant has the advantage of the graft versus lymphoma effect and remains the only curative treatment for FL (see Chapters 35 and 38). Small series of patients with transformed lymphomas treated with either myeloablative or reduced-intensity conditioning regimens have been published, but patient numbers are even smaller than the autologous transplant series (Table 43.1). The largest published series on myeloablative allogeneic transplant in the rituximab era reported a five-year event-free survival (EFS) of 24% and five-year OS of 33%. TRM was very high at 27% at 100 days. Many studies indicate improved survival with ASCT compared to allogeneic transplant (Table 43.1), probably in large part due to significant transplant-related toxicity with the latter. For these reasons, outside a clinical trial, we would favor salvage chemotherapy and ASCT for the patient described above.

Emerging novel therapies offer an additional therapeutic option for patients who have relapsed after ASCT, or for patients who are not candidates for ASCT. Table 43.2 outlines the major novel therapies available for patients with transformed FL. CAR T cell therapy is perhaps the most promising, as it offers an opportunity for durable remission in patients with pretreated transformed lymphoma. Several CAR T trials for DLBCL have included patients with transformed lymphoma, although not all have reported outcomes specifically in the transformed group. The TRANSCEND trial (Lancet; 2020) included 57 patients with transformed FL, and in this group, CR rate was 63.2% with a relatively low incidence of grade 3 or worse toxicity. At least two prior lines of therapy were required for eligibility, including anti-CD20 therapy; candidates were those who had already failed ASCT or were ineligible for transplant. The ZUMA-7 (NEJM; 2022) and TRANSFORM (Lancet; 2022) trials evaluated CAR T-cell therapy in the second-line setting for relapsed/refractory DLBCL, compared to standard of care (ASCT). Both studies showed superior event-free survival with CAR T compared to ASCT. These patients had disease that was refractory or relapsed within 1 year of first-line therapy. About 46 and 11 patients with tFL were included in ZUMA-7 and TRANSFORM, respectively. As a result, CAR T-cell therapy is now approved for treatment of tFL in the second-line setting, and prior failure of ASCT is no longer required. (see also Chapter 40).

Correct Answer: B

Case Study 6

An 84-year-old female with FL treated previously with rituximab and R-CHOP presents with B-symptoms and biopsy-proven transformation to DLBCL.

10) **What is your choice of treatment?**
   A) Supportive or palliative therapy only.
   B) Clinical trial.
   C) CAR T cell therapy.
   D) Polatuzumab vedotin plus bendamustine and rituximab.
   E) Lenalidomide-based therapy.
   F) All of the above.

Expert Perspective: The preferred strategy for transformed FL is an anthracycline-containing regimen, most often R-CHOP. Unfortunately, this isn't an option in this patient because of prior therapy with anthracycline. As discussed in Case study 5, consolidation with high-dose chemotherapy and autologous stem cell transplant is a strategy associated with durable responses in patients with previously treated transformed lymphoma. This approach is not appropriate for this patients because of advanced age. Nonetheless, dis-

Table 43.1 Results of studies of autologous and allogeneic transplantation in transformed lymphoma.

Study	N	Median age (range)	Main conditioning regimen used	Autolo-gous or allogeneic	Median follow-up (yr)	ORR % (CR/PR) after transplant	PFS	OS	TRM/ secondary MDS
Williams et al. (2001)	50	45.8 (28.0–60.6)	Cy/TBI (56%), BEAM (20%)	Auto	4.9	76 (62/14)	20% at 5 years	51% at 5 years	8% at 100 days/ –
Ramadan et al. (2008)	25	49 (29–55)	Cy/TBI (83%), Cy/VP16/ TBI (10%)	Allo	2.1	–	25% at 3 years	32% at 3 years	33% at 1 year/ –
Thomson et al. (2009)	18	46 (23–64)	Fludarabine/ Alemtuzumab (100%)	Allo	4.3	–	60% at 4 years	61% at 4 years	29% at 1 year/ –
Eide et al. (2011)*	47/30*	55 (31–65)	BEAM (100%)	Auto	3.9	83 (60/23)	32% at 5 years	47% at 5 years	7%/0%
Wirk et al. (2014)	108	56	Myeloablative ±TBI (100%)	Auto	7.1	–	35% at 5 years	50% at 5 years	– /4%
	33	49	Myeloablative ± TBI (61%)/RIC ± TBI (33%)/ unknown (6%)	Allo	5.3	–	18% at 5 years	22% at 5 years	36%/ –
Smith et al. (2009)	25	57	CBV (100%)	Auto	2.1	–	64% at 3 years	63% at 3 years	–
Ban-Hoefen et al. (2012) (NCCN Database)	18	58 (40–65)	BEAM (78%), Cy/TBI (17%)	Auto	3.3	94% RR before transplant	59% at 2 years	82% at 2 years	0%/11%

(Continued)

Table 43.1 (Continued)

Study	N	Median age (range)	Main conditioning regimen used	Autolo-gous or allogeneic	Median follow-up (yr)	ORR % (CR/PR) after transplant	PFS	OS	TRM/ secondary MDS
Reddy et al. (2012)	44	55	CBV (88%)	Auto	3.0	–	45% at 5 years	62% at 5 years	–/11%
	7	55	Myeloablative (43%)/RIC (57%)	Allo	3.0	–	46% at 5 years	69% at 5 years	–
Villa et al. (2013)	97	56	–	Auto	7.5	–	55% at 5 years	65% at 5 years	5% at 5 years/–
	22	48	95% myeloablative	Allo	7.5	–	46% at 5 years	46% at 5 years	23% at 5 years/ –
Madsen et al. (2015)	54	56	–	Auto	3.4	–	60% at 5 years	67% at 5 years	–
Heinzelmann et al. (2018)	33	51	BuCyMel ±TBI (27%)/ RIC ±TBI (73%)	Allo	7.1	–	24% at 5 years	33% at 5 years	27% at 100 days/6%
Chin et al. (2020)	49	56	BEAM (20%)/CBV (73%)/ Other myeloablative (6%)	Auto	3.7	–	77% at 4 years	88% at 4 years	–/4%

BuCyMel: busulfan-cyclophosphamide-melphalan; CR: complete response; Cy/TBI: cyclophosphamide and total body irradiation; CBV: cyclophosphamide-etoposide-carmustine; MDS: myelodysplastic syndrome; ORR: overall response rate; OS: overall survival; PFS: progression-free survival; PR: partial response; RIC: reduced intensity conditioning; TRM: treatment-related mortality; VP16: etoposide.
*Only prospective study: 47 patients entered the study, and 30 patients received autologous transplantation.

Table 43.2 Results of studies with novel therapies that have included transformed lymphoma.

Study	N	Median age (range)	Treatment	Median number of prior therapies	Median follow-up (months)	ORR % (CR/PR)	PFS (months)
Kaminski et al. (2001)	23	*60 (38–82)	I[131] tositumomab	4	*47	39 (13/26)	**8.4
Witzig et al. (2002)	9	*60 (29–80)	^{90}Y-ibritumomab tiuxetan	*2	–	56 (NR)	*11.2
Friedberg et al. (2008)	15	*63 (38–84)	Bendamustine 120 mg/m[2] IV every 3 weeks for six cycles	*2	*26	66 (13/53)	4.2
Czuczman et al. (2011)	33	66 (42–84)	Lenalidomide 25 mg days 1–21 of 28 d cycle	4	5.6	46 (21/25)	5.4
Locke et al. (2019)	16	*58–59 (34–69)	Axicabtagene ciloleucel	*3	*27.1	83 (84/101)	*5.9
Hirayama et al. (2019)	13	60	CD19 CAR T-cell immonotherapy	5	38	46 (6/13)	11.2
Abramson et al. (2020)	57	*63	Lisocabtagene maraleucel	*3	*18.8	84.2	*6.8
Salles et al. (2020)	7	—	Tafasitamab 12 mg/kg (days 1, 8, 15, 22 of 28-day cycle), lenalidomide 25 mg daily (day 1–21 of 28-day cycle) × 12 cycles	*2	*13.2	*60 (48/80)	*16.2

(Continued)

Table 43.2 (Continued)

Study	N	Median age (range)	Treatment	Median number of prior therapies	Median follow-up (months)	ORR % (CR/PR)	PFS (months)
Segman et al. (2021)	16	—	Polatuzumab vedotin + rituximab ± bendamustine	*3	*66.1	*61	*5.6
Kalakonda et al. (2020)	31	*67 (35–85)	Selinexor 60 mg on days 1 and 3, weekly.	*2	*11.1	*28 (12/17)	—
Caimi et al. (2021)	29	*66 (56–71)	Loncastuximab tesirine	*3	—	*70 (35/35)	*4.9
Locke et al. (2022)	19	*58 (21–80)	Axicabtagene ciloleucel	—	*24.9	*83 (65/18)	*8.3
Kamdar et al. (2022)	7	*60 (53.5–67.5)	Lisocabtagene maraleucel	—	*6.2	*79 (61/18)	*10.1
Sehgal et al. (2022)	6	*74 (70–78)	Lisocabtagene maraleucel	—	*12.3	*80 (54/26)	*9.03

A: anemia; CR: complete response; N: neutropenia; NR: not reached; ORR: overall response rate; OS: overall survival; PFS: progression-free survival; PR: partial response; T: thrombocytopenia.

*Results of the whole study (the specific data on TL are not reported separately in the study).

**PFS of patients who responded to I[131]-Tositumomab in the whole study (data for TL are not reported).

ease control and even a period of remission may be achieved with alternative therapies. CAR T-cell therapy is approved in the second-line setting for patients who are not eligible for ASCT based on results from the phase II PILOT study (Lancet Oncology; 2022), and would be considered for this patient; although some of its toxicities may preclude its use in an 84-year-old patient, especially if comorbidities are present. Alternative non-anthracycline-containing regimens used in DLBCL would be reasonable options, for example a gemcitabine-containing regimen or rituximab-lenalidomide, among others. If the patient declines treatment or is not a candidate for treatment because of a poor performance status and comorbidities, supportive or palliative care may be appropriate.

There is a rapidly expanding number of second- and third-line treatments for DLBCL, but there is little data specifically for patients with transformed lymphoma. A phase II study of lenalidomide in 33 patients with relapsed or refractory transformed lymphoma showed a response rate of 46% with a median duration of response of 12.8 months and PFS of 5.4 months in the entire cohort. A more recent retrospective analysis of 18 patients with TL treated with lenalidomide (± rituximab) at a single institution showed better outcomes with an ORR of 63%, PFS of 24 months, and OS of 46.7 months. Lenalidomide has also been combined with tafasitamab, an anti-CD19 monoclonal antibody, and the combination is FDA approved for second-line therapy of relapsed/refractory DLBCL in patients ineligible for ASCT. Both the anti-CD19 targeted antibody-drug conjugate loncastuximab tesirine and selinexor, an oral inhibitor of nuclear export protein, are approved for DLBCL that arises from transformation of a low-grade lymphoma or specifically FL, respectively, after two prior lines of therapy. Other therapies for relapsed/refractory DLBCL that have also been used in patients with transformed lymphoma include polatuzumab vedotin, an anti-CD79b-directed antibody-drug conjugate, combined with bendamustine-rituximab (GO29365 study).

It is always important to consider a clinical trial when considering treatment options; many of the new targeted agents are well-tolerated oral formulations (see http://www.clinicaltrials.gov). There are few clinical trials specifically for patients with transformed lymphoma; instead, patients with transformed lymphoma are frequently included on studies evaluating new agents in DLBCL.

Correct Answer: F

Recommended Readings

Al-Tourah, A.J., Gill, K.K., Chhanabhai, M., Hoskins, P.J., Klasa, R.J., Savage, K.J. et al. (2008). Population-based analysis of incidence and outcome of transformed non-Hodgkin's lymphoma. *J Clin Oncol* 26 (32): 5165–5169.

Ban-Hoefen, M., Vanderplas, A., Crosby-Thompson, A.L., Abel, G.A., Czuczman, M.S., Gordon, L.I. et al. (2013). Transformed non-Hodgkin lymphoma in the rituximab era: Analysis of the NCCN outcomes database. *Br J Haematol* 163 (4): 487–495.

Fischer, T., Zing, N.P.C., Chiattone, C.S., Federico, M., and Luminari, S. (2018). Transformed follicular lymphoma. *Ann Hematol* 97 (1): 17–29.

Huet, S., Sujobert, P., and Salles, G. (2018). From genetics to the clinic: a translational perspective on follicular lymphoma. *Nat Rev Cancer* 18 (4): 224–239.

Kamdar M., Solomon S.R., Arnason J., et al. (2022 June). TRANSFORM Investigators. Lisocabtagene maraleucel versus standard of care with salvage chemotherapy followed by autologous stem cell transplantation as second-line treatment in patients with relapsed or refractory large B-cell lymphoma (TRANSFORM): results from an interim analysis of an open-label, randomised, phase 3 trial. *Lancet* 399 (10343): 2294–2308. doi: 10.1016/S0140-6736(22)00662-6. Erratum in: *Lancet* 2022 Jul 16;400(10347):160. PMID: 35717989.

Link, B.K., Maurer, M.J., Nowakowski, G.S., Ansell, S.M., Macon, W.R., Syrbu, S.I. et al. (2013). Rates and outcomes of follicular lymphoma transformation in the immunochemotherapy era: a report from the university of iowa/mayoclinic specialized program of research excellence molecular epidemiology resource. *J Clin Oncol: Off J Am Soc Clin Oncol* 31 (26): 3272–3278.

Sarkozy, C., Maurer, M.J., Link, B.K., Ghesquieres, H., Nicolas, E., Thompson, C.A. et al. (2019). Cause of death in follicular lymphoma in the first decade of the rituximab era: a pooled analysis of french and US cohorts. *J Clin Oncol* 37 (2): 144–152.

Sarkozy, C., Trneny, M., Xerri, L., Wickham, N., Feugier, P., Leppa, S. et al. (2016). Risk factors and outcomes for patients with follicular lymphoma who had histologic transformation after response to first-line immunochemotherapy in the PRIMA trial. *J Clin Oncol* 34 (22): 2575–2582.

Sehn, L.H., Hertzberg, M., Opat, S., et al. (2022 January 25). Polatuzumab vedotin plus bendamustine and rituximab in relapsed/refractory DLBCL: survival update and new extension cohort data. *Blood Adv* 6 (2): 533 543. doi: 10.1182/bloodadvances.2021005794. PMID: 34749395; PMCID: PMC87915 82.

Villa, D., Crump, M., Panzarella, T., Savage, K.J., Toze, C.L., Stewart, D.A. et al. (2013). Autologous and allogeneic stem-cell transplantation for transformed follicular lymphoma: A report of the Canadian blood and marrow transplant group. *J Clin Oncol* 31 (9): 1164–1171.

Wagner-Johnston, N.D., Link, B.K., Byrtek, M., Dawson, K.L., Hainsworth, J., Flowers, C.R. et al. (2015). Outcomes of transformed follicular lymphoma in the modern era: a report from the National LymphoCare Study (NLCS). *Blood* 126 (7): 851–857.

44

Burkitt Lymphoma

Mark Roschewski and Wyndham Wilson

National Cancer Institute, National Institutes of Health, Bethesda, MD

Introduction

Burkitt lymphoma (BL) is a highly aggressive B-cell lymphoma characterized by marked tumor proliferation resulting from a *MYC* translocation on the long arm of chromosome 8 (8q24) and one of three locations on Ig genes: t(8;14), t(2;8), or t(8;22). It is the most common B-cell lymphoma in children but accounts for only ~2% of adult lymphomas. Distinct clinical variants include endemic, sporadic, and immunodeficiency-associated forms with variable association with Epstein-Barr virus. All clinical variants present dramatically characterized by rapidly dividing tumors with a predilection for involvement of extranodal sites, including the intestines, bone marrow, and central nervous system (CNS). Early recognition of "possible BL" represents a medical emergency that should prompt urgent diagnostic procedures and initiation of aggressive supportive care before tissue confirmation to prevent tumor lysis syndrome, electrolyte disturbances, gastric perforation, or multi-system organ dysfunction. BL is highly sensitive to chemotherapy, and most patients treated with highly intensive combination chemotherapy regimens are cured, but treatment-related toxicities remain problematic for older patients and those with comorbid conditions. Younger patients are less susceptible to the acute toxicities but endure long-term risks of treatment, including infertility and secondary malignancies. Dose-adjusted EPOCH-R (DA-EPOCH-R) has less toxicity than pediatric BL regimens with high rates of cure across a diverse range of patients, including those with disseminated disease, advanced age, and HIV. Still, patients with CNS involvement remain at high risk for both treatment failure and early toxic death. Improved therapy for patients with active CNS disease and those with primary resistance to chemotherapy remain major unmet needs. Future studies combining rational targeted agents to DA-EPOCH-R or novel immunotherapy approaches may further improve cure rates.

Case Study 1

A 55-year-old man presents to the emergency department with the sudden onset of severe abdominal pain in his right lower quadrant (RLQ) over the preceding two days. He is afebrile with stable vital signs and slight tachycardia. He has significant point tenderness in his right lower quadrant. Complete blood count reveals a total white blood cell (WBC) count of 8.0×10^9/L, hemoglobin of 10.5 g/dL, and platelets of 110×10^9/L. Serum chemistries are notable for a lactate dehydrogenase (LDH) level of 2500 U/L and uric acid of 12.5 mg/dL with normal renal and hepatic function. A computed tomography (CT) scan of the abdomen and pelvis demonstrates a 6×8 cm abdominal mass arising from the cecum with a moderate amount of ascites. General surgery and medical oncology are consulted for recommendations regarding evaluation and management.

1) **What are the diagnostic considerations in cases of possible Burkitt lymphoma (BL), as in this case?**

Expert Perspective: It is critical to approach patients with possible Burkitt lymphoma (BL) as a medical emergency since these patients are at risk for spontaneous tumor lysis syndrome before the initiation of therapy and early toxic death during the first course of treatment. Further, all variants of BL often involve extranodal anatomic sites including the gastrointestinal tract (GI), bone marrow (BM), and central nervous system (CNS). GI involvement may mimic surgical emergencies such as acute appendicitis as depicted in this case. Medical oncology consultation before biopsy is appropriate to choose the best diagnostic approach. Subclassification of lymphoma relies on clinical, morphologic, and cytogenetic and molecular features, rendering the material obtained with the initial biopsy critical. In general, a fine-needle aspirate is insufficient. In the present case, BL should be suspected due to the location of the mass, the rapid onset of symptoms, and the extreme elevation of LDH. BL is the fastest growing human tumor and can double in size in 24–48 hours. It has a male predilection and is common in children but rare in adults and often overlooked. In most cases, surgery is unnecessary and prompt institution of effective immunochemotherapy is the primary goal, although risk of gastric perforation during therapy is important to recognize. Incisional or excisional biopsy via laparoscopy or adequate CT-guided core needle biopsies with tissue sent for fluorescent in situ hybridization (FISH) testing for rearrangements of the *MYC* oncogene is mandatory. Goal turnaround time from first suspecting BL to initiation of therapy is 48–72 hours, making a high suspicion of "possible BL" critical. Morphologically, BL typically demonstrates a "starry sky" appearance of diffuse and monotonous small to medium-sized B cells with a distinct immunophenotypic profile that is positive for surface IgM with immunoglobulin light chain (kappa > lambda), CD20, CD10, and B-cell lymphoma-6 (BCL6), and negative for BCL2, which distinguishes it from diffuse large B-cell lymphoma (DLBCL; see Chapter 34).

2) **What is the current understanding about the pathogenesis of BL and its relationship to DLBCL?**

Expert Perspective: The normal germinal center B-cell is the cell of origin for BL and many cases of DLBCL, and these malignancies share overlapping clinical and pathologic features. Most cases of BL have demonstrable *MYC* (8q24) rearrangements, in the background of a few other aberrations ("*MYC* simple"). Up to 10% of newly diagnosed

DLBCL cases also harbor *MYC* rearrangements, but these cases are usually associated with other chromosomal abnormalities ("*MYC* complex"). In endemic BL, the breakpoint in chromosome 8 usually lies adjacent to the *MYC* gene, while in sporadic BL it often lies within intron 1 of *MYC*. The 2016 revision of the World Health Organization (WHO) classification introduced two new entities: high-grade B-cell lymphoma, defined by the presence of *MYC* and *BCL2* and/or *BCL6* rearrangements (HGBCL-DH/TH; see Chapter 42) as well as Burkitt-like lymphoma with 11q aberration, which has a gene expression profile similar to BL but lacks *MYC* rearrangements. RNA-resequencing (RNA-seq) analysis of sporadic BL has confirmed the molecular distinction of BL and identified many genes more frequently mutated in BL than DLBCL, including *TCF3*, *ID3*, and *TP53*. The ID3 mutations are seen in up to 38% of BL cases and not seen in DLBCL. Components of the B-cell receptor (BCR) are upregulated by TCF3 but via different mechanisms than seen in *DLBCL*. RNA interference screens demonstrate that knockdown of the BCR subunit *CD79A* and inhibition of PI3K were toxic to BL cell lines, supporting these as cooperative pathways in BL pathogenesis. In support of this hypothesis, Sander et al. (2012) demonstrated that combining constitutive c-MYC expression and PI3K activity in germinal center B-cells of the mouse led to tumors with a striking similarity to BL.

3) How do cofactors such as Epstein-Barr virus (EBV), malaria, and human immunodeficiency virus (HIV) contribute to the pathogenesis of BL?

Expert Perspective: The syndrome of rapidly enlarging tumors of the jaw in children was first described by the Irish surgeon Denis Burkitt while working in Uganda in 1958. Today, we subdivide BL into three clinical variants—endemic (African) BL, sporadic BL, and immunodeficiency (HIV)-associated with important differences in epidemiology, clinical presentation, and biology. Endemic BL, which is the most common subtype, occurs in developing countries such as equatorial Africa and Papua New Guinea. It frequently affects the jaw and is seen almost exclusively in children. Endemic BL is an apparent polymicrobial disease, with clonal EBV found in the neoplastic cells of virtually all patients (positive expression of CD21); cases are also linked to the prevalence of malaria, and the incidence is highest in people with high titers of Plasmodium falciparum. In contrast, EBV occurs in ~40% of sporadic BL and HIV-associated cases. Evidence for the oncogenic role of EBV stems from the fact that cell lines that have lost EBV do not induce tumors in mice, but re-infection with EBV reestablishes a malignant phenotype. EBV contributes to genomic instability in endemic BL. The relationship of HIV and BL was first noted in 1982; it may also increase the risk of BL, possibly via chronic stimulation of B cells, as is suspected in malaria. Interestingly, HIV-associated BL can occur at any CD4 count, suggesting that immunosuppression itself is not the sole contributing factor. Recent studies utilizing whole genome sequencing have suggested that the molecular profile of BL is distinguished mostly by presence of EBV and is not different across age groups or clinical variants.

4) What is the most effective chemotherapy regimen in BL?

Expert Perspective: Patients treated with regimens such as rituximab, cyclophosphamide, doxorubicin, vincristine, and prednisone (R-CHOP) have poor outcomes, and this is clearly inadequate therapy. Multiple other regimens are effective for BL, and many factors must be considered during the initial treatment decision such as age and the presence of comorbidities. The traditional approach to BL in developed countries is high-intensity, short-duration combination chemotherapy given in alternating cycles as originally developed for acute lymphoblastic leukemia (ALL) in children. BL regimens administer therapies directed at the central nervous system (CNS) in all patients without regard to tumor bulk or disease stage. These BL regimens achieve complete remission in 80–90% of patients, but the risk of significant acute toxic effects and long-term toxicities are very high including second malignancies, neurologic dysfunction, and infertility. With these regimens, age is an important consideration since older patients tolerate therapy poorly and are frequently unable to complete the therapy. The infusional regimen dose-adjusted infusional etoposide, vincristine, and doxorubicin with prednisone, cyclophosphamide, and rituximab (DA-EPOCH-R) has been used for both sporadic and HIV-associated BL, and a recent multicenter study demonstrated that a risk-adapted approach can cure most patients with less toxicity. Age or HIV status are not prognostic with the use of DA-EPOCH-R, but the presence of CNS or bone marrow disease is associated with both early toxic death and disease progression. Before therapy, it is critical to assess for cerebrospinal fluid (CSF) disease with flow cytometry if DA-EPOCH-R is considered. Patients who have high-risk disease and are CSF negative on flow cytometry are given intrathecal (IT) therapy for CNS prophylaxis, while patients who are positive for CSF disease by flow cytometry are administered active IT therapy until the CSF is cleared. Risk-adapted approaches may ultimately replace ALL-type regimens if comparable efficacy is demonstrated given the favorable toxicity profile.

5) Are subtypes of BL treated differently?

Expert Perspective: In general, subtypes of BL are not treated differently, but therapy depends on tolerance of toxicity and the ability to administer the necessary supportive care. Because most cases of endemic BL occur in equatorial Africa, where medical resources are scarce, the use of ALL-like regimens is not possible. Dramatic responses to chemotherapy were reported in Africa with as little as a single dose of cyclophosphamide, but most patients relapsed, and the survival of patients was no more than 10–20%. In 2004, the International Network for Cancer Treatment and Research (INCTR) developed joint treatment protocols using a three-drug regimen of cyclophosphamide, methotrexate, and vincristine. These drugs were considered affordable and accessible in low-resource settings. With a uniform treatment protocol, the INCTR reported overall survival rates of 67% and 62% at years 1 and 2, respectively. Similarly, patients with HIV-associated BL are often unable to tolerate the high-intensity ALL-like regimens commonly employed for BL. DA-EPOCH-R is another option since only 3–4 cycles of chemotherapy have proven effective.

At the National Cancer Institute, we initiate therapy with DA-EPOCH-R for patients with sporadic BL regardless of risk status due to our preliminary results and relative lower toxicity compared to R-CODOX-M/IVAC or R-HyperCVAD/R. Patients with HIV-associated BL are given 3–4 cycles of immunochemotherapy, with rituximab given twice per cycle. At this point, the presence of EBV co-infection does not have a known effect on the prognosis or treatment of BL.

6) What is the role of rituximab in BL?

Expert Perspective: Rituximab is a chimeric monoclonal antibody against CD20 that is an essential component of the treatment of both indolent and aggressive B-cell lymphomas. Until recently, the contribution of rituximab to outcomes in BL was not entirely clear because intensive chemotherapy resulted in such high remission rates. Phase II studies have reported the feasibility of rituximab use in BL, and Ribrag et al. (2012) recently reported the results of a randomized study of rituximab added to the backbone of the standard LMBA protocol in HIV-negative adult patients with BL. With rituximab given on days 1 and 6 of the first two courses of chemotherapy, they reported an improvement in event-free survival of 76% versus 64% at a median follow-up of 38 months without any obvious increase in toxicity. The three-year overall survival also favored the use of rituximab (82% vs 71%). Thus, rituximab should be included in the treatment regimen of all patients being treated for BL.

7) What is the most appropriate CNS prophylaxis method in BL?

Expert Perspective: Strategies to prevent CNS disease relapse are important considerations in the treatment of BL since disease relapse within the CNS is a devastating clinical scenario. All patients should have a lumbar puncture with flow cytometry to assess for CNS disease at the time of initial diagnosis. Most regimens include high doses of systemic chemotherapy that crosses the blood-brain barrier (methotrexate and/or cytarabine), intrathecal therapy, or both given to all patients with advanced-stage disease. The toxicities of CNS-directed therapies, however, can be significant, and the most effective approach has not been well studied. The Cancer and Leukemia Group B (CALGB) observed that the use of prophylactic CNS irradiation led to intolerable short- and long-term complications, and it dropped its use from their protocols although this approach is still utilized in Europe. Patients with low-risk disease and CSF that is negative by flow cytometry at diagnosis may not need CNS prophylaxis, but further research is needed to confirm these findings. High doses of cytarabine and methotrexate also contribute to myelosuppression and may not be essential in patients with low tumor burden. A recent retrospective study suggested that CNS relapse is a problem with all regimens used for BL, and improving therapy that prevents and treats active CNS disease is a current unmet medical need.

8) What are the supportive care considerations in patients with newly diagnosed BL?

Expert Perspective: Aggressive supportive care with careful attention to the potential complications is essential. An improvement over the last decade in BL outcomes is likely due to modern supportive care measures. In places in which supportive care is limited, outcomes in BL are inferior including third-world countries. Further, recent retrospective studies demonstrated that patients treated outside of academic centers had worse outcomes. This may reflect a referral bias, limited expertise in highly complex cases, or less availability of intensive supportive care resources including a potential urgent need for hemodialysis. The most important consideration is prompt diagnosis and initiation of chemotherapy without delay. BL cells are rapidly proliferating and, as previously explained, tumor mass can double in 24–48 hours. Due to the rapid doubling, tumor cells may undergo spontaneous tumor lysis syndrome (TLS), and prevention is a major consideration when initiating therapy. Adequate hydration and allopurinol should be instituted in all cases before therapy. Electrolytes such as uric acid, potassium, calcium, and phosphorous should be closely monitored to prevent and recognize signs of TLS. The recombinant urate oxidase, rasburicase, has been used to catalyze the uric acid already produced in cases of BL, but this is not essential in every case. Patients with glucose-6-phosphate dehydrogenase deficiencies should not be treated with rasburicase due to the risk of hemolytic anemia.

Patients treated with BL regimens are also at high risk for severe and prolonged neutropenia. The use of granulocyte colony-stimulating factors is mandatory to limit the duration of neutropenia and the incidence of treatment delay. One should pay close attention for signs of clinical infection, and prompt institution of intravenous antibiotics and antifungals in accordance with published guidelines is mandatory. Indeed, the physician and institution's familiarity with highly intense chemotherapy regimens have profound effects on individual patient outcomes.

Recommended Readings

Thomas, N., Dreval, K., Gerhard, D.S., et al. (2023 February 23). Genetic subgroups inform on pathobiology in adult and pediatric Burkitt lym phoma. *Blood* 141 (8): 904 916. doi: 10.1182/blood.2022016534. PMID: 36201743; PMCID: PMC10023728.

Roschewski M, Staudt LM, Wilson WH. Burkitt's Lymphoma. *N Engl J Med*. 2022 Sep 22;387(12):1111–1122. doi: 10.1056/NEJMra2025746. PMID: 36129999.

Dave, S.S., Fu, K., Wright, G.W. et al. (2006). Molecular diagnosis of Burkitt's lymphoma. *N Engl J Med* 354 (23): 2431–2442.

Evens, A., Danilov, A., Jagadeesh, D. et al. (2021 January 21). Burkitt lymphoma in the modern era: real-world outcomes and prognostication across 30 US cancer centers. *Blood* 137 (3): 374–386.

Molyneux, E.M., Rochford, R., Griffin, B. et al. (2012). Burkitt's lymphoma. *Lancet* 379 (9822): 1234–1244.

Olszewski, A., Jakobsen, L.H., Collins, G. et al. (2021 April 1). Burkitt lymphoma international prognostic index. *J Clin Oncol* 39 (10): 1129–1138.

Panea, R., Love, C., Shingleton, J.R. et al. (November 7). The whole-genome landscape of Burkitt lymphoma subtypes. *Blood*. 134 (19): 1598–1607.

Roschewski, M., Dunleavy, K., Abramson, J. et al. (2020 August 1). Multicenter study of risk-adapted therapy with dose-adjusted EPOCH-R in adults with untreated burkitt lymphoma. *J Clin Oncol* 38 (22): 2519–2529.

Schmitz, R., Young, R.M., Ceribelli, M. et al. (2012). Burkitt lymphoma pathogenesis and therapeutic targets from structural and functional genomics. *Nature* 490 (7418): 116–120.

45

Primary and Secondary CNS Lymphomas

Leon D. Kaulen[1,2], Nicholas A. Blondin[1], Fred H. Hochberg[3], and Joachim M. Baehring[1]

[1] *Yale School of Medicine, Department of Neurology, New Haven, CT*
[2] *Heidelberg University Hospital, Heidelberg University, Heidelberg, Germany*
[3] *University of California at San Diego, Department of Neurosurgery, San Diego, CA*

Introduction

Primary central nervous system lymphoma (PCNSL) is an extranodal non-Hodgkin lymphoma (NHL) confined to the brain, leptomeninges, eye(s), or spinal cord. Excluded from this WHO 2016 definition are lymphomas of the dura, intravascular large B-cell lymphomas, lymphomas with evidence of systemic disease or secondary CNS lymphomas, and all immunodeficiency-associated lymphomas. PCNSL accounts for < 1% of all non-Hodgkin lymphomas and 4% of all brain tumors with an age-adjusted incidence rate of four cases per 1,000,000 persons per year, with patients' median age of 65 years at diagnosis. Since the year 2000, there has been an increase in the overall incidence of PCNSL, especially in the older immunocompetent population.

Case Study 1

Mr. PL is a 66-year-old man who developed progressively worsening headaches and left-sided weakness over a two-week period. He fell at home and was taken to a local hospital. Neurologic examination confirmed a left hemiparesis (4/5 throughout) with normal muscle tone. Brisk tendon stretch reflexes were noted in the left arm and leg. Babinski and Hoffman sign were positive on the left suggestive of an upper motor lesion. A computed tomography (CT) scan of the head demonstrated a mass lesion isodense to gray matter in the right frontal lobe surrounded by a considerable amount of vasogenic cerebral edema (Figure 45.1). After contrast administration, the lesion was noted to enhance homogeneously. A second lesion was seen in the superior right frontal lobe, which also demonstrated homogeneous contrast enhancement. He was admitted to the hospital for further evaluation.

Cancer Consult: Expertise in Clinical Practice, Volume 2: Neoplastic Hematology & Cellular Therapy,
Second Edition. Edited by Syed A. Abutalib, Maurie Markman, James O. Armitage, and Kenneth C. Anderson.
© 2024 John Wiley & Sons Ltd. Published 2024 by John Wiley & Sons Ltd.

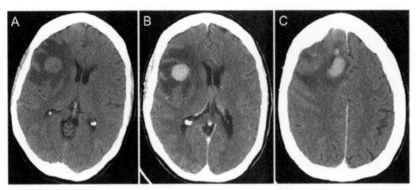

Figure 45.1 Computed tomography scan shows several right frontal mass lesions that are hyperdense prior to (A) and homogeneously enhancing after administration of contrast dye (B and C). The masses are surrounded by a hypodense area with finger-like protrusions consistent with vasogenic edema.

1) **When should central nervous system (CNS) lymphoma be suspected in the differential diagnosis of a patient with brain tumor?**
   A) Presentation with a seizure.
   B) Patient younger than 50.
   C) Presence of multifocal enhancing mass lesions.
   D) Cortical location of the lesions.

Expert Perspective: Primary CNS lymphoma (PCNSL) constitutes a rare aggressive, extranodal variant of non-Hodgkin lymphoma that is confined to the central nervous system (brain, cerebrospinal fluid, spine, leptomeninges, or eyes) at the time of diagnosis. Incidence in North America stands at 0.4/100,000 and it accounts for 2% of primary brain tumors. The median age at diagnosis is 67 with increasing incidence noted in the elderly, although it can occur at any age.

Most patients (70%) present with focal neurologic deficits resulting in prompt diagnostic evaluation. However, in 30–40% of the cases nonspecific behavioral or neuropsychiatric symptoms are found, and diagnostic workup may be delayed. Symptoms or signs of increased intracranial pressure are also common and noted in one third of patients. Seizures are less frequently noted (15%) as the cortex is often spared by PCNSL lesions. Ocular or spinal cord symptoms are only rarely found at presentation.

Common imaging findings on initial CT brain with contrast include the presence of multiple, often periventricular, homogeneously contrast-enhancing lesions with associated cerebral edema and mass effect.

Correct Answer: C

Case Study continued: Following hospital admission, CNS lymphoma was considered the most likely diagnosis, given the history and imaging findings. The differential diagnosis included other primary brain tumors, infection, and demyelinating encephalitis.

2) **What is the most appropriate diagnostic evaluation for a patient with suspected CNS lymphoma?**
   A) 18-fluorodeoxyglucose (FDG) positron-emission tomography (PET) of the brain, biopsy; if positive, body 18-FDG PET, lumbar puncture, serum lactate levels, bone marrow biopsy and aspiration.
   B) Lumbar puncture, bone marrow biopsy, CT scan of the brain, brain biopsy.
   C) MRI of the brain; empiric therapy; if unresponsive, further diagnostic workup.
   D) CT scan of the chest, abdomen, and pelvis; magnetic resonance imaging (MRI) of the brain and spinal cord in all cases; lumbar puncture; and biopsy.
   E) MRI brain; biopsy; if positive, CT scan of the chest, abdomen, and pelvis, lumbar puncture, ophthalmologic exam, serum lactate dehydrogenase, human immunodeficiency virus (HIV) testing, bone marrow biopsy, and aspiration.

Expert Perspective: The International Primary CNS Lymphoma Collaborative Group (IPCG) has published consensus guidelines for the diagnostic evaluation of patients with suspected primary CNS lymphoma. Patients should undergo a comprehensive physical exam, with particular attention to lymph nodes in all patients and testes in older men, and a comprehensive neurologic exam, including evaluation of cognitive function. A dilated fundoscopic exam should be performed to exclude ocular involvement.

Serum tests should include lactate dehydrogenase, as an elevated level has prognostic implications, as well as the determination of adequate hepatic and renal function (in anticipation of possible chemotherapy treatment), and HIV testing, as there is an increased risk of PCNSL in this population and HIV status may have an impact on choice of therapy.

Imaging should include gadolinium-enhanced MRI of the brain; a contrast-enhanced CT is only appropriate in patients with a contraindication to MRI. PCNSL in the immunocompetent host typically appears as solitary or multifocal, homogeneously enhancing lesions adjacent to the ventricular system. Infiltrative growth along the course of white matter tracts is characteristic. Lesions are iso- to hyperintense on T2-weighted imaging and often accompanied by moderate vasogenic edema further increasing mass effect. Due to their high cellularity, the tumor masses display restricted water diffusion with hyperintensity noted on diffusion-weighted imaging (DWI) and corresponding hypointensity on apparent diffusion coefficient (ADC) maps. In the immunodeficient host, PCNSL is more often multifocal, and lesions typically display peripheral contrast enhancement with water diffusion only restricted in the periphery of the lesions. A gadolinium-enhanced MRI of the spine is only required in patients demonstrating spinal symptoms, as involvement of the spinal cord parenchyma is rare. The utility of 18-fluorodeoxyglucose (FDG) positron-emission tomography (PET) of the brain for the diagnosis of PCNSL is limited. PCNSL lesions are FDG-avid, but small lesions in proximity to FDG-avid gray matter may evade detection. However, body PET-CT scan can abrogate the requirement of bone marrow biopsy (Lugano criteria).

If PCNSL is suspected on MRI, definitive diagnosis is typically established by histopathologic evaluation of a stereotactic brain biopsy specimen. Alternatively, in case of ocular involvement, pars plana vitrectomy may be considered. As a lumbar puncture, especially in HIV-infected individuals, should be performed in all cases unless prohibited by increased intracranial pressure and brain herniation, detection of lymphoma cells in the cerebrospinal fluid (CSF) may also be sufficient. CSF studies should include cell count, glucose, protein, cytopathological examination, and flow cytometry and immunoglobulin heavy-chain (IgH) and T-cell receptor (TCR) gene rearrangement analysis for clonality analysis. PCNSL-specific molecular markers in blood and CSF ("liquid biopsy") are subject to ongoing research. A rapid multiplex genotyping assay for characteristic mutations found in PCNSL was recently shown to improve and accelerate the diagnostic yield of CSF studies. The genotyping assay allowed an accurate diagnosis of hematological malignancy with a 100% specificity and 57.6% sensitivity within 80 minutes.

Complete systemic staging is required to exclude occult systemic disease. This includes a CT scan of the chest, abdomen, and pelvis; a bone marrow biopsy with aspirate; and testicular ultrasound in older men to exclude testicular lymphoma. A body 18-FDG PET scan may increase diagnostic sensitivity but is generally not required.

Correct Answer: E

Case Study continued: As CNS lymphoma was considered in the differential diagnosis, our patient underwent an MRI of the brain, which again demonstrated homogeneously enhancing mass lesions in the right frontal lobe (see Figure 45.2). There was no leptomeningeal thickening or enhancement. Restricted water diffusion of the lesion was noted on diffusion-weighted imaging further supporting the clinical suspicion of PCNSL. Stereotactic brain biopsy of the lesion was planned.

3) **Moderate vasogenic edema with mass effect was noted on initial imaging. When should steroid treatment be initiated?**
   A) Treatment with steroids should be initiated immediately.
   B) It is currently recommended to hold steroids until after biopsy.
   C) The use of steroids is contraindicated in patients with PCNSL.
   D) It is currently recommended to hold steroids until after brain imaging.
   E) Treatment with steroids should be initiated after the first cycle of chemotherapy only.

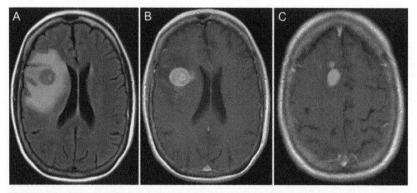

Figure 45.2 The mass lesions are hypointense on fluid attenuated inversion recovery (FLAIR) images (A) and homogeneously enhancing on T1-weighted images after administration of gadolinium (B and C). Surrounding vasogenic edema is hyperintense on FLAIR and hypointense on T1.

Expert Perspective: Corticosteroids cause rapid apoptosis of lymphocytes, disrupting the cellular morphology of the tumor and improving imaging. Steroid therapy can lead to a false-negative biopsy result, as the tissue may appear diffusely necrotic or merely inflammatory with T-cell predominance. While a recent retrospective analysis suggested that corticosteroid administration prior to biopsy does not have a major impact on diagnostic yield, it is currently recommended to hold corticosteroids in a patient with suspected PCNSL until after a biopsy is performed.

    Case Study continued: Patient presented in the clinical case underwent stereotactic brain biopsy as planned, which confirmed a diagnosis of CNS lymphoma (Figure 45.3). Steroid treatment was commenced immediately following surgery. Pathologic findings included infiltration of numerous large CD20-positive and mitotically active lymphoid cells with prominent nucleoli, intermixed with abundant CD3+ T cells consistent with diffuse large B-cell lymphoma (DLBCL). Epstein-Barr virus (EBV), a known driver of lymphomagenesis in immunocompromised patients with PCNSL, was not detected in the specimen. The Hans algorithm using immunohistochemical stainings for CD10, BCL6, and MUM1 is used for subtyping in three molecular groups: Germinal center B-cell like (GCB), nongerminal center (NGC)/activated B-cell like (NGC/ABC), and NGC/type 3 (NGC/type 3).

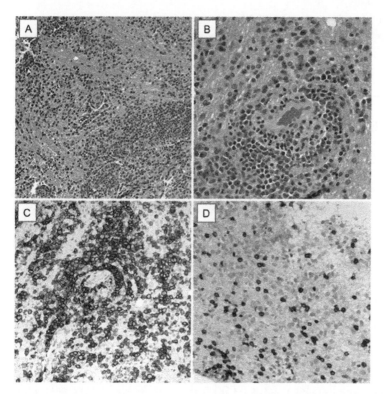

Figure 45.3 (A) Hematoxylin and eosin stain shows a mononuclear cerebral parenchymal cell infiltrate. (B) At higher-power magnification, the angiocentric arrangement of tumor cells is highlighted. (C) Immunohistochemistry using an anti-CD20 antibody identifies the large, atypical cells within the infiltrate as B cells. (D) A CD3-stain shows a reactive T-cellular infiltrate.

The majority of PCNSL (85%) is classified as NGC/ABC correlating with inferior overall survival compared to systemic DLBCL. Mr. PL's tumor was classified as NGC/ABC subtype. To exclude systemic dissemination a CT scan of chest, abdomen, and pelvis as well as a bone marrow biopsy were performed, which were both unremarkable. Testicular ultrasound demonstrated no abnormalities. Lumbar puncture was deferred, given the mass effect visualized on the MRI of the brain. Dilated fundoscopic exam failed to reveal retinal lesions or vitreal cells. Serologic testing for HIV was negative. Lactate dehydrogenase (LDH) was elevated at 264 U/L. Liver function tests were within normal limits, and creatinine was 1.1 mg/dL. A 24-h urine collection was performed, and creatinine clearance was found to be 102 mL/min (24-h urine assessment not always required).

Correct Answer: B

4) **Which of the following are prognostic factors included in commonly used prognostic scoring systems?**
   A) Age, performance status, LDH serum levels, high CSF protein, involvement of deep brain regions.
   B) Performance status, creatinine serum levels, number of lesions, involvement of cortical brain regions.
   C) Age, body weight, CSF cell count, CSF lactate levels, serum lactate levels.
   D) Performance status, ki67 proliferation index, degree of necrosis on pathological evaluation, degree of blood vessel infiltration on pathological evaluation.
   E) *MGMT* promoter methylation status, *IDH* mutation status, 1p/19q co-deletion status.

Expert Perspective: Both the IPCG and MSKCC prognostic scoring systems for PCNSL are simple, statistically powerful, and universally applicable. The introduction of molecular markers (e.g. the molecular classification according to the Hans algorithm) into the prognostic scoring system is still pending and may further improve risk stratification.

The IPCG scoring system includes five variables: age > 60 years, Eastern Co-operative of Oncology Group (ECOG) performance status > 1, elevated LDH levels in the serum, high CSF protein concentration, and deep brain involvement on MRI. Unfavorable variables are assigned a value of 1 whereas favorable variables are assigned a value of 0. Values are then added up to calculate the final prognostic score. The two-year overall survival (OS) ratio of patients with a score of 0–1, 2–3, 4–5 was 85%, 57%, and 24%, respectively.

In contrast the MSKCC prognostic scoring system only includes two variables: age ⩾ 50 years and Karnofsky performance status (KPS) < 70 (more convenient model!). Patients are stratified into three risk groups (I: age ⩽ 50 years; II: age ⩾ 50 years + KPS > 70; III: age ⩾ 50 years, KPS < 70). Median OS for class I, II, and III patients was 5.2 years, 2.1 years, and 0.8 years, respectively.

Correct Answer: A

Case Study continued: Performance status (ECOG 0 /KPS 100%) and absent deep brain involvement on MRI were favorable variables in Mr. PL's case according to both scoring systems. Age of 66 years at diagnosis and elevated LDH serum levels were considered unfavorable markers. With absent CSF data his IPCG score was 2, and he fulfilled MSKCC class II criteria.

5) **Large-scale sequencing studies have recently led to an improved understanding of the genetic landscape of PCNSL. Which of the following are common genetic findings?**
   A) Aberrant somatic hypermutation (aSHM).
   B) *MYD88* hotspot (L265P) mutations.
   C) *CDKN2A* loss.
   D) Amplification of 9p24.1 including immune checkpoint genes PD-L1/PD-L2.
   E) All the above.

Expert Perspective: Recent large-scale genomic sequencing studies have improved the pathogenetic understanding of PCNSL. Common genetic mutations are found in the B-cell receptor (BCR), and toll-like receptor (TLR) signaling pathways resulting in NF-kB pathway activation. *MYD88 L265P* hotspot mutations, detected in up to 76% of samples, were shown to lead to TLR activation. CD79b Y196 hotspot mutations, identified in up to 83% of specimens, as well as CARD11 variants, found in around 20% of cases, activate the BCR pathway. Inactivating mutations or deletion of *TNFAIP3*, a negative regulator of NF-kB, further drive NF-kB pathway activation. Of note, MYD88 and CD79b variants are enriched in immune-privileged lymphoma sites such as the testes and the brain and particularly found in ABC subtype PCNSL. One-third of variants detected in PCNSL are typically a result of aberrant somatic hypermutation (aSHM). Mutations are found in *WRCY* or *RGWY* motifs with known target genes including *PIM1* and *BTG2* among others. aSHM likely results in an overall increase of the mutational load. Common copy number variations include biallelic loss of the tumor suppressor *CDKN2A* on chromosome 9p21 in 60% of cases, which otherwise blocks transition from G1 to S-phase. Amplifications include 9p24 including the PD-L1/PD-L2 immune checkpoint gene locus in 30–50% of patients. Improved understanding of the genetic landscape of PCNSL has opened novel, personalized therapeutic avenues currently subject to clinical investigation. Activation of BCR signaling can be targeted by upstream inhibition of Bruton tyrosine kinase (e.g. ibrutinib) or downstream inhibition of IRF4 using immunomodulatory drugs (e.g. thalidomide or lenalidomide). Amplification of PD-L1 and PD-L2 may serve as a rationale for immune checkpoint inhibition (e.g. nivolumab or pembrolizumab) whereas loss of *CDKN2A* may render lymphomas susceptible to cyclin-dependant kinase inhibitors (e.g. abemaciclib).

Correct Answer: E

Case Study continued: Our patient's tumor was analyzed by whole exome sequencing and revealed a genetic landscape typical for PCNSL including *MYD88* and *CD79b* hotspot mutations, signs of aSHM including multiple PIM1 variants within the RGYW motif, and biallelic loss of *CDKN2A*.

6) **What is the current standard of care for initial treatment of primary CNS lymphoma?**
   A) High-dose (> 3.5 g/m^2) methotrexate (MTX)-based polychemotherapy.
   B) Rituximab, cyclophosphamide, doxorubicin, vincristine, and prednisone (R-CHOP) polychemotherapy.
   C) Whole-brain radiation therapy (WBRT) alone.
   D) Surgical resection of the lesions.
   E) Intrathecal rituximab chemotherapy.

Expert Perspective: The current standard of care for initial treatment of PCNSL consists of systemic high-dose methotrexate-based polychemotherapy. Based on available clinical trials HD-MTX is combined with rituximab, a monoclonal antibody targeting the B-cell surface antigen CD20, and an alkylating agent. Polychemotherapy regimens currently in use include MATRix (HD-MTX, cytarabine, thiotepa, and rituximab), R-MT (rituximab, HD-MTX, and temozolomide), R-MVP (rituximab, HD-MTX, vincristine, procarbazine), and R-MBTP (rituximab, HD-MTX, BCNU, teniposide, prednisone). Results from phase II trials suggest similar overall response rates and two-year progression-free survival of these regimens. Selection of HD-MTX-based polychemotherapy regimen mostly depends on availability of chemotherapy agents and geographical region.

Rituximab in PCNSL: The addition of rituximab to MTX-based polychemotherapy was supported by the recent IELSG32/MATRix trial, which compared three treatment arms (I: HD-MTX + cytarabine; II: HD-MTX + cytarabine + rituximab; III: HD-MTX + cytarabine + rituximab + thiotepa). The addition of rituximab and thiotepa (arm III = MATRix regimen) resulted in an improved complete remission rate (CRR) of 49% compared to 30% (arm II without thiotepa) and 23% (arm I without thiotepa and rituximab). Two-year OS was superior for patients who received the MATRix regimen (69% vs arm II: 56% vs arm I: 42%). Treatment-related hematological toxicity was most prevalent in the MATRix arm while treatment-related mortality was low across all three arms. It is important to note that the IELSG32/MATRix trial was, however, not powered for comparison of the three treatment arms and outcome of the conventional treatment arm (HD-MTX + cytarabine) was inferior to previous cohorts receiving the same regimen.

The benefit of adding rituximab to MTX-based polychemotherapy was recently challenged by the HOVON105 phase III trial, which compared MBTP versus R-MBTP. Event-free survival at one year was not statistically different in both treatment arms (49% without RTX vs 52% with rituximab). A trend toward improved event-free survival was observed for younger patients receiving rituximab. The short follow-up, however, limits conclusions from this study, and rituximab has remained an integral part of PCNSL chemotherapy regimens at most centers so far.

WBRT in PCNSL: Whole-brain radiation therapy (WBRT) with 45 Gray (Gy) alone was the treatment of choice in the pre-HD-MTX era. PCNSL responds well to radiation therapy with a 90% overall response rate. However, median OS is poor (12–18 months) resulting from early relapse. Currently WBRT, therefore, mostly plays a role as palliative treatment for patients with chemoresistant disease or individuals who cannot tolerate chemotherapy. Low-dose WBRT may have a role as consolidation therapy after remission induction with chemotherapy.

Surgical resection in PCNSL: Aggressive surgical resections of PCNSL lesions have not proven beneficial in most clinical studies likely because of the diffusely infiltrative growth pattern of lymphoma cells in the CNS. This notion was recently challenged by a subset analysis of the G-PCNSL-SG1 trial, which suggested improved outcome for patients following subtotal or gross total resection. This benefit was, however, lost following adjustment for additional variables that might have influenced OS. To date, no sufficient evidence, therefore, exists to support extensive surgical resection of PCNSL lesions, and surgical approaches additionally carry the risk of surgery-related neurological deficits.

Intrathecal chemotherapy in PCNSL: Currently available data do not support widespread use of intrathecal chemotherapy in PCNSL. Intrathecal or intraventricular chemotherapy may help to bypass the blood-brain barrier and allow higher CNS drug doses with smaller systemic exposures and fewer systemic adverse effects. Various chemotherapy agents have safely been administered intrathecally including MTX, rituximab, cytarabine, and thiotepa. However, increased toxicity within the CNS and complications related to the mode of application (e.g. infectious ventriculitis and chemical) have limited the use of intrathecal chemotherapy. Systemically administered methotrexate provides for a more favorable pharmacokinetic profile (lower peak concentrations, longer duration of lymphotoxic MTX concentrations in CSF) than intrathecal injection. Multiple retrospective analyses including cases with CSF dissemination of PCNSL have failed to demonstrate a measurable benefit from the addition of intrathecal chemotherapy to conventional MTX-based systemic chemotherapy regimens. At this point, the use of intrathecal chemotherapy in PCNSL is mostly limited to individuals with clinical, neuroimaging, or CSF evidence of meningeal disease dissemination as an adjunct to systemic therapy. Intrathecal rituximab is reserved for patients with refractory meningeal disease along with systemic therapy for PCNSL.

Correct Answer: A

Case study continued: Various treatment options were discussed with our patient. He asked whether there are specific treatment recommendations for patients in his age group.

7) Are there special considerations for treatment in elderly patients with PCNSL?
   A) WBRT should be used as first-line therapy in elderly patients.
   B) High-dose methotrexate can be safely used in the elderly, with dose adjustment for creatinine clearance.
   C) High-dose methotrexate is not an option in elderly patients.
   D) Temozolomide should be used as first-line treatment in elderly patients.
   E) Rituximab is contraindicated in elderly patients.

Expert Perspective: The feasibility of HD-MTX therapy in elderly patients has been demonstrated in numerous studies, although patient exclusion based on comorbidities or chronic renal failure is more common than in younger individuals. High-dose MTX-based therapy is associated with a lower response rate, shorter progression-free survival, and higher mortality in the elderly population compared with younger adults. However, whenever feasible, HD-MTX therapy should be given priority in all individuals with PCNSL.

In the PRIMAIN study only immunocompetent patients older than 65 years at diagnosis were included. R-MP (rituximab, MTX at 3 g/m^2, procarbazine) followed by procarbazine maintenance therapy was feasible and effective in an older PCNSL population, with CR achieved in 31.6% of cases. Two-year progression-free survival and OS rates were 37.3% and 47.7%, respectively. In the NORDIC trial a similar patient cohort was treated with R-MT (rituximab, MTX at 3 g/m^2, and temozolomide) followed by temozolomide maintenance therapy. CR was achieved in 57.7% of patients with an even higher progression-free survival (44.4%) and OS (55.6%) at two years. Another recent phase II clinical trial in the elderly population (ANOCEF-GOELAMS) compared the safety and efficacy of two chemotherapy regimens (MTX and temozolomide vs HD-MTX, procarbazine, vincristine, and cytarabine). The complete response rate (53% vs 38%) and two-year OS rates (58% vs 39%) were superior in patients treated with the latter, more aggressive chemotherapy regimen while treatment-related toxicity was moderate and similar in both treatment arms. While phase III clinical trials powered to compare various polychemotherapy regimens are pending in the elderly population, aggressive MTX-based regimens appear feasible in this cohort with moderate albeit increased toxicity rates. As in younger PCNSL patients, HD-MTX-based treatment selection in the elderly population with acceptable renal function mostly depends on availability of chemotherapy agents and geographical region. Reasonable alternatives are available for individuals with MTX contraindications. A study of elderly patients evaluating temozolomide alone as up-front therapy in the elderly, for example, found a complete response rate of 47% and median OS of 21 months.

Particularly in older PCNSL patients, WBRT with 45 Gy is associated with neurotoxicity (psychomotor slowing, memory, or neurocognitive deficits, etc.). Lower-dose WBRT with 23.4 Gy may be useful as consolidation therapy in the selected elderly patients with acceptable toxicity. To date, like in younger PCNSL cohorts, WBRT is mainly used in the palliative or chemo-refractory relapse setting in elderly patients.

Correct Answer: B

Case Study continued: He learns that his age represents no contraindication for aggressive polychemotherapy, and his normal renal function will allow administration of MTX. He asks whether there are any novel approaches to PCNSL therapy.

8) **What is the role of CAR T Cell therapy or targeted therapy (besides anti-CD20 agents) in the management of primary CNS lymphoma?**
   A) CAR T cell therapy should be considered only in immunodeficient patients.
   B) Ibrutinib constitutes a standard first-line therapy in ABC subtype PCNSL.
   C) Immune checkpoint inhibition is considered a standard first-line therapy.
   D) CAR T cell therapy is preferred over HD-MTX-based polychemotherapy regimen.
   E) CAR T cell therapy has shown promising activity in patients with relapsed and refractory PCNSL.

Expert Perspective: Both targeted and CAR T cell therapy for PCNSL are currently under investigation in numerous clinical trials. Some initial phase I/II trials were encouraging, and both treatments may constitute alternatives to conventional HD-MTX-based polychemotherapy. Comparison with conventional polychemotherapy is, however, pending, and both targeted and CAR T cell therapy are, therefore, currently only offered in the setting of clinical trials.

Genetic characterization of PCNSL paved the way for various targeted therapies. Ibrutinib, a BTK inhibitor, has been studied in phase I trials as monotherapy or in combination with MTX and rituximab or alkylating agents in recurrent or refractory PCNSL. It may prove particularly effective in patients with ABC subtype PCNSL, where activating mutations in the BCR and TLR pathways such as *MYD88 L265P* are enriched. Monotherapy achieved clinical responses in 10 of 13 patients in a phase I trial. CARD11 and CD79b variants were suspected to confer complete or partial resistance to BTK inhibition in PCNSL, which may explain why responses were often short-lived and combination regimens may hence be required. Since PD-L1 and PD-L2 are frequently amplified in PCNSL, immune checkpoint inhibition with nivolumab or pembrolizumab has emerged as a novel therapeutic avenue. In a small series of four recurrent PCNSL treated with nivolumab monotherapy, encouraging progression-free survival ranging between 14 and 17 months was achieved. Larger studies are currently under way to explore the role of immune checkpoint inhibition alone or in combination with other agents. Immunomodulatory drugs such as lenalidomide leading to downregulation of IRF4 and subsequent inhibition of the NF-kB pathway among other mechanisms was also previously shown as safe and effective in recurrent PCNSL. In combination with rituximab a complete response rate of 32% was accomplished with a median progression-free survival of 7.8 months. Other targeted therapy approaches under investigation include PI3K/mTOR signaling pathway inhibition (e.g. PQR309 and copanlisib).

CAR T cell therapy represents another potential novel approach to treat PCNSL. Initial clinical studies demonstrated safety and efficacy in systemic NHL. However, PCNSL patients were initially excluded from these studies out of concern for neurotoxicity and impaired T-cell expansion when disease is confined to the CNS. A recent retrospective study of eight patients with secondary CNS lymphoma treated with off-label CAR T cells reported responses in half of the patients with minimal neurotoxicity and confirmation of successful expansion of T cells. In a large meta-analysis of CNS lymphomas, toxicity of anti-CD19-CAR T-cell therapy was similar to that of registrational studies in systemic LBCL with no increased signal of neurotoxicity observed. Encouraging efficacy was demonstrated in patients with CNS lymphoma with no discernible differences between PCNSL and SCNSL. Study results evaluating CAR T cell therapy for PCNSL are eagerly awaited.

Correct Answer: B

Case Study continued: Mr. PL is informed that targeted (besides anti-CD20 agents) and CAR T cell therapy are currently evaluated in clinical trials. As the role of both treatments for PCNSL needs to be defined and more importantly compared to conventional MTX-based polychemotherapy, targeted and CAR T cell therapy are currently offered in the clinical trial setting only. Based on the favorable data available including the elderly cohort, Mr. PL agrees to pursue HD-MTX-based polychemotherapy.

9) What monitoring is suggested during treatment for primary CNS lymphoma?
   A) MRI every 4–8 weeks during remission induction, every 8–12 weeks during consolidation, and every 3–6 months during post chemotherapy; ophthalmologic examination at least once a year; lumbar puncture needs to be repeated at least once during therapy in patients with meningeal dissemination to document CR in CSF.
   B) MRI, ophthalmologic evaluation, and lumbar puncture every three months.
   C) MRI and lumbar puncture once monthly during induction and consolidation therapy, ophthalmologic exam only when symptoms are present.
   D) MRI and lumbar puncture only in the case of neurologic deterioration, ophthalmologic exam only when symptoms are present.
   E) CT scan every two months; MRI, lumbar puncture, and ophthalmologic exam if relapse is suspected.

Expert Perspective: A gadolinium-enhanced MRI should be obtained every 4–8 weeks during remission induction, every 8–12 weeks during consolidation, and every 3–6 months during post chemotherapy. Ophthalmologic slit lamp examination ought to be performed at least once a year even if patients are asymptomatic and ocular involvement was absent at initial diagnosis. A lumbar puncture needs to be repeated at least once during therapy in patients with meningeal dissemination to document CR in CSF. In addition, patients treated with HD-MTX have their creatinine clearance calculated or measured before each cycle, which is used to adjust the MTX dose. HD-MTX (> 3.5 g/m^2) should not be used if the creatinine clearance is less than 60 mL/min.

Correct Answer: A

Case Study continued: Our patient was started on HD-MTX-based polychemotherapy. After two cycles of high-dose MTX, he reported the new onset of headaches that felt like a constant, dull ache in the forehead. A lumbar puncture was performed to evaluate for CNS dissemination of lymphoma. CSF analysis revealed one red blood cell, 0 nucleated cells, CSF glucose 65 mg/dL, and CSF total protein 32 mg/dL. Neither cytomorphological examination nor flow cytometry nor IgH– and TCR gene rearrangement analyses were indicative of leptomeningeal diseases. The headaches subsequently improved with conservative management. Follow-up MRI scans revealed complete radiologic remission. You discuss how to proceed for consolidation therapy.

10) **What is the standard of care for consolidation therapy of primary CNS lymphoma?**
    A) Chemoimmunotherapy.
    B) High-dose myeloablative chemotherapy followed by autologous stem cell transplantation (HDT-ASCT).
    C) WBRT possibly at lower doses (23.4 Gy) to reduce neurotoxicity with chemoimmunotherapy.
    D) No general standard of care has been established; an individualized selection of any of the options above is typically made.

Expert Perspective: Historically, WBRT was the consolidation therapy of choice in PCNSL. However, particularly in older patients, late neurotoxicity emerged as a relevant side effect of adjuvant radiation therapy following the introduction of HD-MTX-based polychemotherapy. This led to a phase III study (G-PCNSL-SG-1) evaluating omission of WBRT from consolidation strategies in PCNSL. WBRT with 45 Gy was compared to observation only after CR or to cytarabine in the case of partial remission following HD-MTX-based induction therapy. Although the non-inferiority margin was not met, OS was similar (32.4 months) with and without WBRT (37.1 Gy) whereas neurotoxicity was more frequently noted in the WBRT treatment group (49% vs 26%). Long-term neurotoxicity and outcome following lower WBRT consolidation doses (23.4 Gy) are currently being investigated in clinical trials. In a single-arm phase II study, it offered improved disease control with only mild executive and attention dysfunction at three-year follow-up. Additional randomized trials will determine whether lower-dose WBRT represents an applicable alternative especially for younger patients who do not qualify for other more aggressive consolidation treatments.

Neurotoxicity following WBRT led to the exploration of alternative consolidation strategies for PCNSL.

Auto-HCT: High-dose myeloablative chemotherapy followed by autologous stem cell transplantation (HDT-ASCT) offers long-term disease control with lower rates of treatment-related neurotoxicity. It should be considered particularly in young patients with good performance status and without severe comorbidities rendering them unable to tolerate myeloablative chemotherapy. HDT-ASCT was recently compared with WBRT in two randomized phase II trials (IELSG32/MATRix and PRECIS), both of which were not powered for comparison.

- In the IELSG32/MATRix study, after MATRix induction polychemotherapy, patients were assigned to receive either 36 Gy WBRT or HDT-ASCT following thiotepa and carmustine conditioning. Two-year progression-free survival was not statistically different (WBRT: 80%; HDT-ASCT: 69%).
- In the PRECIS study following R-MBVP polychemotherapy patients were treated either with 40 Gy WBRT or HDT-ASCT after thiotepa, busulfan, and cyclophosphamide conditioning. Two-year progression-free survival in this trial appeared slightly improved following HDT-ASCT (87% vs 63%). Overall, both consolidation strategies were considered feasible and effective. Neurotoxicity was more common in patients treated with WBRT while fewer hematological side events were noticed.
- The Alliance for Clinical Trials in Oncology has fully accrued a randomized phase II trial of ASCT versus non-myeloablative consolidation chemotherapy (113 patients). Results are awaited. (As of press time, data has been published in abstract form at https://ascopubs.org/doi/abs/10.1200/JCO.2021.39.15_suppl.7506.)

Selecting the best consolidation therapy in elderly PCNSL patients is especially challenging as they carry a higher risk for neurotoxicity following WBRT and may be unable to tolerate myeloablative chemotherapy. Chemotherapy with alkylating agents may offer a reasonable alternative for consolidation therapy. In the above-mentioned PRIMAIN and NORDIC studies procarbazine and temozolomide were successfully used, respectively, and yielded favorable long-term outcome. Elderly patients with CR after induction therapy or those unable to tolerate additional treatment may also be simply followed up clinically and radiologically or may be started on maintenance therapy especially on a clinical trial.

Overall, no general standard of care has been established for consolidation therapy of PCNSL. Treatment modalities are selected mainly based on age, response to induction therapy, comorbidities, performance status, and institutional and patient preference.

Correct Answer: D

Case Study continued: Given our patient's age and comorbidities, alkylating chemotherapy with temozolomide was considered his best option for consolidation, or more properly stated as "maintenance" strategy. Due to comorbidities, he was considered unable to tolerate HDT-ASCT, and given his age, his risk for late neurotoxicity following WBRT was considered unacceptably high. One year after completion of therapy, he complains of floaters in the left eye. Dilated eye examination reveals abnormal cells in vitreous. A pars plana vitrectomy confirms ocular lymphoma, and IgH gene rearrangement analysis confirms the clonal relationship between the cerebral parenchymal and the ocular tumor.

11) What is the relationship between primary CNS lymphoma and vitreous lymphoma?
   A) Ocular lymphoma complicates more than 50% of cases of primary CNS lymphoma.
   B) There is no clear correlation between primary CNS lymphoma and ocular lymphoma.

C) Ocular lymphoma complicates 20–30% of cases of primary CNS lymphoma.
D) Ocular lymphoma complicates less than 5% of cases of primary CNS lymphoma.
E) Ocular lymphoma complicates nearly all cases of primary CNS lymphoma.

Expert Perspective: Concurrent ocular lymphoma may be present in as many as 30% of PCNSL. Common symptoms are reduced visual acuity, and visual illusions (floaters). In as many as 50% of cases, ocular dissemination is entirely asymptomatic at diagnosis. Primary intraocular lymphoma is exceedingly rare. Of note, 80% of these cases suffer CNS dissemination. Treatment options include orbital radiation, intraocular chemotherapy (MTX and rituximab), or systemic chemotherapy. While dedicated ocular therapy can improve disease control, it has not been found to affect progression-free survival or OS. Localized therapy is often used in patients without concurrent active CNS disease and in those in whom systemic therapy fails to clear the ocular disease component. When both eyes are affected, orbital radiation is commonly used. However, clear consensus guidelines based on prospective randomized studies are unavailable.

Correct Answer: C

Case Study continued: An MRI of the brain is performed after Mr. PL's vitrectomy. A new small enhancing lesion is seen, again in the right frontal lobe, representing relapsed disease. Treatment options for recurrent PCNSL are discussed with PL.

12) What options exist for salvage chemotherapy in primary CNS lymphoma?
   A) High-dose methotrexate rechallenge.
   B) Temozolomide or rituximab, either alone or in combination.
   C) Autologous transplant if not performed as first-line consolidation.
   D) WBRT if not part of first-line therapy.
   E) Clinical trial.
   F) All of the above may be considered.

Expert Perspective: There is a substantial number of patients with PCNSL relapse. Recurrence typically occurs within the CNS and within the first two years after initial diagnosis. Prognosis is poor with a median OS of two months for untreated patients.

A standard of care for disease recurrence has not been established. Often, relapsed disease remains sensitive to high-dose methotrexate-based regimens, which, therefore, is currently chosen in most cases. Retrospective series suggest 85–91% overall response rate and a 12–62 month median OS following HD-MTX rechallenge provided there is decent interval between previous therapy (> 6 months). It may be particularly effective in patients who previously responded to HD-MTX chemotherapy and who experience disease remission after a longer time interval. If HD-MTX is not feasible, treatment with alkylating agents such as temozolomide or rituximab may be considered alone or in combination. WBRT represents an alternative option in patients who did not undergo radiation therapy as part of their first-line treatment. It was associated with overall response rate of 74–79% and median OS of 10–16 months in retrospective case series. As discussed above, lower-dose WBRT may yield improved long-term neurocognitive outcome with several clinical trials pending.

Correct Answer: F

Case Study continued: Our patient is retreated with high-dose MTX and again achieves a complete response. Due to his age, he was again not considered a good candidate for HDT-ASCT or WBRT consolidation therapy. It was decided to follow him expectantly after successful completion of HD-MTX rechallenge given he was not deemed suitable candidate for further intensive therapy. He has been in remission for 15 months.

13) **What is the prognosis for a patient with newly diagnosed CNS lymphoma?**
   A) Less than one-year median survival.
   B) Less than three-year median survival.
   C) Less than one year based on population statistics; 3–6 years based on referral center cohorts.
   D) More than 10-year median survival.
   E) Less than three years based on population statistics; 5–10 years based on the referral center.

Expert Perspective: The prognosis of patients with newly diagnosed PCNSL has markedly improved over the past two decades. For patients treated with HD-MTX-based regimens in prospective studies at tertiary care referral centers, the median survival is up to 60 months. However, population-based statistics continue to draw a less favorable picture with median OS of less than one year. The 10-year survival rate is 21%. Patients between 45 and 64 years of age constitute the age group with the most favorable prognosis (median OS approximately two years, and 10-year survival 27–28%). Prognostic factors that influence OS and are included in the most widely used prognostic scoring systems are discussed in Question 4.

Correct Answer: C

Recommended Readings

Barajas, R.F., Politi, L.S., Anzalone, N. et al. (2021). Consensus recommendations for MRI and PET imaging of primary central nervous system lymphoma: guideline statement from the International Primary CNS Lymphoma Collaborative Group (IPCG). *Neuro Oncol* 23 (7): 1056–1071.

Bromberg, J.E.C., Issa, S., Bakunina, K. et al. (2019). Rituximab in patients with primary CNS lymphoma (HOVON 105/ALLG NHL 24): A randomised, open-label, phase 3 intergroup study. *Lancet Oncol* 20 (2): 216–228.

Cook, M.R., Dorris, C.S., Makambi, K.H., et al. (2023 January 10). Toxic ity and efficacy of CAR T cell therapy in primary and secondary CNS lymphoma: a meta analysis of 128 patients. *Blood Adv* 7 (1): 32 39. doi: 10.1182/bloodadvances.2022008525. PMID: 36260735; PMCID: PMC9813524.

Ferreri, A.J.M., Cwynarski, K., Pulczynski, E. et al. (2022 July). IELSG32 study investigators. Long-term efficacy, safety and neurotolerability of MATRix regimen followed by autologous transplant in primary CNS lymphoma: 7-year results of the IELSG32 randomized trial. *Leukemia* 36 (7): 1870–1878. doi: 10.1038/s41375-022-01582-5. Epub 2022 May 13. PMID: 35562406.

Frigault, M.J., Dietrich, J., Gallagher, K., et al. (2022 April 14). Safety and efficacy of tisagenlecleucel in primary CNS lymphoma: a phase 1/2 clinical trial. Blood 139 (15): 2306 2315. doi: 10.1182/blood.2021014738. PMID: 35167655; PMCID: P MC9012129.

Ferreri, A.J., Cwynarski, K., Pulczynski, E. et al. (2016). Chemoimmunotherapy with methotrexate, cytarabine, thiotepa, and rituximab (MATRix regimen) in patients with primary CNS lymphoma: results of the first randomisation of the International Extranodal Lymphoma Study Group-32 (IELSG32) phase 2 trial. *Lancet Haematol* 3 (5): e217–27.

Fritsch, K., Kasenda, B., Schorb, E. et al. (2017). High-dose methotrexate-based immuno-chemotherapy for elderly primary CNS lymphoma patients (PRIMAIN study). *Leukemia* 31 (4): 846–852.

Fukumura, K., Kawazu, M., Kojima, S. et al. (2016). Genomic characterization of primary central nervous system lymphoma. *Acta Neuropathol* 131 (6): 865–875.

Grommes, C., Nayak, L., Tun, H.W., and Batchelor, T.T. (2019a). Introduction of novel agents in the treatment of primary CNS lymphoma. *Neuro Oncol* 21 (3): 306–313.

Grommes, C., Pastore, A., Palaskas, N. et al. (2017). Ibrutinib unmasks critical role of bruton tyrosine kinase in primary CNS lymphoma. *Cancer Discov* 7 (9): 1018–1029.

Grommes, C., Rubenstein, J.L., DeAngelis, L.M., Ferreri, A.J.M., and Batchelor, T.T. (2019b). Comprehensive approach to diagnosis and treatment of newly diagnosed primary CNS lymphoma. *Neuro Oncol* 21 (3): 296–305.

Houillier, C., Taillandier, L., Dureau, S. et al. (2019). Radiotherapy or autologous stem-cell transplantation for primary CNS lymphoma in patients 60 years of age and younger: results of the intergroup ANOCEF-GOELAMS randomized phase II PRECIS study. *J Clin Oncol* 37 (10): 823–833.

Karschnia, P., Blobner, J., Teske, N. et al. (2021). CAR T-cells for CNS lymphoma: driving into new terrain? *Cancers (Basel)* 13 (10).

Mo, S.S., Cleveland, J., and Rubenstein, J.L. (2023 January). Primary CNS lymphoma: update on molecular pathogenesis and therapy. Leuk Lymphoma 64 (1): 57–65. doi: 10.1080/10428194. 2022.2133541. Epub 2022 Oct 26. PMID: 36286546.

Kaulen, L.D., Erson-Omay, E.Z., Henegariu, O. et al. (2021). Exome sequencing identifies SLIT2 variants in primary CNS lymphoma. *Br J Haematol* 193 (2): 375–379.

Nayak, L., Iwamoto, F.M., LaCasce, A. et al. (2017). PD-1 blockade with nivolumab in relapsed/refractory primary central nervous system and testicular lymphoma. *Blood* 129 (23): 3071–3073.

Omuro, A., Chinot, O., Taillandier, L. et al. (2015). Methotrexate and temozolomide versus methotrexate, procarbazine, vincristine, and cytarabine for primary CNS lymphoma in an elderly population: an intergroup ANOCEF-GOELAMS randomised phase 2 trial. *Lancet Haematol* 2 (6): e251–e259.

Thiel, E., Korfel, A., Martus, P. et al. (2010). High-dose methotrexate with or without whole brain radiotherapy for primary CNS lymphoma (G-PCNSL-SG-1): A phase 3, randomised, non-inferiority trial. *Lancet Oncol* 11 (11): 1036–1047.

46

HIV-Associated Lymphoma

Elif Yilmaz and Kieron Dunleavy

Lombardi Comprehensive Cancer Center, Georgetown University, Washington, DC

Introduction

The pathogenesis of HIV-associated lymphoma is complex and involves the interplay of several biological factors, such as chronic antigen stimulation, co-infecting oncogenic viruses such as Epstein-Barr virus (EBV) and human herpesvirus-8 (HHV8), genetic abnormalities, and cytokine deregulation. Most HIV-associated lymphomas are of B-cell lineage and demonstrate clonal rearrangement of immunoglobulin genes. T-cell lymphomas are uncommonly observed in the setting of HIV infection.

Chronic antigen stimulation, which is associated with HIV infection, can lead to polyclonal B-cell expansion, and this may then promote and result in the emergence of monoclonal B cells. EBV is the most frequently found oncogenic virus in HIV-associated lymphomas and is observed in approximately 40% of cases. All cases of primary central nervous system lymphoma (PCNSL) and most cases of classic Hodgkin lymphoma (cHL) harbor EBV, as do the majority of diffuse large B-cell lymphoma (DLBCL) cases with immunoblastic features. Primary effusion lymphoma (PEL) cases also harbor EBV in addition to HHV8. In contrast, EBV is only variably present in Burkitt lymphoma (BL) (30–40%) and plasmablastic lymphoma (50%), and it is typically absent in centroblastic lymphomas. EBV-positive HIV-associated lymphomas frequently express the EBV-encoding transforming antigen latent membrane protein-1 (LMP1), which activates cellular proliferation through the activation of the nuclear factor kappa B (NF-κB) pathway and may induce B-cell lymphoma-2 (BCL2) overexpression, promoting B-cell survival and lymphomagenesis (see Chapters 37, 39, 43, and 47).

Following the arrival of antiretroviral therapy (ART) and the development of novel therapeutic strategies, most patients with HIV-associated lymphomas are now cured of their disease, in contrast to the pre-ART era. The availability of ART has resulted in a so-called pathobiological shift away from tumors with adverse biological features toward those that are biologically more favorable (Figure 46.1). Most patients with DLBCL and BL have an excellent outcome, with recent studies supporting the role of rituximab in these diseases. The curability of many patients with HIV-associated lymphoma is now like that of their HIV-negative counterparts. New treatment frontiers need to focus on improving the outcome for patients with advanced immune suppression and for those with adverse tumor biology such as the activated B-cell (ABC) type of DLBCL and the virally driven lymphomas.

Cancer Consult: Expertise in Clinical Practice, Volume 2: Neoplastic Hematology & Cellular Therapy,
Second Edition. Edited by Syed A. Abutalib, Maurie Markman, James O. Armitage, and Kenneth C. Anderson.
© 2024 John Wiley & Sons Ltd. Published 2024 by John Wiley & Sons Ltd.

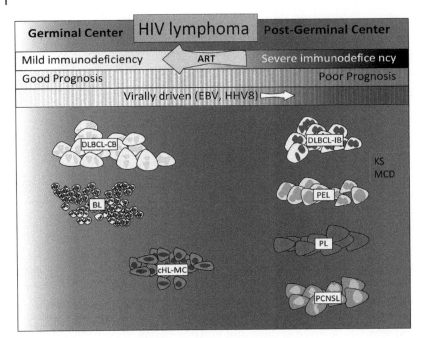

Figure 46.1 Lymphomas that are common in the setting of HIV infection and their relationship to degree of immunosuppression and antiretroviral treatment. Since the advent of antiretroviral therapy, there has been a so-called pathobiologic shift away from lymphomas with more adverse biological factors toward lymphomas with more favorable biology that have a better outcome with therapy. DLBCL–CB = diffuse large B-cell lymphoma, centroblastic type; BL = Burkitt lymphoma; cHL–MC = classical Hodgkin lymphoma–mixed cellularity subtype; DLBCL–IB = diffuse large B-cell lymphoma, immunoblastic type; PEL = primary effusion lymphoma; PL = plasmablastic lymphoma; PCNSL = primary central nervous system lymphoma.

Case study 1

A 35-year-old man with no significant past medical history presents with abdominal pain for three weeks. He also reports night sweats and a 10 lb weight loss over the last six months. Initial laboratory studies including CBC and chemistry were normal except for WBC count of 3,100/μL (with normal differential) and hemoglobin concentration of 10.4 g/dL. Lactate dehydrogenase concentration is high at 986 U/L. CT scan shows a 9.6 cm retroperitoneal mass, moderate splenomegaly, and bilateral inguinal lymphadenopathy. HIV screen comes back positive. Excisional biopsy of the left inguinal lymph node confirms the diagnosis of HIV-associated Burkitt lymphoma. Bone marrow biopsy shows involvement by lymphoma, but CSF cytology and flow cytometry is negative. His CD4 count is 285/μL. Patient is planned to start combination chemotherapy with the DA-EPOCH-R regimen.

1) **Which of the following is most appropriate regarding incorporation of antiretroviral therapy to chemotherapy?**

   A) Defer initiation of antiretroviral therapy until completion of chemotherapy.
   B) Defer initiation of antiretroviral therapy until completion of chemotherapy unless patient develops an opportunistic infection.

C) Initiate antiretroviral therapy immediately.

D) Monitor CD4 count during chemotherapy and start antiretroviral therapy only if CD4 count falls below 100/μL.

Expert Perspective: The risks and benefits of continuing antiretroviral therapy (ART) during curative chemotherapy for aggressive lymphomas were a major therapeutic controversy in the past. When highly active ART first became available, there were concerns regarding potential pharmacokinetic interactions leading to lower steady-state drug concentrations, and/or increased toxicity. In these early days of anti-retroviral availability, it is important to note that the available agents were associated with considerable toxicity and interactions. In contrast to views that advocated suspension of ART, many investigators argued that uncontrolled HIV replication during chemotherapy could worsen immune function and be detrimental to HIV control. Two prospective studies where ART was suspended during chemotherapy (dose-adjusted EPOCH [DA-EPOCH] and short-course EPOCH with dose-dense rituximab [SC-EPOCH-RR]) did not observe a significantly increased risk of infections during therapy. While the HIV viral loads rapidly increased and then plateaued after the first cycle and the CD4 cells decreased over the course of chemotherapy, HIV viral loads returned to baseline by three months, and CD4 cells returned to pretreatment levels by 6–12 months after treatment (Dunleavy et al. 2010). However, another study demonstrated that CD4 counts recovered to pretreatment levels within one month when ART was administered concurrently with chemotherapy (Powles et al. 2002). A meta-analysis of 19 prospective clinical trials of HIV-associated lymphoma also showed that concurrent ART was associated with improved complete remission rates and with a trend toward improved overall survival (OS) (Barta et al. 2013).

Recently, results from a randomized phase II trial evaluating the role of concurrent vs sequential rituximab with DA-EPOCH (AMC 034) showed that patients receiving concurrent ART had lower HIV viral loads and quicker CD4 count recovery compared to patients who did not receive ART (Tan et al. 2018). Additionally, the incidence of grade ≥ 3 infectious, hematologic, or neurological toxicities was similar between both groups. Two recently published multicenter studies, in newly diagnosed patients with Burkitt lymphoma and MYC-rearranged aggressive B-cell lymphoma, included patients who were HIV positive, and they were permitted to receive concomitant antiretroviral therapy. In both studies, the outcome of the HIV-positive group was excellent and non-inferior to HIV-negative patients enrolled. At this point in time, given the much better toxicity profile of ART today compared to the early agents that were used, we recommend concurrent use of ART with chemotherapy in HIV-associated lymphoma as it is safe and results in faster immune reconstitution.

Correct Answer: C

Case study 2

A 42-year-old female with a history of HIV presents with right axillary lymphadenopathy that has grown rapidly over the last two weeks. She reports no history of fevers or night sweats. She is compliant with ART and has undetectable HIV viral load with a CD4 count of 350/μL. Lactate dehydrogenase level is normal. A CT scan of the chest, abdomen, and pelvis shows non-bulky right axillary, b/l supraclavicular, paraaortic, and retroperitoneal lymphadenopathy. FDG PET does not show any evidence of extra-nodal involvement. Excisional biopsy of the right axillary lymphadenopathy shows germinal center B-type (GCB) diffuse large B-cell lymphoma (DLBCL). Fluorescent in situ hybridization (FISH) does not show any *MYC, BCL-2*, or *BCL-6* rearrangements. Bone marrow biopsy does not show any evidence of involvement by lymphoma.

2) Which of the following is the best treatment strategy?

A) R-CHOP with intrathecal methotrexate.
B) DA-EPOCH-R with intrathecal methotrexate.
C) DA-EPOCH (without rituximab).
D) CHOP (without rituximab).
E) Short course of EPOCH-RR.

Expert Perspective: We recommend combined immunochemotherapy. Our first recommendation is therapy with rituximab and DA-EPOCH. The role of rituximab in HIV-associated lymphoma was controversial in the past. This controversy stemmed from an AMC (AMC 010) randomized phase III study of CHOP with or without rituximab in HIV-associated aggressive lymphomas, where it was demonstrated that rituximab was associated with significantly more infectious deaths but only a trend in improved tumor control. On closer evaluation of AMC trial, however, the increased infectious deaths occurred primarily in patients with very low CD4 counts, and many patients received "maintenance" rituximab after chemotherapy, which had not been shown to be useful in HIV-negative DLBCL. To further address the role of rituximab, the AMC performed a follow-up randomized phase II study of concurrent versus sequential rituximab with EPOCH in HIV-associated DLBCL; importantly, in that study, concurrent rituximab was not associated with an increased risk of infectious deaths and resulted higher rate of complete remission (Sparano et al. 2010).

Abbreviated therapy with so-called short-course EPOCH-RR could be administered here. This recommendation is based on results from a phase II study of short-course EPOCH plus dose-dense rituximab where 33 patients with HIV-associated DLBCL received a minimum of three and maximum of six cycles with one cycle beyond CR (Dunleavy et al. 2010). In this study, 80% of patients required just three cycles, and five-year rates of progression-free survival and OS were 84% and 68%, respectively. In a meta-analysis of 1,546 patients from 19 prospective clinical trials, infusional EPOCH was associated with better complete remission rates and improved OS as compared to CHOP (Barta et al. 2013).

Most of the HIV-associated lymphoma cases present at an advanced stage. The risk of CNS involvement is increased due to its tendency for extranodal involvement. Therefore, patients with HIV-associated aggressive B-cell lymphomas **should** have a lumbar puncture for analysis of cerebrospinal fluid by both cytology and flow cytometry to check for the presence of leptomeningeal lymphoma. Indications for CNS prophylaxis are the same as in the HIV-negative cases. Patients with CNS IPI score of 4–6, breast or testicular involvement, and double-hit lymphoma should receive CNS prophylaxis with intrathecal methotrexate and/or cytarabine (see Chapters 36 and 44).

Correct Answer: E

3) **Which of the following statements is accurate regarding the use of fluorodeoxyglucose positron-emission tomography (FDG-PET) for assessment of response to chemotherapy in HIV-associated DLBCL?**

A) Interim FDG-PET after two cycles of combination chemotherapy has a high positive predictive value.
B) Interim FDG-PET after two cycles of combination chemotherapy has a high negative predictive value.
C) Interim FDG-PET after two cycles of combination chemotherapy identifies patients at risk for treatment failure.
D) End-of-treatment FDG-PET following six cycles of combination chemotherapy has a high positive predictive value.

Expert Perspective: Fluorodeoxyglucose positron-emission tomography (FDG-PET) is useful in HIV-negative aggressive lymphomas, but its role in HIV-associated lymphomas has not been well studied and can be confounded by inflammation from HIV-associated nodal reactive hyperplasia, infections, and lipodystrophy. The study of short-course EPOCH-RR in HIV-associated DLBCL showed that FDG-PET obtained following two cycles and at the end of therapy showed a high negative predictive value of 91% and 87%, respectively, but poor or low positive predictive values of only 15% and 7% making choices A, C, and D false and choice B correct.

Correct Answer: B

Case study 3

A 42-year-old man with a history of HIV not on ART presents with a tonic-clonic seizure. On further questioning, the patient reports worsening memory loss, headaches, and 20 lbs weight loss in the last six months. His HIV viral load is 187,000 copies/mL, and CD4 count is 18/µL. MRI brain shows multiple heterogeneously enhancing lesions in the parenchyma. PET-CT does not show any evidence of abnormal hypermetabolic activity in the body. Patient undergoes stereotactic biopsy of the left frontal lobe lesion, and pathology comes back consistent with primary CNS lymphoma (PCNSL).

4) **Which of the following statements regarding HIV-associated PCNSL is correct?**

A) The incidence of HIV-associated PCNSL has increased significantly in ART era.
B) HIV-associated PCNSL harbor HHV-8 approximately in half of the cases.
C) HIV-associated PCNSL is usually seen in patients with CD4 count < 50/µL.
D) HIV-associated PCNSL has a similar prognosis compared to HIV-negative PCNSL.

Expert Perspective: In the setting of HIV infection, PCNSL presents in patients with severe immune suppression, typically with CD4 counts lower than 50/µL. Its incidence has decreased dramatically since the advent of ART. Overall, HIV-associated PCNSL has a worse prognosis compared to HIV-negative PCNSL. Patients frequently present with changes in mental status or focal neurological symptoms and, unlike those with HIV-negative PCNSL, they tend to present with multiple brain lesions. Because these patients are severely immunosuppressed, intracranial opportunistic infections should always be considered in the differential diagnosis when evaluating intracranial lesions on imaging studies. Although the disease remains incurable in most patients, the duration of survival appears to have increased with concurrent use of ART. While most studies in the pre-ART era report a median survival in the range of three months, survival over 1.5 years was reported in patients who responded to ART and were treated with radiation.

Compared to HIV-negative patients, HIV-associated PCNSL is typically EBV positive. A recent study identified distinct immunobiologic features between between EBV+HIV+ and EBV−HIV− PCNSL (Gandhi et al. 2021). EBV+HIV+ PCNSL showed a tolerogenic tumor microenvironment and an increased T-cell signaling whereas EBV−HIV− PCNSL showed a genetic landscape like ABC-DLBCL. These findings might have future therapeutic implications for each subtype such as use of immunotherapy for EBV+HIV+ PCNSL and BTK inhibitors for EBV−HIV− cases.

Until recently, whole brain radiation therapy (WBRT) was the standard approach for most patients with HIV-associated PCNSL. Treatment paradigms have shifted away from WBRT to high-dose methotrexate (HD-MTX)−based combination chemotherapy regimens in the past few years. In a recent prospective phase II study, 12 patients with HIV-associated PCNSL received induction therapy with six cycles of HD-MTX (6 mg/m^2) and rituximab followed by consolidation including two additional cycles of HD-MTX and rituximab in patients who achieved CR or second-line chemotherapy in patients with partial response (Lurain et al. 2020). All patients received ART during chemotherapy. In all, 8 out of 12 patients achieved sustained complete remission without relapse at two years and estimated five-year OS was 67%.

Few studies have been done looking at the biology of primary CNS lymphoma in the setting of HIV and comparing that to PCNSL, in HIV-negative settings. If there are significant biological differences, this is important as we continue to investigate novel targeted agents with promising activity in this disease (see Chapter 46).

Correct Answer: C

Case study 4

A 38-year-old man with HIV on ART presents with a 5 lb weight loss, night sweats, and a right cervical lymphadenopathy. Over the next month, the cervical lymphadenopathy increases in size despite a course of antibiotics. He undergoes an excisional biopsy of the cervical lymphadenopathy, which reveals a diagnosis of nodular sclerosing Hodgkin lymphoma. FDG-PET shows hypermetabolic right cervical, right supraclavicular, bilateral hilar, and retroperitoneal lymphadenopathy with multiple splenic lesions and diffuse uptake in the bone marrow. Laboratory studies show WBC count of 2,400/µL, hemoglobin of 9.8 g/dL, a serum albumin level of 3.5 g/dL, CD4 count of 425/µL, and undetectable HIV viral load. Bone marrow biopsy confirms involvement by classic Hodgkin lymphoma.

5) Which of the following is the best treatment strategy?

   A) Doxorubicin, bleomycin, vinblastine, and dacarbazine (ABVD).
   B) Brentuximab vedotin, doxorubicin, bleomycin, and dacarbazine (A-AVD).

C) Doxorubicin, bleomycin, vinblastine, and dacarbazine (ABVD) followed by consoli-dative involved field radiation therapy (IFRT) to cervical lymph nodes.

D) Brentuximab vedotin, doxorubicin, vinblastine, and dacarbazine (A-AVD) with G-CSF support.

Expert Perspective: In the setting of HIV infection, classic HL (cHL) occurs most frequently in patients with depressed immune function. However, a paradoxical increase in cHL has been observed in the ART era despite an overall improvement in immune function in most patients. This is likely explained by examining the incidence of the two major subtypes of cHL that occur with HIV infection. In the pre-ART era, most cHL was of the mixed-cellularity subtype, which is EBV positive and occurs mostly in immune-suppressed patients, whereas more recently there has been an increased incidence of nodular sclerosis HL, which occurs more commonly at higher CD4 counts. As in the case of HIV-associated non-Hodgkin lymphoma, cHL also presents with high-risk features such as advanced disease, presence of B-symptoms, and extranodal involvement in the majority of the cases. However, studies showed similar outcomes to those with HIV-negative cHL when treated with ABVD regimen. Recently, brentuximab vedotin (BV) was approved in combination with AVD (A-AVD) for treatment of advanced-stage HL in the general population after the ECHELON-1 study showed a higher two-year progression-free survival compared to ABVD regimen (82.1% vs 77.2%; $P = 0.04$). The benefit of BV was more prominent in patients with a high IPS score of 4–7. In a phase I study of six HIV-associated cHL patients, BV in combination with AVD was shown to be well tolerated (Rubinstein et al. 2018). It is important to note that G-CSF should be used in patients receiving brentuximab vedotin to mitigate the risk of febrile neutropenia, especially in patients with bone marrow involvement (see Chapters 31-32).

Correct Answer: D

6) **Which of the following statements is NOT accurate regarding EBV infection in HIV-associated lymphoma?**

A) EBV+ tumors have a worse overall prognosis as compared to EBV− tumors in HIV-positive individuals.

B) Concurrent EBV infection increases the risk of lymphoma development over 60-fold.

C) Concurrent EBV infection is more common in individuals with lower CD4 counts.

D) Almost all cases of primary CNS lymphoma stain positive for EBV tissue markers such has EBER and/or LMP-1.

Expert Perspective: EBV is an oncogenic virus that is acquired by early adulthood in 90–95% of the population. Following primary infection, which is often asymptomatic, EBV establishes latency in B lymphocytes, T lymphocytes, and epithelial cells. It precedes HIV infection in most of the cases. Concurrent EBV and HIV infection increases the risk of lymphomagenesis over 60-fold due to multiple mechanisms involving reduced EBV-directed immunity, T lymphocyte dysfunction, and EBV-mediated immune evasion. EBV associated lymphomagenesis is seen more frequently in individuals with lower CD4 counts, which in part explains the varying degrees of EBV positivity in different HIV-associated lymphomas, ranging from 100% in primary CNS lymphoma to 30–40% in Burkitt lymphoma. Although multiple studies have shown worse outcomes of EBV+ lymphoma as compared to EBV– lymphoma in individuals without HIV infection, the prognostic value of EBV positivity in HIV-associated lymphoma is not clear. A small study of patients from a prospective French cohort of HIV-related lymphomas showed similar two-year progression-free survival between cases with positive pretreatment EBV DNA and negative pretreatment EBV DNA in the plasma or whole blood (Lupo et al. 2019). However, concurrent EBV infection can possibly make patients more prone to chemotherapy-related hematologic toxicities such as febrile neutropenia due to higher degrees of immunosuppression in these cases.

Correct Answer: A

Case study 5

A 58-year-old woman with a history of HIV-associated DLBCL who achieved complete remission following treatment with EPOCH-RR regimen 18 months ago presents with one-month history of abdominal pain and constipation. CT scan shows a 4.4 cm mesenteric lymphadenopathy, 2.2 cm left inguinal lymphadenopathy, and moderate splenomegaly. FDG-PET scan shows increased metabolic activity in these areas with an SUVmax of 14.2. Biopsy of the left inguinal lymphadenopathy confirms relapse of DLBCL. She is compliant with ART with an undetectable HIV viral load and a CD4 count of 535/μL. Other laboratory studies show normal CBC, chemistry, and lactate dehydrogenase level.

7) **Which of the following is the most appropriate treatment strategy for this patient?**

   A) Salvage chemotherapy with 4–6 cycles of rituximab, etoposide, methylprednisolone, high-dose cytarabine, and cisplatin (R-ESHAP).
   B) Salvage chemotherapy with rituximab, ifosfamide, carboplatin, and etoposide (R-ICE) followed by autologous hematopoietic stem cell transplant (auto-ASCT).
   C) Anti-CD-19 chimeric antigen receptor (CAR) T cell therapy.
   D) Salvage chemotherapy with ICE followed by reduced-intensity hematopoietic stem cell transplant.

Expert Perspective: Given the significant improvements in HIV control and immune function, it is reasonable to approach relapsed HIV-associated lymphomas similarly to their HIV-negative counterparts and to pursue aggressive strategies such as autologous stem cell transplant (ASCT) in suitable candidates. Less aggressive strategies, such as ESHAP and CDE, have poor outcomes. ASCT has been shown to be safe and effective in patients with DLBCL whose HIV infection is well controlled. A multicenter phase II trial (AMC 071) evaluated the role of ASCT in 40 relapsed/refractory HIV-associated lymphoma patients with chemo-sensitive disease and showed a two-year OS of 82% at a median follow-up of 24.2 months (Alvarnas et al. 2016). Transplant-related mortality at one year was 5.2%. Another study prospectively evaluated auto-HSCT in 27 patients with relapsed HIV-associated lymphoma (both HL and NHL) who achieved complete response or partial response to salvage chemotherapy and showed a median OS of 33 months. On the contrary, allogeneic hematopoietic stem cell transplantation (allo-HCT) has not been well studied in HIV-associated lymphoma. The only prospective data so far is from a phase II study of allo-HCT in 17 HIV patients with hematologic malignancies that enrolled three patients with NHL. In this study, the two-year OS survival and treatment-related mortality was 52.8% and 18.3%, respectively. Currently, there are only a few case reports of successful treatment of relapsed/refractory HIV-associated DLBCL with anti-CD19 CAR T cell therapy. Patients with HIV have been excluded from anti-CD19 CAR T cell therapy trials.

Correct Answer: B

Recommended Readings

Alvarnas, J.C., Rademacher, J.L., Wang, Y. et al. (2016). Autologous hematopoietic cell transplantation for HIV-related lymphoma: results of the BMT CTN 0803/AMC 071 trial. *Blood* 128 (8): 1050–1058.

Barta, S.K. et al. (2013). Treatment factors affecting outcomes in HIV-associated non-Hodgkin lymphomas: a pooled analysis of 1546 patients. *Blood* 122 (19): 3251–3262.

Dunleavy, K. et al. (2010). The role of tumor histogenesis, FDG-PET, and short-course EPOCH with dose-dense rituximab (SC-EPOCH-RR) in HIV-associated diffuse large B-cell lymphoma. *Blood* 115 (15): 3017–3024.

Gandhi, M.K. et al. (2021). EBV-associated primary CNS lymphoma occurring after immunosuppression is a distinct immunobiological entity. *Blood* 137 (11): 1468–1477.

Louarn, N., Galicier, L., Bertinchamp, R., et al. (2022 April 20). First extensive analysis of 18F labeled fluorodeoxyglucose positron emission tomography computed tomography in a large cohort of patients with HIV Associated Hodgkin lymphoma: baseline total metabolic tumor volume affects prognosis. *J Clin Oncol* 40 (12): 1346 1355. doi: 10.1200/JCO.21.01228. Epub 2022 Jan 24. PMID: 35073166.

Lupo, J. et al. (2019). Epstein–Barr virus biomarkers have no prognostic value in HIV-related Hodgkin lymphoma in the modern combined antiretroviral therapy era. *AIDS* 33 (6): 993.

Lurain, K. et al. (2020). Treatment of HIV-associated primary CNS lymphoma with antiretroviral therapy, rituximab, and high-dose methotrexate. *Blood* 136 (19): 2229–2232.

Powles, T. et al. (2002). Effects of combination chemotherapy and highly active antiretroviral therapy on immune parameters in HIV-1 associated lymphoma. *AIDS* 16 (4): 531–536.

Rubinstein, P.G. et al. (2018). Brentuximab vedotin with AVD shows safety, in the absence of strong CYP3A4 inhibitors, in newly diagnosed HIV-associated Hodgkin lymphoma. *AIDS* 32 (5): 605–611.

Sparano, J.A. et al. (2010). Rituximab plus concurrent infusional EPOCH chemotherapy is highly effective in HIV-associated B-cell non-Hodgkin lymphoma. *Blood* 115 (15): 3008–3016.

Tan, C.R.C. et al. (2018). Combination antiretroviral therapy accelerates immune recovery in patients with HIV-related lymphoma treated with EPOCH: a comparison within one prospective trial AMC034. *Leukemia & Lymphoma* 1851–1860. doi: 10.1080/10428194.2017.1403597.

47

Waldenström's Macroglobulinemia

Morie A. Gertz

Mayo Clinic, Rochester, MN

Introduction

Macroglobulinemia is defined as the presence of lymphoplasmacytic lymphoma in the bone marrow associated with a monoclonal IgM protein of any size. IgM monoclonal gammopathy of undetermined significance is present in 0.5% of all adults over the age of 70. The age-adjusted incidence rate for males is 0.92/100,000 person-years and for females 0.30/100,000 person years. The incidence of the disease rises from 0.5/100,000 at age 50 to 2.2/100,000 at age 90. At diagnosis 28% of patients with macroglobulinemia are smoldering. The median age at diagnosis is 73 years. Most patients present because of their anemia, but occasionally patients will present with symptoms of hyperviscosity. The most reliable signs of hyperviscosity are gingival and nasal bleeding. Less than 20% of patients will have significant lymphadenopathy at diagnosis. Occasionally the lymphoplasmacytic lymphoma will invade the central nervous system, and then it is called Bing Neel syndrome. Rare symptoms associated with the monoclonal IgM protein can be seen and include cold agglutinin hemolytic anemia, type 2 mixed cryoglobulinemia, IgM amyloidosis, and IgM-mediated sensory motor peripheral neuropathy. With current therapies the disease is incurable, and the most important prognostic factor at diagnosis is age. A significant proportion of patients die of causes completely unrelated to the disorder.

1) What is Waldenström's macroglobulinemia, and when should it be suspected?

Expert Perspective: Waldenström's macroglobulinemia (WM) is defined by the World Health Organization as a lymphoplasmacytic lymphoma (LPL) associated with a monoclonal immunoglobulin M (IgM) protein. The classic characteristic pentad of WM is (i) M-protein on serum protein electrophoresis confirmed to be (ii) IgM by immunofixation, with (iii) bone marrow evidence of lymphoplasmacytic lymphoma and, in some patients, evidence of (iv) hyperviscosity syndrome with (v) normocytic anemia. Using the Surveillance, Epidemiology, and End Results (SEER) data, WM represented 1.9% of all non-Hodgkin lymphoma. The median age at diagnosis was 73 years, with a predilection for men (5.4/million/year) as opposed to women (2.7/million), and a racial skewing toward Caucasians (4.1/million) rather than African Americans (1.8/million). First-degree relatives of patients with LPL–WM have a 20-fold increased risk of LPL–WM.

Other IgM-related conditions include IgM monoclonal gammopathy of undetermined significance (IgM < 3 g/dl; no evidence of marrow infiltration > 10%; and without symptoms of tumor mass or infiltrations, e.g. adenopathy, organomegaly, anemia, or IgM-mediated symptoms), smoldering WM (IgM > 3 g/dl; marrow infiltration > 10%; and with no symptoms of tumor mass or infiltration or IgM-mediated symptoms), IgM-related cold agglutinin hemolytic anemia, type II cryoglobulin, neuropathy, and amyloidosis.

2) Which of the following genetic changes is associated with WM?
   A) t(11;18).
   B) *BRAF V600E.*
   C) *MYD88 L265P.*
   D) *NOTCH2.*

Expert Perspective: Using whole-genome sequencing, over 90% of patients with typical WM or non-IgM WM/LPL have been found to have a common mutation, *MYD88 L265P.* This mutation also appears to be useful in differentiating LPL from other B-cell lymphoproliferative disorders such as splenic marginal zone lymphoma. Furthermore, on metaphase cytogenetics, a deletion in the long arm of chromosome 6 (6q −) may be seen in 40–50% patients. Epigenetic dysregulation; aberrations in the phosphatidylinositol-3 kinase–mammalian target of rapamycin (PI3K–mTOR), nuclear factor kappa B, and Janus kinase–signal transducer and activator of transcription (JAK–STAT) signaling pathways; and bone marrow microenvironmental interactions may be other key factors that are involved in the pathogenesis of WM.

Correct Answer: C

Case Study 1

A 62-year-old male is diagnosed with WM. His hemoglobin is 11.4 g/dL, his white blood cell (WBC) count is 10,000/cu mL, and his platelet count is 102,000/cu mL. The IgM level is 6400 g/dL.

3) Based on this information, what is his risk category?
   A) Low risk.
   B) Intermediate.
   C) High.
   D) Need more information.

Expert Perspective: The International Staging System for Waldenström's macroglobulinemia identifies the following five factors associated with prognosis in WM: (i) age > 65, (ii) hemoglobin < 11.5 g/dL, (iii) platelet count < 100,000/cu mL, (iv) beta-2 microglobulin > 3 mg/dL, and (v) monoclonal IgM > 7 g/dL.

Based on the number of risk factors present, the risk category may be low (0 or 1 risk factor, except age), intermediate (age > 65 or two risk factors), or high risk (> 2 risk factors),

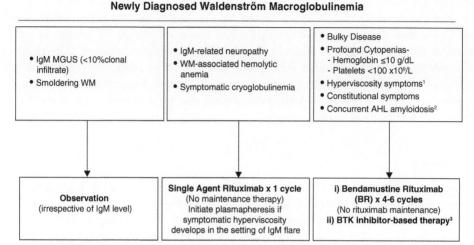

Figure 47.1 The Mayo Clinic approach to Waldenström's macroglobulinemia (WM). IgM, immunoglobulin M; MGUS, monoclonal gammopathy of undetermined significance. (*Source:* Ansell, SM, et al. *Mayo Clin Proc.* 2010;85:824–33. Reproduced with permission of Elsevier).

which are associated with a median survival of 142.5, 98.6, and 43.5 months, respectively. This patients risk can not be determined due to the lack of a beta 2 microglobulin.

The staging system is notable for the absence of lactate dehydrogenase (LDH); however, LDH may have a role in separating the high-risk patients into two distinct categories.

Correct Answer: D

4) The above patient is asymptomatic. His beta-2 microglobulin and LDH are unremarkable; he has 30% involvement of the bone marrow with lymphoma. Does he need treatment?

Expert Perspective: He can be observed (Figure 47.1). Asymptomatic patients without significant cytopenias can be observed. Single-agent rituximab is rarely used but may be indicated for patients with isolated peripheral neuropathy or hemolytic anemia. Single-agent rituximab is inferior to all other published regimens. Patients who need cytotoxic therapy are encouraged to go on clinical trials wherever possible. The standard of care at our institution at the current time is combination chemotherapy with rituximab and bendamustine (Figure 47.1) or zanubrutinib. The discovery of *MYD88* and *CXCR4* mutations in WM has facilitated rational drug development, including the development of BTK inhibitors. Responses to many agents commonly used to treat WM, including the BTK inhibitors are affected by *MYD88* and/or *CXCR4* mutation status. The mutation status of both *MYD88* and *CXCR4* can be used for a precision-guided treatment approach to WM. Patients with *MYD88* mutations who are wild type for *CXCR4* have better outcomes associated with ibrutinib. Patients with both *MYD88* and *CXCR4* mutations exhibit a delay by 4-5 months in attaining a major response to ibrutinib. WM with wild-type *MYD88* treated with ibrutinib rarely respond. In ASPEN trial, extended follow-up results with zanibrutiib confirm improved long-term safety and tolerability of zanubrutinib compared with ibrutinib and support deeper, earlier, and more durable responses in patients with WM regardless of previous treatment or *CXCR4* and *MYD88* mutational statuses.

Case Study 2

A 48-year-old male presents to his primary care doctor with blurred vision. He has had headaches and also notes nose bleeds. Examination reveals retinal venous dilation (Figure 47.2). Further work-up reveals a mild anemia with hemoglobin of 11.5 g/dL and a platelet count of 95,000/mL^3. Chemistry shows normal creatinine and a total protein level of 9 g/dL.

5) What is going on with the patient?
   A) Hyperviscosity syndrome.
   B) Dehydration.
   C) Thrombotic thrombocytopenia purpura.
   D) Amyloidosis.

Expert Perspective: Hyperviscosity is a potentially life-threatening complication of WM that is, fortunately, rarely encountered. The risk of hyperviscosity depends on the IgM level, and it is rare at an IgM level lower than 4 g/dL. Symptoms may be nonspecific, with generalized fatigue, dizziness, and lightheadedness. Bleeding can result with epistaxis, gingival bleeding, and retinal hemorrhages. Classic ophthalmologic findings include sausaging of retinal veins from venous engorgement, as seen on fundoscopic examination. Hyperviscosity syndrome is rare unless the serum viscosity exceeds 4 cpoise (normal ≤ 1.5 cpoise). Hyperviscosity syndrome can be treated immediately by the institution of plasmapheresis, (blood warmers should be used during apheresis in patients with cryoglobulins) followed by the institution of chemotherapy. Elevated viscosity without the presence of symptoms is not an indication for treatment. When single-agent rituximab is used, patients can develop an initial IgM flare that may result in hyperviscosity after the initiation of treatment. It is important to be watchful of the IgM and serum viscosity levels if single-agent rituximab is used with a low threshold for plasmapheresis. The other important implication of this observation is to not change therapy during a flare, as these patients can still respond to treatment. A single plasma exchange is often sufficient to resolve the clinical symptoms of hyperviscosity.

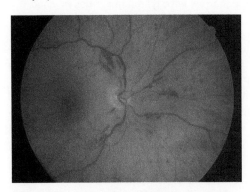

Figure 47.2 Abnormal fundoscopic examination in a patient with acute onset of blurred vision.

Table 47.1 Response criteria to Waldenström's macroglobulinemia (WM) treatment.

Complete response	Disappearance of serum and urine M protein by immunofixation, histologic absence of malignant cells in bone marrow, resolution of lymphadenopathy or organomegaly, and no signs or symptoms attributable to WM
Partial response	≥ 50% reduction in serum M protein by electrophoresis, ≥ 50% decrease in adenopathy and organomegaly, and no new signs or symptoms of active WM
Minor response	≥ 25% but < 50% reduction in serum M protein by electrophoresis; no new signs or symptoms of active WM
Stable disease	< 25% reduction or increase in serum M protein by electrophoresis without progression of adenopathy and organomegaly or symptoms or signs attributable to WM
Progressive disease	≥ 25% increase in serum M protein by electrophoresis (on two measurements) or progression of clinically significant findings; symptoms or signs attributable to WM

Source: Kimby, E, et al. *Clin. Lymphoma Myeloma Leuk* 2006;6:380–3. Reproduced with permission of Elsevier.

6) How is response to treatment measured?

Expert Perspective: Response to treatment, was defined by a consensus panel at the Third International Workshop on Waldenström's macroglobulinemia, shown in Table 47.1. There are a few important caveats to consider: (i) patients may have a delayed response, especially after purine analog and monoclonal antibody therapy, and best response may not be achieved until six months after treatment; and (ii) patients with minor responses may do just as well clinically as patients with better responses.

7) What are the different standard and novel therapies in WM?

Expert Perspective: The standard therapy for WM may be alkylator based (cyclophosphamide) with the anti-CD20 monoclonal antibody rituximab. Newer drugs include the BTK inhibitor, ibrutinib or zanubrutinib or acalabrutinib, alkylator, bendamustine or cyclophosphamide, immunomodulatory drugs lenalidomide or pomalidomide, and proteasome inhibitors bortezomib and carfilzomib. Everolimus, the mTOR inhibitor, has high efficacy in WM with response rates up to 70% when used as a single agent. Ofatumumab, a third-generation anti-CD20 monoclonal antibody, appears to offer no advantages to rituximab. Second-generation BTK inhibitors including acalabrutinib and zanubrutinib have clear-cut activity in macroglobulinemia with fewer off-target effects compared with ibrutinib. Patients treated with second-generation inhibitors have significantly lower rates of diarrhea and atrial fibrillation. Currently most newly diagnosed patients in the united States are treated with either rituximab plus bendamustine or a BTK inhibitor. Patients that progress over three years following cessation of therapy may be re-treated with the original regimen. Early relapses may be treated with second-line therapies, which include bortezomib-, ixazomib-, and cyclophosphamide-based regimens.

8) Is there a role for rituximab maintenance?

Expert Perspective: The benefit of maintenance rituximab therapy is controversial. Based on the East German Lymphoma Study Group 2019 MAINTAIN trial, 218 patients were randomized to rituximab for two years versus observation; there was no difference in progression-free survival in the two groups, and in this largest phase III trial, rituximab maintenance was not beneficial.

9) Should autologous stem cell transplantation be a front-line option?

Expert Perspective: Autologous stem cell transplantation produces durable responses with a low treatment-related mortality rate. Heavily pretreated patients (more than three regimens) and those who are chemorefractory at the time of transplantation are unlikely to benefit. Although autologous stem cell transplantation is still performed regularly in Europe, its use in the United States as an option is in decline despite the fact that it can produce median progression-free survival in excess of four years.

10) How is relapsed disease managed?

Current treatment options for patients with previously treated WM are highly effective. Our suggested treatment algorithm for previously treated WM patients is shown in Figure 47.3. Additionally venetoclax, everolimus and cladribine can be useful in certain circumstances. R-CHOP is preferred in cases of DLBCL transformation.

11) What about allogeneic stem cell transplantation?

Expert Perspective: Allogeneic transplantation is generally used in the investigational setting. As WM tends to occur at older ages, this makes allo-transplantation more difficult. The largest literature supporting allogeneic transplantation in WM comes from the European Bone Marrow Transplantation registry (304 patients, 2000–2011), in which patients who received reduced-intensity conditioning and myeloablative conditioning showed an overall survival of 62% and 66%, and three-year response rates of 21% and 26%, respectively.

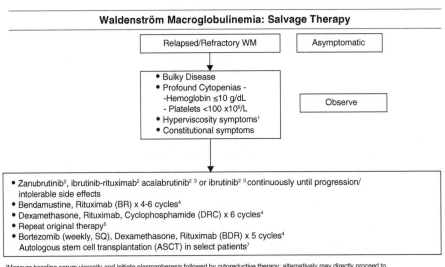

Figure 47.3 The Mayo Clinic approach for salvage therapy in Waldenström's macroglobulinemia. (*Source:* Ansell, SM, et al. *Mayo Clin Proc.* 2010;85:824–33. Reproduced with permission of Elsevier).

Cryoglobulinemia and Related Autoimmune Disorders in WM

12) What are the treatment options for IgM-related autoimmune conditions?

Expert Perspective: The monoclonal IgM protein can result in a number of autoimmune conditions. Type II cryoglobulinemia is common; all of the type II cryoglobulins are composed of the monoclonal IgM protein. Type I cryoglobulinemia may be an incidental finding without symptoms or signs. Type II cryoglobulinemia is composed of monoclonal and polyclonal immunoglobulins. Patients with mixed IgM–IgG cryoglobulinemia can have a variety of symptoms and signs related to cold sensitivity, purpura, arthralgias, and vasculitis. Type II cryoglobulinemia can have a marked effect on serum viscosity owing to the high thermal amplitude of the IgM–IgG cryoglobulin. Patients can also develop a cold agglutinin disease (CAD) from a monoclonal IgM directed against the red cell I or i antigen. Symptoms include acrocyanosis, Raynaud's phenomenon, and an immune hemolytic anemia on cold exposure. Last, the IgM protein can also attack neural proteins, resulting in immune neuropathies (see the "IgM-related neurologic manifestations" section). Type II cryoglobulinemia or CAD can be asymptomatic. Symptomatic patients with IgM-related autoimmune disorders can be treated with single-agent rituximab alone (if without bulky disease, cytopenias, or B-symptoms), as shown in Figure 47.1. Patients with other symptoms related to WM are treated with cytotoxic therapy with rituximab.

Risk of Amyloid Light-chain (AL) Amyloidosis

13) What are the treatment options for IgM amyloidosis?

Expert Perspective: Primary systemic amyloidosis is a rare complication of WM. This should be considered when a patient has symptoms of peripheral neuropathy. This is an important complication to identify, as the development of amyloidosis can cause significant morbidity as well as mortality from organ involvement over the risk of progression of WM. In a series of 22 patients with IgM amyloidosis studied at the Mayo Clinic, patients tend to be older, with more peripheral nerve involvement and a lesser degree of cardiac involvement. Rarely, patients with WM can present with localized AL amyloidosis primarily affecting the lymph nodes. This tends to be a more indolent form of amyloidosis in which the amyloid deposition occurs peri-tumorally at the site of lymphoma cells without affecting distant organs. Treatment of IgM amyloidosis is similar to the treatment of primary systemic AL amyloidosis. There is some anecdotal evidence that treatment directed at the lymphoma cells with drugs such as rituximab may be of benefit. The treatment options vary including BoCyD with rituximab and bendamustine plus rituximab. (see Chapter 56)

IgM-related Neurologic Manifestations

14) What is Bing-Neel Syndrome?

Expert Perspective: The most common neurologic complication of WM is peripheral neuropathy. These may be seen as frequently as in half of all patients. The clinical presentation and neurologic findings are identical to those seen with IgM-MGUS (monoclonal gammopathy of undetermined significance) and are probably related to immune-mediated axonal loss. Known targets against which monoclonal IgM may be directed include myelin-associated glycoprotein (MAG) or sulfatide, but only a minority of patients have these auto-antibodies. Other mechanisms of peripheral nerve damage may include direct infiltration of nerves by tumor cells, IgM directed against unidentified neural proteins, or other known complications of WM such as AL amyloidosis and cryoglobulinemia. Last, chemotherapeutic drugs such as bortezomib can worsen peripheral neuropathy.

The central nervous system can be affected in WM. Separate from hyperviscosity syndrome, rarely WM can involve the meninges, brain, and cerebrospinal fluid (CSF), which is termed Bing–Neel syndrome (BNS). In a review of 31 cases of BNS, patients may or may not have evidence of lymphoplasmacytoid cells within the brain or CSF and presumably have an autoimmune mechanism mediated by IgM. White matter changes are seen on brain magnetic resonance imaging (MRI) in 65% of patients, and spinal fluid syndromes were seen in 67% of patients. Treatment of the WM provided improvement in 42% of patients, with sustained responses from six months to four years. Ibrutinib crosses the blood-brain barrier and is an important therapeutic intervention for these patients.

Survivorship Issues in WM

15) Do patients with WM have increase risk of additional cancers?

Expert Perspective: The long survival and advanced age of presentation of WM have to be considered when selecting the most appropriate treatment. Treatment-associated morbidity is important to consider, with the risk of secondary infections from monoclonal antibody therapy, delayed response from purine analogs, myelodysplasia from fludarabine, and peripheral neuropathy related to bortezomib. Lastly, patients with WM are at an increased risk of developing a second malignancy, including diffuse large B-cell lymphoma, acute myeloid leukemia, and brain cancer.

Recommended Readings

Ansell, S.M., Kyle, R.A., Reeder, C.B. et al. (2010). Diagnosis and management of Waldenstrom macroglobulinemia: mayo stratification of macroglobulinemia and risk-adapted therapy (mSMART) guidelines. *Mayo Clin Proc* 85: 824–833.

Buske , C., Dimopoulos, M.A., Grunenberg, A. et al. (2023 May 10). Bortezomib dexamethasone, rituximab, and cyclophosphamide as first line treatment for waldenström's macroglobulinemia: a prospectively randomized trial of the European Consortium for Waldenström' s Macroglobulinemia. *J Clin Oncol* 41 (14): 2607 2616. doi: 10.1200/JCO.22.01805. Epub 2023 Feb 10. PMID: 36763945.

Buske, C., Jurczak, W., Salem, J.E., and Dimopoulos, M.A. (2023 January). Managing Waldenström's macroglobulinemia with BTK inhibitors. *Leukemia* 37 (1): 35–46. doi: 10.1038/s41375-022-01732-9. Epub 2022 Nov 19. PMID: 36402930; PMCID: PMC9883164.

Castillo J.J., Libby E.N., Ansell S.M., Palomba M.L., Meid K., et al. (2020 Oct). Multicenter phase 2 study of daratumumab monotherapy in patients with previously treated Waldenström macroglobulinemia. *Blood Adv* 4 (20): 5089–5092. doi: 10.1182/bloodadvances.2020003087. PMID: 33085756; PMCID: PMC7594378.

Gertz M.A. (2022 Aug). Waldenstrom Macroglobulinemia: Tailoring Therapy for the Individual. *J Clin Oncol* 40 (23): 2600–2608. doi: 10.1200/JCO.22.00495. Epub 2022 Jun 14. PMID: 35700418; PMCID: PMC9362871.

Gertz, M. (2012). Waldenstrom macroglobulinemia: my way. *Leuk Lymphoma* 54 (3): 464–471.

Issa, G.C., Leblebjian, H., Roccaro, A.M. et al. (2011). New insights into the pathogenesis and treatment of Waldenstrom macroglobuline-mia. *Curr Opin Hematol* 18: 260–265.

Kastritis, E., Kyrtsonis, M.C., Hadjiharissi, E. et al. (2010). Validation of the international prognostic scoring system (IPSS) for Waldenstrom's macroglobulinemia (WM) and the importance of serum lactate dehydrogenase (LDH). *Leuk Res* 34: 1340–1343.

Paludo, J., Abeykoon, J.P., Shreders, A. et al. (2018 August). Bendamustine and rituximab (BR) versus dexamethasone, rituximab, and cyclopho sphamide (DRC) in patients with Waldenström macroglobulinemia. *Ann Hematol* 97 (8): 1417 1425. doi: 10.1007/s00277 018 3311 z. Epub 2018 Apr 3. PMID: 29610969.

Treon, S.P., Patterson, C.J., Sanz, R.G., and Miguel, J.S. (2023 March). Highlights of the 11th International Workshop on Waldenstrom's Macroglobulinemia: what we learned, and how it will impact scientific discovery and patient care. *Semin Hematol* 60 (2): 59 64. doi: 10.1053/j.seminhematol.2023.05.001. Epub 2023 May 10. PMID: 37202255.

Treon S.P., Xu L., Guerrera M.L., et al. (2020 Apr) Genomic Landscape of Waldenström Macroglobulinemia and Its Impact on Treatment Strategies. *J Clin Oncol* 38 (11): 1198–1208. doi: 10.1200/JCO.19.02314. Epub 2020 Feb 21. PMID: 32083995; PMCID: PMC7351339.

Varettoni, M. and Matous, J.V. (2023 August). BTK inhibitors in the frontline management of Waldenström Macroglobulinemia. *Hematol Oncol Clin North Am* 37 (4): 707 717. doi: 10.1016/j.hoc.2023.04.005. Epub 2023 May 26. PMID: 37246088.

Varettoni, M., Tedeschi, A., Arcaini, L. et al. (2012). Risk of second cancers in Waldenstrom macroglobulinemia. *Ann Oncol* 23: 411–415.

48

Primary Cutaneous Lymphomas

Nicholas A. Trum, Jasmine Zain, Steven T. Rosen, and Christiane Querfeld

City of Hope National Medical Center, Duarte, CA

Introduction

Primary cutaneous lymphomas (PCLs) are a clinically, histopathologically, and prognostically heterogenous group of rare non-Hodgkin lymphomas (NHLs) that may originate from either T, NK/T, or B lymphocytes. They are divided by cell-of-origin (COO) into cutaneous T-cell lymphomas (CTCL), NK/T-cell lymphomas, and B-cell lymphomas (CBCL). Unlike nodal lymphomas, they all develop from resident skin lymphocytes without evidence of nodal involvement at the time of diagnosis. Some PCLs are indolent and do not require systemic therapies, while other are aggressive or become more aggressive over time necessitating systemic therapies. Due to their status as "zebras," CBCLs are rarely considered in differential diagnoses, and clinicians unfortunately conflate classic CTCLs (mycosis fungoides [MF] and Sézary syndrome, discussed in Chapter 40) with all CTCL, resulting in longer time to diagnosis, underdiagnosis, and poorer outcomes for these patients. The scope of this chapter includes the epidemiology, key diagnostic pearls and most recent evidence-based management options for PCLs excluding MF, SS, and adult T-cell leukemia/lymphoma (ATLL), referred to here as "rare PCLs."

1) What are the types of rare primary cutaneous lymphomas?

Expert Perspective: Table 48.1 lists all PCLs as classified by the 2018 update of the World Health Organization-European Organization for Research and Treatment of Cancer (WHO-EORTC) system (Willemze et al. 2019). There are 15 recognized rare PCLs (10 CTCL, 5 CBCL) under this classification.

2) What is the epidemiology of rare primary cutaneous lymphomas?

2.1 Incidence

Expert Perspective: Rare PCLs account for approximately one-third of all PCL incidence in the United States (Willemze et al. 2019). CTCLs are more common than CBCLs (~75% vs ~25%) because the most common CTCL (MF, 59% overall PCL, discussed in Chapter 40) constitutes the majority of PCL incidence. The second most common group of CTCLs is the spectrum of CD30+ lymphoproliferative disorders (CD30+ LPDs):

Cancer Consult: Expertise in Clinical Practice, Volume 2: Neoplastic Hematology & Cellular Therapy,
Second Edition. Edited by Syed A. Abutalib, Maurie Markman, James O. Armitage, and Kenneth C. Anderson.
© 2024 John Wiley & Sons Ltd. Published 2024 by John Wiley & Sons Ltd.

Table 48.1 Clinical course of primary cutaneous lymphomas excluding mycosis fungoides and Sézary syndrome. Based on data in the Dutch and Austrian cutaneous lymphoma registries between 2002 and 2017.

WHO-EORTC Classification 2018	Abbreviation	Frequency (%)	5-yr DSS
Cutaneous T-cell lymphoma	**CTCL**		
Indolent course			
Primary cutaneous CD30+ lymphoproliferative disorders	CD30+ LPD		
Primary cutaneous anaplastic large cell lymphoma	pcALCL	8	95
Lymphomatoid papulosis	LyP	12	99
Subcutaneous panniculitis-like T-cell lymphoma	SPTCL	1	87
Primary cutaneous peripheral T-cell lymphoma, rare subtypes			
Primary cutaneous CD4+ small/medium T-cell (pleomorphic) lymphoproliferative disorder (provisional)	CD4+ SMPTC-LPD	6	100
Primary cutaneous acral CD8+ T-cell lymphoma (provisional)	Acral CD8+ TCL	< 1	100
Aggressive course			
Extranodal NK/T-cell lymphoma, nasal type	ENKTCL-NT	< 1	16
Primary cutaneous peripheral T-cell lymphoma, NOS	pcPTCL-NOS	2	15
Primary cutaneous peripheral T-cell lymphoma, rare subtypes			
Primary cutaneous gamma/delta T-cell lymphoma	pcGDTCL	< 1	11
CD8+ aggressive epidermotropic cytotoxic TCL (provisional)	CD8+ AETCL	< 1	31
Chronic active EBV infection	CAEBV		n/a
Cutaneous B-cell lymphoma	**CBCL**		
Indolent course			
Primary cutaneous marginal zone lymphoma	pcMZL	9	99
Primary cutaneous follicle center lymphoma	pcFCL	12	95
EBV+ mucocutaneous ulcer (provisional)	EBVMCU	< 1	100
Aggressive course			
Primary cutaneous diffuse large B-cell lymphoma	pcDLBCL-LT	4	56
Intravascular large B-cell lymphoma	ILBCL	< 1	72

Source: Adapted from the 2018 update of the WHO-EORTC classification for primary cutaneous lymphomas (Willemze et al 2019). Permission conveyed through Copyright Clearance Center, Inc.

lymphomatoid papulosis (LyP, 12% overall PCL) and primary cutaneous anaplastic large cell lymphoma (pcALCL, 8%), followed by CD4+ small/medium pleomorphic T-cell lymphoproliferative disorder (CD4+ SMPTC-LPD, 6%). All other CTCLs are exceedingly rare (≤ 2% overall each).

Incidence varies by continent and region. In a 2020 meta-analysis of 16,953 patients across North America, South America, Europe, and Asia, CTCL was found to occur in 7.5 people per million annually (Dobos et al. 2020). Interestingly, LyP incidence is heterogenous worldwide; its frequency varies between 1% and 26% of reported CTCL cohorts across Europe alone (Dobos et al. 2020). Several are more common in Asia than the United States, including primary cutaneous extranodal NK/T-cell lymphoma, nasal type (ENKTCL-NT), subcutaneous panniculitis-like T-cell lymphoma (SPTCL), chronic active Epstein-Barr virus infection (CAEBV), and primary cutaneous peripheral T-cell lymphoma, not otherwise specified (pcPTCL-NOS) (Dobos et al. 2020). However, other rare CTCLs have a relatively homogenous global incidence, including pcALCL, CD4+ SMPTC-LPD, CD8+ aggressive epidermotropic T-cell lymphoma (CD8+ AETCL; Berti's lymphoma), and primary cutaneous gamma/delta T-cell lymphoma (pcGDTCL) (Dobos et al. 2020). It is currently unknown to what degree unique regional genetics, environmental exposures, and underdiagnosis contribute to the worldwide heterogeneity of rare CTCL incidence.

In the United States, 3.1 people per 1,000,000 annually are diagnosed with CBCL (Bradford et al. 2009). The most common CBCL is primary cutaneous follicle center lymphoma (pcFCL, 12%), followed closely by primary cutaneous marginal zone lymphoma (pcMZL, 9%) and primary cutaneous diffuse large B-cell lymphoma, leg type (pcDLBCL-LT, 4%) (Willemze et al. 2019).

2.2 Race

Although the incidence of MF is higher among black people when compared to other ethnicities in the United States, rare PCLs show the opposite trend; CD30+ LPDs and CBCL are most often diagnosed in non-Hispanic Whites but least in Black, Hispanic, and Asian/Pacific Islander populations (Bradford et al. 2009). Significant data regarding race in other PCLs is not available due to rarity.

2.3 Gender

Men are diagnosed with rare CTCL more often than women by a factor of 1.2–2:1 (Bradford et al. 2009). Notable exceptions to this pattern include SPTCL and pcGDTCL (female predominance) (Bradford et al. 2009, Willemze et al. 2008) and LyP, which has a slight male predominance overall but a bimodal incidence in adults (female) and children (male) (ML G 2010, Wieser et al. 2016).

CBCL patients are also predominantly male [pcFCL (1.5:1); pcMZL (2:1)] (Bradford et al. 2009, Zinzani et al. 2006). Conflicting evidence exists for pcDLBCL; some studies report a strong female predominance (~0.6:1), but the largest study of 3,884 PCL cases in the United States based on Surveillance, Epidemiology, and End Results (SEER) program data reported a male predominance of 1.7:1 (Bradford et al. 2009, Grange et al. 2007, Kodama et al. 2005, Senff et al. 2007, Zinzani et al. 2006).

2.4 Age

Incidence increases with age. Adults are almost exclusively affected in most rare PCLs (Bradford et al. 2009). CBCLs are 40 times less common in children than adults and frequently resolve spontaneously and rarely require treatment in children (Bomze et al. 2021). In contrast, LyP most often affects adults but occurs at a notably wider age range; the youngest case reported was at eight months and oldest at 88 years (Bekkenk et al. 2000).

3) What should be included in the workup for primary cutaneous lymphomas?

Expert Perspective: PCLs all present heterogeneously but may share overlapping features. Additionally, there are no single pathognomonic findings for any rare PCL; however, some features are more specific than others. As a result, diagnosis requires clinicopathologic correlation; that is, the combination of clinical, histologic, genetic, and immunologic features is unique to each PCL, and careful consideration of each "puzzle piece" is ultimately key to the best diagnosis, management, and outcome. To accomplish this goal, a careful history and physical examination must be taken. Clinical pictures are helpful to trend disease and assess whether a change in management is required months or years from the initial assessment, as with most chronic dermatologic disease. One or more biopsies must be taken from involved skin most representative of disease. Definitive diagnosis requires histopathologic analysis in addition to considerate selection of immunophenotypic markers for staining (Tables 48.2a and 2b) according to the clinically suspected lymphoma.

Standard laboratory studies to further assess disease extent include a complete blood count with differential, and complete metabolic panel with lactose dehydrogenase (LDH) should be taken. Should erythrodermic CTCL be in the differential diagnosis, a flow cytometry of peripheral blood focused on Sézary syndrome specific markers should be ordered (Novelli et al. 2015). Relevant markers include high CD4:CD8 ratio (> 6:1), loss of CD5 and/or CD7 expression, and the percentage of CD4+/CD7− and/or CD4+/CD26− cells (Novelli et al. 2015). Appropriate imaging studies of the chest, abdomen, and pelvis are required to exclude skin involvement secondary to systemic disease in most cases, as lesions are confined to the skin by definition (Kempf et al. 2011). If lesions suspicious for extracutaneous disease are discovered, their biopsy and histologic analysis is required to rule out systemic involvement (Willemze 2005). Bone marrow biopsy is indicated if there is suspicion for systemic disease based on imaging and other laboratory data. Identification of a dominant (clonal) T- or B-cell population through determination of T-cell receptor (TCR) or B-cell receptor (BCR) clonality is a helpful yet binary diagnostic tool (Bruggemann et al. 2007, Kansal et al. 2018, Nollet et al. 2019, van Krieken et al. 2007). In the presence of correlative clinicopathologic evidence, positive clonality further supports CTCL or CBCL but does not rule them out if absent. Clonality also does not narrow down the differential diagnosis between PCLs because they each demonstrate clonality to varying degrees. Additionally, lymphocyte clonality is nonspecific to PCLs; benign dermatoses such as pseudolymphomas and reactive lymphoid proliferations may also demonstrate clonality (Arai et al. 2007).

4) How does each primary cutaneous lymphoma present?

Expert Perspective: Rare PCLs are difficult to diagnose in large part because they frequently mimic the most common CTCL (i.e. MF), other PCLs, and common dermatological conditions such as eczematous or autoimmune dermatitides, psoriasis, and other benign reactive infiltrates that mimic arthropod bite reactions (Kartan et al. 2019). Tables 48.2a and 2b summarize key clinicopathologic characteristics of each rare primary cutaneous lymphoma. The following are clinical and histopathologic pearls helpful for their diagnosis.

4.1 Location and quantity

Although exceptions exist for each, lesion locations follow the name: CD8+ acral T-cell lymphoma (acral CD8+ TCL) typically presents at acral sites, pcDLBCL, leg type on legs, and ENKTCL, nasal type in the nasal area. PCLs that are most often solitary are pcALCL, CD4+ SMPTC-LPD, acral CD8+ TCL, pcMZL, EBVMCU, and pcDLBCL-LT. Others are typically multifocal or disseminated (Tables 48.2a, 2b, 3a, and 3b).

4.2 Ulceration

PCLs that ulcerate also typically express cytotoxic granules (Tables 48.2a and 2b), most often in aggressive types; however, ulceration can be observed in the indolent SPTCL.

If an indolent PCL develops ulceration, the diagnosis should be reevaluated. For example, CD8+ pcAETCL often initially presents with MF-like plaques; however, they more frequently ulcerate and unlike MF generally do not respond to skin-directed therapy and ultimately progress (Berti et al. 1999).

4.3 CD30+ lymphoproliferative disorders

LyP and pcALCL represent two polar ends of the CD30+ LPD spectrum. LyP typically presents with recurrent, spontaneously resolving crops of ulceronecrotic, papulonodular lesions that coexist in varying states of evolution (Figure 48.1a), while pcALCL typically presents as a solitary ulceronecrotic tumor (Figure 48.1c). In contrast to LyP, spontaneous remission occurs in only 50% of pcALCL cases and is less often multifocal (20%) (Liu et al. 2003, Weaver et al. 2010). In the middle of this spectrum, borderline lesions share clinicopathologic features of both entities and are initially difficult to differentiate (Figure 48.1b) (Kartan et al. 2019). The true nature of these ambiguous lesions is revealed by their clinical behavior over time.

LyP has six histologic subtypes (Table 48.4) that may present concomitantly in the same patient but have no prognostic significance between them. Each subtype characteristically shares a similar histopathology to another PCL; for example, LyP subtype B resembles patch/plaque-stage MF and subtype D resembles CD8+ pcAETCL. Unlike the PCLs they mimic histologically, all subtypes demonstrate spontaneous remission clinically.

4.4 SPTCL and pcGDTCL

SPTCL presents with painful, subcutaneous nodules or deeply seated plaques (Figure 48.2a) that resolve with lipoatrophy (Figure 48.2b–c) and histopathology that shows malignant lymphocytes either in sheets or rimming adipocytes, often sparing the epidermis and dermis (Table 48.2a) (Willemze et al. 2019). SPTCL was initially characterized by a 1991 11-patient case series with two subtypes based on TCR expression: SPTL-AB (TCR α/β) and SPTL-GD (TCR γ/δ) (Gonzalez et al. 1991). Over time, it was recognized that SPTL-GD patients had a poorer prognosis and lesions that ulcerated more often (Hoque et al. 2003, Salhany et al. 1998, Willemze 2005). A 2008 report suggested a distinction, and a subsequent update to the WHO-EORTC classification clearly distinguished SPTL-AB from SPTL-GD, now SPTCL and pcGDTCL, respectively (Willemze et al. 2019, 2008).

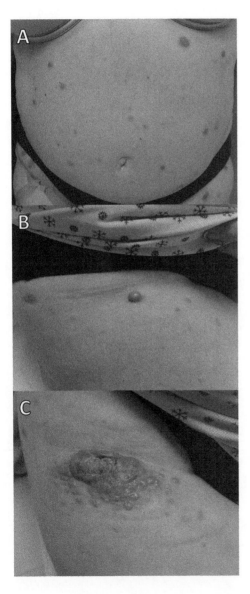

Figure 48.1 Clinical presentation of CD30+ lymphoproliferative disorder (CD30+ LPD) with concomitant lymphomatoid papulosis (LyP) and primary cutaneous anaplastic large cell lymphoma (pcALCL). In LyP (a), crops of papular lesions in different stages of evolution are seen simultaneously. New papules or nodules (b) can demonstrate clinicopathologic features of both LyP and pcALCL. Follow-up clarifies the nature of such lesions; this nodule evolved into a large ulceronecrotic tumor over several months, typical of pcALCL (c).

Figure 48.2 Clinical presentation of subcutaneous panniculitis-like T-cell lymphoma (SPTCL). Subcutaneous nodules represent disease (a), and lipoatrophy may be seen after lesion resolution (b, c).

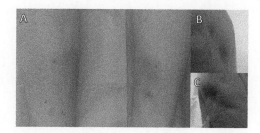

pcGDTCL typically presents as disseminated ulceronecrotic tumors/plaques with B-symptoms, hemophagocytic syndrome, and extracutaneous disease at diagnosis. However, it may alternatively present with an initially indolent course and SPTCL- or MF-mimicking lesions (Figure 48.3a, b) that eventually become aggressive (Figure 48.3c) (Caudron et al. 2011, Endly et al. 2013, Hosler et al. 2008, Vin et al. 2014).

Prognosis is worse for the 15–20% of SPTCL patients with concomitant hemophagocytic syndrome (five-year survival 46% vs 91%), requiring more aggressive treatment (Willemze et al. 2008). In contrast, hemophagocytic syndrome occurs more often in pcGDTCL (50%) but has no effect on its already dismal prognosis (five-year survival: 11%) (Foppoli and Ferreri 2015, Toro et al. 2003, Willemze et al. 2019). It is debated whether pcGDTCL patients with isolated subcutaneous involvement suffer a worse prognosis (Goyal et al. 2021, Khallaayoune et al. 2020, Merrill et al. 2017). Both SPTCL and pcGDTCL should be considered in the differential diagnosis for panniculitides, as they may mimic common panniculitides such as lupus panniculitis and erythema nodosum.

4.5 CD4+ SMPTC-LPD and acral CD8+ TCL

CD4+ SMPTC-LPD usually presents as a solitary plaque/nodule on face, neck, or upper trunk (Figure 48.4). It was recently recategorized from a lymphoma to a lymphoproliferative disorder due to its consistently indolent nature. Likewise, acral CD8+ TCL is also indolent in nature and presents with a solitary papule/nodule but exclusively at acral sites (ears/nose/feet). Both demonstrate an excellent survival rate (five-year OS: 100%) and thus must be differentiated from more aggressive lymphomas that share clinicopathologic features; these include cutaneous follicular T-helper lymphomas and other CD8+ TCLs such as CD8+ pcAETCL (Willemze et al. 2019).

4.6 PTCL-NOS

PTCL-NOS is an umbrella term given to T-cell lymphomas that do not better fit clinical and histopathologic criteria of another PCL entity (Willemze et al. 2019). Four better defined and previously mentioned subtypes of pcPTCL-NOS were recently added as provisional entities to the WHO-EORTC classification: CD8+ AETCL, pcGDTCL, CD4+ SMPTC-LPD, and acral CD8+ TCL. Notably, up to 22% of PTCL-NOS involves the skin as an extranodal site, but its frequency as a primary cutaneous entity (pcPTCL-NOS) is unknown (Oh et al. 2021, Weisenburger et al. 2011). As a diagnosis of exclusion, its histologic and

Table 48.2a Indolent cutaneous T-cell lymphomas: clinical, pathologic, and treatment differences.

| | Indolent CTCL | | | PTCL, NOS group | |
| | CD30+ LPD spectrum | | SPTCL | | |
	LyP	PC-ALCL		PC CD4+ SMPTC-LPD	PC acral CD8+ TCL
Clinical					
Typical Patient	Female adult or male child	Male adult	Female adult	Adult, either sex	Male adult
Lesion Key findings	Chronic, recurrent crops of papules/ nodules; spontaneous resolution in 3–8 weeks	Solitary (80%) or multifocal (20%) rapidly growing nodules/tumors that commonly ulcerate; spontaneous resolution rare	Multiple (80%) or single (20%) painless subcutaneous nodule(s) or poorly circumscribed plaques on extremities, trunk, and/or face; ulceration rare	Solitary, rarely generalized plaque/ tumor on face, neck, upper trunk	Solitary, occasionally multiple/bilateral papule(s)/ nodule(s) on an acral site (ear, nose, foot)
May be associated with	Comorbid lymphoma (20%)		Comorbid autoimmune disease (20%) B symptoms, HLH		
May closely mimic	PC-ALCL(borderline cases)	LyP(borderline cases)	Panniculitides, i.e.:1. Erythema nodosum2. Lupus panniculitis 3. Subacute migratory panniculitis	PTCL, NOS	1. PCFCL2. FMF3. cutaneous B-cell pseudolymphoma

Lymphocyte Pathology						
Histopathology						
Epidermotropism	Varies by subtype	Varies by subtype	Rare	Rare	Negative	Negative with Grenz zone
Key morphology findings	Varies by subtype	Varies by subtype	Dense clusters or sheets of large anaplastic cells	Fat cell rimming with atypical lymphocytes of varying size, typically sparing dermis, epidermis ± fat necrosis, karyorrhexis	Dense, diffuse or nodular dermal ± subdermal infiltrate	Diffuse CD8+ monomorphous medium size blasts in dermis and subcutis
May closely mimic	Varies by subtype	Varies by subtype	CD30+ transformed MF; Systemic ALCL; LyP	PTCL, NOS; Tumor-stage MF; GDTCL	PTCL, NOS	
Immunophenotype						
Typically positive	CD4, CD30, CLA, cytotoxic proteins	CD4, CD30, CLA, cytotoxic proteins	Beta TCR, CD3, CD8, cytotoxic proteins	CD3, CD4, TFH markers	CD3, CD8, TIA-1, CD68	
Positive or negative	Varies by subtype	Varies by subtype	Pan-T cell antigens, TCR	Pan-T cell antigens	Pan-T cell antigens	Pan-T cell antigens, cytotoxic proteins
Typically negative	Varies by subtype	Varies by subtype	EMA, ALK	Delta TCR, CD4, CD56	CD8, CD30, cytotoxic proteins	CD4, granzyme-B, CD30
Molecular						
TCR/BCR clonality	~40–100%	Almost always	Almost always, if expressed	Almost always	Almost always	Almost always
Genetic aberration	DUSP22-IRF4 at 6p25.3	–	–	HAVCR2	–	–
EBV/EBER positivity	–	–	–	–	–	–

(Continued)

Table 48.2a (Continued)

| | Indolent CTCL | | | PTCL, NOS group | |
| | CD30+ LPD spectrum | | | | |
	LyP	PC-ALCL	SPTCL	PC CD4+ SMPTC-LPD	PC acral CD8+ TCL
Treatment	Does not vary by subtype1st line: Low-dose MTX or observationScarring lesions: PUVA, local chemotherapy	Localized: Excision, LRTMultifocal skin lesions: low-dose MTX, brentuximab-vedotinExtracutaneous: multi-agent ChT	Solitary: LRTMultifocal, no HLH: Systemic steroid, immunosuppressive agents (cyclosporin/MTX) Aggressive, refractory, or HLH: multi-agent ChT	Observation LRT or excision	Observation LRT or excision

Abbreviations:

CTCL: cutaneous T-cell lymphoma; LyP: lymphomatoid papulosis; PC: primary cutaneous; LCL: primary cutaneous anaplastic large cell lymphoma; SMPTC-LPD: small/medium pleomorphic T-cell lymphoproliferative disorder; TCL: T cell lymphoma; ENKTCL: extranodal NK/T-cell lymphoma, nasal type; PTCL: peripheral T-cell lymphoma; NOS: not otherwise specified; GDTCL: gamma/delta T-cell lymphoma; AECTCL: aggressive epidermotropic cutaneous T-cell lymphoma; CAEBV: chronic active Epstein Barr virus infection; HV-like LPD: hydroa vacciniforme LPD; HLH: hemophagocytic lymphohistiocytosis; MF: mycosis fungoides; CLA: cutaneous lymphocyte antigen; EMA: epithelial membrane antigen; ALK: anaplastic lymphoma kinase; TCR: T-cell receptor; ChT: chemotherapy; LRT: localized radiotherapy; SMILE: dexamethasone, methotrexate, ifosfamide, L-asparaginase and etoposide; HSCT: hematopoietic stem cell transplant.

Definitions:

Pan-T cell antigens: CD2, CD5, CD7. Antigens that define a T-cell immunophenotype.
TFH (Follicular helper T-cell) antigen profile includes PD-1, CXCL13, BCL-6.
Cytotoxic proteins: granzyme B, perforin, T-cell restricted intracellular antigen 1 (TIA-1).
B-symptoms: Fever, night sweats, weight loss.

ESMO clinical practice guidelines:

D'Amore, F., et al. (2015). "Peripheral T-cell lymphomas: ESMO Clinical Practice Guidelines for diagnosis, treatment and follow-up." *Annals of Oncology 26* (suppl 5): v108–v115.
Willemze, R., et al. (2018). "Primary cutaneous lymphomas: ESMO Clinical Practice Guidelines for diagnosis, treatment and follow-up." *Annals of Oncology 29* (Suppl 4): iv30–iv40.

National Cancer Care Network Guidelines:
National Comprehensive Cancer Care Network. Primary Cutaneous Lymphomas (2021). "Primary Cutaneous Lymphomas (Version 2.2021)." Accessed from https://www.nccn.org/guidelines/guidelines-detail?category=1&id=1491.

Table 48.2b Aggressive cutaneous T-cell lymphomas: clinical, pathologic, and treatment differences.

		Aggressive CTCL				
			PTCL, NOS group			
		PC-ENKTCL, nasal type	PC-PTCL, NOS	PC-GDTCL	CD8+ AECTCL	Cutaneous T-cell CAEBV(HV-like LPD, HMB)
Clinical	Typical patient	Male adult	Male adult	Female adult	Male adult	Female adult
	Lesion / Key findings	Multiple ulcerating plaques/nodules most commonly on the nose	Solitary or multiple plaques, nodules, or tumors at any skin site	Disseminated, ulceronecrotic nodules, plaques, or tumors on extremities; may initially be indolent	Disseminated, rarely solitary1. papules/nodules/tumors ± central ulceronecrosis2. Hyperkeratotic patches/plaques	Cutaneous manifestations:1. Hydroa vacciniforme–like lymphoproliferative disorder2. Hypersensitivity to mosquito bitesMust be 6+ mo. of symptoms
	May be associated with	Nasopharyngeal or visceral involvement		HLH	Prodrome of chronic patches	Systemic manifestations, includingB-symptoms, HLH
	May closely mimic	CAEBV	Any CTCL	1. MF2. SPTCL	MF	Hydroa vacciniforme Allergic reaction to mosquito bite

(Continued)

Table 48.2b (Continued)

	Aggressive CTCL	PTCL, NOS group			
Lymphocyte Pathology	PC-ENKTCL, nasal type	PC-PTCL, NOS	PC-GDTCL	CD8+ AECTCL	Cutaneous T-cell CAEBV(HV-like LPD, HMB)
Histopathology					
Epidermotropism	Negative	Varies	May occur	Positive	Negative
Key morphologyfindings	Diffuse infiltrate of normal and abnormal lymphocytes of varying size ± coagulative necrosis, angiodestruction	Nodular or diffuse infiltrate of variably sized pleomorphic cells ± central ulceration	Epidermal, dermal, or subcutis infiltrate ± angiocentricity/destruction, necrosis	Early: Lichenoid with epidermotropism and subepidermal edemaLate: Diffuse dermal infiltrate ± necrosis, ulceration, angiocentricity/invasion	HV-like LPD: epidermal spongiosis, vesiculation, necrosis over a dense dermal infiltrate of EBER + acute and chronic inflammatory cells HMB: angiocentric infiltrate of EBER + atypical lymphocytes
May closely mimic	NK cell leukemialymphomatoid granulomatosisPTCL, NOS	Any CTCL	PTCL, NOStumor-stage MFSPTCL	LyP type DCD8+ MFPC acral CD8+ TCL	Hydroa vacciniforme angiocentric lymphoma
Immunophenotype					
Typically positive	Cytoplasmic CD3, CD2, CD56, cytotoxic proteins	Varies	Delta TCR, CD2, CD3, CD56, cytotoxic proteins	Beta TCR, CD3, CD8, CD45RA, cytotoxic proteins	Pan T- or NK-cell antigens
Positive or negative	CD4, CD7, CD8, CD30	Varies	Beta TCR	CD2, CD7, CD30, CD45RA	
Typically negative	Surface CD3, CD8, TCR	Varies	CD4, CD5, CD8	CD4, CD5, CD45RO	
Molecular					
TCR/BCR clonality	No	Varies	Almost always	Almost always	Varies
Genetic aberration	No; germline NK cell configuration	Varies	–	–	DDX3X
EBV/EBER positivity	+	Varies	–	–	+

| | Treatment | Frail patient and/or small, solitary lesion: LRTOtherwise: LRT + combined modality therapy with ChT containing L-asparaginase (ex: SMILE) | | | Palliative: High-dose systemic corticosteroid, ganciclovir + HDACi/ bortezomibCurative: HSCTRelapse: Donor-derived virus-specific T cells |

Abbreviations:

CTCL: cutaneous T-cell lymphoma; LyP: lymphomatoid papulosis; PC: primary cutaneous; ALCL: primary cutaneous anaplastic large cell lymphoma; SMPTC-LPD: small/ medium pleomorphic T-cell lymphoproliferative disorder; TCL: T-cell lymphoma; ENKTCL: extranodal NK/T-cell lymphoma, nasal type; PTCL: peripheral T-cell lymphoma; NOS: not otherwise specified; GDTCL: gamma/delta T-cell lymphoma; AECTCL: aggressive epidermotropic cutaneous T-cell lymphoma; CAEBV: chronic active Epstein Barr virus infection; HV-like LPD: hydroa vacciniforme LPD; HLH: hemophagocytic lymphohistiocytosis; MF: mycosis fungoides; CLA: cutaneous lymphocyte antigen; EMA: epithelial membrane antigen; ALK: anaplastic lymphoma kinase; TCR: T-cell receptor; ChT: chemotherapy; LRT: localized radiotherapy; SMILE: dexamethasone, methotrexate, ifosfamide, L-asparaginase, and etoposide; HSCT: hematopoietic stem cell transplant.

Definitions:

Pan-T cell antigens: CD2, CD5, CD7. Antigens that define a T-cell immunophenotype.

TFH (Follicular helper T-cell) antigen profile includes PD-1, CXCL13, BCL-6.

Cytotoxic proteins: granzyme B, perforin, T-cell restricted intracellular antigen 1 (TIA-1).

B-symptoms: Fever, night sweats, weight loss.

ESMO clinical practice guidelines: D'Amore, F., et al. (2015). "Peripheral T-cell lymphomas: ESMO Clinical Practice Guidelines for diagnosis, treatment and follow-up." *Annals of Oncology* 26 (suppl 5): v108–v115.

Willemze, R., et al. (2018). "Primary cutaneous lymphomas: ESMO Clinical Practice Guidelines for diagnosis, treatment and follow-up." *Annals of Oncology* 29 (Suppl 4): iv30–iv40.

National Cancer Care Network Guidelines:
National Comprehensive Cancer Care Network. Primary Cutaneous Lymphomas (2021). "Primary Cutaneous Lymphomas (Version 2.2021)." Accessed from https://www.nccn.org/ guidelines/guidelines-detail?category=1&id=1491.

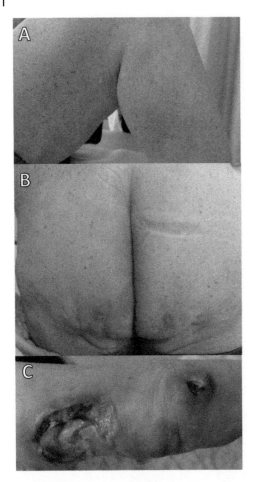

Figure 48.3 Clinical examples of primary cutaneous gamma/delta T-cell lymphoma (pcGDTCL). Lesions are frequently disseminated and initially appear similar to subcutaneous panniculitis-like T-cell lymphoma or mycosis fungoides (a, b). Advanced disease (c) consists of multifocal inflamed, deeply ulcerated, necrotic treatment-refractory nodules.

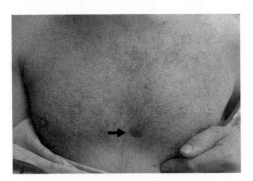

Figure 48.4 Clinical presentation of CD4+ small/medium pleomorphic T-cell lymphoproliferative disorder (CD4+ SMPTC-LPD), showing a small solitary circular plaque with well-demarcated borders.

immunohistochemical studies are nonspecific. However, its clinical course tends to be aggressive and portends a poor prognosis (five-year OS: 15%). They may initially be misdiagnosed as classical CTCL until an uncharacteristically rapid, progressive course is observed (see Chapter 40).

4.7 CD8+ pcAETCL

CD8+ pcAETCL is an exceptionally rare and provisional entity in the WHO-EORTC classification that presents with disseminated nodules and plaques that tend to ulcerate (Figure 48.5). It is most often refractory to treatments typically given for MF and has a poor prognosis (five-year OS: 31%) (Willemze et al. 2019).

4.8 ENKTCL-NT

ENKTCL is an aggressive EBV-associated malignancy that presents with ulcerating plaques/tumors most frequently in the nasopharyngeal and aerodigestive tracts (Figure 48.6). The skin and subcutaneous tissues are common sites for secondary spread; primary cutaneous ENKTCL-NT is rare. Like pcDLBCL-LT, this lymphoma may occur anywhere on the skin despite its name. Prognosis is dismal (five-year OS: 16%) (Willemze et al. 2019).

4.9 CAEBV

CAEBV is a chronic manifestation of Epstein-Barr virus (EBV) infection lasting at least six months (Kimura 2006). It is rare in the United States but primarily reported in East Asia and Latin America, suggesting a genetic component (Kimura and Cohen 2017). Cutaneous

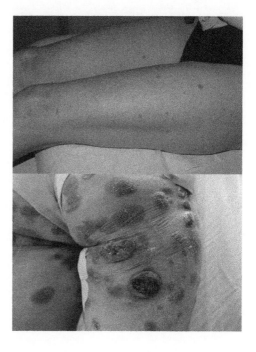

Figure 48.5 Clinical presentation of primary cutaneous aggressive epidermotropic CD8+ T cell lymphoma (AETCL), showing early disseminated papules and small plaques that eventually evolved into occasionally ulceronecrotic plaques, nodules, and tumors.

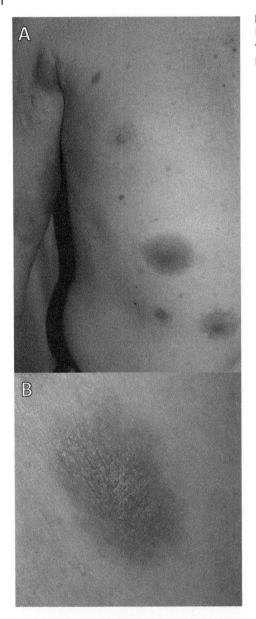

Figure 48.6 Clinical example of extranodal NK/T-cell lymphoma, nasal type (ENKTCL-NT) with disseminated, violaceous nodules (a) and plaques (b) that tend to ulcerate.

manifestations are usually secondary to systemic involvement and include hydroa vacciniforme–like lymphoproliferative disorder (Figure 48.7; HV-like LPD) and hypersensitivity to mosquito bites (HMB). Unlike systemic CAEBV, both primary cutaneous variants have a good prognosis and more often affect young female adults (Miyake et al. 2015). However, they carry a significant risk for systemic progression (Yamada et al. 2021).

Progression to systemic involvement carries a grim prognosis. Presentation may include hemophagocytic syndrome, B-symptoms (fever, night sweats, weight loss), and various

Figure 48.7 Clinical presentation of hydroa vacciniforme–like lymphoproliferative disorder (HV-like LPD), a cutaneous manifestation of chronic active Epstein Barr virus infection (CAEBV) showing small hemorrhagic and/or crusted papules and vesicles.

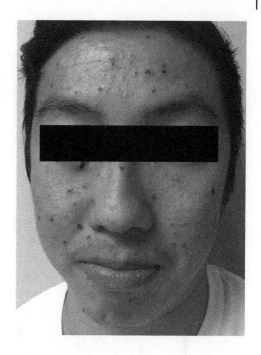

manifestations of atypical EBV+ T-cell tissue infiltration: rapid cognitive decline, neurological deficits, liver failure, and/or coronary artery aneurysm(s) (Kimura and Cohen 2017).

4.10 Cutaneous B-cell lymphomas

pcMZL (Figure 48.8) and pcFCL both present as erythematous-violaceous plaques, nodules, and/or tumors. Both may present on the trunk, but pcMZL is more commonly found multifocally on the extremities, while pcFCL is more commonly found as a solitary lesion on the head (Willemze et al. 2019). Table 48.3a further describes differentiating histologic and immunohistochemical characteristics.

pcDLBCL-LT is aggressive and typically presents as a solitary erythematous/bluish nodule or tumor on the lower legs (Table 48.3b). However, up to 10–15% of cases occur at other sites (Figure 48.9) (Senff et al. 2007). Extracutaneous involvement of pcDLBCL-LT occurs more frequently than pcMZL or pcFCL.

EBVMCU is a self-limiting, localized manifestation of EBV lymphoproliferative disorder that occurs in the setting of iatrogenic, immunosenescent, or primary immunosuppression after local trauma (Roberts et al. 2015). It typically presents as a solitary ulcer in an older patient on common immunosuppressants (methotrexate, steroid-sparing agents, TNF inhibitors, or topical steroids) after local trauma (Dojcinov et al. 2018, Ikeda et al. 2021).

Intravascular large B-cell lymphoma (ILBCL) presents similarly to CAEBV with severe systemic symptoms, rapid cognitive decline, a T-cell phenotype, and EBV positivity.

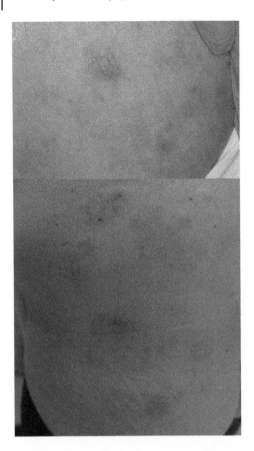

Figure 48.8 Clinical examples of primary cutaneous marginal zone lymphoma (pcMZL). Lesions are typically non-scaling grouped violaceous patches and/or plaques that demonstrate confluency.

However, lesion and histologic morphology differs; small, HV-like lesions with extravasated atypical lymphocytic tissue infiltrates are most often seen in CAEBV, while ILBCL presents with larger, multifocal, violaceous lesions and its eponymous intravascular atypical lymphocytes on histopathology (Kimura and Cohen 2017, Ponzoni et al. 2018).

5) How are rare primary cutaneous lymphomas staged?

Expert Perspective: The de facto staging system for all NHL is the anatomic Ann Arbor system, augmented by the International Prognostic Index (IPI) in 1993 to help guide treatment decisions (International Non-Hodgkin's Lymphoma Prognostic Factors P 1993) However, it under- or overemphasizes the prognostic implications of otherwise aggressive or indolent features in rare PCL, respectively. For example, indolent PCLs that present with multiple lesions (ie, LyP) are erroneously advanced stage (IVB), while an aggressive PCL with one lesion (ie, pcDLBCL-LT) is early stage (IE). The nonspecificity of Ann Arbor-IPI fails to stratify risk and prognosis for accurate comparison between PCLs.

In response to the recognized lack of utlity from previous staging systems, the Tri-Societies [International Society for Cutaneous Lymphomas (ISCL), the United States Cutaneous Lymphoma Consortium (USCLC), and the Cutaneous Lymphoma Task Force of the European Organization for Research and Treatment of Cancer (EORTC)] proposed a standardized TNM staging and clinical trial design system for rare PCLs in 2022, itself an

Table 48.3a Indolent cutaneous B-cell lymphomas: clinical, pathologic, and treatment differences.

		Indolent CBCL		
		PCMZL	PCFCL	EBVMCU
Clinical	Typical patient	Male adult	Elderly male	Elderly female
	Lesion	Solitary/grouped red/violaceous/brown papules, nodules, plaques, or tumors most often on extremities/trunk;frequent relapse, multifocal lesions more frequent	Solitary/grouped red/violaceous papules, nodules, plaques, or tumors most often on head or trunk ± acneiform lesions, erythematous background;multifocal lesions less frequent	Solitary sharply demarcated ulcerating lesion on skin, oropharyngeal mucosa, or GI tract in an immunosuppressed patient; self-limiting, relapse rare
	Key findings			
	May be associated with	*B. burgdorferi/afzelii* infection(strong association)	*B. burgdorferi/afzelii* infection(weak association)	Immunosuppression may be age-related, iatrogenic, or primary
	May closely mimic	PCFCL Reactive or clonal dermatoses Skin involvement of systemic MZL	PCMZL Reactive or clonal dermatosesSkin involvement of systemic FCL	PC-ALCLDDx for skin and mucosal ulcers

(Continued)

Table 48.3a (Continued)

		Indolent CBCL		
		PCMZL	PCFCL	EBVMCU
Lymphocyte Pathology	Histopathology			
	Epidermotropism	Negative with Grenz zone	Negative	Negative
	Key morphologyfindings	Nodular/diffuse infiltrate of small-medium lymphocytes, admixed reactive T cells, peripheral monotypic plasma cells ± reactive germinal centers, lymphoplasmacytoid cells (Dutcher, Russel bodies), monocytoid B cells	Diffuse/perivascular/periadnexal infiltrate of medium-large centrocytes in a follicular and/or diffuse pattern	Ulceration with Hodgkin- or Reed-Sternberg-like EBV+ B cells of all sizes at base sharply rimmed with reactive T cells in a mixed inflammatory background
	May closely mimic	Secondary extranodal B-cell NHL cutaneous lymphoid hyperplasia pseudolymphoma	PCDLBCL, LT secondary extranodal B-cell NHL cutaneous lymphoid hyperplasiapseudolymphoma	EBV+ DLBCL. Hodgkin lymphoma CD30+ T-cell LPD traumatic ulcerative granuloma with stromal eosinophilia
	Immunophenotype			
	Typically positive	CD20, CD22, CD79a, BCL2, cytoplasmic Ig light chain restriction Reactive germinal centers: BCL6, CD10	Pan B-cell antigens,BCL6	PAX5, IRF4/MUM1, CD30
	Positive or negative	CXCR3	CD10, cytoplasmic and monotypic surface Ig	CD20, CD15
	Typically negative	CD3, CD5, CD10, BCL6, CXCR3	BCL2, CD5, IRF4/MUM1	CD10, BCL6
	Molecular			
	TCR/BCR clonality	Almost always	Almost always	May occur
	Genetic aberration	FAS non-class-switched: MYD88	RELDel 14q32.33	None
	EBV/EBER positivity	-	-	+

| Treatment | EORTC/ISCL guidelines:Solitary: LRT, excision, systemic antibiotic against *B. burgdorferi*Multifocal: observational, low-dose LRT, systemic antibiotic against *B. burgdorferi*, intralesional steroids, single-agent rituximabRefractory: Single or combination ChT | Conservative: observation, wound careIatrogenic: reduce immunosuppressive therapy.Persistent/debilitating: CD20 or CD30 antibody therapy, LRT, excision, ChT |

Abbreviations:

CBCL: cutaneous B-cell lymphoma; PCMZL: primary cutaneous marginal zone lymphoma; PCFCL: primary cutaneous follicle center lymphoma; PCDLBCL, LT: primary cutaneous diffuse large B-cell lymphoma, leg type; BCL: B-cell lymphoma; HLH: hemophagocytic lymphohistiocytosis; CNS: central nervous system; MF: mycosis fungoides; CLA: cutaneous lymphocyte antigen; EMA: epithelial membrane antigen; ALK: anaplastic lymphoma kinase; TCR: T-cell receptor; BCR: B-cell receptor; ChT: chemotherapy; LRT: localized radiotherapy; SMILE: dexamethasone, methotrexate, ifosfamide, L-asparaginase, and etoposide; HSCT: hematopoietic stem cell transplant.

Definitions:

B-symptoms: fever, night sweats, weight loss.
Cytotoxic proteins: granzyme B, perforin, TIA-1.
Pan-B cell antigens: CD19, CD20, CD22, CD79a. Antigens that define a B-cell immunophenotype.Beta TCR expression is synonymous with beta-F1 positivity.

ESMO clinical practice guidelines: D'Amore, F., et al. (2015). "Peripheral T-cell lymphomas: ESMO Clinical Practice Guidelines for diagnosis, treatment and follow-up." *Annals of Oncology* 26 (suppl 5): v108–v115.Willemze, R., et al. (2018). "Primary cutaneous lymphomas: ESMO Clinical Practice Guidelines for diagnosis, treatment and follow-up." *Annals of Oncology* 29 (Suppl 4): iv30–iv40.

National Cancer Care Network Guidelines:
National Comprehensive Cancer Care Network. Primary Cutaneous Lymphomas (2021). "Primary Cutaneous Lymphomas (Version 2.2021)." Accessed from https://www.nccn. org/guidelines/guidelines-detail?category=1&id=1491.

Table 48.3b Aggressive cutaneous B-cell lymphomas: clinical, pathologic, and treatment differences.

		Aggressive CBCL	
		PCDLBCL, LT	ILBCL
Clinical	Typical Patient	Elderly adult	Elderly adult
	Lesion	Solitary/clustered red/brown nodules ± ulceration; most often on distal legs but uncommonly other sites	Multiple firm, red/purple/gray-blue ulcerating nodules, plaques, tumors, macules on trunk/thighs with telangiectasia Primary cutaneous form: young females; better prognosis
	Key findings		FUO B-symptoms HLH blood vessel occlusion:rapidly progressive CNS deficits
	May be associated with	B. burgdorferi/afzelii infection(weak association)	
	May closely mimic		Vascular lesionspanniculitidies
Lymphocyte Pathology	Histopathology		
	Epidermotropism	Negative	Negative
	Key morphologyfindings	Diffuse monotonous sheets of centroblasts/immunoblasts with few peripheral reactive T cells ± subcutis involvement	Large lymphoid cells in the lumen/endothelium of capillaries or post-capillary venules in any tissue, most commonly skin and brain
	May closely mimic	PCFCL, diffuse large cell growth pattern	Reactive inflammation endothelial vascular neoplasms intralymphatic histiocytosis
	Immunophenotype		
	Typically positive	Pan B-cell antigens,BCL2, IRF4/MUM1, FOXP1, MYC, cytoplasmic IgM	Pan B-cell antigens;rarely of T or NK cell origin
	Positive or negative	IgD, BCL6	PD-L1, CXCR5, CCR6, CCR7
	Typically negative	CD10	CD29, MMP-2, MMP-9
	Molecular		
	TCR/BCR clonality	May occur	May occur
	Genetic aberration	MYD88, MYC, CDNK2A/B, CARD11, CD79B, TNFAIP3/A20	MYD88, CD79B
	EBV/EBER positivity	–	+ (only in cases with HLH)

| Treatment | Solitary: LRT+ R-CHOPMultifocal: R-CHOP, Disseminated/recurrent: rituximab single agent | Primary cutaneous or systemic:R-CHOP, Solitary lesions or contraindication to ChT: LRT |

Abbreviatios:

CBCL: cutaneous B-cell lymphoma; PCMZL: primary cutaneous marginal zone lymphoma; PCFCL: primary cutaneous follicle center lymphoma; PCDLBCL: LT, primary cutaneous diffuse large B-cell lymphoma, leg type; BCL: B-cell lymphoma; HLH: hemophagocytic lymphohistiocytosis; CNS: central nervous system; MF: mycosis fungoides; CLA: cutaneous lymphocyte antigen; EMA: epithelial membrane antigen; ALK: anaplastic lymphoma kinase; TCR: T-cell receptor; BCR: B-cell receptor; ChT: chemotherapy; LRT: localized radiotherapy; SMILE: dexamethasone, methotrexate, ifosfamide, L-asparaginase, and etoposide; HSCT: hematopoeitic stem cell transplant.

Definitions:B-symptoms: fever, night sweats, weight loss.
Cytotoxic proteins: granzyme B, perforin, TIA-1.
Pan-B cell antigens: CD19, CD20, CD22, CD79a. Antigens that define a B-cell immunophenotype.Beta TCR expression is synonymous with beta-F1 positivity.

ESMO clinical practice guidelines: D'Amore, F., et al. (2015). "Peripheral T-cell lymphomas: ESMO Clinical Practice Guidelines for diagnosis, treatment and follow-up." *Annals of Oncology* 26 (suppl 5): v108–v115.Willemze, R., et al. (2018). "Primary cutaneous lymphomas: ESMO Clinical Practice Guidelines for diagnosis, treatment and follow-up." *Annals of Oncology* 29 (Suppl 4): iv30–iv40.

National Cancer Care Network Guidelines

Table 48.4 Lymphomatoid papulosis histologic subtypes.

LyP type	Relative frequency	Histopathology	Most common phenotype	Histopathologically mimics	Main differential diagnosis
A	> 80%	Initially non-epidermotropic, extensive, diffuse wedge-shaped large atypical lymphocytic infiltrate admixed with small lymphocytes, neutrophils, eosinophils and histiocytes	CD4+ CD8− CD30+	cHL	cHL pcALCLMF, tumor stage MF with CD30+ LCT
B	< 5%	Epidermotropic band-like distribution of small-medium atypical lymphocytes with cerebriform nuclei	CD4+ CD8− CD30-	MF, patch/plaque stage	MF, patch/plaque stage Epidermotropic pcGDTCL
C	10%	Epidermotropic monotonous sheets of large cells with mild mixed inflammatory infiltrate	CD4+ CD8− CD30+	pcALCL	pcALCL or sALCLMF with CD30+ LCT PTCL, NOS ATLL
D	< 5%	Epidermotropic small-medium atypical lymphoid infiltrate	CD4+ CD8+ CD30+ CD45RO+	CD8+ AETCL	CD8+ AETCL pagetoid reticulosis pcGDTCL PLC/PLEVA
E	< 5%	Angiocentric/destructive, pleomorphic small-medium lymphoid infiltrate with scattered large cells	CD4+ CD8+ CD30+ EBER-	ENKTCL	ENKTCL pcGDTCL pcALCL or sALCL

DUSP22-IRF44 rearrangement	< 5%	Biphasic growth pattern:1. Epidermotropic CD30− small-medium cerebriform lymphocytes 2. Dermal/periadnexal CD30+ atypical lymphocytes	CD4- CD8- CD30±	Pagetoid reticulosis	MF with CD30 + LCT LyP type C pcGDTCL ATLL pagetoid reticulosis
Rare subtypes Folliculotropic (proposed F)	N/A	Prominent hair follicle pathology associated with perifollicular infiltrate of atypical lymphocytes	CD4+ CD30+	FMF	FMF follicular mucinosis
Granulomatous		Noncaseating granulomas with perivascular/eccrinotropic/neurotropic mononuclear infiltrate and dermal lymphocytes ± subcutis involvement	CD4+ CD8- CD30+	SPTCL	SPTCL discoid lupus erythematosus Jessner lymphocytic infiltrate arthropod bite reactive dermatosis
Syringotropic		Periglandular infiltrate of eccrine units N/A		STMF	N/A

Abbreviations:

LyP: lymphomatoid papulosis; cHL: classic Hodgkin lymphoma; MF: mycosis fungoides; pcALCL: primary cutaneous anaplastic large cell lymphoma; sALCL: systemic anaplastic large cell lymphoma; PLC: pityriasis lichenoides chronica; PLEVA: pityriasis lichenoides et varioliformis acuta; ENKTCL: extranodal NK/T-cell lymphoma; LCT: large cell transformation; FMF: folliculotropic mycosis fungoides; SPTCL: subcutaneous panniculitis-like T-cell lymphoma; STMF: syringotropic mycosis fungoides; N/A: not available.

Sources:

1) Willemze, R., Cerroni, L., Kempf, W., et al. (2019). "The 2018 update of the WHO-EORTC classification for primary cutaneous lymphomas." *Blood* 133(16): 1703–1714.
2) de Masson, A., Battistella, M., Vignon-Pennamen, M.D., et al. (2014). "Syringotropic mycosis fungoides: clinical and histologic features, response to treatment, and outcome in 19 patients." *J Am Acad Dermatol* 71(5): 926–934.
3) Saggini, A., Gulia, A., Argenyi, Z., et al. (2010). "A variant of lymphomatoid papulosis simulating primary cutaneous aggressive epidermotropic CD8+ cytotoxic T-cell lymphoma. Description of 9 cases." *Am J Surg Pathol* 34(8): 1168–1175.
4) Crowson, A. N., Baschinsky, D.Y., Kovatich, A., et al. (2003). "Granulomatous eccrinotropic lymphomatoid papulosis." *Am J Clin Pathol* 119(5): 731–739.
5) de Souza, A., el-Azhary, R.A., Camilleri, M.J., et al. (2012). "In search of prognostic indicators for lymphomatoid papulosis: a retrospective study of 123 patients." *J Am Acad Dermatol* 66(6): 928–937.
6) Kempf, W., Kazakov, D.V., Baumgartner, H.P., et al. (2013). "Follicular lymphomatoid papulosis revisited: a study of 11 cases, with new histopathological findings." *J Am Acad Dermatol* 68(5): 809–816.
7) Kempf, W. (2017). "A new era for cutaneous CD30-positive T-cell lymphoproliferative disorders." *Semin Diagn Pathol* 34(1): 22–35.
8) Wieser, I., Oh, C.W., Talpur, R., et al. (2016). "Lymphomatoid papulosis: Treatment response and associated lymphomas in a study of 180 patients." *J Am Acad Dermatol* 74(1): 59–67.
9) McQuitty, E., Curry, J.L., Tetzlaff, M.T., et al. (2014). "The differential diagnosis of CD8-positive ('type D') lymphomatoid papulosis." *J Cutan Pathol* 41(2): 88–100.
10) Karai, L. J., Kadin, M.E., His E.D., et al. (2013). "Chromosomal rearrangements of 6p25.3 define a new subtype of lymphomatoid papulosis." *Am J Surg Pathol* 37(8): 1173–1181.

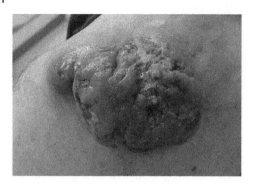

Figure 48.9   Clinical presentation of a large solitary primary cutaneous diffuse large B-cell lymphoma, leg type (pcDLBCL-LT), with ulceronecrotic debris and bleeding.

update to the first staging system for rare PCLs proposed in 2007 (Kim et al. 2007, Olsen et al. 2022). The updated TNM staging system is reproduced in Table 48.5. Moving forward, this collaboratively and internationally developed staging system allows for the collation of future clinical trial data that will ultimately result in the creation and approval of therapies with improved outcomes.

Per the 2022 TNM staging system, the diagnosis of all PCLs other than MF/SS requires clinicopathologic correlation with typical clinical features in the setting of representative skin lesion biopsy with typical histopathologic features. For patients with equivocal clinicopathologic findings, the diagnosis may be confirmed with molecular and/or immunophenotypic studies (clonality, pathogenic genomic variants). Staging with appropriate imaging is recommended for all rare PCL subtypes for clinical trial purposes. Lymph node and visceral lesion size should be initially assessed and reassessed with the same imaging technique for clinical trending and internal validity purposes. Acceptable imaging methods reported by the Tri-Societies include computed tomography (CT), positron emission tomography–computed tomography (PET-CT), magnetic resonance imaging, or ultrasound. In practice outside of clinical trials, staging with imaging is unnecessary for PCLs that typically display indolent behavior and a negligible risk of systemic involvement: CD4+ SMPTC-LPD, acral CD8+ TCL, and typical cases of LyP.

The 2022 updated staging proposal by Olsen et al. is recommended for further reading and information on preferred diagnostic methods, treatment response criteria, and tools for skin/lymph node/viscera assessment.

6) How do rare primary cutaneous lymphomas differ in aggressiveness and survival?

Expert Perspective: Table 48.1 shows five-year disease-specific survival for each PCL, based on patient data in the Dutch registry collected from 2008 to 2017 across participating European clinics (Willemze et al. 2019). Indolent PCLs have an excellent prognosis, with most five-year survival rates well over 90%, the lowest being SPTCL (87%) due to a subgroup that presents with HPS and worse prognosis (Willemze et al. 2008). Aggressive CTCLs demonstrate poorer five-year survival (11–31%) than aggressive CBCLs (53–72%).

Five-year survival rates were found to be stagnant in a 2009 study of 2880 PCL patients in SEER databases (870 of which had rare PCL) diagnosed in the 1990s and early 2000s

Table 48.5 TNM staging system for primary cutaneous lymphomas other than mycosis fungoides and Sézary syndrome.

2022 ISCL/USCLC/EORTC modified staging of non-MF/SS PCLs

T (Tumor)

    T1: Solitary lesion T0: Absence of clinically suspicious lesions[a]

        T1A: < 5 cm diameter

        T1B: ≥ 5 cm diameter

    T2: Regional skin involvement: multiple lesions limited to 1 body region or 2 contiguous body regions

        T2A: All disease encompassing in a < 15 cm diameter circular area

        T2B: All disease encompassing in a > 15 to < 30 cm diameter circular area

        T2C: All disease encompassing in a ≥ 30 cm diameter circular area

    T3: Generalized skin involvement

        T3A: multiple lesions involving 2 noncontiguous body regions

        T3B: multiple lesions involving ≥ 3 body regions

N (Node)

    N0: No clinical or pathologic lymph node involvement[b]

    N1: Involvement of 1 peripheral lymph node region that drains an area of current or prior skin involvement: biopsy positive for lymphoma

    N2: Involvement of ≥ 2 peripheral lymph node regions or involvement of any lymph node region that does not drain an area of current or prior skin involvement: biopsy positive for lymphoma

    N3: Involvement of central lymph nodes: biopsy positive for lymphoma

    Nx: Clinically abnormal peripheral or central LN but no pathologic determination. Other surrogate means of determining involvement may be determined by Tri-Society consensus

M (metastasis)

    M0: No visceral involvement

    M1: Visceral involvement

    Mx: Visceral involvement is neither confirmed nor refuted by available pathologic or imaging assessment

Source: Adapted from Olsen, E.A., Whittaker, S., Willemze, R., et al. (2022). Primary cutaneous lymphoma: recommendations for clinical trial design and staging update from the ISCL, USCLC, and EORTC. Blood 140 (5): 419–437. Permission conveyed through Copyright Clearance Center, Inc.

a) T0 is used for clinical trials in order to track clearance of lesions in the skin compartment. No patient with PCL at time of diagnosis should be T0.

b) Abnormal lymph nodes (LNs) are those now > 1.5 cm in the longest diameter (LDi) according to the Lugano classification and confirmed by imaging. The pathological findings of a representative abnormal LN may apply to all abnormal LNs. The revised nodal drainage areas for determination of classification of skin involvement in non-MF/non-SS PCLs are based on the Ann Arbor classification and thoroughly defined in the source material above.

(Bradford et al. 2009). However, no comprehensive survival study on PCLs has been done in the past five years. We project that five-year survival rates may increase over the next decade due to the recently expanded set of targeted therapy options (e.g. brentuximab-vedotin, durvalumab) with superior response rates to previous therapies for refractory/aggressive PCLs.

7) Have any risk factors or associations been identified for rare primary cutaneous lymphomas?

Expert Perspective: There are no identified risk factors for any PCLs. However, several important associations have been made between PCLs and genetic, environmental, autoimmune, and infectious factors.

7.1 Genetic

A 2019 genetic enrichment study identified rare germline *HAVCR2* mutations (p.Y82C and p.T101I) in patients of Asian ethnicity present in many SPTCL patients (Polprasert et al. 2019). Biallelic inheritance of either mutation leads to a nonfunctional gene product, HAVCR2 (also known as TIM-3), a negative immune checkpoint normally expressed on CD4+ and CD8+ T cells and myeloid cells. Reduced function of this negative feedback cycle may explain the pathophysiology of SPTCL, its response to immunosuppressive therapy, and its association with autoimmune disease and HPS. Thus, SPTCL is now thought to be a congenital disease with autosomal recessive inheritance. However, underlying autoimmune disease and somatic mutations in the PI3K/AKT/mTOR signaling pathway are common in SPTCL and may contribute to its pathogenesis. It is currently unknown if *HAVCR2* mutations are involved in the pathophysiology of other TCLs.

Regional heterogeneity in CAEBV incidence suggests a genetic predisposition (Fujiwara and Nakamura 2020). Two human leukocyte antigen (HLA) alleles common in East Asia and Mexico, A26 and B52, are positively and negatively associated with CAEBV, respectively (Kimura et al. 2012). Both are thought to be involved in its pathogenesis by allowing for or protecting against, respectively, an EBV-specific immunodeficiency that results in unchecked systemic EBV+ lymphoproliferation (Latour and Winter 2018). Germline mutations in several genes including CD27 and CD70 may contribute to dysfunctional EBV defense (Latour and Winter 2018).

7.2 Comorbidity

Preexisting autoimmune disease is seen in 20% of SPTCL patients, particularly systemic lupus erythematosus (Lopez-Lerma et al. 2018, Pincus et al. 2009, Willemze et al. 2008, Yi et al. 2013).

A hematological or non-hematological malignancy develops in 15–50% of patients with LyP, before, during, or after diagnosis, most commonly MF or pcALCL (Melchers et al. 2020). Risk factors may include older age, monoclonal TCR rearrangement, coexistent LyP histologic subtypes, subtypes B and C, fascin expression, or high blood levels of related markers (CD30, CD25, interleukin-6, interleukin-8) (Cordel et al. 2016, de Souza et al. 2012, Kadin et al. 2012, Kempf et al. 2002, Wieser et al. 2016).

7.3 Infectious

Associated infectious agents include Borrelia species, Epstein-Barr virus (EBV), and several other viruses including HIV and hepatitis C virus in case reports and series (Beylot-Barry et al. 1999, Campos and Zago Ferreira 2021, McGregor et al. 1993, Nagore et al. 2000, Peris et al. 1994, Viguier et al. 2002, Watabe et al. 2002).

Borrelia infection has a highly heterogenous regional prevalence and has been significantly associated with pcMZL in European but not American studies (Jelic and Filipovic-Ljeskovic 1999, Li et al. 2003, Wood et al. 2001). Genotypic differences in dominant Borrelia strains may account for regional heterogeneity (Wood et al. 2001).

EBV-associated PCLs include ENKTCL-NT; CAEBV; and some cases of pcPTCL-NOS and ILBCL (Tables 48.2 and 3) and may be secondary to regional, EBV-specific immunodeficiencies (Fujiwara and Nakamura 2020). Barring ATLL (human T-lymphotropic virus-1, HTLV-1), no other viruses have been significantly associated with PCLs outside of case reports.

7.4 Environmental

Environmental risk factors have not been identified for any rare PCL except ENKTCL-NT; a 2006 study demonstrated significantly increased odds ratios in those who work with pesticides and chemical solvents, such as farmers (Xu et al. 2007).

8) Which therapies are used in rare primary cutaneous lymphomas management, and how does the approach differ between indolent and aggressive PCLs?

Expert Perspective: Indolent PCLs often only require observation or skin-directed therapies, frequently including surgical excision or localized radiotherapy (RT). More aggressive or multifocal PCLs necessitate systemic immunotherapies, biologics, and/or multiagent chemotherapy; hematopoietic stem cell transplant is the only curative option. Full guidelines for the diagnosis and treatment of primary cutaneous lymphomas are available from the National Cancer Care Network (NCCN) and the European Society of Medical Oncology (ESMO) and are frequently updated (Network NCC 2021a, Willemze et al. 2018).

8.1 Cutaneous T-cell lymphomas

8.1.1 CD30+ LPDs (LyP and pcALCL)

In LyP, lesions usually spontaneously resolve without intervention over 8–12 weeks. Therefore, most LyP patients do not require treatment (Kluk et al. 2016). Though no therapy is curative or alters disease course, the goal of treatment for symptomatic/widespread LyP is to induce remission and control symptoms. When necessary, commonly used skin-directed options include narrowband (nb-) UVB phototherapy, psoralen and ultraviolet light A (PUVA) photochemotherapy, intralesional interferon-alpha (IFN-α), bexarotene gel, imiquimod, topical chemotherapy, and radiation therapy (Di Raimondo et al. 2020). Topical and intralesional corticosteroids have a transient effect with little benefit. Systemic options include oral low-dose methotrexate (MTX; 15–30 mg weekly), doxycycline (QD, 100 mg). Brentuximab-vedotin (BV) is not recommended in most instances because its potential benefits are outweighed by significant side effects, including peripheral neuropathy (Prince et al. 2017). However, in treatment-refractory cases with extensive involvement, NCCN guidelines recommend BV or clinical trial participation. Patients typically relapse upon cessation of any treatment.

Phototherapy is associated with a lower risk for early cutaneous relapse when compared to other first-line therapies (MTX, corticosteroids) (Fernández-De-Misa et al. 2018).

Compared to nbUVB, PUVA has a superior overall response rate and quicker lesion size reduction but a relatively increased risk of cataract formation, photoaging, and skin cancers (Fernández-De-Misa et al. 2018).

Likewise, no aggressive treatments are typically necessary for pcALCL. First-line and well-tolerated modalities for localized pcALCL treatment include surgical resection, localized RT, and intralesional corticosteroids (Million et al. 2016, Querfeld et al. 2010, Specht et al. 2015). Recommended localized RT dosage varies between 20 and 30 Grays (Gy) (Melchers et al. 2017, Million et al. 2016). Combining excision with LRT is not recommended because it yields no synergistic benefit (Liu et al. 2003).

For multifocal or relapsed pcALCL, options include oral bexarotene, low-dose MTX, or BV. Patients presenting with less than five lesions may be treated with low-dose localized RT (8 Gy over two fractions) (Melchers et al. 2017, Prince et al. 2017). Multiagent chemotherapy has not been proven superior to single-agent chemotherapy for pcALCL; both are reserved for treatment-refractory, aggressive disease (Kempf et al. 2011). Response information for allogeneic hematopoietic stem cell transplantation (allo-HSCT) is limited to small case series (Oka et al. 2016, Saruta et al. 2017, Wehkamp et al. 2015).

8.1.2 CD4+ SMPTC-LPD and acral CD8+ TCL

CD4+ SMPTC-LPD and acral CD8+ TCL both respond exceptionally well to skin-directed therapies due to their indolent nature as solitary lesions (Li et al. 2014, Virmani et al. 2016). Options include LRT, excision, and intralesional steroids. Relapses are uncommon but are successfully retreated with the same skin-directed therapies. Spontaneous remission may occur after biopsy of CD4+ SMPTC-LPD, after which only observation is warranted (Keeling et al. 2017). Excellent prognosis and absence of extracutaneous or disseminated disease suggests that aggressive therapy is not required for either entity.

8.1.3 SPTCL

SPTCL was historically managed with anthracycline-based multiagent chemotherapy, radiation, and/or allo-HSCT, but response rates were poor (Go and Wester 2004). Several studies have since found that patients respond to immunosuppressive therapies, bexarotene, and/or localized RT similarly to or better than multiagent chemotherapy (Willemze et al. 2008).

Oral corticosteroids and/or other immunosuppressive agents (cyclosporine A, low-dose MTX, hydroxychloroquine) have achieved complete responses (CRs) approaching 85%, often significantly superior to multiagent chemotherapy (Lopez-Lerma et al. 2018, Michonneau et al. 2017, Willemze et al. 2008). Responses to corticosteroid monotherapy are short-lived, and relapses frequently occur when tapered. However, durable CRs to cyclosporine A alone have been reported, even in patients with HPS or relapsed/refractory disease (Chen et al. 2010, Jung et al. 2011, Lee et al. 2014, Mizutani et al. 2011, Rojnuckarin et al. 2007). Bexarotene has also demonstrated excellent overall response with little toxicity (Mehta et al. 2012). Multiagent chemotherapy is typically reserved for patients with progressive or treatment-refractory disease and those presenting with hemophagocytic syndrome. Allo-HSCT also shows variable success in case series and reports in this population (Gibson et al. 2015, Jung et al. 2011, Mukai et al. 2003, Sakurai et al. 2013). Individual or localized lesions are sensitive to localized RT and may be considered as adjunctive treatment for multifocal cases (Go and Wester 2004, Lopez-Lerma et al. 2018). Notably, some cases have an MF-like clinical presentation and can be treated similarly to MF. Surveillance is required to monitor for progression in any case.

8.1.4 pcGDTCL

Initial presentation may be clinically indolent (MF-like) and may be successfully managed with systemic therapies suitable for MF. However, clinicopathologic differentiation from MF or initial treatment failure necessitates multiagent chemotherapy based on guidelines for treating systemic T-cell lymphomas (Foss et al. 2020, Network NCC 2021b, Willemze et al. 2019). Few patients achieve durable CRs, with no existing evidence to support one regimen over another (Foss et al. 2020, Willemze et al. 2008). Fortunately, a building body of evidence suggests that allo-HSCT can result in long-term remission and should be considered early in management (Foss et al. 2020, Gibson et al. 2015, Isufi et al. 2020, Koch et al. 2009, Paralkar et al. 2012).

8.1.5 CD8+ AETCL

No standard therapy specific to CD8+ AETCL exists, but treatment usually consists of multiagent chemotherapy and allo-HSCT (Guitart et al. 2017, Nofal et al. 2012). Due to its early clinical mimicry of MF, it may initially be treated similarly; however, it is unresponsive to skin-directed therapies used in MF management (corticosteroids, phototherapy) (Berti et al. 1999, Gormley et al. 2010). The paucity of treatment guidance specific to CD8+ AETCL may be attributed to its rarity and novelty as a recently recognized subtype of PTCL-NOS. Therefore, treatment decisions may otherwise be guided by the NCCN and ESMO guidelines for PTCL-NOS (D'Amore et al. 2015, Network NCC 2021a, Willemze et al. 2018).

8.1.6 PTCL-NOS

Treatment guidelines currently do not distinguish between management for cutaneous and systemic PTCL-NOS (D'Amore et al. 2015, Network NCC 2021a, 2021b). Despite its nonspecific nature, PTCL-NOS has a poor prognosis (Willemze et al. 2019).

NCCN guidelines recommend six cycles of multiagent chemotherapy with or without involved site radiation therapy (ISRT) but strongly encourage clinical trial participation instead (Network NCC 2021b). The best outcomes have been observed with induction anthracycline-based multimodal chemotherapy [typically CHOP or CHOEP (CHOP with etoposide)] (Briski et al. 2014, D'Amore et al. 2015, Kim et al. 2021). Brentuximab-vedotin with or without CHP (cyclophosphamide, doxorubicin, prednisone) is recommended for cases with CD30 overexpression (Network NCC 2021b). Although autologous HSCT is often used initially or as a salvage strategy, significant data regarding its benefit remains scarce (see Chapter 40).

8.1.7 ENKTCL-NT

As outlined in the NCCN guidelines, the mainstay of treatment for localized cutaneous disease is combined modality therapy with localized RT concurrently or sequentially with an L-asparaginase-containing chemotherapy regimen (Li et al. 2017, Network NCC 2021b, Willemze et al. 2018). Widespread cutaneous or extracutaneous disease is best treated with

L-asparaginase-containing chemotherapy regimens followed by stem cell transplantation, which has shown promising activity in relapsed disease.

8.1.8 CAEBV

There are no consensus treatment guidelines for primary cutaneous or systemic CAEBV. A wide range of treatments has been suggested for primary cutaneous variants (HV-like LPD and HMB): topical/systemic corticosteroids, antihistamines, antiviral agents, radiotherapy, chemotherapy, immunomodulatory therapies (IFN-a, IL-2), and allogeneic HSCT (Guo et al. 2019, Yamada et al. 2021). Patients with primary cutaneous disease may forego treatment altogether but should be monitored for progression to systemic CAEBV.

For systemic CAEBV, single institutions have recommended management strategies (Bollard and Cohen 2018). A Japanese group reported a three-step plan, starting with immunosuppressive therapies (prednisolone, cyclosporine A, etoposide) followed by multiagent chemotherapy and allogeneic HSCT (Sawada et al. 2017). Donor-derived virus-specific T-cells may be used for relapses (Perna et al. 2015). Dr. Catherine Bollard, a leading figure in the field, has also recommended bortezomib and antiviral agents (Bollard and Cohen 2018). Concomitant hemophagocytic syndrome is life-threatening and takes management priority before proceeding with CAEBV-directed therapy; its treatment is outside the scope of this chapter.

8.2 Cutaneous B-cell lymphomas

8.2.1 pcFCL and pcMZL

Management is similar for both entities. Surgical excision and localized RT yield the best response rates (Senff et al. 2008). For localized lesions that can fit in one radiation field, NCCN guidelines recommend localized RT monotherapy (Network NCC 2021a). Successful dosages range between 24 Gy and 45 Gy, but one study reported responses with as little as 8 Gy over two fractions (Hamilton et al. 2013, Neelis et al. 2009, Senff et al. 2008). Excision may alternatively be considered for lesions that are poor irradiation candidates. For symptomatic, multifocal disease, other approaches such as intralesional triamcinolone or IFN-a, low-dose localized RT, and excision should be prioritized over systemic chemotherapy to avoid significant toxicity. Relapses are common, and no therapy demonstrates clearly superior relapse rates, varying between approximately 30% and 60%; however, relapses are easily retreated.

Alternatively, systemic treatment with single-agent rituximab or chlorambucil have produced durable remissions in observational studies (Hoefnagel et al. 2005, Kyrtsonis et al. 2006, Penate et al. 2012, Soda 2001). Initial treatment for Borrelia-positive pcMZL and pcFCL may be attempted with cephalosporin or doxycycline monotherapy (Amitay-Laish et al. 2009, Senff et al. 2008, Suárez et al. 2013). This approach is relatively less aggressive than other first-line therapies, but NCCN guidelines do not mention it, and successful antibiotic use is most often reported in Europe (Ferreri et al. 2009, Goodlad et al. 2000, Wood et al. 2001).

8.2.2 pcDLBCL-LT

Management is similar to limited-stage systemic DLBCL and depends on lesion number and patient frailty. Standard therapies include localized RT and anthracycline-based multimodal chemotherapy combined with rituximab (i.e. R-CHOP). Solitary lesions are usually managed with both R-CHOP and localized RT (up to 40 Gy) (Senff et al. 2008). In contrast, multifocal or disseminated disease is managed with R-CHOP only. Frail patients that cannot tolerate multimodal chemotherapy toxicity may be managed with palliative LRT monotherapy for multifocal disease, and solitary lesions can be managed by localized RT with or without single-agent rituximab. Less aggressive regimens are associated with worse five-year survival (Grange et al. 2014).

Targetable, activating mutations in the NF-kB pathway and BCR genes (*MYD88*, *CARD11*, CD79B) are highly prevalent in pcDLBCL-LT and portend a worse prognosis (Pham-Ledard et al. 2012, 2014). Research is ongoing to determine the role of molecular targeted agents in treatment-refractory pcDLBCL-LT and systemic DLBCL, including ibrutinib (Bruton tyrosine kinase [BTK] inhibitor targeting BCR signaling) (Al-Obaidi et al. 2020, Gupta et al. 2015, Pang et al. 2019), lenalidomide (small molecule inhibitor of NF-kB signaling) (Al Dhafiri 2019, Beylot-Barry et al. 2018, Zinzani et al. 2013), venetoclax (BCL-2 inhibitor) (Smith et al. 2020), and bortezomib (NF-kB proteasome inhibitor) (Villacampa et al. 2021). Pembrolizumab has shown similarly promising responses in MF, SS, and other hematological malignancies, but there is a paucity of data for pcDLBLCL, LT (Badros et al. 2017, Di Raimondo et al. 2019). Case studies show promising results for each agent; however, meta-analyses of their use in combination with R-CHOP show significantly increased toxicity in older patients and response benefit only in younger patients (Pasvolsky et al. 2021, Villacampa et al. 2021). Further studies are required to determine the most beneficial molecular therapy augmentation strategy to standard R-CHOP.

8.2.3 EBVMCU

Due to its indolent course, EBVMCU responds well to conservative management. Spontaneous remission may occur, but reduction of immunosuppressive therapies also results in resolution (Obata et al. 2021) Persistent lesions require more aggressive treatment; limited evidence exists supporting IFN-a2b, CD20-, or CD30-directed antibodies; localized RT; surgical excision; and/or single-agent chemotherapy (Magalhaes et al. 2015, Roberts et al. 2015, Xu et al. 2021).

9) What are the most recent advancements and future directions of primary cutaneous lymphomas management?

Expert Perspective: Beyond skin-directed therapies including surgery, intralesional therapy, and radiation, management for PCLs relies on biologic, immunosuppressive, and chemotherapeutic strategies that are extrapolated from systemic lymphoma management evidence. The latter are used mostly for recurrent disease or if the disease is considered to be aggressive with risk for systemic involvement. Unfortunately, outcomes in PCLs are poorly studied, and patients are typically excluded from clinical trials of systemic therapies due to their rarity and unique staging and response criteria.

However, recent molecular studies are improving the understanding of PCL lymphomagenesis, tumor microenvironment as well as resistance mechanisms, opening the door to novel approaches in their management. The most notable include immune checkpoint inhibitors (pembrolizumab, nivolumab in Hodgkin's disease) (Armand et al. 2018, 2020, Chen et al. 2017, 2019, Kuruvilla et al. 2021, Moskowitz et al. 2021, Ramchandren et al.

2019), antibody-based directed treatments (brentuximab vedotin in ALCL) (Duvic et al. 2009, Lewis et al. 2017, Prince et al. 2017, Song et al. 2021), epigenetic agents (romidepsin in PTCL) (Falchi et al. 2021, Reiman et al. 2019, Shimony et al. 2019, Vu et al. 2020), targeted treatments such as BTK inhibitors (Ibrutinib in DLBCL and chronic lymphocytic leukemia [CLL]) (Davids et al. 2019, Denker et al. 2021, Villacampa et al. 2021, Wang et al. 2021), phosphoinositol-3 kinase (PI3K) inhibitors (Duvelisib in CLL) (Flinn et al. 2018a, 2019, 2018b, Huen et al. 2020), and many more that are changing the treatment landscape of lymphomas. Furthermore, bispecific antibodies (mosunetuzumab) (Phillips et al. 2020) and chimeric antigen receptor augmented immune cells such as CAR T-cells (axicabtagene ciloleucel) (Locke et al. 2019, Neelapu et al. 2017) continue to evolve and even challenge stem cell transplant therapies. The future looks bright and will provide improved outcomes for patients with these lymphomas. Hence, it is imperative that patients with PCL be included in trials of these novel approaches to ensure that these patients also continue to benefit from novel treatments.

Conclusion

PCLs are unique diseases with biological features distinct from their systemic counterparts. Given their rarity and heterogeneity, diagnosis is challenging and warrants a high level of suspicion to confirm each diagnosis. Therefore, they need to be approached in a manner that will ensure their timely diagnosis and management. By virtue of their presentation, most patients are first seen and evaluated by a dermatologist. We recommend a multidisciplinary approach consisting of dermatology, hematology/oncology, pathology (dermatopathology and hematopathology), and radiation oncologists with appropriate expertise in managing PCL to provide optimal care. In addition, palliative care, wound care, and social workers are also crucial to ensure adequate support for these patients and should be part of the management team (Garbe et al. 2020, Martinez et al. 2021). Studies to address the pathogenesis, molecular biology, and tumor microenvironment of these diseases need to continue in order to provide mechanistically well-reasoned and individually based treatment approaches in the future.

Recommended Readings

Di Raimondo, C. Parekh, V., Song, J.Y. et al. (2020). Primary cutaneous CD30+ lymphoproliferative disorders: a comprehensive review. *Curr Hematol Malig Rep* 15 (4): 333–342.

Gru, A.A. and E.S. Jaffe (2017). Cutaneous EBV-related lymphoproliferative disorders. *Semin Diagn Pathol* 34 (1): 60–75.

Guitart, J., Martinez-Escala, E.M., Subtil, A. et al. (2017). Primary cutaneous aggressive epidermotropic cytotoxic T-cell lymphomas: reappraisal of a provisional entity in the 2016 WHO classification of cutaneous lymphomas. *Mod Pathol* 30 (5): 761–772.

Krenitsky, A., Klager, S., Hatch, L. et al. (2022). Update in Diagnosis and Management of Primary Cutaneous B-Cell Lymphomas. *Am J Clin Dermatol* 23 (5): 689–706.

National Comprehensive Cancer Care Network. Primary Cutaneous Lymphomas (2021). Primary cutaneous lymphomas (Version 2.2021). https://www.nccn.org/guidelines/guidelines-detail?category=1&id=1491.

Olsen, E.A., Whittaker, S., Willemze, R., et al. (2022). Primary cutaneous lymphoma: recommendations for clinical trial design and staging update from the ISCL, USCLC, and EORTC. *Blood* 140 (5): 419–437.

Welborn, M. and M. Duvic (2019). Antibody-based therapies for cutaneous T-cell lymphoma. *Am J Clin Dermatol* 20 (1): 115–122.

Willemze, R., Jansen, P.M., Cerroni, L. et al. (2008). Subcutaneous panniculitis-like T-cell lymphoma: definition, classification, and prognostic factors: an EORTC cutaneous lymphoma group study of 83 cases. *Blood* 111 (2): 838–845.

Willemze, R., Cerroni, L., Kempf, W. et al. (2019). The 2018 update of the WHO-EORTC classification for primary cutaneous lymphomas. *Blood* 133 (16): 1703–1714.

Zain, J.M. (2019). Aggressive T-cell lymphomas: 2019 updates on diagnosis, risk stratification, and management. *Am J Hematol* 94 (8): 929–946.

49

Mycosis Fungoides and Sézary Syndrome

Robert Stuver, Alison Moskowitz, Sarah Noor, and Steven M. Horwitz

Memorial Sloan Kettering Cancer Center, New York, NY

Introduction

The cutaneous T-cell lymphomas (CTCLs) comprise a group of non-Hodgkin lymphomas primarily presenting with cutaneous involvement, though with capability to involve nodal regions, blood, and visceral organs (Willemze et al. 2019). Mycosis fungoides (MF) is the most common type of CTCL, accounting for nearly 50% of all primary cutaneous lymphomas. Sézary syndrome (SS) is rare, accounting for < 5% of all primary cutaneous lymphomas. Important questions that frequently arise in the clinical care of patients with CTCL are highlighted in our chapter.

1) Early-stage mycosis fungoides: What are the pitfalls of diagnosis?

Expert Perspective: Mycosis fungoides (MF) is the most common subtype of CTCL. The staging of MF follows the T (skin), N (node), M (visceral), and B (blood involvement) classification as defined by the International Society for Cutaneous Lymphomas (ISCL) and European Organisation for Research and Treatment of Cancer (EORTC), as shown in Table 49.1 (Olsen et al. 2007). Early-stage MF is generally considered stage I–IIA disease and is characterized by an absence of tumors and primarily limited to the skin.

Mycosis fungoides is rare, and the major pitfall of early-stage MF is establishing the diagnosis. In early stages and more minimal presentations, the differential diagnosis includes benign reactive conditions (e.g. drug reaction) or inflammatory dermatoses such as eczema or psoriasis. Pathological samples should be reviewed by a hematopathologist or dermatopathologist with experience in CTCL, and the initial evaluation should optimally occur in a multidisciplinary, high-volume referral setting with input from dermatology and hematology/oncology. Treating clinicians must realize that early-stage MF is often an indolent neoplasm with a prolonged clinical course defined by intermittent, stable, or slow progression of disease, and the goal of treatment is to reduce symptoms and minimize the risk of progression while avoiding cumulative or other significant toxicity (Prince et al. 2009) (see Chapter 34).

Cancer Consult: Expertise in Clinical Practice, Volume 2: Neoplastic Hematology & Cellular Therapy,
Second Edition. Edited by Syed A. Abutalib, Maurie Markman, James O. Armitage, and Kenneth C. Anderson.

Table 49.1 Clinical staging of mycosis fungoides and Sézary syndrome.

Clinical Stage	T (skin)	N (Node)[†]	M (Visceral)	B (Blood)[‡]
IA (limited skin)	T1 (< 10% body surface area [BSA])	N0	M0	B0–1
IB (skin only)	T2 (≥ 10% BSA)	N0	M0	B0–1
IIA	T1-2	N1–2	M0	B0–1
IIB (tumor stage)	T3 (≥ 1 tumor [≥ 1 cm in diameter])	N0–2	M0	B0–1
IIIA (erythrodermic)	T4 (confluence of erythema ≥ 80% BSA)	N0–2	M0	B0
IIIB (erythrodermic)	T4	N0–2	M0	B1
IVA$_1$ (Sézary)	T1-4	N0–2	M0	B2
IVA$_2$ (Sézary or non)	T1-4	N3	M0	B0–2
IVB (visceral)	T1-4	N0–3	M1 (visceral involvement)	B0–2

†For N (node) classification, see NCI-VA Lymph Node Classification (Clendenning and Rappaport 1979) and Dutch Criteria for Lymph Nodes (Scheffer et al. 1980).
‡B0: ≤ 5% or < 250/μL peripheral blood lymphocytes are Sézary cells or < 15% of CD4+/CD26− or CD4+/CD7− cells of total lymphocytes; B1: > 5% peripheral blood lymphocytes are Sézary cells or > 15% CD4+/CD26− or CD4+/CD7− cells of total lymphocytes (but not meeting B0/B2 criteria); B2: ≥ 1000 μL Sézary cells or ≥ 1000 CD4+/CD26− or CD4+/CD7− cells/μL. For full definitions see Olsen, E, et al., *Blood* 2007;110:1713–1722.[2]

2) How best to make a diagnosis of mycosis fungoides?

Expert Perspective: The diagnosis is confirmed by biopsy (or biopsies) in combination with an appropriate or at least consistent clinical presentation. The cutaneous manifestations are heterogeneous, and there should be a high degree of suspicion for any lesion in question. The most common initial lesions arise in sun-protected regions and characteristically show a combination of patches (lesion without significant elevation or induration) and plaques (lesions with elevation or induration). Lesions can vary widely in appearance, and the presence or absence of pigmentation, scaling, crusting, and poikiloderma should be noted. Rare variants with different phenotypic presentations include folliculotropic MF (follicular papules and plaques associated with alopecia, usually involving the head and neck (van Doorn et al. 2002), granulomatous slack skin (bulky, pendulous skin folds in flexural areas) (LeBoit et al. 1988), and pagetoid reticulosis (large, usually single-scaling plaque often on extremities) (Haghighi et al. 2000). These variants are rare and have distinct pathological findings that require expert review.

Punch or broad shave biopsies are recommended. and multiple biopsies from different lesions at different points in time may be needed to confidently confirm the diagnosis, as findings may be subtle in early lesions. The initial pathology review should focus on histopathological and immunohistochemical phenotype.

- **Histopathology:** MF lesions generally comprise an infiltrate of small- to medium-sized atypical mononuclear cells with highly indented (cerebriform) nuclei and mild cytologic atypia. Pautrier microabscesses (intraepidermal aggregates of atypical cells) are highly characteristic but not always observed. Epidermotropism (colonization of the epidermis and palisading of cells at the dermal-epidermal junction) is often detected. Epidermotropism may be masked by recent use of topical steroids, and repeat biopsy of a lesion, left untreated for several weeks, may be needed to identify this key finding. At the tumor stage, epidermotropism can be lost, and cells may increase in number and size.

- **Immunophenotype:** The most typical immunophenotype in MF is CD2+, CD3+, CD4+, CD5+, CD7−, CD8−, CD20−, CD26−, PD-1±, and CD30−/+ although variability is seen. Primary cutaneous follicular helper T-cell (TFH) lymphoma may be distinguished by its clinical presentation and expression of TFH markers, such as CXCL13, ICOS, and PD-1 (Bosisio and Cerroni 2015). Molecular analysis should be performed to establish clonality (detection of T-cell gene rearrangements), though clonality alone does not constitute a diagnosis as clonal reactive processes are occasionally seen (and the absence of clonality should not discount the diagnosis).

3) How best to determine the extent of the disease?

Expert Perspective: The initial workup should include a complete physical examination that incorporates a full skin assessment, palpation of peripheral lymph nodes, and palpation of organomegaly. Laboratory studies include a complete blood count, comprehensive metabolic panel with lactate dehydrogenase (LDH), and flow cytometric studies for Sézary cells (considered optional for stage I). Imaging with computed tomography (CT) of the chest, abdomen, and pelvis or whole body positron-emission tomography (PET)-CT should be obtained for T3-4 disease and can be considered on an individualized basis in other cases (Hodak et al. 2021). Biopsy of enlarged nodes or extracutaneous sites should be pursued when possible. Bone marrow biopsy is not required for staging in the absence of hematologic abnormalities. Clinical staging of MF and SS is displayed in Table 49.1.

4) What is the relevance of large-cell transformation in mycosis fungoides?

Expert Perspective: Large-cell transformation is a descriptive histopathological condition in which neoplastic cells undergo transformation from small- to intermediate-sized cerebriform cells to large cell variants. Traditionally, the presence of such large cells at greater than 25% of the total lymphoid infiltrate has been used to define large cell transformation. This entity was first noted by multiple reports over 30 years ago as a histological finding in those who had begun to experience rapid clinical deterioration (Dmitrovsky et al. 1987, Salhany et al. 1988). As such, large cell transformation was recognized as a distinct clinical condition that in general is associated with an accelerated, aggressive phase of disease.

The defining cells of transformed disease are large in diameter (> 4 times that of a small lymphocyte) with large oval nuclei, prominent nucleoli, moderate-abundant amphophilic cytoplasm, and often significant nuclear irregularity (Barberio et al. 2007). Molecular and genetic analyses have shown that large cell transformation represents clonal evolution of the original malignant clone as opposed to a novel clonal process (Wolfe et al. 1995, Wood et al. 1993). The diagnosis can be challenging, especially because the transformed cells may mimic those of other lymphoproliferative disorders, such as lymphomatoid papulosis or anaplastic large-cell lymphoma (ALCL), in particular when CD30-positive. In this scenario, large cell transformation is favored if clinical transformation is seen within a preexisting MF lesion or if cellular pleomorphism is observed with cerebriform T lymphocytes mixed with fewer than 75% of CD30 + large T cells (Barberio et al. 2007). In addition, differentiating large T lymphocytes from histiocyte macrophages (which are more commonly present in granulomatous MF) is problematic unless immunohistochemistry is performed. Cases in question should be reviewed by an experienced pathologist at a high-volume center, as establishing the diagnosis is critical in order to define prognostic implications.

Multiple retrospective series and few prospective reports have described the clinical relevance of large cell transformation. Table 49.2 shows outcomes among four major publications evaluating large cell transformation (Arulogun et al. 2008, Lansigan et al. 2020, Talpur et al. 2016,Vergier et al. 2000). Drawing definitive conclusions from these reports is challenging given varying definitions and intermittent reporting of variables of interest, but in general, large cell transformation is uncommon in early-stage disease and becomes increasingly prevalent with increasing stage. For example, in the Australian report of 297 patients with MF/SS, large cell transformation occurred in a mere 1% of early stage disease but occurred in 58% of patients with stage IV disease (Arulogun et al. 2008). Patients are older (age range 60–65) and may have extracutaneous disease (22–59%) and an elevated LDH (47–53%) at the time of diagnosis. A certain proportion of patients consistently express CD30, but degree of expression can vary from < 10% to > 75%. With the exception of the MD Anderson database (Talpur et al. 2016), survival is typically less than three years from the time of large cell transformation.

Patients with large cell transformation consistently perform worse than their non-transformed counterparts. In the Australian data set, median survival in the transformed versus non-transformed population was 2.2 versus 5.2 years ($P = 0.17$) (Arulogun et al. 2008). This finding was redemonstrated in a large collaboration from the Cutaneous Lymphoma International Consortium, which reported large cell transformation as an independent prognostic marker of worse survival (Scarisbrick et al. 2015). Patients with large cell transformation at diagnosis also potentially fare worse, with median OS of 3.6 years versus 8.8 years ($P = 0.0001$) in the MD Anderson publication (Talpur et al. 2016), though this was not observed in a similar retrospective evaluation from Memorial Sloan Kettering Cancer Center (Pulitzer et al. 2014). The presence of large cell transformation in tumors or nodal regions may portend worse outcomes than large cell transformation within patches or plaques, as seen in the COMPLETE database (Lansigan et al. 2020). Other factors that might be associated with shorter survival are age > 60, elevated LDH, advanced-disease stage, and CD30 negativity, though findings have not been consistent in regard to these variables (Lansigan et al. 2020, Pulitzer et al. 2014, Scarisbrick et al. 2015).

There is no standard of care in treating large cell transformation, and treatment paradigms are hindered by a lack of prospective data and variability of stages at time of large cell transformation. For patients with localized cutaneous large cell transformation, local therapy with radiation therapy (often preferred) or topical chemotherapy should be considered along with concurrent management of additional sites of disease. In fact, localized large cell transformation may not negatively affect prognosis since it can typically be effectively treated with radiation (Talpur et al. 2016). However, for those with generalized cutaneous large cell transformation or extracutaneous disease, treatment paradigms generally

Table 49.2 Reports of large cell transformation in mycosis fungoides.

Reference	No. of Patients	Median Age (Range)	Median Time to LCT^	Stage of MF	Extracutaneous Disease	CD30 Expression	Elevated LDH	PFS[†]	OS[†]
Vergier et al., 2000	45	65 (31–90)	6.5 y	<T3: 11% ≥T3: 89%	45%	Negative: 68% <75%: 16% ≥75%: 16%	NR	NR	2-y: 61% 5-y: 21% median: 36 m
Arulogun et al., 2008	22	64 (44–79)	2.3 y	IA/IB/IIA: 14% IIB: 50% III: 5% IVA: 22% IVB: 9%	NR	41%[‡]	NR	NR	2-y: 51% 5-y: 33% median: 27 m
Talpur et al., 2016	187	60 (22–89)	NR	IA: 9%IB: 8%IIB: 44%III: 1%IVA: 28%IVB: 10%	22%	<10%: 37% ≥10%: 65%[§]	47%	2-y: 78% 5-y: 45% median: NR	2-y: 83% 5-y: 48% median 4.7 y*
Lansigan et al., 2020	17	61 (57–71)	4.4 y	NR	59%	47%[‡]	53%	median: 8.4 m	median: 18.4 m

LCT: large cell transformation; LDH: lactate dehydrogenase; m: month; MF: mycosis fungoides; No.: number; NR: not reported; OS: overall survival; PFS: progression-free survival; y: year.

^ If not present at diagnosis.

[†] From time of diagnosis of LCT.

[‡] Level of expression not reported.

[§] 52 patients were not assessed for CD30 expression.

* Not specified whether survival was from time of MF diagnosis or time of diagnosis of LCT.

mirror that of advanced-stage MF/SS. The CD30-targeting antibody-drug conjugate brentuximab vedotin is effective in CD30-positive CTCL, including large cell transformation. In ALCANZA, the phase III study that demonstrated superiority of brentuximab vedotin over physician's choice in CD30-positive MF, about 35% of patients had large cell transformation, and brentuximab vedotin was effective regardless of large cell transformation status (Duvic et al. 2009, Kim et al. 2021, Prince et al. 2017). Additional data exists for pralatrexate, a novel folate analog, and intermittent low-dose gemcitabine (Awar and Duvic 2007, Foss et al. 2012). Finally, it is worth noting that patients with large cell transformation were excluded from the pivotal phase III trial evaluating the CCR4 monoclonal antibody mogamulizumab versus vorinostat in R/R CTCL (Kim et al. 2018).

In summary, to answer the original question, large cell transformation is relevant in MF. It is a distinct histological finding and generally a harbinger of aggressive disease with worse outcomes compared to non-transformed patients. However, localized large cell transformation may not impact prognosis if it can be treated with local measures. In addition, brentuximab vedotin is effective for CD30-positive large cell transformation and therefore has potentially improved its prognosis. For CD30-negative large cell transformation, there is no dedicated treatment toward large cell transformation to date and management mirrors advanced MF/SS.

5) Mycosis fungoides and Sézary syndrome: The same or distinct entities?

Expert Perspective: As described above, mycosis fungoides is a mature T-cell lymphoma that classically presents in the skin though in higher stages may involve the lymph nodes, blood, and viscera. SS is a distinctive erythrodermic mature T-cell lymphoma defined by leukemic involvement of clonal malignant T cells. Until recently, the distinction between MF and SS has been blurry, and for many years it was thought that SS was an evolution or progression of MF along a continuum from cutaneous disease to leukemic involvement. However, recent investigations have shown that MF and SS are likely distinct clinical entities with different cells of origin, unique mutational profiles, and varied clinical outcomes.

Phenotyping studies within the past decade suggest that MF is a malignancy of skin resident effector memory T cells, whereas SS is a malignancy of central memory T cells. In a small study from the Dana-Farber/Brigham and Women's Cancer Center, monoclonal antibody staining for 12 patients with SS showed variable to low levels of skin-homing molecules, such as CLA (cutaneous-leukocyte associate antigen), CCR6 (chemokine receptor 6), and CCR10 (Campbell et al. 2010). All clones co-expressed CCR7 and L-selectin, both considered necessary for T-cell homing to lymph nodes via the blood, as well as CD27, which is generally expressed by central memory T cells and lost by effector memory T cells. However, in marked contrast to this phenotype, clonal T cells isolated from skin lesions in patients with MF had near absence of CCR7, L-selectin, and CD27, arguing against an identical cell of origin in MF and SS. Furthermore, in biopsies of skin lesions in patients with SS, the L-selectin+/CCR7+ central memory T cell phenotype was maintained, again supporting a unique etiological process.

Deeper cytogenetic and molecular analyses support these phenotypic findings. For example, array-based comparative genomic hybridization to evaluate copy number alterations (gains or losses of segments of DNA) reveal clear differences in patterns observed in

MF versus SS, demonstrating that the molecular oncogenesis of these entities is quite different (van Doorn et al. 2009). Examples include frequent gain of 7q21-6 and 1p36.2 and loss of 5q13 and 9p21 in MF, versus frequent gain of 17q22-25 and 8q22-24 and loss of 17p13 and 10q25 in SS (van Doorn et al. 2009). While heterogeneity exists, several chromosomal aberrations commonly observed in MF are rarely observed in SS, again arguing that SS is not a mere progression of MF. At the gene level, similar discrepancies are observed. Overexpression of multiple genes in SS, such as *CDO1* and *DNM3*, have not been seen in MF (Booken et al. 2008).Taken together, existing phenotypic and molecular analyses point toward different cells of origin and discrete mutational profiles, indicating that MF and SS have different biological roots.

Speaking to this variable biological profile, the clinical outcomes between patients with MF and SS differ. Direct comparisons are challenging because the two are often considered together in retrospective databases, but in general early-stage MF has a favorable, near normal survival (Kim et al. 1996) whereas SS (and stage IV disease in general) consistently demonstrates worse overall survival (Kim et al. 2003, Scarisbrick et al. 2015). Treatment paradigms differ as well, though this is largely based on stage. Skin-directed therapies are employed in early-stage disease with limited skin involvement, whereas systemic therapies, often in combination with continued skin-directed treatment, are needed in advanced-stage disease. These systemic therapies are generally used interchangeably for advanced MF and SS, and most clinical trials have considered advanced MF and SS as both eligible for trials and often reported data based on stage as opposed to subtype (a notable exception being the ALCANZA trial, as referenced above, which excluded patients with concurrent SS or B2 disease) (Prince et al. 2017).

In summary, MF and SS are distinct entities with different clonal origins and particular chromosomal and mutational signatures. Clinical behavior in early-stage MF is favorable compared to SS, though advanced-stage MF and SS have historically been considered together in trials and treatment. As we gain appreciably deeper understanding of the different pathways in lymphomagenesis in MF and SS, targeted treatments aimed at overcoming their unique biologies is warranted.

6) Is allogeneic hematopoietic stem cell transplantation useful in CTCLs?

Expert Perspective: Allogeneic hematopoietic stem cell transplantation (allo-HCT) remains a critical component of treatment for those with advanced MF/SS with relapsed or refractory (R/R) disease. While there are no randomized data evaluating this modality in the R/R setting, multiple retrospective, and very limited prospective series, demonstrate that allo-HCT can be a potentially curative approach in certain patients with resistant disease.

Table 49.3 shows outcomes across six major series of allo-HCT in advanced MF/SS (de Masson et al. 2014, Domingo-Domenech et al. 2021, Hosing et al. 2015, Lechowicz et al. 2014, Mori et al. 2020, Weng et al. 2020). Smaller, single-center series exist as well (Delioukina et al. 2012, Jacobsen et al. 2011, Paralkar et al. 2012). Drawing definitive or specific conclusions from these data sets is challenging given variability in conditioning regimens, graft sources, disease status at the time of allo-HCT, and graft-versus-host disease (GvHD) prophylactic strategies. Within the limits and flaws of these observational data sets, approximately half of all patients appear to relapse after allogeneic allo-HCT,

Table 49.3 Major publications of allogeneic transplantation in cutaneous T-cell lymphoma

Reference	No. of Patients	Conditioning Intensity	Donor Type	Relapse	PFS	OS	NRM	GVHD^
Lechowicz et al., 2014	129	MAC: 46 RIC: 83	Matched sibling: 64, Mismatched related: 9, MUD: 56	1-yr: 50%, 5-yr: 61%	1-yr: 31%, 5-yr: 17%	1-yr: 54%, 5-yr: 32%	1-yr: 19%, 5-yr: 61%	100-d acute: 41%, 1-yr chronic: 42%
de Masson et al., 2014	37	MAC: 12, RIC: 25	Sibling[†]: 17, MUD: 17, MMUD[‡]: 4	1-yr: 49%, 2-yr: 56%	1-yr: 39%, 2-yr: 31%	1-yr: 65%, 2-yr: 57%	1-yr[§]: 18%, 2-yr[§]: 18%	acute: 49% (at any time), 2-yr chronic: 44%
Hosing et al., 2015	47	all RIC	Matched sibling: 21, MUD: 24, MMUD: 2	50% (of all pts)	4-yr: 26%	4-yr: 51%	1-yr: 10.4%, 2-yr: 16.7%	acute: 40% (at any time), chronic: 28%
Mori et al., 2020	48	MAC: 17, RIC: 31	Related[†]: 18, Unrelated[†]: 21, Cord[†]: 9	2-yr: 65.9%	3-yr: 18.8%	3-yr: 30.0%	2-yr[§]: 15.4%	100-d acute: 35%, 1-yr chronic: 32%
Weng et al., 2020[*]	35	all RIC (TSEBT-TLI-ATG)	Sibling[†]: 17, MUD: 22, MMUD: 7	57% (of all pts)	180-d: 73%, 5-yr: 41%	1-yr: 80%, 5-yr: 56%	1-yr: 3%, 2-yr: 14%	180-d acute: 19%, 2-yr chronic: 32% (moderate/severe)
Domingo-Domenech et al., 2021	117	MAC: 28, RIC: 85	Matched sibling: 70, URD[†]: 43	1-yr: 40%, 5-yr: 45%	1-yr: 34%, 5-yr: 26%	1-yr: 56%, 5-yr: 38%	1-yr: 26%, 3-yr: 28%	100-d acute: 47%, 5-yr chronic: 48%

d: day; GVHD: graft-versus-host disease; MAC: myeloablative conditioning; MMUD: mismatched unrelated donor; No.: number; NRM: non-relapse mortality; OS: overall mortality; PFS: progression-free survival; pts: patients; RIC: reduced intensity conditioning; TSEBT-TLI-ATG: total skin electron beam therapy, total lymphoid irradiation, antithymocyte globulin; URD: unrelated donor; yr: year.

^ Acute GVHD reported as grade II–IV.

† Match status not reported.

‡ Includes two cord blood transfers for which match status was not reported.

§ Reported as transplant-related mortality.

* Prospective phase II trial.

with most relapses occurring in the first year. Mortality after relapse is not consistently reported, but in at least one series was as high as 70% (Domingo-Domenech et al. 2021). In addition, non-relapse mortality (NRM) is a significant contributor to overall mortality, with one-year non-relapse mortality ranging from 3 to 26%. GvHD is frequent, with cumulative incidence of acute and chronic GvHD ranging from 19 to 49% and 28 to 48%, respectively (with the caveat that different time frames were used for data reporting). Still, a consistent finding from each of the reports is a subpopulation of patients that has extended, relapse-free survival.

A meta-analysis of 266 patients from five studies was reported in 2020 (Iqbal et al. 2020). This analysis included all studies between 2010 and 2015 that reported outcomes for ≥ 10 patients who underwent allogeneic HCT for the sole purpose of treatment of MF/SS and had at least one year of follow-up. The pooled progression-free and overall survival (OS) was 36% (95% CI 27–45%; $I^2 = 41.7\%$) and 59% (95% CI 50–69%; $I^2 = 47.8\%$). The pooled relapse rate was 47% (95% CI 41–53%; $I^2 = 0\%$) and the pooled non-relapse mortality was 19% (95% CI 13–27%; $I^2 = 38.6\%$). Again, comparable to the results reported in Table 49.3, this analysis highlights the potentially curative effect of HCT in certain patients while also showing a consistently appreciable relapse rate and degree of NRM. Importantly, only 20 patients across this meta-analysis proceeded to HCT in a complete response (though some data was not reported), suggesting that even those with refractory or persistent disease can potentially derive benefit.

Deciding when and in whom to employ allo-HCT requires careful consideration. Disease status at the time of transplant is likely a critical factor. In the European Society for Blood and Marrow Transplantation (EBMT) retrospective registry series of 113 patients, advanced-stage disease at the time of allo-HCT (defined as primary refractory or relapsed/progressive disease in those that had received ≥ 3 lines of therapy, or complete and partial remissions > 3) was an adverse prognostic factor associated with higher relapse (HR 3.38; $P = 0.0013$) and worse progression-free survival (HR 3.23; $P < 0.001$) and OS (HR 2.42; $P = 0.0017$) (Domingo-Domenech et al. 2021). This was similarly reported in the nationwide registry database analysis of the Japan Society for Hematopoietic Cell Transplantation (JSHCT) (Mori et al. 2020) in which three-year PFS for those in complete or partial response at the time of transplant was 40.8% versus just 9.8% for all others ($P < 0.05$). Three-year OS was similarly poor for those not in complete or partial response at allo-HCT (55.0% vs 20.1%; $P < 0.05$). These findings have been consistently observed and suggest that chemosensitivity and/or lower disease burden at the time of allo-HCT is a critical consideration and prognostic factor.

The choice of conditioning regimen is a second influential decision point. In the Center for International Blood and Marrow Transplant Research (CIBMTR) retrospective registry series (Lechowicz et al. 2014) outcomes by intensity of conditioning regimen were reported. Notably, the only statistically significant difference in outcomes was five-year progression-free survival, which favored reduced intensity conditioning over myeloablative conditioning regimens (23% vs 6%; $P = 0.029$). There were no other statistically significant differences. For example, one-year relapse for both myeloablative and reduced intensity conditioning was 50% ($P = 0.982$). Five-year OS for myeloablative versus reduced intensity conditioning was 21% versus 36% ($P = 0.208$), and five-year non-relapse mortality was 27% versus 20% ($P = 0.399$). These data suggest that reduced intensity conditioning may offer increased progression-free survival with no difference (or potentially improved) survival and non-relapse mortality. This finding has been shown elsewhere (Domingo-Domenech et al. 2021) and suggests that myeloablative conditioning regimen has a limited role in this setting (see Chapter 50).

Novel conditioning strategy: The incorporation of total skin electron beam therapy (TSEBT) is a further component that has been recently explored. In a prospective phase II trial from Stanford University, a novel non-myeloablative regimen of TSEBT with total lymphoid irradiation (TLI) and antithymocyte globulin (ATG) was evaluated in 35 patients with relapsed disease (Weng et al. 2020). All patients had active skin disease at the time of conditioning, and the authors hypothesized that the use of skin-directed therapy as a component of conditioning may provide additional reduction in skin disease burden. TSEBT was administered up to nine weeks before TLI-ATG. Initial response rates were high, with 57% global complete remission rate at 90 days and 73% progression-free survival at 180 days. Five-year progression-free survival and OS approached that of other series, reported as 41% and 56%, respectively. However, non-relapse mortality was notably lower than that of other series, at a mere 3% at one year and 14% at two years. The use of TSEBT has been explored at additional centers (Duvic et al. 2010, Thompson et al. 2021) and likely deserves additional evaluation.

Relapse after allo-HCT: This scenario is in desperate need of advanced strategies. Enhancement of graft-versus-lymphoma (GVL) effect via reduction in immunosuppression, donor lymphocyte infusion (DLI), or immunomodulation (such as with low-dose interferon) have been effectively employed but do not have consistent efficacy (Hosing et al. 2015, Weng et al. 2020). A deeper understanding of the mechanisms of relapse is needed so that strategies in this setting can be targeted to overcome these mechanisms.

In conclusion, allo-HCT is indeed useful in some but not all patients with advanced CTCL. Still, a sizeable proportion of patients experience relapse, and non-relapse mortality occurs in approximately one in five patients. Identifying the most appropriate patients for allografting—ideally those with chemosensitive disease—as well as employing the most effective conditioning regimen, are crucial facets in achieving success in this modality.

Recommended Readings

Booken, N., Gratchev, A., Utikal, J. et al. (2008). Sézary syndrome is a unique cutaneous T-cell lymphoma as identified by an expanded gene signature including diagnostic marker molecules CDO1 and DNM3. *Leukemia* 22 (2): 393–399.

de Masson, A., Beylot-Barry, M., Bouaziz, J.-D. et al. (2014). Allogeneic stem cell transplantation for advanced cutaneous T-cell lymphomas: a study from the French Society of Bone Marrow Transplantation and French Study Group on Cutaneous Lymphomas. *Haematologica* 99 (3): 527–534.

Delioukina, M., Zain, J., Palmer, J.M. et al. (2012). Reduced-intensity allogeneic hematopoietic cell transplantation using fludarabine-melphalan conditioning for treatment of mature T-cell lymphomas. *Bone Marrow Transplant* 47 (1): 65–72.

Domingo-Domenech, E., Duarte, R.F., Boumedil, A. et al. (2021). Allogeneic hematopoietic stem cell transplantation for advanced mycosis fungoides and Sézary syndrome. an updated experience of the Lymphoma Working Party of the European Society for Blood and Marrow Transplantation. *Bone Marrow Transplant* 56 (6): 1391–1401.

Duvic, M., Donato, M., Dabaja, B. et al. (2010). Total skin electron beam and non-myeloablative allogeneic hematopoietic stem-cell transplantation in advanced mycosis fungoides and Sezary syndrome. *J. Clin. Oncol.* 28 (14): 2365–2372.

Foss, F., Horwitz, S.M., Coiffier, B. et al. (2012). Pralatrexate is an effective treatment for relapsed or refractory transformed mycosis fungoides: a subgroup efficacy analysis from the PROPEL study. *Clin. Lymphoma Myeloma Leuk.* 12 (4): 238–243.

Horwitz, S.M., Ansell, S., Ai, W.Z . et al. (2022 March). T Cell Lymphomas, Version 2.2022, NCCN clinical practice guidelines in oncology. *J Natl Compr Canc Netw* 20 (3): 285 308. doi: 10.6004/jnccn.2022.0015. PMID: 35276674.

Hodak, E., Sherman, S., Papadavid, E. et al. (2021). Should we be imaging lymph nodes at initial diagnosis of early-stage mycosis fungoides? results from the PROspective Cutaneous Lymphoma International Prognostic Index (PROCLIPI) international study. *Br. J. Dermatol.* 184 (3): 524–531.

Hosing, C., Bassett, R., Dabaja, B. et al. (2015). Allogeneic stem-cell transplantation in patients with cutaneous lymphoma: updated results from a single institution. *Ann. Oncol. Off. J. Eur. Soc. Med. Oncol.* 26 (12): 2490–2495.

Iqbal, M., Reljic, T., Ayala, E. et al. (2020). Efficacy of Allogeneic Hematopoietic Cell Transplantation in Cutaneous T Cell Lymphoma: results of a systematic review and meta-analysis. *Biol. Blood Marrow Transplant.* 26 (1): 76–82.

Kim, Y., Bagot, M., Pinter-Brown, L. et al. (2018). Mogamulizumab versus vorinostat in previously treated cutaneous T-cell lymphoma (MAVORIC): an international, open-label, randomised, controlled phase 3 trial. *Lancet. Oncol* 19 (9).

Kim, Y.H., Liu, H.L., Mraz-Gernhard, S., Varghese, A., and Hoppe, R.T. (2003). Long-term outcome of 525 patients with mycosis fungoides and Sézary syndrome. *Arch. Dermatol.* 139 (7): 857–866.

Kim, Y.H., Prince, H.M., Whittaker, S. et al. (2021). Response to brentuximab vedotin versus physician's choice by CD30 expression and large cell transformation status in patients with mycosis fungoides: an ALCANZA sub-analysis. *Eur. J. Cancer.* 148: 411–421.

Lansigan, F., Horwitz, S.M., Pinter-Brown, L.C. et al. (2020). Outcomes of patients with transformed mycosis fungoides: analysis from a prospective multicenter US cohort study. *Clin. Lymphoma Myeloma Leuk.* 20 (11): 744–748.

Mori, T., Shiratori, S., Suzumiya, J. et al. (2020). Outcome of allogeneic hematopoietic stem cell transplantation for mycosis fungoides and Sézary syndrome. *Hematol. Oncol.* 38 (3): 266–271.

Prince, H.M., Kim, Y.H., Horwitz, S.M. et al. (2017). Brentuximab vedotin or physician's choice in CD30-positive cutaneous T-cell lymphoma (ALCANZA): an international, open-label, randomised, phase 3, multicentre trial. *Lancet (London, England)* 390 (10094): 555–566.

Prince, H.M., Whittaker, S., and Hoppe, R.T. (2009). How I treat mycosis fungoides and Sézary syndrome. *Blood* 114 (20): 4337–4353.

Pulitzer, M., Myskowski, P.L., Horwitz, S.M. et al. (2014). Mycosis fungoides with large cell transformation: clinicopathological features and prognostic factors. *Pathology* 46 (7): 610–616.

Scarisbrick, J.J., Prince, H.M., Vermeer, M.H. et al. (2015). Cutaneous lymphoma international consortium study of outcome in advanced stages of mycosis fungoides and Sézary syndrome: effect of specific prognostic markers on survival and development of a prognostic model. *J. Clin. Oncol.* 33 (32): 3766–3773.

Scheffer, E., Meijer, C.J.L.M., and van Vloten, W.A. (1980). Dermatopathic lymphadenopathy and lymph node involvement in mycosis fungoides. *Cancer* 45 (1): 137–148.

Thompson, L.L., Pan, C.X., Chang, M.S. et al. (2021). Alemtuzumab, total skin electron beam, and non-myeloablative allogeneic haematopoietic stem-cell transplantation in advanced sezary syndrome: a retrospective cohort study. *J. Eur. Acad. Dermatol. Venereol.* 35 (6): e373–e375.

Weng, W.-K., Arai, S., Rezvani, A. et al. (2020). Nonmyeloablative allogeneic transplantation achieves clinical and molecular remission in cutaneous T-cell lymphoma. *Blood Adv* 4 (18): 4474–4482.

Willemze, R., Cerroni, L., Kempf, W. et al. (2019). The 2018 update of the WHO-EORTC classification for primary cutaneous lymphomas. *Blood* 133 (16): 1703–1714.

Wolfe, J.T., Chooback, L., Finn, D.T. et al. (1995). Large-cell transformation following detection of minimal residual disease in cutaneous T-cell lymphoma: molecular and in situ analysis of a single neoplastic T-cell clone expressing the identical T-cell receptor. *J. Clin. Oncol.* 13 (7): 1751–1757.

50

Peripheral T-Cell Lymphoma

Avyakta Kallam and James O. Armitage

University of Nebraska Medical Center, Omaha, Nebraska

Introduction

Peripheral T-cell lymphomas (PTCL) are a group of non-Hodgkin lymphomas (NHL), with varying geographic patterns of incidence and clinical outcomes. The T-cell lymphomas are a heterogenous group of diseases, with the recent WHO classification identifying over 25 different subtypes (Siaghani et al. 2019, Swerdlow 2017). These lymphomas arise from the mature T cells of post-thymic origin and account for about 10% of all NHL. The incidence of peripheral T-cell lymphomas has gradually been increasing in North America over the past decade. T-cell lymphomas were previously approached in a manner similar to the B-cell lymphomas. It was only in the late 1970s that the T-cell lymphomas started to be recognized as separate from the B-cell lymphomas.

With a few exceptions, PTCL are aggressive lymphomas, with a poor prognosis when compared to B-cell lymphomas. These lymphomas often tend to have high relapse rates. The heterogenous nature of this disease makes designing clinical trials challenging. With improved understanding of the disease biology and incorporation of novel agents in the front-line setting, the role of hematopoietic stem cell transplantation in T-cell lymphomas is being redefined. We will review a few clinical scenarios where hematopoietic stem cell transplant is considered in aggressive PTCL.

Aggressive PTCL with nodal presentations can be broadly defined into three main histological categories: (i) Nodal T-cell lymphoma, with nodal T follicular helper phenotype, (ii) anaplastic large cell lymphoma, and (iii) PTCL, not otherwise specified (PTCL-NOS). Rarer subtypes include extra-nodal NK/T-cell lymphomas, hepatosplenic T-cell lymphomas, and intestinal T-cell lymphomas (Wang and Vose 2013).

PTCL-NOS is the most common subtype of PTCL worldwide, followed the adult T-cell leukemia and lymphoma (ATLL), anaplastic large T-cell lymphoma, and extra-nodal natural killer (NK) and T-cell lymphoma. In North America, PTCL-NOS is the most

Cancer Consult: Expertise in Clinical Practice, Volume 2: Neoplastic Hematology & Cellular Therapy,
Second Edition. Edited by Syed A. Abutalib, Maurie Markman, James O. Armitage, and Kenneth C. Anderson.
© 2024 John Wiley & Sons Ltd. Published 2024 by John Wiley & Sons Ltd.

common subtype (34.4%), followed by angioimmunoblastic T-cell lymphoma (AITL, 16%), anaplastic large cell lymphoma (ALCL), ALK-positive (16%), and ALK negative (7.8%) (Wang and Vose 2013).

Case Study 1

A 53-year-old otherwise healthy male presents with drenching night sweats, 30 lbs. weight loss, enlarged cervical lymph nodes. Staging workup shows extensive lymphadenopathy, both above and below the diaphragm, hepatomegaly, and splenomegaly. Excisional biopsy of the cervical lymph node shows effacement of the lymph node architecture, with intermediate to large lymphocytes, with open chromatin and prominent nucleoli. Immunohistochemistry demonstrated lymphocytes that were strongly positive for CD3, CD30 (80%), BCL2, MUM01. CD 4 was focally positive. The Ki-67 was 80%. Molecular studies showed a T-cell receptor (TCR) gamma, beta chain rearrangement. The diagnosis was PTCL-NOS with CD30 expression (80%).

1) What is the standard initial treatment approach for advanced-stage PTCL-NOS?

Expert Perspective: PTCL-NOS refers to a subgroup of lymphomas that are categorized by cytological and phenotypic heterogeneity that cannot fit into any specific definition of PTCL. Morphologically, PTCL-NOS demonstrates paracortical infiltrates, with effacement of the normal lymph node architecture. It is commonly associated with expression of CD3 and CD4 and loss of CD7 and CD5. CD30 is expressed in about 34–64% of cases with PTCL-NOS. EBV is found in 30% of all PTCL-NOS (Broccoli and Zinzani 2017).

PTCL-NOS is the most common PTCL subtype in Western countries. It affects older patients, with a mean age at diagnosis of 60 years. There is a slight male predilection, with a majority of patients presenting with advanced-stage disease (Broccoli and Zinzani 2017).

Given the paucity of clinical trials for T-cell lymphomas, the treatment protocols for all T-cells lymphomas until recently were heavily influenced by that of diffuse large B-cell lymphomas. Patients typically received multiagent chemotherapy, with an anthracycline-containing regimen. In the United States, the most commonly used regimen was CHOP (cyclophosphamide, doxorubicin, vincristine, prednisone). The outcomes of patients with PTCL-NOS were found to be inferior to those of their B-cell counterparts, with long-term survival rates of 20–40%. In an attempt to improve the outcomes, several chemo-immunotherapy regimens were proposed incorporating more chemotherapy drugs into the front-line setting with limited benefit over CHOP.

- A phase III study was conducted comparing an alternating etoposide, ifosfamide, cisplatin (VIP) and adriamycin, bleomycin, vinblastine, dacarbazine (ABVD) to CHOP (Wilhelm et al. 2016, Abouyabis et al. 2011). The study did not show any improvement in the two-year event-free survival when compared to CHOP. Moreover, VIP-ABVD hybrid was noted to have high toxicity when compared to CHOP.

Subsequent studies incorporating novel agents such as lenalidomide with CHOP and alemtuzumab with CHOP have been designed, without a notable benefit.

- The German High-Grade Non-Hodgkin Lymphoma Study Group (DSHNHL) retrospectively analyzed 343 patients with PTCL treated on phase II or III clinical trials (Wilhelm et al. 2016). Patients in this study were treated with CHOP-like regimens. In this study, the three-year event-free survival and OS in patients with PTCL-NOS was 41% and 54%, respectively. It was noted that patients younger than 60 years, with a normal LDH did well with addition of etoposide to CHOP (CHOEP), with a longer event-free survival and OS. In patients older than 60, receiving etoposide with CHOP was associated with poor outcomes.

Presently, the prognosis of patients with PTCL remains significantly inferior to B-cell lymphomas regardless of the chemotherapy approach, as also noted by a meta-analysis of 2,815 patients. These patients were treated with CHOP or a CHOP-like regimen, and the study reported a five-year OS of 38.5% for all PTCL. The five-year OS of patients with PTCL-NOS was 45% (Abouyabis et al. 2011). The majority of studies included in the meta-analysis did not incorporate any consolidation strategies. Only one prospective study included patients who had received front-line auto-HCT consolidation.

Given the suboptimal response to multiagent chemotherapy in the first-line setting, regimens incorporating brentuximab vedotin, a CD30 antibody drug conjugate, were proposed, with good results (Lunning 2015). CD30 is widely expressed on the cell surface of almost all ALCL, some PTCL-NOS, and other entities as enteropathy-associated T-cell lymphoma, making CD30 an ideal target.

- ECHELON-2 was a double-blind, multicenter study comparing brentuximab vedotin +CHP (cyclophosphamide, adriamycin, prednisone) with CHOP in untreated PTCL with CD30+ expression > 10% (Horwitz et al. 2019). Of the 226 patients enrolled, 72 patients had PTCL-NOS. The five-year progression-free survival was 51% in the brentuximab vedotin + CHP arm and 43% in the CHOP arm. The five-year OS rates were 70% with brentuximab vedotin + CHP vs 61% with CHOP. Although ECHELON-2 was not powered to compared brentuximab vedotin + CHP vs CHOP among various subgroups of PTCL, responses were observed in all the major subtypes of PTCL and were statistically significant in both ALK-positive and ALK-negative ALCL. Adverse events were generally similar between treatment arms, with peripheral sensory neuropathy reported in 52% of patients receiving brentuximab vedotin + CHP and 55% of patients receiving CHOP. These findings led to approval of brentuximab vedotin + CHP for the front-line treatment of CD30 +PTCL, which has become a standard of care option for all subsets of CD30 + PTCL, particularly for ALCL.

For a patient with advanced-stage PTCL-NOS that is CD30 positive (any positivity on IHC), we recommend treatment with six cycles of brentuximab vedotin + CHP, followed by a PET-CT scan to assess response.

If the patient was CD30 negative, we would consider treatment with six cycles of CHOEP.

Case Study continued: Patient has a complete response to brentuximab vedotin + CHP.

2) Is there a role for autologous consolidative autologous hematopoietic stem cell transplant in PTCL-NOS?

Expert Perspective: Given the difficulty in sustaining long-term remission with multiagent chemotherapy, consolidation with autologous and allogeneic stem cell transplants have been explored to improve survival in patients with PTCL.

Several retrospective studies have evaluated the role of consolidative autologous stem cell transplantation (auto-HCT), with mixed results. Most of these studies have been done in the pre-ECHELON-2 era, before the incorporation of brentuximab vedotin in the front-line setting (Shustov 2013, Reimer et al. 2009).

- A large multicenter retrospective study evaluated the role of consolidation auto-HCT in 269 patients < 65 years with PTCL (Fossard et al. 2018). The study included patients with PTCL-NOS, AITL, and ALK-negative ALCL. Among the patients who responded to multiagent chemotherapy, 134 received an auto-HCT. The five-year progression-free survival and OS were 45% and 60%, respectively. In the PTCL-NOS subgroup, the five-year OS was 20%. This study did not show a survival advantage with a consolidative auto-HCT for patients after induction. Age of the patients and achievement of a complete response (CR) to chemotherapy showed a survival advantage over other prognostic factors. It must be noted that only 46% of the patients had achieved a CR with multiagent chemotherapy.
- A prospective study evaluated the efficacy of consolidation auto-HCT (32 patients had PTCL-NOS and 27 patients had AITL) (Reimer et al. 2009). Among the 83 patients enrolled, 66% of the patients had a consolidative auto-HCT, with the rest unable to proceed to an auto-HCT due to progressive disease. The overall response rate in these patients was 79%, with a three-year OS of 38%. The three-year OS was 71% for patients who underwent an auto-HCT.
- Based on the results from these data, a prospective phase II study was conducted enrolling 166 patients with PTCL (D'Amore et al. 2012). All patients received six cycles of CHOEP on a biweekly schedule. Patients who responded to therapy received high-dose chemotherapy, followed by a consolidative auto-HCT. Only 58% of the patients were eligible to undergo auto-HCT. The five-year progression-free survival and OS were 44% and 51%, respectively. Both these studies were limited due to lack of direct comparison among patients in CR who received an auto-HCT vs those who did not receive a consolidation auto-HCT.
- COMPLETE study (Park et al. 2019) was a large prospective study comparing the survival outcomes among patients with PTCL who underwent an auto-HCT and those who were monitored (Park et al. 2019). This study evaluated 119 patients who achieved a CR following first-line therapy but failed to demonstrate a statistically significant difference in survival between patients who underwent an auto-HCT and the non-auto-HCT group. However, there was a trend toward improved overall survival noted in the auto-HCT group. The subgroup analysis suggested that patients with high-risk disease (advanced stage, high IPI) and AITL benefit with consolidation auto-HCT.

Based on these studies, high-dose chemotherapy followed by a consolidative auto-HCT has become a preferred treatment approach in transplant-eligible patients who have achieved a CR to induction chemotherapy.

3) Should we consider a consolidative auto-HCT in the brentuximab vedotin era?

Expert Perspective: Exploratory outcomes from the ECHELON 2 study evaluated the patients who underwent an auto-HCT after achieving a CR with brentuximab vedotin + CHP and showed an improved survival benefit for patients who received a consolidative auto-HCT (Savage et al. 2019). However, the results were confounded by the small sample size. It was found that only 33% of the patients who had achieved a CR had a consolidative auto-HCT. Further studies are needed to determine the benefit of an auto-HCT in patients receiving a brentuximab vedotin–based chemotherapy regimen. Based on the data available so far, it appears to be reasonable to consider an auto-HCT in a young patient who achieves a CR to brentuximab vedotin + CHP in the front-line setting.

4) What is the role of adding etoposide to CHP backbone in patients who are not candidates for brentuximab vedotin?

Expert Perspective: Given studies showing superior outcomes of CHOEP over CHOP in younger patients with normal LDH, a multicenter phase II study was conducted evaluating the addition of etoposide to BV + CHP (CHEP-BV) followed by BV consolidation in patients with newly diagnosed CD30-expressing PTCL (Herrera et al. 2019). Patients were then randomized to receive a consolidation auto-HCT. Of the 48 patients enrolled, 18 patients had AITL, 11 had PTCL-NOS, and 11 ALK-negative ALCL. The overall response rate was 91% and CR 81% at the completion of therapy. The one-year PFS was 82% in patients who received auto-HCT when compared to 48% in patients who did not receive auto-HCT. This suggests a superior efficacy of combination targeted- and high-intensity chemotherapy in the front-line setting.

5) What is the role for an allogeneic hematopoietic stem cell transplantation over autologous stem cell transplantation as consolidation therapy?

Expert Perspective: A phase II prospective study was conducted randomizing patients to either receive a consolidative auto-HCT or an allogeneic stem cell transplantation (allo-HCT) in patients who achieved a CR with first-line chemotherapy. One hundred and four patients with PTCL were randomized to receive four cycles of CHOEP, followed by high-dose chemotherapy and auto-HCT or myeloablative conditioning and an allo-HCT (Huang et al. 2017). The primary endpoint was event-free survival at three years. After a median follow-up of 42 months, the three-year event-free survival after allo-HCT was 43%, as compared with 38% after auto-HCT. The OS with allo-HCT at three years was 57% vs 70% after auto-HCT. None of the 21 responding patients proceeding to allo-HCT relapsed, as opposed to 13 of 36 patients (36%) proceeding to auto-HCT. Eight of 26 patients (31%) and none of 41 patients died of transplant-related toxicity after allo- and auto-HCT, respectively. The graft-versus-lymphoma effect after an allo-HCT was counterbalanced by transplant-related mortality. Given the high non-relapse mortality associated with allogeneic transplant, it is generally not recommended at first CR for patients with PTCL-NOS.

In summary, there is room for improvement as PTCL is characterized by substantial induction failures and early relapses. Across studies, approximately 20–40% of patients do not respond to front-line therapies, and the prognosis is poor. More effective induction strategies incorporating novel agents are needed.

Case Study 2

A 45-year-old male presented with fevers, night sweats, and enlarging lymph nodes both above and below the diaphragm. Excisional biopsy of the lymph nodes was consistent with a CD30+ ALK-negative ALCL. Treatment was initiated with brentuximab vedotin + CHP. He had transient improvement in his symptoms following initiation of therapy. However, his symptoms recurred during cycle four of chemotherapy. The end-of-treatment PET-CT scan showed persistent lymphadenopathy in the periportal and inguinal regions. Biopsy confirmed relapsed disease.

6) What is the role of transplantation in this patient's primary refractory disease?

Expert Perspective: Patients with relapsed/refractory PTCL have a poor prognosis, with studies showing a median OS and progression-free survival after relapse of 5.5 and 3.1 months, respectively, with outcomes being marginally better for those who could receive chemotherapy at the time of relapse (OS and progression-free survival of 6 months and 4 months, respectively). Studies have shown the benefit of an allo-HCT at relapse; however, it is important to note that about one-third of the patients do not proceed to transplantation due to rapidly progressing disease and poor performance status at the time of relapse.

- **Second-line chemotherapy before transplant:** Combination chemotherapy using gemcitabine, ifosfamide, carboplatin, cytarabine, and bendamustine–containing regimens are sometimes used as salvage therapies in fit patients as a bridge to stem cell transplantation (Zinzani et al. 2005, Zhang et al. 2016, Zinzani et al. 1998, Lunning and Horwitz 2013, Zelenetz et al. 2003). However, the responses are limited, often of short duration, with a median overall response rate of 55% and CR rate of only 30%.
- **Non-chemotherapy regimen prior to transplant:** Novel agents such as pralatrexate, romidepsin, belinostat, and brentuximab vedotin have been approved in recent years for treatment of relapsed/refractory PTCL (Amengual et al. 2018). Pralatrexate is an antifolate that when evaluated in patients with relapsed/refractory PTCL (PROPEL study) showed an overall response rate of 29% and a CR of 11% (O'connor et al. 2011). The ORR in patients with PTCL-NOS was 32%. The progression-free survival was three months, with a median OS of 14.5 months. Romidepsin and belinostat are histone deacetylase inhibitors that have demonstrated an overall response rate of 25%, with CR of 19% in patients with relapsed/refractory PTCL (Piekarz et al. 2011). In the PTCL-NOS subgroups, the response rates with both romidepsin and belinostat are similar, with an overall response rate of 25% and a CR noted in 14% of the cases.
- **Second-line consolidation with transplant:** Corradini et al. published a report on 52 patients with relapsed/refractory PTCL-NOS, AITL, and ALCL (Dodero et al. 2012). These patients underwent reduced-intensity conditioning with cyclophosphamide, fludarabine, and thiotepa, followed by an allogeneic stem cell transplantation. HLA-identical related donors were the most common, but matched unrelated donors and haplo-identical donors were used as well. The five-year OS and progression-free survival were 50% and 40%, respectively. The type of donor or histological subtype did not influence the outcome. Chemo-refractory disease at the time of transplant was an important risk factor, with the five-year progression-free survival noted to be 8%, compared to 51% for patients with chemosensitive disease.

Several retrospective studies have been conducted evaluating the role of allo-HCT in relapsed/refractory PTCL. The studies are confounded by the heterogeneity in the histological subtypes, conditioning regimens used, disease status at the time of transplant, and the graft-versus-host disease prophylaxis used.

In 2018, a French registry–based study reported a series of 77 transplanted patients with relapsed PTCL (PTCS-NOS 39%, AITL 29%, anaplastic T-cell lymphoma 15%) (Le Gouill et al. 2008). At a median follow-up of 33 months, the two-year OS was 64%. Cumulative incidence of relapse was 22% at two years. For patients transplanted with progressive disease, 50% reached a CR after allo-HCT, confirming the graft-versus-lymphoma effect in T-cell lymphomas. There are no optimal conditioning regimens. Studies have shown reduced-intensity conditioning to have slightly lower non-relapse mortality, and no statistically significant differences were found for progression-free survival and OS. The non-relapse mortality across all studies ranges from 25 to 32%.

The role of allo-HCT is controversial in relapsed/refractory PTCL. Retrospective studies comparing auto-HCT to allo-HCT in the relapsed setting have shown mixed results, with some studies showing benefit with an allo-HCT and other studies failing to show improvement in OS. A retrospective trial evaluated 67 patients with relapsed PTCL and reported a three-year progression-free survival of 49%, three-year OS of 53%, and one-year non-relapse mortality of 18% for patients with allo-HCT. For patients undergoing auto-HCT, the three-year progression-free survival was 20%, three-year OS was 20%, and one-year non-relapse mortality was 7% (Huang et al. 2017). Smith et al. reported a three-year OS of 46%, three-year progression-free survival of 37%, and a three-year non-relapse mortality of 34% in patients with relapsed/refractory PTCL with an allo-HCT, compared to a three-year OS of 59%, three-year progression-free survival of 47%, and a three-year non-relapse mortality of 6% among patients who received an auto-HCT (Smith et al. 2013).

A large meta-analysis evaluated 1,765 patients with relapsed/refractory PTCL who underwent a hematopoietic stem cell transplant and reported that the three-year OS was 50%, three-year progression-free survival was 42%, and transplant-related mortality was 32% among patients undergoing an allo-HCT (Du et al. 2021). The three-year OS was 55%, three-year progression-free survival was 41%, and three-year transplant-related mortality was 7% among patients who received an auto-HCT. These differences were not statistically significant. Patients who had partial response to chemotherapy did significantly better with an allo-HCT when compared to an auto-HCT. Benefit was noted across all histological subtypes.

Our opinion: Auto-HCT may be considered in a certain small number of patients with chemotherapy-sensitive disease at the time of first relapse and whose performance status precludes them from receiving an allo-HCT.

Angioimmunoblastic T Cell Lymphoma

7) How best to treat patients with AITL?

Expert Perspective: AITL is an aggressive subtype of PTCL primarily occurring in older adults. The median age of presentation is 65 years and is more commonly seen in women. It typically presents as an advanced-stage disease and is often associated with autoimmune findings such as positive rheumatoid factor, skin rash, and autoimmune hemolytic anemias, which can often mask the diagnosis.

The cell of origin for AITL is the follicular T helper cell. The morphologic presentation consists of effacement of the follicles of the lymph nodes by a polymorphous infiltrate of immunoblasts, B cells, plasma cells, eosinophils, histiocytes, and epithelioid cells. Irregular proliferation of the follicular dendritic cells and endothelial venules is also present. The malignant follicular T helper cells reside in close proximity to the venules. These cells express CD3, CD4, CD10, and CXCL13. CD30 expression is seen in 20% of the cases. These cells express PD-1 and BCL-6, which distinguishes AITL from benign lymphoproliferative disorders (Lunning and Vose 2017) (see Chapter 34).

The outcomes of patients with AITL remain poor, with a median survival of 32% with conventional multiagent chemotherapy. The disease is characterized by short duration of remissions, even in patients who respond to chemotherapy. There is no gold standard chemotherapy for treatment of AITL. ECHELON-2, which incorporated brentuximab vedotin + CHP in CD30-positive patients with AITL, did not show a statistically significant benefit over CHOP. CHOEP remains to be the preferred approach in younger patients who are CD30 negative as discussed previously. Several studies are ongoing incorporating novel agents such as lenalidomide, azacytidine, and pralatrexate along with CHOP in the frontline setting with a goal of improving the response rates.

A phase III study evaluated CHOP with or without romidepsin in untreated PTCL but failed to meet the primary endpoint of improved progression-free survival. However, the subgroup analysis did show a progression-free survival benefit in patients with AITL and other follicular T helper cell lymphomas (Bachy et al. 2021).

Consolidative auto-HCT at first remission has shown to improve the outcomes in patients with AITL. The European Group for Blood and Marrow Transplantation (EBMT) analyzed the outcomes of patients with AITL who underwent an auto-HCT and noted that 56% of individuals remained disease free at two years. Among patients with chemo-sensitive disease, there was a survival advantage in those who were not in complete remission at the time of transplant (Kyriakou et al. 2008).

In the relapsed/refractory setting, approach to AITL is similar to that of PTCL-NOS. In chemotherapy-sensitive, transplant-eligible patients, outside of a clinical study, an allo-HCT is the preferred treatment approach. The European Group for Blood and Bone marrow Transplantation (EBMT) reported the outcomes of 45 patients with relapsed/refractory AITL in patients and noted that the three-year progression-free survival and OS for all patients were 53% and 64%, respectively, with one-year cumulative incidence of treatment-related mortality of 25%. As noted in other studies, patients with chemosensitive disease had better a three-year OS than those with refractory disease at the time of allo-HCT (81% vs 37%) (Kyriakou et al. 2009).

NK/T-Cell Lymphoma, Nasal Type

Case study 3

A 45-year-old Vietnamese man is referred with a new diagnosis of NK/T-cell lymphoma, nasal type. He presented with a large nasopharyngeal mass, in addition to thoracic lymphadenopathy and axial skeletal lesions. He was noted to have an elevated LDH and low albumin.

8) How best to treat a patient with NK/T-cell lymphoma, nasal type?

Expert Perspective: NK/T-cell lymphoma is commonly seen in Asian and Latin American countries. It constitutes up to 10% of all lymphomas in East Asia. It is less commonly seen in the United States. A majority of cases arise from the nasal cavity and the paranasal sinuses.

Traditionally, the outcomes of patients with disseminated NK/T-cell lymphomas when treated with CHOP-like chemotherapy regimens were poor, with an OS of 20%. Incorporation of peg-asparaginase to chemotherapy regimens has improved the outcomes significantly.

In a phase II study evaluating SMILE regimen (dexamethasone, methotrexate, ifosfamide, L-asparaginase, etoposide), 38 patients with newly diagnosed stage IV disease, relapsed disease, and refractory disease were enrolled. All patients received two cycles of SMILE regimen (Yamaguchi et al. 2011). Twenty-one patients underwent a consolidative auto-HCT or an allo-HCT. The overall response rate for patients with stage IV was 80%, with a CR of 40%. The ORR for patients with relapsed disease was 93%, with a CR of 64%. The response in primary refractory disease was poor, with an overall response rate of 25% and a no CR. The median one-year OS was 55%, which was significantly higher than with non-asparaginase-based regimens. In another prospective study that evaluated 86 patients with NT/T-cell lymphoma, the five-year OS with SMILE was 52%, with a four-year PFS of 64%. Newly diagnosed, advanced-stage patients as well as patients with relapsed/refractory NK/T-cell lymphoma were enrolled this study (Kwong et al. 2012). Twenty-four patients underwent a consolidative autologous/allogeneic stem cell transplant.

The data supporting the role of an auto-HCT in the setting of regimens such as SMILE is less clear. It is best tested in clinical trials. A retrospective study analyzed 12 patients with NK/T-cell lymphomas receiving allo-HCT as consolidation at remission (Murashige et al. 2005). At a median follow-up of 16 months, the three-year OS and progression-free survival were 55% and 53%, respectively. The transplant-related mortality was 8%. With limited data available, patients with chemotherapy-sensitive disease or relapsed disease may be offered an allogeneic stem cell transplantation. However, the time of the transplant remains controversial in this disease.

CAR T Cell Therapy

9) What are the limitations in development of CAR T cell therapy against T-cell NHLs?

Expert Perspective: Chimeric antigen receptor T cells, targeting CD19, have significantly improved outcomes in B-cell lymphomas (see Chapter 40). CAR T therapy has since been expanded into treatment of other hematological malignancies such as multiple myeloma (see Chapters 55 and 57). Studies have been ongoing to determine whether CAR T cells could be used to treat T-cell lymphomas.

Designing CAR T cells to target T-cell neoplasms has been challenging due to the following complications (Safarzadeh Kozani et al. 2021). CAR-T fratricide, due to endogenous expression of T-cell antigens that CAR T cells are designed against, limits T-cell expansion. Preclinical studies are ongoing, investigating manipulating the CAR antigen target in order to bypass the fratricide (Safarzadeh Kozani et al. 2021). T-cell aplasia is a potential complication. Unlike B-cell aplasia, which is encountered with CD 19 CARs, T-cell aplasia has a risk of permanent immunosuppression, resulting in life-threatening infections. CAR T cells targeting CD 30 are being developed, with preclinical studies showing good cell expansion and cytotoxic activity against PTCL xenograft tumors (Wu et al. 2022). CAR T cells targeting CD4, CD5, and CD7 are also being developed. Allogeneic T cells and use of alternate cell sources such as CAR-macrophages are also in early-phase clinical trials. Cellular therapy may have the potential to improve outcomes in chemotherapy-refractory PTCL and could potentially lead to improved outcomes.

Conclusion

PTCL remains a challenging set of heterogenous diseases, with poor outcomes. Advances in genomic and molecular diagnostic methods have helped categorize the diseases and identify key pathways. Incorporation of novel agents into the front-line setting may reduce primary refractory disease and improve the OS outcomes. The role of transplantation will be better defined and could possibly take a backseat with the advent of newer targeted agents and cellular therapy. The future for T-cell lymphomas looks exciting with several new exciting novel agents and targeted therapies on the horizon such as valemtostat (EZH inhibitor), duvelisib (PI3 kinase inhibitor), ruxolitinib (JAK-STAT inhibitor) and CAR T cell therapy

Recommended Readings

Bachy, E., Camus, V., Thieblemont, C., Sibon, D., Casasnovas, R., Ysebaert, L. et al. (2021). Romidepsin plus CHOP versus CHOP in patients with previously untreated peripheral T-cell lymphoma: results of the Ro-CHOP phase III study (conducted by LYSA). *J Clin Oncol* JCO. 21.01815.

D'Amore, F., Relander, T., Lauritzsen, G.F., Jantunen, E., Hagberg, H., Anderson, H. et al. (2012). Up-front autologous stem-cell transplantation in peripheral T-cell lymphoma: NLG-T-01. *J Clin Oncol* 30 (25).

Du, J., Yu, D., Han, X., Zhu, L. and Huang, Z. (2021). Comparison of allogeneic stem cell transplant and autologous stem cell transplant in refractory or relapsed peripheral T-cell lymphoma: a systematic review and meta-analysis. *JAMA Netw Open* 4 (5): e219807.

Herrera, A.F., Zain, J., Savage, K.J., Feldman, T.A., Brammer, J.E., Chen, L. et al. (2019). Preliminary results from a phase 2 trial of brentuximab vedotin plus cyclophosphamide, doxorubicin, etoposide, and prednisone (CHEP-BV) followed by BV consolidation in patients with CD30-positive peripheral T-cell lymphomas. *Blood* 134: 4023.

Horwitz, S., O'Connor, O.A., Pro, B. et al. (2022 March). The ECHELON-2 Trial: 5-year results of a randomized, phase III study of brentuximab vedotin with chemotherapy for CD30-positive peripheral T-cell lymphoma. *Ann Oncol* 33 (3): 288–298. doi: 10.1016/j.annonc.2021.12.002. Epub 2021 Dec 16. PMID: 34921960; PMCID: PMC9447792.

Horwitz, S., O'connor, O.A., Pro, B., Illidge, T., Fanale, M., Advani, R. et al. (2019). Brentuximab vedotin with chemotherapy for CD30-positive peripheral T-cell lymphoma (ECHELON-2): a global, double-blind, randomised, phase 3 trial. *The Lancet* 393 (10168): 229–240.

Kwong, Y., Kim, W.S., Lim, S.T., Kim, S.J., Tang, T., Tse, E. et al. (2012). SMILE for natural killer/T-cell lymphoma: analysis of safety and efficacy from the Asia Lymphoma Study Group. *Blood J Am Soc Hematol* 120 (15): 2973–2980.

Kyriakou, C., Canals, C., Goldstone, A., Caballero, D., Metzner, B., Kobbe, G. et al. (2008). High-dose therapy and autologous stem-cell transplantation in angioimmunoblastic lymphoma: complete remission at transplantation is the major determinant of outcome-lymphoma working party of the. *J Clin Oncol* 26 (2): 218–224.

Leca, J., Lemonnier, F., Meydan, C. et al. (2023 February 13). IDH2 and TET2 mutations synergize to modulate T Follicular Helper cell functional interaction with the AITL microenvironment. *Cancer Cell* 41 (2): 323–339.e10. doi: 10.1016/j.ccell.2023.01.003. Epub 2023 Feb 2. PMID: 36736318.

O'connor, O.A., Pro, B., Pinter-Brown, L., Bartlett, N., Popplewell, L., Coiffier, B. et al. (2011). Pralatrexate in patients with relapsed or refractory peripheral T-cell lymphoma: results from the pivotal PROPEL study. *J Clin Oncol: Offic J Am Soc Clin Oncol* 29 (9): 1182–1189.

Park, S.I., Horwitz, S.M., Foss, F.M., Pinter-Brown, L.C., Carson, K.R., Rosen, S.T. et al. (2019). The role of autologous stem cell transplantation in patients with nodal peripheral T-cell lymphomas in first complete remission: report from COMPLETE, a prospective, multicenter cohort study. *Cancer* 125 (9): 1507–1517.

Piekarz, R.L., Frye, R., Prince, H.M., Kirschbaum, M.H., Zain, J., Allen, S.L. et al. (2011). Phase 2 trial of romidepsin in patients with peripheral T-cell lymphoma. *Blood* 117 (22): 5827–5834.

Reimer, P., Rüdiger, T., Geissinger, E., Weissinger, F., Nerl, C., Schmitz, N. et al. (2009). Autologous stem-cell transplantation as first-line therapy in peripheral T-cell lymphomas: results of a prospective multicenter study. *J Clin Oncol* 27 (1): 106–113.

Safarzadeh Kozani, P., Safarzadeh Kozani, P. and Rahbarizadeh, F. (2021). CAR-T cell therapy in T-cell malignancies: is success a low-hanging fruit? *Stem Cell Res Ther* 12 (1): 1–17.

Savage, K.J., Horwitz, S.M., Advani, R. et al. (2022 October 11). Role of stem cell transplant in CD30+ PTCL following frontline brentuximab vedotin plus CHP or CHOP in ECHELON-2. Blood Adv 6 (19): 5550–5555. doi: 10.1182/bloodadvances.2020003971. PMID: 35470385; PMCID: PMC9647727.

Savage, K.J., Horwitz, S.M., Advani, R.H., Christensen, J.H., Domingo-Domenech, E., Rossi, G. et al. (2019). An exploratory analysis of brentuximab vedotin plus CHP (A CHP) in the frontline treatment of patients with CD30 peripheral T-cell lymphomas (ECHELON-2): impact of consolidative stem cell transplant. *Blood* 134: 464.

Smith, S.M., Burns, L.J., Van Besien, K., Lerademacher, J., He, W., Fenske, T.S. et al. (2013). Hematopoietic cell transplantation for systemic mature T-cell non-Hodgkin lymphoma. *J Clin Oncol* 31 (25): 3100.

Wilhelm, M., Smetak, M., Reimer, P., Geissinger, E., Ruediger, T., Metzner, B. et al. (2016). First-line therapy of peripheral T-cell lymphoma: extension and long-term follow-up of a study investigating the role of autologous stem cell transplantation. *Blood Cancer J* 6 (7): e452.

Part 8

Plasma Cell Neoplasms and Related Disorders

51

Monoclonal Gammopathy of Undetermined Significance and Smoldering Multiple Myeloma

Francesco Maura, Dickran Kazandjian, and Ola Landgren

Sylvester Comprehensive Cancer Center, University of Miami, Miami, FL

Introduction

MGUS is defined as the presence of a serum monoclonal (M) protein < 3 g/dL, fewer than 10% monoclonal plasma cells in the bone marrow, no other B-cell proliferative disorders, and, most importantly, the absence of end organ damage that can be attributed to the plasma cell proliferative disorder (Kyle et al. 2006, Kyle and Rajkumar 2007, Rajkumar et al. 2014). End organ damage is characterized by the presence of CRAB (hypercalcemia, renal insufficiency, anemia, or bone lesions), which is related to the plasma cell proliferative disorder. Additionally, with the revised International Myeloma Working Group diagnostic criteria, patients must not have myeloma-defining events (bone marrow plasmacytosis $\geq$ 60%, serum free light chain ratio $\geq$ 100, or $\geq$ 2 focal lesions on MRI) (Rajkumar et al. 2014). Multiple myeloma (MM) is the second most common hematological malignancy. This aggressive tumor is consistently preceded by detectable and asymptomatic expansion of clonal plasma cells in the bone marrow, clinically recognized as monoclonal gammopathy of undetermined significance (MGUS) or smoldering myeloma (SMM) (Landgren et al. 2009a).

Case Study 1

A 58-year-old overweight African American male with a history of mild hypertension and hypercholesterolemia was evaluated by his primary care physician during a wellness check appointment. On routine laboratory evaluations, the serum total protein was noted to be slightly above normal at 9.1 g/dL, prompting the physician to check a serum protein electropheresis with immunofixation, which showed a monoclonal protein of 1.8 g/dL of the IgA kappa isotype. On routine labs, hemoglobin, calcium, and renal function were all within normal limits. The doctor assured the patient that he "just" had monoclonal

Cancer Consult: Expertise in Clinical Practice, Volume 2: Neoplastic Hematology & Cellular Therapy, Second Edition. Edited by Syed A. Abutalib, Maurie Markman, James O. Armitage, and Kenneth C. Anderson. © 2024 John Wiley & Sons Ltd. Published 2024 by John Wiley & Sons Ltd.

gammopathy of undetermined significance (MGUS) and that he should have his myeloma labs checked occasionally.

One year after his diagnosis, repeat laboratory evaluations revealed normal hemoglobin, calcium, and renal function and a monoclonal protein of 2.4 g/dL. Subsequent evaluations were ordered showing a serum free light chain kappa of 111 mg/dL and lambda of 0.9 mg/dL, a bone marrow biopsy showing 65% clonal plasma cells, and a normal skeletal survey. The patient was again reassured that he "just" had smoldering myeloma and that treatment is not needed. However, the patient decided to receive another opinion from a myeloma expert.

The myeloma expert ordered a PET/CT, which showed diffuse FDG-avid osteolytic lesions and diagnosed the patient with multiple myeloma (MM). The patient was started on novel immunomodulatory and proteosome inhibitor–based triplet therapy.

Comment: This patient initially did not receive an appropriate evaluation. The patient should have initially had his serum free light chains evaluated, and given the amount of serum monoclonal protein and non-IgG istotype, a bone marrow biopsy and PET/CT would have been indicated. These additional tests might have shown early detection of MM. A year later, given his testing results, he was incorrectly diagnosed as having smoldering MM. Given the patient's amount of bone marrow plasmacytosis and serum free light chain ratio, the patient had MM. Furthermore, poor sensitivity of skeletal surveys did not reveal osteolytic bone destruction later seen on PET-CT scan.

1) What is MGUS?

Expert Perspective: MGUS was introduced over five decades ago when monoclonal and polyclonal gammapathies were being evaluated in terms of clinical disease by Waldonstrom, Kyle, and others (Heremans et al. 1961, Kyle 1978, Kyle and Greipp 1980, Waldenstrom 1984). Kyle believed that patients with initial asymptomatic gammopathies over time developed MM, while Waldenström believed the two were unrelated entitities. It was in 1978 that Kyle first published his characterization of a retrospective cohort of 241 patients diagnosed with monoclonal gammopathy at the Mayo clinic (Kyle 1978). After five years of follow-up, he observed that the monoclonal protein remained stable in approximately half the patients, but in 9% it increased by ≥ 50% and in 11%, multiple myeloma, Waldenström's macroglobulinemia, or amyloid light-chain amyloidosis developed.

2) How is MGUS recognized?

Expert Perspective: Most cases are recognized when a myeloma laboratory evaluation is initiated in patients who present with no symptoms but are found to have an abnormal laboratory evaluation (e.g. elevated total protein) or when patients are evaluated for nondescript symptoms (e.g. mild neuropathy). Screening for an M protein should be performed even if there is a low clinical suspicion of MM, Waldenström's macroglobulinemia (WM), amyloid light-chain (AL) amyloidosis, or a related disorder. An adequate evaluation for MGUS would necessitate both a serum protein electrophoresis (SPEP) and immunofixation (IFE) regardless of SPEP findings, as IFE is more sensitive in detecting occult M proteins. In addition, serum free light chain assay, which has largely replaced 24-hour urine electrophoresis, is required especially in cases of light-chain–only disease. A small subset of suspected MGUS cases in reality represent an oligo/polyclonal non-malignant plasmacytosis, seen in a variety of chronic inflammatory conditions including HIV and rheumatologic disease. In these cases, the SPEP is unable to define with sufficient resolution the presence of multiple antibodies, and the only definitive diagnosis would be from a bone marrow biopsy. This limitation is likely to be solved in the near future with the development and incorporation of mass spectrometry to detect individual M proteins (Murray et al. 2019). The decision to further evaluate patients with MGUS by bone marrow biopsy and imaging should be determined based on risk prognostication at the time of evaluation. However, this risk in some patients is dynamic, and therefore this risk needs to be reevaluated in every patient at least annually, including assessing the need for bone marrow biopsy and imaging based on any evolving risk. Currently, people are not uniformly screened for MGUS as part of primary prevention guidelines. However, an ongoing prospective screening trial being performed as part of a national initiative in Iceland, iStopMM, has preliminarly showed that active screening identifies significantly higher number of individuals with MM and SMM, suggesting that early detection and intervention is achievable (Kristinsson et al. 2021). Although these early findings are encouraging, a more mature follow-up is needed before supporting MGUS screening in healthy individuals outside of clinical trials.

3) **What is the prevalence of MGUS in people ≥ 70 years of age in Olmsted County, Minnesota?**
   A) < 1%.
   B) 2%.
   C) 5%.
   D) 10%.

Expert Perspective: MGUS has been historically reported in 1–2% of adults in multiple studies. The mean age at diagnosis is approximately 70 years, with fewer than 2% recognized before the age of 40 years (Kyle et al. 2006, Landgren et al. 2017). The prevalence increases with older age. In Olmsted County, Minnesota, a seminal population-based study involving 77% of residents who were 50 years of age or older was performed. MGUS was found in 694 (3.2%) of this population (Kyle et al. 2006). The prevalence was 5.3% in persons 70 years of age or older and 8.9% in men older than 85 years. The size of the M protein was < 1.5 g/dL in 80% of the MGUS patients, and ≥ 2 g/dL in only 4.5%. Overall, patients with MGUS had shorter survival than was expected in the control population of Minnesota residents of matched age and sex (median, 8.1 vs 12.4 years; P < 0.001) (Kyle et al. 2018).

The development of novel high-sensitivity mass spectrometry assays has made it possible to accurately detect monoclonal protein in the blood with an unprecedented resolution. Leveraging this approach, MGUS was detected in 887 of 17,367 persons across the entire Olmsted County cohort, translating into a prevalence of 5.1% among persons 50 years of age and older (Murray et al. 2019). This data suggest that MGUS prevalence is likely higher than previously reported (Murray et al. 2019).

Correct Answer: C

4) What is the cause of MGUS?

Expert Perspective: The cause of MGUS is not known. Radiation exposure, pesticides, obesity, environmental disasters (e.g. 9/11 World Trade Center attack), certain ethnic background (e.g. African Americans), and a familial element (which may be genetic or a shared environmental effect) have been reported to be associated with an increased risk of MGUS development (Landgren et al. 2017, 2009b, 2015, 2018, Landgren and Weiss 2009, Maura et al. 2020, 2021). Recent next-generation sequencing (NGS) studies linked the origin of MGUS and other MM precursor conditions to a B-cell aberrantly exposed to the germinal center mutational machinery (Rustad et al. 2020). While the MM and MGUS genomic background has been progressively better understood, the reason why these B cells acquired certain initiating genomic aberrations is still unknown. Furthermore, analyses of populations at increased risk of MGUS (e.g. Gaucher's disease) suggest the possible existence of a polyclonal phase preceding the development of MGUS (Nair et al. 2016, 2018).

5) What are the different classes of MGUS?

Expert Perspective: IgG constitutes about 70%, IgA accounts for about 10%, IgM is found in 15–20%, 3–5% have biclonal gammopathy of undetermined significance (two mono-clonal proteins), and < 1% are IgD (Kyle et al. 2018). The clinical features of biclonal gam-mopathy are similar to those of MGUS. Kappa accounts for about two-thirds. The risk of progression of IgM MGUS is approximately 1.5% per year similar to other types of MGUS. Light-chain MGUS is defined as the presence of an abnormal FLC ratio with no heavy-chain expression and an increased concentration of the involved light chain. The preva-lence of light-chain MGUS is 0.8% in Olmsted County.

6) What is the natural history of MGUS?

Expert Perspective: In a referral population of 241 patients seen at Mayo Clinic from the years 1956–1970, the actuarial risk of progression was 17% at 10 years, 34% at 20 years, and 39% at 25 years, for a progression rate of approximately 1.5% per year. More than two-thirds of those who progressed developed myeloma. The interval from recognition of MGUS to the diagnosis of MM ranged from 1 to 32 years (median: 10.6 years). Only 6% were alive with no substantial increase of M protein after 3,579 person-years of observation (Kyle 1978).

Risk of Progression of Myeloma Precursor Conditions

In order to eliminate the bias that occurs with referral populations, a population-based study of 1384 patients with MGUS from 11 counties of southeastern Minnesota were eval-uated from 1960 to 1994 (Kyle et al. 2003). During a total of 11,009 person-years follow-up (median: 15.4 years; range: 0–35 years), MM, AL amyloidosis, WM, lymphoma with IgM monoclonal protein, plasmacytoma, or chronic lymphocytic leukemia developed in 8%. At 10 years, 10% had progressed; at 20 years, 21% had progressed; and at 25 years, 26% had progressed, for a rate of approximately 1% per year (Figure 51.1).

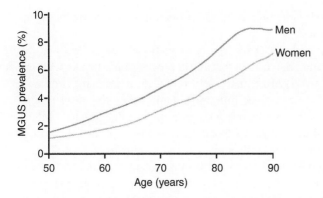

Figure 51.1 Prevalence of MGUS according to age. Years of age greater than 90 have been collapsed to 90 years (*Source:* Figure adapted from: Kyle, RA, et al. *NEJM.* 2006;354:1362–9).

7) What are the disease burden–related risk factors for MGUS progression?

Expert Perspective:

A) *Size of the M protein.* The size of the M protein at the time of recognition of MGUS is an important predictor of progression. Twenty years after recognition of MGUS, the risk of progression to myeloma or a related disorder was 14% for patients with an initial M protein value ≤ 0.5 g/dL and 49% in those with an initial M spike of 2.5 g/dL.

B) *Type of serum M protein.* Patients who had an IgM or an IgA monoclonal protein had an increased risk of progression compared to those patients who had an IgG monoclonal protein ($P = 0.001$) (Kyle and Rajkumar 2007).

C) *Bone marrow plasma cells.* The presence of more than 5% bone marrow plasma cells was an independent risk factor for progression; another study reported progression in 37% of those with an initial bone marrow plasmacytosis of 10–30%, compared to 6.8% when the plasma cell level was < 10% (Baldini et al. 1996, Cesana et al. 2002, Kyle and Rajkumar 2011).

D) *Serum FLC ratio.* In a study of 1,148 of the 1,384 MGUS patients from southeastern Minnesota, an abnormal FLC ratio was found in 33%. The risk of progression in patients with an abnormal FLC ratio was higher than in patients with a normal ratio (hazard ratio = 3.5), and this was independent of the concentration and type of M protein (Rajkumar et al. 2005).

Other features helpful in prognosis include the presence of abnormal plasma cells in the peripheral blood (Sanoja-Flores et al. 2018). A marked preponderance of abnormal plasma cells in the bone marrow as determined by flow cytometry is also associated with a significantly greater risk of progression to MM, as is reduction of uninvolved immunoglobulins (Perez-Persona et al. 2007). Finally, there is emerging evidence that clonal plasma cells' gene expression profiling and immune microenviroment composition predicts the risk of progression (Dhodapkar et al. 2014, Zavidij et al. 2020).

In the Mayo cohort of patients with elevated serum M protein ≥ 1.5 g/dL, the presence of IgA or IgM monoclonal protein and an abnormal serum FLC ratio had an absolute risk of progression at 20 years of 58% (high risk) compared to a risk of only 5% when none of these risk factors were present (low risk) (Kyle and Rajkumar 2007). Plasma cell disorders developed in 10% of our southeastern Minnesota MGUS patients after 20 years of follow-up, while 72% had died of other causes.

In the longitudinal follow-up NCI PLCO study, a cross-sectional marker analysis was conducted identifying the following risk factors for MGUS progression: M-spike with IgA isotype, M-spike concentration of 1.5 g/dL or more, serum FLC ratio less than 0.1 or more than 10, and immunoparesis ($\geq$ 1 uninvolved immunoglobulin below the lower level of normal) (Landgren et al. 2019). In this study, restricting the analysis to light-chain MGUS (i.e. MGUS without monoclonal protein in the blood), serum FLC ratio less than 0.1 or more than 10 and immunoparesis were significantly associated with an increased risk of MGUS progression. Combining these features into a scoring system, 53% and 70% of progressing MGUS and light-chain MGUS, respectively, were defined as high risk. Most patients who developed MM after a preceding state of high-risk MGUS had converted from low- or intermediate-risk stages within five years before MM diagnosis. Furthermore, only 21% of patients with MGUS progression fulfilled the blood-based criteria for smoldering MM before diagnosis of MM, highlighting the importance of stratifying MGUS patients according to their risk of progression over time.

8) What are the disease burden–related risk factors for progression of MGUS?

Expert Perspective: Most of the prognostic markers for MGUS progression have been based on indirect measurement of the disease burden (Maura et al. 2020). Patients with a high tumor burden and systemic dissemination will likely progress earlier compared to the others. Recent advances in the field of genomics have shown that using distinct genomic aberrations (i.e. myeloma genomic defining events), it is possible to distinguish MGUS that will progress from MGUS that will not (Bolli et al. 2018, Bustoros et al. 2020, Mikulasova et al. 2017, Misund et al. 2020, Oben et al. 2021). These experimental approaches have the potential to radically change our approach to MGUS and MM, allowing a more accurate and biologically based definition of the risk of progression.

9) What is the differential diagnosis of a patient with a monoclonal gammopathy?

Expert Perspective: A bone marrow aspirate and biopsy as well as a radiographic imaging, preferably PET/CT or low-resolution whole body CT, are recommended (i) in all patients with more than one risk factor including an M protein $\geq$ 1.5 g/dL, abnormal serum free light chain ratio, and/or non-IgG isotype; and (ii) in all patients who have abnormalities suggestive of a malignant plasma cell disorder based on their hemoglobin, calcium, or creatinine levels, including minor criteria such as chronic infections from immunoparesis or significant osteopenia. While outdated technologies like fluorescence in situ hybridization (FISH) do not help differentiate MGUS and MM because they share many of the same abnormalities, whole exome and genome sequencing approaches have shown high potential in segregating the two phenotypes based on the molecular and genetic pathways activated (Bolli et al. 2018, Bustoros et al. 2020, Mikulasova et al. 2017, Misund et al. 2020, Oben et al. 2021). The presence of distinct drivers is strongly predictive of progressive precursor conditions; in contrast, their absence is usually associated with indolent clinical course. This scenario suggests the existence of two biologically and clinically distinct myeloma precursor entities that are either progressive or stable.

10) How frequently is MGUS present prior to the diagnosis of multiple myeloma?

   A) 20%.

   B) 50%.

   C) 80%.

   D) 100%.

Expert Perspective: Myeloma was recognized in 71 of 77,469 healthy adults enrolled in the nationwide population-based prospective prostate, lung, colorectal, and ovarian (PLCO) cancer screening trial in which serially collected serum samples were obtained 2 to 9.8 years before the diagnosis of MM. MGUS was present in 100% two years before the diagnosis of MM. At five years before the diagnosis of MM, 95% had MGUS, whereas 82% had a recognizable MGUS for eight or more years before the recognition of MM. Therefore, the NCI PLCO prospective observational study showed that all cases of MM were at some point preceded by MGUS and that MM does not develop *de novo* (Landgren et al. 2019).

Correct Answer: D

11) How often is MGUS recognized in an 80-year-old person in routine clinical practice at Mayo Clinic, Olmsted County, Minnesota?

   A) 20%.

   B) 30%.

   C) 60%.

   D) 90%.

Expert Perspective: At age 50 years, only 8% of the population with MGUS was recognized clinically. At 80 years of age, 33% of patients were recognized during routine clinical practice. Most of these MGUS cases will never progress and likely reflect processes of bone marrow stroma aging.

Correct Answer: B

12) What is the duration of MGUS before it is recognized clinically?

   A) Less than one year.

   B) Three years.

   C) Five years.

   D) Ten years.

   E) Fifteen years.

Expert Perspective: In the Mayo Clinic cohort, the incidence of MGUS was first determined by using the MGUS prevalence data from Olmsted County, Minnesota, as well as follow-up of a large cohort of patients with clinically detected MGUS. The annual incidence of MGUS in men was 120/100,000 population at the age of 50 years, and increased to 530/100,000 at age 90 years. It was estimated that 55% of men 70 years of age diagnosed as having MGUS had the condition for more than 10 years and that 31% had MGUS for more than 20 years (Kyle et al. 2006, Kyle and Rajkumar 2007).

Recent mathematical estimations using whole-genome sequencing have shown that the first multiple myeloma cell is initiated 30–40 years before the diagnosis (Rustad et al. 2020).

These estimates are in line with recent work from Mayo Clinic in which high-sensitivity mass spectrometry assays detected monoclonal protein up to 10 years before the MGUS diagnosis (Murray et al. 2019). This scenario suggests that MGUS and MM development span over decades.

It is apparent that the increased prevalence of MGUS in older patients is not simply an accumulation of cases but rather that the incidence of MGUS increases with advancing age. The clinician should know that the presence of a mild MGUS is usually unrelated to the patient's current medical problem.

Correct Answer: E

13) How best to manage patients with MGUS?

Expert Perspective: At diagnosis of MGUS as well as at follow-up, the physician should be on alert for any symptoms or findings that suggest symptomatic WM, AL amyloidosis, or MM. A CBC, serum calcium, and creatinine should be performed. If proteinuria is present, a 24-hour urine collection followed by electrophoresis and immunofixation is needed. Serum protein electrophoresis should be repeated 3–6 months after recognition, since the M protein may represent an early MM or WM.

In patients with low-risk MGUS (serum M protein < 1.5 g/dL, IgG type, and a normal free light chain ratio), the absolute risk of progression at 20 years is 5%, compared to 58% for the high-risk group (Kyle and Rajkumar 2007). Initially, recommendations for monitoring low-risk patients at time of risk determination were 3–5-year intervals; however, the recent PLCO data suggests that categorizing risk as a single snapshot is not satisfactory, as the risk may evolve over time, requiring clinicians to reevaluate risk at least annually (Landgren et al. 2019).

Patients with high-risk MGUS have a serum M protein > 1.5 g/dL, an IgA or IgM isotype, or an abnormal FLC ratio. A bone marrow aspirate and biopsy and a metastatic bone survey should be performed. If the results of these tests are satisfactory, the patient should be followed with serum protein electrophoresis and a CBC in 3–4 months and, if stable, annually for life. Patients must always be told to contact their physician if there is any change in their clinical condition. Treatment is not indicated unless it is part of a clinical trial.

In the future, an improved understanding of the MGUS and MM genomic and immune dysregulation will allow to better define these entities and their risk of progression to clinical symptomatic disease (Maura et al. 2021).

Smoldering (Asymptomatic) Multiple Myeloma (SMM)

Case Study 2

A 60-year-old male was found to have a hemoglobin value of 12.1 g/dL, an SPEP demonstrating an M-protein in the gamma region of 3.4 g/dL with an IFE confirming an IgG kappa isotype, and a serum kappa (50 mg/dL) to lambda free light chain ratio of 80. Total serum IgG was elevated, while total IgM was below normal (immunoparesis). The bone marrow biopsy demonstrated 35% CD138 kappa-restricted plasma cells, and flow cytometry showed that 98% of the plasma cells had aberrantly expressed antigens. PET/

CT showed no lytic lesions but diffuse heterogenous radiotracer uptake in the marrow. Patient was diagnosed with smoldering multiple myeloma, given the lack of CRAB symptoms. He was told that standard-of-care management for SMM was evaluation of MM blood markers every three months. The patient was not satisfied with a watch-and-wait approach, given his five-year risk of developing symptomatic MM of > 70%. He, therefore, self-referred to an MM research institute to be evaluated for a high-risk smoldering MM interventional clinical trial. As part of the screening evaluation for the trial, he underwent a diffusion-weighted whole-body MRI, which demonstrated two focal lesions > 1 cm in the femur and humerus. He was told that he didn't qualify for the trial based on these findings.

Comment: The patient's initial evaluation was consistent with high-risk smoldering MM based both on the PETHEMA (immunoparesis, ≥ 95% aberrant plasma cells) and Mayo (≥ 20% plasma cells, M protein ≥ 2 gm/dL, light chain ratio ≥ 20) criteria. However, the last piece of the initial MM diagnostic evaluation (MRI) was not completed. The new IMWG criteria incorporate myeloma-defining events, in this case more than one focal lesion. Albeit, a whole-body MRI may not be feasible for all patients at time of diagnosis, this is the perfect case where it is warranted. All other MM criteria were negative, and the patient was a motivated young patient. This patient had newly diagnosed MM and should be treated with standard-of-care triplet-based combination therapy for newly diagnosed MM.

14) What is the definition of SMM?

Expert Perspective: The differentiation between SMM and MGUS is clinical and arbitrarily created, based on indirect measurement of the disease burden introduced four decades ago (Kyle and Greipp 1980). According to these criteria, SMM was defined by the presence of an M protein ≥ 3 g/dL and/or ≥ 10% monoclonal plasma cells in the bone marrow, with no evidence of end organ damage known as CRAB (calcium elevation, renal insufficiency, anemia, and bone lesions). In a series of 276 patients with SMM, 59% developed SMM or AL amyloidosis during follow-up. The risk of progression was 10% per year for the first five years, 3% per year for the next five years, and 1–2% for every year at 10 years and after (Figure 51.2) (Kyle and Rajkumar 2007).

In 2014 the International Myeloma Working Group updated criteria for the diagnosis of MM (Rajkumar et al. 2014). Following these criteria, a fraction of high-risk SMM are now defined as MM and therefore eligible for treatment, despite the absence of organ damage and/or symptoms. The crietria for defining these patients are: clonal bone marrow plasma cell percentage ≥ 60%, involved:uninvolved serum free light chain ratio ≥ 100, and more than one focal lesion on MRI studies.

15) How best to manage patients with SMM?

Expert Perspective: At diagnosis, a CBC, calcium, creatinine, SPEP and IFE, and serum free light chains (largely replacing 24-hour urine collection) should be performed. A bone marrow biopsy and aspirate and preferably a PET/CT or whole-body low-resolution CT are also required. In select cases, a whole-body MRI is also required to exclude MM. The blood tests should be repeated in 2–3 months and, if stable, should be repeated every 4–6 months

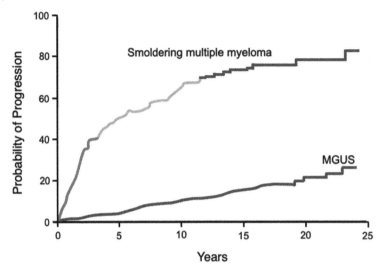

Figure 51.2 Myeloma precursor conditions' clinical outcome can follow three main trajectories: (1) the SMM/MGUS is already progressing into MM but have not reached enough disese burden to cause organ damage (medium gray); (2) the SMM/MGUS dominant clone has high predisposition to acquire new driver events and progress over the time (light gray); (3) SMM/MGUS has a low risk of progression and indolent clinical course (dark gray). *Source:* Figure adapted from Kyle, RA, et al. *NEJM.* 2007; 356(25):2582–90).

for one year; if still stable, the interval between evaluations can be lengthened to every 6–12 months.

Currently, the standard of care is observation, but patients at high risk of progression to symptomatic disease may benefit from early treatment strategies (Kazandjian et al. 2021, Lonial et al. 2020, Mateos and San Miguel 2013). Nevertheless, early treatment should not be performed outside of clinical trials.

16) How best to predict progression of SMM?

Expert Perspective: In addition to the size of the serum M protein and number of bone marrow plasma cells, the serum FLC ratio (≤ 0.125 or ≥ 8) was an independent additional risk factor for progression in the original Mayo risk model (Kyle et al. 2006). Patients with one, two, or three risk factors (bone marrow plasma cells $\geq 10\%$, serum M protein ≥ 3 g/dL, and/or an abnormal FLC ratio) had progression rates of 25%, 51%, and 76%, respectively, at five-year follow-up. In a parallel study by the Spanish PETHEMA group (n $= 93$), immunoparesis and $\geq 95\%$ aberrant plasma cells by bone marrow flow cytometry were identified as independent risk factors (Perez-Persona et al. 2007). Patients who had none, one, or both factors had a five-year risk of progressing to overt MM of 4%, 46%, and 72%, respectively. In an updated larger patient cohort analysis by the Mayo Clinic in 2018, $\geq 20\%$ bone marrow plasma cells, M protein ≥ 2 g/dL, and serum FLC ratio of ≥ 20 (involved chain must be ≥ 10 mg/dL) were determined to be risk factors. Patients who had 0, 1, and 2–3 factors had a risk of progression at two years of 6.2%, 17.9%, and 44.2%, respectively.

In addition, other risk models using gene expression profiling and imaging have been developed based on small number of patients (Dhodapkar et al. 2014). However, it has been shown that these risk models are significantly discordant in identifying high-risk patients (Table 51.1) (Hill et al. 2021). This discrepancy is not surprising, as these criteria are based on tumor load and not underlying molecular pathology and in addition are heavily affected by lead time bias, as initial diagnosis in patients is only a snapshot in time and sporadic (Maura et al. 2020). For example, patients at diagnosis may have signicantly elevalted levels of M protein and/or serum free light chains but in fact have indolent disease where it may have taken many years for it to slowly reach that point before being diagnosed.

Different from MGUS, the relatively high risk of progression of SMM requires the development of a more accurate prognostic model. In the last 20 years, several prognostic scores have been developed leveraging indirect measurement of the disease burden (Kyle et al. 2006, Perez-Persona et al. 2007). These scores perform relatively well in identifying patients with a high risk of progression but because of their dependency on disease burden, are not accurate among all other patients. In this scenario, whole exome and genome sequencing have shown high accuracy in predicting patients who will progress, independently from their disease burden and systemic dissemination (Bustoros et al. 2020, Mikulasova et al. 2017, Misund et al. 2020, Oben et al. 2021). The integration of current prognostic features with those identified from next-generation sequencing has the potential to redefine myeloma precursor conditions, not according to the disease burden (i.e. MGUS vs MGUS) but rather based on underlying biology and risk of progression.

Table 51.1 Comparison between the three risk models, Mayo Clinic 2008 and 2018 and PETHEMA, for the identification of patients with high-risk SMM[†].

		PETHEMA Risk Model			
Risk Category n = 145		**Low**	**Intermediate**	**High**	**Overall agreement**
Mayo 2008 risk model	Low	13 (9%)	24 (17%)	23 (16%)	42/145 (29%)
	Intermediate	8 (6%)	21 (14.5%)	47 (32%)	
	High	0 (%)	1 (1%)	8 (6%)	
Mayo 2018 risk model	Low	13 (9%)	17 (12%)	10 (7%)	72/145 (50%)
	Intermediate	5 (3%)	13 (9%)	22 (15%)	
	High	3 (2%)	16 (11%)	46 (32%)	
Risk agreement		11 (8%)	5 (4%)	8 (6%)	24/145 (17%)

Adapted from Hill et al. (2021).
[†]Blue and orange boxes reflect the proportion of concordance and discordance, respectively, between the three models. In this study, the risk of progression for each of the risk categories was established using the two Mayo Clinic risk models and PETHEMA risk model.

Recommended Readings

*Dhodapkar, M.V. et al. (2014). Clinical, genomic, and imaging predictors of myeloma progression from asymptomatic monoclonal gammopathies (SWOG S0120). *Blood* 123: 78–85.

*Hill, E. et al. (2021). Assessment of discordance among smoldering multiple myeloma risk models. *JAMA Oncol* 7: 132–134.

*Kazandjian, D. et al. (2021). Carfilzomib, lenalidomide, and dexamethasone followed by lenalidomide maintenance for prevention of symptomatic multiple myeloma in patients with high-risk smoldering myeloma: a phase 2 nonrandomized controlled trial. *JAMA Oncol* 7: 1678–1685.

*Kristinsson, S. et al. (2021). Screening for monoclonal gammopathy of undetermined significance: a population-based randomized clinical trial. First results from the iceland screens, treats, or prevents multiple myeloma (iStopMM) study. *Blood* 138: 156.

*Kyle, R.A. et al. (2006). Prevalence of monoclonal gammopathy of undetermined significance. *N Engl J Med* 354: 1362–1369.

*Kyle, R.A. et al. (2018). Long-term follow-up of monoclonal gammopathy of undetermined significance. *N Engl J Med* 378: 241–249.

*Kyle, R.A. and Rajkumar, S.V. (2007). Monoclonal gammopathy of undetermined significance and smouldering multiple myeloma: emphasis on risk factors for progression. *Br J Haematol* 139: 730–743.

* Landgren, O. et al. (2017). Prevalence of myeloma precursor state monoclonal gammopathy of undetermined significance in 12372 individuals 10–49 years old: a population-based study from the National Health and Nutrition Examination Survey. *Blood Cancer J* 7: e618.

*Landgren, O. et al. (2018). Multiple myeloma and its precursor disease among firefighters exposed to the world trade center disaster. *JAMA Oncol* 4: 821–827.

*Landgren, O. et al. (2019). Association of immune marker changes with progression of monoclonal gammopathy of undetermined significance to multiple myeloma. *JAMA Oncol* 5: 1293–1301.

*Landgren, O. and Weiss, B.M. (2009). Patterns of monoclonal gammopathy of undetermined significance and multiple myeloma in various ethnic/racial groups: support for genetic factors in pathogenesis. *Leukemia* 23: 1691–1697.

*Lonial, S. et al. (2020). Randomized trial of lenalidomide versus observation in smoldering multiple myeloma. *J Clin Oncol* 38: 1126–1137.

*Mateos, M.V. and San Miguel, J.F. (2013). Treatment for high-risk smoldering myeloma. *N Engl J Med* 369: 1764–1765.

*Maura, F. et al. (2020). Moving from cancer burden to cancer genomics for smoldering myeloma: a review. *JAMA Oncol* 6: 425–432.

*Mikulasova, A. et al. (2017). The spectrum of somatic mutations in monoclonal gammopathy of undetermined significance indicates a less complex genomic landscape than that in multiple myeloma. *Haematologica* 102: 1617–1625.

*Murray, D. et al. (2019). Detection and prevalence of monoclonal gammopathy of undetermined significance: a study utilizing mass spectrometry-based monoclonal immunoglobulin rapid accurate mass measurement. *Blood Cancer J* 9: 102.

*Rustad, E.H. et al. (2020). Timing the initiation of multiple myeloma. *Nat Commun* 11: 1917.

52

Risk Stratification Including Measurable Residual Disease in Multiple Myeloma

Charalampos Charalampous and Shaji Kumar

Division of Hematology, Mayo Clinic, Rochester, MN

1) What are the factors that determine prognosis of MM patients at diagnosis?

Expert Perspective: As with every malignancy, the interactions between biological aspects of the disease and host factors play a cumulative role in the overall outcome. Broadly, the prognostic factors can be grouped into factors specific to the tumor clone, factors related to the host, and factors that reflect the interaction between the host and tumor (Table 52.1).

The initial attempt at disease staging, which also had prognostic implications, was the Durie Salmon staging system. The Durie-Salmon staging is a diverse tumor assessment tool as it incorporates both clinical and tumor burden factors. Briefly, stratification is based on combining cell mass estimates with myeloma symptoms, such as CRAB (elevated calcium, renal failure, anemia, bone disease). Moreover, the amount of monoclonal

Table 52.1 Prognostic factors.

Host factors	Tumor clone–related factors	Factors reflecting host-tumor interaction
Age	Tumor burden	Immunosuppression
Frailty: performance status	Cytogenetic aberrations	Hypoalbuminemia
	Gene mutations	Renal insufficiency
Comorbidities	Gene expression profile	Serum LDH
Transplant eligibility	Tumor cell proliferation	$\beta2$ microglobulin
	Circulating tumor cells	
	Extramedullary disease	
	Plasma cell immunophenotype (plasmablastic morphology)	
	Marrow microvessel density (angiogenesis)	

Cancer Consult: Expertise in Clinical Practice, Volume 2: Neoplastic Hematology & Cellular Therapy,
Second Edition. Edited by Syed A. Abutalib, Maurie Markman, James O. Armitage, and Kenneth C. Anderson.
© 2024 John Wiley & Sons Ltd. Published 2024 by John Wiley & Sons Ltd.

protein found in blood and urine is used to evaluate disease burden. Its primary disadvantage, however, is the subjective nature of disease assessment, particularly pertinent to the measurement of the lytic lesions on bone scans. Hence, its regular use has been abandoned, especially with the emergence of more objective methods capable of accurately determining the prognostic profile of newly diagnosed patients.

The International Staging System (ISS) was subsequently developed using a large cohort of patients and focusing on easily available laboratory tests. The ISS stratified patients based on the levels of β2-microglobulin and albumin into three groups:

1. Stage I: β_2 microglobulin < 3.5 mg/L and serum albumin ≥ 3.5 g/dL
2. Stage II: Neither stage I nor stage III
3. Stage III: β_2 microglobulin ≥ 5.5 mg/L

Despite being very robust in identifying patients with worse outcomes, this staging system does not take into account the differences in tumor biology such as the genetic abnormalities, and importantly both measures can also be affected by patient factors such as concurrent renal failure and general frailty. In addition, it does not consider the overall performance status in terms of eligibility for intensified treatment regimens, such as high-dose chemotherapy and subsequent transplantation. Furthermore, the ISS staging has not provided definitive evidence supporting disease management approaches based on initial risk.

2) What are the important genetic factors that affect outcomes?

Expert Perspective: The recurrent genetic abnormalities observed in the myeloma cells are the major drivers of the outcomes in this disease. Early assessment of genetic aberrations in the plasma cells relied on metaphase cytogenetics that demonstrated an abnormality in less than a third of the patients, primarily related to the low proliferative nature of the plasma cells. Currently, the therapeutic approach in patients with MM is predominantly guided by interphase fluorescence in situ hybridization (FISH) performed at diagnosis. The primary abnormalities can be grouped into translocations involving the immunoglobulin heavy-chain region on chromosome 14 and five recurrent partner chromosomes (4, 6, 11, 16, and 20) or trisomies typically involving the odd-numbered chromosomes. These aberrations are often considered the initiating events leading to the clone establishment, and thus are present in nearly all cells of the involved malignant population. In addition, with disease progression myeloma cells can acquire additional (secondary) abnormalities involving chromosomes 1, 13, and 17. Compared to primary abnormalities, these changes can be overlapping (two concurrent abnormalities present in the same clone), and they are typically subclonal, with varying proportions of cells harboring each abnormality. The two major subcategories based on FISH studies are standard-risk [trisomic myeloma, t(6;14), t(8;14), t(11;14)] and high-risk myeloma [defined by the presence of t(4;14), t(14;16), t(14;20), gain/amplification 1q21, del(17p)]. The FISH stratification model allows for accurate detection of high-risk patients (25%); their median overall survival is shorter compared to standard-risk patients (3–5 years compared to 7–10 years). Of note, there is evidence that the simultaneous presence of both abnormalities (a trisomy and a high-risk abnormality) may diminish the negative impact conferred by the high-risk alteration.

One additional benefit of this stratification approach is that it may influence treatment selection according to FISH results. For example, patients with t(4;14) translocation benefit significantly from the early use of bortezomib-containing regimens and up-front autologous transplantation, with studies showing at least partial abrogation of the otherwise unfavorable outcome. This is also true in the relapsed disease setting, with the anti-myeloma activity shown by the drug venetoclax in patients with t(11;14) translocation.

The most controversial high-risk marker is t(14;16), with some studies showing independent association with worse outcomes in multivariate analyses with other high-risk factors. It is possible that the prognostic value of this translocation derives from its common coexistence with other high-risk abnormalities, namely deletions on chromosome 17, as well as high levels of light chain that can contribute to renal failure at diagnosis. The presence of del(17) has been well established as the most detrimental genetic MM variation. This deletion, especially when associated with biallelic *TP53* gene locus mutations, confers the worst prognostic outcome (median OS three years), with several multidrug regimens failing to reverse the disease course. Notably, for the detrimental effect to be observed, the abnormality must be present in 55% or more of the clonal cells. These abnormalities should also be assessed in the post-treatment phase, as there is growing evidence that acquiring these abnormalities later in the disease course yields crucial prognostic significance.

In an attempt to integrate the tumor's inherent disease aggressiveness into the ISS staging system, the Revised ISS (R-ISS) was developed. In addition to incorporating high-risk genetic abnormalities, R-ISS also includes the serum LDH level to the model, based on the biochemical principle that increased LDH serum levels signify either accelerated necrosis in the tumor microenvironment or upregulation of the anaerobic glycolysis undertaken by plasma cells, signifying increased disease burden (Warburg effect). Multiple studies have validated this observation for MM patients. Most recently, the second revision of ISS (R2-ISS) was published. It stems from the work of the European Myeloma Network within the European Union–funded HARMONY project (n = 10,843). The impact on overall survival (OS) of widely available prognostic tools, such as ISS, serum lactate dehydrogenase (LDH) levels, deletion(17p), translocation(4;14), and 1q gain/amplification (1q+), was used to define R2-ISS. Four risk groups predicting different OS and progression-free survival (PFS) rates were identified. Compared with the R-ISS, the R2-ISS is an improved and simple prognostic staging system that includes the independent poor prognostic factors 1q gain (three copies of 1q) or amplification (at least four copies of 1q) resulting in better stratification of especially the large group of patients with intermediate-risk newly diagnosed multiple myeloma.

A value was assigned to each risk feature according to their OS impact. Patients were stratified into four risk groups according to the total additive score:

- Low in case of 0 points;
- Low-intermediate in case of 0.5–1 points;
- Intermediate-high in case of 1.5–2.5 points; and
- High in case of 3–5 points.

Median OS was not reached versus 109.2 versus 68.5 versus 37.9 months, and median PFS was 68 versus 45.5 versus 30.2 versus 19.9 months, respectively. The score was validated in an independent validation set of 3,771 patients of whom 1,214 had complete data to calculate R2-ISS maintaining its prognostic value.

Apart from structural changes, nearly a dozen recurrent mutations have been identified in MM and have prognostic implications. The most commonly mutated genes belong to the DNA repair enzymes pathway and have an association with the primary and secondary cytogenetic abnormalities mentioned above. For instance, cyclin D dysregulation is directly involved in t(11;14) and t(6;14) and thus signifies standard-risk disease. This is also true for mutations affecting the *MYC* proto-oncogene and trisomic MM. Of note, *MYC* mutations are associated with higher disease burden and inferior survival outcomes, regardless of initial cytogenetic classification (high/standard risk). For high-risk abnormalities, *FGFR3-MMSET* and *PRKD2* gene mutations are primarily seen in patients with t(4;14) and *c-MAF* and *MAF-B* mutations seen in t(14;16) and t(14;20), respectively. Clinically MAF mutations are associated with high free light chains in the serum and acute renal failure. The most commonly dysregulated pathway in MM cells is the MAPK signaling pathway, involved in cell growth and survival. This pathway is primarily disrupted with mutations affecting the *KRAS* (20–25%), *NRAS* (23–25%), and *BRAF* (6–15%) genes. Drugs that target these signaling cascades (e.g. MEK-ERK inhibitors, *BRAF* inhibitors) are currently being tested, but due to the mutations' subclonal presence, modest results are seen thus far. Nevertheless, combinations of drugs targeting specific mutations harbored in the malignant clone, with the standard-of-care treatment, portray a valid portal toward personalized interventions and improved outcomes for MM. Other genomic abnormalities such as microRNA alterations and epigenetic mutations can also be prognostically valuable.

3) What other aspects of disease biology affect outcomes?

Expert Perspective: Despite the excellent relationship observed between unfavorable outcomes and high R-ISS stage or high-risk FISH abnormalities, these measurements are only able to account for ~60% of the variability we see in the outcomes. It is clear that additional disease characteristics may help predict the disease course more accurately, highlighting the heterogeneous nature of MM. For example, extramedullary myeloma, a disease continually on the rise since the emergence of effective treatment options, can be best assessed by PET-CT scan or MRI. The incidence of extramedullary disease (EMD) in MM ranges from 1.7 to 4.5% for bone-unrelated lesions (e.g. organ infiltration) and 6–34% for bone-related (cortical breakthrough and soft tissue extension). While both types of EMD are associated with heavy tumor burden and unfavorable outcomes, the presence of lesions at sites distant to the primary bone niche constitutes a unique biologic entity with a particularly aggressive course and dismal prognosis. Aside from EMD, the role of imaging in terms of staging has been extensively validated in MM, and recent studies have identified PET-CT parameters that can effectively determine the tumor burden in the diagnostic evaluation. More specifically, the presence of more than three hypermetabolic focal lesions, a SUVmax > 4.2, and the occurrence of extramedullary plasmacytomas can independently influence MM progression and survival, even when analyzed with known risk factors.

Circulating tumor cells (CTC), detected by immunophenotypic methods, have been recognized as an independent risk factor for aggressive tumor biology. Although originating from the original BM clone, it is assumed that these tumor cells exhibit a rather autonomous behavior, with varying levels of integrin expression concordance with the cells in the marrow. In 2005, Nowakowski et al. showed that the presence of > 10 circulating CD38 +/CD45– plasma cells (indicate malignant origin) per 50,000 mononuclear cells is associated with 22 months decrease in median survival, compared with the patients with < 10 plasma cells (37 months vs 59 months, respectively). More recently, *Garces JJ et al.* revealed that for newly diagnosed patients eligible for autologous transplantation and consolidation, the presence of CTCs was the most relevant biomarker for prognosis. Importantly, unpredictable outcomes found with the traditional prognostic systems (R-ISS) (i.e. Stage 1 patients exhibiting high-risk trajectories) can be consistently explained by the detection of plasma cells in the blood, highlighting a previously unknown element of the disease complexity. The prognostic value of CTCs may be correlated with upregulation of bone marrow angiogenesis and the density of the microvessel environment, which was shown to be relevant independently in one study (77, 30, and 14 months median survival for low, intermediate, and high angiogenesis, respectively).

Other plasma cells features are also being evaluated for disease prognostication. Calculation of the proliferation rate in the marrow by the percentage of tumor cells in the S phase of the cell cycle by flow cytometry has been studied as a potential adverse marker for MM. Albeit an increased rate (proliferation index > 2%) has been associated with inferior outcomes, recent data question whether this high proliferation rate can independently improve risk assessment when age and R-ISS are also evaluated. Tumor aggressiveness is also determined by cell morphology, with worse outcomes seen in patients with plasmablastic (8% of MM patients) compared to reactive, normal-appearing plasma cells.

Lastly, tumor gene expression profiling (GEP) on purified CD138(+) plasma cells has shown great promise in identifying patients with adverse outcomes. While not routinely tested, several commercially available GEP signatures have been validated in clinical trials, whose implementation, along with the traditional prognostic markers, should be the future approach to risk assessment in MM. More specifically, signatures developed from the University of Arkansas for Medical Sciences (UAMS) experts (model of 70 signature genes), the Erasmus Medical Center (EMC92) in the Netherlands (model of 92 signature genes), and Intergoupe Francophone du Myelome IFM studies (model of 15 genes) were consistently associated with inferior OS outcomes, especially when combined with high-risk FISH aberrations and high ISS score. In a cohort of 532 newly diagnosed MM patients, the UAMS70 model identified 13% of patients as high risk, and patients harboring these mutations had an HR of 4.75 ($P < 0.001$) for OS in the test cohort. Of note, 30% of the upregulated genes and 50% of the downregulated genes related to inferior outcomes in the UAMS70 model were mapped in chromosome 1. The EMC92 model was validated on patients from the HOVON65/GMMG-HD4 trial, with significantly reduced PFS and OS seen in the high-risk group and prognostic significance retained in multivariable analysis. Future studies are needed to further delineate the most predictive set of genes, as the published models have nonoverlapping gene repertoires with significant variability among the signatures used (Table 52.2).

Table 52.2 Gene expression profile (GEP) models and associated outcomes.

GEP model	Overall survival (OS)	Percentage of genes with high-risk signature
UAMS 70-gene signature	5-year OS: 28% vs 78% for high and low-risk signatures, respectively	13%
	Median OS: 19 vs unreached for high- and low-risk signatures, respectively (HR = 14.1)	16%
Centrosome index (CI)	Median OS: 11.5 vs 20.9 for high and low-risk CI in patients enrolled in bortezomib trials, respectively	15%
IFM 15-gene signature	3-year OS: 47.4% vs 90.5% for high- and low-risk signatures, respectively	Not provided
EMC 92-gene signature	UAMS-TT2 data set: HR = 3.4 for high-risk signatures (95% CI 2.19–5.29)	19.4%
	UAMS-TT3 data set: HR = 5.23 high-risk signatures (95% CI 2.46–11.13)	16.2%
	MRC-IX data set: HR = 2.38 high-risk signatures (95% CI 1.65–3.43)	20.2%

Abbreviations:

UAMS: University of Arkansas for Medical Science; EMC92: Erasmus Medical Center; IFM: Intergoupe Francophone du Myelome; OS: overall survival.

4) What is the impact of host factors and factors reflecting the impact of the tumor on the host?

Expert Perspective: Another aspect that needs to be considered when evaluating the drivers of prognosis for MM is patient characteristics, such as age at diagnosis and comorbidities. Age has been linked to inferior outcomes as data show consistently decreasing survival with advancing diagnostic age, starting at 40 years (median OS 6.3 years compared to 2.6 years for older than 80 years). This is partially due to the enhanced toxicities these patients experience in response to intensified treatment and subsequent discontinuation of therapy. Treatment options are further restricted by significant comorbidities (e.g. patients with concomitant renal failure are typically not treated with lenalidomide) and increased general frailty, as transplant therapy is generally withheld due to increased morbidity. The International Myeloma Working group (IMWG) created a scoring system that assesses aging and physiological age as markers of prognosis for MM (Chapter 54). The IMWG evaluated 869 transplant-ineligible MM patients with a median age at diagnosis of 74 years. Physiological age and frailty assessment were estimated by the validated ADL (activity of daily living), IADL (instrumental activity of daily living), and CCI (Charlson comorbidity index). This score distinguished three groups (fit, intermediate, frail) and comparisons between frail and fit patients led to significant differences in OS, PFS, rates of treatment discontinuation, and non-hematologic toxicities (Figure 52.1). It is unclear whether this association between age and adverse outcomes is related to more aggressive disease manifestation in older patients (e.g. studies have shown a higher percentage of plasma cells in the S phase) or failure to withstand high-dose therapy due to declining functional status. These patients constitute a unique group among MM with consistently poor outcomes

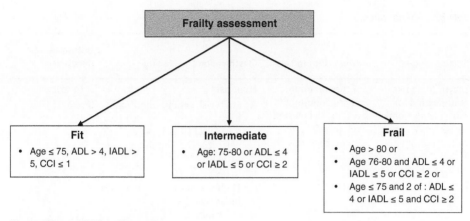

Figure 52.1 IMWG frailty score.

ADL: activities of daily living; IADL: instrumental activities of daily living; CCI: Charlson comorbidity index

irrespective of favorable disease biology, and future prospective trials need to account for the impact of this complex interaction on primary outcomes and eventually to patient care.

Table 52.3 summarizes the prognostic systems currently in use.

Table 52.3 Prognostic systems in use.

Staging system	Prognostic markers	Classification and staging	Outcomes (Median OS)
International staging system (ISS)	Serum albumin and β2-microglobulin	Stage I: β2 microglobulin < 3.5 mg/L and serum albumin ≥ 3.5 g/dl	62 months
		Stage II: neither I nor III	44 months
		Stage III: β2-microglobulin ≥ 5.5 mg/L	29 months
Revised international staging system for Myeloma (R-ISS)	Serum albumin, LDH, β2-microglobulin, FISH results	Stage I: ISS stage I, standard-risk FISH, and normal LDH	Not reached
		Stage II: neither I nor III	83 months
		Stage III: ISS stage III, and either a high-risk abnormality [del(17p) or t(14;16) or t(4;14)] or high LDH levels (defined as higher than upper limit of normal)	43 months
International Myeloma Working Group (IMWG) risk staging	Serum albumin, β2 microglobulin, FISH results and age	Low risk: ISS I or II, age < 55 years, no del(17p), gain(1q), t(4;14)	> 10 years
		Standard risk: not low or high risk	7 years
		High risk: ISS II or III, and t(4;14) or del(17p)	2 years

(Continued)

Table 52.3 (Continued)

Staging system	Prognostic markers	Classification and staging	Outcomes (Median OS)
Mayo Clinic risk stratification for multiple myeloma (mSMART), (www.msmart.org)	Serum albumin, β2 microglobulin, FISH results and plasma cell proliferation index, high-risk GEP profile	High risk: A) High-risk genetic abnormalities: t(4;14), t(14;16), t(14;20), del(17p), *TP53* mutation, gain(1q) B) R-ISS stage III C) High plasma cell proliferation index (cutoffs vary) D) GEP: high-risk signature double-hit myeloma: any 2 concurrent high-risk abnormalities triple-hit myeloma: 3 or more concurrent high-risk abnormalities	Approximately: 3 years
		Standard risk: trisomies, t(11;14), t(6;14), and all others	Approximately: 8–10 years
Cytogenetic prognostic index (PI), developed by IFM	FISH results; PI = 0.4 × t(4;14) + 1.2 × del(17p) − 0.3 × trisomy 5 + 0.3 × trisomy 21 + 0.5 × 1q gain + 0.8 × del(1p32)	Low-risk: PI ≤ 0	5-year survival: > 75%
		Intermediate-risk = 0–1	5-year survival: 50–75%
		High-risk > 1	5-year survival: < 50%

Abbreviations:
OS: overall survival; FISH: fluorescence in situ hybridization; GEP: gene expression profile.

5) Is there a role of reassessing the risk stratification after diagnosis?

Expert Perspective: Risk stratification in MM is a dynamic process as the disease evolves over time. Patients considered standard risk may behave clinically in an aggressive manner and should be regarded as high risk, even in the absence of the previously detailed abnormalities. For instance, patients who acquire high-risk features [e.g. del(17p) or other secondary abnormalities] during relapse or progression should be considered high risk, since most of these changes retain prognostic significance. Many factors used as prognostic indicators at diagnosis (e.g. R-ISS) can also be used in the relapsed setting, along with additional information based on clinical course. More specifically, both lack of adequate response to the initial therapy (primary refractory disease) and early relapse denote aggressive disease manifestation. Duration of response is particularly relevant for patients undergoing autologous stem cell transplantation (ASCT), as early progression (12–18 months) or failure to achieve a deep response (very good partial response or better) is associated with inferior outcomes. Of note, patients with high-risk features are more likely to achieve deep responses early in their treatment course. Still, these responses are not correlated with improved outcomes, since most lack long-term sustainability. In addition to biochemical evaluation, persistent PET-CT positivity with more than 10 focal lesions or new extramedullary disease at relapse strongly correlates with adverse prognosis. Therefore, comprehensive risk stratification of MM patients requires serial assessment of both cytogenetic and clinical information, both at diagnosis and follow-up.

6) What is the role of measurable residual disease (MRD) evaluation in multiple myeloma?

Expert Perspective: Traditionally, treatment response in MM has been followed by measuring the changes in the monoclonal protein produced by the plasma cells, either by protein electrophoresis or the more sensitive immunofixation. The bone marrow residual plasma cells were evaluated with immunohistochemistry, and the percentage of abnormal cells detected on biopsy was reported. Per the IMWG criteria published in 2016, a standard complete response was defined as the complete resolution of any residual M protein found on serum/urine with immunofixation and electrophoresis, plus the detection of less than 5% of plasma cells in the bone marrow aspirate. Stringent complete response was defined as complete response plus normalization of the free light chain ratio and no detectable plasma cells in the marrow. These categories, albeit prognostically valuable to this day, have failed to accurately depict the underlying plasma cell progression potential, since many of these patients were relapsing early in their treatment follow-up. It is now clear that the prognostic benefit conferred by the achievement of deep conventionally defined responses lies in the absence of measurable residual disease in the marrow. Up to 25% of patients with complete response have measurable disease, detected by sensitive multicolor flow cytometry techniques (detection of one tumor cell in 10^4 assayed). The intuitive rationale of the correlation between the depth of response and prolonged survival rates has recently become highly relevant due to the advent of novel therapeutic regimens and the regular achievement of complete or near-complete responses.

Multiple groups have explored the prognostic significance of attaining an MRD-negative state, and valuable results are now at our disposal. In a recent meta-analysis, the largest to date, Munshi et al. evaluated 44 studies with eligible MRD data for PFS and 23 for OS. The results showed that achieving MRD negativity led to improved PFS (HR 0.33; 95% CI 0.29–0.37; $P < 0.001$) and OS (HR 0.45; 95% CI 0.39–0.51; $P < 0.001$). The robustness of the results is denoted by the sustainability of the MRD prognostic utility across multiple disease variables. More specifically, MRD-negative patients enjoyed prolonged survival rates, regardless of the method utilized for detection, treatment differences, initial cytogenetic risk, and time of MRD evaluation. The ability of MRD negativity to at least partly overcome the impact of the high risk characteristics (not necessarily in "ultra high-risk genetics" e.g. as defined in MASTER trial) has shifted the management paradigm, with many clinicians opting for multidrug regimens in order to accomplish the deepest response possible up front.

Furthermore, the prognostic utility of MRD negativity is not strictly restricted to newly diagnosed patients. This was also demonstrated in a pooled analysis of the CASTOR and POLLUX trials by Avet-Loiseau et al., which showed durable MRD(−) response rates with the daratumumab-based regimens (anti CD-38 antibody). Evidently, establishing an effective prognostic model even at later stages will aid in assessing the recently introduced immunotherapy options for MM, especially the highly effective CAR T therapies.

7) What are the current approaches to MRD detection in the bone marrow?

Expert Perspective: The two methods currently utilized for the detection of MRD in the bone marrow are next-generation flow cytometry (NGF), using distinctive cell surface and cytoplasmic markers for aberrant plasma cell detection, and next-generation sequencing (NGS), using specific V(D)J rearrangements for clonality identification. These two methods are considered next generation due to their ability to detect minute quantities of residual tumor cells in the marrow, with a sensitivity of 1 in 10^5–10^6. Additionally, these methods are thoroughly standardized for widespread homogenous reporting across different trials.

Multicolor flow cytometry (MFC), the method traditionally used for MRD quantification, can accurately detect malignant plasma cells in a bone marrow aspirate with sensitivities of 10^{-4}. Most older studies operated with this threshold to define MRD positivity and negativity. As mentioned above, the large meta-analysis from Munshi et al. included studies that defined MRD negativity with these detection limits and still found prognostic significance. However, the IFM2009 study of lenalidomide-bortezomib-dexamethasone (VRd) with consolidative vs salvage autologous stem transplant (ASCT) therapy showed that patients with double negativity with the MFC (sensitivity of 1 cell in 10^4) and NGS (sensitivity of 1 cell in 10^6) had superior PFS than those who tested negative only for the MFC method. This finding underscores the importance of quantitative reporting of the MRD status (when analytically feasible) across the spectrum of detectable sensitivities rather than a more arbitrary dichotomous approach (positive/negative). Another aspect that needs to be emphasized is the importance of sequential MRD assessment across the phases of treatment (post-induction, pre-maintenance, etc.). More specifically, while even a single MRD measurement holds significant prognostic value for a given patient, continuous, sequential, and standardized approaches have been shown to yield more accurate information about the disease course through serial assessment during follow-up. To support this claim, there is evidence that high-risk patients who achieve MRD negativity early in the disease management and then quickly relapse have worse outcomes than those with unremitting, low MRD positive rates.

The relatively unstandardized reporting of MRD assessment observed in older clinical studies led to a consensus effort to accurately define the thresholds and methods to be used by clinicians and researchers in terms of MRD evaluation. According to the panel of experts, the MRD negative state is defined as the absence of phenotypically aberrant clonal plasma cells, assessed by NGF on bone marrow aspirates, using the EuroFlow standard operation procedure (or a validated equivalent method) with a minimum sensitivity of 1 in 10^5 nucleated cells or higher. The same sensitivity level is required for the NGS method. Although the sensitivity of 10^{-5} is an important prognostic landmark, the threshold was primarily based on the available efficacy data and reliable technological detection limits at the time. Since 2016 both methods have been adequately optimized to identify residual cells at much higher sensitivities.

Both methods have their respective advantages and disadvantages, with most laboratories operating based on convenience rather than prognostic superiority. The Euroflow next-generation assay is easy to use, has high applicability to nearly all samples (99%), and due to the prespecified panel of antibodies used, the results can be safely generalized. In addition, flow cytometry can address the presence of hemodilution by measuring the non-plasma cell populations in the sample (i.e. mast cells). This integrative assessment of the bone marrow microenvironment may help identify additional abnormalities for high-risk patients, thus expanding the prognostic value. Major disadvantages include the relatively high number of cells required to achieve a 10^{-5} sensitivity (~5–10 million cells) and the need for urgent sample analysis. Typically, the sample needs to be analyzed within 24–48 hours and cannot be stored for future use. On the other hand, NGS sample can be cryopreserved and analyzed at future time points. However, the need for a baseline sample at diagnosis and the possibility of failure to detect the clone after extensive somatic hypermutation can limit the use in the general population (90–92% detection rate in the MRD assessment).

8) What methods are required to complement bone marrow studies for MRD?

Expert Perspective: While the methods mentioned above carry significant prognostic value regarding MRD assessment in the marrow, they are inherently constrained by the nature of their target tissue. For instance, these assays cannot monitor EMD, making them inadequate sole estimators of disease extent for these patients. In addition, the spatial heterogeneity of bone marrow infiltration exhibited in the post-treatment setting has introduced the possibility of false-negative results, especially when blind marrow pulls are utilized. This created the need for a multidimensional evaluation of residual disease, which will meticulously assess all the different behavioral patterns of MM progression.

Relying on existing data, the IMWG defined the deepest response attainable as MRD negativity in the marrow and resolution of all PET-CT hypermetabolic lesions for at least a year. PET-CT negativity is described as the disappearance of every area of increased tracer uptake found at baseline or a preceding PET-CT or decrease to less mediastinal blood pool SUV or decrease to less than that of surrounding normal tissue. This definition is based on the biologically logical and clinically significant correlation between the response's depth and corresponding sustainability.

The inability of conventional MRI to accurately differentiate healthy bone remodeling from residual disease has limited its utility in the post-treatment setting. A novel imaging modality, diffusion-weighted MRI (DWI-MRI), has emerged as a potential substitute to the gold-standard PET-CT, with recent data showing comparable, if not more sensitive, detection rates in the treatment efficacy assessment. Of note, a recent study found that although DWI-MRI was more sensitive in detecting residual lesions, not all PET-CT signals were correlated with the ones found on MRI. As a result, additional studies are needed to investigate if DWI-MRI should be used complementarily to the PET-CT or as an independent, solitary method.

Liquid biopsies can, in theory tackle the limitations mentioned above. They permit real-time estimation of the disease burden, with no additional invasive procedures for the patients. The two main targets of liquid biopsies are cell free tumor DNA or malignant plasma cells, while mass spectrometry can detect very small amounts of residual monoclonal protein. Both tumor-based methods have exhibited non-conclusive results in efficiently substituting the BM standard, as regular discordances are seen between the detected cells in the plasma and the marrow. Many patients are found positive on bone marrow biopsies and negative in the circulation, and thus, at this point, it is not time to advocate for any change in the MRD assessment method.

Mass spectrometry is conceptually based on each monoclonal protein's particular amino acid sequence and thus distinct mass. Measurement of this mass can, with great precision, identify and quantify the protein of interest. Many studies have highlighted the superiority of this method compared to standard immunofixation, with mass spectrometry being 100 times more sensitive in detecting M protein. However, when evaluating the complete resolution of malignant residues, the prolonged half-life of M protein in the serum has a critical confounding effect, with the patients found positive for mass spectrometry and negative in BM not typically following aggressive disease courses.

Much as further optimization is required for standard clinical incorporation, MRD assessment with blood-based tests adds a potentially feasible alternative for clinicians and patients. One option would be to check for blood-based abnormalities frequently and extend the periods of laborious procedures between prespecified time intervals (e.g. every two years) or when the blood test is positive. That way, we will significantly lower the burden of invasive procedures at the patient level and at the same time have an elaborate approach toward disease detection.

9) How can we use MRD in myeloma?

Expert Perspective: The fortuitous advancement in the treatment landscape of MM has bestowed many critical dilemmas for clinicians and patients. The progress seen in the development of immunotherapy (e.g. anti-BCMA CAR T) and targeted antibody therapy, along with the increased PFS and OS, will soon render these definitions practically irrelevant within the context of a limited trial timeline. Implementing MRD as a legitimate surrogate marker for these traditional measures is of utmost importance. This will eventually allow for the timely detection of disease re-aggravation before overt biochemical or clinical signs and also help determine the true therapeutic efficacy of novel agents. Efforts on this front are currently being made with investigators and regulatory agencies working together to achieve a consensus agreement.

On the other hand, the role of MRD assessment in the clinical setting is not yet clearly defined. Due to a lack of studies, the overwhelming prognostic impact of MRD negativity has not correlated with evidence of benefit in guiding treatment decisions. For instance, an option would be to investigate the possibility of stopping extended maintenance therapy when durable imaging and MRD resolutions are achieved over prolonged periods (e.g. three years). Another question is whether there is a critical time point when MRD negative status should be vigorously pursued or if intensifying the therapeutic regimen in patients who do not achieve these resolutions is clinically useful (as opposed to withholding treatment for the first relapse).

In conclusion, MRD assessment will eventually become an indispensable tool in evaluating myeloma patients' response to treatment. The methods currently used are adequately standardized, and future studies should focus on solidifying MRD's role in treatment modification strategies through a multifaceted evaluation of the remarkably heterogenous multiple myeloma.

Recommended Readings

Cavo, M. et al (2017). Role of (18)F-FDG PET/CT in the diagnosis and management of multiple myeloma and other plasma cell disorders: A consensus statement by the International Myeloma Working Group. *Lancet Oncol* 18 (4): e206–e217.

Costa, L.J., Chhabra, S., Medvedova, E. et al. (2023 September 27). Minimal residual disease response-adapted therapy in newly diagnosed multiple myeloma (MASTER): final report of the multicentre, single-arm, phase 2 trial. *Lancet Haematol.* S2352–3026(23)00236-3. doi: 10.1016/S2352-3026(23)00236-3. Epub ahead of print. PMID: 37776872.

Costa, L.J. et al (2021). International harmonization in performing and reporting minimal residual disease assessment in multiple myeloma trials. *Leukemia* 35 (1): 18–30.

D'Agostino, M., Cairns, D.A., Lahuerta, J.J. et al. (2022 October 10). Second revision of the International Staging System (R2-ISS) for overall survival in multiple Myeloma: a European Myeloma Network (EMN) report within the HARMONY project. *J Clin Oncol* 40 (29): 3406–3418. doi: 10.1200/JCO.21.02614. Epub 2022 May 23. PMID: 35605179.

Diamond, B.T. et al (2021). Defining the undetectable: the current landscape of minimal residual disease assessment in multiple myeloma and goals for future clarity. *Blood Rev* 46: 100732.

Ferreira, B. et al (2020). Liquid biopsies for multiple myeloma in a time of precision medicine. *J Mol Med* 98 (4): 513–525.

Kumar, S. et al (2016). International Myeloma Working Group consensus criteria for response and minimal residual disease assessment in multiple myeloma. *Lancet Oncol* 17 (8): e328–e346.

Kumar, S.K. and Rajkumar, S.V. (2018). The multiple myelomas - current concepts in cytogenetic classification and therapy. *Nat Rev Clin Oncol* 15 (7): 409–421.

Munshi, N.C. et al (2020). A large meta-analysis establishes the role of MRD negativity in long-term survival outcomes in patients with multiple myeloma. *Blood Adv* 4 (23): 5988–5999.

Palumbo, A. et al (2015). Geriatric assessment predicts survival and toxicities in elderly myeloma patients: an International Myeloma Working Group report. *Blood* 125 (13): 2068–2074.

Rajkumar, S.V. (2020). Multiple myeloma: 2020 update on diagnosis, risk-stratification and management. *Am J Hematol* 95 (5): 548–567.

Vicentini, J.R.T. and Bredella, M.A. (2021). *Role of FDG PET in the Staging of Multiple Myeloma*. Skeletal Radiology.

53

Newly Diagnosed Multiple Myeloma: Transplant Eligible

Sagar Lonial

Emory University, Atlanta, GA

Introduction

Multiple myeloma is a clonal plasma cell disorder that can present with multiple end organ findings including bone disease, renal insufficiency, anemia, and/or electrolyte abnormalities. Myeloma is characterized by proliferation of clonal plasma cells in the bone marrow that not only replace normal hematopoiesis but also results in profound immune dysfunction as manifest by reduced humoral immunity that can cause frequent infections, recurrent episodes of pneumonia or sinusitis, and poor responses to vaccination strategies. The typical age for presentation for patients with plasma cell disorders is 65 years, with increasing incidence as the population ages. Additionally, the incidence of myeloma or any of the plasma cell disorders is higher among persons of African descent, with almost a 2:1 incidence in the black population. Black patients who present with myeloma present almost a decade younger than European descent patients, though interestingly, the incidence of high-risk genetics is lower among Black patients. This difference in age of presentation and genetics is challenging to reconcile with large SEER data sets showing that survival for Black patients is worse than survival for patients of European ancestry, suggestive of problems with access to new or aggressive treatments that may be at fault here. In our most recent RVD 1,000 data set (Joseph et al. 2020), we have demonstrated similar PFS and OS for Black and White patients, supporting the notion that access to aggressive therapy can equalize outcomes between these populations. Also of note, the median OS and median PFS for all 1,000 patients was 10 years and 65 months, respectively, after RVD induction followed by high-dose therapy and autologous transplant and then risk-adapted maintenance therapy. This data supports the role for aggressive induction and consolidation for medically fit patients, which can have a significant impact on remission duration and overall survival.

Case Study 1

A 59-year-old female is newly diagnosed with multiple myeloma (MM). Laboratory results show anemia, calcium and renal function that are normal, and an immunoglobulin A (IgA) kappa monoclonal protein that is 3.5 g/dL. The patient's β2-microglobulin (β2 m) is 3.1 mg/L, and the albumin is 2.2 g/dL, LDH is normal, and FISH testing shows hyperdiploidy only, so she has Revised International Staging System stage II myeloma.

1) **What is the role of the Revised International Staging System (R-ISS) in the era of new drugs in MM?**
   A) It provides prognostic information.
   B) It is necessary in making therapeutic choices.
   C) It is considered to predict higher-risk disease.
   D) A and C.

Expert Perspective: Multiple myeloma is a heterogeneous disease with variable disease courses, responses to therapy, and survival outcomes that range from less than one year in patients with aggressive disease to more than 10 years in patients with indolent disease presentation. Many studies have focused on the description of prognostic factors capable of predicting this heterogeneity in survival. Analysis of prognostic factors is essential to compare outcomes within and between clinical trials.

The Durie-Salmon staging system (DSS) was used in patients with newly diagnosed MM to determine tumor burden and estimate survival. However, there are significant shortcomings with this system, and one of them is it does not incorporate biology-associated predictors of outcome.

The DSS was replaced with the International Staging System (ISS), which stratifies patients into three groups based on serum albumin and β2 m levels: Stage I with β2 m < 3.5 mg/L and serum albumin ≥ 3.5 g/dL (median survival: 62 months); stage II, which is neither stage I nor stage III (median survival: 44 months); and stage III with β2 m ≥ 5.5 mg/L (median survival: 29 months).

Compared with the DSS, the ISS is more reproducible and easier to compute, and it reflects both patient and tumor factors, with β2 m being a measure of tumor bulk and renal function, while albumin is associated with the general state of the patient.

For the most part, the ISS replaced the Durie-Salmon staging system, as it did represent a better way to assess outcomes. However, the ISS has some important limitations. A recent study demonstrated that in patients who are aggressively treated using up-front autologous stem cell transplantation (auto-SCT), the ISS did not improve the prediction of post-transplant outcomes compared with the DSS. The use of ISS to determine choice of therapy for individual patients remains unproven, and its validity with combination novel agent therapy still needs to be confirmed. We think the ISS should be supplemented and not necessarily supplanted. There is a clear need and consensus to add other markers to the ISS for predicting patient outcome. Avet-Loiseau et al. (2013) demonstrated that the combination of immunofluorescent in situ hybridization (iFISH) data with ISS significantly improves risk assessment in myeloma versus ISS staging alone. Boyd et al. (2012) showed that by integrating the ISS and FISH abnormalities that are associated with short survival, it is possible to better identify a group of patients with a very poor outcome.

These observations led to the creation of the revised international staging system (R-ISS), which is a way to add biologic characteristics into the ISS. The R-ISS requires the β2 m and albumin similar to the ISS but also adds the absence of high-risk FISH abnormalities [del(17p), t(4;14), t(14;16), or t(14;20) and LDH above or below the normal range]. In aggregate, this revised staging better defines differences in outcomes between three groups of patients, and incorporates genetics and biology (LDH) in a way that previous systems did not. Of note, patients can have high-risk genetics but still not be R-ISS stage III. This suggests that high-risk disease is an amalgamation of not only genetics but also other biologic features that impact proliferation and drug resistance. While the notion of del(17p) patients who are not considered high risk is somewhat controversial, there is data suggesting that the percentage of cells with a specific abnormality does impact PFS1. However, it is also important that these high-risk factors are likely to be enriched in subsequent relapse, ultimately affecting OS.

Prior to the initiation of therapy, risk stratification of the MM helps predict the clinical course. For example, there is now emerging data suggesting that patients with high-risk disease benefit from more intensive induction therapy. Our group adopted the use of KRD as induction therapy for patients with high-risk disease over two years ago, and most recently there is data from the FORTE trial suggesting improved outcomes for high-risk patients who receive KRD induction, followed by transplant, KRD consolidation, and maintenance. The improved outcomes are assessed as improved PFS as well as sustained MRD negativity, which clearly favors the use of early transplant. The concept of how to best use genetics identified at the time of initial diagnosis likely also plays a major role when considering how to approach maintenance therapy. All patients (standard or high risk) can achieve a major response following effective induction therapy; however, the durability of that remission is what may be risk dependent. As such, our group has adopted a risk-adapted maintenance strategy to prolong duration of remission and survival based on the genetic risk at the time of diagnosis (Nooka et al. 2014). With the more recent switch to KRD induction for these patients, our maintenance course is now KRD consolidation and maintenance using weekly dosing of carfilzomib for patient convenience.

Age, performance status, and comorbidities are prognostic factors and affect therapeutic decision-making. It has been recently shown that, despite being enriched for higher-risk genetic subtypes, younger patients live longer, presumptively because of their ability to better tolerate treatments. Results of phase II GMMG-CONCEPT and final result of MASTER trial were reported most recently. In the GMMG-CONCEPT trial isatuximab (Isa) plus KRD was tested in transplant-eligible and transplant-noneligible patients with exclusively high-risk disease (ISI stage II/III combined with del17p, t(4;14), t(14;16), or more than three 1q21 copies) aiming to induce MRD (<10-5, next-generation flow) negativity. Patients received Isa-KRD induction/consolidation and Isa-KR maintenance. Transplant-eligible patients received high-dose melphalan. Transplant-noneligible patients received two additional Isa-KRD cycles postinduction. The trial met its primary end point with MRD negativity rates after consolidation of 67.7% (transplant-eligible) and 54.2% (transplant-noneligible) of patients. Eighty-one of 99 transplant-eligible-intention-to-treat-interim analysis patients reached MRD negativity at any time point (81.8%). MRD negativity was sustained for ≥1 year in 62.6% of patients. With a median follow-up of 44 (transplant-eligible) and 33 (transplant-noneligible) months, median PFS was not reached in either arm. In the final analysis of the MASTER trial (transplant eligible) of daratumumab,-KRD (Dara-KRd) therapy MRD status was used to modulate treatment duration and cessation. The primary endpoint was reaching MRD negativity (NGS<10-5). Participants who reached MRD negativity after or during two consecutive phases stopped treatment and began observation with MRD surveillance (MRD-SURE); participants who did not reach two consecutive MRD-negative results received maintenance lenalidomide. For the 84 participants reaching MRD-SURE, the 24-month cumulative incidence of progression from cessation of therapy was 9% (95% CI 1-19) for participants with no high risk cytogenetic abnormalities [t(4;14); t(14;16); or del(17p)], 9% (1-18) for those with one high risk cytogenetic abnormality, and 47% (23-72) for those with two or more high risk cytogenetic abnormalities (ultra high risk) Outcomes for patients with ultra-high-risk MM remain unsatisfactory, and these patients should be prioritized for trials with early introduction of therapies with novel mechanisms of action.

Baseline sFLC concentration may also provide useful prognostic information. Usmani et al. (2012) showed that extramedullary disease is more prevalent in genomically defined high-risk MM and is associated with shorter PFS, even in the era of novel agents. Other features considered significant as individual prognostic factors are IgA, renal failure, and plasma cell leukemia; however, their general prognostic applicability is unknown, and there is a consensus that no change from conventional treatment is currently indicated based on such single higher-risk features.

Correct Answer: D

2) What is the role of imaging in prognostication of patients with myeloma?

Expert Perspective: Fluorine-18 fluorodeoxyglucose positron-emission tomography (FDG-PET) and magnetic resonance imaging (MRI) probably contribute meaningfully to prognostication. A recent study has reported that the presence of more than three fluorodeoxyglucose-avid focal lesions is the leading independent parameter associated with inferior overall and event-free survival. Walker et al. (2007) showed that the presence of focal lesions on MRI independently affected survival and that achieving MRI-directed complete remission has prognostic significance. Additionally, the new imaging guidelines from the IMWG (International Myeloma Working Group) no longer consider skeletal survey as a baseline imaging study in MM. They suggest the use of whole-body low-dose CT scan, MRI, or PET-CT as baseline imaging. It is clear from large data sets that resolution of PET-CT abnormalities over time also correlates with improved PFS and OS.

3) What is the minimal FISH panel to stratify newly diagnosed patients with myeloma ?
   A) t(4;14), del(17p), and del(13q14).
   B) t(4;14), t(14;16), and del(17p).
   C) t(4;14), del(17p), +1q21, and t(11;14).

Expert Perspective: There is a consensus that both cytogenetics and FISH play important and independent roles in risk stratification of myeloma. The general purpose of risk stratification is not to decide time of therapy but to prognosticate, and so it is applicable to newly diagnosed patients. Most myeloma experts recommend that either FISH or conventional cytogenetics, or preferably both, should be done at diagnosis in all patients.

t(11;14): Among all newly diagnosed myeloma patients, 15% harbor t(11;14), and in most series tested it seems to be associated with a favorable outcome; however, this effect is not strong enough to be statistically significant, and it may relate to heterogeneity within patients with t(11;14). In fact, some cases of MM with t(11;14) manifest with an aggressive phenotype such as plasma cell leukemia. Then, the global effect of t(11;14) on prognosis remains neutral.

t(4;14): This abnormaility is noted in about 15% of MM patients and has been associated with adverse prognosis in a variety of clinical settings. It does appear from an analysis performed by an Italian group that the use of bortezomib and an immunomodulatory agent at the time of diagnosis and in the setting of consolidation therapy (VTD) is able to overcome what has traditionally been the poor risk set of patients with t(4:14). This was also noted in an analysis of the Total Therapy 3 (TT3) series from Barlogie et al. (2007), where a much more intense treatment approach appeared to overcome the poor risk features of t(4;14).

t(14;16): The significance of t(14;16) has recently been questioned. Although the Intergroupe Francophone du Myelome (IFM) group did not correlate this translocation with adverse survival, several groups have shown that t(14;16) is associated with poor prognosis.

Del(17p) is the most important molecular cytogenetic factor for prognostication, and in all series tested, it confers a very negative effect on survival.

Del(13q): The prognostic influence of deletion 13 by iFISH was shown to disappear in the IFM study when patients with simultaneous t(4:14) or del(17p) were excluded, indicating that the prognostic value of iFISH-detected deletion 13 was due to its frequent association with other known high-risk genetic abnormalities.

It is generally accepted that t(4;14), t(14;16), and del(17p) abnormalities demonstrated by FISH confer an adverse outcome in myeloma. It has therefore been proposed that these abnormalities define "high-risk" myeloma and that a FISH panel for MM should at a bare minimum include testing for t(4;14), t(14;16), and del(17p). There are some reports that the gain of 1q21 has been linked to adverse prognosis in a patient treated with tandem transplantation; however, its value as an independent FISH biomarker of adverse prognosis has not been validated by other groups. Recently, many studies have proposed that 1q analysis should be added to the diagnostic panel of FISH probes used in the routine assessment of prognosis in patients with MM. Boyd et al. (2012) demonstrated that t(4;14), t(14;16), t(14;20), +1q21, and del(17p) can be used to define adverse prognosis in myeloma and that those patients with the worst clinical outcome are identified by the cosegregation of more than one of these lesions. Another study recommended that the FISH panel should include testing for del(17p), chromosome 13 abnormalities, the five recurrent IgH translocations, and trisomy of any of the odd-numbered chromosomes; the latter trisomies ameliorate the poor prognosis in patients with high-risk cytogenetics.

The expansion of a minimal panel to other probes may be desirable, as it provides a more comprehensive assessment of the disease biology, clinical biology, clinical features, and likely outcome. Additionally, it is important that FISH testing include some method for identifying plasma cells in the mixed bone marrow aspirate. This can be done using light-chain staining to colocalize the FISH analysis on plasma cells or using CD138 selection of plasma cells before performing FISH analysis. If unselected FISH is performed, one runs the risk of incomplete staging, as a negative result may be a false negative. The use of some plasma cell selection should be mandatory when assessing the risk status in a newly diagnosed myeloma patient.

Recent reports suggested that novel approaches based on microarray technology should be used to achieve a more powerful prediction. Shaughnessy et al. (2007) have identified a set of 70 genes linked to shorter durations of complete remission, event-free survival, and overall survival in 532 newly diagnosed myeloma patients. Decaux et al. (2008) also demonstrated a set of 15 genes in 182 patients that was able to identify the patients with the poorest prognosis. Although both these studies have included patients undergoing high-dose therapy, the 70 and 15 gene models do not share common genes. Novel gene expression profiling could be developed in the future and may be useful in risk stratification.

Correct Answer: B

Case Study 2

A 61-year-old male patient is newly diagnosed with symptomatic MM due to the presence of bone disease detected by body X-ray and MRI. His laboratory results show an IgG kappa monoclonal protein that is 3.7 g/dL and a free light chain (FLC) ratio that is 131. After completing six cycles of bortezomib-based therapy, his M-component protein has fallen to 0.5 g/dL, and his FLC ratio is normal.

4) Should serum FLC assay be used to assess response to therapy in patients with myeloma?

Expert Perspective: The European Group for Blood and Bone Marrow Transplant (EBMT), International Bone Marrow Transplant Registry (IBMTR), and American Bone Marrow Transplant Registry (EBMT–IBMTR–ABMTR) criteria were updated by the International Myeloma Working Group (IMWG) in 2006, and further modifications were subsequently proposed. The IMWG recognized the need for uniformity and published uniform response criteria that are to be used in future clinical trials.

Changes in the M-component level are the principal indicators used for response evaluation. The IMWG uniform response criteria were developed similarly to the EBMT criteria, and the major response categories including complete response (CR), partial response (PR), stable disease (SD), and progressive disease (PD) were maintained.

CR is defined as a negative immunofixation on the serum and urine, the absence of any plasmacytoma, and < 5% bone marrow plasma cells. PR is a reduction larger than 50% of serum M-component and a reduction in 24-hour urinary M-protein greater than 90%, or it is less than 200 mg in 24-hour urine collection. The PD criteria require more than a 25% increase in the M-spike in monoclonal protein, at least 0.5 g/dL serum M-spike, and at least 200 mg/24-hour urine M-spike. The development of new bone disease or the observation of a new plasmacytoma and the development of hypercalcemia are also criteria for progression of disease. SD includes not meeting the criteria for CR, PR, or PD. The IMWG added two new response categories: very good partial remission (VGPR) and stringent complete response (sCR). The VGPR category is a useful measure of depth response. It identifies patients with excellent responses that may have outcomes like those of patients considered to be in CR compared to those who merely have 50% reduction in their serum M-spike. This requires a serum and urine M-protein detectable by immunofixation but not electrophoresis, or a reduction in serum M-protein > 90% and in 24-hour urine sample less than 100 mg. The sCR category arises from the need to assess the exact magnitude of response in the era of new drugs, whereas CR was rarely observed with old conventional therapy. sCR is defined as CR plus a normal serum FLC ratio and the total absence of plasma cells in bone marrow by immunohistochemistry or immunofluorescence. This category has been refined recently to incorporate the use of flow cytometry to detect mesurable residual disease (MRD) on the basis of the presence of an aberrant immuno-phenotype. Low levels of residual disease may also be demonstrated using allele-specific polymerase chain reaction (PCR), and a further new category of molecular CR is proposed that is defined as the absence of disease by sequence-specific PCR methods with a sensitivity of 10^{-5}. The minimal response (MR) category should be also reported separately in clinical trials for patients with relapsed or refractory myeloma.

Another important issue is the addition of response criteria for the patients with oligo-secretory or nonsecretory myeloma using the FLC assay. It is important to note that the FLC assay should not be used to assess response in patients with measurable levels of M-protein in either serum or urine. It has been shown that FLC response after two months of therapy is superior to early M-protein measurement to predict overall response, but it does not predict for overall or progression-free survival, and serial measurements of FLC do not appear to have added value in patients who have M-proteins measurable by electrophoresis. Additionally, for patients with high-risk disease or heavily pretreated mye-loma, there is a phenomenon known as light-chain escape whereby patients' tumor cells no longer make a heavy chain, and disease can only be followed by FLC measurement. For this reason, adding serum FLC testing with each disease assessment (we do this monthly) is a way to assess if disease is relapsing.

The IMWG included a new category of clinical relapse that reflects the fact that PD as defined does not necessarily indicate a need for further therapy but should be evaluated by the presence of CRAB features (calcium elevation, renal insufficiency, anemia, and bone abnormalities) to identify progression requiring intervention.

Over time, these assessments may be replaced with the use of mass spectometry, a much more sensitive measure for protein production that may also have the advantage of being useful for MRD assessment as well as response criteria.

5) Is there a role for functional imaging methods in the response assessment for patients with myeloma?

Expert Perspective: In MM, the introduction of novel agents has allowed the achievement of unprecedented high rates of CR in patients, especially in young patients, which has translated into extended PFS and OS. As a consequence, interest in the evaluation of the depth of response beyond the conventionally defined CR level has progressively grown. At present, magnetic resonance imaging (MRI) and positron-emission tomography with computed tomography (PET-CT) have increasingly important roles in the diagnosis and management of patients with MM, and whole-body X-ray has been replaced by these more sensitive techniques. In addition, these functional imaging methods have been proposed as an additional tool to increase the definition level of CR and to identify the persistence of residual disease outside of the bone marrow.

MRI is the elective imaging technique for assessing the degree of bone marrow plasma cell infiltration. By using MRI in MM, it is possible to recognize five different patterns of marrow involvement, with focal and diffuse patterns associated with a higher tumor burden and reduced OS in MM patients. Moulopoulos et al. (1994) reported that a change in MRI pattern may correlate with response to therapy. Lecouvet et al. (2001) showed a significant correlation between an index for the assessment of spine MRI changes after transplant and treatment response. Walker et al. (2007) demonstrated that the resolution of lesions in MRI after total therapy is associated with a better prognosis. Hillengass et al. (2012) found a correlation between serological response and post-transplant number of focal lesions detected by MRI.

PET-CT is an excellent imaging tool to monitor the response to treatment, due to its ability to distinguish between active disease and fibrotic lesion. Recent studies have demonstrated that normalization of PET-CT correlated well with high-quality responses to therapy and that PET negativity preceded the achievement of conventionally defined CR, before normalization of the MRI pattern. Combining PET-CT with laboratory data improves the accuracy of prediction of relapse and progression, compared with each test alone.

Importantly, based on the currently available evidence, the IMWG agreed that MRI and PET-CT findings will be incorporated formally into the response criteria for the purposes of assessing depth of response; thus imaging is now included in the response criteria for CR in myeloma.

Case Study 3

A 63-year-old male patient, newly diagnosed with symptomatic MM is treated with four cycles of bortezomib, lenalidomide, and dexamethasone and achieves a CR. After induction, he procedes to auto-SCT. He achieves a sCR and declines maintenance therapy. After nine months, he experiences symptomatic relapsed disease with anemia and new bone disease.

6) What is the current role of measurable residual disease (MRD) assessment in MM?
   A) It is useful to assess the depth of response.
   B) It provides prognostic information.
   C) It is necessary to evaluate the potential benefits of consolidation therapies.
   D) It is an exploratory endpoint in myeloma.

Expert Perspective: In most hematologic malignancies, the quality of response to treatment, particularly achieving CR, is strongly associated with longer survival. However, duration of CR may be a more useful metric, given that high-risk and standard-risk patients may achieve CR with similar rates but duration of CR is shorter with high-risk patients. This is especially the case when no or limited duration maintenance is adminsitered.

For many years, the major goal of MM therapy was to achieve PR or SD. With the introduction of high-dose therapy plus auto-SCT (HDT–auto-SCT) and novel agents incorporated into induction, the new goal became the achievement of CR. CR may be viewed as a surrogate marker for predicting outcome, and in the context of transplant or in elderly patients treated with novel agents, the achievement of CR is associated with prolonged PFS and survival. Nevertheless, the current definition of CR is not fully satisfactory, and it presents limitations including low sensitivity; in fact, the amount of M-component does not directly reflect the residual tumor burden, as it only measures the product of secreting clone, and not all MM-plasma cells are secretory. Another pitfall of using the M-component to define CR is the prolonged clearance of residual immunoglobulins.

MRD monitoring is defined as any approach aimed at detecting and possibly quantifying residual tumor cells beyond the sensitivity level of routine imaging and laboratory techniques. MRD can be assessed using several different approaches such as qualitative and real-time quantitative polymerase chain reaction (PCR), multiparameter flow cytometry (MFC), or more recently the use of next-generation sequencing (NGS).

Ladetto et al. (2010) demonstrated that the achievement of MRD negativity, assessed by real-time quantitative PCR (RQ-PCR), following consolidation therapy is associated with better outcomes in terms of PFS and OS and conversely, that a dynamic increase in molecular tumor burden detectable by RQ-PCR predicts late-disease relapses several months before clinical recurrence. It is also important to note that the major predictive value of RQ-PCR is after consolidation but not at diagnosis or after auto-SCT, probably because the response level obtained at the end of the whole treatment is the most important outcome predictor. This suggests that even patients not achieving a maximum cytoreduction after auto-SCT may have a good outcome if they achieve a major reduction in tumor burden after consolidation.

Paiva et al. (2008) showed, in a large series of uniformly treated patients with MM, that MRD evaluation by MFC 100 days after auto-SCT was the most relevant prognostic factor and that the PFS and OS of patients with residual tumor plasma cells was shorter than those of patients with no detectable residual tumor cells. A recent study has also evaluated the clinical impact of the immunophenotypic CR in the context of patients with high-risk cytogenetic disease: a Spanish group has reported that the presence of baseline t(4;14), t(14;16), or del(17p) by FISH, along with persistent MRD detected by MFC 100 days after auto-SCT, allows one to identify patients in CR at risk of early progression after HDT–auto-SCT. These were the only two independent factors that predicted unsustained CR.

Most recently, several groups have adopted the use of NGS using a patient-specific sequence to identify whether there are any residual clones present in the sampled marrow. As with other mechanisms of MRD assessment, the readout of the test is in large part dependent on the quality of the marrow, as hemodilute samples may under-represent the disease burden by NGS or other testing modalities. The advantage of NGS is that it is often faster, easier to standardize, and provides sensitivity down to 1×10^{-6} in the setting of an adequate sample. Many trials have demonstrated that achieving this level of MRD assessment is associated with an improvement in PFS or OS, but whether this is prognostic or predictive remains the focus of ongoing studies.

In conclusion, MRD evaluation by NGS or MFC seems to be a very useful technique for assessing depth of response to a greater sensitivity than can be observed using SPEP or serum FLC assessments. Moreover, this analysis can contribute to the evaluation of the potential benefits of consolidation therapies. Soon, understanding if/how to change therapy based on MRD assessments, attention to sustained MRD, and depth of response (10^{-5} vs 10^{-6}) are all the subject of ongoing trials to inform therapy and duration based on depth of response.

Correct Answer: D

Case Study 4

A 65-year-old male presents with R-ISS stage II myeloma with bone disease and anemia. Genetics shows del(13q) and hyperdiploidy. He is started on RVD in combination with daratumumab induction therapy (similar to Griffin study), achieves a stringent CR after four cycles of therapy, and has tolerated treatment well.

7) At this point, which of the following is best supported by evidence for a treatment recommendation.

A) Collect cells for transplant, and continue treatment with RVD + daratumumab.

B) Continue RVD + daratumumab, and do not collect cells for transplant.

C) Collect cells, and proceed to transplant.

D) Stop treatment as the patient has already achieved a CR.

Expert Perspective: The question and role of HDT–auto-SCT is one that continues to be challenged, as new treatments emerge and can induce deep responses when incorporated into standard induction therapy. However, to date, the evidence supporting its continued use remains very strong. HDT–auto-SCT provides not only the longest PFS1 but is also associated with the highest rates of sustained MRD negativity. In the two trials testing transplant vs no transplant, the group that received transplant had a longer PFS. In the IFM 2009 study that randomized patients to either RVD followed by transplant or continued RVD, the PFS for the transplant group was superior while OS was equal. However, in the most recent update of this trial that evaluated the importance of achieving MRD negativity, it was clear with longer follow-up that those patients who received an initial transplant and achieved MRD negativity had a longer PFS1 than patients who just received RVD and achieved MRD negativity. A similar story was noted in the FORTE study, which was a three-arm randomized trial comparing KCD followed by auto-transplant vs KRD followed by auto-transplant vs KRD and no transplant. All patients were subsequently randomized to receive either R or KR maintenance. In the most recent update of this trial, the group that received KCD was inferior in all measured endpoints. However, while the overall response rate, CR rates, and MRD negativity rates were similar between the KRD transplant and the KRD no transplant arms, the sustained MRD negativity rate (either at 6 or 12 months) was superior for the KRD transplant arm, which translated into a superior PFS for patients who received transplant as part of their treatment. This benefit was seen for all risk groups and further supports the use of transplant, even when using modern induction regimens.

Correct Answer: C

8) The patient proceeds with collection of hematopoietic stem cells and then autologous transplant. At day + 100 he is in stringent CR and MRD negative (10^{-5}) using NGS testing.

What is the next best management strategy?

A) A second or tandem transplant.

B) Consolidation with RVD + daratumumab.

C) No consolidation at all, proceed to lenalidomide maintenance.

D) Stop therapy as the patient has achieved MRD negativity.

Expert Perspective: The role of tandem transplant and consolidation is an area of considerable discussion and research. Much of the data supporting the use of tandem transplant and/or consolidation stems from large European trials where the induction regimens utilize either thalidomide (VTD) or cyclophosphamide (VCyD or KCyD) as part of a triplet regimen. When these regimens are used in the absence of risk-adapted maintenance (triplet maintenance for high-risk patients as discussed previously or continuous lenalidomide maintenance for standard-risk patients), the use of consolidation with a tandem transplant or intensive therapy may be a valuable part of the treatment program. In the STAMINA trial, a three-arm randomized trial performed in the US that tested the relative benefit of tandem transplant, RVD consolidation, or no consolidation, all of which were followed by continuous lenalidomide maintenance, there was no benefit for either consolidation approach. Thus, for patients in the US who receive RVD/KRD or a quadruplet induction regimen, the relative benefit of either a tandem transplant or consolidation before starting maintenance does not appear to offer any benfit, no matter what genetic risk group the patient is in. Over the past two decades of evolving MM treatment, the use of more chemotherapy was never demonstrated to improve the outcomes for high-risk patients, so this situation should be no different. It is the use of more intensive combination or maintenance using new drugs and targets that has had the greatest impact on high-risk MM, and our focus should be on those approaches, rather than continued use of alkylating agents beyond a single cycle of HDT and autologous transplant.

Correct Answer: C

Recommended Readings

Attal, M., Lauwers-Cances, V., Hulin, C., Leleu, X., Caillot, D., Escoffre, M. et al. (2017 April 6). IFM 2009 study. Lenalidomide, bortezomib, and dexamethasone with transplantation for myeloma. *N Engl J Med* 376 (14): 1311–1320.

Avet-Loiseau, H., Durie, B.G., Cavo, M., Attal, M., Gutierrez, N., Haessler, J., Goldschmidt, H., Hajek, R., Lee, J.H., Sezer, O., Barlogie, B., Crowley, J., Fonseca, R., Testoni, N., Ross, F., Rajkumar, S.V., Sonneveld, P., Lahuerta, J., Moreau, P., Morgan, G. (2013 March). International Myeloma Working Group. Combining fluorescent in situ hybridization data with ISS staging improves risk assessment in myeloma: an International Myeloma Working Group collaborative project. *Leukemia* 27 (3): 711–717. doi: 10.1038/leu.2012.282. Epub 2012 Oct 3. PMID: 23032723; PMCID: PMC3972006.

Boyd, K.D., Ross, F.M., Chiecchio, L., Dagrada, G.P., Konn, Z.J., Tapper, W.J., Walker, B.A., Wardell, C.P., Gregory, W.M., Szubert, A.J., Bell, S.E., Child, J.A., Jackson, G.H., Davies, F.E., Morgan, G.J. (2012 February). NCRI Haematology Oncology Studies Group. A novel prognostic model in myeloma based on co-segregating adverse FISH lesions and the ISS: analysis of patients treated in the MRC Myeloma IX trial. *Leukemia* 26 (2): 349–355. doi: 10.1038/leu.2011.204. Epub 2011 Aug 12. PMID: 21836613; PMCID: PMC4545515.

Cavo, M., Rajkumar, S.V., and Palumbo, A. (2011). International Myeloma Working Group (IMWG) consensus approach to the treatment of multiple myeloma patients who are candidates for autologous-stem cell transplantation. *Blood* 117 (23): 6063–6073.

Costa, L.J., Chhabra, S., Medvedova, E., et al. (2022 September 1). Daratumumab, carfilzomib, lenalidomide, and dexamethasone with minimal residual disease response-adapted therapy in newly diagnosed multiple myeloma. *J Clin Oncol* 40 (25): 2901–2912. doi: 10.1200/ JCO.21.01935. Epub 2021 Dec 13. PMID: 34898239.

D'Agostino, M., Cairns, D.A., Lahuerta, J.J. et al. (2022 October 10). Second revision of the international staging system (R2-ISS) for overall survival in multiple myeloma: a European

Myeloma Network (EMN) report within the HARMONY project. *J Clin Oncol* 40 (29): 3406–3418. doi: 10.1200/JCO.21.02614. Epub 2022 May 23. PMID: 35605179.

Dimopoulos, M., Terpos, E., Comenzo, R.L. et al. (2009). International Myeloma Working Group consensus statement and guidelines regarding the current role of imaging techniques in the diagnosis and monitoring of multiple myeloma. *Leukemia* 23: 1545–1556.

Fonseca, R., Bergsagel, P.L., Drach, J. et al. (2009). International Myeloma Working Group molecular classification of multiple myeloma: spotlight review. *Leukemia* 23 (12): 2210–2221.

Goel, U., Usmani, S., Kumar, S. (2022 May). Current approaches to management of newly diagnosed multiple myeloma. *Am J Hematol* 97 (Suppl 1): S3–S25. doi: 10.1002/ajh.26512. Epub 2022 Mar 10. PMID: 35234302.

Gupta, V.A., Joseph, N.S., Nooka, A.K. (2020 January). Approaches to Treating Multiple Myeloma, Now and Moving Forward. *JCO Oncol Pract* 16 (1): 15–16. doi: 10.1200/JOP.19.00560. PMID: 32039661.

Joseph, N.S., Kaufman, J.L., Dhodapkar, M.V., Hofmeister, C.C., Almaula, D.K., Heffner, L.T. et al. (2020 June 10). Long-term follow-up results of lenalidomide, bortezomib, and dexamethasone induction therapy and risk-adapted maintenance approach in newly diagnosed multiple myeloma. *J Clin Oncol* 38 (17): 1928–1937.

Leypoldt, L.B., Tichy, D., Besemer, B., et al. (2023 September 27). Isatuximab, carfilzomib, lenalidomide, and dexamethasone for the treatment of high-risk newly diagnosed multiple myeloma. *J Clin Oncol.* JCO2301696. doi: 10.1200/JCO.23.01696. Epub ahead of print. PMID: 37753960.

Ludwig, H., Durie, B.G., Bolejack, V. et al (2008). Myeloma in patients younger than age 50 years presents with more favorable features and shows better survival: an analysis of 10,549 patients from the International Myeloma Working Group. *Blood* 111: 4039–4047.

Nooka, A.K., Kaufman, J.L., Muppidi, S., Langston, A., Heffner, L.T., Gleason, C., Casbourne, D., Saxe, D., Boise, L.H., Lonial, S. (2014 March). Consolidation and maintenance therapy with lenalidomide, bortezomib and dexamethasone (RVD) in high-risk myeloma patients. *Leukemia* 28 (3): 690–693. doi: 10.1038/leu.2013.335. Epub 2013 Nov 13. PMID: 24220275.

Raje, N.S., Anaissie, E., Kumar, S.K. et al. (2022 February). Consensus guidelines and recommendations for infection prevention in multiple myeloma: a report from the International Myeloma Working Group. *Lancet Haematol* 9 (2): e143-e161. doi: 10.1016/S2352-3026(21)00283-0. PMID: 35114152.

Richardson, P.G., Jacobus, S.J., Weller, E.A. et al. (2022 July 14). DETERMINATION Investigators. Triplet Therapy, Transplantation, and Maintenance until Progression in Myeloma. *N Engl J Med* 387 (2): 132-147. doi: 10.1056/NEJMoa2204925. Epub 2022 Jun 5. PMID: 35660812.

Stadtmauer, E.A., Pasquini, M.C., Blackwell, B., Hari, P., Bashey, A., Devine, S. et al. (2019 March 1). Autologous transplantation, consolidation, and maintenance therapy in multiple myeloma. results of the BMT CTN 0702 trial. *J Clin Oncol* 37 (7): 589–597.

Usmani, S.Z., Heuck, C., Mitchell, A., Szymonifka, J., Nair, B., Hoering, A., Alsayed, Y., Waheed, S., Haider, S., Restrepo, A., Van Rhee, F., Crowley, J., Barlogie, B. (2012 November). Extramedullary disease portends poor prognosis in multiple myeloma and is over-represented in high-risk disease even in the era of novel agents. *Haematologica* 97 (11): 1761–1767. doi: 10.3324/haematol.2012.065698. Epub 2012 Jun 11. PMID: 22689675; PMCID: PMC3487453.

54

Newly Diagnosed Multiple Myeloma: Transplant Ineligible

Daniele Derudas[1] and Claudio Cerchione[2]

[1] *Ospedale Oncologico di Riferimento Regionale "A. Businco", Cagliari, Italy*
[2] *Hematology Unit, Istituto Scientifico Romagnolo per lo Studio e la Cura dei Tumori (IRST) IRCCS, Meldola, Italy*

Introduction

Multiple Myeloma (MM) is a malignant plasma cell disorder that accounts for 15% of annually reported cases of hematological malignancies in the Western countries. It is strongly associated with advancing age: about 70% of newly diagnosed myeloma patients are older than 65 years, with 40% older than 75 years. The introduction of high-dose therapy and autologous stem cell transplant (ASCT) and novel agents including immunomodulatory drugs (IMIDs), proteasome inhibitors (IPs), and monoclonal antibodies (MoAbs), in association with advancements in the diagnosis, monitoring and supportive care, have resulted in a dramatic improvement in progression-free survival (PFS) and overall survival (OS). However, this improvement is less marked in the elderly population due to a less extensive use of ASCT and a more conservative approach.

Furthermore, older patients with comorbidities are underrepresented in clinical trials, and there are few studies designed for frail patients.

For this reason, we need to achieve a balance in daily clinical practice between efficacy and toxicity in managing myeloma, considering the growing aging population.

1) What is the myeloma diagnostic criteria, and how best to risk-stratify myeloma patients?

Expert Perspective: In 2014 the International Myeloma Working Group (IMWG) revised the diagnostic criteria for plasma cell disorders and MM with the introduction of the concept of "ultra-high-risk multiple myeloma," characterized by the presence of myeloma-defining events (Table 54.1) in addition to CRAB features as an indication for treatment. Those criteria are applicable to both transplant-eligible and transplant-ineligible MM patients. The diagnostic workup includes a history and physical examination, laboratory evaluation, imaging, and bone marrow studies with cytogenetics and fluorescence in situ hybridization (FISH) to assess for recurring chromosomal translocations and deletions/duplications seen in MM. The genetic assessment of standard versus high risk can be useful in fit patients in order to define transplant eligibility or the best intensive treatment but may be less useful in the very old or frail population in whom the treatment goal is disease control and achievement of a good quality of life. Moreover, establishing the diagnosis in this setting of patients can be challenging because comorbidities and illnesses may

Cancer Consult: Expertise in Clinical Practice, Volume 2: Neoplastic Hematology & Cellular Therapy,
Second Edition. Edited by Syed A. Abutalib, Maurie Markman, James O. Armitage, and Kenneth C. Anderson.
© 2024 John Wiley & Sons Ltd. Published 2024 by John Wiley & Sons Ltd.

Table 54.1 2014 IMWG definition of multiple myeloma*.

Definition of multiple myeloma

Clonal bone marrow plasma cells ≥ 10% or biopsy-proven bony or extramedullary plasmacytoma*
and any one or more of the following myeloma defining events:

Myeloma defining events:

1. Evidence of end organ damage that can be attributed to the underlying plasma cell
   proliferative disorder, specifically:

   A. Hypercalcemia: serum calcium > 0.25 mmol/L (> 1 mg/dL) higher than the upper limit of
      normal or > 2.75 mmol/L (> 11 mg/dL)

   B. Renal insufficiency: creatinine clearance < 40 mL† per min or serum creatinine > 177
      μmol/L (> 2mg/dL)

   C. Anemia: hemoglobin value of > 20 g/L below the lowest limit of normal, or a hemoglobin
      value < 100 g/L

   D. Bone lesions: one or more osteolytic lesions on skeletal radiography, CT, or PET-CT††

2. Any one or more of the following biomarkers of malignancy:

   A. Clonal bone marrow plasma cell percentage* ≥ 60%

   B. Involved:uninvolved serum free light chain ratio§ ≥ 100

   C. > 1 focal lesions on MRI studies

PET-CT: 18F-fluorodeoxyglucose PET with CT. *Clonality should be established by showing kappa/lambda
light-chain restriction on flow cytometry, immunohistochemistry, or immunofluorescence. Bone marrow
plasma cell percentage should preferably be estimated from a core biopsy specimen; in case of disparity
between the aspirate and core biopsy, the highest value should be used. †Measured or estimated by
validated equations. †† If bone marrow has less than 10% clonal plasma cells, more than one bone lesion is
required to distinguish from solitary plasmacytoma with minimal marrow involvement §These values are
based on the serum Freelite assay (The Binding Site Group, Birmingham, UK). The involved free light
chain must be ≥ 100 mg/L. Each focal lesion must be 5 mm or more in size.
*From International Myeloma Working Group updated criteria for the diagnosis of multiple myeloma,
Rajkumar, SV, et al. *Lancet Oncol* 2014; 15: e538–48

confound the evaluation. For example, anemia, peripheral neuropathies, and renal impairment can be associated with a number of other causes, and it is essential to manage or rule out other etiologies (Table 54.2).

Following the diagnosis and the choice of treatment needed, the International Staging System (ISS), based on serum albumin and β2 microglobulin, represents a simple tool to determine the staging of disease. ISS is useful in defining prognosis in transplant even in transplant-ineligible MM patients, regardless of frailty status and treatment goal. The Revised-International Staging System (R-ISS), which incorporates serum lactate dehydrogenase levels and high-risk cytogenetics, seems to be useful in the fit setting undergoing a more curative therapy. The IMWG has also established uniform criteria for assessing response to disease based on clinical factors, myeloma blood profiling, and imaging. Most recently, measurable residual disease (MRD) assessment by next-generation flow cytometry and/or next-generation sequencing (NGS) can be considered for the monitoring of response and informing treatment primarily in the context of clinical trials (see Chapter 52).

Table 54.2 Clinical features of multiple myeloma and its differential diagnosis.

Clinical features of myeloma	Alternate diagnoses that can mimic myeloma
Hypercalcemia (13% at diagnosis): increased osteoclastic bone resorption, increased renal tubular calcium resorption	Hypercalcemia: primary hyperparathyroidism, tertiary hyperparathyroidism (CKD, vitamin D deficiency), malignancy (e.g. bone metastases), drugs (e.g. thiazides, lithium, vitamin D, vitamin A), endocrine conditions (e.g. thyrotoxicosis, Addison's disease), granulomatous conditions (e.g. sarcoidosis, tuberculosis), other (e.g. prolonged immobilization, milk-alkali syndrome)
Renal failure (19% at diagnosis): light chain cast nephropathy; hypercalcemia; monoclonal immunoglobulin deposition disease; plasma cell infiltration of the kidneys; concurrent amyloidosis, drug-induced (NSAIDs, bisphosphonate)	Renal failure AKI (acute kidney injury): prerenal causes (e.g. dehydration, sepsis); renal causes (e.g drug-induced, infections); postrenal causes (e.g. acute urinary retention); CKD (chronic kidney disease), which affects 60% of > 80 years; age-related decrease in eGFR; hypertension; diabetic nephropathy, drug-induced (e.g. diuretic, NSAIDs); obstructive uropathy (e.g. due to BPH); glomerulonephrities
Anemia (35% at diagnosis): bone marrow infiltration by plasma cells, cytokine-mediated suppressive effect on erythropoiesis, renal failure (decreased erythropoietin production)	Anemia (25% of > 80 years): anemia of chronic disease, iron deficiency (dietary and/or blood loss), vitamin B12 or folate deficiency, chronic kidney disease, myelodysplasia, others (e.g. hemolytic anemia, thalassemia)
Bone pain (58% at diagnosis): increased osteoclast activity causing lytic bone lesions, osteoporosis, pathological fractures, plasmacytomas affecting the bone	Bone Pain Nonmalignant causes: osteoporosis, osteomalacia, osteomyelitis, Paget's disease, injury (e.g. fractures) Malignant causes: primary bone cancer, bony metastases (e.g breast, prostate, lung, thyroid, kidney, testicular, ovarian)

BPH: benign prostatic hypertrophy; NSAIDs: nonsteroidal anti-inflammatory drugs; eGRF: estimated glomerular filtration rate.

2) How to define the transplant eligibility in older adults?

Expert Perspective: The up-front ASCT intensification following induction therapy remains to date the standard of care in newly diagnosed myeloma patients. For this reason, the definition of transplant eligibility is the cornerstone for the treatment plan. Historically, patients older than 65 years have been considered ineligible for ASCT due to an increased risk of treatment-related mortality from comorbidities resulting in reduced drug tolerance. In recent years the improvement of supportive care and increasing of the incidence of MM in the elderly population has allowed for this strategy to be applied more widely. Although the quality of the evidence is limited, the cumulative literature based on on retrospective studies and few clinical trials does favor an ASCT approach for improving overall survival and complete response rates. However, this treatment plan should be reserved for very fit patients with adequate organ function, evaluated for fitness through multiple parameters (Table 54.3). Among these parameters, the hematopoietic cell transplant comorbidity index (HCT-CI) can help estimate non-relapse treatment-related

Table 54.3 Assessment of suitability for autologous transplant in patients with myeloma.

Assessment for ASCT	Test in MM patients	Criteria
Performance status	History and physical exam	ECOG 2 or better, or KPS > 70%
Transplant comorbidity index	HCT-CI	HCT-CI score 1 or better
Disease status	Reduction in M-spike at least 50%	At least 50%
Cardiac function	Echocardiogram or MUGA scan	EF > 40%
Pulmonary function	Spirometry and DLCO diffusion	DLCO/FEV1 > 40–80%
Liver function	Liver function tests	Bilirubin < 2–3 times upper limit of normal
Renal function	Creatinine clearance	eGFR > 40 mL/min
Psychosocial/economic evaluation	Family support	Must be compliant and have caregiver/support throughout

mortality and fitness for ASCT. To decrease mortality and morbidity associated with transplant, the use of reduced dose of melphalan (100–140 mg/m^2) is suggested in selected patients with comorbidities. Moreover, clinical trials have demonstrated the efficacy and safety of combination therapy with anti-CD38 monoclonal antibodies (daratumumab), IMIDs, and IPs, which could in the future represent an alternative to ASCT, particularly in the fit and intermediate fit population.

3) How to plan the anti-myeloma therapy in older patients?

Expert Perspective: The caring of elderly MM population is complex and challenging, with patients ranging from extremely fit to severely frail. Aging is associated with numerous comorbidities that may further impair organ function. Although the novel agents introduced for the treatment of MM have improved the outcome of patients in this setting, on the other hand they cause several side effects and an increased rate of hematologic and non-hematologic toxicities, treatment discontinuation, impairment of quality of life, and high risk of mortality, particularly in the very frail population with comorbidities.

For this reason, it is mandatory to tailor the treatment plan in terms of goal, schedule, and duration and dosage of therapy according to frailty and fitness score, rather than merely the chronologic age, which does not always coincide with biological age and frailty status.

Frailty is a complex clinical constellation associated with increased vulnerability, distinct from disability and comorbidities, due to cumulative deficit in activities of daily living, resulting in reduced resistance to stressors and worse survival.

The geriatric assessment is a valuable tool based on various features (comorbidities, daily functions, cognition, polypharmacy, social support, depression, psychosocial distress) that allow for the identification of frailty status taking into consideration occult health factors in this population. The geriatric assessment is effective in predicting mortality, and its components are cornerstones for decision-making, tailoring interventions, and predicting future outcomes.

Table 54.4 Frailty scores for Multiple Myeloma.

IMWG frailty score

1. Age

2. Comorbidities

    Charlson Comorbidity Index

3. Patient-reported functional status

    Katz index of independence in Activities of Daily Living (ADL)

    Lawton Instrumental Activities of Daily Living (IADL)

Categories:

fit: score 0;   intermediate fit: score 1;   frail: score > 2

R-MCI

1. Age

2. Comorbidities

    Renal function

    Pulmonary function

3. Frailty evolution

4. Karnofsky performance status

5. Cytogenetics

Categories:

fit: score ≤ 3;   intermediate fit: score 4–6;   frail: score > 6

MAYO CLINIC SCORE

1. Age

2. ECOG performance status

3. Circulation NTproBNP levels

Categories:

Stage I: score 0;   Stage II: score 1:   Stage III: score 2;   Stage IV: score 3

EVALUATION OF SARCOPENIA

1. Muscle mass: CT 3rd lumbar vertebra area

2. Muscle function: grip strength

3. Physical performance: gait speed, etc.

SIMPLIFIED FRAILTY SCORE

1. Age

2. Comorbidities

    CCI

3. ECOG Performance Status

Categories:

non-frail: score 0–1;   frail: score ≥ 2

Different geriatric assessments (GAs) have been designed for the MM population and validated either retrospectively or prospectively (Table 54.4). The two most used GAs are the IMWG frailty score (http://www.myelomafrailtyscorecalculator.net) and Revised Myeloma Comorbidity Index (https://www.myelomacomorbidityindex.org/en_calc.html). These GAs categorize the elderly population into fit, intermediate, and frail patients, each with different goals and approaches to therapy.

4) How to tailor the medication dosage according to the fitness status?

Expert Perspective: One approach to minimize the side effects and treatment discontinuation is the dose modulation (or adjustment) of drugs based on the fitness and frailty status of the patient (Table 54.5). Full-dose therapy should be reserved for fit patients with the goal to achieve a deep response, an MRD-negative complete response. The intermediate population may require reduction to dosage level −1 to minimize the side effects while achieving a good response and decreasing symptoms. A dosage reduction at level −2 may be required for frail patients in whom the goal is to achieve a good quality of life and control of disease with the lowest toxicity.

Table 54.5 Dosage of drugs according with frailty status.

Risk factors
Age > 75 years
Comorbidities (pulmonary, renal, cardiac, and hepatic dysfunction) and Geriatric Assessment with IMWG—frailty index and/or R-MCI in order to define fit, intermediate-fit, and frail patients for adaptive antimyeloma therapy

	FIT	INTERMEDIATE-FIT	FRAIL
IMWG-frailty index	0	1	≥ 2
R-MCI	1–3	4–6	7–9
DOSE LEVEL	0	−1	−2

Treatment doses	Level 0	Level −1	Level −2
Prednisone	2 mg/kg days 1–4 of a 4–6-week cycle or 60 mg/m² days 1–4 of a 6-week cycle	1 mg/kg days 1–4 of a 4–6-week cycle or 30 mg/m² days 1–4 of a 6-week cycle	0.5 mg/kg days 1–4 of a 4–6-week cycle or 15 mg/m² days 1–4 of a 6-week cycle

(Continued)

Table 54.5 (Continued)

Dexamethasone	40 mg day 1, 8, 15, 22 of a 28-day cycle	20 mg day 1, 8, 15, 22 of a 28-day cycle	10 mg day 1, 8, 15, 22 of a 28-day cycle
Melphalan	0.25 mg/kg days 1–4 of a 4–6-week cycle	0.18 mg/kg days 1–4 of a 4–6-week cycle	0.13 mg/kg days 1–4 of a 4–6-week cycle
Thalidomide	100 (–200) mg/day	50 (–100) mg/day	50 mg every other day (–50 mg/day)
Lenalidomide	25 mg days 1–21 of a 28-day cycle	15 mg days 1–21 of a 28-day cycle	10 mg days 1–21 of a 28-day cycle
Pomalidomide*	4 mg days 1–21 of a 28-day cycle	3 mg days 1–21 of a 28-day cycle	2 mg days 1–21 of a 28-day cycle
Bortezomib	1.3 mg/m^2 twice weekly day 1, 4, 8, 11 every 3 weeks	1.3 mg/m^2 twice weekly day 1, 8, 15, 22 every 5 weeks	1.0 mg/m^2 twice weekly day 1, 8, 15, 22 every 3 weeks
Carfilzomib*	20 mg/m^2 d 1, 2, 8, 9, 15, 16 cycle 1; 27 mg/m^2 cycle 2 every 4 weeks	20 mg/m^2 cycle 1; 27 mg/m^2 d 1, 8, 15, 22 cycle 2 every 4 weeks	20 mg/m^2 d 1, 8, 15 once weekly every 4–5 weeks
Ixazomib*	4 mg d 1, 8, 15 every 4 weeks	3 mg d 1, 8, 15 every 4 weeks	2.3 mg d 1, 8, 15 every 4 weeks
Daratumumab*	16 mg/kg cycle 1–8: weekly; cy 9–24: d + 15; week 25 onwards: every 4 weeks	16 mg/kg cycle 1–8: weekly; cy 9–24: d + 15; week 25 onwards: every 4 weeks Consider splitting the dose on 2 consecutive days in the first cycle	16 mg/kg cycle 1–8: weekly; cy 9–24: d + 15; week 25 onwards: every 4 weeks Consider splitting the dose on 2 consecutive days in the first cycle
Elotuzumab*	10 mg/kg d 1, 8, 15, 22 cy 1 + 2, cy 3: d1 + 15	10 mg/kg d 1, 8, 15, 22 cy 1 + 2, cy 3: d1 + 15	10 mg/kg d 1, 8, 15, 22 cy 1 + 2, cy 3: d1 + 15
Panobinostat*	20 mg d 1, 3, 5, 8, 10, 12 every 4 weeks	15 mg d 1, 3, 5, 8, 10, 12 every 4 weeks	10 mg d 1, 3, 5, 8, 10, 12 every 4 weeks

*No known dose adaptation in elderly and/or frail patients were reported; carfilzomib dose in the ENDEAVOR study was 56 mg/m^2 weekly, and no dose modifications according to age were reported.

5) How to manage the newly diagnosed elderly fit patents?

Expert Perspective: Elderly fit patients potentially can reach a normal life expectancy and tolerate a full-dose treatment. To achieve a high overall response rate and a deep response that translates into an improved PFS and OS, various treatment strategies can be utilized. Importantly, clinical trials with immunotherapeutic agents (daratumumab) for newly diagnosed transplant-ineligible MM patients have recently shown a high rate of MRD negativity (see Chapter 52).

According to National Comprehensive Cancer Network (NCCN) 2021 and European Hematology Association/European Society for Medical Oncology (EHA/ESMO) 2021

Table 54.6 Fragility assessment and myeloma therapy.

FRAILTY ASSESSMENT IMWG Frailty Score		
FIT PATIENTS (score 0)	INTERMEDIATE-FIT PATIENTS (score 1)	FRAIL PATIENTS (score ≥ 2)
age ≤ 75 + ADL > 4 + IADL > 5 CCI ≤ 1	age 76–80 + ADL ≤ 4 or IADL ≤ 5 + CCI > 1	age > 80; age 76–80 + ADL ≤ 4 or IADL ≤ 5 or CCI > 1; age ≤ 75 + at least 2 ADL ≤ 4 or IADL ≤ 5 or CCI > 1

MAIN GOALS		
Life expectancy Efficacy sCR/MRD negativity	Efficacy/safety Good response	Quality of life Safety Low toxicity

APPROVED REGIMENS		
Daratumumab-VMP Daratumumab-Rd VRd ASCT in pts ≦ 70 years old	Daratumumab-weekly VMP Daratumumab-Rd VRd-lite Vd	Dose-adjusted Rd ± daratumumab Dose-adjusted Rd Palliative care

Table 54.7 Regimens in multiple myeloma.

Regimen	Usual Dosing Schedule
Daratumumab-lenalidomide-dexamethasone (DRd)	Daratumumab 16 mg/kg intravenously weekly × 8 weeks, and then every 2 weeks, for 4 months, and then once monthly lenalidomide 25 mg oral days 1–21
	Dexamethasone 40 mg intravenous days 1, 8, 15, 22 (given oral on days when no daratumumab is being administered), lenalidomide-dexamethasone repeated in usual schedule every 4 weeks
Daratumumab-bortezomib-melphalan-dexamethasone (D-VMP)	Daratumumab 16 mg/kg intravenously weekly × 6 wk. (cycle 1), every 2 weeks, cycle 2–9, then once monthly from cycle 10
	Bortezomib 1.3 mg/m² subcutaneous twice weekly at weeks 1, 2, 4, and 5 for the first 6-week cycle (cycle 1), once weekly weeks 1, 2, 4, and 5 for 8 more 6-week cycles (cycles 2–9)
	Melphalan 9 mg/m² and prednisone 60 mg/m² oral on days 1 to 4 of the 9 6-week cycles (cycles 1–9)

(Continued)

Table 54.7 (Continued)

Bortezomib-lenalidomide-dexamethasone (VRd)	Bortezomib 1.3 mg/m^2 subcutaneous days 1, 4, 8, 11
	Lenalidomide 25 mg oral days 1–14
	Dexamethasone 20 mg oral on day of and day after bortezomib (or 40 mg days 1, 4, 8, 11)
	Repeated every 3 weeks
Bortezomib-lenalidomide-dexametasone (VRd lite)	Induction (9 cycles):
	Bortezomib 1.3 mg/m^2 subcutaneous days 1, 8, 15, 22
	Lenalidomide 15 mg oral days 1–21
	Dexamethasone 20 mg oral on day of and day after bortezomib (or 20 mg days 1, 8, 15, 22 for patients older than 75 years)
	Repeated every 35 days
	Consolidation (6 cycles):
	Bortezomib 1.3 mg/m^2 subcutaneous days 1, 15, cycle 1–9
	Lenalidomide 15 mg oral days 1–21
	Repeated every 28 days
Bortezomib-melphalan-prednisone (wVMP)	Bortezomib 1.3 mg/m^2 subcutaneous days 1, 8, 15, 22
	Melphalan 9 mg/m^2 oral days 1–4
	Prednisone 60 mg oral on days 1–4
	Repeated every 35 days
Lenalidomide-dexamethasone (Rd)	Lenalidomide 25 mg oral days 1–21 every 28 days Dexamethasone 40 mg oral days 1, 8, 15, 22 every 28 days Repeated every 4 weeks

guidelines, the most effective regimens available for these patients are represented by DRd (daratumumab, lenalidomide, dexamethasone), D-VMP (daratumumab, bortezomib, melphalan, prednisone), and VRd (bortezomib, lenalidomide, dexamethasone). Other regimens with a lower level of efficacy include VMP Vista (bortezomib, melphalan, prednisone) and Rd (lenalidomide, dexamethasone) (see Tables 54.6 and 7).

The phase III label MAIA study compared continuous DRd with Rd every 28 days treatment until progression. Daratumumab was administrated at dosage of 16 mg/kg once weekly during cycles 1 and 2, then every two weeks during cycles 3 to 6, and every four weeks thereafter. The most frequent side effects of this combination are cytopenia (particularly neutropenia), respiratory infections, and infusion-related reactions. Before the daratumumab administration, requirements include: (i) an accurate study of pulmonary function and HBV status; (ii) a pre-infusion premedication with steroids, paracetamol/acetaminophen, and antihistamines; (iii) thromboprophylaxis according to the risk status of the patients; and (iv) an accurate evaluation of white cell count, with use of G-CSF and antibiotics as needed to prevent or treat infections. It is also important to collaborate with the blood bank to manage the interference of daratumumab with the direct antiglobulin test in case red cell transfusion is needed (see Chapter 53). Another warning is the interference of the monoclonal antibody with the definition of complete response; for this reason, the laboratory needs to know of daratumumab treatment to avoid incorrect evaluation of monoclonal component. The dermatologic and gastrointestinal toxicities need specific treatment and reduction of dosage (see Table 54.8). Diarrhea and nausea can be very common in this setting and lead to an increased risk of morbidity and mortality, compromising the ability to administer an effective continuous treatment. The lenalidomide dose must be managed according with the renal function of the patient.

D-VMP is the association of daratumumab with subcutaneous bortezomib, oral melphalan, and prednisone. Unlike DRd, this regimen is characterized by nine cycles of daratumumab with VMP at different frequency, followed by monthly administration of monoclonal antibody.

Cytopenias and gastrointestinal side effects are correlated with bortezomib and melphalan, and antiviral prophylaxis is mandatory to avoid the recurrence of herpes-zoster infection. In this regimen, only the melphalan dosage must be reduced in case of renal impairment. Although the subcutaneous administration of bortezomib has reduced the rate of peripheral neuropathy, an accurate neurologic assessment before the start of therapy (to rule out other causes of lesions) and aggressive management of this toxicity is warranted to minimize its impact on quality of life and limit treatment discontinuation.

The VRd combination is widely used outside Europe and only recently used (and only for transplant-ineligible patients) in European countries. According to the SWOG-S0777 trial, this regimen is administered in 21-day cycles with bortezomib twice weekly subcutaneous, lenalidomide 25 mg from day 1 to 14 plus 20 mg dexamethasone twice weekly for eight cycles, followed by continuous Rd until progression. The most frequent toxicities described consist of cytopenias and peripheral neuropathy. To improve the safety profile, it was modified with dose adjustment to "VRd lite," which is given in 35-day cycles with bortezomib weekly subcutaneous, lenalidomide 15 mg from day 1 to day 21 and dexamethasone 20 mg weekly. This regimen included nine cycles, followed by six cycles of consolidation with bortezomib and lenalidomide without maintenance. This last regimen is not available in European countries.

Overall, according with clinical data, DRd seems to represent the best regimen for the transplant-ineligible newly diagnosed multiple myeloma (transplant-ineligible, or nontransplant-eligible, NDMM) patients in terms of efficacy and tolerability. Moreover, subgroups of patients could take advantage from a specific association of drugs. For example, in case of renal impairment and extramedullary masses, the D-VMP combination may work better and VRd treatment may play a role in the patients with chronic inflammatory lung disease (COPD) or another contraindication to anti-CD38 monoclonal antibody.

In case of logistic problems, clinical contraindications, comorbidities, and unavailability of monoclonal antibodies, the VMP regimen according to the VISTA trial schedule (but with a subcutaneous administration of bortezomib) or Rd in the FIRST trial fashion represent optimal alternatives. Although the results of VMP and Rd are less impressive in comparison with D-VMP, DRd, and VRd, the impact on PFS and OS remains of good quality in this patient setting.

6) How to manage the newly diagnosed intermediate-fit and frail patients?

Expert Perspective: Regardless of the geriatric assessment tools used to define the frailty of the newly diagnosed transplant-ineligible MM patients, the intermediate-fit and frail population are more vulnerable subgroups compared with the fit subset and need a different caring approach. The prevention of toxicity and the preservation of quality of life are essential for those patients, and a less intensive treatment is mandatory to achieve the goals of management.

To spare toxicity and treatment discontinuation three options are possible: two-drug regimens, reduction of dose intensity over time, and choice of "non-frail drugs" (drugs included in standard regimens for fit patients) in less toxic combinations.

The goal of management of intermediate-fit patients is to achieve increased overall response rate and progression-free-survival, together with relief of symptoms. The best reduced-intensity regimens for this population with multiple or severe comorbidities are weekly VMP/weekly VCD, VRD-lite, full-dose Rd, or full-dose Vd. In the absence of major contraindications, low-dose immuno-chemotherapy DRd or D-VMP may be useful.

The frail population has severe comorbidities with a very low life expectancy. Consequently, it is mandatory to control the symptoms and to ensure a good quality of life. The low-dose two-drug treatments, such as low-dose lenalidomide and dexamethasone and low-dose bortezomib and dexamethasone, represent the best regimens in the majority of patients, while palliation and supportive care remain the optimal approach in the very vulnerable populations.

7) How to manage the elderly patients with relapsed/refractory myeloma?

Expert Perspective: The goal of treatment of relapsed/refractory (R/R) MM is to induce a deep response and achieve an improved progression-free survival (see Chapters 55 and 57). Sequencing of therapy at each subsequent relapse is individualized based on patient status, comorbidities, previous treatment adverse events, prior therapies, time and aggressiveness of relapse, duration of previous responses, availability of drugs, and cytogenetic abnormalities. Regarding transplant-ineligible MM patients, treatment is limited by comorbidities, with different goals regarding the frail, intermediate-frail, and fit populations. Moreover, patients aged 75 years or older represent a minority of study populations (10–15%) in the clinical trials on R/R MM, and data of frailty assessment have not been collected.

When re-treatment is needed, repeating the frailty assessment can help to inform the best therapy. The new combinations incorporating carfilzomib, ixazomib, elotuzumab, and daratumumab can be considered for all the transplant-ineligible patients with R/R MM, but the dosage must be modified on the basis of the frailty status, with two-drug regimens preferred for the more vulnerable patients. The main side effects of the drugs could be evaluated to minimize the toxicities and to tailor the treatment. For example, an accurate cardiologic assessment (arterial pressure monitoring and echocardiogram, lipid metabolism study), correction of cardiovascular risks, and appropriate management of underlying cardiac conditions is required before administering carfilzomib-based therapy.

Patients not refractory to IPs and progressing during or following lenalidomide could receive Kd (carfilzomib, dexamethasone), PVD (pomalidomide, bortezomib, dexamethasone), Dara-Vd (daratumumab, bortezomib, dexamethasone), or Dara-Kd (daratumumab, carfilzomib, dexamethasone). In the population not-refractory to bortezomib and lenalidomide, carfilzomib (KRd), daratumumab (DRd), ixazomib (IxaRd), and elotuzumab (EloPd) could be added to Rd. The last two options are very useful in frail and intermediate-frail patients, particularly in non-aggressive relapse, due to a low rate of toxicities. Moreover, IxaRd is an all-oral treatment and represents an option when it is difficult to travel. The combinations incorporating daratumumab and elotuzumab are not associated with an additional toxicity if compared with doublets, and for this reason can be considered in intermediate-fit and frail patients.

From the third relapse, in case of exposition to PIs and IMIDs, the association with pomalidomide (i.e. isatuximab-pomalidomide-dexamethasone or elotuzumab-pomalidomide-dexamethasone) or belantamab mafodotin single agent or selinexor-dexamethasone could be effective options (see Chapter 55).

The very frail patients may benefit from palliative therapies and low-dose oral cyclophosphamide or melphalan.

8) How to manage the very old patients?

Expert Perspective: Because of the increasing population life span and availability of effective and feasible MM treatment options in very old patients, the incidence and prevalence of octogenarians with MM will continue to expand. According to the IMWG frailty index, patients older than age 80 are frail by definition; however, although chronologic aging is accompanied by age-related physiologic changes, there is a pronounced heterogeneity in physiologic and functional age. Therefore, it is questionable whether age of 80 years should be a sole definition of frailty in patients with MM. An important consideration for treatment decisions in octogenarians is life expectancy based on age in relation to general health status since this affects the expected survival benefit. According to recent data from clinical trials and epidemiology studies, it is important to distinguish between MM octogenarians without geriatrics impairment (< 10% of newly diagnosed transplant-ineligible MM enrolled in clinical trials) and octogenarians with geriatric impairments. The former population could benefit from new treatments (e.g. monoclonal antibodies) that can be safely delivered continuously for a long period of time, are better tolerated, and have a lower discontinuation risk, potentially improving their outcome. The latter population must be considered very frail with an excess of early toxic deaths and high risk of drugs discontinuation, which can be reduced by dose de-escalation strategies in the first months after diagnosis.

9) How to treat the high-risk elderly patients?

Expert Perspective: The high-risk (HR) status of MM patients is influenced by multiple prognostic factors (included factors that are identified later in the disease course); for this reason, the definition of HR patients is based on the predicted OS and is made when OS is less than two years in ASCT-ineligible population. These prognostic factors can be primarily patient-related, tumor-related, and those that reflect the impact of cancer on the host. Within the first group, the general performance status, comorbidities, and enhanced toxicity of the anti-myeloma treatment represent the main factors that affect survival. In non-transplant eligible NDMM patients, the frailty status itself acts as a risk factor. Cytogenetic abnormalities including t(4;14), t(14;16), t(14;20), del(17p), and all types of gain(1q) represent the most potent prognostic tumor-related factor. The serum lactate dehydrogenase (LDH), serum free light chain ratio, serum albumin, and serum β2-microglobulin level is also associated with tumor mass and are widely used as components of the ISS and R-ISS (see Table 54.8). Clinical manifestations linked to adverse prognosis include the presence of extramedullary disease and plasma cell leukemia. Renal function is a factor that reflects interaction between the host and MM (see Chapter 52).

Among all prognostic factors, genetic aberrations evaluated with interphase fluorescence in situ hybridization (iFISH) appear to have the widest practical use. Subgroup and post hoc analyses suggest that older patients are less likely to have HR cytogenetic

Table 54.8 Widely used prognosis models in multiple myeloma.

ISS	R-ISS
Stage I All of the following: • Serum albumin ≥ 3.5 g/dL • Serum β2-microglobulin < 3.5 mg/L	Stage I All of the following: • Serum albumin ≥ 3.5 g/dL • Serum β2-microglobulin < 3.5 mg/L • No high-risk cytogenetics • Normal serum lactate dehydrogenase level
Stage II • Serum β2-microglobulin < 3.5 mg/L but serum albumin < 3.5 mg/L • Serum β2-microglobulin 3.5–5.5 mg/L irrespective of serum albumin level	Stage II • Not fitting Stage I or III
Stage III Serum β2-microglobulin ≥ 5.5 mg/L	Stage III Both of the following: • Serum β2-microglobulin > 5.5 mg/L • High-risk cytogenetics [t(4;14), t(14;16), or del(17p)] or elevated serum lactate dehydrogenase level

abnormalities compared to younger patients, but these subgroup analyses could be under-powered. In fact, the data from clinical trials involving transplant-ineligible MM patients have failed to detect statistically significant differences in outcomes between interventional vs control arm within the HR subgroup. Based on the observations that bortezomib, lenalidomide, and daratumumab could partially abrogate the prognostic factor of HR cyto-genetics, it is reasonable to conclude that this particular population should receive therapy including three agents (DRd, D-VMP, VRd).

10) What are preferred supportive care strategies?

Expert Perspective: Appropriate and adequate supportive care and early identification of complications and toxicity are crucial in the management of transplant-ineligible MM patients, due to the high incidence of adverse events and drug discontinuation.

The elderly population is characterized by a high rate of infections and death secondary to infection in the first three months after diagnosis due to immune compromise. Antimicrobial prophylaxis should be initiated during induction. A one-time pneumococcal vaccine should be evaluated at diagnosis in addition to yearly influenza vaccination. Prophylactic antiviral therapy for herpes-zoster is indicated in case of PIs and daratumumab treatment. Anemia related to MM can be managed with red cell transfusion and erythropoietin-stimulating agents. Radiotherapy, analgesics (according to the World Health Organization guidelines), vertebroplasty, kyphoplasty, and rarely other orthopedic interventions are indicated in patients with symptomatic lytic lesions and pathologic fractures.

Bisphosphonates reduce the risk of skeletal-related events, decrease mortality, and pro-long progression-free survival when given along with anti-myeloma agents. Zoledronic acid or pamidronate administered intravenously every four weeks should be continued for two years in all patients with active disease. Preventive strategies and dosage reduction should be considered to avoid renal toxicity and osteonecrosis of the jaw, and supplementation with calcium and vitamin D is advised to maintain calcium homeostasis and prevent hypocalcemia. Denosumab, a receptor activator of nuclear factor kappa B ligand (RANKL) inhibitor, represents an alternative to bisphosphonates, particularly if kidney dysfunction is present. The presence of spinal cord compression requires emergent short course of radiotherapy and high dose of dexamethasone administration, even before a definitive treatment plan. In case of acute myeloma-related kidney failure, dexamethasone, and bortezomib-based therapy, as well as daratumumab, is effective therapy.

Elderly patients may suffer chronic pain mainly due to myeloma bone disease and chemotherapy-induced neuropathy. Bisphosphonates, denosumab, and analgesics such as opioids, acetaminophen, and corticosteroids are administered to treat pain related to skeletal disease. Neuropathic pain can be treated with tricyclic antidepressants, serotonin/norepinephrine reuptake inhibitors such as duloxetine, and gabapentin.

Recommended Readings

Dimopoulos, M.A., Moreau, P., Terpos, E., Mateos, Mv., Zweegman, S., Cook, G. et al. (2021 February 3). Multiple myeloma: EHA-ESMO clinical practice guidelines for diagnosis, treatment and follow-up. *Hemasphere* 5 (2): e528. doi:10.1097/HS9.0000000000000528. eCollection 2021 Feb.PMID: 33554050.

Grant, S.J., Mian, H. S., Giri, S., Boutin, M., Dottorini, L., Neuendorff, N. R. et al. (2021 May). Transplant-inelegible newly diagnosed multiple myeloma: Current and future approaches to clinical care: A young international society of geriatric oncology review paper. *J Geriatr Oncol* 12 (4): 499–507. doi:10.1016/j.jgo.2020.12.001. Epub 2020 Dec 17.PMID: 33342724.

Kumar, S.K., Callander, N. S., Adekola, K., Anderson, L., Baljevic, M., Campagnaro, E. et al. (2020 December 2). Multiple myeloma, version 3.2021, NCCN practice guidelines in oncology. *J Natl Compr Canc Netw* 18 (12): 1685–1717. doi:10.6004/jnccn.2020.0057. PMID: 3328552.

Rajkumar, S.V. (2020 May). Multiple myeloma: 2020 update on diagnosis, risk-stratification and management. *Am J Hematol* 95 (5): 548–567. doi:10.1002/ajh.25791. PMID: 32212178.

van de Donk, N.W.C.J., Pawlyn, C., and Yong, K. L. (2021 January 30). Multiple myeloma. *Lancet* 397 (10272): 410–427. doi:10.1016/S0140-6736(21)00135-5. PMID: 33516340.

Zweegman, S., and Larocca, A. (2019 March). Frailty in multiple myeloma: The need for harmony to prevent doing harm. *Lancet Haematol* 6 (3): e117–e118. doi:10.1016/S2352-3026(19)30011-0. Epub 2019 Feb 6.PMID: 30738833.

55

Relapsed/Refractory Multiple Myeloma

Neha Korde and Saad Z. Usmani

Memorial Sloan Kettering Cancer Center and Department of Medicine, Weill Cornell Medical College, NY, USA

Introduction

Despite advances in therapies for multiple myeloma, a majority of the patients relapse after front-line therapy. The management of relapsed/refractory multiple myeloma has become quite challenging in clinical practice, as one must pay attention to patient related factors (age, comorbidities, preferences, social support and financial support, etc.), disease and treatment related factors (pace of disease relapse, high risk cytogenetics, prior treatment history and side effects, etc.). Furthermore, triple class (proteasome inhibitor, immuno-modulatory drugs, anti-CD38 monoclonal antibody) exposed/refractory MM is becoming an area of unmet need with a median PFS of 2.8 months and median OS of 8.6 months (Bal S et al., *Leukemia* 2021). The current chapter will attempt to address some difficult clinical scenarios in relapsed/refractory multiple myeloma.

Case Study 1

Asian female, 76 y.o. with past medical history of hypertension, atrial fibrillation, and hypo-thyroidism was diagnosed with IgG lambda Multiple Myeloma after presenting to her primary doctor with anemia symptoms of fatigue, dyspnea on exertion, and a hemoglo-bin of 8.2 g/dL. A bone marrow biopsy and aspiration demonstrated 70% plasma cells by CD138 + immunohistochemistry stains. Flow cytometry showed an abnormal lambda restricted plasma cell population. FISH studies on bone marrow biopsy were positive for t(4,14) and del(13q). Initial serum studies demonstrated monoclonal protein (m-protein) of 5.15 g/dL and serum free lambda of 96.3 mg/dL with a K/L ratio < 0.01. Her Revised International Staging System (R-ISS) score was stage III. She was given dose-reduced lenalidomide, bortezomib, and dexamethasone (RVD – lite) for eight cycles, reaching a very good partial response (VGPR) with < 5% plasma cells on bone marrow biopsy. She

Cancer Consult: Expertise in Clinical Practice, Volume 2: Neoplastic Hematology & Cellular Therapy,
Second Edition. Edited by Syed A. Abutalib, Maurie Markman, James O. Armitage, and Kenneth C. Anderson.
© 2024 John Wiley & Sons Ltd. Published 2024 by John Wiley & Sons Ltd.

transitioned to oral lenalidomide maintenance and remained on it for two years until she had progression of disease with rising m-protein of a nadir 0.1 g/dL to 2.25 g/dL and worsening cytopenias. Repeat bone marrow biopsy demonstrated over 40% plasma cells.

1. The best term to define the patient's current disease state:
   A) Primary refractory myeloma.
   B) Relapsed/refractory myeloma.
   C) Relapsed myeloma.
   D) Complete response with minimal residual disease positivity.

Expert Perspective: According to the International Myeloma Working group criteria outlined by Kumar et al., progressive disease is defined as an > 25% increase in nadir from one or more of the following: serum m-protein (absolute m-protein increase should be > 0.5 g/dL in serum; if lowest M-protein is > 5 g/dL, the absolute increase should be > 1.0 g/dL), urine m-protein (absolute m-protein increase > 200 mg/24 hr in urine), or difference between involved and uninvolved free light chains (absolute increase must be > 10 mg/dL) in patients without serum and/or urine m-protein. In patients without serum and/or urine m-protein or measurable serum free light chains, progressive disease is defined as a > 25% increase in nadir bone marrow plasma-cell percentage (absolute increase must be > 10%), appearance of new lesion(s), or worsening of old lesions [> 50% increase from nadir in SPD (sum of the products of the maximal perpendicular diameters) of > 1 measured lesion, or > 50% increase in the longest diameter of a previous lesion > 1 cm in short axis], or increase in circulating plasma cells (> 50% increase [minimum of 200 cells/µL] (Kumar et al. 2016). The two types of refractory myeloma disease are "primary refractory myeloma," defined as progressing or non-progressing disease where patients have never achieved > minimal response (MR) with any therapy, and "relapsed/refractory myeloma," defined as a disease that is nonresponsive while on salvage therapy or progressing within 60 days of last therapy after achieving at least an MR. "Relapsed myeloma" is defined as previously treated multiple myeloma that progresses but does not meet the criteria for primary refractory myeloma or relapsed/refractory myeloma (Rajkumar et al. 2011). Since the patient achieved a VGPR response with the first line of therapy and progressed while on lenalidomide maintenance, the patient meets the definition for relapsed/refractory Multiple Myeloma (MM).

2. What treatment options could be considered for the next line of therapy?
   A) Daratumamab–based therapy.
   B) Carfilzomib-based therapy.
   C) Isatuximab-based therapy.
   D) Bortezomib-based.
   E) Pomalidomide-based therapy.
   F) Any of the above.

Expert Perspective: In the case above, the patient is considered lenalidomide refractory. The clinician and patient have several options to choose from in the early relapsed/refractory MM disease setting (one to three lines of therapy), including anti-CD38 monoclonal antibodies (MoABs), proteasome inhibitors (PIs), immunomodulatory agents (IMiDs), and other classes of agents. Several factors, including lenalidomide refractoriness, side effect profile, and prior exposures (PI or anti-CD38 MoAB) may influence the next line of therapy. Furthermore, the nature of clinical relapse (slow vs rapid, presence of renal failure, presence of extramedullary plasmacytomas, previous history of autologous stem cell transplant (ASCT), time of remission since last ASCT, pre-existing side effects, and degree of cytopenias) would also potentially play a factor in treatment selection. (Figure 55.1).

Pomalidomide, dexamethasone (Pd) is a key backbone regimen in the early relapsed setting and served as a basis to several early relapsed/refractory MM studies: pomalidomide, bortezomib, dexamethasone (PVd) in OPTIMISMM; elotuzumab, pomalidomide, dexamethasone (EPd) in ELOQUENT-3; and daratumamab, pomalidomide, dexamethasone (DPd) in APOLLO (Miguel et al. 2013; San Miguel et al. 2015). PVd combination (n = 281) was compared to bortezomib, dexamethasone (Vd) (n = 278) in the OPTIMISMM study where enrolled patients were previously treated with one to three prior lines therapy, received more than two consecutive cycles of lenalidomide, and were not allowed to be progressing on a twice-weekly bortezomib-containing regimen. Approximately 70% of patients were lenalidomide refractory. Overall, PVd demonstrated improved median PFS over Vd (median PFS 11.2 months vs 7.1 months; HR 0.61; 95% CI 0.49–0.77; $P < 0.0001$), and the benefit remained in the lenalidomide refractory patients (median PFS 9.5 months vs 5.6 months; HR 0.65; 95% CI 0.50–0.84) (Richardson et al. 2019). In ELOQUENT-3, EPd demonstrated a benefit over Pd among MM patients who received more than two lines of therapy including a PI and IMiD and > 84% of patients were refractory to lenalidomide (median PFS 10.3 months vs 4.7 months; HR 0.54; 95% CI 0.34–0.86; $P = 0.008$). Again, subgroup analysis still favored EPd over Pd in lenalidomide and PI refractory MM patients (HR 0.56; 95% CI 0.33–0.97) (Dimopoulos et al. 2018).

In addition to the bortezomib-containing (PVd) regimen studied in OPTIMISMM, PI-combination therapies make logical sense to consider in an early relapsed/refractory MM patient that is lenalidomide refractory given the usual desire to class switch change. The phase III ENDEAVOR trial evaluated carfilzomib, dexamethasone (Kd) against Vd in relapsed/refractory MM patients who had received one to three prior lines of therapy (median PFS 18.7 months vs 9.4 months; HR 0.53; 95% CI 0.44–0.65; $P < 0.0001$) (Dimopoulos et al. 2016a). Interim survival analysis favored Kd over Vd [median overall survival (OS) 47.6 months vs 40.0 months; HR 0.79; 95% CI 0.65–0.96; $P = 0.01$), although prior IMiD exposure did not necessarily offer a benefit of one PI over another (Dimopoulos et al. 2017). Other potential PI combinations include cyclophosphamide, bortezomib, dexamethasone (CyBord), carfilzomib, pomalidomide, and dexamethasone (KPd), and ixazomib, pomalidomide, and dexamethasone (IxaPd), and additional studies below show the benefit of PI combination with anti-CD38 MoABs.

Both anti-CD38 MoABs, daratumumab and isatuximab, demonstrate superior efficacy when combined with PIs or IMiDS. Daratumamab is a targeted IgG1k monoclonal antibody that targets CD38, a cell surface glycoprotein highly expressed on myeloma plasma cells. It can be administered as two different formulations, Darazalex (intravenous) or Darazalex Faspro (subcutaneous). The phase III CASTOR study, comparing daratumumab, bortezomib, dexamethasone (DVd) to Vd in patients with > 1 line of therapy, showed improved outcomes (median PFS 16.7 months vs 7.1 months; HR 0.31; 95% CI 0.25–0.40; $P < 0.0001$) in the DVd arm (Mateos et al. 2020; Palumbo et al. 2016). DVD was favored in IMiD refractory disease (HR 0.50; 95% CI 0.31–0.80). Similarly, in both the

APOLLO (DPd) and CANDOR [daratumamab, carfilzomib, dexamethasone (DKd)] studies, daratumumab-containing regimens demonstrated improved efficacy over their doublet counterparts. In APOLLO, DPd significantly improved overall response rates (ORR) and median PFS over Pd in relapsed/refractory MM patients previously treated with more than one line of therapy including lenalidomide and PI (median PFS 12.4 months vs 6.9 months; HR 0.63; 95% CI 0.47–0.85; P = 0.0018) while demonstrating a favorable profile in lenalidomide refractory disease (HR 0.66; 95% CI 0.49–0.90). Approximately 80% of patients treated in APOLLO were lenalidomide refractory (Dimopoulos et al. 2021). In the phase III CANDOR study, DKd improved median PFS over carfilzomib and dexamethasone (Kd) in relapsed/refractory MM patients (n = 466) with one to three prior lines of therapy and > partial response (PR) to at least one previous line of therapy (median PFS not reached vs 15.8 months; HR 0.63; 95% CI 0.46–0.85; P = 0.0027) (Dimopoulos et al. 2020). Additional analysis demonstrated significant deeper response rates in the DKd arm (10^{-5} MRD negative complete response rates at 12 months: 13% vs 1%; P < 0.0001) and benefit across several pre-specified subgroups, including IMiD and lenalidomide refractory disease (Dimopoulos et al. 2020). Isatuximab is another anti-CD38 MoAb that binds to a different epitope on CD38 compared to daratumamab (Martin et al. 2019). In the phase III ICARIA study, relapsed/refractory MM patients with more than two lines of therapy, refractory to prior IMiD and PI, and progressing on the last line of therapy were treated with either isatuximab, pomalidomide, dexamethasone (IsaPd) or Pd. Patients refractory to anti-CD38 therapy or pomalidomide exposed were excluded. IsaPd demonstrated better median PFS compared to Pd (median PFS 11.53 months vs 6.47 months; HR 0.60; 95 CI 0.436–0.814; P < 0.001). Patients refractory to lenalidomide had a favorable outcome to IsaPd (HR 0.59; 95% CI 0.43–0.82) including those that were refractory to lenalidomide in the last line of therapy (HR 0.50; 95% CI 0.34–0.76) (Attal et al. 2019). Similarly, the IKEMA study, evaluating isatuximab, carfilzomib, dexamethasone (IsaKd) versus carfilzomib, dexamethasone (Kd) demonstrated superior PFS results with IsaKd (median PFS not reached vs 19.2 months; HR 0.53; 99% CI 0.32–0.89; P = 0.0007) in relapsed refractory MM patients with one to three prior lines of treatment and no prior carfilzomib exposure (Moreau et al. 2021).

Case Study 2

African American male, 62 y.o. was diagnosed with IgG Kappa MM, ISS Stage I. Initial bone marrow demonstrated 60% kappa restricted plasma cell neoplasm, and FISH/cytogenetics were notable for deletion 13, + t(11,14) and normal male XY karyotype. Labs demonstrated anemia with a hemoglobin of 10.2 g/dL and an initial m-protein of 1.7 g/dL. A skeletal survey showed multiple lytic lesions in the pelvis, ribs, and spine. He received 4 cycles of induction therapy with RVd followed by ASCT. After ASCT, serum markers and a re-staging day 100 bone marrow showed an sCR/MRD negative (10^{-6}) response by next-generation sequencing. He was placed on lenalidomide maintenance, but it was discontinued after 1.5 years for uncontrolled diarrhea. At the time, serum markers confirmed a durable sCR response, and the patient opted for no maintenance therapy. After five years of no treatment, he reported symptoms of posterior left shoulder back pain. Imaging by FDG

PET-CT scan demonstrated new FDG-avid lytic lesions in the left scapula, right proximal femur, and left ninth rib, and serum markers demonstrated a measurable m-protein of 2.3 g/dL, IgG kappa.

3. What treatment options could be considered for the next line of therapy in this patient?

A) Carfilzomib, lenalidomide, dexamethasone (KRd).

B) Daratumamab, lenalidomide, dexamethasone (DRd).

C) Elotuzumab, lenalidomide, dexamethasone (ERd).

D) Ixazomib, lenalidomide, dexamethasone (IxaRd).

E) Any of the above

Expert Perspective: In addition to the combination therapies mentioned in the prior section, this patient could also still benefit from a lenalidomide-based treatment regimen. In the ASPIRE trial (n = 792), KRd therapy was compared to lenalidomide and dexamethasone (Rd) in relapsed MM after receiving one or more lines of therapy (median PFS 26.3 months vs 17.6 months; HR 0.69; 95% CI 0.57–0.83; P = 0.0001) (Stewart et al. 2015). A more recent update on ASPIRE demonstrates KRd improved overall survival (median OS 48.3 months vs 40.4 months; HR 0.79; 95% CI 0.67–0.95; P = 0.0045) (Siegel et al. 2018). The efficacy of DRd was shown in the phase III study POLLUX, where DRd (n = 283) compared to Rd (n = 286) showed superior efficacy and good tolerability in relapsed patients with more than one line of therapy (median PFS 44.5 months vs 17.5 months; HR 0.44; 95% CI 0.35–0.54; P = 0.012) (Kaufman and San-Miguel et al. 2019). Of note, depth of response was significantly higher in the DRd arm (>CR 43.1% vs 19.2, P < 0.001; 10^{-5} MRD neg 22.4% vs 4.6%, P < 0.001) (Dimopoulos et al. 2016b). In ELOQUENT-2, ERd was compared to Rd (median PFS 19.4 months vs 14.9 months; HR 0.70; 95% CI 0.57–0.85; P = 0.0004) (Lonial et al. 2015). An all-oral IxaRd regimen demonstrated improved PFS over Rd in TOURMALINE (median PFS 20.6 months vs 14.7 months; HR 0.74; 95% CI 0.59–0.94; P = 0.012) (Moreau et al. 2016); however, subsequent update after median follow-up of 85 months demonstrates that the PFS was not enough to improve OS (median OS 53.6 months vs 51.6 months; HR 0.94; P = 0.50) (Richardson et al. 2021). (Figure 55.1).

4. What are the ASTCT/IMWG guidelines for use of stem cell transplant in this patient?

A) Consider single autologous stem cell transplant as consolidation.

B) Consider tandem autologous stem cell transplant as consolidation.

C) Consider single autologous stem cell transplant as consolidation followed by an allogeneic stem cell transplantation.

D) Consider an allogeneic stem cell transplantation.

E) Any of the above.

F) None of the above.

Expert Perspective: The ASTCT/IMWG guidelines recommend a second transplant at relapse for eligible patients who have had at least 24 months of remission duration from the first transplant [Giralt S et al., Biol Blood Marrow Transplant 2015;21(12):2039–2051].

The patient was subsequently treated with KRd induction for four cycles followed by second autologous stem cell transplant and then lenalidomide as maintenance for 2.5 years before biochemical progression. He then received DaraKd achieving VGPR after eight cycles, he began progressing again with a rising M-protein and worsening anemia two years after starting DaraKd. He underwent a bone marrow biopsy demonstrating 40% plasmacytosis. FISH demonstrated presence of + t(11,14) in > 60% of CD138 selected plasma cells.

5. What is the median overall survival in anti-CD38 refractory disease?
A) 2.1 months.
B) 8.6 months.
C) 18.3 months.
D) 32.4 months.

Expert Perspective: The large retrospective study, MAMMOTH, included 275 patients across 14 different institutions to determine outcomes on anti-CD38 refractory MM patients (Gandhi et al. 2019). The median number of prior lines of therapy was four (range 1–16). In the study 54% were triple refractory or quad-refractory (CD38 MoAB + 1 PI + 1 or 2 IMiDs or CD38 MoAB + 1 or 2 PI + 1 IMiDS), 21% was non-triple refractory (CD38 MoAB but not both PI and IMiD), and 25% was penta-refractory (CD38 MoAB, 2 PIs, and 2 IMiDS). The median OS was 8.6 months (95% CI 7.5 – 9.9 mo) in anti-CD38 refractory disease. The median OS also varied according to the level of refractoriness, 11.2 months in non-triple refractory, 9.2 months in triple or quadruple refractory, and 5.6 months in penta-refractory disease. Up-and-coming anti-BCMA therapies and developing novel agents will likely change these outcomes in the future.

6. Which of the following therapeutic agents demonstrates selective activity in t(11;14) MM patients?
A) Selinexor.
B) Venetoclax.
C) Panobinostat.

Expert Perspective: Venetoclax is an oral BCL-2 inhibitor that demonstrates selective activity in + t(11,14) and high BCL-2 expressing MM. In a randomized phase III study comparing venetoclax, bortezomib, and dexamethasone (VenVd) to placebo, bortezomib, and dexamethasone (PlacVd) in relapsed or refractory MM patients with one to three prior therapies, VenVd demonstrated superior deep responses in patients with translocation t(11,14)/high BCL-2 expression compared to the overall venetoclax intention-to-treat group (>CR response rate 45%/36% vs 26%; *P* = 0.00024) (Kumar et al. 2020). Importantly, for the overall cohort, while PFS improved in the VenVd arm compared to PlacVd group (median PFS 22.4 months vs 11.5 months; HR 0.63; *P* = 0.10), an increased mortality rate (4%) seen in the VenVd obviated the PFS benefit seen. A subgroup PFS analysis still favored patients with MM patients with t(11,14) (NR vs 9.5 months; HR 0.11; 95% CI 0.02–0.56) and high BCL2 expression by IHC (NR vs 12.2 months; HR 0.50; 95% CI 0.29–0.89).

While venetoclax is not yet approved by the FDA for treatment of relapsed/refractory MM, further investigation of venetoclax in t(11,14) and high BCL2 expressing MM patients is currently underway.

Selinexor is an oral therapy that inhibits nuclear export protein, exportin-1 (XPO1). XPO1 regulates the transport of proteins, including tumor-suppressing proteins, across the nucleus and cytoplasm, thereby effectively controlling the translation of cellular oncoproteins and promoting tumorigenesis. In a phase 2 study including 122 penta-exposed relapsed/refractory MM patients, combination selinexor and dexamethasone (Sd) demonstrated an overall response rate (ORR) of 26%, median PFS 3.7 months, and median OS 8.6 months, while penta-refractory patients showed an ORR of 25.3% (Chari et al. 2019). Additionally, based on the phase III BOSTON study, anobinos, bortezomib, and dexamethasone (SVd) showed benefit over twice weekly Vd in relapsed/refractory MM patients who have received one to three prior lines of therapy (median PFS 13.9 months vs 9.5 months; HR 0.70; 95% CI 053–0.93; $P = 0.0075$) (Grosicki et al. 2020). Selinexor is FDA approved in combination with dexamethasone for penta-refractory relapsed refractory MM patients who have received at least four prior therapies or in combination bortezomib and dexamethasone for patients who had received at least one prior line of therapy. Selinexor often causes fatigue and thrombocytopenia that can be managed with supportive care and once-weekly dosing schedules.

Panobinostat is a histone deacetylase inhibitor demonstrated to be effective when combined with bortezomib and dexamethasone. In the phase II PANORAMA study, anobinostat, bortezomib, and dexamethasone (PanoVd) was tested in relapsed MM patients who received more than two prior lines of therapy, including IMiDS and those progressing on bortezomib. The PanoVd combination showed an ORR of 34.5% and a median PFS of 5.4 months (Richardson et al. 2013). In the phase II PANORAMA 3 study, oral Panobinostat (20 mg vs 10 mg three times weekly vs 20 mg twice weekly) was investigated in combination with subcutaneous bortezomib and dexamethasone. Results demonstrated improved overall response rates with both the 20 mg dosing cohorts (three times weekly and twice weekly) compared to the 10 mg three times weekly schedule, showing ORR 62.2–65.1% vs 50.6%. Importantly, grade 3 and 4 adverse events (75–91%) along with serious adverse events (44–54%) were high across all treatment cohorts (Laubach et al. 2021). While overcoming PI resistance is promising, side effects such as thrombocytopenia, fatigue, and diarrhea often prohibit tolerability of the combination and require supportive care.

Case Study 3

71 year-old, female with IgG lambda relapsed/refractory MM female has received a total of four prior lines of therapy, including two PIs, two IMiDS, anti-CD38 MoAB, and an autologous stem cell transplant. She has a good performance status and no medical comorbidities. Blood counts and renal function are adequate. She is contemplating an anti-BCMA therapeutic for her next line of therapy.

7. Which of the following therapeutic platforms have been utilized to target BCMA?

A) Antibody-drug conjugate

B) Chimeric antigen receptor T-cells (CAR T-cell)

C) Bi-specific antibody

D) All of the above

Expert Perspective: B-cell maturation antigen (BCMA) is widely expressed on MM plasma cells and has been therapeutically targeted using all three platforms – antibody-drug conjugate, chimeric antigen receptor T-cell (CAR-T) therapies, and bi-specific antibody therapies. Belantamab mafodotin is an antibody-drug conjugate that uses a cytotoxic payload, mafodotin, to disrupt MM cellular activity while enhancing antibody-directed cellular toxicity. It is FDA approved for the use of relapsed/refractory MM in patients that have received at least four prior therapies, including anti-CD38 MoAB, PIs, and IMiDS. The DREAMM-2 randomized phase II study assessed two different dosing levels (2.5 or 3.4 mg/kg) (n = 196 mm). Overall response rates were 31% at the 2.5 mg/kg dose (97.5% CI 20.8–42.6) and 34% at the 3.4 mg/kg dose (97.5% CI 23.9–46) (Lonial et al. 2020). In DREAMM-1, the phase I/II study showed an ORR of 60% (95% CI 42.1–76.1) and median PFS of 12.0 months (95% CI 3.1–not estimable) in a less advanced MM population (prior alkylators, PIs, and IMiDs and refractory to the last line of therapy) (Trudel et al. 2019).

In March of 2021, idecabtagene vicleucel (IDE-cel), targeting BCMA, was the first CAR T-cell therapy, approved for the treatment of relapsed/refractory MM who have received at least 4 therapies, including IMiDS, PIs, and anti-CD38 MoABs. The decision was made based on the KARMMA-2 trial (n = 128) that showed a 73% ORR with a depth of response reaching 26% MRD negativity (10^{-5}) among all patients. The median PFS was 8.8 months (95% CI 5.6–11.6), and cytokine release syndrome was noted in 84% of all patients with 5% CRS being grade 3 or higher (Munshi et al. 2021). Other promising CAR T-cell therapies are being investigated, including ciltacabtagene autoleucel of CARTITUDE-1 Phase Ib/II study demonstrating at most recent follow-up an ORR rate of 98%, sCR rate of 80.4% with 92% being MRD negative 10^{-5} and 18-month PFS rate of 66% and OS rate of 81% (Usmani et al. 2021). Most recently, CARTITUDE-4 study demonstrated that a single infusion of ciltacabtagene autoleucel resulted in a lower risk of disease progression or death than standard care in lenalidomide-refractory patients with multiple myeloma who had received one to three previous therapies. (see Chapter 56).

Finally, several bispecific antibodies targeting BCMA and CD3 are currently under investigation and demonstrating promising results with ORRs ranging from 62.5–80% in heavily pre-treated patients with relapsed/refractory MM (Usmani et al. 2021–34). The administration, durability, and general application of the bi-specific anti-BCMA/CD3 therapeutics compared to CAR T-cell therapy remains an open-ended question but remains critical to the field.

8. What black box warning is included on the drug label for belantamab mafodotin?

A) Cardiac toxicity.

B) Cytokine release syndrome.

C) Ocular toxicity.

D) Neurological toxicity.

Expert Perspective: Ocular toxicity commonly occurs in patients receiving belantamab mafodotin. In a pooled safety analysis (n = 218), ocular toxicity was reported in up to 77% of patients with adverse reactions including keratopathy (76%), changes in visual acuity (55%), blurred vision (27%), and dry eyes (19%). Serious grade 3 or higher keratopathy, according to the keratopathy and visual acuity (KVA) scale, occurred in 45.5%, while a significant decrease in visual acuity occurred in 19% of patients [35]. Given this toxicity profile, belantamab mafodotin was available through a risk evaluation and mitigation strategy (REMS) program, requiring ophthalmology examinations by an eye care professional at baseline and at least one week after the previous dose and within two weeks before the next dose. Nonetheless, the drug was withdrawn from the market following the request of the FDA. This request was based upon the previously announced outcome of the DREAMM-3 phase III confirmatory trial which did not meet the requirements of the FDA Accelerated Approval regulations.

Case Study 4

African American female, 68 year-old African American female, has had IgA lambda MM for 5.5 years. She was initially diagnosed and treated with RVD therapy x 4 cycles followed by ASCT and lenalidomide maintenance. She had progressive disease 2 years later, and received DKd for 13 months, followed by CyBorD for seven months, and EPd for four months. After her last relapse, she received CAR T-cell therapy with idecabtagene vicleucel, and the duration of response lasted 15 months. Her most recent labs demonstrated an increase in m-protein of 1.35 g/dL but adequate blood counts. New imaging demonstrates several new FDG-avid lesions on PET-CT. She has an excellent performance status with no comorbidities.

9. What would be your next preferred line of therapy?

Expert Perspective: The patient should consider a clinical trial. While she has the aforementioned standard of care treatment options remaining, the current number of promising novel therapeutics being investigated in the post-BCMA exposed disease space make clinical trials an important option for this patient to consider. These include other bi-specific antibodies, such as talquetamab, and novel CAR T-cell therapies (MCARH109) targeting GPRC5D, as well as cevostamab, a bi-specific antibody directed against FCRh5. Other potential mechanisms of action being investigated are immune-regulatory based, such anti-TIGIT and anti-LAG-3 therapies, anti-CD47 antibodies, platform studies such as MyCheckpoint and MyImmune, and small molecule pathway inhibitors, such as cereblon modulators (CelMoDs) are currently under development aimed at targeting essential cellular functions such as protein degradation. (Table 55.1; also see Chapter 57)

Table 55.1 Options at relapse based on prior treatments.

Len Naïve or Sensitive / Bort Naïve or Sensitive	Len Refractory / Bort Naïve or Sensitive	Bort Refractory / Len Naïve or Sensitive	Len and Bort Refractory	Len / Bort Refractory but Carfilzomib and Pomalidomide Naïve / Sensitive	Len / Carfilzomib Refractory, Pomalidomide Naïve or Sensitive	Pom / Bort Refractory but Carfilzomib Naïve or Sensitive	Pom / Carfilzomib Refractory
Len-Based • DRd • KRd • ERd • IRd	Pom-Based • DPd • KPd • PVd • PCd PI-Based • DVd • DKd • KCd • SVd • VCd • Kd†	Len-Based • DRd • KRd • ERd	Pom-Based • DPd • IsaPd • KPd • PCd • EPd Carfilzomib-Based • DKd • IsaKd • KCd	Dara Naïve / Sensitive • DPd • KPd • DKd • EPd • PCd • KCd Dara Refractory • KPd • EPd • PCd • KCd • Kd†	Dara Naïve / Sensitive • DPd • IsaPd • EPd • PCd Dara Refractory • EPd • PCd	Dara Naïve / Sensitive • DKd • IsaKd • KCd • Dara for frail patient • DPd Dara Refractory • KCd • Kd†	Dara Naïve / Sensitive • DPd • IsaPd • DKd • IsaKd • Dara for frail patient Dara Refractory • PanoKd • PanoVd • teclistamab or elranatamab or talquetamab • Selid • Ide-cel or cilta-cel • Vtxd [t(11;14)+

Autologous Stem Cell Transplant Candidate?
- SCT not performed as part of frontline therapy
- Durable remission after 1st SCT (≥18-24 months)

†Triplet combinations have outperformed doublet therapy consistently in phase III clinical trials and can be used in frail patients with appropriate dose / schedule modifications. As such, the Kd doublet should rarely be used and only in exceptional circumstances.

††Only for patients with disease refractory to pomalidomide and daratumumab in separate lines of therapyCarfilzomib, lenalidomide, dexamethasone (KRd), daratumamab, lenalidomide, dexamethasone (DRd), isatuximab, carfilzomib, dexamethasone (IsaKd), pomalidomide, bortezomib, dexamethasone (PVd), daratumamab, pomalidomide, dexamethasone (DPd), daratumamab, bortezomib, dexamethasone (DVd), cyclophosphamide, bortezomib, dexamethasone (CyBord), ixazomib, lenalidomide, dexamethasone (IxaRd), elotuzumab, lenalidomide, dexamethasone (ERd), elotuzumab, pomalidomide, dexamethasone (EPd), venetoclax, dexamethasone (Vtxd), selinexor, bortezomib, dexamethasone (SVd), panobinostat, bortezomib, and dexamethasone (PanoVd), cyclophosphamide, carfilzomib dexamethasone (KCd), panobinostat, carfilzomib, and dexamethasone (PanoKd), selinexor, dexamethasone (Selid), idecabtagene vicleucel (Ide-cel) ciltacabtagene autoleucel (cilta-cel)

Table 55.2 Regimens with dosing and schedules.

Trial	Regimen	Dosing/Schedule	Overall Response Rate	PFS vs. Control arm (months)
ENDEAVOR[1]	Kd	Carfilzomib 20/56mg/mg^2 IV days1,2,8,9,15,16; Dexamethasone	76%	18.7 vs. 9.4
PANORAMA[2]	PanoVd	Panobinostat 20mg oral days1,2,4,5,8,9,11,12; Bortezomib 1.3mg/mg^2 days1,4,8,11; Dexamethasone	61%	12 vs. 8
CASTOR[3]	DVd	Daratumamab 16mg/kg IV days weekly days1,8,15 (C1-3), once every 3 weeks day 1 (C4-8), and then once every 4 weeks; Bortezomib 1.3mg/mg^2 days1,4,8,11 (C1-8); Dexamethasone	85%	16.7 vs. 7.1
OPTIMISSM[4]	PVd	Pomalidomide 4mg oral days 1-14; Bortezomib 1.3mg/mg^2 days1,4,8,11 (C1-8), days1,8 (after C8); Dexamethasone	82.2%	11.2 vs. 7.1
ASPIRE[5]	KRd	Carfilzomib 20/27mg/mg^2 IV days1,2,8,9,15,16 (C1-12), days1,2,15,16 (C13-18); Lenalidomide 25mg oral days1-21; Dexamethasone	87%	26.3 vs 17.6
TOURMALINE3[6]	IRd	Ixazomib 4mg oral days1,8,15; Lenalidomide 25mg oral days1-21; Dexamethasone	78%	20.6 vs 14.7
ELOQUENT2[7]	ERd	Elotuzumab 10mg/kg days1,8,15,22 (C1-2), days1,15 (after C3); Lenalidomide 25mg oral days1-21; Dexamethasone	79%	19.4 vs 14.9
POLLUX[8]	DRd	Daratumamab 16mg/kg IV days weekly days1,8,15,22 (C1-2), every 2 weeks days1,15 (C3-6), every 4 weeks (after C6); Lenalidomide 25mg oral days1-21; Dexamethasone	93%	44.5 vs 17.5
APOLLO[9]	DPd	Daratumamab 16mg/kg IV days weekly days1,8,15,22 (C1-2), every 2 weeks days1,15 (C3-6), every 4 weeks (after C6); Pomalidomide 4mg oral days1-21; Dexamethasone	69%	12.4 vs 6.9
ICARIA[10]	IsaPd	Isatuximab 10mg/kg weekly days1,8,15,22 (C1), every 2 weeks days1,15 (after C1); Pomalidomide 4mg oral days1-21; Dexamethasone	60%	11.5 vs 6.5
ELOQUENT3[11]	EPd	Elotuzumab 10mg/kg days1,8,15,22 (C1-2), days1,15 (after C3); Pomalidomide 4mg oral days1-21; Dexamethasone	53%	10.3 vs 4.7
CANDOR[12]	DKd	Daratumamab 16mg/kg IV days weekly days1,8,15 (C1-3), once every 3 weeks day 1 (C4-8), and then once every 4 weeks; Carfilzomib 20/56mg/mg^2 IV days1,2,8,9,15,16; Dexamethasone	84%	28.6 vs 15.2

(Continued)

Table 55.2 (Continued)

Trial	Regimen	Dosing/Schedule	Overall Response Rate	PFS vs. Control arm (months)
IKEMA[13]	IsaKd	Isatuximab 10mg/kg weekly days1,8,15,22 (C1), every 2 weeks days1,15 (after C1); Carfilzomib 20/56mg/mg^2 IV days1,2,8,9,15,16; Dexamethasone	87%	NR* vs 19.2
GEM-KyCyDex[14]	KCd	Cyclophosphamide 300 mg/m^2 IV days1,8,15; Carfilzomib 20/70mg/mg^2 IV days1,8,15; Dexamethasone	78%	20.7 vs 15.2

Carfilzomib, lenalidomide, dexamethasone (KRd), daratumamab, lenalidomide, dexamethasone (DRd), daratumamab, carfilzomib, dexamethasone (DKd), isatuximab, carfilzomib, dexamethasone (IsaKd), pomalidomide, bortezomib, dexamethasone (PVd), daratumamab, pomalidomide, dexamethasone (DPd), daratumamab, bortezomib, dexamethasone (DVd), cyclophosphamide, bortezomib, dexamethasone (CyBord), ixazomib, lenalidomide, dexamethasone (IxaRd), elotuzumab, lenalidomide, dexamethasone (ERd), elotuzumab, pomalidomide, dexamethasone (EPd), venetoclax, dexamethasone (Vtxd), selinexor, bortezomib, and dexamethasone (SVd), panobinostat, bortezomib, and dexamethasone (PanoVd), cyclophosphamide, carfilzomib dexamethasone (KCd).

[1.]Dimopoulos MA, et al. *Lancet Oncol.* 2016;17(1):27-38; 2. San Miguel JF, et al. *Lancet Oncol.* 2014;5(11):1195–1206; 3. Mateos M-V et al. Clinical Lymphoma, Myeloma and Leukemia 2019; 4. Richardson P et al Lancet Oncol 2019; 5. Stewart AK, et al. *N Engl J Med.* 2015;372(2):142-152; 6. Moreau P, et al. *N Engl J Med.* 2016;374:1621-1634; 7. Lonial S, et al. *N Engl J Med.* 2015;373(7):621-631; 8. Bahlis NJ, et al. *Leukemia* 2020 [online ahead of print]; 9. Dimopolus et al *Lancet Oncol* 2021; 10. Attal et al *Lancet* 2019; 11. Dimopolus et al *NEJM* 2018; 12. Dimopolus et al *Lancet* 2020; 13. Moreau et al. *Lancet* 2021; 14. Mateos MV et al *ASH* 2020.

Recommended Readings

Dimopoulos, M. et al. (2020). Carfilzomib, dexamethasone, and daratumumab versus carfilzomib and dexamethasone for patients with relapsed or refractory multiple myeloma (CANDOR): results from a randomised, multicentre, open-label, phase 3 study. *Lancet* 396 (10245): 186–197.

Dimopoulos, M.A. et al. (2016b). Daratumumab, lenalidomide, and dexamethasone for multiple myeloma. *N Engl J Med* 375 (14): 1319–1331.

Dimopoulos, M.A. et al. (2017). Carfilzomib or bortezomib in relapsed or refractory multiple myeloma (ENDEAVOR): an interim overall survival analysis of an open-label, randomised, phase 3 trial. *Lancet Oncol* 18 (10): 1327–1337.

Dimopoulos, M.A. et al. (2021). Daratumumab plus pomalidomide and dexamethasone versus pomalidomide and dexamethasone alone in previously treated multiple myeloma (APOLLO): an open-label, randomised, phase 3 trial. *Lancet Oncol* 22 (6): 801–812.

Kaufman, J.L., San-Miguel, J. et al. (2019). Four year follow-up of the phase 3 POLLUX study of daratumamab plus lenalidomide and dexamethasoen (D-Rd) versus lenalidomide and dexamethasone (Rd) alone in relapsed and refractory multiple myeloma. *Blood* 134 (suppl 1): 1866.

Kumar, S. et al. (2016). International myeloma working group consensus criteria for response and minimal residual disease assessment in multiple myeloma. *Lancet Oncol* 17 (8): e328–e346.

Kumar, S.K. et al. (2020). Venetoclax or placebo in combination with bortezomib and dexamethasone in patients with relapsed or refractory multiple myeloma (BELLINI): a randomised, double-blind, multicentre, phase 3 trial. *Lancet Oncol* 21 (12): 1630–1642.

Laubach, J.P. et al. (2021). Efficacy and safety of oral panobinostat plus subcutaneous bortezomib and oral dexamethasone in patients with relapsed or relapsed and refractory multiple myeloma (PANORAMA 3): an open-label, randomised, phase 2 study. *Lancet Oncol* 22 (1): 142–154.

Lonial, S. et al. (2015). Elotuzumab therapy for relapsed or refractory multiple myeloma. *N Engl J Med* 373 (7): 621–631.

Mateos, M.V. et al. (2020). Daratumumab, bortezomib, and dexamethasone versus bortezomib and dexamethasone in patients with previously treated multiple myeloma: three-year follow-up of CASTOR. *Clin Lymphoma Myeloma Leuk* 20 (8): 509–518.

Miguel, J.S. et al. (2013). Pomalidomide plus low-dose dexamethasone versus high-dose dexamethasone alone for patients with relapsed and refractory multiple myeloma (MM-003): a randomised, open-label, phase 3 trial. *Lancet Oncol* 14 (11): 1055–1066.

Munshi, N.C. et al. (2021). Idecabtagene vicleucel in relapsed and refractory multiple myeloma. *N Engl J Med* 384 (8): 705–716.

Palumbo, A. et al. (2016). Daratumumab, bortezomib, and dexamethasone for multiple myeloma. *N Engl J Med* 375 (8): 754–766.

Richardson, P.G. et al. (2013). PANORAMA 2: panobinostat in combination with bortezomib and dexamethasone in patients with relapsed and bortezomib-refractory myeloma. *Blood* 122 (14): 2331–2337.

Richardson, P.G. et al. (2019). Pomalidomide, bortezomib, and dexamethasone for patients with relapsed or refractory multiple myeloma previously treated with lenalidomide (OPTIMISMM): a randomised, open-label, phase 3 trial. *Lancet Oncol* 20 (6): 781–794.

Richardson, P.G. et al. (2021). Final overall survival analysis of the TOURMALINE-MM1 phase III trial of ixazomib, lenalidomide, and dexamethasone in patients with relapsed or refractory multiple myeloma. *J Clin Oncol* JCO2100972.

San Miguel, J.F. et al. (2015). Impact of prior treatment and depth of response on survival in MM-003, a randomized phase 3 study comparing pomalidomide plus low-dose dexamethasone versus high-dose dexamethasone in relapsed/refractory multiple myeloma. *Haematologica* 100 (10): 1334–1339.

San Miguel, J., Dhakal, B., Yong, K., et al. (2023 July 27). Cilta cel or standard care in Lenalidomide refractory multiple myeloma. N Engl J Med 389 (4): 335 347. doi: 10.1056/NEJMoa2303379. Epub 2023 Jun 5. PMID: 37272512.

Siegel, D.S. et al. (2018). Improvement in overall survival with carfilzomib, lenalidomide, and dexamethasone in patients with relapsed or refractory multiple myeloma. *J Clin Oncol* 36 (8): 728–734.

Stewart, A.K. et al. (2015). Carfilzomib, lenalidomide, and dexamethasone for relapsed multiple myeloma. *N Engl J Med* 372 (2): 142–152.

Usmani, S.Z. et al. (2021). Updated cartitude-1 results of ciltacabtagene autoleucel, A B-cell maturation antigen-directed chimeric antigen receptor T cell therapy in relapsed/refractory multiple myeloma. *EHA* Annual Meeting; *June 9-17*.

56

Light-chain (AL) Amyloidosis

Vaishali Sanchorawala

Amyloidosis Center, Boston University Chobanian & Avedisian School of Medicine and Boston Medical Center, Boston, MA, USA

Introduction

Amyloidosis encompasses a heterogeneous group of disorders, each classified according to an underlying precursor protein. At present, 36 human proteins are known to have the potential to misfold and form extracellular amyloid aggregates. The most commonly recognized disease class has historically been systemic immunoglobulin light chain (AL) amyloidosis in association with a plasma cell dyscrasia or, less commonly, multiple-myeloma or a lymphoproliferative disorder. Other classes, including hereditary transthyretin variant (ATTRv) and wild-type transthyretin (ATTRwt) amyloidosis, previously termed senile systemic amyloidosis, have been seen less commonly due in part to the challenges of establishing diagnosis and a paucity of treatments.

Due to the multiple types of amyloidosis and the complexity of this multi organ-system disease, accurate diagnosis including typing of the precursor protein is imperative to offer correct treatments. An advent of cutting-edge biochemical analysis techniques and cardiac imaging modalities has recently transformed how amyloidosis is detected and accurately typed. Specialized amyloidosis centers in all the countries around the world have experienced an upsurge of referrals for ATTR amyloidosis due to ease of non-biopsy diagnosis, increased awareness, and an emerging and expanding therapeutic landscape.

Case Study 1

An 80-year-old man is referred for evaluation and treatment. The patient had been noted by his primary care doctor to have a monoclonal gammopathy of uncertain significance (MGUS) 10 years prior. Over the past year, the patient has developed dyspnea on exertion and signs of congestive heart failure, and he was placed on a diuretic and an angiotensin-converting enzyme inhibitor by his cardiologist. The cardiac evaluation has revealed increased wall thickness on echocardiography with diastolic dysfunction, and a cardiac magnetic resonance (CMR) study showed delayed gadolinium enhancement of the subendocardium consistent with amyloidosis. The cardiologist and primary care doctor have concluded the patient has light chain amyloidosis (AL), and they are referring the patient to you for treatment. The performance status of the patient is good.

Cancer Consult: Expertise in Clinical Practice, Volume 2: Neoplastic Hematology & Cellular Therapy,
Second Edition. Edited by Syed A. Abutalib, Maurie Markman, James O. Armitage, and Kenneth C. Anderson.
© 2024 John Wiley & Sons Ltd. Published 2024 by John Wiley & Sons Ltd.

1) What is the next best step in the management?
A) Start the patient on treatment with daratumumab.
B) Start the patient on melphalan and dexamethasone.
C) Start the patient on treatment with CyBorD (cyclophosphamide, bortezomib, and dexamethasone).
D) Refer the patient to a colleague for consideration of autologous stem cell transplantation.
E) Carry out additional diagnostic studies.

Expert Perspective: Systemic AL amyloidosis is a disease that can progress rapidly and is fatal without treatment. Cardiac involvement and its severity remain the driver of survival in AL amyloidosis. However, it would not be appropriate to treat this patient with chemotherapy without confirmation of accurate diagnosis.

There are two essential steps in diagnosing AL amyloidosis: Proving that amyloid fibrils/deposits are present in a tissue biopsy and proving that a plasma cell dyscrasia is responsible for the deposits. The demonstration of amyloidosis can be accomplished by biopsy of the involved organ, in this case the heart, or by a less invasive aspiration under local anaesthesia of abdominal fat, which is stained with Congo red dye and examined under polarized light microscopy to demonstrate apple green birefringence (Figure 56.1). Abdominal fat pad aspiration is positive in 75–80% of patients with systemic AL amyloidosis.

Correct Answer: E

Case Study 1 Continues: An abdominal fat aspirate is performed, dried on a slide, stained with Congo red dye, and examined under polarized light microscopy, demonstrating characteristic green birefringence.

2) What is the next best step in the management?
A) Start the patient on treatment with daratumumab.
B) Start the patient on melphalan and dexamethasone.
C) Start the patient on treatment with CyBorD (cyclophosphamide, bortezomib, and dexamethasone).
D) Refer the patient to a colleague for consideration of autologous stem cell transplantation.
E) Carry out additional diagnostic studies.

Expert Perspective: You still have not established the diagnosis of AL amyloidosis. MGUS is not uncommon in an 80-year-old man; it occurs in about 7% of 80-year-old White males (data from Olmstead County, Minnesota; see Chapter 51), and the incidence in African Americans is 2–3 times higher. It is important to recognize that older men can develop an entity of wild-type transthyretin (TTR) amyloidosis (ATTRwt), most commonly affecting the heart. It is important to distinguish it from a hereditary form of amyloidosis due to production of a mutant TTR, ATTRv, a subtype of familial amyloidosis. These patients should not be treated with chemotherapy directed toward plasma cell dyscrasia. The TTR is synthesized in the liver, and chemotherapy would have no benefit. Moreover, abdominal fat pad aspiration can have Congophilia in 25% of patients with ATTRwt amyloidosis.

Correct Answer: E

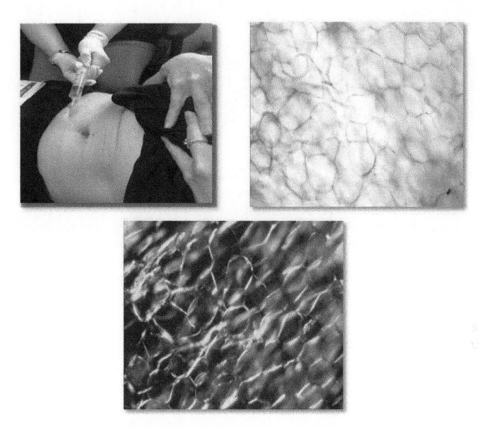

Figure 56.1 (a–c) (a) Abdominal fat pad aspiration (b) stained with Congo red, under light microscopy and (c) under polarized light microscopy.

3) How do you go about proving this is AL amyloidosis due to aggregation and deposition of clonal immunoglobulin light chains produced by clonal bone marrow plasma cells?

Expert Perspective: The clinical presentation and family history can favor one or the other (e.g. a patient whose parent had ATTRv probably has the same diagnosis as it is inherited as autosomal dominant but with variable penetrance, whereas a patient who has multiorgan disease, or macroglossia, with a plasma cell dyscrasia undoubtedly has AL amyloidosis).

- **Immunohistochemistry:** In many cases, the clinical diagnosis should be confirmed using immunochemical or molecular testing. Most pathology laboratories can perform immunohistochemistry. However, amyloid fibrils can bind antibodies nonspecifically, and if multiple antibodies are positive, the immunohistochemistry results are not helpful. Moreover, commercial antibodies in an inexperienced center can lead to false typing in 50–60% of cases of AL amyloidosis.
- **Immunoelectron microscopy:** has more specificity but is not widely available. Many cases can be sorted out with mass spectrometric analysis of fibrils harvested from

tissue sections using laser capture microdissection, which is available as a commercial test. If the patient in question has TTR deposition (not light chain derived amyloid!) by an immunochemical technique, gene sequencing should be done to distinguish a TTR variant, versus the wild-type TTR.

Based on clinical presentation, there is a real possibility that this patient has two unlinked age-related conditions, MGUS and ATTRwt amyloidosis. In that case, management would be supportive care to reduce heart failure symptoms and specific treatment for stabilization of TTR with tafamidis or diflunisal.

4) **If the diagnostic evaluation including mass spectrometry reveals light chain as precursor protein to amyloid fibrils consistent with the diagnosis of AL amyloidosis, then which of the following is the best answer?**
   A) Start the patient on treatment with daratumumab plus CyBorD (cyclophosphamide, bortezomib, and dexamethasone).
   B) Start the patient on melphalan and dexamethasone.
   C) Start the patient treatment with CyBorD (cyclophosphamide, bortezomib, and dexamethasone).
   D) Refer the patient to a colleague for consideration of autologous hematopoietic stem cell transplantation.
   E) Tailor treatment based on the patient's performance status and comorbidities.

Expert Perspective: There are no evidence-based guidelines for treatment of AL amyloidosis in patients older than 70 years. Most centers would no longer consider autologous stem cell transplantation for patients older than 70 years of age, particularly with cardiac involvement which is a risk for high treatment-related mortality and morbidity. CyBorD (cyclophosphamide, bortezomib, and dexamethasone) is a highly effective three-drug combination regimen and should be used with weekly low-dose dexamethasone at 10–20 mg and subcutaneous bortezomib weekly. The recently completed clinical trial ANDROMEDA and accelerated approval of subcutaneous daratumumab plus CyBorD in the treatment of newly diagnosed AL amyloidosis leading to very high hematologic deep responses and organ responses imply that this could be the treatment of choice for this patient with AL amyloidosis.

Correct Answer: A

Case Study 2

A patient is referred from primary care because of a small "M spike," a monoclonal gammopathy, of 0.4 g/dL. The patient is a 50-year-old woman who has had significant fatigue over the past year, which has been attributed to menopause. To risk-stratify her disease, you carry out appropriate testing, including a bone marrow biopsy, immunofixation electrophoresis (IFE) of serum and urine, and serum free light chains. These studies reveal 15% lambda monotypic plasma cells in the bone marrow, an immunoglobulin G lambda and free lambda monoclonal bands on serum IFE, and both albumin and lambda light chains in the urine. Lambda serum free light chains are elevated at 70 mg/L (normal: 5.7–26.3 mg/L) with a kappa of 5.0 mg/L (normal: 3.3–19.4 mg/L); the calculated kappa:lambda free light chain ratio (FLCR) is 0.07 mg/L (normal: 0.26–1.65). The patient is not anemic or hypercalcemic, and she has no lytic lesions on a skeletal survey. The serum creatinine is reported as normal.

5) What is the diagnosis for this patient?

A) MGUS; no further workup is necessary currently. Non-invasive studies should be repeated in six months and, if unchanged, every 1–2 years.

B) Smoldering myeloma; no further workup is necessary currently. Non-invasive studies should be repeated every 3–4 months.

C) Unclear. Additional diagnostic studies should be done.

Expert Perspective: This patient does not have MGUS, as the percentage of bone marrow plasma cells exceeds 10%. Could this patient have smoldering myeloma? Smoldering myeloma is diagnosed when the serum M protein is ⩾ 3 g/dL or clonal bone marrow plasma cells are ⩾ 10%, without the CRAB features (hypercalcemia, renal failure, anemia, or lytic bone lesions). Hematologically, the patient's plasma cell dyscrasia fits this diagnosis (see Chapter 51). However, for either MGUS or smoldering myeloma, there should be no end organ disease or symptoms associated with the plasma cell dyscrasia.

Correct Answer: C

6) What should the next best step in her management?

A) 24-hour urine collection to assess urinary protein excretion and UPEP.

B) Electrocardiogram and echocardiogram.

C) Measurement of NT-proBNP and/or BNP, and troponin levels.

D) Referral to a psychiatrist.

E) A, B, and C.

Expert Perspective: Patients with MGUS or smoldering myeloma should have NO SYMPTOMS AND NO ORGAN DYSFUNCTION associated with their disease. A patient who appears to have MGUS or smoldering myeloma but has significant fatigue, dyspnea on exertion, edema, lightheadedness, peripheral neuropathy, gastrointestinal symptoms, periorbital ecchymoses, hoarseness, macroglossia, or jaw or buttock claudication MUST be evaluated for amyloidosis. Delay in diagnosis of AL amyloidosis, particularly with cardiac involvement, can be fatal. As we have learned earlier, this patient should have an abdominal fat aspiration performed, with Congo red staining.

Correct Answer: E

In view of nephrotic syndrome, the patient had renal biopsy and typing by immunofluorescence showing AL-lambda amyloidosis. She has 8 g/24-hour albuminuria, and her estimated glomerular filtration rate is normal at 90 mL/min/1.73 m². She is asking about prognosis with respect to development of end-stage renal disease (ESRD) and the need for dialysis.

7) Which of the following is the correct response?

A) Stage I renal disease with two-year risk of dialysis 0–3%.

B) Stage II renal disease with two-year risk of dialysis 11–25%.

C) Stage III renal disease with two-year risk of dialysis 60–75%.

Expert Perspective: Renal staging system in AL amyloidosis has been developed and validated in large cohort of patients which can predict two-year and annual risk of dialysis (Table 56.1). This staging system is based on 24-hour urine total protein excretion and estimated glomerular filtration rate. Of note, the majority of patients in this study were treated with oral melphalan and dexamethasone treatment and not contemporary treatment regimens.

Table 56.1 Renal staging system in AL amyloidosis.

Renal stage	eGFR (mL/min/1.73m²)		24 hr urine protein (g/24-hr)	2-year risk of dialysis	Annual risk of dialysis after 2 years
I	≥ 50	and	< 5	0–3%	0–1%
II	< 50	or	≥ 5	11–25%	< 5%
II	< 50	and	≥ 5	60–75%	0–15%

Correct Answer: B

The patient would like to know her survival probability from AL amyloidosis. She has cardiac involvement, and her cardiac biomarkers are elevated; BNP 250 pg/mL and troponin I < 0.006 ng/mL. Echocardiogram shows interventricular septum to be 12 mm and grade I diastolic dysfunction with a normal LV ejection fraction.

8) Which of the following is correct response?
   A) Stage I disease with median overall survival not reached with median follow-up 12 years.
   B) Stage II disease with median overall survival of 9.4 years.
   C) Stage III disease with median overall survival of 4.2 years.
   D) Stage IIIb disease with median overall survival of one year.

Expert Perspective: Cardiac staging system predicting overall survival was first developed in 2004 and was updated in 2012 by Mayo Clinic.

- Mayo 2004 staging system used NTproBNP and troponin biomarkers (NTproBNP > 332 pg/mL, cTnT > 0.035 pg/mL, TnI > 0.1 ng/mL,) and Mayo 2012 staging system incorporated dFLC (difference between abnormal to normal free light chains), NTproBNP and troponin T levels (dFLC > 180 mg/L, NTproBNP > 1800 pg/mL, cTnT > 0.025 pg/mL).
- European investigators added stage IIIb for those with NTproBNP of > 8,500 pg/mL and the median survival of these patients is approximately six months.
- Boston University staging system with BNP and troponin I and through strong correlation with the well-validated and well-studied Mayo 2004 scheme (BNP > 81 pg/mL, TnI > 0.1 ng/mL).

Institutions without access to serum NT-proBNP testing could instead use BNP (Boston University staging system) with reasonable confidence for application in stratifying and prognosticating patients with AL amyloidosis.

Correct Answer: B

Case Study 2 Continues: She has renal stage II and cardiac stage II AL amyloidosis with a good functional status. She was treated with four cycles of daratumumab plus CyBorD with good tolerability as induction therapy leading to hematologic partial response.

9) What is the best treatment options for her?
   A) Oral melphalan and dexamethasone.
   B) High-dose melphalan and autologous stem cell transplantation.

C) Give four more cycles of daratumumab plus CyBorD (cyclophosphamide, bortezomib, and dexamethasone).

D) Any of the above choices.

Expert Perspective: High-dose melphalan and autologous stem cell transplantation achieves a high durable hematologic response with long term survival of 30% at 20 years. However, only 20–25% of highly selected patients with newly diagnosed AL amyloidosis are eligible to receive this aggressive treatment. Eligibility criteria vary based on the experience of the treating team. Treatment-related early mortality could range from 5–10% and has decreased with refinement in patient selection from prior years. A recently completed and published trial led to accelerated approval of daratumumab plus CyBorD for the treatment of newly diagnosed patients with AL amyloidosis (except for those with NYHA class III and IV CHF, NTproBNP > 8,500 pg/mL and eGFR < 20 mL/min/1.73 m^2) achieving unprecedented high hematologic responses. However, long-term data with respect to survival are lacking; therefore, autologous transplant remains an important strategy in suitable patients with AL amyloidosis.

The European Hematology Association (EHA) and International Society of Amyloidosis (ISA) guidelines (2022) recommend 2–4 cycles of induction therapy with proteasome inhibitor–based treatment regimen prior to autologous transplant for patients with bone marrow plasma cells of > 10% at the time of diagnosis. These guidelines do not recommend use of maintenance therapy post-transplant unless AL amyloidosis is associated with myeloma. However, patients with medically refractory pleural effusions, advanced cardiac involvement with stage IIIb disease, orthostatic hypotension refractory to medical therapy, acquired factor X deficiency with active bleeding, and gastrointestinal involvement with gastrointestinal bleeding are not eligible to receive transplant. For patients achieving hematologic complete response after induction therapy, transplant should be delayed and be offered at the time of hematologic relapse if organ function permits. Stem cell mobilization should be performed with granulocyte colony-stimulating factor (G-CSF) alone either as a single dose or split dose, and plerixafor could be used to reduce capillary leak syndrome associated with G-CSF.

Correct Answer: B

Case Study 3

A 56-year-old woman with kappa light chain multiple myeloma diagnosed in 2013 when she presented with anemia and back pain due to a compression fracture of the T12 vertebral body. She had multiple myeloma with 50% kappa-restricted plasmacytosis, normal cytogenetics, fluorescence in situ hybridization (FISH) study with t(11;14); serum and urine electrophoresis and immunofixation did not detect monoclonal protein. A serum-free kappa light chain level of 1,200 mg/L, serum lambda light chain level of 10 mg/L, and ratio of 120 were noted.

Treatment was initiated with four cycles of lenalidomide, bortezomib, and dexamethasone (RVD) followed by high-dose melphalan at 200 mg/m^2 and autologous hematopoietic cell transplantation. The patient was then started on lenalidomide maintenance in early 2014. She developed easy bruising around her eyes in the summer of 2014 (Figure 56.2), and after a routine visit with her myeloma specialist, she was referred to a dermatologist. She was diagnosed as having contact dermatitis from eye makeup products. She stopped applying eye makeup without complete resolution of the bruising.

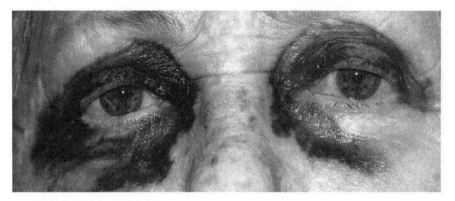

Figure 56.2 Patient with periorbital bruising while on therapy for multiple myeloma.

Meanwhile, the patient remained on lenalidomide maintenance. She started to experience gradual worsening of her breathing and shortness of breath with leg swelling in early 2015. An echocardiogram showed increased left-ventricular wall thickness, interventricular septum measurement of 13 mm, and left-ventricular ejection fraction of 60%. Her cardiac biomarkers were elevated: N-terminal–pro B-type natriuretic peptide (NT-proBNP) was 1,200 pg/mL, BNP was 400 pg/mL, and troponin I was 0.1 ng/mL.

In addition to worsening dyspnea, she started to experience frequent spontaneous periorbital bruising despite not applying eye makeup. A year after easy bruising around the eyes, consideration for AL amyloidosis was given in the summer of 2015. An abdominal fat pad aspiration was performed and subjected to Congo red staining, which showed congophilic amyloid deposits (i.e. readily stained by Congo red).

10) What is the final diagnosis?
   A) Light chain myeloma.
   B) AL amyloidosis.
   C) Myeloma-associated secondary AA amyloidosis.
   D) Myeloma-associated AL amyloidosis.

Expert Perspective: AL amyloidosis, like multiple myeloma, is associated with a plasma cell dyscrasia. However, in AL amyloidosis, there is deposition of amyloid fibrils, derived from immunoglobulin light chains, into a multitude of organs and soft tissues, leading to a plethora of clinical symptoms and eventually vital organ dysfunction. It has been estimated that overt organ dysfunction from AL amyloidosis occurs in approximately 10% of patients with multiple myeloma; however, subclinical, or occult AL amyloidosis is higher and may occur in 30–40% of patients with multiple myeloma.

Despite the known relationship between the two disorders, namely myeloma and AL amyloidosis, delays in the diagnosis of AL amyloidosis in patients with existing myeloma remains a major problem. Such delays invariably are associated with needless physical, mental, and financial distress to patients and their families.

AA amyloidosis, historically known as secondary amyloidosis, is related to infections or inflammatory conditions and is caused by misfolding of serum amyloid A protein, which is upregulated in the setting of infection/inflammation. AA amyloidosis leads to renal, liver, and spleen involvement and is treated with the therapies for the underlying inflammatory conditions.

Correct Answer: D

Case Study 4

A 68-year-old man of African descent presented with new onset heart failure in 2015. Echocardiogram showed interventricular septal diameter in end-diastole (IVSd) 18 mm (normal 6-11mm) and left ventricular ejection fraction of 35%. He then underwent unremarkable left-heart catheterization. The final diagnosis of non-obstructive coronary artery disease was established. Additional investigations are listed below:

1) Cardiac MRI (April 2016): late gadolinium enhancement
2) Serum and urine immunofixation studies: presence of IgG kappa monoclonal gammopathy
3) Serum free light chains: kappa 45 mg/L, lambda 23 mg/L, kappa/lambda ratio 1.99
4) Bone marrow biopsy: 5% plasma cells with kappa predominance
5) Abdominal fat pad aspirate revealed amyloid deposits

11) What is the diagnosis, and what should be done?

Expert Perspective: He was diagnosed with systemic AL amyloidosis (without additional studies) and treated with four cycles of CyBorD. Due to lack of response to treatment, he was referred to a center of excellence for consideration of treatment options for refractory AL amyloidosis. The following investigations were performed at the center of excellence.

1) ^{99m}Technetium pyrophosphate scan with increased cardiac uptake (Figure 56.3)
2) Endomyocardial biopsy, Congo red staining, and mass spectrometry showing amyloid deposits and TTR as the precursor amyloid protein (Figure 56.4)
3) Genetic testing showing V122I TTR variant

The final diagnosis of this patient is ATTRv amyloidosis with an unrelated monoclonal gammopathy of unknown significance (MGUS), and the treatment should focus on TTR gene silencer or TTR stabilizer, rather than plasma cell dyscrasia–directed therapy.

Cardiac amyloidosis due to V122I ATTRv amyloidosis is underdiagnosed, especially in underrepresented populations. It is important to recognize cardiac amyloidosis due to valine to isoleucine substitution at position 122 of the *TTR* gene, which is present in 3–4% of Black Americans and up to 12% of Afro-Caribbean patients over the age of 60 with heart failure.

The hallmark of AL amyloidosis is the finding of a monoclonal protein, present in greater than 90% (not 100%!) of patients with systemic AL amyloidosis and usually associated with an abnormal serum free light chain assay. As emphasized earlier, the diagnosis of AL amyloidosis requires evidence of organ dysfunction related to a monoclonal paraprotein. However, a monoclonal gammopathy can be present as an MGUS in patients with ATTR amyloidosis, posing a diagnostic challenge.

The prevalence of MGUS in V122I ATTRm amyloidosis is reported with disproportionately higher rate in ~50% of patients, for reasons that are currently unclear. Therefore, an assumption to diagnosis of AL amyloidosis in patients with cardiomyopathy and MGUS should be avoided.

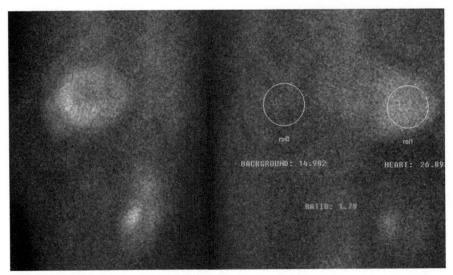

Figure 56.3 ^{99m}Technetium pyrophosphate scan with increased cardiac uptake.

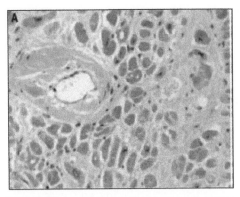

Figure 56.4 Endomyocardial biopsy with eosinophilic material with Congo red stain under light microscopy.

Recommended Readings

Gillmore, J.D., Maurer, M.S., Falk, R.H., Merlini, G., Damy, T., Dispenzieri, A. et al. (2016). Nonbiopsy diagnosis of cardiac transthyretin amyloidosis. *Circulation* 133: 2404–2412.

Merlini, G., Dispenzieri, A., Sanchorawala, V., Schönland, S.O., Palladini, G., Hawkins, P.N. et al. (2018). Systemic immunoglobulin light chain amyloidosis. *Nat Rev Dis Primers* 4: 38.

Lilleness, B., Ruberg, F.L., Mussinelli, R., Doros, G., and Sanchorawala, V. (2019). Development and validation of a survival staging system incorporating BNP in patients with light chain amyloidosis. *Blood* 133: 215–223.

Palladini, G., Hegenbart, U., Milani, P., Kimmich, C., Foli, A., Ho, A.D. et al. (2014). A staging system for renal outcome and early markers of renal response to chemotherapy in AL amyloidosis. *Blood* 124: 2325–2332.

Mendelson, L., Shelton, A., Brauneis, D., and Sanchorawala, V. (2020). AL amyloidosis in myeloma: red flag symptoms. *Clin Lymphoma Myeloma Leuk* 20: 777–778.

Muchtar E., Dispenzieri A., Wisniowski B., et al. (2022). Graded Cardiac Response Criteria for Patients With Systemic Light Chain Amyloidosis. *J Clin Oncol* 2023 Mar 1;41 (7): 1393–1403. doi: 10.1200/JCO.22.00643. Epub 2022 Oct 10. PMID: 36215675.

Staron, A., Connors, L.H., Ruberg, F.L., Mendelson, L.M., and Sanchorawala, V. (2019). A new era of amyloidosis: the trends at a major US referral centre. *Amyloid* 26: 192–196.

Sanchorawala, V. (2020). High-dose melphalan and autologous peripheral blood stem cell transplantation in AL amyloidosis. *Acta Haematol* 143 (4): 381–387.

Sarosiek, S. and Sanchorawala, V. (2019). Treatment options for relapsed/refractory systemic light-chain (AL) amyloidosis: current perspectives. *J Blood Med* 10: 373–380.

Phull, P., Sanchorawala, V., Connors, L.H., Doros, G., Ruberg, F.L., Berk, J.L. et al. (2018). Monoclonal gammopathy of undetermined significance in systemic transthyretin amyloidosis (ATTR). *Amyloid* 25: 62–67.

Sanchorawala, V., Boccadoro, M., Gertz, M., Hegenbart, U., Kastritis, E., Landau, H., Mollee, P., Wechalekar, A., and Palladini, G. (2022 March). Guidelines for high dose chemotherapy and stem cell transplantation for systemic AL amyloidosis: EHA-ISA working group guidelines. *Amyloid* 29 (1): 1–7.

57

Bispecific T Cell Engager and Cell Based Immune Therapy in Multiple Myeloma

Meera Mohan, Parameswaran Hari, and Saurabh Chhabra

Division of Hematology Oncology, Medical College of Wisconsin, USA

Introduction

Despite the enormous advances in therapeutics, multiple myeloma (MM) remains largely incurable. Newer immunotherapeutic approaches have been developed over recent years to break the vicious circle of tumor-induced immunosuppression and harness the patient's immune system to destroy malignant plasma cells. Among the plethora of game-changing immunotherapy options, the most encouraging developments include chimeric antibody therapy T cells (CAR-T) and bispecific antibodies (bsAb). Early trials in the relapsed/refractory setting have demonstrated significant single-agent activity with manageable side effect profiles. These promising results have led to clinical trials investigating these agents in earlier lines of therapy. Taken together, these immunotherapy agents are likely redefining the existing treatment paradigm in MM. In the current chapter, we discuss the various clinical trials that have been carried out to date and potential future innovations that could enhance the efficacy and/or reduce the toxicities associated with T cell–directed therapies.

The past five years have seen amazing progress in the long sought-after goal of safe and effective immunotherapy in multiple myeloma (MM), an effort that started more than two decades ago with such therapeutic modalities as interferon and allogeneic HCT (Bruno et al. 2007, Schaar et al. 2005). In this chapter, we attempt to capture the state of the art and controversies in the modern era of immunotherapy for MM.

1) What is Chimeric Antigen Receptor (CAR) T Cell therapy?

Expert Perspective: Chimeric antigen receptor (CAR) T cell therapy is a highly promising cellular immunotherapeutic option that has dramatically changed the treatment landscape of B-cell malignancies. CAR T cell therapy combines the advantage of the target specificity of monoclonal antibodies (mAbs) and the cytotoxicity of T cells. CARs are artificial fusion proteins with a modular design that confer antigen-specificity to T cells in a human

Cancer Consult: Expertise in Clinical Practice, Volume 2: Neoplastic Hematology & Cellular Therapy,
Second Edition. Edited by Syed A. Abutalib, Maurie Markman, James O. Armitage, and Kenneth C. Anderson.
© 2024 John Wiley & Sons Ltd. Published 2024 by John Wiley & Sons Ltd.

leukocyte antigen (HLA)-independent manner and provide intracellular stimulatory signals to promote T cell survival and proliferation and induce cytokine production, thus enhancing the cytolytic activity of T cells. CAR T cells can circumvent the limitations of T-cell receptor (TCR)-induced immunity, including major histocompatibility complex (MHC) loss on tumor cells and weak antigen-binding affinity of T cells. CARs are comprised of extracellular antigen recognition and binding domain (short chain variable fragment; scFv), hinge; a modified spacer, CD28 or CD8, which redirects CAR T cells to recognize malignant cells; transmembrane domains which link the antigen-binding domain to the intracellular signaling domain, which in turn, consists of T cell activation domain; CD3ζ, and one or two co-stimulatory domains (4-1BB, CD28) to promote efficient CAR T-cell signaling, persistence, and efficacy. Engagement of the cognate antigens by CAR T cells initiates signaling cascade in the T cells stimulating the production and release of pro-inflammatory cytokines such as IL2, IL6, TNF-α, and IFN-γ, resulting in target cell lysis. The US Food and Drug Administration in March 2021 approved the first autologous CAR T cell therapy, idecabtagene autoleucel (previously bb2121, Abecma®, Bristol Myers Squibb™), for treatment of patients with relapsed/refractory multiple myeloma (R/R MM) after four or more prior therapies, including an immunomodulatory drug (IMiD), a proteasome inhibitor (PI), and an anti-CD38 mAb.

2) How are CAR T cells manufactured?

Expert Perspective: Multiple CAR T manufacturing processes are involved before CAR T cells can be infused. Commercial scale manufacturing is a laborious process that takes a range of 2–4 weeks for completion in a good manufacturing practice (GMP) facility. CAR T cell therapy is currently autologous, and the manufacturing process begins with the collection of peripheral blood mononuclear cells (PBMCs) to obtain CD3+ T cells from patients with MM via leukapheresis. T-cell population enrichment followed by gene modification results in expression of CARs on the T cells. Viral transduction (using γ-retrovirus or lentivirus) has been the method for gene delivery in frontrunner clinical trials and commercially available CAR T products. Non-viral transfer technology (DNA transposon or mRNA transfection) has also been attempted in some clinical trials. This step is followed by immunophenotyping analyses to ensure successful endowment of T cells with CARs and their cytolytic activity. These CAR T cells subsequently undergo *ex vivo* expansion in growth factor–enriched media, before finally being cryopreserved for storage or immediately transported to the clinic for administration. Once the CAR T cells are ready for infusion, patients are subjected to a conditioning lymphodepleting chemotherapy usually consisting of fludarabine and cyclophosphamide to set the stage for proliferation of the infused CAR T cells.

3) What is most common target antigen for CAR T generation in multiple myeloma?

Expert Perspective: The most widely studied myeloma CAR target is B-cell maturation antigen (BCMA), a transmembrane glycoprotein member of the tumor necrosis factor receptor superfamily member 17 (TNFRSF17), which is encoded by the BCMA gene located on chromosome 16. It is considered an ideal target due to its exclusive expression on plasmablasts and plasma cells and upregulation during B-cell differentiation. It is not expressed on CD34$^+$ hematopoietic cells or naive and memory B cells. BCMA is an important regulator of B cell proliferation and survival, as well as maturation and differentiation into plasma cells. BCMA promotes growth and proliferation of plasma cells in the bone marrow after binding to its ligands, B-cell activating factor (BAFF) and A proliferation-inducing ligand (APRIL). Although BCMA expression is heterogeneous, it is universally present on MM cells; moreover, its increased expression is considered to be prognostic, but not predictive, of response based on data available from autologous CAR T therapy studies in relapsed/refractory MM. Other targets including GPRC5D, SLAMF7, CD38, or multi-targeting approaches are currently experimental.

4) BCMA CAR T therapies—what is the current level of evidence in MM?

Expert Perspective: The first-in-human phase I clinical trial to test the safety of BCMA-targeted CAR T cells in relapsed/refractory MM was conducted by National Cancer Institute (NCI) group. BCMA-specific CAR T with a CD28 costimulatory domain (murine scFv) was employed in heavily pretreated patients. At the highest CAR T dose (9×10^6 cells/kg), 13 of 16 patients (81%) had a response with a median event-free survival of 31 weeks. The University of Pennsylvania developed a BCMA CAR with a fully human scFv and 4-1BB costimulatory molecule and investigated it in a phase I clinical trial, which enrolled 25 heavily pretreated relapsed/refractory MM patients. Safety data showed that cytokine release syndrome (CRS) was observed in 88% patients including 32% developing grade 3–4, all of whom received the highest dose of CAR T cells. Immune effector cell-associated neurotoxicity syndrome (ICANS) was seen in 32%; severe (grade ≥ 3 in 12%) ICANS was associated with high tumor burden, high dose of CAR T cells, and concurrent grade 3–4 CRS. The ORR was 48%. The median PFS (mPFS) was 1.9–4.2 months depending on the cohort, and the median OS (mOS) was 11.8 months to not reached. Responses were associated with higher premanufacturing $CD4^+/CD8^+$ T cell ratio and frequency of $CD45RO^-CD27^+CD8^+$ T cells, suggesting that enrichment of less differentiated, more naive or stem cell memory–like T cells is needed for improved outcomes. There was no correlation between baseline BCMA expression and CAR T expansion or response. In patients responding to the treatment, a decrease in BCMA expression was observed that subsequently increased upon progression.

Idecabtagene vicleucel (ide-cel; previously bb2121) and now FDA approved as Abecma™ is a second-generation CAR T incorporating an anti-BCMA scFv with 4-1BB co-stimulatory domain and CD3ζ signaling domain, which showed potent cytotoxicity against MM cells regardless of the ratio of BCMA expression in MM cells or the presence of soluble BCMA. The first-in-human study with ide-cel (CRB-401) evaluated escalating doses of CAR T (50×10^6, 150×10^6, 450×10^6, or 800×10^6 followed by an expansion phase with 150×10^6–450×10^6 dose) in extensively pretreated MM (median of six prior therapy lines: 69% triple-class refractory) (Raje et al. 2019). The former phase enrolled RRMM patients with $\geq 50\%$ BCMA expression on plasma cells, while in the latter phase patients with less than 50% BCMA expression could also be included. Thirty-six patients were enrolled, and a total of 33 patients received CAR T therapy (three patients discontinued after apheresis due to MM progression). Twelve patients in the dose expansion phase received 150×10^6 to 450×10^6 CAR T cells. For the entire cohort ORR was 85%, with 45% patients achieving complete response (CR) or better. At doses $\geq 150 \times 10^6$ (n = 30) ORR was 90%, with 50% patients achieving $\geq$ CR. Responses appeared independent of soluble BCMA (sBCMA) levels or tumor BCMA expression levels. After a median follow-up of 11.3 months, the mPFS in the $\geq 150 \times 10^6$ cohort was 11.8 months. All patients who had a response (partial response or better) had MRD negativity at 10^{-4}. Patients who received 450×10^6 CAR T cells attained a similar response rate, independent of tumor BCMA expression levels < 50% or > 50% in plasma cells (100% vs 91%, respectively). There was a trend toward lower response in patients who received $\leq 150 \times 10^6$ CAR T, in those with less in vivo CAR T expansion, and in those with high-risk cytogenetic abnormalities. Persistence of CAR T cells at 6 and 12 months was detected in 57% and 20% of patients, respectively, and blood CAR T cell levels were higher in patients who achieved a response. Safety signal was significant for CRS in 76% patients, mostly grade 1–2 and $\geq$ grade 3 in 7% patients (no grade 4 or 5), which was treated with tocilizumab or corticosteroids effectively. The CRS incidence correlated with CAR T dose. Other common adverse events included neutropenia (92%), leukopenia (61%), anemia (58%), and thrombocytopenia (58%). Neurotoxicity including ICANS occurred in 42% patients, including only one patient (3%) developing grade 4 ICANS.

Based on the promising results in the phase I trial, a phase II trial (KarMMa) was conducted to evaluate ide-cel in a larger cohort of relapsed MM patients who were previously exposed to IMiD, a PI, and an anti-CD38 mAb (Munshi et al. 2021). In this study, 140 patients were enrolled with a manufacturing success of 99%, and 128 (91%) patients received CAR T. Patients were treated at target dose levels of $150–450 \times 10^6$ CAR T cells, and 84% were triple-class refractory (refractory to PI, IMiD, and anti-CD38 mAb). ORR was 73%, including $\geq$ CR in 33% and MRD-negative CR in 26%. As in the phase I trial, baseline BCMA expression did not correlate with response to ide-cel. At a median follow-up of 13.3 months ORR was 73%, including 33% patients with $\geq$ CR. Median PFS was 8.8 months. PFS increased with higher CAR T dose, with a mPFS of 12.1 months for patients who received the target dose of 450×10^6 CAR T. Patients who achieved at least CR experienced better PFS ($\geq$ CR: mPFS of 20.2 months; VGPR: mPFS of 11.3 months; PR: mPFS of 5.4 months; no response: 1.8 months). Median OS was 19.4 months. Durable CAR T persistence was observed up to one year: CAR T were detected in 59% and 36% patients at 6 and 12 months, respectively, after infusion. Out of 128 patients enrolled in the trial, 107 patients experienced CRS (84%), while only seven patients (5%) had a CRS grade $\geq$ 3. One patient had grade 5 CRS. Most patients required at least one dose of tocilizumab for CRS. Eighteen percent reported ICANS, which was mostly grade 1/2. However, 4 patients (3%) had grade 3 ICANS and none with grade 4 or 5.

Ciltacabtagene autoleucel (Cilta-cel), also known as JNJ-4528, is another CAR T cell containing a 4-1BB costimulatory domain and two binding sites that attach to BCMA to confer greater antigen binding affinity (Berdeja et al. 2021). JNJ-4528 takes after the exact construct of LCAR-B38M that was evaluated in China in the LEGEND-2 trial (Zhao et al. 2018) and showed deep and durable responses in patients with RRMM. In the LEGEND-2 trial, different conditioning regimens were used, as well as variable CAR T infusion methods (split vs single infusion). The Xi'an site, which used cyclophosphamide as lymphodepletion chemotherapy and three dose of CAR T for infusion ($0.07–2.1 \times 10^6$/kg; median dose of 0.50×10^6/kg) enrolled 57 patients. These patients had received a median of three prior lines of therapy. ORR was 88%, with CR in 74% patients. At a median follow-up of 25 months, mPFS was 19.9 months, although it was 28.2 months for those patients in CR. Median OS was 36.1 months.

The phase Ib/II CARTITUDE-1 study evaluated cilta-cel in R/R MM patients who had received more than three prior lines of therapy or were double refractory to PIs or IMiDs and received anti-CD38 mAb. Sixteen of 113 patients who underwent apheresis were not dosed because of consent withdrawal (n = 5), progressive disease (n = 2), or death (n = 9). The remaining 97 patients received cilta-cel (target dose of $0.5–1.0 \times 10^6$ CAR + T /kg), and had received a median of six prior lines of therapy. Ninety-seven percent of patients achieved ORR, with sCR in 67%. Forty-eight of 57 patients who were evaluable for MRD (93%) were MRD negative at the level of 10^{-5}. Response was independent of baseline BCMA expression. After a median follow-up of 12.4 months, 12-month PFS and OS were 77% and 85%, respectively. CRS was reported in 94.8% patients, including 4% grade > 3, with a median onset of seven days after CAR-T infusion. Neurotoxicity occurred in 21% patients, including 10% grade > 3 events. Recently, the results of CARTITUDE-4, a phase 3, randomized, open-label trial were reported. The patients with lenalidomide-refractory multiple myeloma received ciltacabtagene autoleucel or the physician's choice of effective standard care. A total of 419 patients underwent randomization (208 to receive ciltacabtagene autoleucel and 211 to receive standard care). At a median follow-up of 15.9 months (range, 0.1 to 27.3), the median PFS (primary endpoint) was not reached in the ciltacabtagene autoleucel group and was 11.8 months in the standard-care group (hazard ratio, 0.26; 95% CI, 0.18 to 0.38; P<0.001). More patients in the ciltacabtagene autoleucel group than in the standard-care group had an overall response (84.6% vs. 67.3%), a CR or better (73.1% vs. 21.8%), and an absence of MRD (60.6% vs. 15.6%). Death from any cause was reported in 39 patients and 46 patients, respectively (hazard ratio, 0.78; 95% CI, 0.5 to 1.2). Most patients reported grade 3 or 4 adverse events during treatment. Among the 176 patients who received ciltacabtagene autoleucel in the as-treated population, 134 (76.1%) had CRS (grade 3 or 4, 1.1%; no grade 5), 8 (4.5%) had ICAN (all grade 1 or 2), 1 had movement and neurocognitive symptoms (grade 1), 16 (9.1%) had cranial nerve palsy (grade 2, 8.0%; grade 3, 1.1%), and 5 (2.8%) had CAR-T-related peripheral neuropathy (grade 1 or 2, 2.3%; grade 3, 0.6%).

Despite the current FDA label for ide-cel in relapsed/refractory MM patients with four or more prior therapies (including PI, IMiD, and CD38 mAb), the optimal timing of CAR T cell therapy in the sequence of anti-myeloma therapy remains an important open question. The unprecedented response rates obtained with CAR T cell therapy trials in heavily pre-treated relapsed and/or refractory MM patients have prompted the question of whether CAR T cells should be considered as an earlier line therapy. The lower biologic risk of relapse in the newly diagnosed or early-stage MM may represent an opportunity to utilize CAR T therapy with higher probability of achieving deeper and more durable remissions. In addition, it is hypothesized that due to prior therapy and T cell dysfunction, CAR T cell products generated in the relapsed/refractory setting could be of inferior potency compared with products generated from patients earlier in the disease course. The inclusion of CAR T cell therapy within earlier lines of MM treatment needs to be evaluated in clinical trials. In an ongoing phase III study, ide-cel is compared with standard-of-care regimens in patients with 2–4 prior regimens, including IMiD, PI, and CD38 mAb (KarMMa-3). Ide-cel is also being evaluated in the ongoing multicohort KarMMa-2 study in patients with early relapse after first-line therapy or patients with suboptimal response after autologous transplant (less than very good partial response [VGPR]), and in first-line (KarMMa-4) treatment in high-risk MM patients. Cilta-cel is being evaluated in a phase III study (CARTITUDE-4) comparing CAR T vs current standard-of-care treatment (pomalidomide, bortezomib, and dexamethasone or daratumumab, pomalidomide, and dexamethasone) in relapsed and lenalidomide-refractory MM. In addition, the ongoing CARTITUDE-2 study is evaluating cilta-cel in multiple patient populations, including those with early relapse after front-line therapy, prior exposure to a BCMA-targeting therapy, and those with < CR post-autologous transplant.

5) What are the most relevant toxicities after CAR T therapy?

Expert Perspective: CAR T cell therapy can induce unique on-target and off-tumor toxicity, including CRS and neurotoxicity such as immune effector cell–associated neurotoxicity syndrome (ICANS). CRS is the most frequent and potentially serious acute CAR T cell–related toxicity, with an absolute incidence of 30–100%, and 10–30% for CRS grade ≥ 3. CRS is a systemic inflammatory response observed after adoptive T cell therapy. It is the result of secretion of cytokines IL-2, IL-6, IL-10, IFN-γ, tumor necrosis factor-α (TNF-α), and production of granzyme and perforin, triggered by the activation and expansion of the CAR T cells and lysis of normal and tumor cells. This toxicity is non-antigen specific, is related to high immune activation, and in some patients CRS-related clinical and laboratory findings are like macrophage activation syndrome/hemophagocytic lymphohistiocytosis (MAS/HLH). The common clinical features of CRS include fever, hypotension, tachycardia, hypoxia, and rigor: the clinical presentation can range from flu-like symptoms to life-threatening manifestations (hypotension requiring pressors, capillary leak, coagulopathy, and organ dysfunction). The treatment of CRS is supportive care with antipyretics, intravenous hydration, vasopressor support, supplemental oxygen, and in severe cases IL-6 receptor antagonist, tocilizumab, and corticosteroids.

ICANS is the second most frequent serious adverse event after CAR T cell infusion. Symptoms are variable, ranging from toxic encephalopathy with word-finding difficulty, aphasia, and confusion, to more severe cases with coma, seizures, and cerebral edema. ICANS usually occurs during or after CRS and may manifest a biphasic course, in about 10% of cases up to four weeks after CAR T infusion. A 10-point neurologic assessment, at least twice a day, using the ICE screening tool is recommended for early detection. Importantly, a broad consensus statement offering updated comprehensive recommendations for the management of ICANS associated with immunotherapies has been recently published by ASTCT (Lee et al. 2019). The treatment is supportive care, and corticosteroids are generally reserved for grade 3–4 ICANS. The use of tocilizumab is recommended only if there is concurrent CRS. High-grade (grade 3–4) ICANS sometimes requires prolonged hospitalization and intensive care in a subset of patients with delayed recovery. Cerebral edema is the most common finding of MRI in patients with ICANS, followed by leptomeningeal enhancement and multifocal microhemorrhage. Although the pathogenesis of ICANS has not been clearly elucidated yet, several factors including high tumor burden and a higher peak of CAR T cells by in vivo expansion have been implicated. Delayed neurologic events including facial palsy, movement disorders, and neurocognitive dysfunction observed in CARTITUDE 1 study are thought to be associated with higher tumor burden at the time of CAR T therapy.

BCMA is also co-expressed on normal B-lymphocytes, and BCMA CAR T cell therapy could therefore also cause on-target/off-tumor effects of B-cell aplasia, hypogammaglobulinemia, and neutropenia, which lead to increased risk of infection. Hemophagocytosis and prolonged cytopenias may also occur. Most cases are reversible and are shortly resolved with tocilizumab, anakinra, and corticosteroids treatment.

6) What are the important limitations and barriers of CAR T cell therapy?

Expert Perspective:

1) The manufacturing of autologous CAR T cells may limit the number of patients who can benefit from this therapy. It can be difficult to collect sufficient numbers of autologous $CD3^+$ T cells through leukapheresis because of lymphopenia related to the disease or use of prior therapies. The use of high doses of steroids, alkylators, or bendamustine immediately before apheresis could lead to low T cell numbers.

2) The generation of autologous CAR T cell products is a time-consuming, logistically complex, labor- and resource-intensive procedure in general. Availability of manufacturing slots and current turnaround times may render CAR T cell therapy access difficult or unsuitable for patients with rapidly progressing disease. Rapid or near-patient manufacturing, off-the-shelf approaches, and use in earlier lines of therapy may alter this situation.

3) Antigen evasion (expression of different form of antigen lacking the target epitope) or antigen loss or downregulation mechanisms can lead to resistance or lack of durability of response after CAR T. Heterogeneously expressed BMCA at the intra-tumor level can lead to preferential targeting of cells with high BCMA while sparing those with low/no BCMA expression, resulting in selection of the latter clones. BCMA may lose its expression upon disease relapse after the CAR T therapy, suggesting selection for BCMA-negative MM clones (Samur et al. 2020). BCMA antigen escape can be caused by inadvertent transfer from malignant clone to T cells in a process called trogocytosis causing T-cell fratricide or it can be shed into the blood circulation (sBCMA) mediated by γ-secretase. The use of γ-secretase inhibitors to increase target antigen density on plasma cells is being explored in clinical trials.

4) The current BCMA-directed autologous CAR T cell therapy products have scFv derived from nonhuman species (murine for ide-cel and camelid for cilta-cel) (Gazeau et al. 2021). Nonhuman scFv can induce immunogenicity from an adaptive immune response after CAR T cell therapy: the resulting anti-CAR antibodies may limit the persistence of the CARs, thereby increasing the risk of relapse. The development of anti-scFv antibodies in patients relapsing following BCMA-CAR-T cell therapy requires the strategy of employing humanized or fully human scFv.

7) What is the status on safety and efficacy of bispecific antibody (bsAb) therapy in MM?

Expert Perspective: Currently available bsAb in MM are T-cell engaging antibodies that bind to specific targets on the plasma cells and the CD3 antigen on T cells, thus facilitating cytolytic T cell activation and tumor cell death. Some of the agents targeting the plasma cell–specific antigens include BCMA, CD38, GPRC5D, and FcRH5. Structurally, bsAb are fusion molecules composed of Fab variable regions of the two separate target antigen recognition motifs (Lancman et al. 2020). Differences between the various agents arise from the various conformations of the fusion antibody and formulation differences. These agents

Table 57.1 Comparison of current data on bispecific T cell engager agents.

Molecule	Teclistamab	Elranatamab	REGN 5448	TNB-383B	Talquetamab	CC93269	Cevostamab(BFCR4350A)	AMG701
Company	Janssen	Pfizer	Regeneron/Sanofi	Tenebio/Abbvie	Janssen	Celgene	Genentech	Amgen
Administration	SC and IV	SC	IV	IV	SC and IV	SC and IV	IV	IV
Target	BCMA/CD3	BCMA/CD3	BCMA/CD3	BCMA/CD3	CPRC5D/CD3	BCMA/CD3	FcRH5/CD3	BCMA/CD3
Dosing	QW	QW/Q2W	QW/Q2W	Q3W	QW/Q2W	Q4W	Q3W	QW
MTD	1550 µg/kg sc	215–1000 µg/kg SC	96 mg	40–60 mg	405 µg/kg SC		3.6-90 mg	12 mg
Pts treated with MTD or highest dose / ITT	22/65 (SC)	20/30	8/49	15/58	13/55 (SC)	9/30 (IV)	18/53	6/82
Median number of prior lines	5	8	5	6	4.5	5	6	6
ORR/ ≥ CR	73%/23%	80%/20%	62.5%/0%	80%/13.3%	69%/15%	89%/44%	61%/17%	83%/33%
CRS/ Neurotoxicity all grades	64%/3%	90%/20%	38%/NA	80%/NA	68%/5%	77%/NA	76%/28%	65%/NA
CRS/ Neurotoxicity grade ≥ 3	0%/0%	0%/0%	0%/0%	0%/0%	0%/0%	5%/NA	2%/0%	9%/0%
Median PFS	94% at 3.9 months mFU	NR	DOR: 6 months	NR	NR at 3.7 months mFU	NR	NR at 10.3 months mFU	NR at 6.5 months mFU

lead to an immunological synapse formation independent of MHC (between CD3 on T cells and target antigen on plasma cells), recruitment of alpha beta T cells, cytolytic T cell activation, and transient expansion. Endogenous T cell numbers, phenotype, and function are critical to success. Compared to the initial generation of bsAbs, agents in development for MM have longer half-lives and a superior dosing schema.

Efficacy Data:

Recently presented data pertain to their efficacy and safety in relapsed and refractory multiple myeloma with at least three lines of therapy including an IMiD, PI, and anti-CD38 monoclonal antibodies (Table 57.1). Usmani S et al. reported a large phase I–II study assessing the single agent activity of the BCMA targeted bsAb, teclistamab (Usmani et al. 2021). The ORR at the recommended phase II dose was 65%, with 58% patients achieving a very good partial response or better and 40% patients a CR or better. At a median follow-up of 6.1 months, the median duration of response was not reached. Other BCMA targeted bsAb in clinical trial include PF-3135, REGN 5448, and TNB-383B. Early-phase studies with these are summarized in Table 57.1. Depending on dose level and dosing schema, ORR ranges from 36 to 89%, with ongoing responses. The majority of these responses are deep and durable, with bone marrow MRD negativity (10^{-5}) attained in a significant proportion of trial patients. Durability of responses, PFS, and OS are immature for the majority of these early-phase trials. On October 25, 2022, the FDA granted accelerated approval to teclistamab, the first BCMA-directed CD3 T-cell engager, for adult patients with relapsed or refractory multiple myeloma who have received at least four prior lines of therapy, including a proteasome inhibitor, an immunomodulatory agent, and an anti-CD38 monoclonal antibody. Elranatamab, another BCMA-directed CD3 T-cell engager, was approved by FDA on August 14, 2023 for similar indication as teclistamab and talquetamab. The latter is a a bispecific antibody against CD3 and GPRC5D (not BCMA) was approved on August 9, 2023.

Side Effect Profile:

The incidence of CRS (all grade) ranges from 65 to 75% across the various trials, and neurotoxicity (all grades) ranges from 5 to 28%. Most CRS is seen with the first cycle, and mitigation measures such as initial inpatient hospitalization with step-up dosing schedule and premedication with steroids were employed depending on study protocols. Additionally, modification of the construct, as in TNB-3838, to have a lower affinity for CD3 is also a strategy to minimize CRS. Subcutaneous route of administration seems to influence side effects and CRS, as the rates of both were lower with PF-3135, teclistamab, and talquetamab. Common hematological complications included anemia, neutropenia, lymphopenia, leukopenia, and thrombocytopenia, which were self-limiting. Infectious complications are of concern particularly with BCMA targeting bsAb, and incidence range from 21 to 52% across various trials of BCMA, with serious infections ranging from 8 to 30%. Overall, there is a lower risk of immune-mediated toxicities such as high-grade CRS or ICANS, and thus less-fit patients could be considered a candidate for treatment. The bsAbs are a desirable off-the-shelf treatment option especially in rapidly progressing relapsed refractory MM and preclude the need for bridging therapy required in CAR T therapy. Given the overall favorable tolerability, these agents are suitable candidates for combination therapy with naked antibodies or other novel therapies. The need for continuous dosing (weekly to every three

Table 57.2 Current BCMA targeted therapies—a comparison.

Antibody-drug conjugate	CAR T-cells	Bispecific antibody
E.g. Belantamab	E.g. Idecel; Ciltacel	E.g. Teclistamab
Off-the-shelf	Personalized	Off-the-shelf
Targeted cytotoxicity not dependent on T-cell health encouraging responses in triple class exposed pts	Targeted immuno-cytotoxicity: unprecedented ORR incl. MRD-neg in heavily pretreated pts	Targeted immuno-cytotoxicity. rapid and deep responses in ongoing trials
No lymphodepletion no steroids	Single infusion ("one and done"); long "chemo holiday"	No lymphodepletion minimal steroids
Outpatient administration; can be given in the community	Potentially persistent	Can be given in the community after 1st cycle (once approved)
Currently requires REMS/close collaboration with ophthalmology	Manufacturing time makes impractical for pts with rapidly progressive disease	Dosing/schedule/combinations to be determined
Modest ORR and PFS in TCR pts	Accredited center, with required infrastructure	Initial hospitalization required until low CRS risk
Requires continuous treatment until progression or intolerance	CRS and ICANS: hospitalization likely required; safety in frail elderly?	CRS and neurotoxicity possible but low risk; limited severe cases
	Dependent on T-cell health manufacturing success	Dependent on T-cell health (T-cell exhaustion)
	Requires significant social support; caregiver required	Requires continuous treatment

weeks), lack of treatment-free periods, and feasibility of outpatient administration espe-cially in a community clinic setting are limitations. Additionally, there is currently limited experience in patients with renal failure, as well as in advanced-disease settings such as extramedullary disease, plasma cell leukemia, and central nervous system disease. One of the major attractions of CAR T cells is their single-use approach, while bsAb are continu-ously dosed till progression in R/R MM, at least in the currently ongoing studies. The risk of persistent hypogammaglobulinemia and secondary immune deficiency with ongoing therapy is a factor that might distinguish CAR T immunotherapy vs bsAb (Table 57.2).

8) How are immune-based therapies such as CAR T cells and bsAbs redefining the role of autologous stem cell transplantation (ASCT) in MM?

Expert Perspective: Currently the primary use of ASCT in MM is as consolidative therapy following initial induction in patients with newly diagnosed transplant-eligible patients. There are no randomized studies comparing any form of immunotherapy versus ASCT as consolidative therapy after induction. There is considerable enthusiasm for the use of CAR T therapy earlier in the disease course of myeloma, given the high MRD negativity rates and possibility that post CAR T remissions could be even longer-lasting in the context of newly diagnosed disease. Current phase I–II studies are exploring the role of CAR T cell therapy instead of ASCT in high-risk disease (Idecel; KarMMa 4 trial; NCT 04196491) and in standard-risk or high-risk cohorts with Ciltacel in the CARTITUDE 2 study (NCT 04133636). The Blood and Marrow Transplant Clinical Trials Network (BMT-CTN) is initi-ating 2 multicenter phase II clinical trials to evaluate ide-cel in the post-ASCT context to augment suboptimal responses (< VGPR) after ASCT (BMT CTN 1902) or as additional consolidation for high-risk MM after ASCT (BMT CTN 1901). The recently concluded US State of the Science in cellular therapy symposium recommended that the network under-take studies that explore the use of CAR T and bsAb in sequential fashion after ASCT in high-risk MM, which is an area of unmet medical need in MM (Heslop et al. 2021).

Recommended Readings

Berdeja, J.G., Madduri, D., Usmani, S.Z., Jakubowiak, A., Agha, M., Cohen, A.D. et al. (2021). Ciltacabtagene autoleucel, a B-cell maturation antigen-directed chimeric antigen receptor T-cell therapy in patients with relapsed or refractory multiple myeloma (CARTITUDE-1): A phase 1b/2 open-label study. *Lancet* 398: 314–324.

Bruno, B., Rotta, M., Patriarca, F., Mordini, N., Allione, B., Carnevale-schianca, F. et al. (2007). A comparison of allografting with autografting for newly diagnosed myeloma. *N Engl J Med* 356: 1110–1120.

Gazeau, N., Beauvais, D., Yakoub-Agha, I., Mitra, S., Campbell, T.B., Facon, T., and Manier, S. (2021). Effective anti-BCMA retreatment in multiple myeloma. *Blood Adv* 5: 3016–3020.

Heslop, H.E., Stadtmauer, E.A., Levine, J.E., Ballen, K.K., Chen, Y.B., Dezern, A.E. et al. (2021 November). Blood and marrow transplant clinical trials network state of the science symposium 2021: looking forward as the network celebrates its 20th year. *Transplantat Cell Ther* 27 (11): 885–907. ISSN 2666–6367.

Lancman, G., Richter, J., and Chari, A. (2020). Bispecifics, trispecifics, and other novel immune treatments in myeloma. *Hematology* 2020: 264–271.

Lee, D.W., Santomasso, B.D., Locke, F.L., Ghobadi, A., Turtle, C.J., Brudno, J.N. et al. (2019 April). ASTCT consensus grading for cytokine release syndrome and neurologic toxicity associated with immune effector cells. *Biol Blood Marrow Transplant* 25 (4): 625–638. doi: 10.1016/j.bbmt.2018.12.758. Epub 2018 Dec 25. PMID: 30592986.

Munshi, N.C., Anderson, L.D., Shah, N., Madduri, D., Berdeja, J., Lonial, S. et al. (2021). Idecabtagene vicleucel in relapsed and refractory multiple myeloma. *N Engl J Med* 384: 705–716.

Raje, N., Berdeja, J., Lin, Y., Siegel, D., Jagannath, S., Madduri, D. et al. (2019). Anti-BCMA CAR T-cell therapy bb2121 in relapsed or refractory multiple myeloma. *N Engl J Med* 380: 1726–1737.

Samur, M.K., Fulciniti, M., Aktas-samur, A., Bazarbachi, A.H., Tai, Y.-T., Campbell, T.B. et al. (2020). Biallelic loss of BCMA triggers resistance to anti-BCMA CAR T cell therapy in multiple myeloma. *Blood* 136: 14-14.

San Miguel, J., Dhakal, B., Yong, K., Spencer, A., Anguille, S., Mateos, M.V., Fernández de Larrea, C., Martínez López, J., Moreau, P., Touzeau, C., Leleu, X., Avivi, I., Cavo, M., Ishida, T., Kim, S.J., Roeloffzen, W., van de Donk, N.W.C.J., Dytfeld, D., Sidana, S., Costa, L.J., Oriol, A., Popat, R., Khan, A.M., Cohen, Y.C., Ho, P.J., Griffin, J., Lendvai, N., Lonardi, C., Slaughter, A., Schecter, J.M., Jackson, C.C., Connors, K., Li, K., Zudaire, E., Chen, D., Gilbert, J., Yeh, T.M., Nagle, S., Florendo, E., Pacaud, L., Patel, N., Harrison, S.J., and Einsele, H. (2023 July 27). Cilta cel or standard care in Lenalidomide refractory multiple myeloma. *N Engl J Med* 389 (4): 335 347. doi: 10.1056/NEJMoa2303379. Epub 2023 Jun 5. PMID: 37272512.

Schaar, C.G., Kluin-nelemans, H.C., Te Marvelde, C., Le Cessie, S., Breed, W.P., Fibbe, W.E. et al. (2005). Interferon-alpha as maintenance therapy in patients with multiple myeloma. *Ann Oncol* 16: 634–639.

Usmani, S.Z., Garfall, A.L., Van De Donk, N., Nahi, H., San-Miguel, J.F., Oriol, A. et al. (2021). Teclistamab, a B-cell maturation antigen × CD3 bispecific antibody, in patients with relapsed or refractory multiple myeloma (MajesTEC-1): A multicentre, open-label, single-arm, phase 1 study. *Lancet* 398: 665–674.

Zhao, W.H., Liu, J., Wang, B.Y., Chen, Y.X., Cao, X.M., Yang, Y. et al. (2018). A phase 1, open-label study of LCAR-B38M, a chimeric antigen receptor T cell therapy directed against B cell maturation antigen, in patients with relapsed or refractory multiple myeloma. *J Hematol Oncol* 11: 141.

Part 9

Special Issues in Neoplastic Hematology and Cellular Therapy

58

Treatment of Lymphomas During Pregnancy

Kieron Dunleavy[1], Emanuele Zucca[2], and Fedro A. Peccatori[3]

[1] *Lombardi Cancer Center, Georgetown University, Washington, DC, USA*
[2] *Oncology Institute of Southern Switzerland, Ente Ospedaliero Cantonale, and Institute of Oncology Research, Bellinzona, Switzerland and Università della Svizzera Italiana, Lugano, Switzerland*
[3] *European Institute of Oncology IRCCS, Milan, Italy*

Introduction

Lymphoma is the fourth most common type of cancer encountered in pregnancy with Hodgkin lymphoma occurring at the highest frequency, followed by non-Hodgkin lymphomas such as primary mediastinal B-cell lymphoma (Brenner et al. 2012; Dunleavy and McLintock 2020; Froesch et al. 2008). The setting of pregnancy presents us with many unique therapeutic challenges, the most important of which is to carefully balance the delivery of optimal curative therapy with mitigation of risks to the pregnant mother and developing fetus (Peccatori et al. 2013). Pregnancy represents a unique therapeutic setting where the collaborative expertise of a multidisciplinary team including specialists from maternal-fetal medicine, neonatology, anesthesiology, and hematology is critical for best outcomes (Cubillo et al. 2021). While the clinical and histological aggressiveness of the lymphoma are key determinants of the need for urgent treatment initiation, therapeutic approach may be significantly affected by the trimester in which the lymphoma diagnosis occurs (Lishner et al. 2016). There is a paucity of data and experience using many anti-lymphoma drugs in both pregnancy and the postpartum period. This is particularly true with respect to novel agents, which are increasingly incorporated in up-front standard regimens for these diseases (Luttwak et al. 2021). In this chapter, we focus on some of the unique challenges that treating lymphoma in pregnancy presents and through case-based discussions, provide perspectives on how these can be optimally tackled.

Case Study 1

A 37-year-old female was diagnosed with stage IVA, diffuse large B-cell lymphoma (DLBCL) four months following delivery of her first infant. She was successfully breastfeeding her baby girl when she noticed an enlarged supraclavicular lymph node, the biopsy of which demonstrated DLBCL, and imaging confirmed stage IV disease. Her hematologist expediently started treatment with R-CHOP. She was reluctant to interrupt breastfeeding and inquired about the safety of continuing this during chemotherapy plus rituximab. She was also concerned about the safety of whole-body FDG-PET imaging while breastfeeding.

1) **In your opinion, is breastfeeding during chemotherapy a safe option for the patient and her daughter?**
   A) Yes, breastfeeding is safe while receiving chemotherapy.
   B) Yes, but only if she expresses milk by pumping and bottle-feeds her daughter.
   C) No, anthracyclines and cyclophosphamide may pass in human milk and possibly harm a developing infant.
   D) No, breastfeeding may increase the risk of lymphoma progression during chemotherapy.

Expert Perspective: Breastfeeding, for at least six months, is highly recommended to improve maternal-fetal health and promote successful bonding within the baby/mother dyad. Nonetheless, several issues need consideration when a breastfeeding mother receives chemotherapy. While not all anticancer therapies pass into breast milk, some do, and this is of particular concern for the infant, who has immature and developing drug detoxifying systems (Pistilli et al. 2013). Moreover, chemotherapy may alter the normal microbiome and chemical makeup of breastmilk. The amount of drug taken up by the baby (the so-called infant dose) depends on the levels of that specific drug in the milk, the volume of milk ingested, and the gastric absorption. Few data are available regarding breast milk concentrations of doxorubicin, cyclophosphamide, vincristine, and rituximab in nursing mothers (Codacci-Pisanelli et al. 2019). According to the Internet Drugs and Lactation Database (LactMed) [accessible from https://www.ncbi.nlm.nih.gov books/ NBK501922/] doxorubicin and cyclophosphamide are both contraindicated during breastfeeding due to their long half-life and adverse events (mainly neutropenia) described in infants. In one study, toxic metabolites of doxorubicin and cyclophosphamide were found in breast milk up to 21 days following their administration to the mother (Codacci-Pisanelli et al. 2019). On the contrary, the passage of rituximab in milk is probably very low and delivered infant dose negligible because of its high molecular weight and destruction in the infant's gastrointestinal tract (Codacci-Pisanelli et al. 2019). While the American College of Rheumatology guidelines do not contraindicate breastfeeding during rituximab treatment, the number of reported cases is low and caution is recommended (Bragnes et al. 2017; Sammaritano et al. 2020).

Correct Answer: C

2) **Whole-body FDG-PET scans are frequently used in lymphoma patients. How should you advise this patient about breastfeeding after FDG-PET?**
   A) She should immediately stop breastfeeding and avoid intimate contact with her daughter for at least 48 hours.
   B) She could continue breastfeeding and avoid intimate contact with her daughter for 6–12 hours.
   C) She could continue breastfeeding until the start of chemotherapy, without further precautions.
   D) She should interrupt breastfeeding because of its psychological burden.

Expert Perspective: Radioactive fluorodeoxyglucose (18-FDG) is a positron emitter tracer used in PET scans for its high affinity with neoplastic tissue. The physical half-life of 18-FDG is 0.89 hours, and radioactive levels in human milk after diagnostic examination are very low (Leide-Svegborn et al. 2016). Thus, most guidelines suggest continuation of breastfeeding after 18-FDG PET scan. Nonetheless, 18-FDG may accumulate in the lactating breast tissue, and this should be considered in the nuclear medicine report. To keep infant exposure as low as possible, nursing mothers might want to avoid close contacts with their infants for 6–12 hours after 18-FDG PET scans and discard the pumped milk to avoid breast engorgement and allow subsequent recovery of breastfeeding.

Correct Answer: B

Case Study 2

A 30-year-old woman underwent an abdominal ultrasound for investigation of vague pelvic symptomatology and fatigue lasting a few months following her first pregnancy. Enlarged para-aortic and iliac lymph nodes (6.0 × 4.0 cm) were detected, together with a 6-week uterine gestational chamber. The patient was counseled regarding pregnancy termination to enable lymph node biopsy and staging, but she sought a second opinion as she was reluctant to terminate the pregnancy. An ultrasound-guided retroperitoneal biopsy confirmed a grade 1 follicular non-Hodgkin lymphoma, with low proliferative index.

A follow-up disease surveillance plan with abdominal ultrasound and whole-body MRI was set up, and it was decided to withhold therapy in the absence of clear disease progression. Whole-body MRI performed at 16, 25, and 32 weeks of pregnancy confirmed enlarged retroperitoneal lymph nodes that remained stable during the pregnancy, and the patient spontaneously delivered a healthy baby girl at 38 + 1 weeks of gestation.

Following delivery, she was restaged with whole-body CT scan and FDG-PET, and treatment with bendamustine-rituximab was instituted with complete radiological remission. At 30 months following the initial diagnosis, she remains asymptomatic and in continued complete remission.

3) In your opinion, was the management of this patient's gestational lymphoma appropriate?

Expert Perspective: Yes; follicular lymphoma is an infrequent diagnosis during pregnancy. In the rare occurrence of an indolent lymphoma diagnosed during pregnancy, a watch-and-wait strategy can be proposed, and treatment, if required, can be deferred until after delivery.

In this case, pregnancy termination was not mandatory. Ultrasound-guided nodal biopsies can be safely performed during pregnancy, and the pregnancy itself does not accelerate the growth of non-Hodgkin or Hodgkin lymphomas. The so-called pregnancy-induced immunosuppression has no impact on the clinical course of most neoplasms diagnosed during pregnancy and should not be a reason to terminate the pregnancy.

Whole-body diffusion-weighted MRI has been effectively used to stage and follow up pregnant patients with cancer and is preferred to FDG-PET for the absence of ionizing radiations and contrast media (Table 58.1). Retroperitoneal disease can be difficult to visualize with ultrasounds in the second and third trimester, but echography is an excellent diagnostic mean in case of superficial nodes (Shah et al. 2020; Woitek et al. 2016).

Table 58.1 This table outlines the common imaging modalities that are used in the diagnosis and staging of patients with lymphoma. The table indicates estimated effective radiation doses that the fetus and mother receive according to the study used.

Imaging Modality	Radiation Dose to Fetus (mSv)	Radiation Dose to Mother (mSv)
CT chest	0.01–0.66	4–18
CT abdomen and pelvis	13–25	3–45
Chest X-ray	0.0005–0.01	0.02
^{18}FDG-PET	1.4–5.2	3–9
^{18}FDG-PET-CT	10–22	13–32
Abdominal ultrasound	None	None
Body MRI	None	None

Estimated delivered radiation doses to mother and fetus for standard imaging modalities used in lymphoma assessment (*Source:* Costello et al. 2013; Pahade et al. 2009; Tirada et al. 2015; Zanotti-Fregonara and Stabin, 2017).

Case Study 3

A 38-year-old female, who was at 16 weeks gestation, had chest imaging following a presentation of chest discomfort and cough that was persistent and worsening over two weeks. Imaging (chest X-ray followed by a confirmatory chest CT scan) revealed a large anterior mediastinal mass measuring 18 cm in maximal diameter. She underwent a core biopsy of the mass, and this revealed a diagnosis of classic Hodgkin lymphoma (cHL). Reed-Sternberg cells were present, and the tumor cells were CD15 and CD30 positive and negative for CD20 and EBER—consistent with nodular sclerosing subtype. She had no B-symptoms but had an elevated LDH level. She went on to have a whole-body MRI scan, and this revealed a moderate conglomerate of lymph nodes in the mesenteric area, and hence her clinical stage was IIIA. Her desire was to continue her pregnancy.

4) **Given that the diagnosis of cHL is very early in the second trimester and she desires continuation of pregnancy, should initiation of therapy be deferred?**

Expert Perspective: No. As the patient has a large mediastinal mass that is already causing significant symptoms, deferral of therapy is not an option. If the diagnosis occurred in late pregnancy, early induction/delivery of the baby might be a feasible option. While deferral of therapy during pregnancy may be an option with gestational indolent lymphoma, this is rarely the case with Hodgkin lymphoma and primary mediastinal B-cell lymphoma, which are relatively common in females of childbearing age.

5) **Which of the following approaches would you favor in the management of this patient?**
   A) Six cycles of brentuximab with AVD.
   B) Six cycles of ABVD (AVD following ABVD × 2 if in complete remission).
   C) Escalated BEACOPP.
   D) Standard-dose BEACOPP.

Expert Perspective: The ECHELON-1 randomized study demonstrated that patients with stage III or IV cHL had a superior outcome (they had improved modified progression-free survival) when brentuximab-vedotin (an anti-CD30 monoclonal antibody conjugated to a highly active antitubulin agent) replaces bleomycin in the standard ABVD regimen (doxorubicin, bleomycin, vinblastine, and dacarbazine) (Connors et al. 2018). Therefore, given her stage, if this patient were not pregnant, it would be reasonable to consider this regimen; however, she is pregnant (16 weeks gestation), and there is a paucity of data using brentuximab-vedotin or indeed other antibody drug conjugates in pregnancy. There is no data evaluating the ability of antibody drug conjugates to cross the placental barrier, and these agents have high potential for harming the fetus and affecting delivery. Indeed, CD30 is expressed by multiple organs during organogenesis and brentuximab-vedotin is embryo-toxic and teratogenic in animals (Gurevich-Shapiro and Avivi 2019; Moshe et al. 2017). As we have no data as to their potential toxicity in pregnancy, all ADCs should be avoided at this point in time, until more safety data is attained (Dunleavy and McLintock 2020; Luttwak et al. 2021). BEACOPP (standard or escalated) is significantly more toxic than ABVD and has demonstrated significant risk for the development of myelodysplastic syndrome (Eichenauer et al. 2014). Hence, it is likely to have higher teratogenicity than ABVD and should be avoided in pregnancy. In conclusion, we would treat this patient with ABVD, and if she is in remission following two cycles of treatment, drop the bleomycin for further cycles (Johnson et al. 2016).

Interim FDG-PET imaging is now considered a standard and critical response assessment tool in the management of patients with cHL (Barrington et al. 2016). The RATHL study (Barrington et al. 2016; Johnson et al. 2016) demonstrated that bleomycin can be safely omitted from subsequent cycles in patients with a negative PET-CT after two cycles of ABVD. However, there are no data as to whether treatment de-escalation can be safely implemented based on interim MRI, and this is a consideration in a case like this.

Correct Answer: B

6) **Which of the following strategies is best to assess interim response after two cycles (weeks 23 and 24 of gestation)?**
   A) FDG-PET scan.
   B) CT body scan.
   C) MRI body scan.
   D) Response assessment should be deferred until the completion of therapy.

Expert Perspective: Interim response assessment in lymphoma typically uses modalities such as CT imaging or (Eichenauer et al. 2014) F-flurodeoxyglucose positron-emission tomography (FDG-PET). Whole-body magnetic resonance imaging (MRI) is much less frequently used. In the setting of pregnancy, exposure to any type of ionizing radiation is problematic and poses a risk to the developing fetus—in that regard, there is no defined safe level of radiation exposure (see Table 58.1, which lists materno-fetal exposure doses of ionizing radiation with different imaging modalities) (Goldberg-Stein et al. 2011). While FDG-PET is the preferred imaging modality for cHL interim response assessment in non-pregnant patients, we know that the radiotracer used in PET imaging crosses the placenta and the effective, delivered dose of radiation is higher in the first and second trimesters (Shah et al. 2020; Woitek et al. 2016). We, therefore, recommend that FDG-PET imaging be avoided during pregnancy and MRI used alternatively for interim response assessment.

Correct Answer: C

Case Study 4

A 36-year-old woman who was 32 weeks pregnant presented with a two-week history of progressive chest discomfort and dyspnea associated with palpitations. Initially, there was concern for a pulmonary embolus, and she underwent a CT pulmonary angiogram; there was no evidence of embolus, but there was a large anterior mediastinal mass that measured approximately 11.5 × 8 cms in diameter—additionally a small pericardial effusion was observed. Clinically, she also had early evidence of superior vena caval obstruction. She underwent a core biopsy of the mass, and this revealed a B-cell lymphoma that was strongly CD20 positive, weakly CD30 positive, and negative for CD15. The clinicopathologic diagnosis was primary mediastinal B-cell lymphoma.

7) Which of the following is the most appropriate next step?
   A) Emergency cesarean section and initiation of therapy post partum.
   B) Initiate immunochemotherapy as soon as possible.
   C) Initiate high-dose steroids, and defer immunochemotherapy until delivery.

Expert Perspective: As with Case Study 3, this patient has a highly curable lymphoma and is already starting to demonstrate signs and symptoms of disease such as evidence of early hemodynamic compromise and early superior vena caval obstruction (Dunleavy and Gross 2018). Deferral of therapy is not an option (Figure 58.1). High-dose steroids may be somewhat effective anti-lymphoma therapy as a short temporizing measure but are unlikely to be effective for a significant duration of time and should not replace initiation of curative therapy. The question of emergency cesarean section can be considered, and engagement of the patient's obstetrician in decision-making is critical—however, emergent cesarean section at 32 weeks gestation is associated with many risks, and this needs to be balanced with the risk/benefit of instituting immunochemotherapy immediately.

   In this case, the patient received first cycle of therapy (DA-EPOCH-R) at 33 weeks following earlier initiation of high-dose steroids and clinically responded very well (Dunleavy et al. 2013). Induction of labor was conducted at 36 weeks, and she received the second cycle of immunochemotherapy in the early post-partum period.

   In our opinion, it was considered vital to institute therapy expediently due to early hemodynamic compromise, and cesarean section would have been very challenging and risky. Reducing the size of the mediastinal mass with immunochemotherapy relieved the early SVC obstruction, making delivery at 36 weeks much safer (and exposure of the fetus to immunochemotherapy was limited to one cycle). Delivery at or after 36 weeks is considered low risk for complications of prematurity, so this strategy enabled effective urgent therapy of the lymphoma and safe delivery of the fetus.

Correct Answer: B

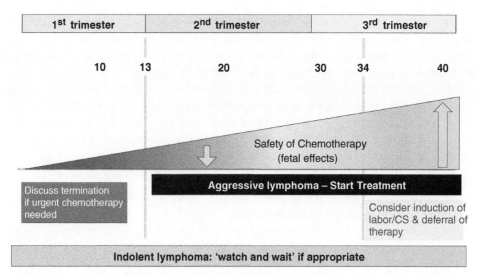

Figure 58.1 Summary of proposed approach to gestational lymphoma. Management of lymphoma during pregnancy may differ according to the trimester at diagnosis. Therapy needs to consider not only disease histology and stage but also maternal factors and potential fetal effects of treatment.

8) Is the use of granulocyte colony-stimulating factor (GCSF) safe in pregnancy?

A) G-CSF may be used based on available data and experience.

B) G-CSF should always be avoided.

Expert Perspective: Granulocyte-colony stimulating factor (G-CSF) is frequently used following certain lymphoma regimens to limit duration of post-chemotherapy-induced neutropenia. Animal models have demonstrated that G-CSF crosses the placenta and causes neutrophilia, but there is no evidence to suggest that it has adverse outcomes when given during pregnancy. An international registry that captured the use of G-CSF during pregnancy for the treatment of severe chronic neutropenia reported no increased incidence of adverse outcomes https://www.drugs.com/pregnancy/filgrastim.html. As this patient received a regimen that includes the use of growth factors, she received G-CSF without any compications.

Correct Answer: A

Case Study 5

A 37-year-old female, who is 20 weeks pregnant, presents for evaluation. Approximately three years previously, she had a diagnosis of diffuse large B-cell lymphoma (DLBCL), non-germinal center B-cell (GCB) subtype. At that time, she had stage IIA disease (bilateral cervical and mediastinal lymphadenopathy) and received six cycles of R-CHOP immunochemotherapy. An end-of-treatment FDG-PET scan demonstrated a complete metabolic remission. A few weeks into her current pregnancy, she noticed a right breast mass. This was biopsied and demonstrated recurrent non-GCB, DLBCL. By immunohistochemistry studies, this was a triple-expressor lymphoma with high protein expression of BCL2, BCL6, and c-MYC; FISH testing demonstrated absence of any genetic rearrangements. Her physician was concerned about the triple-expressor findings and recommended pregnancy termination to enable complete staging (by FDG-PET imaging) and prompt institution of salvage chemotherapy followed by autologous stem cell transplantation. However, the patient wanted to consider alternative options that would allow continuation of the pregnancy without compromising curability of her lymphoma. She is seeking your expert opinion on starting therapy that offers a high probability of eradicating her lymphoma but minimizing risk of any possible fetal toxicity.

9) What are your recommendations regarding next steps?

A) Proceed with termination of pregnancy and urgent institution of salvage chemotherapy and autologous transplantation.

B) Perform staging MRI scan followed by 2–3 cycles of immunochemotherapy with rituximab, doxorubicin, vincristine, and prednisone. Following delivery, treatment would be completed with a more appropriate regimen.

C) Following staging, if the MRI confirms localized right breast disease only, surgical removal of the tumor as a temporizing strategy before proceeding to definitive chemotherapy following delivery.

D) Immediate initiation of salvage therapy with regimens such as R-DHAP (rituximab, dexamethasone, cytarabine, cisplatin) (Gisselbrecht et al. 2010; Crump et al. 2014), R-GDP (rituximab, gemcitabine, dexamethasone, cisplatin) (Crump et al. 2014), or R-ICE (rituximab, ifosfamide, carboplatin, etoposide) (Gisselbrecht et al. 2010). After delivery, proceed with an autologous transplant.

Expert Perspective: Albeit not directly related to the question above, the case raises an important point that involvement of the breast or other reproductive organs (ovary, uterus, placenta) is observed in nearly 50% of gestational NHL where information on extranodal involvement is available. The pathophysiological basis for this is unclear (Kumar and De Jesus 2022). Let's now address the treatment choices. Even if standard R-CHOP regimen (rituximab, cyclophosphamide, doxorubicin, vincristine, and prednisone) could be administered safely in the third trimester (Maggen et al. 2019), its curative potential in the salvage setting case is low; some experts do not avoid cyclophosphamide at this stage in pregnancy but treatment with rituximab, doxorubicin, vincristine, and prednisone, sparing alkylating agent administration, may be a safer choice, albeit limited data. This combination (also referred as APO regimen) has been effectively used for initial debulking and chemosensitivity testing in autologous transplant procedures for high-risk lymphoma patients (Brenner et al. 2012).

There is a paucity of data on the use of salvage regimens for relapsed/refractory aggressive lymphomas in pregnancy. The physiological changes of pregnancy can have a major impact on pharmacokinetics: changes in albumin levels, volume of distribution, and clearance of drugs in the second and third trimesters are well-recognized phenomena (Anderson 2005). Indeed, studies of anthracyclines, cisplatin, and ifosfamide suggest that, during pregnancy, optimal or ideal dosing may differ from standard dosing (Germann et al. 2004; Köhler et al. 2015; Mir et al. 2012). In addition, these regimens are highly myelotoxic (Crump et al. 2014; Gisselbrecht et al. 2010) causing severe thrombocytopenia, neutropenia, and infections. Therefore, they can potentially cause harmful sequelae for both mother and the child.

G-CSF: It should be additionally noted that the efficacy and safety profile of granulocyte colony-stimulating factor (G-CSF) in pregnancy has not been definitively studied or determined (Mir and Berveiller 2012); however, most of the available evidence suggests it can be safely given for treatment of neutropenia (Berends et al. 2021; Shah et al. 2020).

The very limited data available on the use of salvage high-grade lymphoma regimens in pregnancy mainly derives from treatment experience with other tumors (leukemias, sarcomas, and solid tumors).

Cytarabine: This has low protein binding and broad tissue distribution, including the amniotic cavity. Available data on cytarabine use in acute myeloid leukemia (AML) in the second and third trimester demonstrates that combinatorial approaches with anthracyclines are feasible (Lishner et al. 2016); however, there is a non-negligible risk of intrauterine growth restriction, intrauterine fetal death, preterm delivery, and neonatal myelosuppression (Azim et al. 2010). Nevertheless, these patients typically received concomitant daunorubicin, with cytarabine given at lower doses (100–200 mg/m^2 intravenous continuous infusion over 24 hours for seven days) and different schedules (Murphy and Yee 2017) compared to the DHAP regimen (2000 mg/m^2 intravenous infusion over three hours once every 12 hours for two doses) (Crump et al. 2014; Gisselbrecht et al. 2010).

Etoposide: The use of etoposide in pregnancy (usually in combination with cisplatin with or without bleomycin) has been described in gynecological tumors and appears to be safe for women in the second and third trimesters; however, the number of cases is small (Amant et al. 2019). The information on the long-term effects is particularly limited. A preclinical study on murine gonadal tissue found that etoposide damages female germ cells in the developing ovary and may impair future fertility of female fetuses exposed to this agent (Stefansdottir et al. 2016).

Platinums: The administration of platinum derivatives appears feasible during the second and third trimesters. In gynecological cancers, carboplatin is nowadays preferred over cisplatin (except for germ cell tumors), which may be nephrotoxic and carries the risk of dose-dependent ototoxicity in the neonate (Amant et al. 2019; Benoit et al. 2021). However, how to calculate the optimal dose of carboplatin in pregnancy is unclear (Amant et al. 2019; Benoit et al. 2021). Notably, the transplacental transfer of cisplatin and carboplatin can increase in late pregnancy with potential short- and long-term toxicity that remains unknown (Berveiller et al. 2016; Mir et al. 2008).

Gemcitabine: Therapeutic doses of gemcitabine may be given in late pregnancy without major developmental toxicities to the fetus; however, the evidence is based only on four cases reported (Wiesweg et al. 2014).

Anthracycline: Doxorubicin and epirubicin are usually considered safe in the second and third trimester, with limited fetal toxicity (Benoit et al. 2021; Berveiller et al. 2016). More than 300 patients have been treated with anthracyclines during pregnancy, and their babies have been followed up in time with normal cardiac and neurocognitive function (Germann et al. 2004). Dose should be calculated according to the actual maternal weight, considering the altered pharmacokinetics due to pregnancy (Anderson 2005).

Vincristine: Vinca alkaloid have a very low transplacental transfer and are considered safe during pregnancy (Benoit et al. 2021). In a retrospective study of patients treated for cHL during pregnancy, 72 patients received vinca alkaloid-based chemotherapy without major fetal toxicities (Maggen et al. 2019).

In addition to these agents, for patients who present with relapsed/refractory Hodgkin lymphoma in pregnancy, brentuximab-vedotin, which has been already discussed (see Case 3), and the immune checkpoints inhibitors, pembrolizumab and nivolumab may be appropriate therapies. The latter immunotherapeutic agents are monoclonal antibodies that block binding of PD-L1/PD-L2 to PD-1, restoring tumor immunosurveillance. Pregnancy and fetal outcomes following PD1 inhibitors have been reported in a limited number of women, mainly with melanoma. Cases of uncomplicated pregnancy with birth of normal newborns, but also a case of congenital hypothyroidism were reported in patients treated with pembrolizumab or nivolumab (Anami et al. 2021; Hutson et al. 2022; Le-Nguyen et al. 2022; Xu et al. 2019). However, some preclinical data indicate an increased risk of pregnancy loss with these agents, and the evidence to support their use in pregnancy remains limited (Luttwak et al. 2021).

Case Study continued: Although cyclophosphamide has been safely administered in the third trimester, it was not included here due to concern about additive toxicity (see text above for details). She had two cycles of R-APO (rituximab, doxorubicin, vincristine, and prednisone—dosing as per the R-CHOP regimen) during the third trimester and achieved an almost complete clinical remission of the breast mass. As she had received a cumulative doxorubicin dose of 400 mg/m^2, treatment was discontinued and labor induced at week 36. She had a normal vaginal delivery with no maternal or neonatal complications and gave birth to a healthy girl (weight at birth 2,650 g). Following delivery, she had two cycles of salvage treatment with the DHAP regimen. Restaging breast MRI was consistent with a complete remission. After successful autologous stem cell harvest, consolidation with high-dose chemotherapy (BEAM) and autologous rescue was administered, with no major complications. At day 100 post-transplant, an FDG-PET-CT scan demonstrated a complete metabolic remission (Deauville score 2).

Correct Answer: B

Case Study 6

A 36-year-old woman (married, with three children, no relevant medical history) presented to the emergency room complaining of acute onset swelling of the left arm. She also had a history of fatigue and worsening shortness of breath over two weeks. She was afebrile, tachycardic at 115 b.p.m., and normotensive (125/72). Oxygen saturation on room air was 96%. Clinical examination demonstrated a slightly swollen left arm and bilateral jugular venous distension. A left supraclavicular lymph node was palpable (approx. 2 cm in diameter). Chest auscultation was normal. Breast and abdominal examinations were normal. Electrocardiogram demonstrated sinus tachycardia and a chest X-ray showed an enlarged mediastinum. CBC did not show major abnormalities (hemoglobin 12.4 g/dL, WBC 5.1 G/L with normal differential counts, and PLT 219 G/L). The metabolic panel showed increased CRP (33 mg/L; reference range < 5), ESR (38 mm/hr; reference range < 20), LDH (967 U/l, reference range 211–425), and D-dimers (1042 ng/mL, reference range < 250). The remaining blood chemistry was normal. The patient underwent upper extremity Doppler ultrasonography that revealed an occlusive thrombosis in the left internal jugular and left subclavian veins. A subsequent contrast-enhanced CT of the chest showed an anterior mediastinal bulky mass (measuring 14 × 11 × 10 cm) with compression of central vessels and a mild pericardial effusion. A CT-guided biopsy of the mediastinal tumor revealed a diagnosis of a B-cell lymphoma, characterized by medium to large polymorphic cells with clear cytoplasm, and evident sclerosis with fine compartmentalizing fibrosis. Following biopsy, she commenced prednisone 100 mg/d and underwent a low-dose PET-CT—this demonstrated hypermetabolism in the mediastinal mass (SUVmax of 32) with no other FDG-avid lesions. Steroid treatment led to rapid improvement of respiratory symptoms and was promptly followed by the administration of a cycle of chemotherapy (R-CHOP regimen). Within a week, a final diagnosis of PMBCL was made based on the morphologic, immunohistochemical (strong expression of CD20+, CD79a, BCL2, PAX5, CD45; heterogeneous expression of CD30; no expression of CD15, CD10, MUM1, cyclin D1) and molecular (no rearrangement of MYC and BCL2) characteristics of the tumor. The patient had been using contraception and denied any risk of pregnancy when she underwent imaging investigations. However, she later became concerned about a 10-day delay in her menstrual period and underwent a pregnancy test, which was inconclusive. A repeat test three and five days later confirmed pregnancy.

10) What are your recommendations regarding next steps?
   A) Given that she has received chemotherapy during the first trimester (embryonic phase), teratogenicity has likely occurred and termination of pregnancy is indicated with subsequent post-delivery resumption of aggressive treatment (such as DA-EPOCH-R).
   B) Assuming that there is no spontaneous miscarriage, chorionic villus sampling should be obtained between weeks 10 and 12 of pregnancy. If a normal fetal karyotype is demonstrated, termination of pregnancy can be avoided. She can then receive intensive chemotherapy during the second and third trimester.
   C) She should receive supradiaphragmatic irradiation with a 42 Gy total dose administered in 2-Gy fractions (Kumar and De Jesus 2022). With state-of-the-art equipment and modern techniques, supradiaphragmatic radiotherapy with abdominopelvic shielding is safe in pregnancy and the above-mentioned dose and schedule can eradicate her lymphoma enabling continuation of pregnancy with no significant risk to mother or child.

Expert Perspective: Even where pregnancy termination appears to be the most feasible solution, possible alternatives should be discussed with the individual patient. In PMBCL, promptly instituted, aggressive treatment should be administered without delay. In this case, the lymphoma presentation was potentially life-threatening. This is a distinct disease entity with specific clinicopathological and molecular characteristics. Patients are most frequently young females in their third to fourth decade of life. PMBCL is typically characterized by a rapidly progressive anterior mediastinal mass, with local invasion and compressive symptoms, and by occasional dissemination to unusual extranodal sites. The response to aggressive combination chemotherapy is generally excellent, and consolidation radiotherapy may be spared in patients with complete metabolic remission. Since the addition of rituximab, long-term overall survival rates over 85% have been consistently reported. These outcomes are better than in other DLBCL types; however, when initial treatment fails, the results of salvage chemotherapy and autologous transplant are poor. Hence, there is a critical need to maximize cure rates with initial therapy (that has led to controversy over type and extent of treatment). In this context, it is important to point out that there is no evidence of a curative role of radiotherapy alone in primary mediastinal B-cell lymphoma.

Similar considerations may be applied to Burkitt and lymphoblastic lymphoma arising in the setting of early pregnancy. Despite historical data, which indicate that supradiaphragmatic radiotherapy can be feasible and safe in pregnancy, there are no data on the safety of newer radiotherapy modalities (such as intensity-modulated radiotherapy and volumetric modulated arc therapy). These techniques aim at delivering high and conformal doses of radiation to the tumor while avoiding irradiation of non-target organs, However, even refined radiation techniques may lead to lower radiation doses to larger volumes of tissue, which may be problematic in pregnancy (Cubillo et al. 2021).

The current evidence for the feasibility and safety of intensity-modulated RT and other modern radiotherapy techniques in pregnant women is very limited, and their potential role remains uncertain, with no data on short- and long-term health effects of fetal exposure (Mazzola et al. 2019). Therefore, these advanced techniques should be used with caution in pregnancy. We believe that radiotherapy in general should be avoided whenever possible in pregnancy or deferred to the postpartum period. Only in very selected cases, it may have a role (e.g. to control localized low-grade lymphoma, when a watch-and-wait approach is not possible).

Case Study continued: AShe decided to undergo immediate medical abortion. She then had five additional courses of DA-EPOCH-R. PET-CT after the end of immunochemotherapy showed a partial metabolic response, with a PET-positive (Deauville score 4) residual lesion (4 × 2 × 2 cm) in the anterior upper mediastinum. She had consolidation involved-field radiotherapy (30 Gy in 2-Gy fractions) followed by a booster dose to the residual lesion (10 Gy in 2-Gy fractions, for a total dose of 40 Gy). At day 100 post radiotherapy a PET-CT showed a complete metabolic response (Deauville score 2). At her last follow-up visit, eight years after the diagnosis, there was no evidence of disease, and no late adverse events were reported.

Answer unclear: This case illustrates the need for shared decision-making with the patient (and her family) following clear communication and discussion of risks and benefits. (see discussion).

Conclusions

While the development of lymphoma in pregnancy is rarely encountered, increasing gestational age, particularly in Western countries, has led to its rising incidence. Its optimal management requires attention to maternal and fetal health, necessitating an experienced multidisciplinary team. Currently, the outcome for patients with gestational lymphoma is excellent. Based on available evidence, standard therapeutic approaches are typically appropriate but individualization of treatment, with consideration of maternal and fetal characteristics is needed. Management of lymphoma not only needs to consider therapy selection but also factors such as optimal and safe staging of disease during pregnancy and lactation needs following delivery of the baby. Among the most difficult challenges in management of these patients are treatment of lymphoma during the first trimester and determining optimal time of delivery in the third trimester. As the lymphoma therapeutic landscape evolves and outcomes improve for patients, it is critical that experience and safety data with new approaches and novel agents in the setting of pregnancy is captured in order to inform on their optimal application to this patient population.

Recommended Readings

Benoit, L., Mir, O., Vialard, F., and Berveiller, P. (2021). Cancer during pregnancy: a review of preclinical and clinical transplacental transfer of anticancer agents. *Cancers (Basel)* 13 (6).

Berends, C., Maggen, C., Lok, C.A.R. et al. (2021). Maternal and neonatal outcome after the use of G-CSF for cancer treatment during pregnancy. *Cancers (Basel)* 13 (6).

Bragnes, Y., Boshuizen, R., de Vries, A., Lexberg, Å., and Østensen, M. (2017). Low level of Rituximab in human breast milk in a patient treated during lactation. *Rheumatology (Oxford)* 56 (6): 1047–1048.

Codacci-Pisanelli, G., Honeywell, R.J., Asselin, N. et al. (2019). Breastfeeding during R-CHOP chemotherapy: please abstain! *Eur J Cancer* 119: 107–111.

Cubillo, A., Morales, S., Goñi, E. et al. (2021). Multidisciplinary consensus on cancer management during pregnancy. *Clinical and Translational Oncology* 23 (6): 1054–1066.

Dunleavy, K. and McLintock, C. (2020). How I treat lymphoma in pregnancy. *Blood* 136 (19): 2118–2124.

Froesch, P., Belisario-Filho, V., and Zucca, E. (2008). Hodgkin and non-Hodgkin lymphomas during pregnancy. *Recent Results Cancer Res* 178: 111–121.

Germann, N., Goffinet, F., and Goldwasser, F. (2004). Anthracyclines during pregnancy: embryo-fetal outcome in 160 patients. *Ann Oncol* 15 (1): 146–150.

Gurevich-Shapiro, A. and Avivi, I. (2019). Current treatment of lymphoma in pregnancy. *Expert Rev Hematol* 12 (6): 449–459.

Horowitz, N.A., Benyamini, N., Wohlfart, K., Brenner, B., and Avivi, I. (2013). Reproductive organ involvement in non-Hodgkin lymphoma during pregnancy: a systematic review. *Lancet Oncol* 14 (7): e275–282.

Hutson, J.R., Eastabrook, G., and Garcia-Bournissen, F. (2022). Pregnancy outcome after early exposure to nivolumab, a PD-1 checkpoint inhibitor for relapsed Hodgkin's lymphoma. *Clin Toxicol* 60 (4): 535–536. Doi: 10.1080/15563650.2021.1981361.

Johnson, P., Federico, M., Kirkwood, A., Fosså, A., Berkahn, L., Carella, A., d'Amore, F., Enblad, G., Franceschetto, A., Fulham, M., Luminari, S., O'Doherty, M., Patrick, P., Roberts, T., Sidra, G., Stevens, L., Smith, P., Trotman, J., Viney, Z., Radford, J., Barrington, S. (2016 June 23). Adapted treatment guided by interim PET-CT scan in advanced Hodgkin's lymphoma. *J N Engl J Med* 374 (25): 2419–2429. doi: 10.1056/NEJMoa1510093.PMID: 27332902.

Köhler, C., Oppelt, P., Favero, G. et al. (2015). How much platinum passes the placental barrier? Analysis of platinum applications in 21 patients with cervical cancer during pregnancy. *Am J Obstet Gynecol* 213 (2): 206.e201–205.

Luttwak, E., Gurevich-Shapiro, A., Azem, F. et al. (2021). Novel agents for the treatment of lymphomas during pregnancy: a comprehensive literature review. *Blood Rev* 49: 100831.

Maggen, C., Dierickx, D., Lugtenburg, P. et al. (2019). Obstetric and maternal outcomes in patients diagnosed with Hodgkin lymphoma during pregnancy: a multicentre, retrospective, cohort study. *Lancet Haematol* 6 (11): e551–e561.

Mir, O., Berrada, N., Domont, J. et al. (2012). Doxorubicin and ifosfamide for high-grade sarcoma during pregnancy. *Cancer Chemother Pharmacol* 69 (2): 357–367.

Peccatori, F.A., Azim, H.A., Jr., Orecchia, R. et al. (2013). Cancer, pregnancy and fertility: ESMO clinical practice guidelines for diagnosis, treatment and follow-up. *Ann Oncol* 24 (Suppl 6): vi160–170.

Woitek, R., Prayer, D., Hojreh, A., and Helbich, T. (2016). Radiological staging in pregnant patients with cancer. *ESMO Open* 1 (1): e000017.

59

Complications and Management of CAR T Cell Therapy

Radowan A. Elnair and Matthew A. Lunning

Division of Hematology/Oncology at the University of Nebraska Medical Center, Omaha, Nebraska, USA

Introduction

Treatment with CAR T cell therapy can be associated with significant risks, ranging from less serious infusion reactions to potentially life-threatening complications such as cytokin release syndrome (CRS) and neurotoxicity. Those risks are a reason why the FDA requires a Risk Evaluation and Mitigation Strategy (REMS) program to mitigate the risks associated with such therapy and to ensure that centers where patients are treated have the knowledge and capability to manage these and other potentially life-threatening complications and have readily available access to lifesaving interventions such as tocilizumab.

With the landscape of CAR T cell therapy changing quickly, our understanding of the potential risks and complications associated with this modality of therapy will continue to evolve. Many limitations exist in the current approach for treatment of those complications, as many of the currently adopted interventions and preventive/prophylactic approaches are not based on high-level evidence, but institutaional approaches.

The risk for each of those complications is dependent on factors that can be divided into three categories:

1) CAR T product–related factors (e.g. CAR T cells construct, costimulatory domain, CAR T cell dose and expansion kinetics, lymphodepleting chemotherapy regimen).
2) Patient-related factors (e.g. age, performance status, underlying comorbidities, concurrent infection).
3) Disease-related factors (e.g. malignancy being treated, previous lines of therapy, disease volume/burden).

It is thus difficult to design a one-size-fits-all approach for managing those complications given the multitude of available CAR T cell products on the market and even logrithmically more in the development pipeline.

Given all the above factors, we will focus herein on the recognition of these complications and the approach to managing each of those in our practice, primarily in the context of the currently FDA approved CAR T cell products (idecabtagene vicleucel, lisocabtagene maraleucel, brexucabtagene autoleucel, tisagenlecleucel, and axicabtagene ciloleucel).

Cancer Consult: Expertise in Clinical Practice, Volume 2: Neoplastic Hematology & Cellular Therapy,
Second Edition. Edited by Syed A. Abutalib, Maurie Markman, James O. Armitage, and Kenneth C. Anderson.
© 2024 John Wiley & Sons Ltd. Published 2024 by John Wiley & Sons Ltd.

Case Study 1

Mr. E is a pleasant 56-year-old male who is seen is in consultation for consideration of treatment with CAR T cell therapy per the standard of care for relapsed diffuse large B-cell lymphoma. He was initially diagnosed with stage IV disease three years ago with an IPI of 3, with a point each for stage, elevated LDH, and number of extra-nodal sites of disease. At that time, he was treated with six cycles of R-CHOP and achieved a complete response and had been followed expectantly since then. He recently presented to his local oncologist with new B-symptoms with PET-CT imaging showing diffuse nodal FDG uptake in the chest, axilla, and retroperitoneum along with several bony lesions. He felt to be a autologous transplant candidate and was started on second-line chemotherapy with R-ICE, but a restaging PET-CT after two cycles was consistent with a Deauville score of 5 (refractory disease).

His past medical history is notable for hypertension, coronary artery disease, and type II DM, which were all controlled on oral agents. He works as a long-distance truck driver. Mr. E is now being considered for treatment with a CD19 CAR T cell product depending on insurance approval.

1) **What should he be counseled about regarding the CAR T cell infusion process and the earliest complications that may be seen?**
    A) **Infusion reactions**

      Expert Perspective: Infusion reactions seen with CAR T cell therapy range from upper digestive symptoms such as nausea and vomiting, hypotension, and even more severe infusion reaction such as anaphylaxis. Those reactions can be attributed to the premedications used, the DMSO cryo-preservative, or potentially to some of the other residual compounds in the product such as gentamicin or dextran. Most of the currently available commercial CAR T cell products recommend premedication with paracetamol/acetaminophen and diphenhydramine. The prophylactic use of steroids is not generally recommended at this point as it may interfere with the activity and expansion of CAR T cells. Fortunately, infusion reactions are infrequent and when seen are generally of mild degree.

    B) **Tumor lysis syndrome (TLS)**

      Expert Perspective: Although rare, TLS has been observed in patients treated with CAR T cell therapy. The reported incidence in the DLBCL populations is estimated at 1% and is slightly higher in the pre-B ALL population at 6%. Nonetheless, TLS prophylaxis in patients with an elevated uric acid and those with significant disease burden was used in the registrational trials for CAR T cell products and remains a standard of care in our opinion in that population given the low risk of toxicity seen with prophylaxis and the potential for further complications if TLS were to develop. When seen in this population, the standard treatment for TLS is employed (often a cominbination of IV fluids resuscitation, allopurinol, or a non-allopurinol alternative such as febuxostat, and rasburicase in severe cases).

Cytokine release syndrome (CRS)

Case Study continued: After a long discussion about the risks and benefits, he consents to treatment with axicabtagene ciloleucel (axi-cel). He received lymphodepleting chemotherapy with cyclophosphamide and fludarabine, followed by infusion of the CAR T cell product. On the second day, he developed a fever of 39.7°C with mild hypotension, which responded to IV fluid resuscitation. He additionally developed new oxygen needs (2L via nasal canula).

2) What are the best next steps to pursue?

Expert Perspective: CRS is a well-known consequence described with CAR T cell therapy. The definition has evolved through the years. The incidence of CRS varies among studies and reports and has been estimated to be anywhere between 30% and 90% (depending on product, patient, and disease-related factors). Symptoms of CRS usually develop within the first week after infusion, butcan occur as early as few hours after CAR T cells infusion.

The first system used to grade CRS was the Lee criteria developed by a group of pediatric oncologists. Earlier studies used varying methods to define and grade CRS, but rigorous efforts have been made to standardize the definition, grading, and reporting of CRS in clinical studies and in real-life practice, culminating in the ASTCT consensus grading for CRS (and ICANS). Table 59.1 summarizes some of the published CRS grading systems.

The ASTCT consensus guidelines defines CRS as a supraphysiologic response that may include symptoms of hypotension, hypoxia, and end organ dysfunction (Table 59.2). The definition requires the presence of fever at the onset. The development of fever in those patients should sound the alarm for consideration of CRS but also note that infection in this vulnerable population, in which cytopenias, prior chemotherapy, presence of lines/catheters, and frequent hospitalization all raise this risk. Indeed, many of the symptoms of CRS can be confused with an infection. Workup with blood cultures, imaging (CXR, CT as indicated, etc.), and evaluation as indicated by the clinical scenario should be pursued and empiric antimicrobial treatment should be promptly started.

As previously stated; the risk for CRS is variable, and some of the factors that have been described to influence this risk include tumor burden, CAR T cells dose, CAR T cell construct, and concurrent infectious illness. Peak levels of CAR T cells, along with levels of inflammatory markers and cytokines (CRP, ferritin, IL-6) correlate with the development of CRS. Table 59.3 highlights the reported incidence of CRS and ICANS in the landmark CAR T cell trials.

In line with its role in the pathogenesis of CRS, blockage of IL-6 with tocilizumab (a monoclonal antibody against IL-6 receptor) has been adopted as the mainstay treatment for CRS. This agent appears to not affect the antitumor effect of CAR T cells, and durable remissions have been seen in patients who were treated with tocilizumab for CRS with response rates comparable to those who were not. It has also been demonstrated that the use of tocilizumab does not impair expansion of CAR T cells in peripheral blood and bone marrow.

Tocilizumab received FDA approval for this indication in adults and pediatric patients two years of age and older at the time of the approval of the first CAR T product, tisagenlecleucel,

Table 59.1 Previous CRS grading systems.

Grading system	Grade 1	Grade 2	Grade 3	Grade 4
Lee criteria	Symptoms are not life-threatening and require symptomatic treatment only (e.g. fever, nausea, fatigue, headache, myalgias, malaise)	Symptoms require and respond to moderate intervention: oxygen requirement < 40% FiO2, or hypotension responsive to IV fluids or low dose of one vasopressor, or grade 2 organ toxicity (per CTCAE 4.03)	Symptoms require and respond to aggressive intervention: oxygen requirement ≥ 40% FiO2, or hypotension requiring high dose or multiple vasopressors, or grade 3 organ toxicity, or Grade 4 transaminitis	Life-threatening symptoms: requirement for ventilator support, or grade 4 organ toxicity (excluding transaminitis)
Penn criteria	Mild reaction: treated with supportive care such as antipyretic, antiemetics	Moderate reaction: some signs of organ dysfunction (grade 2 creatinine or grade 3 LFTs) related to CRS and not attributable to any other condition Hospitalization for management of CRS-related symptoms (not including fluid resuscitation for hypotension)	More severe reaction: hospitalization required for management of symptoms related to organ dysfunction, including grade 4 LFTs or grade 3 creatinine, related to CRS and not attributable to any other condition hypotension treated with multiple fluid boluses or low-dose vasopressors coagulopathy requiring FFP, cryo or fibrinogen concentrate hypoxia requiring supplemental oxygen (nasal canula, high flow oxygen, CPAP, or BIPAP)	Life-threatening complications such as hypotension requiring high-dose vasopressors hypoxia requiring mechanical ventilation

Table 59.2 ASTCT CRS Consensus Grading.

Parameter	Grade 1	Grade 2	Grade 3	Grade 4
Fever	Temp ≥ 38°C	Temp ≥ 38°C With	Temp ≥ 38°C With	Temp ≥ 38°C With
Hypotension	None	Not requiring vasopressin and/or	Requiring a vasopressor ± vasopressin and/or	Requiring multiple vasopressors (excluding vasopressin) and/or
Hypoxia	None	Requiring low flow nasal cannula (≤ 6L/ minute) or blow by	Requiring high flow nasal cannula, facemask, non-rebreather or venturi	Requiring positive pressure (e.g. CPAP, BIPAP, mechanical ventilation)

Table 59.3 Reported incidence of CRS and neurotoxicity in landmark CAR T cell trials.

Trial	ZUMA-1 (Axi-cel) Neelapu et al., *NEJM* 2017	JULIET (Tisa-Cel) Schuster et al., *NEJM* 2019	TRANSCEND (Liso-cel) Abramson et al., *The Lancet* 2020	ZUMA-2 (Brexu-cel) Wang et al., *NEJM* 2020	KarMMa (Ide-Cel) Munshi et al., *NEJM* 2021
Population studied	R/R Large B-cell lymphoma	R/R Large B-cell lymphoma	R/R Large B-cell lymphoma	Mantle cell lymphoma	R/R Multiple Myeloma
CRS of any grade	93% (13% grade ≥ 3) Lee criteria	58% (22% grade ≥ 3) Penn criteria	47% (2% ≥ grade 3) Lee criteria	91% (15% ≥ grade 3) Lee criteria	84% (5% ≥ grade 3) Lee criteria
Neurological toxicity	64% (28% grade ≥ 3)	21% (12% grade ≥ 3)	30% (10% grade ≥ 3)	63% (31% grade ≥ 3)	18% (3% grade ≥ 3)

for pediatric and young adult patients with relapsed/refractory B-cell precursor ALL. The approved dose is 8 mg/kg for patients with weight > 30 kg with a maximum of 800 mg per dose and can be repeated with doses being separated by at least eight hours.

The optimal timing for the use of tocilizumab is an area of ongoing research with earlier reports suggesting no decremental effect on CAR T efficacy. A safety expansion cohort of the ZUMA-1 trial of axi-cel in relapsed/refractory aggressive NHL suggested a beneficial effect in reducing the incidence of severe CRS but not neurologic events. Other reports have suggested worsened ICANS with the use of prophylactic tocilizumab though the data in this space is conflicting. The pathophysiology for potentially worsened ICANS has been attributed to tocilizumab's poor penetration of the blood-brain barrier and utilization may lead to higher CSF levels of IL-6, one of the primary mediators of neurotoxicity, occurring from tocilizumab's competition with IL-6 for the IL-6R. On the other hand, siliturimab—a chimeric monoclonal IL-6 antibody that binds directly to IL-6—is unlikely to have this effect. Siltuximab is now being studied in prospective clinical trials. However, prospective trials comparing the two agents are lacking, and toclilizumab remains the agent most commonly used in practice at this time.

Given all of the above; the use of prophylactic tocilizumab was adopted by some centers but is not yet accepted as an agreed-upon standard of care, and the role of tocilizumab in prophylaxis and whether to add single dose corticosteroids in the early grade CRS management of CRS is likely to evolve in the future.

Corticosteroids are generally added for treatment of those patients who do not demonstrate a rapid response to tocilizumab. Almost half the patients treated in early CAR T cell trials required management in the intensive care unit. This rate, however, has steadily declined with better understanding and more experience in management of CRS, and requirement for ICU level of care is now the exception rather than the norm in experienced centers. Most recently, FDA approved an update to the prescribing information for axicabtagene ciloleucel to include use of prophylactic corticosteroids across all approved indications.

In patients who are refractory to tocilizumab and corticosteroids, no standard approach exists as to the best next step. Some of the agents used in this space include anakinra (IL-1 antagonist), the etanercept (TNF-α blocker), siltuximab (IL-6 blocker), or ATG.

Immune effector cell-associated neurotoxicity syndrome (ICANS)

Case Study continued: On day four, the nursing staff notes intermittent confusion. Mr. E is found to be alert and oriented to time and person but not to place. He had no focal neurological deficits on motor and sensory exam but has clear difficulty in naming objects. His family was in the room and were worried that he may be having a stroke.

3) What would be the best approach, and what's the extent of workup that should be pursued?

Expert Perspective: The development of neurological symptoms after CAR T cell therapy can be seen within the first few days. Those symptoms are encompassed in the term "immune effector cell–associated neurotoxicity syndrome" (ICANS), reflecting that the syndrome can also be seen with other T-cell engaging therapies such as blinatumomab.

Akin to CRS, higher cell dose and increased peak CAR T cell expansion is also associated with an increased ICANS incidence. The pathogenesis of the syndrome is not fully understood but is thought to be related to blood-brain barrier disruption and a CNS inflammatory phenomenon that follows. Early onset and severe degree of CRS along with high levels of inflammatory cytokines have also been shown to be associated with increased risk for ICANS. There has also been a correlation demonstrated for higher-grade CRS with higher grade of ICANS, though there are exceptions where severe cases of ICANS have developed in patients with milder degrees or no lead-in CRS. An ongoing rise in inflammatory markers can be a helpful hint of a higher risk for development of either condition but may lag behind clinical symptoms.

The clinical spectrum of ICANS can range from subtle symptoms such as language dysfunction, dysgraphia, and fine tremors, to profound encephalopathy with confusion, visual/auditory hallucinations, cerebral edema, coma, or even death.

Early recognition of the syndrome depends mostly on high clinical vigilance especially in patients at higher risk, with frequent screening for symptoms such as orientation and dysgraphia. Building on prior effort of the CARTOX consensus group, the ASTCT developed an updated encephalopathy screening tool, the Immune Effector Cell-Associated Encephalopathy (ICE) score (Table 59.4).

Table 59.4 ICE (Immune Effector Cell Encephalopathy) Score.

Assessment	Points
Orientation: orientation to year, month, city, hospital	4 points
Naming: name 3 objects (e.g. point to clock, pen, button)	3 points
Following commands: e.g. show me 2 fingers, close your eyes and stick out your tongue	1 point
Writing: Ability to write a standard sentence (e.g. our national bird is the bald eagle)	1 point
Attention: Count backward from 100 by 10	1 point

The scoring system has the potential of 10 points and assesses several domains; however, the grading of ICANS requires the additional incorporation of other variables such as consciousness, motor symptoms, seizures, and signs or symptoms of cerebral edema, and those can occur independent of the presence of encephalopathy (Table 59.5).

Brain imaging and EEG: In the vast majority of patients who develop ICANS, brain imaging with CT or MRI is unrevealing. Nevertheless, findings of white matter changes and diffuse cerebral edema can be seen in patients with severe degrees of ICANS. Routine brain imaging is thus not routinely recommended in milder degrees of ICANS and should be reserved for the appropriate clinical context, such as patients who have focal symptoms or those with severe ICANS. Obtaining an EEG to rule out any seizure-like activity in those cases is prudent, as this can be subtle. The most commonly noted pattern on EEG is diffuse slowing, which is a nonspecific indicator of encephalopathy and commonly seen in critically ill patients.

Table 59.5 ASTCT ICANS Score.

Neurotoxicity Domain	Grade 1	Grade 2	Grade 3	Grade 4
ICE Score	7–9	3–6	0–2	0 (patient is unarousable and unable to perform ICE)
Depressed level of consciousness	Awakens spontaneously	Awakens to voice	Awakens only to tactile stimulus	Patient is unarousable or requires vigorous or repetitive tactile stimuli to arouse. Stupor or coma
Seizure	N/A	N/A	Any clinical seizure focal or generalized that resolves rapidly or nonconvulsive seizures on EEG that resolve with intervention	Life-threatening prolonged seizure (> 5 minutes) Or Repetitive clinical or electrical seizures without return to baseline in between
Motor findings	N/A	N/A	N/A	Deep focal motor weakness such as hemiparesis or paraparesis
Elevated ICP/ Cerebral edema	N/A	N/A	Focal/local edema on neuroimaging	Diffuse cerebral edema on neuroimaging, or decerebrate or decorticate posturing, or cranial nerve IV palsy, or papilledema, or Cushing's triad

Steroids and antiseizure medications: The mainstay for treatment of ICANS is with glucocorticoids, antiseizure medications, and supportive care measures. The ideal use of glucocorticoids in this setting is an ongoing area of research, given concern about the potential for steroids to limit the expansion and efficacy of CAR T cells. The generally recommended dose and frequency is dependent on the grade of toxicity. With improvement, the steroids can be tapered quickly. Those who experience a slower response or who have worsening symptoms on tapering steroids may be considered for a slower taper.

Lumbar puncture: Patients who fail to improve quickly within a day or two should be considered for lumbar puncture and CSF sampling to rule out other etiologies. Brain imaging in this setting should be strongly considered as many of these patients will require transfer to an intensive care unit and more supportive measures (e.g. vasopressors for BP support with concurrent severe CRS, mechanical ventilation for depressed consciousness) where obtaining brain imaging is likely more challenging at least from a logistics standpoint. It is important to realize that the findings on CSF specimen in ICANS are nonspecific. The CSF protein is typically abnormal with median levels of 80–110. CAR T cells have been detected in CSF of all patients with ICANS in a pediatric study of CD19 CAR T cells for ALL. However, the incidence of finding CAR T cells in patients without ICANS was as high as 90%, limiting the utility of such assessment, which is not readily available for routine clinical practice.

Other approaches: While efficacious in the prevention and treatment of CRS, tocilizumab has little efficacy in ICANS, which has been attributed at least in part to its inability to cross the blood-brain barrier.

In patients who have refractory neurotoxicity, no standard approach is available. Some of the agents used based on case reports and case series include intrathecal chemotherapy (methotrexate, cytarabine, hydrocortisone), rabbit ATG, siltuximab, and anakinra.

Aggressive supportive care with use of mannitol, hypertonic saline, and consideration of extra ventricular drain placement should all be considered in patients with severe neurotoxicity and radiographic evidence of cerebral edema. Close management with an experienced multidisciplinary team that includes ICU, neurology, and neurosurgery is of great importance.

Cardiotoxicity

4) How would you factor Mr. E's previous cardiac history into the risk/benefit balance of treatment with CAR T cell therapy?

Expert Perspective: Some of the adverse cardiovascular events reported with CAR T cell therapy include arrhythmias, elevated serum troponin levels, new onset heart failure, or death. The most prominent of those is profound hypotension requiring vasopressors support, as can be seen with CRS. The pathophysiology can be attributed to a similar mechanism to that seen in cardiomyopathy associated with sepsis due to the inflammatory cytokines surge, or due to autoimmunity with off-target activity against some cardiac muscle proteins. In one registry study, a higher-grade CRS (Grade ⩾ 3) was associated with a five-fold higher rate of major adverse cardiac events, highlighting the relationship between the pathophysiology of CRS and cardiovascular toxicity. Cardiomyopathy with a drop in ejection fraction of more than 10% from baseline to less than 50% has also been reported.

A multidisciplinary approach in managing and counseling these patients prior to CAR T cell therapy is essential in predicting and preventing such complications. It is recommended to obtain a transthoracic echocardiographic as part of the workup pre-CAR T cell therapy infusion. Those found to have abnormal testing should ideally be referred to a cardio-oncology team to be optimized as best as possible before infusion of CAR T cells.

Consultation with a cardiologist and further workup of cardiac dysfunction should be sought in patients with higher grades of CRS who experience refractory hypotension despite adequate fluid resuscitation, tocilizumab, and vasopressor support. Patients in the midst of CRS are at a higher risk of fluid overload and fluid third spacing, and clinicians should be vigilant for an inherently higher risk of heart failure exacerbation in those with a known cardiomyopathy.

Infections

5) What are the generally accepted prophylactic antimicrobial agents used following CAR T cell therapy, and what is the ideal duration for use of those regimens?

Expert Perspective: Some of the infections reported in recipients of CAR T cell therapy include C. difficile, catheter-associated infections, cellulitis, meningitis, mucormycosis, aspergillosis, and urinary tract infections. Upper respiratory tract infections and bloodstream infections are among the commonly seen events, while reactivation of CMV, EBV, or HHV-6 are rare occurrences but have been reported.

High-level data for infectious prophylaxis and monitoring (such as CMV monitoring) are lacking and are an area of unmet need. Therefore, most of the current practice in the field is based on institutional guidelines.

Before the administration of CAR T cell therapy, screening for HIV and viral hepatitis (HBV and HCV) is recommended. There is no standard of care for testing and monitoring CMV, EBV, or HHV-6 given the rarity of such reactivation events, although it should be considered in the right clinical scenario, such as patients with a prior history of CMV or EBV viremia or reactivation events with prior lines of therapy.

The use of tocilizumab and steroids in management of CRS and ICANS both contribute to a higher risk of infection. We recommend that patients be on fluoroquinolone prophylaxis (or alternative antibiotics for neutropenic prophylaxis) while neutropenic, and the use of acyclovir and PCP prophylaxis is generally recommended for at least six months after CAR T cell therapy infusion. While some clinicians advocate for incorporating measuring CD4+ T cells priort to the time of discontinuation of the latter two agents (with ideally CD4+ count of > 200), we generally consider assessment of the CD4+ T cells count when theabsolute lymphocyte count is > 500. In those with prolonged neutropenia, antifungal prophylaxis should be started, keeping in mind local patterns of resistance and incidence of invasive mold infections. We additionally consider antifungal prophylaxis with anti-mold activity in those expected to need high-dose steroids for more than two weeks, heavily pretreated patients (four or more prior lines of therapy), and those with prior history of an invasive fungal infection.

The SARS-CoV-2 infection (declared a pandemic in March 2020) continues as of this writing to be an active issue with several ramifications affecting not only access to CAR T cell therapy but also adding to the complexity of caring for patients post CAR T cell therapy given the higher risk of severe disease and mortality with the immune dysregulation seen with this therapy. As an example, a study by the European Society for Blood and Marrow Transplantation (EBMT) Infectious Diseases Working Party and the European Hematology Association (EHA) Lymphoma Group of COVID-19 infection in patients treated with CAR T cell therapy for B-cell malignancies reported a COVID-19 attributed mortality of 41%. We thus recommend SARS-CoV-2 vaccination for all patients post CAR T cell therapy (as detailed below), and strongly consider treatment with monoclonal antibodies (e.g. sotrovimab) for those who are diagnosed with COVID-19 even with mild disease and regardless of the number of days post CAR T cell therapy their diagnosis was made.

The FDA in December 2021 granted emergency use authorization (EUA) for ctixagevimab co-packaged with cilgavimab (Evusheld)—a combination of two monoclonal antibodies—for the pre-exposure prophylaxis of COVID-19 in patients aged 12 years of age and older with moderate to severely compromised immune systems or those in whom vaccination is not recommended due to a history of an adverse reaction to a COVID-19 vaccine or a component of those vaccines, with one dose administered as two separate consecutive intramuscular injections potentially providing protection for six months. We know consistently provide Evushled to post CAR T cell therapy patients every 6 months as access allows

Cytopenias

6) How do you manage cytopenias in the post-CAR T cell setting? And what is the extent of the workup that should be pursued?

Expert Perspective: While hematologic toxicity is a common occurrence in this patient population, prolonged grade 3–4 cytopenias persisting up until two years from CAR T cell infusion has been reported in about 10% of patients based on retrospective series, and opportunistic infections such as herpes zoster and PJP pneumonia have been reported in this population, highlighting the importance of prolonged antimicrobial prophylaxis in those patients. Development of myelodysplastic syndrome (MDS) in those with prolonged cytopenia should be suspected, as many of those patients had been exposed to many lines of therapy and a number of agents that carry a risk for development of secondary hematologic malignancies. We generally provide supportive transfusions per institutional guidelines and would routinely consider G-CSF in those with persistent grade 4 neutropenia beyond 30 days. We consider the use of ESA and TPO on a case-by-case basis.

As a majority of patients experience hematologic recovery by 90 days, we consider a bone marrow biopsy in those with prolonged cytopenias beyond that timeline, those with consistent immature forms on CBC differential, lack of response to myeloid growth factors, and inappropriately low reticulocyte count. Peripheral smear evaluation should be pursued in each of these situations, if not already done. (Figure 59.1)

Hypogammaglobulinemia

7) How do you manage hypogammaglobulinemia following CAR T cell therapy?

Expert Perspective: The frequency of monitoring and replacement of immunoglobulins after CAR T cell therapy is a dilemma commonly encountered in practice. However, there remains no high-level evidence to guide IVIG replacement specifically in this population.

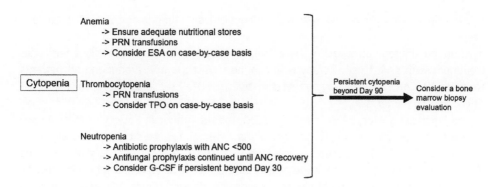

Figure 59.1 Approach to cytopenias following CAR T Cell therapy.

The use of IVIG is associated with significant cost and often on supply shortage, which may pose a significant challenge, and thus a thoughtful discussion about risks and benefits is vital while awaiting higher-level evidence.

Reduced immunoglobulin levels can develop a few weeks after CAR T cell therapy infusion and can last for months to years. Extrapolation of data from other contexts (such as CLL-related hypogammaglobulinemia) suggests that prophylactic IgG replacement may reduce rates of serious bacterial infections. Nonetheless, the notion that such a benefit will translate in the context of CAR T cell patients is yet to be proven.

It is perceived that the level at which the risk of recurrent infections appears to be increased is an IgG level of < 400 mg/dL, and this is the level at which we consider a discussion with patients about risks and benefits of immunoglobulin replacement when they're asymptomatic. We recommend replacement in those with a level of < 500 mg/dL with recurrent sinopulmonary infections and/or a history of an infection requiring hospitalization or IV antibiotic therapy with adjustment of the dosing and frequency of administration to maintain a nadir IgG level of 500 mg/dL.

Immunizations

8) When is it safe for Mr. E to consider the seasonal flu, SARS-CoV-2 vaccination, and other routine vaccinations?

Expert Perspective: Recommendations for vaccination following CAR T cell therapy have generally been based on the expected kinetics of immune reconstitution following CAR T cell infusion, the type of vaccine in question (killed/inactivated vs live vaccine, mRNA based), and in light of studies of vaccine responses in other immunocompromised populations (post autologous/allogeneic stem cell transplant, post anti-CD 20 monoclonal antibodies, etc.).

The optimal timing for vaccination following CAR T cell therapy is complicated by the negative compounding factors such as hypogammaglobulinemia, persistent cytopenias, type of lymphodepleting chemotherapy, and the response of the underlying malignancy.

We generally recommend that killed/inactivated vaccines be considered only after at least six months of CAR T cell therapy, while live vaccines (e.g. MMR) not be administered for at least 12 months, with assessment of Ab titers for seroconversion and sero-protection in a multidisciplinary approach with our colleagues from immunology and infectious diseases.

Although limited retrospective data suggest that the loss of protective titers after treatment with CAR T cell therapy is uncommon, we currently recommend all patients treated with CAR T cell therapy be revaccinated with DTaP, seasonal influenza, and hep B (if considered higher risk).

The American Society of Hematology (ASH) and the American Society of Transplantation and Cellular Therapy (ASTCT) strongly supported early access to mRNA SARS-CoV-2 vaccination for CAR T cell therapy recipients, and this can be offered as early as three months from therapy with the hope of preventing severe disease and mortality despite some potential of a suboptimal vaccine response with such timing. No preference for a vaccine formulation is recommended at this time, and readers are encouraged to continue following ASH/ASTCT guidance, which is likely to be updated as more data becomes available. Additionally, we recommend SARS-CoV-2 revaccination or variant boosters following CAR T therapy for those previously vaccinated pre-CAR T cell therapy (as recommended by ASTCT and CIBMTR).

Conclusion

CAR T cell therapy is a rapidly evolving field, and as more products get approved and used, our knowledge and understanding of how to best approach the complications that can arise post therapy will similarly evolve, though it's inevitable that some delay will be seen. The experience of seeing CAR T cell therapy evolve strongly highlights the need for a team-based approach in caring for these patients. Our institution has established a working group that is tasked with regularly updating the institutional guidelines for caring for CAR T cell therapy patients, including the recommended length of stay, antimicrobial prophylaxis, and approach to treating CRS and ICANS. The group includes physicians and advanced practice providers who care for CAR T cell therapy patients along with pharmacists and infectious disease specialists, and we work closely with a cardio-oncologists and our colleagues from neurology when caring for patients with severe CRS and/or ICANS. As is the case in caring for any cancer patient, a team-based group approach is the key. However, the pace at which the data in all aspects of CAR T cell therapy is evolving and the complexity of care patients in this setting require a dynamic yet systemic approach to providing high-quality care in a multidisciplinary approach for a population that is oftentimes faced with a disease having progressed on many lines of therapy and in need of timely access to care.

Recommended Readings

Frey, N., and Porter, D. (2019). Cytokine release syndrome with chimeric antigen receptor T cell therapy. *Biol Blood Marrow Transplant* 25 (4): e123–e127.

Gutierrez C, Neilan TG, Grover NS. How I approach optimization of patients at risk of cardiac and pulmonary complications after CAR T-cell therapy. *Blood* 2023 May 18;141(20):2452–2459. doi: 10.1182/blood.2022017579. PMID: 36827628; PMCID: PMC10329189.

Lee, D.W., Santomasso, B.D., Locke, F.L. et al. (2019). ASTCT consensus grading for cytokine release syndrome and neurologic toxicity associated with immune effector cells. *Biol Blood Marrow Transplant* 25 (4): 625–638.

Ludwig, H., Terpos, E., van de Donk, N. et al. (2023 June). Prevention and management of adverse events during treatment with bispecific antibodies and CAR T cells in multiple myeloma: a consensus report of the European Myeloma Network. *Lancet Oncol* 24 (6): e255–e269. doi: 10.1016/S1470-2045(23)00159-6. PMID: 37269857.

Morris, E.C., Neelapu, S.S., Giavridis, T. et al. (2021). Cytokine release syndrome and associated neurotoxicity in cancer immunotherapy. *Nat Rev Immunol*.

Santomasso, B.D., Gust, J., and Perna, F. (2023 May 18). How I treat unique and difficult-to-manage cases of CAR T-cell therapy-associated neurotoxicity. *Blood* 141 (20): 2443–2451. doi: 10.1182/blood.2022017604. PMID: 36877916; PMCID: PMC10329188.

Spanjaart, A.M., Ljungman, P., de La Camara, R. et al. (2021). Poor outcome of patients with COVID-19 after CAR T-cell therapy for B-cell malignancies: results of a multicenter study on behalf of the European Society for Blood and Marrow Transplantation (EBMT) Infectious Diseases Working Party and the European Hematology Association (EHA) Lymphoma Group. *Leukemia* 35: 3585–3588.

Teachey, D.T., Lacey, S.F., Shaw, P.A. et al. (2016). Identification of predictive biomarkers for cytokine release syndrome after chimeric antigen receptor T-cell therapy for acute lymphoblastic leukemia. *Cancer Discov* 6 (6): 664–679.

60

Acute Graft-versus-Host Disease

Aaron Etra, Uroosa Ibrahim, Jacques Azzi, and John E. Levine

Tisch Cancer Institute, Icahn School of Medicine at Mount Sinai, New York, NY, USA

Introduction

Acute GvHD (aGvHD) is seen after allogeneic hematopoietic cell transplantation (allo-HCT) and the incidence of aGvHD is between 40% and 60% depending on numerous factors. This transplant complication typically occurs between the time of engraftment through 100 days after transplant, with few cases occurring later, and can have devastating consequences on the skin, gastrointestinal tract, and liver. Chronic GvHD typically occurs after 100 days, although this temporal distinction is blurring with strategies such as reduced-intensity conditioning. Overlap syndrome refers to GvHD that shares features of both aGvHD and cGvHD. Initial therapy for aGvHD is steroids. Prognosis is poor in aGvHD patients not responding to steroids, particularly if gastrointestinal tract involvement is present. Efforts to prevent this complication with careful HLA matching, donor selection, and prophylactic immunosuppression are not always successful. As such, aGvHD prevention and treatment remain an area of intense active research. In the following chapter, we will discuss risk factors for developing aGvHD, the pathogenesis of this condition, methods of minimizing risk, and treatment strategies.

You are consulting on a 54-year-old man for consideration of allogeneic hematopoietic cell transplantation (allo-HCT) as therapy for high-risk acute myeloid leukemia. He asks how you plan to collect stem cells for his transplant and how that may affect his risk for post-transplant complications. He has read about graft-versus-host disease (GvHD) and is particularly fearful of this transplant complication.

1) Which of the following statements about acute GvHD is correct?
   A) Peripheral blood stem cell grafts causes higher rates of acute GvHD when compared to marrow grafts.
   B) BMT CTN 0201 trial demonstrated no difference in grade II–IV acute GvHD between marrow and peripheral blood stem cell grafts from unrelated donors.
   C) Clinically significant acute GvHD (grade II–IV) usually occurs in as many as 90% of related HLA-haploidentical transplants.
   D) Umbilical cord blood grafts are associated with an increased risk for acute GvHD when compared to haploidentical peripheral blood grafts.

Cancer Consult: Expertise in Clinical Practice, Volume 2: Neoplastic Hematology & Cellular Therapy,
Second Edition. Edited by Syed A. Abutalib, Maurie Markman, James O. Armitage, and Kenneth C. Anderson.
© 2024 John Wiley & Sons Ltd. Published 2024 by John Wiley & Sons Ltd.

Expert Perspective: Although some initial studies suggested that PBSC grafts imparted greater risk for aGvHD, larger randomized studies have shown no difference between bone marrow and peripheral blood grafts with rates of aGvHD. The incidence is usually lower using HLA-identical sibling donors. Following are highlights of major studies comparing marrow to PBSC grafts,

- The randomized BMT CTN 0201 clinical trial (Anasetti et al. 2012) showed that HLA-matched unrelated bone marrow recipients were more likely to experience graft failure (9% vs 3%; $P = 0.002$), less likely to develop chronic GvHD (41% vs 53%; $P = 0.01$), and have no significant differences in grade II–IV acute GvHD compared to PBSC recipients (46% vs 47%, $P = 0.87$). The two-year incidence of relapse (approximately 25%) and rates of overall survival (approximately 50–55%) were comparable between graft sources.
- A meta-analysis by Holtick et al. (2014) of nine randomized trials published between 1999 and 2012 confirmed that recipients of peripheral blood stem cell transplants were not more likely to develop acute GvHD grade II–IV than recipients of bone marrow (hazard ratio 1.03; 95% CI 0.89–1.21; $P = 0.67$) or grade III–IV (HR 0.75; 95% CI 0.55–1.02; $P = 0.07$).

Haploidentical transplants: Bone marrow and peripheral blood transplants with multiple HLA mismatches conferred too great a risk of aGvHD to be widely used until recent advances in GvHD prophylaxis such as post-transplant cyclophosphamide and αβ-T cell depletion. Most recent reports, albeit retrospective, have shown that HLA-haploidentical related donors using one of these GvHD prevention strategies result in similar rates of GvHD, relapse, and overall survival as transplants from related or unrelated donors. As a result, haploidentical donors have largely replaced cord blood donors. Unrelated donor transplants require additional expense and logistical complexity compared to related donors. Haploidentical donors may become the preferred donor source following HLA-identical sibling donors if randomized studies show equivalent outcomes between haploidentical related and unrelated donor transplants.

Umbilical cord blood offers a potential graft source for patients who do not have suitably matched donors. Transplants using single umbilical cord blood units, even with multiple HLA mismatches, confer decreased risk for GvHD when compared to marrow or PBSC grafts (HR 0.49–0.59) (Eapen et al. 2010). The decreased absolute number of T cells and the predominance of naive T-cells in the graft may explain why cord blood grafts are more tolerant of HLA disparity than marrow or PBSC grafts; this may also explain the delayed count recovery and increased infectious complications observed after cord blood transplantation. The cell dose available from a single cord blood unit is often insufficient for adult patients; the minimum acceptable pre-cryopreservation cell dose is 2.5×10^7 TNC/kg, and lower cell doses have been associated with poor engraftment and high non-relapse mortality. Transplantation of two cord blood units can overcome this limitation but result in GvHD and survival rates similar to those seen with other stem cell sources. The use of UCB in adults with neoplastic diseases has been declining, especially after acceptance of haploidentical transplants in adults with neoplastic diseases.

Correct Answer: B

Case Study continued: You have identified the patient's brother as a haploidentical donor. He asks you if the choice of conditioning regimen affects GvHD risk.

2) Which of the following conditioning regimens has the highest risk for acute GvHD?

A) High-dose chemotherapy myeloablative conditioning regimen.
B) Total-body irradiation-based myeloablative conditioning.
C) Reduced-intensity conditioning regimen.
D) Nonmyeloablative conditioning regimen.

Expert Perspective: The intensity of conditioning regimens affects the risk of aGvHD.

Pathophysiology of aGvHD is based on the activation of immunocompetent T cells from the donor graft against host antigens. Host tissue damage caused by the conditioning regimen is thought to be the first step affording interaction between T cells and host antigen-presenting cells (APCs) via MHC-T-cell receptor binding and costimulatory signals. This leads to expansion and differentiation into various subtypes of T cells, which traffic to target organs, where they cause host tissue destruction through pathways such as perforin/granzyme and cytokine release (e.g., tumor necrosis factor alpha [TNFα] and interferon gamma [IFNʊ]).

Some studies have shown decreased rates of aGvHD with reduced-intensity conditioning and non-myeloablative conditioning, presumably by decreasing host tissue damage and proinflammatory cytokines. In one study comparing myeloablative to reduced-intensity conditioning regimens, the cumulative incidence of grade II–IV aGvHD at day 100 was lower after reduced-intensity conditioning regimens (31.6% vs 44.7%; $P = 0.024$) (Scott et al. 2017). Additionally, total body irradiation-based myeloablative conditioning has been shown to consistently increase the risk for aGvHD above the level of other myeloablative conditioning regimens (HR ≥ 1.3). Myeloablative doses of total body irradiation also increase the risk of mucositis and gastroenteritis following allo-HCT, which may play a role in further provoking aGvHD.

Case Study continued: You have decided to perform the haploidentical transplant using reduced-intensity conditioning. The patient asks if there are other risk factors for developing GvHD that need to be considered.

3) Besides intensity of conditioning regimen and myeloablative doses of total body irradiation, what are some of the other risk factors for developing acute GvHD?

A) The degree of HLA disparity.
B) Donor age.
C) Multiparous female donor to a male host.
D) All of the above.

Expert Perspective: The most important risk factor is the degree of HLA disparity between the donor and the recipient. Stem cell source, GvHD prophylasis, female donor and male recipient, multiparous female donors, increased age of both the recipient and the donor and pre-transplant comorbidity are additional risk factors for developing aGvHD.

Correct Answer: D

4) What are the immunosuppressive strategies used for GvHD prophylaxis?

Expert Perspective: Acute GvHD is considered a T-cell-mediated disease. Thus, common GvHD prophylaxis strategies focus on the manipulation of T cells, through either diminishing or limiting T-cell numbers or modulating their activity. Chemotherapeutic agents such as methotrexate induce T-cell apoptosis. Cyclophosphamide adminsistered in the post-transplant setting decreases the population and function of effector T cells, while preserving regulatory T cells. Calcineurin inhibitors such as tacrolimus and cyclosporine inhibit T-cell activation and proliferation, primarily through the inhibition of interleukin-2 (IL-2) gene activation. Mycophenolate mofetil inhibits purine metabolism essential to lymphocyte proliferation. Sirolimus inhibits response to IL-2, thus preventing the activation of T cells. For more in-depth discussion of these medications and other less commonly used strategies, please see the recent review by Martinez-Cibrian et al. (2021).

There is no universal consensus on the best GvHD prophylaxis regimen. A clinician must consider multiple factors when determining which medications to use including risk of GvHD, graft rejection, conditioning regimens, and relapse risks, as well as the patient's underlying medical conditions and medications.

In HLA-matched transplants, a calcineurin inhibitor in combination with either mycophenolate mofetil or methotrexate is reasonable. Two randomized controlled trials established that the combination of tacrolimus with methotrexate was significantly superior to the combination of cyclosporin and methotrexate in the prevention of aGvHD. Additionally, another study showed that in matched unrelated HCT, tacrolimus and methotrexate were more effective in preventing aGvHD than tacrolimus and mycophenolate mofetil.

Methotrexate has hepatic, renal, and mucous membrane toxicities, so it should be used with caution in patients with evidence of liver or kidney dysfunction. Furthermore, methotrexate should be avoided in patients with large pleural effusions or ascites because these fluid collections can act as reservoirs for the drug, which can lead to prolonged exposure and increased toxicity. For patients who cannot receive methotrexate, many clinicians will administer mycophenolate mofetil or sirolimus in concert with the calcineurin inhibitors. Mycophenolate mofetil is often favored following reduced-intensity or non-myeloablative conditioning regimens or when using umbilical cord blood or haploidentical grafts.

Several prospective studies have investigated the role of sirolimus in combination with other immunosuppressive drugs. The BMT CTN 0402 was a phase III multicenter study that compared tacrolimus and sirolimus to tacrolimus and methotrexate as GvHD prophylaxis. Although it showed equivalent GvHD-free survival when both prophylactic regimens were compared, tacrolimus and sirolimus were associated with more endothelial toxicities (Cutler et al. 2014). Another multicenter randomized controlled trial (Armand et al. 2016) evaluated the addition of sirolimus to GvHD prophylaxis regimen. They reported a significant reduction in aGvHD in the triple-arm therapy (sirolimus, tacrolimus, and methotrexate) when compared to the standard GvHD regimen at the expense of toxicity. Sirolmus should be avoided with busulfan-based myeloablative conditioning given increased risk of sinusoidal obstructive syndrome (SOS).

While the use of *ex vivo* T-cell depleted grafts has not been as promising mainly due to poor engraftment and higher rate of disease relapse (although αβ-T cell depletion may be an exception), the introduction of post-transplant cyclophosphamide particularly in the setting of haploidentical transplantation showed significant benefits. In vivo T-cell depletion options also include antithymocyte globulin as part of the conditioning regimen with reduction in acute GvHD observed in randomized trials (Finke et al. 2009; Soiffer et al. 2017). ATG may decrease the risk of graft failure and is an integral part of the conditioning regimen for diseases such as aplastic anemia. ATG use differs geographically. For example, in Europe, patients receiving myeloablative conditioning will commonly receive antithymocyte globulin, and some transplant centers administer ATG to all transplant recipients.

5) What are the data for post-transplant cyclophosphamide in haploidentical transplants?

Expert Perspective: Cyclophosphamide administered early post HCT preferentially kills allo-reactive T cells while sparing resting, non allo-reactive T cells leading to suppression of GvHD as well as graft rejection. The effectiveness of cyclophosphamide as a GvHD prophylaxis agent was first discovered in the 1980s by scientists at Johns Hopkins Hospital. There is some debate regarding the exact mechanism, but it has been proposed that cyclophosphamide preferentially spares cells that contain high levels of the enzyme aldehyde dehydrogenase (ALDH) as is the case for non allo-reactive T cells and regulatory T cells.

Post-transplant cyclophosphamide as GvHD prophylaxis was initially developed for haploidentical marrow transplantation after non-myeloablative conditioning but, recently, several studies have extended the approach to peripheral blood stem cell transplantation. Hypothetically, this may result in greater risk of aGvHD and cGvHD due to the 5–10-fold higher number of T cells in the allograft. A recent large analysis compared clinical outcomes in 481 patients receiving haploidentical marrow grafts versus 190 patients receiving haploidentical PBSC grafts (Bashey et al. 2017). There were no significant differences in OS or non-relapse mortality, but patients receiving marrow had a lower risk of acute (25% vs 42%; $P < 0.001$) and chronic GvHD (20% vs 41%; $P < 0.001$). Other studies have also shown lower rates of acute GvHD with bone marrow compared to PBSC grafts in the haploidentical setting. Accordingly, until randomized trials are reported, bone marrow is the preferred stem cell source for haploidentical transplants using post-transplant cyclophosphamide.

6) What are the data for using post-transplant cyclophosphamide GvHD prophylaxis outside of haploidentical transplant setting?

Expert Perspective: Post-transplant cyclophosphamide has also been studied as GvHD prophylaxis when using matched related and unrelated donors. The BMT CTN 1301 study, a phase III multicenter GvHD prophylaxis trial, compared two calcineurin inhibitor-free approaches, post-transplant cyclophosphamide and CD34$^+$ positive selection vs a standard regimen of tacrolimus and methotrexate among patients with acute leukemia or myelodysplasia using matched related or matched unrelated donors. Post-transplant cyclophosphamide on days +3 and +4 post transplant without any other GvHD prophylaxis showed GvHD and survival outcomes similar to tacrolimus and methotrexate and better survival compared to CD34$^+$ cell selection strategy.

As a result of this, interest in extending post-transplant cyclophosphamide to the matched PBSC transplantation setting continues to grow. A randomized multicenter phase III BMT

CTN 1703 study of tacrolimus and methotrexate versus post-transplant cyclophosphamide on days +3 and +4 followed by tacrolimus and mycophenolate mofetil in non-myeloablative or reduced-intensity conditioning allogeneic PBSC transplant demonstrated significantly less severe (grade III/IV) acute GVHD and chronic GVHD resulting in superior one-year GVHD-free, relapse-free survival (GRFS) in the post-transplant cyclophosphamide arm.

Case Study continued: You have decided to use post-transplant cyclophosphamide, tacrolimus, and mycophenolate mofetil for GvHD prophylaxis. Despite this, the patient develops nausea, vomiting, and diarrhea 30 days after his transplant. He asks what needs to be done to evaluate his symptoms.

7) **Which of the following causes of gastrointestinal symptoms are difficult to distinguish from acute GvHD on biopsy?**
   A) Mycophenolate mofetil use.
   B) Cytomegalovirus enteritis.
   C) Total body irradiation effect.
   D) Proton pump inhibitor use.
   E) All of the above.

Expert Perspective: Acute GvHD is diagnosed clinically. Biopsies provide supportive evidence for the diagnosis. Apoptosis is the hallmark histologic finding of acute GvHD, but biopsies can frequently be interpreted as normal or equivocal; thus, a clinician should initiate therapy when there is sufficient pretest probability for GvHD, even in the absence of a tissue diagnosis.

Differential diagnosis: Bacterial and parasitic infections must be ruled out in patients with post-transplant gastrointestinal symptoms. In the absence of a compelling diagnosic alternative, post-transplant gastrointestinal symptoms should be evaluated via esophago-gastroduodenoscopy (EGD) and/or colonoscopy/sigmoidoscopy with accompanying biopsy. There is a risk of false-negative (and sometimes false-positive) results, both regarding endoscopic visual inspection and histopathologic evaluation. Gastrointestinal mucosa may have a normal appearance despite the presence of GvHD, and areas of active GvHD may be missed due to sampling error. Furthermore, several other common post-transplant toxicities can cause apoptosis histologically mimicking GvHD. In the about three weeks following transplant, chemotherapy- and radiation-induced apoptosis complicate evaluation. Proton pump inhibitor use may cause apoptosis observed on gastric biopsies. Brincidofovir or mycophenolate mofetil toxicity is difficult to histologically differentiate from GvHD, although distribution may afford some clues. Both cytomegalovirus and cryptosporidium infections can cause apoptosis in the gut mucosa, although immunologic staining for these pathogens can help differentiate. Immunohistochemical stains for viral infections often are not available immediately, and careful follow-up of all relevant data is critical. Thus, contextual interpretation of histologic findings is essential for transplant patients.

Correct Answer: E

Case Study continued: The endoscopic report states the mucosa was unremarkable, and biopsies come back with rare apoptotic cells. However, the pathologist cannot definitively make the diagnosis of acute GvHD. The patient continues to have multiple episodes of watery diarrhea each day without rash or hyperbilirubinemia. You elect to admit him to initiate systemic corticosteroid therapy for acute GvHD. He states that he has had seven or eight bouts of diarrhea daily for the past 4–5 days and asks if the amount of diarrhea affects his likelihood of survival from acute GvHD.

8) Which acute GvHD onset characteristics are associated with poor outcomes?

Expert Perspective: aGvHD severity is assessed by the degree of involvement of three target organs: skin, liver, and GI tract. Although some centers utilize different GvHD scoring systems, the Mount Sinai Acute Graft vs Host Disease International Consortium (MAGIC) approach has been endorsed by the BMT Clinical Trials Network (BMT CTN), the NIH, the CIBMTR, and the European Society for Blood and Marrow Transplantation (EBMT) (see Table 60.1).

- Skin aGvHD classically manifests as an erythematous maculopapular rash (Figure 60.1), and severity is scored by extent of skin involvement as well as the presence of bullae or desquamation.
- Liver aGvHD presents as cholestatic jaundice, with increased severity ascribed to higher levels of hyperbilirubinemia.
- Gastrointestinal aGvHD can affect the upper gastrointestinal tract, causing nausea, vomiting, and/or anorexia, and/or it can affect the lower gastrointestinal tract, resulting in secretory diarrhea or, in its most severe form, severe pain, ileus, and gastrointestinal hemorrhage.

Table 60.1 MAGIC acute GvHD Target Organ Staging (Harris et al. 2016).

Stage	Skin (active erythema only)	Liver (Bilirubin)	Upper GI	Lower GI (stool output/day)
0	No erythematous rash	< 2 mg/dL	No or intermittent nausea, vomiting, or anorexia	Adult: < 500 mL/day or < 3 episodes/day child: < 10 mL/kg/day or < 4 episodes/day
1	Maculopapular rash < 25% BSA	2–3 mg/dL	Persistent nausea, vomiting, or anorexia	Adult: 500–999 mL/day or 3–4 episodes/day child: 10–19.9 mL/kg/day or 4–6 episodes/day
2	Maculopapular rash 25–50% BSA	3.1–6 mg/dL		Adult: 1000–1500 mL/day or 5–7 episodes/day child: 20–30 mL/kg/day or 7–10 episodes/day
3	Maculopapular rash > 50% BSA	6.1–15 mg/dL		Adult: > 1500 mL/day or > 7 episodes/day child: > 30 mL/kg/day or > 10 episodes/day
4	Generalized erythroderma (> 50% BSA) plus bullous formation and desquamation > 5% BSA	> 15 mg/dL		Severe abdominal pain with or without ileus or grossly bloody stool (regardless of stool volume)

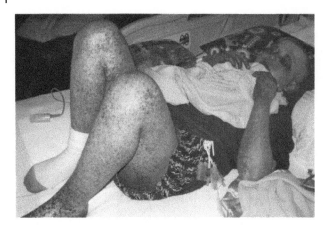

Figure 60.1 Patient with diffuse acute graft-versus-host disease (aGvHD) rash. *Source:* Courtesy of M. Hartwell.

Grade 0: no stage 1–4 of any organ

Grade I: Stage 1–2 skin without liver, upper GI, or lower GI involvement

Grade II: Stage 3 skin and/or stage 1 liver and/or stage 1 upper GI and/or stage 1 lower GI

Grade III: Stage 2–3 liver and/or stage 2–3 lower GI, with or without stage 0–3 skin and/or stage 0–1 upper GI

Grade IV: Stage 4 skin, liver, or lower GI involvement

Limited skin and isolated upper gastrointestinal GvHD do not appear to strongly influence non-relapse mortality and are often treated with topical therapy alone (Dignan et al. 2012; Nikiforow et al. 2018). Severe (grade III–IV) GvHD has reproducibly been associated with increased risk for mortality (HR 1.5–2.6). Severe lower gastrointestinal and/or liver involvement frequently occurs in grade III–IV GvHD; thus, it is unsurprising that involvement by these organs at GvHD onset increases the risk for non-relapse mortality (HR 2.4–4).

9) Which additional tests are available in making the diagnosis of acute GvHD? How about markers for risk stratification?

Expert Perspective: No additional clinical tests are currently available to help with making the diagnosis of aGvHD. However, clinical and biomarker criteria have been validated as prognostic tools and are as follows:

- The Minnesota Acute GvHD Risk Score stratifies patients based on target organ staging at diagnosis. High-risk patients are far less likely to respond to treatment with systemic steroids (odds ratio 0.5) and have higher rates of two-year non-relapse mortality (odds ratio 1.5) as compared to standard-risk patients (MacMillan et al. 2015).
- The MAGIC algorithm probability (MAP), calculates risk of non-relapse mortality on the basis of serum ST2 and REG3α concentrations. These two proteins quantify the extent of gastrointestinal crypt damage during aGvHD. Because gastrointestinal aGvHD is the driver of GvHD-related mortality, the MAGIC algorithm probability is more accurate than clinical symptoms for predicting non-relapse mortality at aGvHD diagnosis and during treatment (Major-Monfried et al. 2018, Srinagesh et al. 2019).

10) What is the appropriate first-line therapy for acute GvHD?

Expert Perspective: There is a paucity of medical literature surrounding the management and natural history of aGvHD that presents as isolated skin aGvHD with ≤ 50% body surface area involvement (grade I GvHD). Many patients are treated with topical steroids. Similarly, patients who present with isolated upper gastrointestinal aGvHD are often treated with non-absorable steroids such as budesonide. Nonethess, many clinicians elect to treat grade I GvHD systemically, especially if they perceive an increased risk for progression to more severe aGvHD as in the setting of early onset or a HLA-mismatched allograft (or other risk factors).

For patients with grade II–IV aGvHD, treatment with 2 mg/kg or methylprednisolone (or equivalent dosing of other corticosteroids) is the most widely used first-line therapy, although some centers prefer to start patients on lower steroid doses (≥ 1 mg/kg) and increase to 2 mg/kg if their aGvHD is unresponsive or progressive. Large studies report response rates (complete or partial) of 55–65% at four weeks of therapy. Currently clinical trials are testing biomarker-based risk (e.g. MAGIC algorithm probability scores) as a way to determine aGvHD treatment intensity.

11) Have any additional agents been proven to improve outcomes in acute GvHD?

Expert Perspective: No single therapy when added to steroids has improved response and/or survival when compared to steroids alone in randomized clinical trials. Treatments investigated in randomized controlled trials include IL2 blockade (daclizumab or basiliximab), TNFα blockade (infliximab), and antithymocyte globulin. A phase III, multicenter, randomized, double-blind clinical trial performed by the BMT Clinical Trials Network investigating the addition of mycophenolate mofetil to systemic steroid therapy was halted due to futility (Bolaños-Meade et al. 2014). Agents that have shown promise in phase II trials, but have not been definitively tested in phase III trials, include etanercept (a 69% CR rate), denileukin diftitox (a 41–50% CR rate in steroid-refractory GvHD), and pentostatin (a 63% CR rate in steroid-refractory GvHD); sirolimus monotherapy has shown potential efficacy in a retrospective report (50% CR rate in some series).

12) What are the therapeutic options for steroid-refractory acute GvHD?

Expert Perspective: Despite GvHD prophylactic therapy, a significant number of patients will develop aGvHD. Approximately 30–50% of these patients will experience steroid-refractory GvHD, whereby they will not respond to systemic corticosteroids. Recently, ruxolitinib was approved by the US Food and Drug Administration for the treatment of steroid-refractory aGvHD based on a randomized phase III REACH2 trial that showed superiority of ruxolitinib to best available therapy in day 28 treatment responses (62% vs 39%; $P = < 0.001$) (Zeiser et al. 2020). No other agents have been approved for the treatment of steroid-refractory aGvHD, and there is no consensus for treatments for patients intolerant or non-responsive to ruxolitinib. Other therapies commonly used for steroid-refractory aGvHD include alemtuzumab, α-1 antitrypsin, abatacept, vedolizumab, etanercept, and rituximab. Additional discussion of steroid-refractory aGvHD treatment may be found in a recent review by Kasikis et al. (2021).

Although few studies report the use of extracorporeal photopheresis (ECP) for acute GvHD, the initial results show some potential benefit for patients with steroid-resistant or -dependent GvHD, with response rates of 50–70% at three months after initiation of ECP and improved survival. Although not clearly elucidated, the leading theory on ECP's mechanism of action is through three main effects: (i) induction of apoptosis of activated T cells, (ii) phagocytosis of the apoptotic T cells by APCs resulting in a switch from proinflammatory to immunotolerant cytokine production, and (iii) induction of regulatory T cells.

The patient develops steroid-refractory acute GvHD. He asks whether this a life-threatening complication.

13) **Which of the following may be the cause of mortality in this patient with steroid-refractory acute GvHD?**
   A) Unresponsive acute GvHD.
   B) Infection.
   C) Chronic GvHD.
   D) All of the above.

Expert Perspective: Steroid-refractory GvHD confers a high risk of death, up to 80% in some published series, due to the toxicity of the disease itself, its treatment, and long-term sequelae. Steroid-refractory GvHD can cause death from GI hemorrhage or other organ failure. Intense immunosuppression to treat GvHD can lead to life-threatening and fatal infections. Acute GvHD is a major risk factor for chronic GvHD, which is a significant contributor to late morbidity and mortality following allo-HCT.

Correct Answer: D

Recommended Readings

Anasetti, C., Logan, B.R., Lee, S.J. et al. (2012 October 18). Peripheral-blood stem cells versus bone marrow from unrelated donors. *N Engl J Med* 367 (16): 1487–1496.

Armand, P., Kim, H.T., Sainvil, M.M. et al. (2016 April). The addition of sirolimus to the graft-versus-host disease prophylaxis regimen in reduced intensity allogeneic stem cell transplantation for lymphoma: a multicentre randomized trial. *Br J Haematol* 173 (1): 96–104.

Bashey, A., Zhang, M.J., McCurdy, S.R. et al. (2017 September 10). Mobilized Peripheral Blood Stem Cells Versus Unstimulated Bone Marrow As a Graft Source for T-Cell-Replete Haploidentical Donor Transplantation Using Post-Transplant Cyclophosphamide. *J Clin Oncol* 35 (26): 3002–3009.

Bolaños-Meade, J., Hamadani, M., Wu, J. et al. (2023 June 22). BMT CTN 1703 Investigators. Post-transplantation cyclophosphamide-based graft-versus-host disease prophylaxis. *N Engl J Med* 388 (25): 2338–2348. doi: 10.1056/NEJMoa2215943. PMID: 37342922.

Bolaños-Meade, J., Logan, B.R., Alousi, A.M. et al. (2014 November 20). Phase 3 clinical trial of steroids/mycophenolate mofetil vs steroids/placebo as therapy for acute GVHD: BMT CTN 0802. *Blood* 124 (22): 3221–3227.

Cutler, C., Logan, B., Nakamura, R. et al. (2014 August 21). Tacrolimus/sirolimus vs tacrolimus/methotrexate as GVHD prophylaxis after matched, related donor allogeneic HCT. *Blood* 124 (8): 1372–1377.

Dignan, F.L., Clark, A., Amrolia, P. et al. (2012 July). Diagnosis and management of acute graft-versus-host disease. *Br J Haematol* 158 (1): 30–45.

Eapen, M., Rocha, V., Sanz, G. et al. (2010 July). Effect of graft source on unrelated donor haemopoietic stem-cell transplantation in adults with acute leukaemia: a retrospective analysis. *Lancet Oncol* 11 (7): 653–660.

Ferrara, J.L.M. and Chaudhry, M.S. (2018). GVHD: biology matters. *Hematology* 2018 (1): 221–227.

Finke, J., Bethge, W.A., Schmoor, C. et al. (2009 September). Standard graft-versus-host disease prophylaxis with or without anti-T-cell globulin in haematopoietic cell transplantation from matched unrelated donors: a randomised, open-label, multicentre phase 3 trial. *Lancet Oncol* 10 (9): 855–864.

Gyurkocza, B. and Sandmaier, B.M. (2014). Conditioning regimens for hematopoietic cell transplantation: one size does not fit all. *Blood* 124 (3): 344–353.

Harris, A.C., Young, R., Devine, S. et al. (2016 January). International, Multicenter Standardization of Acute Graft-versus-Host Disease Clinical Data Collection: A Report from the Mount Sinai Acute GVHD International Consortium. *Biol Blood Marrow Transplant* 22 (1): 4–10.

Holtick, U., Albrecht, M., Chemnitz, J.M. et al. (2014 April 20). Bone marrow versus peripheral blood allogeneic haematopoietic stem cell transplantation for haematological malignancies in adults. *Cochrane Database Syst Rev* 2014 (4): CD010189. doi: 10.1002/14651858. CD010189.pub2. PMID: 24748537.

Kasikis, S., Etra, A., Levine, J.E. et al. (2021 January). Current and emerging targeted therapies for acute graft-versus-host disease. *BioDrugs* 35 (1): 19–33.

Lee, S.J., Logan, B., Westervelt, P. et al. (2016 December 1). Comparison of patient-reported outcomes in 5-year survivors who received bone marrow vs peripheral blood unrelated donor transplantation: long-term follow-up of a randomized clinical trial. *JAMA Oncol* 2 (12): 1583–1589.

MacMillan, M.L., Robin, M., Harris, A.C. et al. (2015 April). A refined risk score for acute graft-versus-host disease that predicts response to initial therapy, survival, and transplant-related mortality. *Biol Blood Marrow Transplant* 21 (4): 761–767.

Major-Monfried, H., Renteria, A.S., Pawarode, A. et al. (2018 June 21). MAGIC biomarkers predict long-term outcomes for steroid-resistant acute GVHD. *Blood* 131 (25): 2846–2855.

Martinez-Cibrian, N., Zeiser, R., Perez-Simon, J.A. et al. (2021 July). Graft-versus-host disease prophylaxis: pathophysiology-based review on current approaches and future directions. *Blood Rev* 48: 100792.

Nikiforow, S., Wang, T., Hemmer, M et al. (2018 October). Upper gastrointestinal acute graft-*versus*-host disease adds minimal prognostic value in isolation or with other graft-*versus*-host disease symptoms as currently diagnosed and treated. *Haematologica* 103 (10): 1708–1719.

Scott, B.L., Pasquini, M.C., Logan, B.R. et al. (2017 April 10). Myeloablative Versus Reduced-Intensity Hematopoietic Cell Transplantation for Acute Myeloid Leukemia and Myelodysplastic Syndromes. *J Clin Oncol* 35 (11): 1154–1161.

Soiffer, R.J., Kim, H.T., McGuirk, J. et al. (2017 December 20). Prospective, Randomized, Double-Blind, Phase III Clinical Trial of Anti-T-Lymphocyte Globulin to Assess Impact on Chronic Graft-Versus-Host Disease-Free Survival in Patients Undergoing HLA-Matched Unrelated Myeloablative Hematopoietic Cell Transplantation. *J Clin Oncol* 35 (36): 4003–4011.

Srinagesh, H.K., Özbek, U., Kapoor, U. et al. (2019 December 10). The MAGIC algorithm probability is a validated response biomarker of treatment of acute graft-versus-host disease. *Blood Adv* 3 (23): 4034–4042.

Symons, H.J., Zahurak, M., Cao, Y. et al. (2020 August 25). Myeloablative haploidentical BMT with posttransplant cyclophosphamide for hematologic malignancies in children and adults. *Blood Adv* 4 (16): 3913–3925.

Zeiser, R., Bubnoff, N., Butler, J. et al. (2020 May 7). Ruxolitinib for glucocorticoid-refractory acute graft-versus-host disease. *N Engl J Med* 382 (19): 1800–1810. doi: 10.1056/ NEJMoa1917635. Epub 2020 Apr 22. PMID: 32320566.

61

Chronic Graft-versus-Host Disease

Andrew Trunk and Daniel R. Couriel

Huntsman Cancer Institute, Salt Lake City, UT, USA

Introduction

Clinical outcomes for patients undergoing allogeneic hematopoietic cell transplantation continue to improve, but chronic graft-versus-host disease (cGvHD) remains a major long-term complication, with profound effects on morbidity, quality of life, and non-relapse mortality. Historically, treatment of cGvHD involved broad, systemic immunosuppression mainly with corticosteroids. As our understanding of the immune and cellular processes underlying cGvHD have improved, more focused therapies have evolved. Targeting signaling pathway effectors such as JAK1/2, ROCK2, BTK, and SYK have led to three new FDA approved therapies for steroid-refractory (SR) cGvHD, including two (ruxolitinib and belumosudil) in 2021. Numerous other agents and combinations of therapies are being investigated, with the cGvHD field progressing at a rate that it has never seen before. The focus of this chapter is to review recent advances in the treatment of cGvHD. We also incorporate some preventive strategies that we believe have or may contribute to change the landscape of the field.

1) What is the incidence of chronic graft-versus-host disease after allogeneic hematopoietic stem cell transplantation?

Expert Perspective: Chronic graft-versus-host disease (cGvHD) is a serious long-term complication affecting 30–60% of patients following an allogeneic hematopoietic stem cell transplant (allo-HSCT) (Lee et al. 2003). Chronic GvHD has profound effects on quality of life and functional status and is the leading cause of non-relapse mortality (MacDonald et al. 2018). Advances in performance of HSCT have reduced the incidence of acute GvHD but unfortunately have not consistently translated into decreased incidence or severity of cGvHD (Jagasia et al. 2015).

2) How is chronic graft-versus-host disease defined, and what is the pathogenesis?

Expert Perspective: The disease is classically defined as having an onset of 100 days after infusion of allogeneic hematopoietic stem cells. Though some degree of graft-versus-leukemia (GvL) effect is desired, cGvHD involves donor T- and B-lymphocytes derived from the graft recognizing and attacking tissues and antigens of the host. This complex molecular

Cancer Consult: Expertise in Clinical Practice, Volume 2: Neoplastic Hematology & Cellular Therapy,
Second Edition. Edited by Syed A. Abutalib, Maurie Markman, James O. Armitage, and Kenneth C. Anderson.
© 2024 John Wiley & Sons Ltd. Published 2024 by John Wiley & Sons Ltd.

interplay first involves an inflammatory cytokine release by host tissues as a consequence of the preparative chemotherapy regimen, namely interleukin-1 (IL-1), tumor necrosis factor alpha (TNF-α), interferon gamma (IFN-γ), and platelet-derived growth factor (PDGF) (Saidu et al. 2020). As a result, by way of macrophages and other antigen-presenting cells (APCs), the donor T-lymphocyte progenitors and mature donor lymphocytes become activated against the host tissue. This initiates a proinflammatory cascade involving natural killer (NK) cells, cytotoxic T cells, and helper T cells (Alexander et al. 2014; Hotta et al. 2019). An optimal transplant outcome requires the donor immune system to develop tolerance to the recipient alloantigens, while maintaining the ability to defend against foreign, non-self-stimuli (Cutler et al. 2017).

3) Which organs are affected by chronic graft-versus-host disease?

Expert Perspective: cGvHD has an insidious onset primarily involving mucocutaneous and connective tissues (Figures 61.1–3). Two broad categories exist by which cGvHD is classified: lichen planus-like, or lichenoid, and sclerodermatous. The lichenoid form clinically resembles lichen-planus and most commonly involves the oral and genitourinary mucosae. The scleroder-matous form is a more fibroprolifera-tive process, with potentially profound effects on the skin and joints. It should be noted that both forms can coexist, and virtually any organ can be involved in cGvHD, including the gastrointes-tinal, pulmonary, hepatic, and musculo-skeletal systems (Table 61.1). The most recent NIH Consensus Conference iden-tified a group of more morbid clinical manifestations without effective organ-specific approaches due to "irreversible" fibrotic sequelae (Wolff et al. 2021).

Though many patients may be in remission or cured of their primary dis-ease, the physical, psychological, and economic impacts that result from cGvHD remain substantial. Much

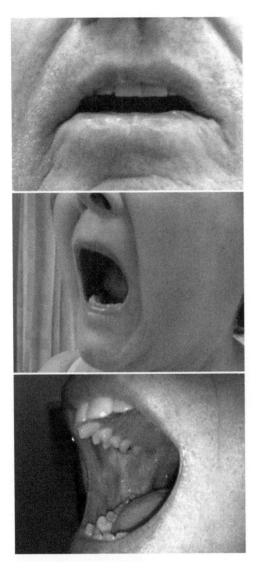

Figure 61.1 Diagnostic oral manifestations of chronic graft-versus-host disease (cGVHD). Top: Lichenoid cGVHD of the lips. Middle: Restricted mouth opening due to sclerotic cGVHD. Bottom: Lichenoid changes to buccal mucosa consistent with cGVHD.

interest and investigation has been undertaken recently for both prevention and management of cGvHD. This review will highlight the current landscape and promising emerging interventions for cGvHD.

4) What is the standard therapy for chronic graft-versus-host disease?

Expert Perspective: For many decades, corticosteroids have been the mainstay of treatment for moderate/severe chronic GvHD due to their broadly immunosuppressive and anti-inflammatory properties (Carpenter et al. 2015; Flowers and Martin 2015), in addition to focused, organ-specific therapies. These interventions may be topical and/or systemic. Steroids to date are still superior to any other treatment when used alone or in combination, although the effect of newer, more active therapies have not yet been evaluated as single agents, or in steroid-free combinations.

Prednisone is usually initiated at a dose of 1 mg/kg, with a slow taper over a prolonged period of time. Consequently, additional steroid-related morbidity

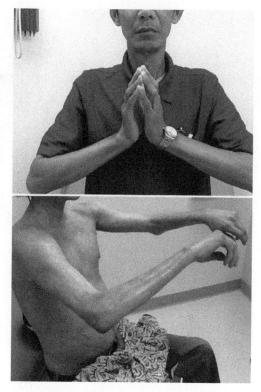

Figure 61.2 Diagnostic musculoskeletal manifestations of chronic graft–versus–host disease (cGVHD). Top: Fasciitis and restriction of the range of motion (ROM). Bottom: Sclerotic cGVHD of the skin with restricted ROM.

develops, such as avascular necrosis of the bone, hyperglycemia and diabetes, and weight gain, to name a few (Koc et al. 2002). These manifestations eventually blend into the syndrome and become as problematic as cGvHD itself.

5) What are the alternative treatment options after steroid failure or intolerance?

Expert Perspective: Unfortunately, more than 50% of patients will require a second-line treatment within two years of steroid initiation (Wolff et al. 2011). This poses a challenge for clinicians, as current National Comprehensive Cancer Network (NCCN) and European Society for Blood and Marrow Transplantation (EBMT) guidelines from 2020 do not define a preferred second-line agent for these steroid-refractory (SR) or steroid-resistant patients (Penack et al. 2020). Thus, clinicians are strongly encouraged to enroll patients in clinical trial when available. Of this relatively large number of options, three have been recently approved by the FDA: ibrutinib, belumosudil, and ruxolitinib, the latter two in 2021. Other secondary therapy options under evaluation and used off-label can be found on Tables 61.2 and 3 and Figure 61.4. These promising developments for steroid-sparing therapies highlight the fact that the standard approach to cGvHD management may soon be changing.

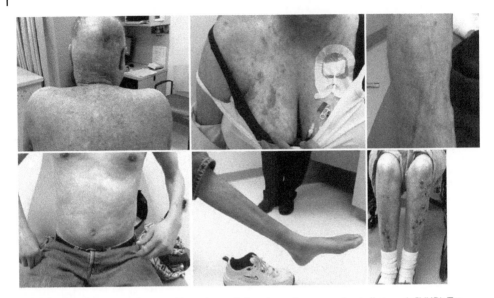

Figure 61.3 Diagnostic skin manifestations of chronic graft–versus–host disease (cGVHD). Top left: Lichen sclerosus. Top middle: Lichen planus–like changes, surrounded by lichen sclerosus. Top right: Lichen planus–like rash. Bottom left: Subcutaneous clerosis. Bottom middle: Sclerosis of the dermis and subcutaneous tissues, with a "pipe stem" appearance to the leg. Bottom right: Severe sclerosis with overlying erosions and ulcerations.

Table 61.1 Selected phase I trials in chronic GvHD.

Agent(s)/Strategy	Mechanism	ClinicalTrials.gov
Leflunomide	Dihydroorotate dehydrogenase (DHODH) inhibitor	NCT04212416
Belimumab, for cGvHD prophylaxis	Anti-B-cell activating factor (BAFF)	NCT03207958
Ruxolitinib, in pediatrics	JAK1/2 inhibitor	NCT05121142
Fostamatinib	Syk inhibitor	NCT02611063
Abatacept	Costimulatory modulator: binds CD80, CD86	NCT01954979
Treg + low-dose IL-2	See text	NCT01937468
Donor Treg	See text	NCT03683498
Ibrutinib, in pediatrics	BTK inhibitor	NCT03790332

6) What are the strategies to prevent and treat chronic graft-versus-host disease?

Expert Perspective: The 2020 Treatment of Chronic GvHD Report from the NIH Consensus Conference proposes a change in our treatment paradigm, where clinical trials exploring an initial steroid-free approach with more novel therapies could lead to new insights into the associations between clinical characteristics of chronic GvHD, pathophysiologic mechanisms of disease, and both clinical and biological effects of novel therapeutic agents, allowing for a more individualized approach (DeFilipp et al. 2021).

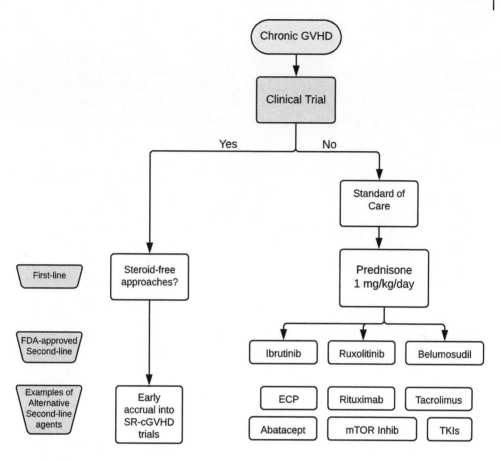

- **CD34 selection:** As donor-derived effector T cells are key mediators in the tissue damage that drives the incidence and severity of cGvHD, another approach is to positively select for CD34+ stem cells. This involves *ex-vivo* use of clinical-grade magnetic bead columns for cell separation and has been shown to result in a 4 to 5 log reduction in T-cell content (Pasquini et al. 2012). Pasquini et al. demonstrated that CD34+ selection resulted in a lower two-year rate of cGvHD (19% vs 50%; $P < 0.001$) without affecting graft rejection, relapse rates, treatment-related mortality, or disease-free or overall survival rates. Though costly, this prophylactic intervention can significantly reduce the incidence of both acute and chronic GvHD.
- **Mesenchymal stem cells (MSCs)** are a heterogeneous population of stromal cells found primarily in the bone marrow but also in the umbilical cord, fallopian tubes, and other fetal tissues. MSCs have the ability to self-renew and differentiate into numerous different tissue types, including adipose and muscle, but can also differentiate to have immunosuppressive and immunomodulatory effects. Though MSCs can suppress mixed lymphocyte reactions in vitro and ameliorate GvHD in in vivo mouse models, clinical trials to date have shown mixed results in treatment of acute GvHD (aGVHD; see Chapter 60) and cGvHD (Kebriaei and Robinson 2011). Multiple phase II trials are ongoing to

Table 61.2 Phase II trials in chronic GvHD.

Agent(s)/Strategy	Mechanism	ClinicalTrials.gov
Itacitinib	*JAK1* inhibitor	NCT04200365
Ibrutinib as front line	*BTK* inhibitor	NCT04294641
Axatilimab, dose-range (AGAVE-201)	*CSF-1R* inhibitor	NCT04710576 (I/II)
SCM-CGH	Allogeneic mesenchymal stem cells	NCT04189432
Itacitinib + ECP	*JAK1* inhibitor	NCT04446182
ECP using Theraflex device	See text	NCT03083574
Acalabrutinib	*BTK* inhibitor	NCT04198922
MSC with glucocorticoids and cyclosporine	See text	NCT04692376
Hydrogen-rich water	See text	NCT02918188
Belumosudil, dose-range (ROCKstar)	*ROCK1/2* inhibitor	NCT03640481
Donor Treg + rapamycin + low-dose IL-2	See text	NCT01903473
Multiple donor Treg donor lymphocyte infusions	See text	NCT02749084 (I/II)
TQ05105	*JAK2* inhibitor	NCT04944043 (Ib/II)
Modification of ECP in cGVHD, or CTCL	Use ALA instead of 8-MOP	NCT03109353 (I/II)
Ibrutinib + rituximab	BTK inhibitor + anti-CD20	NCT04235036
Ruxolitinib cream, for non-sclerotic cutaneous cGVHD	*JAK1/2* inhibitor	NCT03954236 NCT03395340
Glasdegib	Hedgehog inhibitor	NCT04111497 (I/II)
BN101	*ROCK2* selective inhibitor	NCT04930562
ATG + PTCy	See text	NCT04202835
Umbilical cord mesenchymal stem cells	See text	NCT05152160 (I/II)
Amniotic fluid eye drops, for ocular cGvHD	See text	NCT03298815 (I/II)
Ixazomib, for cGvHD prophylaxis	Proteosome inhibitor	NCT03225417 (I/II)
Alvelestat, for bronchiolitis obliterans	Neutrophil elastase inhibitor	NCT02669251 (I/II)
ATG + PTCy, for cGvHD prophylaxis	See text	NCT03357159
Dexamethasone solution in Mucolox, for oral cGvHD	See text	NCT04540133
Umbilical cord mesenchymal stem cell derived exosomes, for ocular cGvHD	See text	NCT04213248 (I/II)
Nintedanib, for bronchiolitis obliterans	Tyrosine kinase inhibitor, including *PDGFR*, *FGFR*, and *VEGFR*	NCT03805477
Reduced dose PTCy, for cGvHD prophylaxis in older/unfit patients	See text	NCT04959175 (I/II)
Obinutuzumab	Anti-CD20	NCT02867384
Chemotherapy + PTCy + TBI, for cGvHD prophylaxis	See text	NCT03192397

(Continued)

Table 61.2 (Continued)

Agent(s)/Strategy	Mechanism	ClinicalTrials.gov
Vorinostat, for cGVHD prophylaxis, in pediatrics	Histone deacetylase (HDAC) inhibitor	NCT03842696 (I/II)
ECP + low-dose aldesleukin	Recombinant human IL-2	NCT03007238 NCT02340676
Low-dose aldesleukin	Recombinant human IL-2	NCT01366092
Ibrutinib, in pediatrics	*BTK* inhibitor	NCT03790332
Ofatumumab	Anti-CD20	NCT01680965 (I/II)
AMG 592 (efavaleukin alfa)	IL-2 mutein-Fc fusion protein	NCT03422627
Baricitinib	*JAK1/2* inhibitor	NCT02759731 (I/II)
SNDX-6352 (axatilimab)	*CSF-1R* inhibitor	NCT03604692 (II/II)
Ruxolitinib	*JAK1/2* inhibitor	NCT03616184
Belumosudil	*ROCK1/2* inhibitor	NCT02841995
Tocilizumab, for cGvHD prophylaxis	*IL-6* inhibitor	NCT03699631
Ruxolitinib, in pediatrics	*JAK1/2* inhibitor	NCT03774082
Pro-ocular 1%, for ocular cGvHD	Progesterone gel	NCT03990051
Cyclophosphamide + tacrolimus + MMF, for cGvHD prophylaxis	See text	NCT03128359

Abbreviations:
cGvHD: chronic graft-versus-host disease; MSC: mesenchymal stem cells; ECP: extracorporeal photopheresis; ATG: antithyroglobulin: PTCy: post-transplantation cyclophosphamide.

Table 61.3 Phase III trials in chronic GvHD.

Agent(s)/Strategy	Mechanism	ClinicalTrials.gov
Corticosteroids + itacitinib, as front-line therapy (GRAVITAS-309)	*JAK1* inhibitor	NCT03584516 (II/III)
Ruxolitinib (REACH3)	*JAK1/2* inhibitor	NCT03112603
Ibrutinib extension study	*BTK* inhibitor	NCT01804686

investigate the role of MSCs, particularly umbilical cord derived, in treatment and prevention of cGvHD (NCT04189432, NCT05152160, NCT04213248; 1–3).

T-cell Strategies

- **Depletion of allo-reactive T cells:** Antithymocyte globulins (ATG) are cytotoxic antibodies against certain antigens expressed on human T lymphocytes. They are produced by immunizing either rabbits (with the T-lymphoblastic Jurkat cell line) or horses (with human thymus lymphocytes). When administered in humans, they result in T-cell depletion via direct cell lysis. ATG may promote engraftment and prevent acute GvHD. The use of ATG has been explored in prevention of cGvHD and indicates some potential benefit (Kroger et al. 2016; Walker et al. 2016). However, differences in study design, target population, ATG preparation, scheduling, and dosages have led to inconsistent results across studies (Soiffer et al. 2017). Multiple phase II studies of ATG in combination with post-transplantation cyclophosphamide are currently recruiting (NCT04202835, NCT03357159).

- **Additional cGvHD prevention strategies** have involved depleting CD6+ T cells and naive T cells (Bleakley et al. 2015; Soiffer et al. 1997, 2001) Selective *ex vivo* depletion of T cells expressing αβ receptors is another approach to isolate CD34+ cells for transfusion (Bertaina et al. 2014; Schumm et al. 2013). Finally, *in vivo* T-cell depletion with the use of post-transplant cyclophosphamide (PTCy), particularly in haploidentical and HLA-mismatched donors, is increasingly used for prevention of cGvHD.

Inhibition of T-cell Signaling

JAK1/2 Inhibitors

JAK 1 and 2: Janus kinase (JAK) is a family of intracellular, nonreceptor tyrosine kinases that, via the JAK-STAT pathway, transduce cytokine-mediated signals. These signals result in immune cell division, survival, and activation (Murray 2007). This broad immune regulation by *JAKs* seems to underlie autoimmunity and GvHD, with involvement of T cells, B cells, and antigen-presenting cells (APCs). The JAK proteins seem to play a role in tissue inflammation, T-cell/APC interaction, and immune cell mitigation. *JAK* blockade seemed to reduce GvHD while at the same time preserving graft-versus-leukemia (GvL) effect, making them an appealing target for GvHD treatment (Carniti et al. 2015; Choi et al. 2014; Schroeder et al. 2018; Spoerl et al. 2014).

- Ruxolitinib is an oral selective *JAK1/2* inhibitor, initially FDA approved in 2011 for treatment of myelofibrosis. Early studies showed an 80% overall response rate, in both mucocutaneous and visceral cGvHD, with 36% cGvHD recurrence at one year (Jagasia et al. 2018; Zeiser et al. 2015). The REACH3 trial demonstrated that ruxolitinib had high 24-week response rates (49.7%), longer median failure-free survival compared to control (> 18.6 mo. vs 5.7 mo.; HR 0.37; $P < 0.001$), and higher symptom response (24.2% vs 11.0%; overall response 2.62; $P = 0.001$) (Zeiser et al. 2021). Notably, this drug also has activity in pediatric bronchiolitis obliterans (Schoettler et al. 2019). A recent meta-analysis reported a 62% overall response rate (27% complete response [CR], 45% partial response) of cGvHD symptoms in response to ruxolitinib in steroid-refractory patients (Hui et al. 2020). In light of these results, the FDA approved ruxolitinib (Jakafi) for second-line cGvHD in September 2021. Grade 3 and 4 adverse events include thrombocytopenia and anemia. Phase I and II trials are currently underway in the pediatric population and for topical ruxolitinib (NCT05121142, NCT03954236 NCT03395340, NCT03616184, NCT03774082).
- Several other *JAK* inhibitors are also under investigation. Itacitinib, a selective *JAK1* inhibitor, has been used in other connective tissue disorders and showed some promise in a phase I study for aGvHD treatment (Schroeder et al. 2020). Itacitinib is currently

being investigated in phase II both as a single agent and in combination with ECP as second-line cGvHD treatment (NCT04200365, NCT04446182). The GRAVITAS-309 phase II/III study of itacitinib with steroids as front-line therapy is currently recruiting (NCT03584516).

- Baricitinib is an additional *JAK1/2* inhibitor, which showed promise in the preclinical setting for prevention of aGvHD and reversal of cGvHD without disturbing the GvL effect (Choi et al. 2018). A phase I/II trial for treatment of cGvHD with baricitinib is planned (NCT02759731).

ROCK2 Inhibitor

- Belumosudil (Rezurock) is an oral selective inhibitor of rho-associated coiled-coil-containing protein kinase 2 (ROCK2). This results in diminished T helper cells (Th17 and follicular type), and increased numbers of regulatory T cells (Tregs). As these are central players in cGvHD, targeting this pathway was logical. The recently completed phase II ROCKstar trial (n = 65) by Cutler and colleagues (2021) demonstrated overall response rate of 75% (95% CI 63–85); 6% of patients achieved a CR, and 69% achieved a partial response. The median time to first response was 1.8 months (95% CI 1.0–1.9). The median duration of response, calculated from first response to progression, death, or new systemic therapies for chronic GvHD, was 1.9 months (95% CI 1.2–2.9). In patients who achieved response, no death or new systemic therapy initiation occurred in 62% (95% CI 46–74%) of patients for at least 12 months since response. All affected organs showed complete responses, which were durable with a median duration of response of 54 months. Symptom reduction was subjectively reported in roughly 60% of patients. Given this overwhelmingly positive study, belumosudil received FDA approval for treatment of steroid-refractory cGvHD in July 2021 (NCT02841995, NCT03640481).

Proteasome Inhibition

- Proteosome inhibitors, which are often used in treatment of multiple myeloma, work by blocking NF-kappa B-activation, which in turn inhibits T-cell activation, proliferation, and survival. Blocking this activity in alloreactive donor T lymphocytes rationalized their investigation in cGvHD. In a phase II trial by Herrera et al., bortezomib + prednisone was used in the front line. The ORR was 80%, with most significant improvements in skin and gastrointestinal (GI) GvHD, and the regimen was well tolerated (Herrera et al. 2014). As a single agent, bortezomib may also stabilize lung function in long-standing bronchiolitis obliterans (Jain et al. 2018) and improve cutaneous and sclerodermatous cGvHD (Pai et al. 2014).
- Ixazomib, which is a reversible 20S binder, has been investigated in cGvHD. In a phase II trial, ixazomib had an ORR of 34% at six months, with a lower treatment failure at that time compared to benchmark (28% vs 44%; $P = 0.01$) (Pidala et al. 2020). A phase II clinical trial of ixazomib for cGvHD prophylaxis is recruiting (NCT03225417).

IL-6 Blockade

- The IMID group of drugs act by inhibiting the production of IL-6, a cytokine notably involved in the proliferation of myeloma cells. IMIDs also directly induce apoptosis and cell death via the caspase-8 pathway. Due to the role of interleukin cytokines in the pathogenesis of cGvHD, thalidomide was studied. Though thalidomide was active, the toxicities of neutropenia, somnolence, and neuropathy discouraged its use (Linhares et al. 2013). Pomalidomide, another IMID, is significantly more potent than thalidomide in terms of blocking TNF-α production and increasing Th-1 cells; it is also significantly less toxic. A phase I/II study of pomalidomide showed some activity against mucocutaneous cGvHD (Pusic et al. 2016). However, these drugs are not often used early in the second line.

Costimulatory Blockade

- Two costimulatory blocking agents are currently under investigation for steroid-refractory cGvHD treatment. Abatacept is a fusion protein made of extracellular human cytotoxic T-lymphocyte antigen-4 (CTLA-4) linked to the modified Fc portion of human immunoglobulin G1 (IgG1). This drug blocks T-cell activation by interfering with CD80 and CD86 expressed on APCs. Early studies of abatacept showed a PR in 44% of patients and significant reduction in steroid dose (Nahas et al. 2018). (NCT01954979). Alefacept is a CD-2-directed fusion protein comprised of leukocyte-function-associated antigen 3 (LFA-3) and the Fc hinge region of IgG1. Though alefacept was shown to be effective in treating cGvHD with 66% of patients responding, responses were not durable, and significant adverse events occurred (Shapira et al. 2009).

Hedgehog Inhibitors

- The hedgehog family of proteins, which includes Sonic (Shh), Indian (Ihh), and Desert (Dhh), are involved in early embryonic development, but activation in adults may lead to carcinogenesis and fibrinogenesis (Zerr et al. 2012a). Beyond direct reduction of collagen production by myofibroblasts, hedgehog signaling may also influence pathogenic B cell and macrophage responses to augment disease (Radojcic et al. 2021). Several Shh agents were considered for early investigation, including glasdegib, sonidegib, and vismodegib. In a phase I study of sonidegib, 47% of patients with sclerodermatous or skin cGvHD had a PR (DeFilipp et al. 2017). The phase II trial of vismodegib showed responses in all six patients treated but was terminated early due to toxicity, mainly muscle cramps and secondarily dysgeusia (Radojcic et al. 2021). The phase I/II trial of glasdegib is currently recruiting (NCT04111497).

Tyrosine Kinase Inhibitors

- Tyrosine kinases are involved in cell differentiation, proliferation, anti-apoptosis, and B- and T-cell signaling. By binding upstream to ATP-binding catalytic sites of receptor tyrosine kinases (RTKs), they prevent phosphorylation and subsequent intracellular signaling events, including those involved in pro-inflammatory cytokine signaling. As TKIs have been used in other hematologic conditions and malignancies, they are appealing drugs for treatment of cGvHD. Imatinib is a first-generation TKI, which, in addition to targeting *BCR::ABL1*-mutated cells, has been shown to inhibit PDGFR and TGF-β pathways, important for sclerodermatous cGvHD pathogenesis (Ghofrani et al. 2005). Studies by Olivieri and Magro showed roughly 50% ORR with sclerodermatous, pulmonary, and GI cGvHD (Magro et al. 2008, 2009; Olivieri et al. 2009). Further reports of imatinib 400 mg daily in sclerodermatous cGvHD showed a partial response of 36%, with stable disease in 50% of patients, though dose reductions were often necessary (Baird et al. 2015), with other similar reports (Osumi et al. 2012). Nilotinib, a second-generation TKI with higher PDGFR affinity, has been a recent drug of interest in cGvHD. Preclinical work was promising for prevention and treatment of sclerodermatous cGvHD in mice (Zerr et al. 2012b). A recent phase I/II dose-escalating trial had overall response rate ranging from 22.2 to 55.6% for higher dose, OS was 75% at 48 months, and the drug was well tolerated (Marinelli Busilacchi et al. 2020; Olivieri et al. 2020). Failure-free survival was 25–30%.

Adoptive Regulatory T Cell (Treg) Products

- The direct transfer of highly purified CD4 Tregs is an appealing intervention to prevent development of cGvHD. In one study, infusion of Tregs that had been isolated by immunomagnetic bead purification resulted in a low incidence of GvHD and enhance immune reconstitution in haploidentical stem cell transplant (Di Ianni et al. 2011). Tregs have also been harvested from umbilical cord blood and expanded *ex vivo*, with post-harvest modifications including genetic modification of Tregs against alloantigen receptors, expansion of minor histocompatibility antigen-specific Tregs, and focusylation to improve engraftment (MacDonald et al. 2016; Parmar et al. 2014; Veerapathran et al. 2013). Limitations of this therapy are the complex methods for cell purification and expansion, in addition to the small fraction of circulating lymphocytes that Tregs represent.

Enhancement of CD4 Treg

- **Extracorporeal Photopheresis (ECP)**: ECP, initially FDA approved in the 1980s for refractory cutaneous T-cell lymphoma, has been one of the most extensively studied interventions for patients with steroid-refractory cGvHD. ECP involves ultraviolet A (UVA) irradiation of leukapheresed cells after exposure to 8-MOP photosensitizer. Though the exact mechanism in GvHD has not been elucidated, it is theorized that ECP-induced lymphocyte apoptosis stimulates dendritic cells (DCs), which develop tolerance of self after uptake of the dead lymphocytes (Bastien et al. 2010; Bruserud et al. 2014; Hart et al. 2013). Couriel et al. reported an overall response rate of 60% in steroid-refractory cGvHD, with durable responses at six months, and 22% steroid discontinuation at one year (Couriel et al. 2006). A randomized, phase II study demonstrated that ECP with best available therapy resulted in greater steroid-sparing effect and higher efficacy, particularly in cutaneous GvHD (Flowers et al. 2008). Numerous intriguing studies are underway involving combination of ECP with IL-2, the *JAK1* inhibitor itacitinib, cyclosporine, and tacrolimus, and one study examining 5-aminolevulinic acid (5-ALA) instead of 8-MOP (NCT04446182, NCT03083574, NCT03109353, NCT03007238, NCT02340676).

Interleukin-2 Administration

- Interleukin-2 (IL-2; aldesleukin) is a critical homeostatic cytokine responsible for Treg survival, expansion, development, and activity (Chinen et al. 2016; Nelson 2004). Administration of "low-dose" (1×10^6 IU/m; MacDonald et al. 2018) IL-2 was found to selectively enhance CD4+ Tregs and provide clinical response in 52% of patients in a phase I study (Koreth et al. 2011; Matsuoka et al. 2013). Therefore, a phase II study was conducted, which demonstrated a 61% overall response rate in virtually all organ systems, and 66% of patients remained on therapy for two years, though no CRs were observed (Koreth et al. 2016).
- Additional studies have been conducted using ultra-low-dose IL-2 for cGvHD prophylaxis, with demonstrated Treg enhancement (Ito et al. 2014; Kennedy-Nasser et al. 2014). Numerous clinical trials are currently recruiting, involving IL-2 combination with ECP, as a fusion protein, and combined with Tregs with and without rapamycin (NCT03007238, NCT02340676, NCT01366092, NCT03422627, NCT01937468, NCT01903473).

Additional Strategies

- Alternative immunosuppressive agents have been or are being investigated for cGvHD treatment. The mTOR inhibitor sirolimus (rapamycin) can promote the reconstitution of Tregs, and has been investigated for the prevention of aGvHD as well as treatment of cGvHD (Zeiser et al. 2008). Sirolimus has been shown to have benefit in cutaneous cGvHD, particularly the sclerodermatous form (Couriel et al. 2005; Johnston et al. 2005). Mycophenolate mofetil (MMF), an inosine-5-monophosphate dehydrogenase inhibitor, has also been shown to promote Treg reconstitution, though a phase III trial of first-line steroids with MMF showed no benefit and potentially greater toxicity (Martin et al. 2009). MMF is being studied in a three-drug cocktail for cGvHD prophylaxis in a planned phase II trial (NCT03128359).
- Axatilimab (SNDX-6352) is a humanized IgG4 monoclonal antibody that binds colony-stimulating factor 1 receptor (CSF-1R), important in macrophage production, differentiation, and function (Alexander et al. 2014). Blocking this process may treat cGvHD particularly of the lungs and skin. Promising phase I results were shown at ASH 2022, and phase Ib/II is now recruiting (NCT04710576).

B-cell Strategies

Signal Inhibition

- **BTK Inhibition:** Ibrutinib is an inhibitor of Bruton tyrosine kinase (BTK), acting predominantly in B cells but also on IL-2-inducible T-cell kinase (ITK) in T cells (Jaglowski and Blazar 2018). Consequently, immunoglobulin cannot be produced, and humoral responses are not mounted. Ibrutinib was the first drug to receive FDA approval for treatment of steroid-refractory cGvHD in 2017. This came after a landmark phase II study showed an overall response rate of 67% at 13.9 months, with 71%

sustained response ≥ 20 weeks, and significant reductions in steroid doses (Miklos et al. 2017). At two-year follow-up, 31% had achieved CR, and 38% a partial response, with responders having durable and sustained effects (Waller et al. 2019). Clinically, a large proportion of patients reported significant functional improvements also (King-Kallimanis et al. 2020). Ibrutinib is currently being investigated in the front line, in pediatrics, and in combination with rituximab (NCT01804686, NCT03790332, NCT04294641, NCT03790332, NCT04235036).

- **SYK Inhibition:** SYK is another cytoplasmic tyrosine kinase involved in immune receptor signaling in B cells more so than T cells, with particular involvement in B-cell proliferation and survival, innate immune recognition, and cell migration. Inhibiting SYK also prevents cytokine and chemokine production necessary for activation of CD4+ T cells. Preclinical data with the SKY inhibitor fostamatinib indicates SYK is crucial for development of cGvHD (Flynn et al. 2015; Le Huu et al. 2014). As such, a phase I dose-range study of fostamatinib for prevention of treatment of cGvHD is underway (NCT02611063). Another SYK inhibitor, entospletinib, preclinically showed positive effects on prevention of cutaneous and ocular GvHD, but this has not translated to a clinical trial (Poe et al. 2018).

B-cell Depletion

- **Rituximab**, an anti-CD20 monoclonal antibody, acts by depleting B cells via a potent cell- and complement-mediated cytotoxicity, consequently preventing B-cell clonal expansion. Cutler et al. demonstrated an overall response rate of 70%, including 9% CR, though with 42% grade 3/4 adverse events, and other studies were inconsistent (Cutler et al. 2006; Kharfan-Dabaja et al. 2009). Rituximab has been shown to be effective at preventing cGvHD and steroid need (Cutler et al. 2013) and when used in combination with the TKI nilotinib, displayed markedly higher overall response rate (63% partial response, 8% CR) with one-year survival of 96.6% in patients with sclerodermatous cGvHD (van der Wagen et al. 2018). As such, Solomon et al. conducted a phase II study investigating rituximab as part of first-line treatment, reporting a cumulative incidence of cGvHD resolution of 41%, 69%, and 77% at one, two, and three years, respectively, and disease-free survival of 36%, 55%, and 57% at those same time points (Solomon et al. 2019). A phase II trial is underway combining rituximab with ibrutinib (NCT04235036).

- **Ofatumumab,** another fully human anti-CD20 monoclonal antibody, works in a similar fashion to rituximab by depleting B lymphocytes. However, it targets a unique epitope, resulting in greater affinity and complement-dependent cytotoxicity, as well as macrophage-mediated phagocytosis. A phase I study showed steroid dose reduction in 90% of patients, and a six-month overall response rate of 72%, including 36% CR (Pidala et al. 2015). The phase I/II trial is ongoing (NCT01680965).

- **Obinutuzumab:** This potent, fully human anti-CD20 monoclonal antibody, exhibits some superiority over rituximab in other hematologic conditions. Obinutuzumab is currently enrolling for phase II trial for administration at 3, 6, 9, and 12 months post-allogeneic stem cell transplant for prevention of cGvHD (NCT02867384).

Conclusion

After decades without clear, significant progress in the management of both primary and steroid-refractory chronic graft-versus-host disease, improved understanding of the underlying immunologic mechanisms and cellular pathways has greatly invigorated and advanced the therapeutic armament for cGvHD management. All active clinical trials reinforce the breadth of investigation into this morbid disease. Through these investigations, within the last year, we have two new FDA approved therapies (belumosudil, ruxolitinib) for steroid-refractory cGvHD. Though other recent clinical studies are promising, larger multicenter phase III studies will be needed to further identify efficacy, toxicity, and long-term effects, both for prevention and treatment of GvHD.

Recommended Readings

Bolaños-Meade, J., Hamadani, M., Wu, J. et al. (2023 June 22). BMT CTN 1703 Investigators. Post-transplantation cyclophosphamide-based graft-versus-host disease prophylaxis. *N Engl J Med* 388 (25): 2338–2348. doi: 10.1056/NEJMoa2215943. PMID: 37342922.

Couriel, D.R., Hosing, C., Saliba, R., EJ, S., Anderlini, P., Rhodes, B. et al. (2006). Extracorporeal photochemotherapy for the treatment of steroid-resistant chronic GVHD. *Blood* 107 (8): 3074–3080.

Cutler, C., Lee, S.J., Arai, S., Rotta, M., Zoghi, B., Lazaryan, A. et al. (2021). Belumosudil for chronic graft-versus-host disease after 2 or more prior lines of therapy: The ROCKstar study. *Blood* 138 (22): 2278–2289.

Cutler, C.S., Koreth, J., and Ritz, J. (2017). Mechanistic approaches for the prevention and treatment of chronic GVHD. *Blood* 129 (1): 22–29.

Cutler, C., Miklos, D., Kim, H.T., Treister, N., Woo, S.B., Bienfang, D. et al. (2006). Rituximab for steroid-refractory chronic graft-versus-host disease. *Blood* 108 (2): 756–762.

Flowers, M.E., Apperley, J.F., van Besien, K., Elmaagacli, A., Grigg, A., Reddy, V. et al. (2008). A multicenter prospective phase 2 randomized study of extracorporeal photopheresis for treatment of chronic graft-versus-host disease. *Blood* 112 (7): 2667–2674.

Flowers, M.E. and Martin, P.J. (2015). How we treat chronic graft-versus-host disease. *Blood* 125 (4): 606–615.

Jagasia, M., Zeiser, R., Arbushites, M., Delaite, P., Gadbaw, B., and Bubnoff, N.V. (2018). Ruxolitinib for the treatment of patients with steroid-refractory GVHD: An introduction to the REACH trials. *Immunotherapy* 10 (5): 391–402.

Kroger, N., Solano, C., and Bonifazi, F. (2016). Antilymphocyte globulin for chronic graft-versus-host disease. *N Engl J Med* 374 (19): 1894–1895.

Lee, S.J., Vogelsang, G., and Flowers, M.E. (2003). Chronic graft-versus-host disease. *Biol Blood Marrow Transplant* 9 (4): 215–233.

MacDonald, K.P.A., Betts, B.C., and Couriel, D. (2018). Emerging therapeutics for the control of chronic graft-versus-host disease. *Biol Blood Marrow Transplant* 24 (1): 19–26.

Miklos, D., Cutler, C.S., Arora, M., Waller, E.K., Jagasia, M., Pusic, I. et al. (2017). Ibrutinib for chronic graft-versus-host disease after failure of prior therapy. *Blood* 130 (21): 2243–2250.

Olivieri, A., Locatelli, F., Zecca, M., Sanna, A., Cimminiello, M., Raimondi, R. et al. (2009). Imatinib for refractory chronic graft-versus-host disease with fibrotic features. *Blood* 114 (3): 709–718.

Schroeder, M.A., Choi, J., Staser, K., and DiPersio, J.F. (2018). The role of Janus Kinase signaling in graft-versus-host disease and graft versus leukemia. *Biol Blood Marrow Transplant* 24 (6): 1125–1134.

Walker, I., Panzarella, T., Couban, S., Couture, F., Devins, G., Elemary, M. et al. (2016). Pretreatment with anti-thymocyte globulin versus no anti-thymocyte globulin in patients with haematological malignancies undergoing haemopoietic cell transplantation from unrelated donors: A randomised, controlled, open-label, phase 3, multicentre trial. *Lancet Oncol* 17 (2): 164–173.

Zeiser, R., Polverelli, N., Ram, R., Hashmi, S.K., Chakraverty, R., Middeke, J.M. et al. (2021). Ruxolitinib for glucocorticoid-refractory chronic graft-versus-host disease. *N Engl J Med* 385 (3): 228–238.

Index

Note: Page numbers followed by "*f*" refer to figures and "*t*" refer to tables.